MEDICAL
MICROBIOLOGY

MEDICAL
MICROBIOLOGY

THIRD EDITION

with 602 illustrations, 535 in color

PATRICK R. MURRAY, PhD

Professor, Departments of Pathology and Medicine
Washington University School of Medicine;
Director, Clinical Microbiology Laboratory
Barnes-Jewish Hospital
St. Louis, Missouri

KEN S. ROSENTHAL, PhD

Professor
Department of Microbiology and Immunology
Northeastern Ohio Universities College of Medicine
Rootstown, Ohio

GEORGE S. KOBAYASHI, PhD

Professor, Departments of Medicine and Molecular Microbiology
Washington University School of Medicine;
Associate Director, Clinical Microbiology Laboratory
Barnes-Jewish Hospital
St. Louis, Missouri

MICHAEL A. PFALLER, MD

Professor
Department of Pathology
University of Iowa College of Medicine
Iowa City, Iowa

Mosby

A Harcourt Health Sciences Company

St. Louis   London   Philadelphia   Sydney   Toronto

Editor: Michael Brown
Developmental Editors: Christy Wells, Linda Caldwell
Project Manager: Carol Sullivan Weis
Designer: Jen Marmarinos
Manufacturing Manager: David Graybill

Third Edition

Mosby, Inc.
11830 Westline Industrial Drive
St. Louis, Missouri 63146

Library of Congress Cataloging-in-Publication Data

Medical microbiology / Patrick R. Murray . . . [et al.]. — 3rd ed.
    p.   cm.
    Includes bibliographical references and index.
    ISBN 0-8151-9035-2
    1. Medical microbiology. I. Murray, Patrick R.
    [DNLM: 1. Microbiology. 2. Parasitology. QW 4 M4862 1997]
   QR46.M4683 1997
   616′ .01—dc21
   DNLM/DLC

97-18902
CIP

00 01 02 / 9 8 7 6 5 4

TO OUR STUDENTS AND FELLOW TEACHERS

Preface

Medical microbiology can be a bewildering field to the novice. The complex nomenclature, spectrum and pathophysiology of diseases, and therapeutic options—all can be overwhelming. What information is important for the student of medicine? What information can be used to diagnose and manage an infected patient? Certainly there are a number of theories about what a student needs to know. Although we do not claim to have a monopoly on the one right system (there is truly no one perfect approach to medical education), we have drawn on our experience gained through years of teaching medical students, residents, and fellows, as well as the work devoted to the two previous editions of this textbook. We have tried to address the question of student needs by presenting the basic concepts of medical microbiology in a succinct, clear manner. The material included in this text—and maybe more important, the material excluded—can be a subject for debate, but we have used our perception of the practical needs of the student as our guide.

As with any science, new discoveries and understandings continue to add to our foundation of knowledge. As authors and teachers, we are forced to decide what information is important and should be added to this textbook and what information has proved to be less important and can be deleted. With that in mind, we have expanded our coverage while attempting to limit the total length of this work. We continue to search for the right presentation of the fundamental aspects of medical microbiology (Sections I to III). The chapters in these sections—Basic Principles of Medical Microbiology, Basic Concepts in the Immune Response, and General Principles of Laboratory Diagnosis—have been extensively revised. In contrast the changes may be less obvious in the individual chapters of the sections, Bacteriology, Virology, Mycology, and Parasitology; however, each chapter has been carefully updated and expanded to include new, medically relevant discoveries. In each of these chapters, we have attempted to present the material that we feel will help the student gain a clear understanding of the significance of the individual microbes and their diseases.

How can the student digest what appear to be innumerable facts? On first impression, success in medical microbiology would seem to depend on memorization. Although memorization is an important part of microbiology, understanding the basic principles and developing a system for storing this information play an important role in mastering this science. We suggest that the student concentrate on learning what is important by thinking like a physician. Continue to ask seven basic questions as you approach this material: who, what, where, when, why, which, and how. For example: Who is at risk for disease? What diagnostic tests should be performed? Where does this organism cause infections (both body site and geographical area)? When is isolation of this organism important? Why is this organism able to cause disease? Which species and genera are medically important? How is this infection managed? Each organism that is encountered can be systematically examined. Know the specifics about how the organism grows, the virulence properties of the organism, and the diseases it causes; understand the epidemiology of infections; know what specimens should be collected and the basic identification tests that should be performed; and be familiar with preventive and therapeutic strategies. Learn three to five words or phrases that are associated with the microbe—words that will stimulate your memory and organize the diverse facts into a logical picture. Develop alternative associations. For example, this textbook presents organisms in a systematic taxonomic structure (frequently called a *bug parade*). Take a given virulence property (e.g., toxin production) or type of disease (e.g., meningitis) and list the organisms that share this property. In other words do not simply attempt to memorize page after page of facts; rather, use techniques that stimulate your mind and challenge your understanding of the facts presented throughout the text.

No textbook of this magnitude would be successful without the contributions of numerous individuals. We are grateful for the help provided by the staff at Mosby Year–Book, Inc., particularly Emma Underdown, Linda Caldwell, Pat Joiner, Bob Boehringer, and Alyssa Naumann. We also want to thank the many students and professional colleagues who have offered their advice and constructive criticism throughout the development of this third edition of *Medical Microbiology*. Every effort has been made to obtain permission for copyrighted material used in this book. In instances where this may not have been possible, please bring this to the attention of the publisher, who will ensure that full acknowledgment is made in future reprints and editions.

Specific medical students and faculty we would like to acknowledge as reviewers are:

Catherine Durishin, BS
Northeastern Ohio Universities
  College of Medicine
Rootstown, Ohio

Ryokei Imai
Baltimore, Maryland

Richard Wang
New York, New York

Remo Morelli, PhD
Department of Biology
San Francisco State University
San Francisco, California

Heather D. Mayor, DSc, PhD
Department of Microbiology
  and Immunology
Baylor College of Medicine
Houston, Texas

Richard E. Depew, PhD
Department of Microbiology and
  Immunology
Northeastern Ohio Universities
  College of Medicine
Rootstown, Ohio

PATRICK R. MURRAY

KEN S. ROSENTHAL

GEORGE S. KOBAYASHI

MICHAEL A. PFALLER

Contents

MEDICAL
MICROBIOLOGY

Introduction to Medical Microbiology

Imagine the excitement felt by the Dutch biologist Anton van Leeuwenhoek in 1674 as he peered through his carefully ground microscopic lenses at a drop of water and discovered a world of millions of tiny "animicules." As fascinating as it was for him to see this population of protozoa and bacteria, he could hardly imagine the far-reaching effects of his first observations. His meticulous drawings, documenting the diversity of this microscopic community, formed the basis of microbiology. Almost 100 years later the Danish biologist Otto Müller extended van Leeuwenhoek's studies and organized bacteria into genera and species according to the classification methods of Linnaeus. This was the beginning of the taxonomic classification of microbes—an exercise that now frustrates microbiologists and physicians (as you will unfortunately learn). In 1840 the German pathologist Friedrich Henle proposed criteria for proving that microorganisms were responsible for causing human disease (the "germ theory" of disease). Koch and Pasteur confirmed this theory in the 1870s and 1880s with a series of elegant experiments proving that microorganisms were responsible for causing anthrax, rabies, plague, cholera, and tuberculosis. Pasteur has been called the *Father of Modern Medicine* and Koch, the *Founder of Diagnostic Microbiology*. Other brilliant scientists went on to prove that a diverse collection of microbes was responsible for causing human disease. The era of chemotherapy was begun in 1910 when the German chemist Paul Ehrlich discovered the first antibacterial agent, a compound effective against the spirochete that causes syphilis. This was followed by Alexander Fleming's discovery of penicillin in 1928, Gerhard Domagk's discovery of sulfanilamide in 1935, and Selman Waksman's discovery of streptomycin in 1943. Fortunately or unfortunately, as the case may be, the ensuing years have witnessed the introduction of hundreds of antimicrobial agents, some potently effective and some just potently toxic. In 1946 the American microbiologist John Enders was the first to cultivate viruses in cell cultures, leading the way to the large-scale production of virus cultures for vaccine development. Thousands of scientists have followed these pioneers, each building on the foundation established by his or her predecessors and each adding an observation that expanded our understanding of microbes and their role in disease.

COMPLEXITY OF THE MICROBIAL WORLD

The world that van Leeuwenhoek discovered was complex, consisting of protozoa and bacteria of all shapes and sizes. However, the complexity of medical microbiology we know today rivals the limits of the imagination. We now know that there are thousands of different types of microbes that live in, on, and around us—and hundreds that cause serious human diseases. To understand this information and organize it in a useful manner, it is important to understand some of the basic aspects of medical microbiology. To start, the microbes can be subdivided into four groups: viruses, bacteria, fungi, and parasites, each having its own level of complexity.

Viruses

Viruses are the smallest infectious particles, ranging in diameter from 18 nm to almost 300 nm (particles less than 200 nm cannot be seen with a light microscope). More than 40 genera of viruses have been implicated in human disease, and certainly more will be discovered each year. Viruses consist of either DNA or RNA (but not both) and proteins required for replication and pathogenesis. These components are then enclosed in a protein coat with or without a lipid membrane coat. These organisms are true parasites, requiring host cells for replication. The cells they infect and the outcome of the infection dictate the nature of the clinical presentation. Infection can lead either to rapid replication of the organisms and destruction of the cell or to a long-term latent relationship with integration of the viral genetic information into the host genome. The factors that determine which of these takes place are only partially understood. For example, infection with the human immunodeficiency virus, the etiological agent of acquired immunodeficiency syndrome (AIDS), can result in the latent infection of CD4 lymphocytes or the active replication and destruction of these immunologically important cells. Likewise, infection can spread to other susceptible cells, such as the microglial cells of the brain, resulting in the neurological manifestations of AIDS. Thus the diseases caused by viruses can range from the common cold to gastroenteritis to fatal catastrophies such as rabies, smallpox, and AIDS.

Bacteria

Bacteria are relatively simple in structure. They are **prokaryotic** organisms—a simple unicellular organism with no nuclear membrane, mitochondria, Golgi bodies, or endoplasmic reticulum that reproduces by asexual division. Although the cell wall encircling bacteria is itself complex, there are only two basic forms: a gram-positive cell wall with a thick peptidoglycan layer and a gram-negative cell wall with a thin peptidoglycan layer and an overlying outer membrane (additional information about this structure is presented in Chapter 3). Some bacteria lack this cell wall structure and compensate by surviving only inside host cells or in a hypertonic environment. The size (1 to 20 μm or longer), shape (spheres, rods, spirals), and spatial arrangement (single cells, chains, clusters) of the cells are used for the preliminary classification of bacteria, and the phenotypic and genotypic properties of the bacteria form the basis for the definitive classification. The human body is inhabited by thousands of different bacterial species—some living transiently, others in a permanent parasitic relationship. Likewise the environment that surrounds us, including the air we breathe, water we drink, and food we eat, is inhabited by bacteria, many of which are relatively avirulent and some of which are capable of producing life-threatening disease.

Fungi

In contrast with bacteria, the cellular structure of fungi is more complex. These are **eukaryotic** organisms that contain a well-defined nucleus, mitochondria, Golgi bodies, and endoplasmic reticulum. Fungi can exist either in a unicellular form (**yeast**) that can replicate asexually or in a filamentous form (**mold**) that can replicate asexually and sexually. Most fungi exist as either yeasts or molds; however, some can assume either morphology. These are known as **dimorphic** fungi and consist of such organisms as *Histoplasma* and *Blastomyces*.

Parasites

Possibly the most complex microbes are parasites. Although all parasites are classified as eukaryotic, some are unicellular, and others are multicellular. They range in size from tiny protozoa as small as 1 to 2 μm in diameter to arthropods and tapeworms that can measure up to 10 meters in length. Indeed, considering the size of some of these parasites, it is hard to imagine how these organisms came to be classified as microbes. Their life cycles are equally complex, with some parasites establishing a permanent relationship with humans and others going through a series of developmental stages in a progression of animal hosts. One of the difficulties confronting students is not only an understanding of the spectrum of diseases caused by parasites, but also an appreciation of the epidemiology of these infections, which is vital for such infections to be controlled.

MICROBIAL DISEASE

One of the most important reasons for studying microbes is to understand the diseases they cause and the ways to control them. Unfortunately, however, the relationship between organisms and their diseases is not simple. Specifically, organisms rarely cause a single well-defined disease, although there are certainly ones that do (e.g., *Treponema pallidum,* syphilis; poliovirus, polio; *Plasmodium* species, malaria). Instead it is more common for a particular organism to produce many manifestations of disease (e.g., *Staphylococcus aureus,* endocarditis, pneumonia, wound infections, food poisoning) or for many organisms to produce the same disease (e.g., meningitis caused by viruses, bacteria, fungi, and parasites). In addition, relatively few organisms can be classified as always pathogenic, though some do belong in this category (e.g., rabies virus, *Brucella* species, *Sporothrix schenckii, Plasmodium* species). Instead, most are able to establish disease only under well-defined circumstances (e.g., the introduction of an organism with a potential for causing disease into a normally sterile site such as the brain, lungs, or peritoneal cavity). Some diseases arise when a person is exposed to organisms from external sources. These are known as **exogenous** infections, and examples include diseases caused by influenza virus, *Neisseria gonorrhoeae, Coccidioides immitis,* and *Entamoeba histolytica.* Most human diseases, however, are produced by organisms in the person's own microbial flora that spread to body sites where disease can ensue (**endogenous** infections).

The interaction between an organism and the human host is complex. Sometimes there is only a transient colonization, sometimes there is a long-term symbiotic relationship, and sometimes disease occurs. The outcome of this interaction is determined by the virulence of the organism, the site of exposure, and the host's ability to respond to the organism. Thus the manifestations of disease can range from mild symptoms to organ failure and death. The role of microbial virulence and the host's immunological response is discussed in depth in subsequent chapters.

Although the human body is remarkably adapted to controlling exposure to pathogenic microbes, the physical barriers that prevent invasion by the organism and the immunological response to infection are frequently inadequate. To improve the human body's ability to prevent infection, the immune system can be augmented either through the passive transfer of antibodies present in immune globulin preparations or through active immunization with microbial antigens. Infections can also be controlled with a variety of chemotherapeutic agents. Unfortunately, microbes can alter their antigenic complexion and develop resistance to even the most potent antibiotics. Thus the battle for control between microbe and host continues, with neither side yet able to claim victory.

DIAGNOSTIC MICROBIOLOGY

The clinical microbiology laboratory plays an important role in the diagnosis and control of infectious diseases. However, the ability of the laboratory to perform these functions is limited by the quality of the specimen collected from the patient, the means by which it is transported from the patient to the laboratory, and the techniques used to demonstrate the microbe in the sample. Because most diagnostic tests are based on the ability of the organism to grow, transport conditions must ensure the viability of the pathogen. In addition, the most sophisticated testing protocols are of little value if the collected specimen is not representative of the site of infection. This seems obvious, but many specimens sent to laboratories for analysis are contaminated during collection with the organisms that colonize the mucosal surfaces. Because most infections are caused by endogenous organisms, it is virtually impossible to interpret the testing results with contaminated specimens.

The laboratory is also able to determine the antimicrobial activity of selected chemotherapeutic agents, although the value of these tests is limited. The laboratory must test only organisms capable of producing disease and only medically relevant antimicrobials. To test all isolated organisms or an indiscriminate selection of drugs can yield misleading results, with potentially dangerous consequences. Not only can a patient be treated inappropriately with unnecessary antibiotics, but the true pathogenic organism may not be recognized among the plethora of organisms isolated and tested. Finally, the in vitro determination of an organism's susceptibility to a variety of antibiotics is only one aspect of a complex picture. The virulence of the organism, site of infection, and patient's ability to respond to the infection influence the host-parasite interaction and must also be considered when planning treatment.

SUMMARY

It is important to realize that our knowledge of the microbial world is continually evolving. Just as the early microbiologists built their discoveries on the foundations established by their predecessors, so too will we and future generations continue to discover new microbes, new diseases, and new therapies. The following chapters are intended as a foundation of knowledge that can be used to enrich your understanding of microbes and their diseases.

SECTION 1

Basic Principles of Medical Microbiology

CHAPTER 2

Bacterial Classification

For the student of bacteriology, understanding the relevance and complex nomenclature of literally hundreds of "important" organisms can certainly be challenging. The mastery of this exercise depends on the systematic organization of the bewildering array of different organisms into logical relationships (i.e., the taxonomic classification of the organisms). Historically, organisms have been classified by examination of their phenotypic characteristics (Box 2-1).

The microscopic and macroscopic **morphologies** of bacteria were the first characteristics used to identify bacteria and are the cornerstones for most identification algorithms used today. For example, bacteria can be classified by their ability to retain the Gram stain (gram positive or gram negative) and by the shape of the individual organisms (cocci, bacilli, curved, or spiral). The macroscopic appearance of colonies of bacteria can also be used to identify bacteria (e.g., hemolytic properties on agar containing blood, pigmentation of the colonies, size and shape of the colonies). Thus *Streptococcus pyogenes* is a gram-positive bacterium that forms long chains of cocci and appears as small, white, hemolytic colonies on blood agar plates. Because many organisms can appear very similar on microscopic and macroscopic examination, morphological characteristics are used to provide a tentative identification of the organism and to select more discriminating classification methods.

Biochemical typing is the most commonly used method for the definitive identification of bacteria. With the use of carefully selected biochemical tests, most clinically significant isolates can be identified with a high degree of precision. Biotyping has also been used for subdividing groups of organisms beyond the species level, primarily for epidemiological purposes (e.g., to determine whether a group of organisms from the same genus and species is from a common source or from distinct sources).

Serological typing is used to identify organisms that are inert in biochemical testing (e.g., *Francisella*, the organism that causes tularemia), are difficult or impossible to grow (e.g., *Treponema pallidum*, the organism responsible for syphilis), are associated with specific disease syndromes (e.g., *Escherichia coli* serotype O157, responsible for hemorrhagic colitis), or need to be identified rapidly (e.g., *S. pyogenes*, responsible for streptococcal pharyngitis). Serotyping is also used to classify bacteria below the species level for epidemiological purposes.

Other phenotypic characteristics used to classify bacteria include **analysis of antibiogram patterns** (patterns of susceptibility to different antibiotics), **pyocin typing** (susceptibility to pyocins, a group of low-molecular weight bactericidal proteins), and **phage typing** (susceptibility to bacteriophages or viruses). Analysis of antibiogram patterns has only limited use for bacterial identification or epidemiological classification, and pyocin and phage typing are primarily restricted to reference laboratories.

Analysis of the analytic characteristics of bacteria has also been used to classify bacteria at the genus, species, or subspecies level (Box 2-2). The chromatographic pattern of **cell wall** mycolic acids is unique for many of the individual species of mycobacteria and has been used for more than 20 years to identify the most commonly isolated species. Analysis of the **lipids in the entire cell** has also proved to be a useful method for characterizing many bacterial species, as well as yeasts. Commercial systems are available for performing these types of analyses. Analyses of the **whole-cell proteins** and **cellular enzymes** (enyzme typing) are also techniques that have been used to characterize bacteria, most typically at the subspecies level for epidemiological investigations. Although these analytic methods are accurate and reproducible, they are labor intensive, and the instrumentation is expensive. For these reasons the analyses are used primarily in reference laboratories.

The most precise method for classifying bacteria is by analysis of their genetic material (Box 2-3). Organisms were initially classified by the ratio of guanine to cytosine; however, this procedure has largely been forsaken for more discriminating methods. DNA hybridization was used initially to determine the relationship among bacterial isolates (e.g., to determine whether two isolates were in the same genus or species). More recently, this technique has been exploited for the rapid identification

---

BOX 2-1   Classification of Bacteria by Phenotypic Characteristics

Morphological characteristics
Biotyping
Serotyping
Antibiogram patterns
Pyocin typing
Phage typing

BOX 2-3   Classification of Bacteria by Genotypic Characteristics

Guanine plus cytosine ratio
DNA hybridization
Nucleic acid sequence analysis
Plasmid analysis
Ribotyping
Chromosomal DNA fragment analysis

BOX 2-2   Classification of Bacteria by Analytic Characteristics

Cell-wall analysis
Whole-cell lipid analysis
Whole-cell protein analysis
Enzyme typing

BOX 2-4   Aerobic, Gram-Positive Bacilli

CATALASE-POSITIVE COCCI	CATALASE-NEGATIVE COCCI
Staphylococcus species	*Streptococcus* species
Micrococcus species	*Enterococcus* species
Stomatococcus species	*Aerococcus* species
	Leuconostoc species
	Pediococcus species
	Alloiococcus species
	Gemella species
	Globicatella species
	Helcococcus species
	Lactococcus species
	Tetragenococcus species
	Vagococcus species

---

of organisms by use of molecular probes. That is, DNA from an organism to be identified is extracted and exposed to species-specific molecular probes. If the probe binds to the DNA, then the organism's identity is confirmed. This technique has also been used to detect organisms directly in clinical specimens, thus avoiding the need to grow the organisms. DNA hybridization has proved to be a valuable tool for the rapid detection and identification of slow-growing organisms such as mycobacteria and fungi.

An extension of the hybridization method is nucleic acid sequence analysis. Probes are used to localize specific nucleic acid sequences that are unique to a genus, species, or subspecies. These sequences are amplified so that millions of copies are produced, and then the amplified genetic material is sequenced to define the precise identity of the isolate. This method primarily analyzes sequences of ribosomal DNA (because highly conserved [family- or genus-specific] sequences and highly variable [species- or subspecies-specific] sequences are present). It has also been used to define the evolutionary relationship among organisms and to identify organisms that are difficult or impossible to grow. Most of the recent changes in taxonomic nomenclature were determined by nucleic acid sequence analysis.

Various other methods have been used, primarily to classify organisms at the subspecies level for epidemiological investigations: plasmid analysis, ribotyping, and analysis of chromosomal DNA fragments. Each method is relatively sophisticated and is performed in reference laboratories or research laboratories. The use of these methods for routine identification is currently limited.

Boxes 2-4 through 2-8 provide a useful classification scheme for organizing the many bacteria that inhabit or infect the human body. The precise arrangement of bacteria in families, genera, and species continues to change. In Section IV, Bacteriology, we identify newly defined relationships among bacteria and predict where reorganization of the bacteria will occur. The listing of bacteria in these tables is not exhaustive, which may be of little comfort to the student. Rather, only the most commonly isolated or important bacteria are included.

BOX 2-5   **Aerobic, Gram-Positive Bacilli**

ACTINOMYCETES WITH CELL-WALL MYCOLIC ACIDS

Corynebacteriaceae
  Corynebacterium species
Nocardiaceae
  Nocardia species
  Rhodococcus species
  Tsukamurella species
  Gordona species
Mycobacteriaceae
  Mycobacteria

ACTINOMYCETES WITH NO CELL-WALL MYCOLIC ACIDS

Actinomadura species
Dermatophilus species
Nocardiopsis species
Oerskovia species

ACTINOMYCETES WITH NO CELL-WALL MYCOLIC ACIDS—cont'd

Rothia species
Streptomyces species
Tropheryma species
Thermophilic actinomycetes
  Saccharomonospora species
  Saccharopolyspora species
  Thermoactinomyces species

MISCELLANEOUS GRAM-POSITIVE BACILLI

Arcanobacterium species
Bacillus species
Erysipelothrix species
Gardnerella species
Listeria species

BOX 2-6   **Aerobic, Gram-Negative Cocci and Bacilli**

COCCI

Neisseriaceae
  Neisseria species
Moraxella
  Moraxella species
  Branhamella species

BACILLI

Enterobacteriaceae
  Citrobacter species
  Enterobacter species
  Escherichia species
  Klebsiella species
  Morganella species
  Proteus species
  Salmonella species
  Shigella species
  Serratia species

BACILLI—cont'd

  Yersinia species
Vibrionaceae
  Vibrio species
Aeromonadaceae
  Aeromonas species
Plesiomonadaceae
  Plesiomonas species
Campylobacteriaceae
  Campylobacter species
  Arcobacter species
Pasteurellaceae
  Haemophilus species
  Actinobacillus species
  Pasteurella species
Legionellaceae
  Legionella species
Miscellaneous genera

BACILLI—cont'd

  Acinetobacter species
  Bartonella species
  Bordetella species
  Brucellae
  Burkholderia species
  Calymmatobacterium species
  Cardiobacterium species
  Eikenella species
  Francisella species
  Helicobacter species
  Kingella species
  Pseudomonas species
  Stenotrophomonas species
  Spirillum species
  Streptobacillus species

BOX 2-7   **Anaerobic Gram-Positive and Gram-Negative Bacteria**

GRAM-POSITIVE COCCI

Peptostreptococcus species

GRAM-POSITIVE BACILLI

Actinomyces species
Bifidobacterium species
Clostridium species
Eubacterium species
Lactobacillus species
Mobiluncus species
Propionibacterium species

GRAM-NEGATIVE COCCI

Megasphaera species
Veillonella species

GRAM-NEGATIVE BACILLI

Bacteroides species
Bilophila species
Fusobacterium species
Porphyromonas species
Prevotella species

BOX 2-8   **Miscellaneous, Medically Important Bacteria**

Mycoplasmataceae
  Mycoplasma species
  Ureaplasma species
Spirochaetaceae
  Borrelia species
  Treponema species
Leptospiraceae
  Leptospira species

Chlamydiaceae
  Chlamydia species
Other bacteria
  Coxiella species
  Ehrlichia species
  Rickettsia species

QUESTIONS

1. Name three examples each of phenotypic, analytic, and genotypic characteristics used to classify bacteria.
2. Describe the microscopic morphology (e.g., Gram stain characteristic, shape of organism) of the following bacteria: *Staphylococcus, Escherichia, Neisseria, Clostridium, Enterococcus,* and *Pseudomonas* species.
3. Which of the following organisms have mycolic acids in their cell walls: *Staphylococcus, Nocardia, Mycobacterium,* and *Klebsiella* species?

Bibliography

Balows A et al, editors: *The prokaryotes,* ed 2, New York, 1992, Springer-Verlag.

Baron EJ, Peterson L, Finegold S: *Bailey and Scott's diagnostic microbiology,* ed 9, St Louis, 1995, Mosby.

Murray PR: *Pocket guide to clinical microbiology,* Washington, DC, 1996, American Society for Microbiology.

Murray PR et al, editors: *Manual of clinical microbiology,* ed 6, Washington, DC, 1995, American Society for Microbiology.

Bacterial Morphology and Cell Wall Structure and Synthesis

Cells are the fundamental units of living things, from the smallest bacterium to the largest of the plants and animals. Bacteria, the smallest cells, are visible only with the aid of the microscope. The smallest bacteria *(Chlamydia* and *Rickettsia)* are only 0.1 to 0.2 μm in diameter, whereas larger bacteria may be many microns in length. However, a newly described species is hundreds of times larger than the average bacterial cell and is visible to the naked eye. Most species, however, are approximately 1 μm in diameter and are therefore visible using the light microscope, which has a resolution of 0.2 μm. In comparison, animal and plant cells are much larger, ranging from 7 μm (the diameter of a red blood cell) to several feet (the length of certain nerve cells).

Each cell contains the genetic basis for reproduction in its DNA genome, the biochemical machinery for transcribing genetic information into messenger RNA and translating the mRNA into proteins, and the machinery for energy production and biosynthesis, which is all packaged by a membrane. The mechanisms and machinery for accomplishing these functions are basically similar, but the specifics may be different for bacteria and for the higher-order organisms. These differences are influenced by the structure of the cell, the environment in which the cell lives, the source and means of the cell's energy production, and the nature of and requirement for cell interaction (or lack thereof).

Bacteria can survive and in some cases grow in hostile environments in which the osmotic pressure outside the cell is so low that most eukaryotic cells would lyse at temperature extremes (both hot and cold), with dryness, and with very dilute and diverse energy sources. Bacteria have evolved the structures and functions to adapt to these conditions.

Differences Between Eukaryotes and Prokaryotes

Cells from animals, plants, and fungi are **eukaryotes** (Greek for "true nucleus"), whereas bacteria and the blue-green algae belong to the **prokaryotes** (Greek for "primitive nucleus"). In addition to lacking a nucleus and other organelles, prokaryotes use a smaller ribosome, the 70S ribosome, and in most bacteria a meshlike peptidoglycan cell wall surrounds the membranes to protect it against the environment. Bacteria can live in hostile environments under nonphysiological conditions and in very dilute solutions of energy sources. These and other distinguishing features are depicted in Figure 3-1 and outlined in Table 3-1. Several of these distinctions provide the basis for antimicrobial action.

Differences Among Prokaryotes

Bacteria can be distinguished from one another by their morphology (size, shape, and staining characteristics) and metabolic, antigenic, and genetic characteristics. Although bacteria are difficult to differentiate by size, they do have different shapes. A spherical bacterium, such as *Staphylococcus,* is a **coccus**; a rod-shaped bacterium, such as *Escherichia coli,* is a **bacillus;** and the snakelike treponeme is a **spirillium**. In addition, *Escherichia* and *Actinomyces* species have **branched filamentous** appearances similar to those of fungi. Some bacteria form aggregates such as the grapelike clusters of *S. aureus* or the **diplococcus** (two cells together) observed in *Streptococcus* or *Neisseria* species.

Gram stain is a powerful, easy test that allows clinicians to distinguish between the two major classes of bacteria and initiate therapy (Figure 3-2). Bacteria that are heat fixed or otherwise dried onto a slide are stained with **crystal violet** (Figure 3-3); this stain is precipitated with **Gram iodine** and then unbound, and excess stain is removed by washing with the acetone-based **decolorizer**. A counterstain, **safranin**, is added to stain any decolorized cells red. This takes less than 10 minutes.

For **gram-positive** bacteria, which turn **purple,** the stain gets trapped in a thick, cross-linked, meshlike structure, the peptidoglycan layer, which surrounds the cell. **Gram-negative bacteria** have a thin peptidoglycan layer that does not retain crystal violet stain, so the cells must be counterstained with safranin and turned **red** (Figure 3-4). A mnemonic device that may help is "P—Purple—Positive." Gram stain is not dependable for bacteria that are starved (e.g., old or stationary phase cultures).

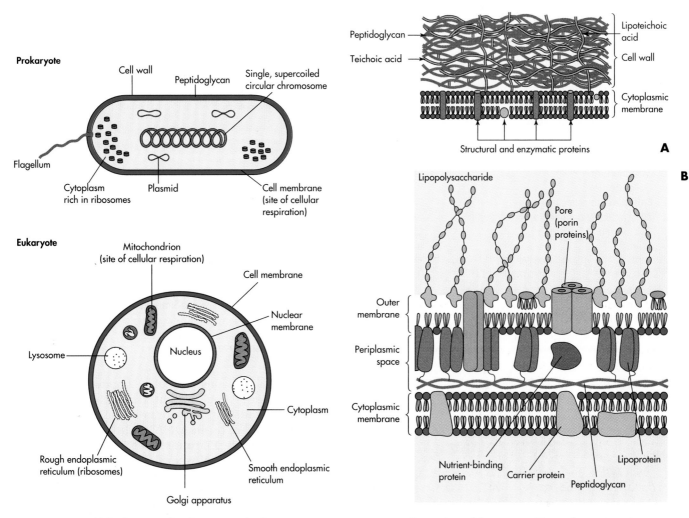

Prokaryote

Cell wall

Peptidoglycan

Single, supercoiled circular chromosome

Flagellum

Cytoplasm rich in ribosomes

Plasmid

Cell membrane (site of cellular respiration)

Eukaryote

Mitochondrion (site of cellular respiration)

Cell membrane

Nuclear membrane

Nucleus

Lysosome

Cytoplasm

Rough endoplasmic reticulum (ribosomes)

Smooth endoplasmic reticulum

Golgi apparatus

FIGURE 3-1 Major features of prokaryotes and eukaryotes.

Peptidoglycan

Teichoic acid

Lipoteichoic acid

Cell wall

Cytoplasmic membrane

Structural and enzymatic proteins

A

B

Lipopolysaccharide

Pore (porin proteins)

Outer membrane

Periplasmic space

Cytoplasmic membrane

Nutrient-binding protein

Carrier protein

Peptidoglycan

Lipoprotein

FIGURE 3-2 Comparison of the gram-positive and gram-negative bacterial cell walls. **A,** A gram-positive bacterium has a thick peptidoglycan layer that contains teichoic and lipoteichoic acids. **B,** A gram-negative bacterium has a thin peptidoglycan layer and an outer membrane that contains lipopolysaccharide, phospholipids, and proteins. The periplasmic space between the cytoplasmic and outer membranes contains transport, degradative, and cell wall synthetic proteins. The outer membrane is joined to the cytoplasmic membrane at adhesion points and is attached to the peptidoglycan by lipoprotein links.

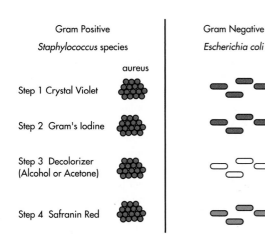

Gram Positive

Staphylococcus species

aureus

Gram Negative

Escherichia coli

Step 1 Crystal Violet

Step 2 Gram's Iodine

Step 3 Decolorizer (Alcohol or Acetone)

Step 4 Safranin Red

FIGURE 3-3 Gram stain. The crystal violet of Gram stain is precipitated by Gram iodine and is trapped in the thick peptidoglycan layer in gram-positive bacteria. The decolorizer disperses the gram-negative outer membrane and washes the crystal violet from the thin layer of peptidoglycan. Gram-negative bacteria are visualized by the red counterstain.

TABLE 3-1	**Major Characteristics of Eukaryotes and Prokaryotes**	
CHARACTERISTC	**EUKARYOTE**	**PROKARYOTE**
Major groups	Algae, fungi, protozoa, plants, animals	Bacteria
Size (approximate)	>5 μm	0.5 to 3 μm
Nuclear structures		
Nucleus	Classic membrane	No nuclear membrane
Chromosomes	Strands of DNA	Single, circular DNA
	Diploid genome	Haploid genome
Cytoplasmic structures		
Mitochondria	Present	Absent
Golgi bodies	Present	Absent
Endoplasmic reticulum	Present	Absent
Ribosomes (sedimentation coefficient)	80S (60S + 40S)	70S (50S + 30S)
Cytoplasmic membrane	Contains sterols	Does not contain sterols
Cell wall	Is absent or is composed of chitin	Is a complex structure containing protein, lipids, and peptidoglycans
Reproduction	Sexual and asexual	Asexual (binary fission)
Movement	Complex flagellum, if present	Simple flagellum, if present
Respiration	Via mitochondria	Via cytoplasmic membrane

From Holt S. In Slots J, Taubman M, editors: *Contemporary oral microbiology and immunology*, St Louis, 1992, Mosby.

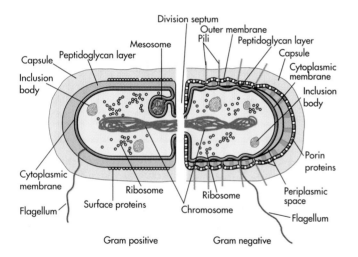

FIGURE 3-4 Gram-positive and gram-negative bacteria. A gram-positive bacterium has a thick layer of peptidoglycan *(left)*. A gram-negative bacterium has a thin peptidoglycan layer and an outer membrane *(right)*.

Bacteria that cannot be classified by Gram stain include mycobacteria, which have a waxy outer shell and are distinguished with the acid-fast stain, and mycoplasmas, which have no peptidoglycan.

BACTERIAL ULTRASTRUCTURE
Cytoplasmic Structures

Gram-positive and gram-negative bacteria have similar internal but very different external structures. The cytoplasm of the bacterial cell contains the DNA chromosome, the mRNA, ribosomes, proteins, and metabolites (Figure 3-4). Unlike eukaryotes, the **bacterial** chromosome is a single, double-stranded circle that is contained not in a nucleus but in a discrete area known as the **nucleoid**. Histones are not required to maintain the conformation of the DNA, and the DNA does not form nucleosomes. **Plasmids**, which are smaller, circular extrachromosomal DNAs, may also be present. Plasmids are most commonly found in gram-negative bacteria, and although not usually essential for cellular survival, they often provide a selective advantage: Many confer resistance to one or more antibiotics.

The lack of a nuclear membrane simplifies the requirements and control mechanisms for the synthesis of proteins. In this case, transcription and translation are coupled; in other words, ribosomes can bind to the mRNA, and protein can be made as the mRNA is being synthesized and still attached to the DNA.

The bacterial ribosome consists of 30S + 50S subunits, forming a 70S ribosome. This is unlike the eukaryotic 80S (40S + 60S) ribosome. The proteins and RNA of the bacterial ribosome are significantly different from eukaryotic ribosomes and are major targets for antibacterial drugs.

The **cytoplasmic membrane** has a lipid bilayer structure similar to the eukaryotic membranes, but it contains **no steroids** (e.g., cholesterol); mycoplasmas are the exception to this rule. The cytoplasmic membrane is responsible for many of the functions attributable to organelles in eukaryotes. These tasks include electron transport and energy production, which are normally achieved in the mitochondria (Figure 3-5). In addition, the membrane contains transport proteins that allow the uptake of metabolites and the release of other substances, ion pumps to maintain a membrane potential, and synthetic enzymes. A coiled cytoplasmic membrane,

FIGURE 3-5 The cytoplasmic membrane contains the machinery for the production of adenoside triphosphate *(ATP)* (electron transport system, cytochromes, F1–adenosine triphosphatase *[F1–ATPase]*) and membrane potential. The membrane potential provides electrochemical energy for transport proteins and the flagellum "motor." *NAD,* Nicotine adenine dinucleotide; *NADH,* reduced form of nicotine adenine dinucleotide; *FAD,* flavin adenine dinucleotide; *Pi,* phosphate.

TABLE 3-2	**Bacterial Membrane Structures**
STRUCTURE	**CHEMICAL CONSTITUENTS**
Plasma membrane	Phospholipids, proteins, and enzymes involved in generation of energy, membrane potential, and transport
Cell wall	
Gram-positive bacteria	
Peptidoglycan	Glycan chains of GlcNAc and MurNAc cross-linked by tetrapeptide bridge
Teichoic acid	Polyribitol phosphate or glycerol phosphate cross-linked to peptidoglycan
Lipoteichoic acid	Lipid-linked teichoic acid
Gram-negative bacteria	
Peptidoglycan	Thinner version of that found in gram-positive bacteria
Periplasmic space	Enzymes involved in transport, degradation, and synthesis
Outer membrane	Phospholipids with saturated fatty acids
Proteins	Porins, lipoprotein, transport proteins
LPS	Lipid A, core polysaccharide, O antigen
Other structures	
Capsule	Polysaccharides (disaccharides and trisaccharides) and polypeptides
Pili	Pilin, adhesions
Flagellum	Motor proteins, flagellin
Proteins	M protein of streptococci (as an example)

GlcNAc, N-Acetylglucosamine; *MurNAc,* N-acetylmuramic acid; *LPS,* lipopolysaccharide.

the **mesosome**, acts as an anchor to bind and pull apart daughter chromosomes during cell division.

Cell Wall

The structure (Table 3-2), components, and functions (Table 3-3) of the cell wall distinguish gram-positive from gram-negative bacteria. The important differences in membrane characteristics are outlined in Table 3-4. The cytoplasmic membranes of most prokaryotes are surrounded by rigid **peptidoglycan** *(murein)* layers. The exceptions are *Archaeobacteria* organisms (which contain pseudoglycans or pseudomureins related to peptidoglycan) and mycoplasmas (which have no cell walls

at all). Because the peptidoglycan provides rigidity, it also determines the shape of the particular bacterial cell. Gram-negative bacteria are also surrounded by outer membranes.

Gram-Positive Bacteria

A gram-positive bacterium has a *thick, multilayered cell wall consisting mainly of* ***peptidoglycan*** (150 to 500 Å) surrounding the cytoplasmic membrane (Figure 3-6). The peptidoglycan is a meshlike exoskeleton similar in function to the exoskeleton of an insect. However, unlike the exoskeleton of the insect, the peptidoglycan of the cell is sufficiently porous to allow diffusion of metabolites to the plasma membrane. The peptidoglycan is **essential** for the structure, for replication, and for survival in the normally hostile conditions in which bacteria grow. During infection, the peptidoglycan can interfere with phagocytosis, is mitogenic (stimulates mitosis of lymphocytes), and has pyrogenic activity (induces fever).

The peptidoglycan can be degraded by treatment with **lysozyme**. Lysozyme, an enzyme in human tears and mucus, is also produced by bacteria and other organisms. Lysozyme degrades the glycan backbone of the peptidoglycan. Without the peptidoglycan, the bacteria succumb to the large osmotic pressure differences across the cytoplasmic membrane and lyse. Removal of the cell wall produces a **protoplast** that lyses unless it is osmotically stabilized.

The gram-positive cell wall may also include other components such as teichoic and lipoteichoic acids and complex polysaccharides (usually called *C polysaccharides*). Proteins such as the M protein of streptococci and R protein of staphylococci also associate with the peptidoglycan. **Teichoic acids** are water-soluble polymers of polyol phosphates, which are covalently linked to the peptidoglycan. **Lipoteichoic acids** have a fatty acid and are anchored in the cytoplasmic membrane. These molecules are common surface antigens that distinguish bacterial serotypes and promote attachment to other bacteria as well as to specific receptors on mammalian cell

TABLE 3-3	Functions of the Bacterial Envelope

FUNCTION	COMPONENT
Structural rigidity	All
Packaging of internal contents	All
Permeabililty barrier	Outer membrane or plasma membrane
Metabolic uptake	Membranes and periplasmic transport proteins, porins, permeases
Energy production	Plasma membrane
Adhesion to host cells	Pili, proteins, teichoic acid
Immune recognition by host	All outer structures
Escape from host immune recognition	Capsule, M protein
Antibiotic sensitivity	Peptidioglycan synthetic enzymes
Antibiotic resistance	Outer membrane
Motility	Flagella
Mating	Pili
Adhesion	Pili

TABLE 3-4	Membrane Characteristics of Gram-Positive and Gram-Negative Bacteria

CHARACTERISTIC	GRAM POSITIVE	GRAM NEGATIVE
Outer membrane	—	+
Cell wall	Thicker	Thinner
LPS	—	+
Endotoxin	—	+
Teichoic acid	Often present	Absent
Sporulation	Some strains	None
Capsule	Sometimes present	Sometimes present
Lysozyme	Sensitive	Resistant
Antibacterial activity of penicillin	More susceptible	More resistant
Exotoxin production	Some strains	Some strains

LPS, Lipopolysaccharide.

surfaces **(adherence).** Teichoic acids are important factors in virulence. Lipoteichoic acids are shed into the media and host and, although weaker, can initiate endotoxic-like activities (see later section).

Gram-Negative Bacteria

Gram-negative cell walls are more complex than gram-positive cell walls, both structurally and chemically (Figure 3-2). Structurally, a gram-negative cell wall contains two layers external to the cytoplasmic membrane. Immediately external to the cytoplasmic membrane is a thin peptidoglycan layer, which accounts for only 5% to 10%

of the gram-negative cell wall by weight. There are *no teichoic or lipoteichoic acids in the gram-negative cell wall.* External to the peptidoglycan layer is the **outer membrane,** which is unique to gram-negative bacteria. The area between the external surface of the cytoplasmic membrane and the internal face of the outer membrane is referred to as the **periplasmic space.** This space is actually a compartment containing a variety of hydrolytic enzymes, which are important to the cell for the breakdown of large macromolecules for metabolism. These enzymes typically include proteases, phosphatases, lipases, nucleases, and carbohydrate-degrading enzymes. In the case of pathogenic gram-negative species, many of the lytic virulence factors such as collagenases, hyaluronidases, proteases, and beta-lactamase are in the periplasmic space. This space also contains components of the sugar transport systems and other binding proteins to facilitate the uptake of different metabolites and other compounds. Some binding proteins can be components of a chemotaxis system, which senses the external environment of the cell.

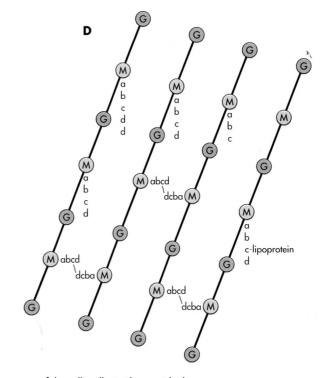

= Peptide linkage

FIGURE 3-6 General structure of the peptidoglycan component of the cell wall. **A,** The peptidoglycan forms a meshlike layer around the cell. **B,** The peptidoglycan mesh consists of a polysaccharide polymer that is cross-linked by peptide bonds. **C,** Peptides are cross-linked through a peptide bond between the terminal D-alanine (D-ala) from one chain and a lysine (lys) (or another diamino amino acid) from the other chain. A pentaglycine bridge (gly$_5$) expands the cross-link in *S. aureus* (as shown). **D,** Representation of the *E. coli* peptidoglycan structure. Diaminopimelic acid, the diamino amino acid in the third position of the peptide, is directly linked to the terminal alanine of another chain to cross-link the peptidoglycan. Lipoprotein anchors the outer membrane to the peptidoglycan. M, *N*-Acetylmuramic acid; G, *N*-acetylglucosamine; *Glu,* glucosamine; *gly,* glycine. (**D** based on Joklik KJ et al, editors: *Zinsser microbiology,* Norwalk, Conn, 1988, Appleton & Lange.)

As mentioned previously, outer membranes (Figure 3-2) are unique to gram-negative prokaryotes. The outer membrane is like a stiff canvas sack around the bacteria. It maintains the bacterial *structure* and is a *permeability barrier* to large molecules (e.g., proteins such as lysozyme and hydrophobic molecules). It also provides protection from adverse environmental conditions such as the digestive system of the host (important for Enterobacteriaceae organisms). The outer membrane has a lipid bilayer structure but differs from any other biological membrane in the structure of the outer leaflet of the membrane. The inner leaflet contains phospholipids normally found in bacterial membranes. However, the outer leaflet is composed primarily of an amphipathic molecule (meaning that it has both hydrophobic and hydrophilic ends) called a **lipopolysaccharide (LPS).** Except for those LPS molecules in the process of synthesis, the outer leaflet of the outer membrane is the only location where LPS molecules are found. Thus this membrane is asymmetrical, with phospholipids located in the inner leaflet and the LPS substituting for the phospholipids in the outer leaflet.

LPS is also called **endotoxin**, a powerful stimulator of immune responses. LPS activates B cells and induces macrophage and other cells to release interleukin-1 and interleukin-6, tumor necrosis factor, and other factors. LPS causes fever and can cause shock. The **Shwartzman reaction** (disseminated intravascular coagulation) follows the release of large amounts of endotoxin into the bloodstream. LPS is shed from the bacteria into the media and host. *N. meningitidis* sheds large amounts of a related compound, lipooligosaccharide, resulting in fever and symptoms.

The variety of proteins found in gram-negative outer membranes is limited, but several of the proteins are present in high concentration, resulting in a total protein content higher than that of the cytoplasmic membrane. Many of the proteins traverse the entire lipid bilayer and are thus transmembrane proteins. A group of these proteins are known as **porins** because they form pores that **allow the diffusion of hydrophilic molecules less than 700 d in size** through the membrane. *The outer membrane and the porin channel allow passage of metabolites and small hydrophilic antibiotics, but the outer membrane is a barrier for large or hydrophobic antibiotics and proteins such as lysozyme.*

The outer membrane also contains structural proteins and receptor molecules for bacteriophages and other ligands. The outer membrane is connected to the cytoplasmic membrane at **adhesion sites** and is tied to the peptidoglycan by **lipoprotein.** The lipoprotein is covalently attached to the peptidoglycan and is anchored in the outer membrane. The adhesion sites provide a membranous route for the delivery of outer membrane components newly synthesized to the outer membrane.

The outer membrane is held together by divalent cation (Mg^{+2} and Ca^{+2}) linkages between phosphates on LPS molecules and hydrophobic interactions between the LPS and proteins. These interactions produce a stiff, strong membrane that can be disrupted by antibiotics (e.g., polymyxin) or by the removal of Mg and Ca ions (chelation with ethylenediaminetetraacetic acid). Disruption of the outer membrane weakens the bacteria and allows the permeability of large, hydrophobic molecules. The addition of lysozyme to cells treated in this manner produces **spheroplasts**, which like protoplasts, are osmotically sensitive.

External Structures

Some bacteria (gram positive or negative) are closely surrounded by loose polysaccharide or protein layers called **capsules** (Figure 3-7). In cases in which it is loosely adherent and nonuniform in density or thickness, the material is referred to as a **slime layer.** The capsule and slime layers are also called the **glycocalyx.** *Bacillus anthracis,* the exception to this rule, produces a polypeptide capsule. The capsule is hard to see in a microscope but can be visualized by the exclusion of India ink particles.

FIGURE 3-7 Transmission electron photomicrographs of *Porphyromonas* (formerly *Bacteroides*) *gingivalis* and *Pseudomonas aeruginosa* revealing the surface-associated capsule. Both strains were isolated from human patients, *P. gingivalis* from an adult with periodontis and *P. aeruginosa* from a patient with cystic fibrosis. *C,* Capsule; *OM,* outer membrane; *PG,* peptidoglycan; *CM,* cytoplasmic membrane; *R,* ribosome; *PP,* polyphosphate. Bar = 0.1 μm. (From Slots J, Taubman MA, editors: *Contemporary oral microbiology and immunology,* St Louis, 1992, Mosby.)

Capsules and slimes are unnecessary for the growth of bacteria but are very important for survival in the host. *The capsule is poorly antigenic and antiphagocytic and is a major virulence factor (e.g., S. pneumoniae).* The capsule can also act as a barrier to toxic hydrophobic molecules, such as detergents, and can promote **adherence** to other bacteria or to host tissue surfaces. For *S. mutans,* the dextran and levan capsules are the means by which the bacteria attach and stick to the tooth enamel. Synthesis of the capsule takes energy and will not be made by the bacteria after continued growth under laboratory conditions away from the selective pressures of the host.

Flagella are ropelike propellers composed of helically coiled protein subunits (**flagellin**) that are anchored in the bacterial membranes through hook and basal body structures and that are driven by membrane potential. Bacterial species may have one or several flagella on their surfaces, and they may be anchored at different parts of the cell. Flagella provide motility for bacteria, allowing the cell to swim (**chemotaxis**) toward food and away from poisons. Bacteria approach food by swimming straight and then tumbling in a new direction. The swimming period becomes longer as the concentration of chemoattractant increases. The direction of flagellar spinning determines whether the bacteria swim or tumble. Flagella also express antigenic and strain determinants.

Fimbriae (pili) (Latin for "fringe") are hairlike structures on the outside of bacteria; they are composed of protein subunits (**pilin**). Fimbriae can be morphologically distinguished from flagella because they are smaller in diameter (3 to 8 nm vs. 15 to 20 nm) and usually are not coiled in structure. Generally, several hundred fimbriae are arranged peritrichously (uniformly) over the entire surface of the bacterial cell. They may be as long as 15 to 20 μm, or many times the length of the cell.

Fimbriae promote adherence to other bacteria or to the host (alternative names: adhesins, lectins, evasins, and aggressins). As an adherence factor (**adhesin**), fimbriae are an important virulence factor for *N. gonorrhoeae* and other bacteria. The tips of the fimbriae contain proteins (lectins) that bind to specific sugars (e.g., mannose). Adherence is essential for *E. coli* colonization and infection of the urinary tract. **F pili (sex pili)** promote the transfer of large segments of bacterial chromosomes between bacteria. These pili are encoded by a plasmid (F).

Bacterial Exceptions

Mycobacteria have a peptidoglycan layer (slightly different structure), which is intertwined with and covalently attached to an arabinogalactan polymer and surrounded by a waxlike lipid coat of mycolic acid (large alpha-branched beta-hydroxy fatty acids), cord factor (glycolipid of trehalose and two mycolic acids), waxD (glycolipid of 15 to 20 mycolic acids and sugar), and sulfolipids. These bacteria are described as **acid-fast staining**. The coat is responsible for virulence and is antiphagocytic. *Corynebacterium* and *Nocardia* organisms also produce mycolic acid lipids. The **mycoplasmas** are also exceptions in that they have no peptidoglycan cell wall and they incorporate steroids from the host into their membranes.

....

STRUCTURE AND BIOSYNTHESIS OF THE MAJOR COMPONENTS OF THE BACTERIAL CELL WALL

The cell wall components are large structures made up of polymers of subunits. This type of structure facilitates their synthesis. Like astronauts building a space station in space, bacteria face problems assembling their cell walls. Synthesis of the peptidoglycan, LPS, teichoic acid, and capsule occurs on the outside of the bacteria, away from the synthetic machinery and energy sources of the cytoplasm and in an inhospitable environment. For both the space station and the bacteria, prefabricated precursors and subunits of the final structure are assembled in a factory-like setting on the inside, attached to a conveyor belt–like structure, brought to the surface and then attached to the preexisting structure. For bacteria, the molecular conveyor belt–like structure is a large hydrophobic phospholipid called **bactoprenol (undecaprenol, C_{55} isoprenoid)**. The prefabricated precursors must also be activated with high energy bonds (e.g., phosphates) or other means to power the attachment reactions occurring outside the cell. For gram-negative bacteria, the outer membrane components are delivered through **adhesion sites.**

Peptidoglycan (Mucopeptide, Murein)

The peptidoglycan is a rigid mesh made up of ropelike linear polysaccharide chains cross-linked by peptides. The polysaccharide is made up of repeating disaccharides of **N-acetylglucosamine** (*GlcNAc, NAG, G*) and **N-acetylmuramic acid** (*MurNAc, NAM, M*) (Figures 3-6 and 3-8).

A tetrapeptide is attached to the MurNAc. The peptide is unusual because it contains both D and L amino acids (D amino acids are not normally used in nature) and the peptide is produced enzymatically. The first two amino acids attached to the MurNAc may vary for different organisims.

The diamino amino acids in the third position are essential for the cross-linking of the peptidoglycan chain. Examples of diamino amino acids include lysine and diaminopimelic and diaminobutyric acids. The peptide cross-link is formed between the free amine of the diamino amino acid in the third position of the peptide and the D-alanine in the fourth position of another chain. *S. aureus* and other gram-positive bacteria use a (glycine)$_5$ bridge between these amino acids to lengthen the cross-link. The precursor form of the peptide has an extra D-alanine, which is released during the cross-linking step.

The peptidoglycan in gram-positive bacteria forms multiple layers and is often cross-linked in three dimensions, providing a very strong, rigid cell wall. In contrast,

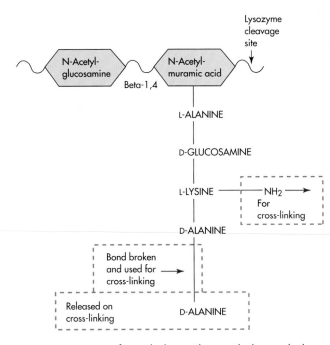

FIGURE 3-8 Precursor of peptidoglycan. The peptidoglycan is built from prefabricated units that contain a pentapeptide attached to the MurNAc. The pentapeptide contains a terminal D-alanine–D-alanine unit. This dipeptide is required for cross-linking the peptidoglycan and is the basis for the action of beta-lactam and vancomycin antibiotics.

the peptidoglycan in gram-negative cell walls is usually only one molecule (layer) thick. The rigidity of the peptidoglycan mesh is determined by the number of cross-links and the length of the cross-link. The site where lysozyme cleaves the glycan of the peptidoglycan is shown in Figure 3-8.

Peptidoglycan Synthesis

Peptidoglycan synthesis occurs in four steps (Figure 3-9). First, inside the cell, glucosamine is enzymatically converted into MurNAc and then energetically activated by a reaction with uridine triphosphate (UTP) to produce uridine diphosphate–N-acetylmuramic acid (UDP-MurNAc). The UDP-MurNAc-pentapeptide precursor is assembled in a series of enzymatic steps:

UDP-MurNAc–AA–AA–AA–D-ALA–D-ALA

Second, the UDP-MurNAc pentapeptide is attached to the **bactoprenol** "conveyor belt" in the cytoplasmic membrane through a pyrophosphate link with the release of uridine monophosphate (UMP). *GlcNAc* is added to make the disaccharide building block of the peptidoglycan. Some bacteria (e.g., *S. aureus*) add a pentaglycine or another chain to the diamino amino acid at the third position of the peptide chain to lengthen the cross-link. Third, the bactoprenol molecule translocates the disaccharide pentapeptide precursor to the outside of the cell. The GlcNAc-MurNAc disaccharide is then attached to a peptidoglycan chain using the pyrophosphate link between itself and the bactoprenol as energy to drive

FIGURE 3-9 Peptidoglycan synthesis. **A,** Peptidoglycan synthesis occurs in three phases. *(1)* Peptidoglycan is synthesized from prefabricated units constructed and activated for assembly and transport inside the cell. *(2)* At the membrane, the units are assembled onto the undecaprenol phosphate conveyor belt, and assembly is completed. *(3)* The unit is translocated to the outside of the cell, where it is attached to the polysaccharide chain, and the peptide is cross-linked to finish the construction. Such a construction can be compared with the assembly of a space station. **B,** The cross-linking reaction is a transpeptidation. One peptide bond (produced inside the cell) is traded for another (outside the cell) with the release of D-alanine. The enzymes that catalyze the reaction are called D-*alanine, D-alanine transpeptidase-carboxypeptidases*. These enzymes are the targets of beta-lactam antibiotics and are called *penicillin-binding proteins*.

the reaction. The pyrophosphobactoprenol is converted back to a phosphobactoprenol and recycled. Fourth, outside the cell but near the membrane surface, peptide chains from adjacent glycan chains are cross-linked to each other by a peptide bond exchange (**transpeptidation**) between the free amine of the amino acid in the third position of the pentapeptide (e.g., lysine), or the N-terminus of the attached pentaglycine chain, and the D-alanine at the fourth position of the other peptide

FIGURE 3-10 Teichoic acid. Teichoic acid is a polymer of chemically modified ribitol (**A**) or glycerol phosphate (**B**). The nature of the modification (e.g., sugars, amino acids) can define the serotype of the bacteria. Teichoic acid may be covalently attached to the peptidoglycan. Lipoteichoic acid is anchored in the cytoplasmic membrane by a covalently attached fatty acid.

chain, releasing the terminal D-alanine of the precursor. This step requires no additional energy because peptide bonds are "traded."

The cross-linking reaction is catalyzed by membrane-bound **transpeptidases.** Related enzymes, DD-**carboxypeptidases,** remove extra terminal D-alanines, which limit the extent of cross-linking. Both of these enzymes are called **penicillin-binding proteins (PBPs)** because they are targets for penicillin and other beta-lactam antibiotics. Penicillin and related beta-lactam antibiotics resemble the "transition state" conformation of the D-ALA–D-ALA unit when bound to these enzymes. Different PBPs are used for extending the peptidoglycan, creating a septum for cell division, and curving the peptidoglycan mesh (cell shape).

The peptidoglycan is constantly being synthesized and degraded. **Autolysins** such as lysozyme are important for determining bacterial shape but continue to degrade the peptidoglycan even if peptidoglycan synthesis is inhibited. Inhibition of synthesis or the cross-linking of the peptidoglycan does not stop the autolysins, and their action weakens the mesh and the bacterial structure and leads to lysis and cell death. New peptidoglycan syn-

FIGURE 3-11 The LPS of the gram-negative cell envelope. **A,** Segment of the polymer showing the arrangements of the major constituents. **B,** Stucture of lipid A of *Salmonella typhimurium.* **C,** Polysaccharide core. **D,** Typical repeat unit (*S. typhimurium*). (Redrawn from Brooks GF, Butel JS, Ornston LN, editors: *Jawetz, Melnick and Aldenberg's medical microbiology,* ed 19, Norwalk, Conn, 1991, Appleton & Lange.)

thesis does not occur during starvation, which leads to a weakening of the peptidoglycan and a loss in the dependability of Gram stain.

An understanding of the biosynthesis of peptidoglycan is essential in medicine because these reactions are unique to bacterial cells and hence can be inhibited with little or no adverse effect on host (human) cells. A number of antibiotics target one or more steps in this pathway (see Chapter 20).

Teichoic and **lipoteichoic acid** are polymers of chemically modified ribose or glycerol connected by phosphates (Figure 3-10). Sugars, choline, or D-alanine may be attached to the hydroxyls of the ribose or glycerol, providing antigenic determinants. These can be distinguished by antibodies and may determine the bacterial serotype. Lipoteichoic acid has a fatty acid and is anchored in the membrane. Teichoic acid is covalently attached to the peptidoglycan. Teichoic acid is synthesized in a manner similar to peptidoglycan.

LPS (endotoxin) *consists of three structural sections: Lipid A, core polysaccharide (rough core), and O antigen* (Figure 3-11). **Lipid A** is an essential component of LPS and is essential for bacterial viability. *Lipid A is responsible for the endotoxin activity of LPS.* It has a phosphorylated glucosamine disaccharide backbone with fatty acids attached to anchor the structure in the outer membrane. The phosphates connect LPS units into aggregates. One carbohydrate chain is attached to the disaccharide backbone and extends away from the bacteria. The basic structure of lipid A is similar for all gram-negative Enterobacteriaceae and identical for related bacteria. The **core polysaccharide** is a branched polysaccharide of 9 to 12 sugars. Most of the core region is also essential for LPS structure and bacterial viability. The **core region** contains an unusual sugar, 2-keto-3-deoxy-octanoate (KDO), and is phosphorylated. The core region is the same for a species of bacteria. The **O antigen** is a long, linear polysaccharide consisting of 50 to 100 repeating saccharide units of 4 to 7 sugars per unit. The O antigen is attached to the core and extends away from the bacteria. It distinguishes serotypes (strains) of a bacterial species.

The lipid A and core portions are enzymatically synthesized in a sequential manner on the inside surface of the cytoplasmic membrane. The repeat units of the O antigen are assembled on a bactoprenol molecule and then transferred to a growing O antigen chain. The finished O antigen chain is transferred to the core lipid A structure. The LPS molecule is translocated through adhesion sites to the outer surface of the outer membrane.

CELL DIVISION

The replication of the bacterial chromosome also triggers the initiation of cell division (Figure 3-12). The production of two daughter bacteria requires the growth and extension of the cell wall components followed by the production of a **septum** (cross wall) to divide the daughter bacteria into two cells. The septum consists of

FIGURE 3-12 Electron photomicrographs of gram-positive cell division (*B. subtilis*) (*left*) and gram-negative cell division (*E. coli*) (*right*). **A** to **C** represent a progression in cell division. *CW*, Cell wall; *CM*, cytoplasmic membrane; *S*, septum; *N*, nucleoid; *OM*, outer membrane. Bar = 0.2 μm. (From Slots J, Taubman MA, editors: *Contemporary oral biology and immunology*, St Louis, 1992, Mosby.)

two membranes separated by two layers of peptidoglycan. Septum formation is initiated at the cell membrane; the septum grows from opposite sides toward the center of the cell, causing cleavage of the daughter cells. This process requires special transpeptidases and other enzymes. New peptidoglycan is synthesized in a defined growth zone, usually in a ring on either side of the growing septum. For streptococci, the growth zone is at 180 degrees from each other, producing linear chains of bacteria. In contrast, the growth zone of staphylococci is at 90 degrees. Incomplete cleavage of the septum can cause the bacteria to remain linked, forming chains (e.g., streptococci) or clusters (e.g., staphylococci).

SPORES

Some *gram-positive, but never gram-negative,* bacteria such as members of the genera *Bacillus* and *Clostridium* (soil bacteria) are spore formers. Under harsh environmental conditions, such as the loss of a nutritional requirement, these bacteria can convert from a **vegetative state** to a **dormant state,** or **spore.** The location of the spore within a cell is a characteristic of the bacteria and can assist in identification of the bacterium.

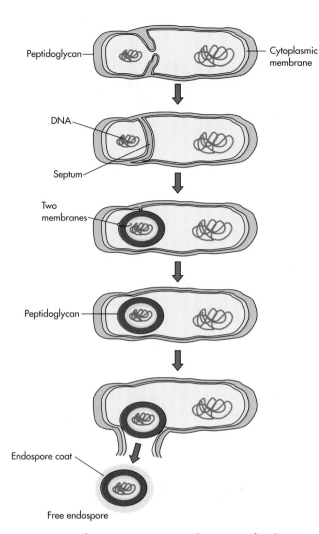

FIGURE 3-13 Endospores. Sporogenesis, the process of endospore formation.

rounded by the peptidoglycan and membrane of the septum. This wraps the DNA in the two layers of membrane and peptidoglycan that would normally divide the cell. The **core** of the spore is surrounded by the **cortex,** which is made up of a thin inner layer of tightly cross-linked peptidoglycan surrounding the cytoplasmic membrane and a loose outer peptidoglycan layer. The cortex is surrounded by the keratin-like protein **coat.**

The germination or transformation of spores into the vegetative state is stimulated by disruption of the outer coat by mechanical stress, pH, heat, or another stressor and requires water and a triggering nutrient (e.g., alanine). The process takes about 90 minutes. Once the germination process has begun, the spore will take up water, swell, shed its coats, and produce one new vegetative cell identical to the original vegetative cell, thus completing the entire cycle. Once germination has begun and the spore coat has been compromised, the spore is weakened and can be inactivated like other bacteria.

QUESTIONS

1. How does each of the differences between prokaryotes and eukaryotes (Table 3-1) influence bacterial infection and treatment?
2. How do the differences between gram-positive and gram-negative cell walls influence the cells' clinical behavior? Detection? Treatment?
3. List the cell wall components that contribute to virulence by protecting the bacteria from immune responses. By eliciting toxic responses in the human host.
4. When peptidoglycan synthesis is inhibited, what processes kill the bacteria? List the precursors that would build up within the bacteria if recycling of bactoprenol were inhibited by vancomycin or bacitracin.
5. Why are spores more resistant to environmental stresses?
6. The laboratory would like to eliminate gram-positive bacteria from a mixture of gram-positive and gram-negative bacteria. Which of the following procedures would be more appropriate and why? Or why not?
   a. Treatment with ethylenediaminetetraacetic acid (a divalent cation chelator)
   b. Treatment with mild detergent
   c. Treatment with lysozyme
   d. Treatment with transpeptidase
   e. Treatment with ampicillin (a hydrophilic beta-lactam antibiotic)

The spore is a dehydrated, multishelled structure that protects and allows the bacteria to exist in "suspended animation" (Figure 3-13). It contains a complete copy of the chromosome, the bare minimum concentrations of essential proteins and ribosomes, and a high concentration of calcium bound to dipicolinic acid. The spore has an inner membrane, two peptidoglycan layers, and an outer keratin-like protein coat. The spore looks refractile (bright) in the microscope. The structure of the spore protects the genomic DNA from desiccation, intense heat, radiation, and attack by most enzymes and chemical agents. In fact, bacterial spores are so resistant to environmental factors that they can exist for centuries as viable spores. Spores are also difficult to decontaminate with standard disinfectants.

Depletion of specific nutrients (e.g., alanine) from the growth medium triggers a cascade of genetic events (comparable to differentiation) leading to the production of a spore. The process requires 6 to 8 hours for completion. After duplication of the chromosome, one copy of DNA and cytoplasmic contents **(core)** are sur-

Bibliography

Davis BD et al, editors: *Microbiology,* ed 4, Philadelphia, 1990, Lippincott.
Slots J, Taubman MA, editors: *Contemporary oral microbiology and immunology,* St Louis, 1992, Mosby.
Stanier RY, Doudoroff M, Adelberg EA: *The microbial world,* ed 4, Englewood Cliffs, NJ, 1976, Prentice Hall.
Talaro K, Talaro AI, editors: *Foundations in microbiology,* ed 2, Dubuque, Iowa, 1996, Wm C Brown.

Bacterial Metabolism and Growth

METABOLIC REQUIREMENTS

Bacterial growth requires a source of energy and the raw materials to build the proteins, structures, and membranes that make up the structure and biochemical machines of the cell. Bacteria must obtain or synthesize the amino acids, carbohydrates, and lipids used as building blocks of the cell.

Although all living cells share the same basic nutritional needs, different cells or cell types have different specific requirements, depending on their biosynthetic repertoire. *In general, bacteria require a source of carbon and nitrogen, an energy source, water, and various ions for growth.* The essential elements and their functions are listed in Table 4-1. Oxygen (O_2 gas), although essential for the human host, is actually a poison for many bacteria. **Iron** is so important that many bacteria secrete special proteins (siderophores) to sequester iron from dilute solutions.

Although some bacteria (such as chemotrophs) can derive energy directly from the oxidation of metal ions such as iron and other bacteria (such as blue-green algae) are capable of photosynthesis, pathogenic bacteria derive their energy by metabolizing sugars, fats, and proteins. Some bacteria, such as certain strains of *Escherichia coli* (a member of the intestinal flora), can synthesize all the amino acids, nucleotides, lipids, and carbohydrates necessary for growth and division when provided with the inorganic nutrients listed in Table 4-1 plus a simple source of carbon, such as glucose. At the other extreme are bacteria, such as the causative agent of syphilis, *Treponema pallidum,* whose growth requirements are so complex that a defined laboratory medium capable of supporting its growth has yet to be developed.

Because of this diversity, growth requirements may be used as a convenient means of classifying different bacteria. For example, unlike animal cells, not all bacteria require oxygen for growth. Some organisms, such as *Clostridium perfringens,* which causes gas gangrene, cannot grow in the presence of oxygen. Such bacteria are referred to as **obligate anaerobes.** Other organisms, such as *Mycobacterium tuberculosis,* which causes tuberculosis, require the presence of molecular oxygen for growth and are therefore referred to as **obligate aerobes.** Most bacteria, however, grow in either the presence or the absence of oxygen. These bacteria are referred to as **facultative anaerobes.**

Bacteria may also be classified on the basis of the predominant source of carbon. Those that can rely entirely on inorganic chemicals for their energy and source of carbon (CO_2) are referred to as **autotrophs (lithotrophs),** whereas many bacteria and animal cells that require organic carbon sources are known as **heterotrophs (organotrophs).**

METABOLISM AND THE CONVERSION OF ENERGY

All cells require a constant supply of energy to survive. This energy, typically in the form of adenosine triphosphate (ATP), is derived from the controlled breakdown of various organic substrates (carbohydrates, lipids, and proteins). This process of substrate breakdown and conversion into usable energy is known as **catabolism.** The energy produced may then be used in the synthesis of cellular constituents (cell walls, proteins, fatty acids, and nucleic acids), a process known as **anabolism.** Together these two processes, which are interrelated and tightly integrated, are referred to as **intermediary metabolism.**

The metabolic process generally begins with the hydrolysis of large macromolecules in the external cellular environment by specific enzymes or exoenzymes (Figure 4-1). The small subunit molecules produced (monosaccharides, short peptides, and fatty acids) are transported across the cell membranes into the cytoplasm by **active** or **passive transport** mechanisms specific for the metabolite. These mechanisms may use specific carrier or membrane transport proteins to help concentrate metabolites from the medium. The metabolites are converted by one or more pathways to one common universal intermediate, **pyruvic acid.** From pyruvic acid the carbons may be channeled toward energy production or the synthesis of new carbohydrates, amino acids, lipids, and nucleic acids.

Catabolism

FIGURE 4-1 Catabolism of proteins, polysaccharides, and lipids produce glucose, pyruvate, or intermediates of the tricarboxylic acid *(TCA)* cycle and ultimately energy in the forms of ATP or the reduced form of nicotinamide adenine dinucleotide *(NADH)*.

TABLE 4-1	**Essential Elements, Their Sources, and Functions in Prokaryotes**

ELEMENT	SOURCE	FUNCTION IN METABOLISM
MAJOR ESSENTIAL ELEMENTS		
C	Organic compounds, CO_2	
O	O_2, H_2O, organic compounds	
H	H_2, H_2O, organic compounds	Major components of cellular material
N	NH_4^+, NO_3^-, N_2, organic compounds	
S	SO_4^{-2}, HS^-, S^0, organic sulfur compounds	Constituent of S-containing amino acids, cysteine, methionine, thiamine pyrophosphate, coenzyme A, biotin, and alpha-lipoic acid
P	HPO_4^{-2}	Constitutent of nucleic acids, phospholipids, nucleotides
K	K^+	Major inorganic cation, cofactor (e.g., pyruvate kinase)
Mg	Mg^{2+}	Cofactor of many enzymes (e.g., kinases); component of cell walls, membranes, ribosomes, and phosphate esters
Ca	Ca^{2+}	Component of exoenzymes (amylases, proteases) and cell walls: major component of endospores as Ca-dipicolinate
Fe	Fe^{2+}, Fe^{3+}	Present in cytochromes, ferredoxins, and other iron-sulfur proteins; cofactor (dehydratases)
Na	Na^+	Transport
Cl	Cl^-	Important inorganic anion
MINOR ESSENTIAL ELEMENTS		
Zn	Zn^{2+}	Component of the enzymes alcohol dehydrogenase, alkaline phosphatase, aldolase, RNA and DNA polymerase
Mn	Mn^{2+}	Present in superoxide dismutase; cofactor of the enzymes PEP carboxykinase, isocitrate synthase
Mo	MoO_4^{-2}	Present in nitrate reductase, nitrogenase, xanthine dehydrogenase, and formate dehydrogenase
Se	SeO_3^{-2}	Component of glycine reductase and formate dehydrogenase
Co	Co^{2+}	Required element in coenzyme B_{12}–containing enzymes (glutamate mutase, methylmalonyl coenzyme A mutase)
Cu	Cu^{2+}	Present in cytochrome oxidase and nitrite reductase
Ni	Ni^{2+}	Present in urease, hydrogenase, and factor F_{430}
W	WO_4^{-2}	Present in some formate dehydrogenases

Modified from Gottschalk E: *Bacterial metabolism,* ed 2, New York, 1985, Springer-Verlag.

Metabolism of Glucose

For the sake of simplicity, this section presents an overview of the pathways by which the model carbohydrate glucose is metabolized to produce energy or other usable substrates. Instead of releasing all the molecule's energy as heat (as for burning), the bacteria break down the glucose in discrete steps to allow the energy to be captured in usable forms. *Bacteria can produce energy from glucose by—in order of increasing efficiency—fermentation or anaerobic respiration (both of which occur in the absence of oxygen) or aerobic respiration.* For a discussion of the metabolism of other organic compounds, including proteins and lipids, see a textbook on biochemistry.

Embden-Meyerhof-Parnas Pathway

Bacteria use three major metabolic pathways in the catabolism of glucose. Most common among these is the glycolytic, or Embden-Meyerhof-Parnas (EMP), pathway (Figure 4-2). This pathway represents the primary means in both bacteria and eukaryotic cells for the conversion of glucose to pyruvate, which as noted previously, is central to a variety of other cellular metabolic pathways. These reactions, which occur under both **aerobic** and **anaerobic** conditions, begin with the "activation" of glucose to form glucose-6-phosphate. This reaction, as well as the third reaction in the series, in which fructose-6-phosphate is converted to fructose-1,6-diphosphate, requires 1 mole of ATP per mole of glucose and represents an initial investment of cellular energy stores.

Energy is produced during glycolysis in two different forms, chemical and electrochemical. In the first, the high-energy phosphate group of one of the intermediates in the pathway is used under the direction of the appropriate enzyme (a **kinase**) to generate **ATP** from adenosine diphosphate (ADP). This type of reaction is termed **substrate-level phosphorylation** and occurs at two different points in the glycolytic pathway (i.e., conversion of 3-phosphoglycerol phosphate to 3-phosphoglycerate and 2-phosphoenolpyruvic acid to pyruvate). Four ATP molecules per molecule of glucose are produced in this manner. Two ATP molecules are consumed in the initial reactions, and the glycolytic conversion of glucose to two molecules of pyruvic acid results in the net production of two molecules of ATP. The reduced form of nicotinamide adenine dinucleotide **(NADH)** that is produced represents the second form of energy, which may then be converted to ATP in the presence of oxygen by a series of oxidation reactions.

In the absence of oxygen, substrate-level phosphorylation represents the primary means of energy production. The pyruvic acid produced from glycolysis is then converted to a variety of end products characteristic of the bacterial species in question in a process known as **fermentation.** Many bacteria are identified on the basis of their fermentative end products (Figure 4-3). These organic molecules, rather than oxygen, are used as electron acceptors to recycle the reduced form of NADH,

which is produced during glycolysis, to nicotinamide adenine dinucleotide (NAD). In yeast, fermentative metabolism results in the conversion of pyruvate to ethanol. Alcoholic fermentation is uncommon in bacteria, which most commonly use the one-step conversion of pyruvic acid to lactic acid. This process is responsible for making milk into yogurt and cabbage into sauerkraut. Other bacteria use more complex fermentative pathways, producing various acids, alcohols, and often gases (many of

FIGURE 4-2 Embden-Meyerhof-Parnas (EMP) glycolytic pathway results in conversion of glucose to pyruvate. The sum of glucose + 2 ADP + 2 Pi + 2 NAD → 2 pyruvate + 4 ATP + 2 NADH + 2 H⁺. Double arrows denote 2 moles reacting per mole of glucose. *ADP,* Adenosine diphosphate; *Pi,* phosphate; *NAD,* nicotinamide adenine dinucleotide; *NADH,* reduced form of NAD.

which have vile odors). These products lend flavors to various cheeses and wines.

Tricarboxylic Acid Cycle

In the presence of oxygen, the pyruvic acid produced from glycolysis, as well as from the metabolism of other substrates, may be completely oxidized (controlled burning) to H_2O and CO_2 using the tricarboxylic acid (TCA) cycle (Figure 4-4), which results in the production of additional energy. The process begins with the oxidative decarboxylation of pyruvate to the high-energy intermediate, acetyl coenzyme A (acetyl-CoA); this reaction also produces NADH. The two remaining carbons derived from pyruvate then enter the TCA cycle by condensation with oxaloacetate, with the formation of citrate. In a stepwise series of oxidative reactions, the citrate is converted back to oxaloacetate, with the net production of 2 moles of CO_2, 3 moles of NADH, 1 mole of flavin adenine dinucleotide ($FADH_2$), and 1 mole of guanosine triphosphate (GTP). GTP is produced via substrate-level phosphorylation in a reaction in which succinyl-CoA is converted to succinate.

The TCA cycle allows the organism to generate substantially more energy per mole of glucose than is possible with glycolysis alone. In addition to the GTP (an ATP equivalent) produced by substrate-level phosphorylation, the NADH and $FADH_2$ produced may enter the electron transport chain. In this chain, the electrons carried by NADH (or $FADH_2$) are passed in a stepwise fashion through a series of donor-acceptor pairs and ultimately to oxygen (Figure 4-5). This process, known as **aerobic respiration,** results in the generation of 3 moles of ATP per mole of NADH and 2 moles of ATP per mole of $FADH_2$. The energetics of aerobic glucose metabolism are depicted in Figure 4-5.

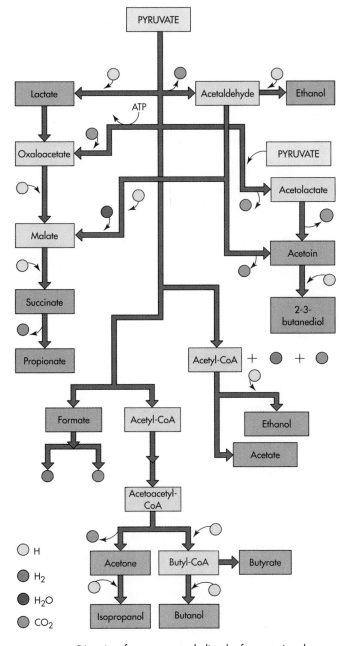

FIGURE 4-3 Diversity of pyruvate metabolism by fermentation demonstrated by microorganisms. The diverse metabolic products have been exploited in the clinical laboratory as phenotypic markers for the differential classification of microbial isolates. *CoA,* Coenzyme A.

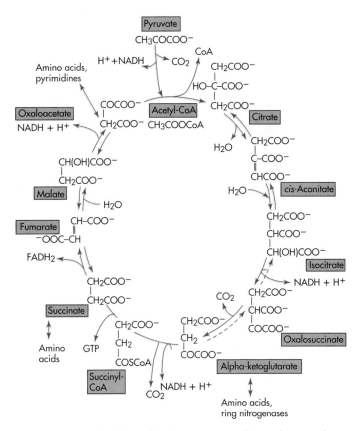

FIGURE 4-4 Tricarboxylic acid cycle occurs in aerobic conditions and is an amphibolic cycle. Precursors for the synthesis of amino acids and nucleotides are also shown. *CoA,* Coenzyme A; *GTP,* guanosine triphosphate; *FADH₂,* flavin adenine dinucleotide.

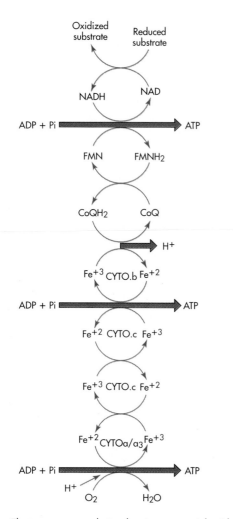

FIGURE 4-5 Electron transport chain, showing sequential oxidation and energy-generating steps. Electron transfer is accompanied by the flow of protons (H^+) from NADH through coenzyme Q *(CoQ)* but not in later steps involving cytochromes *(CYTO)*. Three ATPs are formed per molecule of NADH reoxidized, but only two ATPs are formed per molecule of $FADH_2$ reoxidized. (Modified from Slots J, Taubman MA, editors: *Contemporary oral microbiology and immunology,* St Louis, 1992, Mosby.)

FIGURE 4-6 Aerobic glucose metabolism.

Some bacteria can use compounds other than oxygen (e.g., NO_3^-, SO_4^{2-}, CO_2) as terminal electron acceptors during **anaerobic respiration.** Although this approach is more efficient than fermentation, which uses organic molecules as electron acceptors, it is less efficient than aerobic respiration is because it produces less ATP.

Aerobic organisms are more efficient than anaerobic organisms in which there is no aerobic electron transport or no complete TCA cycle. Fermentation produces 2 ATPs per glucose glycolysis, whereas aerobic metabolism can generate 19 times more energy (38 ATP molecules) from the same starting material (and it is much less smelly) (Figure 4-6).

In addition to the efficient generation of ATP from glucose (and other carbohydrates), the TCA cycle represents a means by which carbons derived from **lipids** (in the form of **acetyl-CoA**) may be shunted toward either energy production or the generation of biosynthetic precursors. Similarly, the cycle includes several points at which **deaminated amino acids** may enter (Figure 4-4). For example, deamination of glutamic acid yields alpha-ketoglutarate, whereas deamination of aspartic acid yields oxaloacetate, both of which are TCA cycle intermediates. The TCA cycle therefore serves the following functions:

1. It is the major mechanism for the generation of ATP.

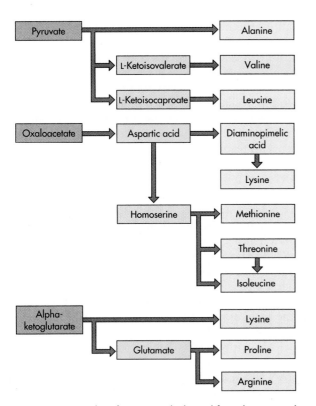

FIGURE 4-7 Examples of amino acids derived from the intermediates of the tricarboxylic acid cycle.

2. It serves as the final common pathway for the complete oxidation of amino acids, fatty acids, and carbohydrates.

3. It supplies key intermediates (i.e., alpha-ketoglutarate, succinyl-CoA, oxaloacetate) for the ultimate synthesis of amino acids (Figure 4-7), lipids, purines, and pyrimidines.

The last two functions make the TCA cycle a so-called **amphibolic cycle** (i.e., it may function in the anabolic and the catabolic functions of the cell).

Pentose Phosphate Pathway

The final pathway of glucose metabolism considered here is known as the *pentose phosphate pathway,* or the **hexose monophosphate shunt** (Figure 4-8). The function of this pathway is to provide precursors and reducing power in the form of nicotinamide-adenine dinucleotide phosphate (reduced form) **(NADPH)** for use in biosynthesis. In the first half of the pathway, glucose is converted to ribulose-5-phosphate, with consumption of 1 mole of ATP and generation of 2 moles of NADPH per mole of glucose. The ribulose-5-phosphate may then be converted to ribose-5-phosphate (a precursor in nucleotide biosynthesis) or alternatively to xylulose-5-phosphate. The remaining reactions in the pathway use enzymes known as *transketolases* and *transaldolases* to generate a variety of sugars, which may function as biosynthetic precursors or may be shunted back to the glycolytic pathway for use in energy generation.

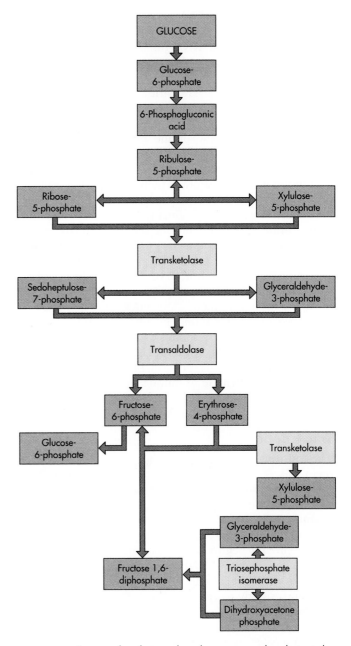

FIGURE 4-8 Pentose phosphate cycle or hexose monophosphate pathway. The enzymes transketolase and transaldolase are central to the cycle's activity.

BIOSYNTHESIS

To this point, we have discussed primarily the catabolic pathways of the bacterial cell, pathways that result in the generation of ATP, NADH, NADPH, and a variety of chemical intermediates. These products may be used for synthesizing major cellular constituents (i.e., peptidoglycan, lipopolysaccharide, proteins, nucleic acids). The following sections describe the important points of the synthesis of each macromolecule from component subunits. DNA and RNA are discussed more fully in Chapter 5.

Nucleic Acid Synthesis

As already discussed, nucleotides not only serve as components of DNA and RNA but also are crucial in the biosynthetic reactions in the growing cell by serving as activators of precursors in the synthesis of polysaccharides, including lipopolysaccharide and peptidoglycan. In addition, nucleotides serve as a usable form of metabolic energy.

The synthesis of the purine nucleotides (adenosine monophosphate and guanosine monophosphate) begins with ribose-5-phosphate formed as a product of the pentose monophosphate shunt. The bicyclic purine ring system is constructed in a stepwise fashion on the sugar phosphate moiety. The product of this series of reactions is the purine nucleotide, inosine monophosphate, which may then be converted to guanosine or adenosine monophosphate. In contrast, the pyrimidine nucleotides are produced by the synthesis of the pyrimidine orotate, which is then attached to the ribose phosphate, forming orotidine monophosphate. This nucleotide may then be converted to cytidine monophosphate or uridine monophosphate. The corresponding deoxynucleotides for use in DNA are synthesized by direct reduction at the 2′ carbon atom of the sugar portion of the ribonucleotide. Production of thymine, a unique nucleotide for DNA, requires the tetrahydrofolate pathway, which makes this pathway a target for antibiotic action.

Transcription

The information carried in the genetic memory of the DNA is transcribed into a useful messenger RNA (mRNA) for subsequent translation into protein. RNA synthesis occurs in a manner similar to that of DNA replication, using a specific DNA-dependent RNA polymerase instead of a DNA polymerase.

The process begins when a component of the multisubunit polymerase recognizes a particular sequence of nucleotides in the DNA (the *promoter;* see Chapter 5) and binds tightly to this site. Promoter sequences occur just before the start of the DNA that actually encodes a protein. Once the polymerase has bound to the appropriate site on the DNA, RNA synthesis proceeds with the sequential addition of ribonucleotides complementary to the sequence in the DNA. Once an entire gene or group of genes (**operon;** see Chapter 5) has been transcribed, the RNA polymerase dissociates from the DNA, a process mediated by signals within the DNA. The bacterial DNA-dependent RNA polymerase is inhibited by rifampin, an antibiotic often used in the treatment of tuberculosis. The transfer RNA (tRNA), which is used in protein synthesis, and ribosomal RNA (rRNA), a component of the ribosomes, are produced in a similar manner.

Translation

Translation is the process by which the **genetic code,** in the form of mRNA, is converted into a sequence of amino acids, the protein product. For the purposes of translation, the nucleotide sequence of the mRNA is divided into groups of three consecutive nucleotides. Each set of three nucleotides is known as a *codon* and encodes a particular amino acid. Because there are four different nucleotides, 4^3, or 64, combinations of 3 are possible, each codon coding for only a single amino acid (or termination signal). However, because there are only 20 amino acids, each may be encoded by multiple triplet codons. This feature is known as the *degeneracy of the genetic code* and may function in protecting the cell from the effects of minor mutations in the DNA or mRNA. The tRNA molecules each contain a three-nucleotide sequence complementary to one of the codon sequences. This tRNA sequence is known as the **anticodon;** it allows base pairing and binds to the codon sequence on the mRNA. Attached to the opposite end of the tRNA is the amino acid that corresponds to the particular codon-anticodon pair.

The process of protein synthesis (Figure 4-9) begins with the formation of the so-called **initiation complex,** in which the two ribosomal subunits, mRNA and initiator tRNA with attached amino acid corresponding to the first codon, are bound together. The ribosome contains two tRNA binding sites, the **A (aminoacyl) site** and the **P (peptidyl) site,** each of which allows base pairing between the bound tRNA and the codon se-

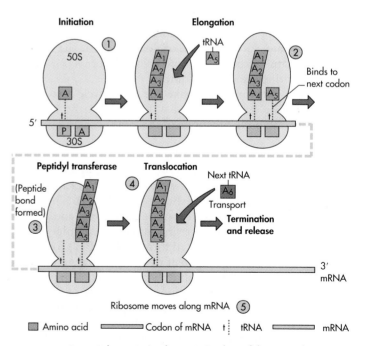

FIGURE 4-9 Bacterial protein synthesis. *1,* Binding of the 30S subunit to the mRNA with the formylmethionine transfer RNA (fmet-tRNA) at the AUG start codon allows assembly of the 70S ribosome. The fmet-tRNA binds to the peptidyl site *(P). 2,* The next tRNA binds to its codon at the A site and, *3,* "accepts" the growing peptide chain. *4,* Before translocation to the peptidyl site. The process is repeated until a stop codon and the protein are released.

quence in the mRNA. The tRNA corresponding to the second codon occupies the A site. The amino group of the amino acid attached to the A site forms a peptide bond with the carboxyl group of the amino acid in the P site in a reaction that is known as **transpeptidation.** This process leaves the tRNA in the P site uncharged (without an attached amino acid), allowing it to be released from the ribosome. The ribosome then moves down the mRNA exactly three nucleotides, thereby transferring the tRNA with attached nascent peptide to the P site and bringing the next codon into the A site. The appropriate charged tRNA is brought into the A site, and the process is then repeated. Translation continues until the new codon in the A site is one of the three termination codons, for which there is no corresponding tRNA. At that point the translation complex is disassembled, and the new protein is released to the cytoplasm.

The process of protein synthesis represents an important target of antimicrobial action. The aminoglycosides (e.g., streptomycin and gentamicin), as well as the tetracyclines, act by binding to the small ribosomal subunit and inhibiting normal ribosomal function. Similarly, the macrolide and lincosamide groups of antibiotics (e.g., erythromycin and clindamycin) act by binding to the large ribosomal subunit.

BACTERIAL GROWTH

Bacterial replication is a coordinated process in which two equivalent daughter cells are produced. For growth to occur, there must be sufficient metabolites to support the synthesis of the bacterial components and especially the nucleotides for DNA synthesis. A cascade of regulatory events (synthesis of key proteins and RNA), much like a countdown at the Kennedy Space Center, must occur on schedule to initiate a replication cycle. *However, once it is initiated, DNA synthesis must run to completion, even if all nutrients have been removed from the medium.*

Chromosome replication is initiated at the membrane, and each daughter chromosome is anchored to a different portion of membrane. In some cells the DNA associates with mesosomes. As the bacterial membrane grows, the daughter chromosomes are pulled apart. The commencement of chromosome replication also initiates the process of cell division, which can be visualized by the start of septum formation between the two daughter cells (Figure 4-10; see also Chapter 3). New initiation events may occur before completion of the chromosome replication and cell division.

Depletion of metabolites (starvation) or a buildup of toxic byproducts (e.g., ethanol) triggers the production of chemical **alarmones,** which cause synthesis to stop, but degradative processes continue. DNA synthesis continues until all initiated chromosomes are completed, despite the detrimental effect on the cell. Ribosomes are cannibalized for deoxyribonucleotide precursors, peptidoglycan and proteins are degraded for metabolites, and the cell shrinks. Septum formation may be initiated, but cell division may not occur. Many cells die. Similar signals may initiate **sporulation** in species capable of this process (see Chapter 3).

Cell wall

Cell membrane

Chromosome 1

Chromosome 2

FIGURE 4-10 Bacterial cell division. Replication requires extension of the cell wall as well as replication of the chromosome and septum formation. Membrane attachment of the DNA pulls each daughter strand into a new cell.

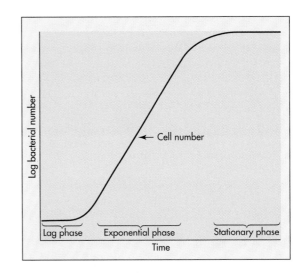

FIGURE 4-11 Phases of bacterial growth, starting with an inoculum of stationary phase cells.

Population Dynamics

When bacteria are added to a medium, they require a period of time to adapt to the new environment before they begin dividing (Figure 4-11). This period is known as the **lag phase** of growth. The bacteria will grow and divide at a **doubling time** characteristic of the strain and the conditions during the **log** or **exponential phase.** During the log phase, the number of bacteria will increase to 2^n, in which n is the number of generations (doublings). Eventually the culture runs out of metabolites, or a toxic substance builds up in the medium; the bacteria then stop growing and enter the **stationary phase.**

QUESTIONS

1. How many moles of ATP are generated per mole of glucose in glycolysis, the TCA cycle, and electron transport? Which of these occur in anaerobic and which in aerobic conditions? Which is most efficient?
2. What products of anaerobic fermentation would be detrimental to host (human) tissue (e.g., *Clostridium perfringens*)?

3. If the number of bacteria during log phase growth can be calculated by the following equation:

$$N_t = N_o \times 2^{t/d}$$

where N_t is the number of bacteria after time (t), t/d is the amount of time divided by the doubling time, and N_o is the initial number of bacteria, how many bacteria will be in the culture after 4 hours if the doubling time is 20 minutes and the initial bacterial inoculum contained 1000 bacteria?

Bibliography

Davis BD et al, editors: *Microbiology,* ed 4, Philadelphia, 1990, JB Lippincott.

Jawetz E et al: *Review of medical microbiology,* ed 16, Los Altos, Calif, 1984, Lange.

Lehninger AL: *Principles of biochemistry,* New York, 1982, Worth.

Mandell GL et al, editors: *Principles and practice of infectious diseases,* ed 3, New York, 1990, Churchill Livingstone.

Slots J, Taubman MA, editors: *Contemporary oral microbiology and immunology,* St Louis, 1992, Mosby.

CHAPTER 5

Bacterial Genetics

DNA: THE GENETIC MATERIAL

The bacterial genome is the **total collection of genes** carried by a bacterium both on its chromosome and on its extrachromosomal genetic elements, if any. The bacterial chromosome differs in several ways from the human chromosome. The chromosome of a typical bacterium such as *Escherichia coli* is a single, double-stranded, circular molecule of DNA containing approximately 5 million base pairs (or 5000 kilobase pairs), an approximate length of 1.3 mm (i.e., about 1000 times the diameter of the cell). The smallest bacterial chromosomes (from **mycoplasmas**) are about one quarter this size. In comparison, humans have two copies of 23 chromosomes, which represent 2.9×10^9 base pairs 990 mm in length. Each genome contains many **operons,** which are made up of **genes.** Eukaryotes usually have two distinct copies of each chromosome (they are therefore **diploid**). Bacteria usually have only one copy of their chromosomes (they are therefore **haploid**). Because bacteria have only one chromosome, alteration of a gene (mutation) will have a more obvious effect on the cell. In addition, the structure of the bacterial chromosome is maintained by polyamines, such as spermine and spermidine, rather than by histones.

Bacteria may also contain extrachromosomal genetic elements such as **plasmids** or **bacteriophages** (bacterial viruses). These elements are independent of the bacterial chromosome and in most cases can be transmitted from one cell to another.

Genes are sequences of nucleotides that have a biological function; examples are protein-structural genes (**cistrons,** which are coding genes), ribosomal RNA genes, and recognition and binding sites for other molecules (promoters and operators). **Promoters and operators** are nucleotide sequences that control the expression of a gene by influencing which sequences will be transcribed into mRNA (more discussion follows).

Operons are groups of one or more structural genes expressed from a particular promoter and ending at a transcriptional terminator. Thus all the genes coding for the enzymes of a particular pathway can be coordinately regulated. Operons with multiple structural genes are **polycistronic.** The *E. coli lac* **operon** for lactose use includes all the genes necessary for lactose metabolism, as well as the control mechanisms for turning off (in the presence of glucose) or turning on (in the presence of galactose or an inducer) these genes only when they are needed. The *lac* operon includes a repressor sequence, a promoter sequence and structural genes for the beta-galactosidase enzyme, a permease, and an acetylase (Figure 5-1). The lac operon is discussed later in this chapter.

REPLICATION OF DNA

The bacterial chromosome is a storehouse of information by which the characteristics of the cell are defined and by which all cellular processes are carried out. It is therefore essential that this molecule be duplicated without errors. Replication of the bacterial genome is triggered by a cascade of events linked to the growth rate of the cell. Replication of bacterial DNA is initiated at a specific sequence in the chromosome called *OriC*. The replication process requires an enzyme (**helicase**) to unwind the DNA at the origin to expose the DNA, an enzyme (**primase**) to synthesize primers to start the process, the enzyme or enzymes (**DNA-dependent DNA polymerases**) that copy the DNA but only in the 5′ to 3′ direction, and other enzymes.

New DNA is synthesized **semiconservatively**, using both strands of the parental DNA as templates. New DNA synthesis occurs at **growing forks** and proceeds bidirectionally. One strand (the leading strand) is copied continuously in the 5′ to 3′ direction, whereas the other strand (the lagging strand), which must also be extended in the 5′ to 3′ direction as its template becomes available, must be synthesized as many pieces of DNA using RNA primers (Okazaki fragments). Then the pieces are ligated together by the enzyme **DNA ligase** (Figure 5-2). To maintain the high degree of accuracy required for replication, the DNA polymerases possess "proofreading" functions, which allow the enzyme to confirm that the appropriate nucleotide was inserted and to correct any errors that were made. Multiple initiations of chromosomal replication may occur before cell division, during log-phase growth in rich medium. This process produces a series of nested bubbles of new daughter

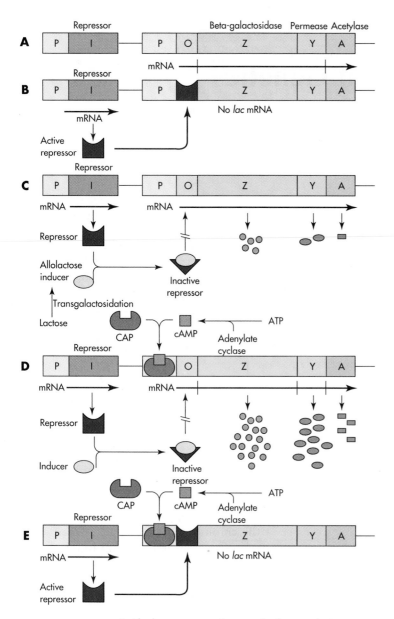

FIGURE 5-1 A, The lactose operon is transcribed as a polycistronic messenger RNA (mRNA) from the promoter *(P)* and translated into three proteins: beta-galactosidase *(Z)*, permease *(Y)*, and acetylase *(A)*. The *lacI* gene encodes the repressor protein. **B,** The lactose operon is not transcribed in the absence of an allolactose inducer, since the repressor competes with the RNA polymerase at the operator site *(O)*. **C,** The repressor, complexed with the inducer, does not recognize the operator because of a conformation change in the repressor. The *lac* operon is thus transcribed at a low level. **D,** *E. coli* is grown in a poor medium in the presence of lactose as the carbon source. Both the inducer and the CAP-cAMP complex are bound to the promoter, which is fully "turned on," and a high level of *lac* mRNA is transcribed and translated. **E,** Growth of *E. coli* in a poor medium without lactose will result in the binding of the CAP-cAMP complex to the promoter region and binding of the active repressor to the operator sequence, since no inducer is available. The result will be that the *lac* operon will not be transcribed. *CAP,* Catabolite gene-activator protein; *cAMP,* cyclic adenosine monophosphate; *ATP,* adenosine triphosphate.

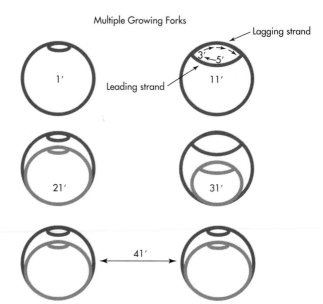

FIGURE 5-2 Assuming 40 minutes to complete one round of replication and assuming new initiation every 20 minutes, initiation of DNA synthesis precedes cell division. Multiple growing forks may be prevented in a cell before complete septum formation and cell division. The daughter cells are "born pregnant."

chromosomes, each with its pair of growth forks of new DNA synthesis. The polymerase moves down the DNA strand, incorporating the appropriate (complementary) nucleotide at each position. Replication is complete when the two replication forks meet 180 degrees from the origin. The process of DNA replication puts great torsional strain on the chromosomal circle of DNA; this strain is relieved by **topoisomerases.** The topoisomerase is essential to the bacteria and is a target for the quinolone antibiotics.

For a more complete description of DNA replication, transcription, and translation, see the textbooks listed in the bibliography.

TRANSCRIPTIONAL CONTROL
Regulation of Gene Expression

Bacteria have developed mechanisms to adapt quickly and efficiently to changes in concentrations of nutrients in their environment. The bacteria turn on a complete set of enzymes when necessary and avoid making the enzyme or enzymes of a pathway when the substrate is absent.

First, the organization of the genes of a biochemical pathway into an **operon,** with appropriate genetic control mechanisms, allows coordinated production of the necessary enzymes in response to a nutritional stimulus. Second, the transcription of the gene is regulated directly by repressor proteins (which bind to operators) in response to nutritional signals within the cell. Third, the rate of protein synthesis by the ribosome can regulate transcription in prokaryotes. The absence of a nuclear membrane in prokaryotes to separate the two processes allows the ribosome to bind to the messenger RNA (mRNA) as it is being transcribed from the DNA.

Transcriptional Regulation

Initiation of transcription may be under positive or negative control. Genes under **negative control** are expressed unless they are switched off by a repressor protein. This **repressor protein** prevents gene expression by binding to a specific DNA sequence, called the **operator,** making it impossible for the RNA polymerase to initiate transcription at the promoter. Inversely, genes whose expression is under **positive control** are not transcribed unless an active regulator protein, called an **apoinducer,** is present. The apoinducer binds to a specific DNA sequence and assists the RNA polymerase in the initiation steps by an unknown mechanism.

Operons can be **inducible** or **repressible.** Introduction of a substrate **(inducer)** into the growth medium may induce an operon to increase the expression of the enzymes necessary for its metabolism. The end products **(corepressors)** of a pathway may signal that a pathway should be shut down or repressed by reducing the synthesis of its enzymes.

The lactose (*lac*) operon responsible for the degradation of the sugar lactose is an inducible operon under positive and negative regulation (Figure 5-1). Normally the bacteria use glucose and not lactose. In the absence of lactose, the operon is repressed by the binding of the repressor protein to the operator sequence, thus impeding the RNA polymerase function. In the absence of glucose, however, the addition of lactose reverses this repression. Full expression of the *lac* operon also requires a protein-mediated, positive-control mechanism. In *E. coli,* a protein called the catabolite gene-activator protein (CAP) forms a complex with cyclic adenosine monophosphate (cAMP), acquiring the ability to bind to a specific DNA sequence present in the promoter. The CAP-cAMP complex enhances binding of the RNA polymerase to the promoter, thus allowing an increase in the frequency of transcription initiation. The CAP-cAMP complex may increase the operon transcription by protein-protein interaction with the RNA polymerase or by protein-DNA interaction.

Although tryptophan is essential for protein synthesis, too much tryptophan in the cell can be toxic; therefore its synthesis must be regulated. The tryptophan operon (*trp* operon) contains the structural genes necessary for tryptophan biosynthesis and is under dual transcriptional control mechanisms (Figure 5-3). At the DNA level, the repressor protein is activated by increased intracellular concentration of tryptophan to prevent transcription. At the protein synthesis level, rapid translation of a "test peptide" at the beginning of the mRNA in the presence of tryptophan promotes the formation of a double-stranded loop in the RNA, which terminates transcription. The same loop is formed if no protein synthesis is

occurring, a situation in which tryptophan synthesis would similarly not be required. This regulates tryptophan synthesis at the mRNA level in a process termed **attenuation,** in which mRNA synthesis is prematurely terminated.

Posttranscriptional or Translational Regulation

Translational control can occur with monocistronic and polycistronic mRNA. With polycistronic mRNA, **translational control** refers to differences in the copy number of each protein expressed from each gene. For example, for the *lac* operon, beta-galactosidase, galactoside permease, and acetylase are produced at a ratio of 10:5:2. The translational process may also be regulated by factors other than their intrinsic structures. In other words, translational initiation may be controlled by a regulator molecule, which will act directly or indirectly to determine whether an initiation site for a coding region is available to the ribosomes.

MUTATION, REPAIR, AND RECOMBINATION

DNA conveys genetic information; therefore there is no molecule in a living organism whose integrity is as vital to the cell as its DNA. Cells must be able to replicate DNA accurately. Furthermore, accidental damage to DNA must be minimized by the elaboration of efficient DNA repair systems. These damage-containment systems are so important for the life of a cell that a bacterium may devote a large percentage of its genome to specify and control the enzymes involved.

Mutations Affecting the DNA

A **mutation** is any change in the base sequence of the DNA. A single base change can result in a **transition,** in which one purine is replaced by another purine or in which a pyrimidine is replaced by another pyrimidine. A **transversion,** in which, for example, a purine is replaced by a pyrimidine and vice versa, may also result. A **silent mutation** is a change at the DNA level that does not result in any change of amino acid in the encoded protein. This type of mutation occurs because more than one codon may encode an amino acid. A **missense mutation** results in a different amino acid being inserted in the protein. Finally, a **nonsense mutation** changes a codon encoding an amino acid to a stop codon (e.g., TAG [thymine-adenine-guanine]), which will cause the ribosome to fall off the mRNA.

More drastic changes can occur in proteins when multiple bases are involved. For example, a small deletion or insertion that is *not in multiples of three* produces a **frameshift mutation.** This results in a change in the reading frame, usually leading to a nonsense peptide and premature truncation of the protein. **Null mutations,** which completely destroy gene function, arise when there is an extensive insertion, deletion, or gross rearrangement of the chromosome structure. The aberrant action of DNA recombination processes or the insertion

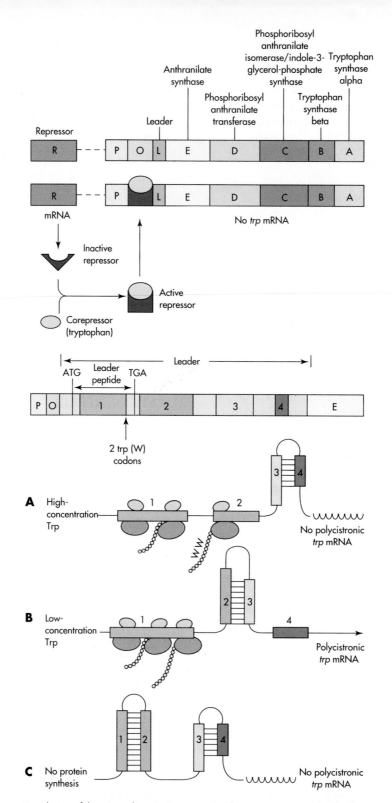

FIGURE 5-3 Regulation of the tryptophan *(trp)* operon. **A,** The *trp* operon encodes the five enzymes necessary for tryptophan biosynthesis. This *trp* operon is under dual control. **B,** The conformation of the inactive repressor protein is changed after its binding by the corepressor tryptophan. The resulting active repressor *(R)* binds to the operator *(O)*, blocking any transcription of the *trp* mRNA by the RNA polymerase. **C,** The *trp* operon is also under the control of an attenuation-antitermination mechanism. Upstream of the structural genes are the promoter *(P)*, the operator, and a leader *(L)*, which can be transcribed into a short peptide containing two tryptophans *(W)* near its distal end. The leader mRNA possesses four repeats *(1, 2, 3,* and *4)*, which can pair differently according to the tryptophan availability, leading to an early termination of transcription of the *trp* operon or its full transcription. In the presence of a high concentration of tryptophan, regions 3 and 4 of the leader mRNA can pair, forming a terminator hairpin, and no transcription of the *trp* operon occurs. However, in the presence of little or no tryptophan, the ribosomes stall in region 1 when translating the leader peptide because of the tandem of tryptophan codons. Then regions 2 and 3 can pair, forming the antiterminator hairpin and leading to transcription of the *trp* genes. Finally, the regions 1:2 and 3:4 of the free leader mRNA can pair, also leading to the cessation of transcription before the first structural gene *trpE*. *A,* Adenine; *G,* guanine; *T,* thymine.

of long sequences of DNA (many thousands of base pairs) by transposition or during genetic engineering can produce null mutations by separating the parts of a gene and preventing the gene's expression.

Many mutations occur spontaneously in nature; however, mutations can also be induced by physical or chemical agents. Among the physical agents used to induce mutations in bacteria are heat, which results in deamination of nucleotides; ultraviolet light, which causes pyrimidine dimer formation; and ionizing radiation, such as x-rays, which may be responsible for opening a ring of a base or single- or double-strand breaks in the DNA.

Chemical agents that also are mutagens can be grouped into three classes. The first class is **nucleotide-base analogues;** they are incorporated into the DNA during replication and lead to mispairing and frequent mistakes during DNA replication. The similarity of 5-bromouracil to thymidine allows the former's incorporation into DNA. However, a structural rearrangement of the molecule allows 5-bromouracil to bind to guanine instead of adenine, changing a T-A base pair to a G-C base pair.

The second class is polycyclic flat molecules, such as ethidium bromide or acridine derivatives; they are examples of *frameshift mutagens.* They insert (or intercalate) between the bases as they stack with each other in the double helix and cause the addition or deletion of a single base. These intercalating agents increase the spacing of successive base pairs, destroying the regular sugar-phosphate backbone and decreasing the pitch of the helix. These changes lead to frequent mistakes during DNA replication.

The third class is **DNA-reactive chemicals;** they act directly on the DNA, resulting in a modification of the normal base into a chemically different structure. The modified bases may pair abnormally or may not pair at all. The damage may cause the removal of the base from the DNA backbone. These include nitrous acid (HNO_2) and alkylating agents, including nitrosoguanidine and ethyl methane sulfonate, which are known to add methyl or ethyl groups to the rings of the DNA bases.

Mutations can also occur in other genes to eliminate the effects of a mutation in the original gene. Such a phenomenon is termed **suppression.** An extragenic suppressor usually involves a mutation in an anticodon of transfer RNA (tRNA). This mutated tRNA reads a mutated codon in the sense of the original codon or gives an acceptable substitute. Intragenic suppression is achieved by a second compensating mutation within the gene, which restores the original reading frame of a gene containing a frameshift mutation.

Repair Mechanisms of DNA

A number of repair mechanisms have evolved in bacterial cells to minimize damage to DNA. These repair mechanisms can be divided into five groups:

1. **Direct DNA repair** is the enzymatic removal of damages, such as pyrimidine dimers and alkylated bases.

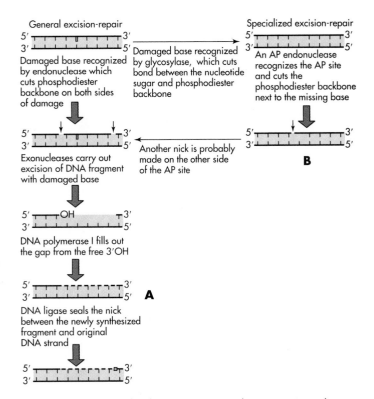

FIGURE 5-4 A, Generalized excision repair mechanism. **B,** Specialized excision repair mechanism. *AP,* Apurinic (endonuclease).

2. **Excision repair** is the excision of a DNA segment containing the damage, followed by synthesis of a new DNA strand (Figure 5-4). Two types of excision-repair mechanisms, generalized and specialized, exist.

3. Recombinational or **postreplication repair** is the retrieval of missing information by genetic recombination when both DNA strands are damaged.

4. The **SOS response** is the induction of many genes (approximately 15) after DNA damage or interruption of DNA replication.

5. **Error-prone repair** is the last resort of a bacterial cell before it dies. It is used when a DNA template is not available for directing an accurate repair.

GENE EXCHANGE IN PROKARYOTIC CELLS

Many bacteria, especially many pathogenic bacterial species, are quite promiscuous with their DNA. The exchange of DNA between cells allows the exchange of genes and characteristics between cells, thus producing new strains of bacteria. This exchange may be advantageous for the recipient, especially if the exchanged DNA encodes antibiotic resistance. The transferred DNA can be integrated into the recipient chromosome or stably maintained as an extrachromosomal element (**plasmid**) or a bacterial virus (**bacteriophage**) and passed on to daughter bacteria as an autonomously replicating unit.

FIGURE 5-5 Plasmids. The pBR322 plasmid was one of the plasmids used for cloning DNA. This plasmid encodes resistance to ampicillin (*amp*) and tetracycline (*tet*) and an origin of replication (*ori*). Different restriction enzyme cleavage sites are indicated. The pGEM plasmid has multiple cloning sites within the beta-galactosidase gene (*lacZ*), which is flanked by bacteriophage promoters to allow directional mRNA expression of the cloned sequence.

FIGURE 5-6 Bacteriophage lambda.

FIGURE 5-7 Lysogenic infection of bacterium with temperate bacteriophage. **A,** The phage infects a sensitive bacterium, and the phage DNA is injected. **B,** The phage DNA becomes integrated into the bacterial chromosome. **C,** The bacterium multiplies, apparently unaffected by the infection. It has been lysogenized. **D,** Occasionally the phage DNA is excised from the bacterial chromosome, takes control of the cell, and replicates. **E,** An individual cell (or, by induction, all the cells) produces phage components. **F,** The components are then later assembled into phage particles. **G,** Ultimately the cell lyses and releases mature phage particles.

Plasmids are small genetic elements that replicate independently of the bacterial chromosome. Most plasmids are circular, double-stranded DNA molecules varying from 1500 to 400,000 base pairs. However, *Borrelia burgdorferi,* the causative agent of Lyme disease, and the related *B. hermsii* are unique among all eubacteria because they possess linear plasmids. Like the bacterial chromosomal DNA, they can autonomously replicate and as such are referred to as **replicons.** Some plasmids,

such as the *E. coli* F plasmid, are **episomes,** which means that they can integrate into the host chromosome.

Plasmids usually do not encode essential functions for bacteria and are thus unnecessary for the growth of the microorganism. However, plasmids carry additional genetic information, which may provide a selective advantage to the bacteria. For example, plasmids may confer high levels of antibiotic resistance, encode the production of bacteriocins or toxins, and contain genes that

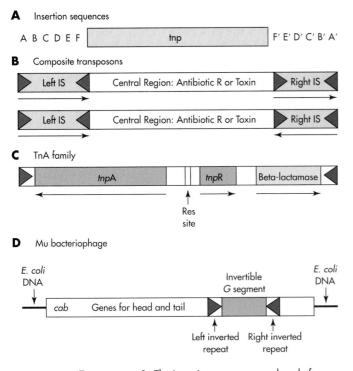

A   Insertion sequences

A B C D E F [tnp] F' E' D' C' B' A'

B   Composite transposons

[Left IS] [Central Region: Antibiotic R or Toxin] [Right IS]

[Left IS] [Central Region: Antibiotic R or Toxin] [Right IS]

C   TnA family

[tnpA] [tnpR] [Beta-lactamase]

Res
site

D   Mu bacteriophage

E. coli
DNA   Invertible   E. coli
                                 G segment   DNA

[cab   Genes for head and tail]

Left inverted   Right inverted
repeat   repeat

FIGURE 5-8 Transposons. **A,** The insertion sequences code only for a transposase *(tnp)* and possess inverted repeats (15 to 40 basepairs) at each end. **B,** The composite transposons contain a central-region coding for antibiotic resistances or toxins, flanked by two insertion sequences *(IS)*, which can be either directly repeated or reversed. **C,** Tn3, a member of the TnA transposon family. The central region encodes three genes—a transposase *(tnpA)*, a resolvase *(tnpR)*, and a beta-lactamase—conferring resistance to ampicillin. A resolution site *(Res site)* is used during the replicative transposition process. This central region is flanked on both ends by direct repeats of 38 basepairs. **D,** Phage-associated transposon is exemplified by the bacteriophage mu.

may provide the bacteria with a unique advantage in metabolizing some substrates (Figure 5-5). The number of copies of plasmid produced by a cell is determined by the particular plasmid. The copy number is the ratio of copies of the plasmid to the number of copies of the chromosome. This may be as few as 1 in the case of large plasmids or as many as 50 in smaller plasmids.

Large plasmids (20 to 120 kb), such as the fertility factor F found in *E. coli* or the resistance transfer factor (80 kb), can often mediate their own transfer from one cell to another by a process called **conjugation** (see the section on conjugation). These conjugative plasmids encode all the necessary factors for their transfer. Other plasmids can be transferred into a bacterial cell by means other than conjugation, such as **transformation, transduction,** and **integration** in the cellular chromosome. These terms will be discussed later in the chapter.

Bacteriophages are bacterial viruses. These extrachromosomal genetic elements can survive outside of a host cell because the nucleic acid genome (which may be DNA or RNA), is **protected by a protein coat** (Figure 5-6).

Bacteriophages infect bacterial cells and either replicate to large numbers and cause the cell to lyse (**lytic** infection) or in some cases integrate into the host genome without killing the host (the **lysogenic** state), such as the *E. coli* **bacteriophage lambda** (Figure 5-7). Some lysogenic bacteriophages carry toxin genes (e.g., **Corynephage** beta carries the gene for the diphtheria toxin). Bacteriophage lambda remains lysogenic as long as a repressor protein is synthesized and prevents the phage from becoming unintegrated and replicating independent of the host chromosome. This reaction can be triggered if the host cell DNA is damaged by radiation or by another means or if the cell can no longer make the repressor protein, a signal that the host cell is unhealthy and is no longer a good place for "freeloading."

Transposons are mobile genetic elements that are dependent replicons (Figure 5-8). They can move from one position to another in the genome or between different molecules of DNA. The simplest transposons are called **insertion sequences.** Complex transposons carry other genes, such as genes that provide resistance against antibiotics. Because these transposons can jump in and out of genes, an antibiotic resistance gene would make the transposon an asset to the cell and therefore would be more likely to be maintained within the chromosome. Sometimes transposons insert into genes and inactivate those genes. If insertion and inactivation occur in a gene that encodes an essential protein, the cell will die.

MECHANISMS OF GENETIC TRANSFER

The exchange of genetic material between bacterial cells may occur by one of three mechanisms: (1) **conjugation,** which is the mating or quasisexual exchange of genetic information from one bacterium (the donor) to another bacterium (the recipient); (2) **transformation,** which results in the acquisition of new genetic markers by the incorporation of exogenous or foreign DNA; or (3) **transduction,** which is the transfer of genetic information from one bacterium to another by a bacteriophage. Conjugation occurs with most, if not all, eubacteria. Conjugation usually occurs between members of the same species but has also been demonstrated to occur between prokaryotes and cells from plants, animals, and fungi.

Transformation is the process by which bacteria take up fragments of naked DNA and incorporate them into their genomes. Transformation was the first mechanism of genetic transfer to be discovered in bacteria. In 1928, Griffith made the observation that pneumococcus virulence was related to the presence of a surrounding polysaccharide capsule and that extracts of encapsulated bacteria producing smooth colonies could transmit this trait to nonencapsulated bacteria, normally appearing with rough edges. Griffith's studies led to Avery, MacLeod, and McCarty's identification of DNA as the transforming principle some 15 years later.

Gram-positive and gram-negative bacteria can take up and stably maintain exogenous DNA (Figure 5-9). Certain species are naturally capable of taking up exogenous DNA (such species are then said to be **competent**), including *Haemophilus influenzae, Streptococcus pneumoniae, Bacillus* species, and *Neisseria* species. Competence develops toward the end of logarithmic growth, some time before a population enters the stationary phase. Most bacteria do not exhibit a natural ability for DNA uptake. Chemical methods or electroporation (the use of high-voltage pulses) is used to introduce plasmid and other DNA into *E. coli* and other bacteria.

Conjugation

Genetic transfer in *E. coli* was first reported by Lederberg and Tatum in 1946, when they observed sexlike exchange between two mutant strains of *E. coli* K12. **Conjugation** is the process by which DNA is passed directly by cell-to-cell contact during the mating of the bacteria. Conjugation results in the one-way transfer of DNA from a donor (or male) cell to a recipient (or female) cell through the sex pilus. The mating type (sex) of the cell depends on the presence (male) or absence (female) of a **conjugative plasmid,** such as the **F plasmid of *E. coli*.** The conjugative plasmid contains genes that convey donor properties, including the ability to make **sex pili** and to initiate DNA synthesis at the **transfer origin (OriT)** of the plasmid. In addition to *E. coli*, conjugation occurs with *Bacteroides* organisms, streptococci, streptomyces, and clostridia. Many of the large conjugative plasmids specify colicins or antibiotic resistances.

FIGURE 5-9 Bacterial transformation. Foreign DNA can be taken up or forced into bacteria and incorporated into the chromosome or maintained as a plasmid. This "transforms" the bacterium into a new organism.

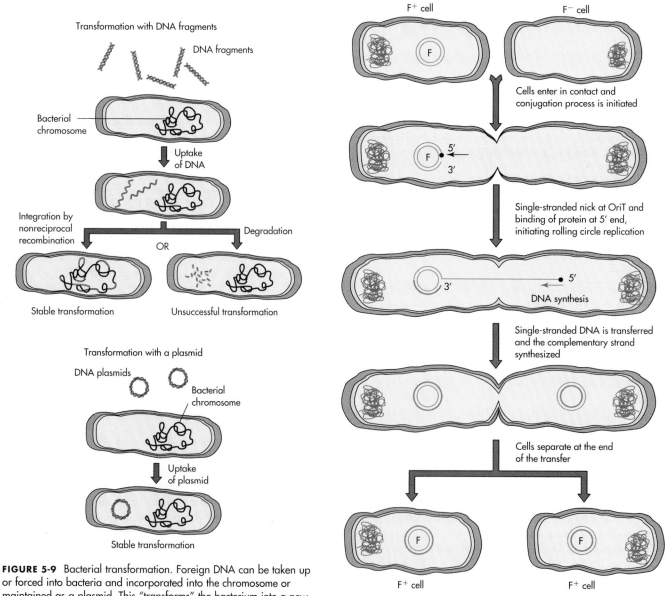

FIGURE 5-10 Genetic transfer of the F plasmid by conjugation.

As an independent plasmid, the F plasmid transfers itself, converting recipients into **F⁺** male cells (Figure 5-10). If a fragment of chromosomal DNA has been incorporated into the plasmid, it is designated an **F prime (F′)** plasmid. When it transfers into the recipient cell, it carries that fragment with it and also converts them into F′ males. If the F plasmid sequence is integrated into the bacterial chromosome, the cell is designated an **Hfr** cell. An Hfr (which stands for *high frequency of recombination*) cell transfers chromosomal genes in an order determined by the position and orientation of the integrated *OriT.* Conjugation *rarely* causes recipients to become Hfr males and then only if the conjugation has first transferred the entire bacterial chromosome.

The DNA that is transferred by conjugation is not a double helix but a single-stranded molecule. **Mobilization** begins when a plasmid-encoded protein makes a single-stranded, site-specific cleavage at the OriT. The nick initiates rolling circle replication, and the displaced linear strand is probably the intermediate structure directed to the recipient cell. However, little is known about how the DNA or DNA-protein complex leaves the donor and enters the recipient cell. Finally, the transferred, single-stranded DNA is recircularized and its complementary strand synthesized. The F plasmid is defined as conjugative because it carries all the genes necessary for its own transfer. However, some plasmids such as ColE1 and ColK are not conjugative plasmids. They are mobilizable, however. These plasmids may be mobilized by some conjugative plasmids cohabiting the same cell.

An important property of the F plasmid is its ability to integrate into the bacterial chromosome, generating an Hfr cell. Such integration of the F plasmid involves breakage and rejoining of both molecules of DNA. Many sites of exchange exist in the F plasmid and an *E. coli* chromosome, leading to Hfr strains. Analysis of some of the Hfr strains indicates that they result from a recombination process between a homologous insertion sequence present on both the F plasmid and the chromosome. Indeed, three types of insertion sequences—IS2, IS3, and TN1000 (gamma-delta)—have been found in the F plasmid.

In Hfr strains, the F plasmid ceases its autonomous replication, but its genes involved in mobilization and transfer are still expressed. Thus conjugation can still be initiated by a nick at the OriT site. However, because F is integrated into the chromosome, only part of the plasmid sequence is initially transferred, followed by chromosomal DNA and sometimes, but only rarely, the remainder of the F plasmid. It would take 100 minutes at 37° C to transfer the complete male genome to the female recipient. However, the fragile connection between the mating pairs is usually broken and the transfer aborted before being completed, explaining why usually only the chromosomal sequences adjacent to the integrated F are transferred. Therefore a mating between an Hfr strain and an F⁻ strain usually leaves the recipient F⁻. Artificial interruption of a mating between an Hfr and an

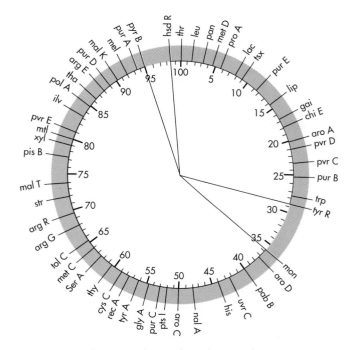

FIGURE 5-11 Chromosomal map of *E. coli* genes. The time (minutes) to transfer DNA segments from the origin of the first Hfr strain is represented by the numbers. (Modified from Bachmann BJ, Low KB, Taylor AL: *Bacterial Rev* 40:116-167, 1976.)

F⁻ pair has been helpful in constructing a consistent map of the *E. coli* chromosomal DNA. In such maps the position of each gene is given in minutes according to its time of entry into a recipient cell in relation to a fixed origin (Figure 5-11).

Conjugative R (antibiotic resistance) plasmids have been found in gram-positive bacteria such as streptococci, streptomyces, and clostridia. However, conjugation in gram-positive bacteria does not seem to rely on the presence of pili. Instead the mating pair is brought together by the presence of an adhesin molecule present on the surface of the donor cell. Moreover, some bacteria, such as *Streptococcus faecalis,* produce a peptide sex pheromone, which is thought to elicit a mating response leading to the expression of the adhesin in the donor cells.

Transduction

Genetic transfer by **transduction** is mediated by bacterial viruses (**bacteriophages**) (Figure 5-12). Fragments of DNA packaged into bacteriophage particles are delivered to infected cells and become incorporated into the bacterial genomes. Transduction can be classified as **specialized** if the phages in question transfer particular genes (usually those adjacent to their integration sites in the genome) or **generalized** if the selection of the sequences is random because of accidental packaging of host DNA into the phage capsid.

Generalized transducing particles should contain primarily bacterial DNA and little or no phage DNA. For

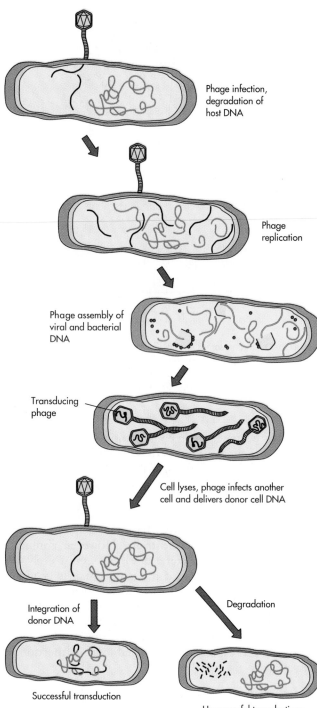

Phage infection, degradation of host DNA

Phage replication

Phage assembly of viral and bacterial DNA

Transducing phage

Cell lyses, phage infects another cell and delivers donor cell DNA

Integration of donor DNA

Degradation

Successful transduction

Unsuccessful transduction

FIGURE 5-12 Transduction by bacteriophages. Bacteriophage infection can deliver genes into the target cell if the cell survives.

DNA. Generalized transducing particles are valuable in the **genetic mapping** of bacterial chromosomes. The closer two genes are within the bacterial chromosome, the more likely they will be cotransduced.

Conjugative Transposons

Transposons can transfer DNA within a cell from one position to another in the genome or from the chromosomal DNA to a plasmid or the reverse. The transposons found in bacteria can be divided into three classes: insertion sequences, complex transposons, and phage-associated transposons. The **insertion-sequence** elements are the simplest transposons; they range in length from 150 to 1500 base pairs and possess inverted repeats of 15 to 40 base pairs at their ends (Figure 5-8). The insertion sequences carry only the genetic information necessary for their own transfer (i.e., the gene coding for the transposase). The insertion sequences can be detected if they insert into a gene and interrupt or inactivate the gene or turn on the expression of adjacent genes.

RECOMBINATION

Incorporation of the DNA into the chromosome occurs by recombination. There are two types of recombination: homologous and nonhomologous. **Homologous (legitimate) recombination** occurs between closely related DNA sequences and generally substitutes one sequence for another. The process requires a set of enzymes produced (in *E. coli*) by the *rec* genes. **Nonhomologous (illegitimate) recombination** occurs between dissimilar DNA sequences and generally produces insertions or deletions or both. This process usually requires specialized (sometimes site-specific) recombination enzymes, such as those produced by many transposons and lysogenic bacteriophages.

GENETIC ENGINEERING

Genetic engineering, also known as **recombinant DNA technology,** uses the techniques and tools developed by the bacterial geneticists to purify, amplify, modify, and express specific gene sequences. The use of genetic engineering and "cloning" has revolutionized biology and medicine. The basic tools of genetic engineering are (1) **cloning vectors,** which can be used to deliver the DNA sequences into receptive bacteria and amplify the desired sequence; (2) **restriction enzymes,** which are used to cleave DNA reproducibly at defined sequences to provide the DNA to be amplified and the means of inserting the DNA into the vector (Table 5-1); and (3) **DNA ligase,** the enzyme that completes the cloning vector.

Cloning vectors must allow foreign DNA to be inserted into them but still must be able to replicate normally in the bacterial host. Many types of vectors are currently used. **Plasmid vectors,** such as pUC, pBR322, and pGEM (Figure 5-5), are used for DNA fragments up

example, the P1 phage of *E. coli* encodes a nuclease that degrades the host *E. coli* chromosomal DNA. A small percentage of the resultant phage particles packages the DNA fragments into their capsids. The encapsulated DNA instead of phage DNA is injected into a new host cell, where it can recombine with the homologous host

TABLE 5-1 **Common Restriction Enzymes Used in Molecular Biology**

MICROORGANISM	ENZYME	RECOGNITION SITE
Acinetobacter calcoaceticus	AccI	5′ G T | (A/C) (G/T) | A C C A (T/G) (C/A) | T G
Bacillus amyloliquefaciens H	BamHI	5′ G|G A T C C C C T A G|G
E. coli RY13	EcoRI	5′ G|A A T T C C T T A A|G
H. influenzae Rd	HindIII	5′ A|A G C T T T T C G A|A
H. influenzae serotype c, 1160	HincII	5′ G T (C/T) | (G/A) A C C A (G/A) | (C/T) T G
Providencia stuartii 164	PstI	5′ C T G C A|G G|A C G T C
Serratia marcescens	SmaI	5′ C C C|G G G G G G|C C C
Staphylococcus aureus 3A	Sau3AI	5′ |G A T C C T A G|
Xanthomonas malvacearum	XmaI	5′ C|C C G G G G G G C C|C

to 20 kb. Bacteriophages, such as lambda, are used for larger fragments up to 25 kb. More recently, **cosmid vectors** have combined some of the advantages of plasmids and phages for fragments up to 45 kb.

Most cloning vectors have been "engineered" to have a site for insertion of foreign DNA; a means of selection, such as antibiotic resistance, for bacteria that have incorporated the vector; and a means of distinguishing the bacteria that have incorporated plasmids containing inserted DNA. Some plasmid vectors contain special sequences that aid in sequencing the cloned DNA or that promote expression of the gene or genes contained within the cloned DNA, either in prokaryotic or eukaryotic cells (e.g., prokaryote or eukaryote promoter sequences to precede the cloned DNA).

For cloning a foreign piece of DNA, both the vector and the DNA must be cleaved with **restriction enzymes** (Figure 5-13). Restriction enzymes recognize a site-specific sequence and make a staggered cut, which generates sticky ends, or a blunt cut, which generates blunt ends (Table 5-1). Most cloning vectors have a sequence that can be cleaved by many restriction enzymes called the *multiple cloning site*. Ligation of the vector with the DNA fragments generates a molecule capable of replicating the inserted sequence called **recombinant DNA** (Figure 5-9). The total number of recombinant vectors obtained when cloning chromosomal DNA is known as a **genomic library** because there should be at least one representative of each gene in the library. An alternative approach to cloning the gene for a protein is to convert

the **mRNA** for the protein into DNA using a retrovirus enzyme called **reverse transcriptase** (RNA-dependent DNA polymerase) to produce a **complementary DNA (cDNA)**.

The recombinant DNA is then transformed into a bacterial host, usually *E. coli*, and the plasmid-containing bacteria are selected for antibiotic resistance (e.g., ampicillin resistance). The library can then be screened to find an *E. coli* clone possessing the desired DNA fragment. Various screening techniques can be used to identify the bacteria containing the appropriate recombinant DNA. Often the multiple cloning site used for inserting the foreign DNA is part of the *lacZ* gene of the *lac* operon. Insertion of the foreign DNA into the *lacZ* gene inactivates the gene (acting almost like a transposon) and prevents the plasmid-directed synthesis of beta-galactosidase in the recipient cell and its cleavage of a chromophore to produce blue colonies. Recombinant plasmid-containing bacteria would produce normal, white colonies. Recombinant plasmid that expresses a protein in bacteria can be screened by immunological means.

Genetic engineering has been used to isolate and express the genes for useful proteins such as insulin, interferon, growth hormones, and interleukin and to allow the production of sufficient quantities of the proteins to allow their purification and use in therapy. **Recombinant vaccines** have been prepared by expression of the surface antigens of pathogens in bacteria, yeast, or even insect cells. In addition to producing large amounts of pure immunogen for the vaccine, this

FIGURE 5-13 Cloning of foreign DNA in vectors. The vector and the foreign DNA are first digested by a restriction enzyme. Insertion of foreign DNA into the *lacZ* gene inactivates the beta-galactosidase gene, allowing subsequent selection. The vector is then ligated to the foreign DNA, using bacteriophage T4 DNA ligase. The recombinant vectors are transformed into competent *E. coli* cells. The recombinant *E. coli* are plated onto agar containing antibiotic, an inducer of the *lac* operon, and a chromophoric substrate that turns blue in cells having plasmid but not insert and white in those cells with plasmid containing insert.

approach also eliminates the need to work with the intact disease organisms.

The development of a vaccine against **hepatitis B** represents the first success of recombinant DNA vaccines approved for human use by the U.S. Food and Drug Administration. The hepatitis B surface antigen is produced by the yeast *Saccharomyces cerevisiae*. In the future, it may be sufficient to inject plasmid DNA capable of expressing the desired immunogen (**DNA vaccine**) into an individual to let the host cells express the immunogen and generate the immune response. Recombinant DNA technology has also become essential to laboratory diagnosis, forensic science, agriculture, and many other disciplines.

QUESTIONS

1. What are the principal properties of a plasmid?
2. Give two mechanisms of regulation of bacterial gene expression. Use specific examples.
3. What types of mutations affect DNA and what agents are responsible for such mutations?
4. What mechanisms may be used by a bacterial cell for the exchange of genetic material? Briefly explain each mechanism.
5. Discuss the applications of molecular biotechnology to medicine, including contributions and uses in diagnosis.

Bibliography

Alberts B et al: *Molecular biology of the cell,* ed 3, New York, 1994, Garland.
Cooper GM: *The cell: a molecular approach,* Washington, DC, 1997, ASM.
Lehninger AL, Nelson DL, Fox MM: *Principles of biochemistry,* ed 2, New York, 1993, Worth.
Lewin B: *Genes VI,* Oxford, England, 1997, Oxford University.
Lodish H et al: *Molecular cell biology,* ed 3, New York, 1995, Scientific American.
Stryer L: *Biochemistry,* ed 4, New York, 1995, Freeman.
Voet D, Voet JG: *Biochemistry,* ed 2, New York, 1995, Wiley.
Watson JD et al: *Molecular biology of the gene,* ed 4, Menlo Park, Calif, 1987, Benjamin-Cummings.

CHAPTER 6

Viral Classification, Structure, and Replication

Viruses were first described as "filterable agents." Their small size allows them to pass through filters that are designed to retain bacteria. Unlike most bacteria, fungi, and parasites, **viruses are obligate intracellular parasites** that depend on the biochemical machinery of the host cell for replication. In addition, *reproduction of viruses occurs by assembly of the individual components rather than by binary fission* (Boxes 6-1 and 6-2).

The simplest viruses consist of a genome of DNA or RNA packaged in a protective shell of protein and sometimes a membrane (Figure 6-1). Viruses lack the capacity to make energy or substrates, cannot make their own proteins, and cannot replicate their genome independent of the host cell. The virus therefore must be adapted to the biochemical rules of the cell to use the cell's biosynthetic machinery.

The physical structure and genetics of viruses have been optimized by mutation and selection to infect human and other hosts and to interact with the biochemical machinery of the host cell. The virus may also have to endure harsh environmental conditions, traverse the skin or other protective barriers of the host, and escape elimination by the host immune response. A knowledge of the structural (size and morphology) and genetic (type and structure of nucleic acid) features of a virus provides insight into how the virus replicates, spreads, and causes disease. The concepts presented in this chapter will be repeated in greater detail in the discussions of specific viruses in later chapters.

CLASSIFICATION

Viruses range from the structurally simple and small parvoviruses and picornaviruses to the large and complex poxviruses and herpesviruses. Their names may describe viral characteristics, the diseases they are associated with, or even the tissue or geographical locale where they were first identified. Names such as *picornavirus* (*pico*, "small"; *rna*, "ribonucleic acid") or *togavirus* (*toga*, Greek for "mantle," referring to a membrane envelope surrounding the virus) describe the structure of the virus, whereas the name *papovavirus* describes the members of its family (*pa*pilloma, *po*lyoma, and *va*cuolating *viruses*). The name *retrovirus* (*retro*, "reverse") refers to the virus-directed synthesis of DNA from an RNA template, whereas the *poxviruses* are named for the disease smallpox, caused by one of its members. The *adenoviruses* (*aden*oids) and the reoviruses (*r*espiratory, *e*nteric, *o*rphan) are named for the body site from which they were first isolated. *Reovirus* was discovered before it was associated with a specific disease, and thus it was designated an "orphan" virus. Coxsackievirus is named for Coxsackie, New York, and many of the togaviruses, arenaviruses, and bunyaviruses are named after African places where they were first isolated.

BOX 6-1	**Definition and Properties of a Virus**

Viruses are filterable agents.

Viruses are obligate intracellular parasites.

Viruses cannot make energy or proteins independent of a host cell.

Viral genomes may be RNA or DNA but not both.

Viruses have a naked capsid or envelope morphology.

Viral components are assembled and do not replicate by "division."

BOX 6-2	**Consequences of Viral Properties**

Viruses are not living.

Viruses must be infectious to endure in nature.

Viruses must be able to use host cell processes to produce their components (viral messenger RNA, protein, and identical copies of the genome).

Viruses must encode any required processes not provided by the cell.

Viral components must self-assemble.

FIGURE 6-1 Components of the basic virion.

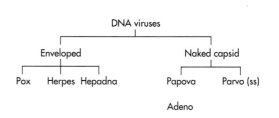

FIGURE 6-2 The DNA viruses and their morphology. The viral families are determined by the structure of the genome and the morphology of the virion.

FIGURE 6-3 The RNA viruses, their genome structure, and their morphology. The viral families are determined by the structure of the genome and the morphology of the virion.

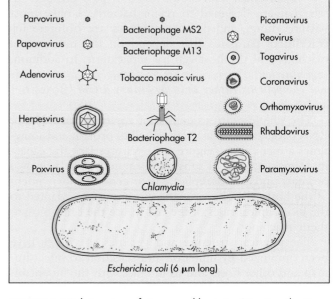

FIGURE 6-4 Relative sizes of viruses and bacteria. (Courtesy the Upjohn Company, Kalamazoo, Mich.)

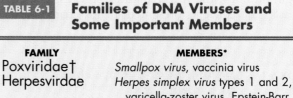

BOX 6-3 Means of Classification and Naming of Viruses

Structure: size, morphology, and nucleic acid (e.g., picornavirus [small RNA], togavirus [cloak])
Biochemical characteristics: structure and mode of replication*
Disease: encephalitis and hepatitis viruses, for example
Means of transmission: arbovirus spread by insects, for example
Host cell (host range): animal (human, mouse, bird), plant, bacteria
Tissue or organ (tropism): adenovirus and enterovirus, for example

*Current means of taxonomic classification of viruses.

TABLE 6-1 Families of DNA Viruses and Some Important Members

FAMILY	MEMBERS*
Poxviridae†	Smallpox virus, vaccinia virus
Herpesvirdae	Herpes simplex virus types 1 and 2, varicella-zoster virus, Epstein-Barr virus, cytomegalovirus, human herpesviruses 6, 7, and 8
Adenoviridae	Adenovirus
Hepadnavirdea	Hepatitis B virus
Papovaviridae	JC virus, BK virus, SV40, papilloma virus
Parvovirdae	Parvovirus B19, adeno-associated virus

*The italicized virus is the important or prototype virus for the family.
†The size of type is indicative of the relative size of the virus.

TABLE 6-2   Properties of Virions of Human DNA Viruses

	GENOME*		VIRION		
FAMILY	**MOLECULAR WEIGHT (×10⁶ DALTONS)**	**NATURE**	**SHAPE**	**SIZE (nm)**	**DNA POLYMERASE†**
Poxviridae	85-140	ds, linear	Brick shaped, enveloped	300 × 240 × 100	+‡
Herpesviridae	100-150	ds, linear	Icosahedral, enveloped	Capsid, 100-110 Envelope, 120-200	+
Adenoviridae	20-25	ds, linear	Icosahedral	70-90	+
Hepadnaviridae	1.8	ds, circular§	Spherical, enveloped	42	+‡‖
Papovaviridae	3-5	ds, circular	Icosahedral	45-55	−
Parvoviridae	1.5-2.0	ss, linear	Icosahedral	18-26	−

ds, Double stranded; *ss*, single stranded.
*Genome invariably a single molecule.
†Polymerase encoded by virus.
‡Polymerase carried in the virion.
§Circular molecule is double stranded for most of its length but contains a single-stranded region.
‖Reverse transcriptase.

TABLE 6-3   Families of RNA Viruses and Some Important Members

FAMILY	MEMBERS*
Paramyxoviridae†	Parainfluenza virus, Sendai virus, *measles virus,* mumps virus, respiratory syncytial virus
Orthomyxoviridae	*Influenza virus types A, B, and C*
Coronaviridae	*Coronavirus*
Arenaviridae	*Lassa fever virus,* Tacaribe virus complex (Junin and Machupo viruses), lymphocytic choriomeningitis virus
Rhabdoviridae	*Rabies virus,* vesicular stomatitis virus
Filoviridae	*Ebola virus,* Marburg virus
Bunyaviridae	*California encephalitis virus,* LaCrosse virus, sandfly fever virus, hemorrhagic fever virus, Hanta virus
Retroviridae	Human T-cell leukemia virus types I and II, *human immunodeficiency virus,* animal oncoviruses
Reoviridae	*Rotavirus,* Colorado tick fever virus
Picornaviridae	Rhinoviruses, *poliovirus,* echoviruses, coxsackievirus, encephalomyocarditis virus
Togaviridae	*Rubella virus;* Western, Eastern, and Venezuelan equine encephalitis virus; Ross River virus; Sindbis virus; Semliki Forest virus
Flaviviridae	*Yellow fever virus,* dengue virus, St. Louis encephalitis virus
Caliciviridae	Norwalk virus
Delta	Delta agent

*The italicized virus is the important or prototype virus for the family.
†The size of the type is indicative of the relative size of the virus.

Viruses can be grouped by characteristics such as disease (e.g., hepatitis), target tissue, means of transmission (e.g., enteric, respiratory), or vector (arboviruses; *ar*thropod-*bo*rne virus) (Box 6-3). *The most consistent and current means of classification is by physical and biochemical characteristics such as size, morphology (e.g., presence or absence of a membrane envelope), type of genome, and means of replication* (Figures 6-2 and 6-3). DNA viruses associated with human disease are divided into six families (Tables 6-1 and 6-2). The RNA viruses may be divided into at least 13 families (Tables 6-3 and 6-4).

VIRION STRUCTURE

The units for measurement of virion size are nanometers (nm). The clinically important viruses range from 18 nm (parvoviruses) to 300 nm (poxviruses) (Figure 6-4). The latter are almost visible with a light microscope and are approximately one fourth the size of a staphylococcus. *Larger virions can hold a larger genome that can encode more proteins, and they are generally more complex.*

The **virion** (the virus particle) consists of a nucleic acid **genome** packaged into a protein coat (**capsid**) or a membrane (**envelope**) (Figure 6-5). The virion may also contain certain essential or accessory enzymes or other proteins. Capsid or nucleic acid–binding proteins may associate with the genome to form a **nucleocapsid,** which may be the same as the virion or surrounded by an envelope.

The **genome** of different viruses consists of either DNA or RNA. The *DNA can be single stranded or double stranded, linear or circular. The RNA can be either positive sense (+) (like messenger RNA [mRNA]) or negative sense (−) (analogous to a photographic negative), double stranded (+/−) or ambisense (containing + and − regions of RNA attached end to end). The* RNA

TABLE 6-4 **Properties of Virions of RNA Human Viruses**

| | GENOME | | | VIRION | | | |
FAMILY	MOLECULAR WEIGHT ($\times 10^6$ DALTONS)	NATURE	SHAPE*	SIZE (nm)	POLYMERASE IN VIRION	ENVELOPE
Paramyxoviridae	5-7	ss, −	Spherical	150-300	+	+
Orthomyxoviridae	5	ss, −, seg	Spherical	80-120	+	+
Coronaviridae	6	ss, +	Spherical	80-130	−	+†
Arenaviridae	3-5	ss, −, seg	Spherical	50-300	+	+†
Rhabdoviridae	4	ss, −	Bullet shaped	180 × 75	+	+
Filoviridae	4	ss, −	Filamentous	800 × 80	+	+
Bunyaviridae	4-7	ss, −	Spherical	90-100	+	+†
Retroviridae	2 × (2-3)‡	ss, +	Spherical	80-110	+§	+
Reoviridae	11-15	ds, seg	Icosahedral	60-80	+	−
Picornaviridae	2.5	ss, +	Icosahedral	25-30	−	−
Togaviridae	4	ss, +	Icosahedral	60-70	−	+
Flaviviridae	4	ss, +	Spherical	40-50	−	+
Caliciviridae	2.6	ss, +	Icosahedral	35-40	−	−

ss, Single stranded; *ds*, double stranded; *seg*, segmented; + or −, polarity of single-stranded nucleic acid.

*Some enveloped viruses are very pleomorphic (sometimes filamentous).

†No matrix protein.

‡Genome has two identical single-stranded RNA molecules.

§Reverse transcriptase.

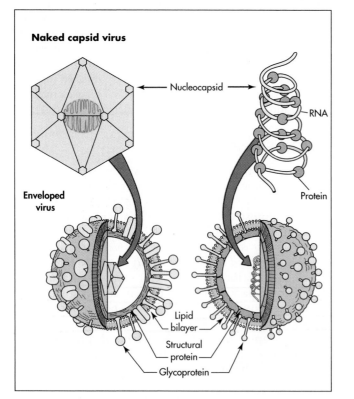

FIGURE 6-5 The structures of a naked capsid virus *(top left)* and enveloped viruses with an icosahedral *(left)* nucleocapsid or a helical *(right)* ribonucleocapsid. The helical ribonucleocapsid is formed by viral proteins associated with an RNA genome.

genome may also be *segmented* into pieces, with each piece encoding an individual gene.

The outer layer of the virion is the **capsid** or **envelope.** These structures are the package, protection, and delivery vehicle during transmission of the virus from one host to another and for spread within the host to the target cell. The surface structures of the capsid and envelope mediate the interaction of the virus with the target cell. Removal or disruption of the outer package inactivates the virus. Antibodies generated against the components of these structures prevents virus infection.

The **capsid** is a rigid structure able to withstand harsh environmental conditions. Viruses with naked capsids are generally resistant to drying, acid, and detergents, including the acid and bile of the enteric tract. Many of these viruses are transmitted by the fecal-oral route and can endure transmission even in sewage.

The **envelope** is a membrane composed of lipids, proteins, and glycoproteins. The membranous structure of the envelope can be maintained only in aqueous solutions. It is readily disrupted by drying, acidic conditions, detergents, and solvents such as ether, resulting in the inactivation of the virus. As a result, enveloped viruses must remain wet and are generally transmitted in fluids, respiratory droplets, blood, and tissue. Most cannot survive the harsh conditions of the gastrointestinal tract. The influence of virion structure on viral properties is summarized in Boxes 6-4 and 6-5.

Capsid Viruses

The viral capsid is assembled from individual proteins associated into progressively larger units. All of the com-

---

COMPONENT

Protein.

PROPERTIES

Is environmentally stable to the following:
 Temperature
 Acid
 Proteases
 Detergents
 Drying
Is released from cell by lysis.

CONSEQUENCES

Can be spread easily (on fomites, from hand to hand, by dust, by small droplets).
Can dry out and retain infectivity.
Can survive the adverse conditions of the gut.
Can be resistant to detergents and poor sewage treatment.
Antibody may be sufficient for immunoprotection.

COMPONENTS

Membrane
Lipids
Proteins
Glycoproteins

PROPERTIES

Is environmentally labile—is disrupted by the following:
 Acid
 Detergents
 Drying
 Heat
Modifies cell membrane during replication
Is released by budding and cell lysis

CONSEQUENCES

Must stay wet
Cannot survive the gastrointestinal tract
Spreads in large droplets, secretions, organ transplants, and blood transfusions
Does not need to kill the cell to spread
May need antibody and cell-mediated immune response for protection and control
Elicits hypersensitivity and inflammation to cause immunopathogenesis

---

ponents of the capsid have chemical features that allow them to fit together and to assemble into a larger unit. Individual structural proteins associate into **subunits,** which associate into **protomers, capsomeres** (distinguishable in electron micrographs), and finally a recognizable **procapsid** or **capsid** (Figure 6-6). A procapsid requires further processing to the final, transmissible capsid. For some viruses, the capsid forms around the genome; for others, the capsid forms as an empty shell (procapsid) to be filled by the genome.

The simplest viral structures that can be built stepwise are symmetrical and include **helical** and **icosahedral** structures. Helical structures appear as rods, whereas the icosahedron is an approximation of a sphere assembled from symmetrical subunits (Figure 6-7). Nonsymmetrical capsids are complex forms and are associated with certain bacterial viruses (phages).

The classic example of a virus with helical symmetry is the tobacco mosaic virus. Its capsomeres self-assemble on the RNA genome into rods extending to the length of the genome. The capsomeres cover and protect the RNA. Helical nucleocapsids are observed within the envelope of many negative-strand RNA viruses (see Figure 55-1).

Simple icosahedrons are used by small, simple viruses such as the picornaviruses and parvoviruses. The icosahedron is made of 12 capsomeres, each with fivefold symmetry (**pentamer** or penton). Every pentamer of the picornaviruses is made up of five protomers, each of which is composed of three subunits of four separate proteins (Figure 6-6). X-ray crystallography and image analysis of cryoelectron microscopy have defined the

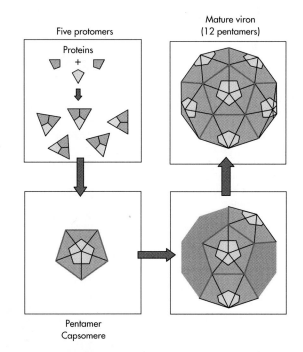

FIGURE 6-6 Capsid assembly of the icosahedral capsid of a picornavirus. Individual proteins associate into subunits, which associate into protomers, capsomeres, and an empty procapsid. Inclusion of the (+) RNA genome triggers its conversion to the final capsid form.

structure of the picornavirus capsid to the molecular level. These studies have depicted a canyonlike cleft, which is a "docking site" for the receptor on the surface of the target cell (see Figure 54-2).

Larger icosahedral virions are constructed by inserting structurally distinct capsomeres between the pentons at the vertices. These capsomeres have six nearest neighbors **(hexons).** This extended icosahedron is called an **icosadeltahedron,** and its size is determined by the number of hexons inserted along the edges and planes between the pentons. *A soccer ball is an icosadeltahedron.* For example, the herpesvirus nucleocapsid has 12 pentons and 150 hexons. The herpesvirus nucleocapsid is also surrounded by an envelope. The adenovirus capsid is composed of 252 capsomeres, with 12 pentons and 240 hexons. A long fiber is attached to each penton of adenovirus to serve as the viral attachment protein (VAP) to target cells and contains the type-specific antigen (see Figure 50-1). The reoviruses have an icosahedral double capsid with fiberlike proteins partially extended from each vertex. The outer capsid protects the virus and promotes its uptake across the gastrointestinal tract and into target cells, whereas the inner capsid contains enzymes for the synthesis of RNA (see Figures 6-7 and 57-1).

Enveloped Viruses

The virion envelope is composed of lipids, proteins, and glycoproteins (Figure 6-5 and Box 6-5). It has a membrane structure similar to cellular membranes. Cellular proteins are rarely found in the viral envelope, even though the envelope is obtained from cellular membranes. Most enveloped viruses are round or pleomorphic. (See Figures 6-2 and 6-3 for the complete listing of enveloped viruses.) Two exceptions are the poxvirus, which has a complex internal and a bricklike external structure, and the rhabdovirus, which is bullet shaped.

Most viral glycoproteins have asparagine-linked (*N*-linked) carbohydrate and extend through the envelope and away from the surface of the virion. For many viruses, these can be observed as spikes (Figure 6-8). Most glycoproteins act as **viral attachment proteins** (VAPs) capable of binding to structures on target cells. VAPs that also bind to erythrocytes are termed **hemagglutinins (HAs).** Some glycoproteins have other functions, such as the neuraminidase of orthomyxoviruses (influenza) and the Fc receptor and the C3b receptor associated with herpes simplex virus glycoproteins or the fusion glycoproteins of paramyxoviruses. Glycoproteins are also major antigens for protective immunity.

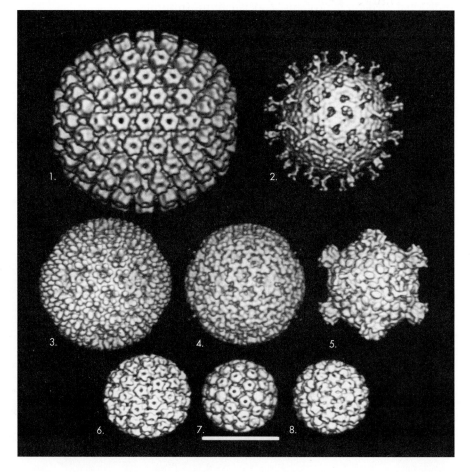

FIGURE 6-7 Cryoelectron microscopy and computer-generated three-dimensional image reconstructions of several icosahedral capsids. These images show the symmetry of capsids and the individual capsomeres. During assembly, the genome may fill the capsid through the holes in the herpesvirus and papovavirus capsomeres. *1,* Equine herpesvirus nucleocapsid; *2,* simian rotavirus; *3,* reovirus type 1 (Lang) virion; *4,* intermediate subviral particle (reovirus); *5,* core (inner capsid) particle (reovirus); *6,* human papilloma virus type 19 (papovavirus); *7,* mouse polyoma virus (papovavirus); *8,* cauliflower mosaic virus. (Bar = 50 nm.) (Courtesy Dr. Tim Baker, Purdue University.)

The envelope of the togaviruses surrounds an icosahedral nucleocapsid containing a positive-strand RNA genome. The envelope contains spikes consisting of two or three glycoprotein subunits anchored to the virion's icosahedral capsid. This causes the envelope to adhere tightly and conform (shrink-wrap) to an icosahedral structure discernible by cryoelectron microscopy.

All of the negative-strand RNA viruses are enveloped. Components of the viral RNA-dependent RNA polymerase associate with the (−) RNA genome of the orthomyxoviruses, paramyxoviruses, and rhabdoviruses to form helical nucleocapsids (Figure 6-5). These enzymes are required to initiate virus replication, and their association with the genome ensures their delivery into the cell. **Matrix** proteins lining the inside of the envelope facilitate the assembly of the ribonucleocapsid into the virion. Influenza A (orthomyxovirus) is an example of a (−) RNA virus with a segmented genome. Its envelope (is lined with matrix proteins and has two glycoproteins: the hemagglutinin (HA) which is the VAP, and a neuraminidase (NA). Bunyaviruses do not have matrix proteins.

The herpesvirus envelope is a baglike structure that encloses the icosadeltahedral nucleocapsid. Depending on the specific herpesvirus, the envelope may contain as many as 11 glycoproteins. The interstitial space between the nucleocapsid and the envelope is called the *tegument* and contains enzymes and proteins that facilitate the viral infection.

The poxviruses are enveloped viruses with large, complex, bricklike shapes. The envelope encloses a dumb-bell-shaped, DNA-containing nucleoid structure; lateral bodies; fibrils; and many enzymes and proteins, including the enzymes and transcriptional factors required for mRNA synthesis.

VIRAL REPLICATION

The major steps in viral replication are the same for all viruses (Figure 6-10 and Box 6-6). The cell acts as a factory, providing the substrates, energy, and machinery necessary for the synthesis of viral proteins and replication of the genome. Processes not provided by the cell must be encoded in the genome of the virus. The manner in which each virus accomplishes these steps and

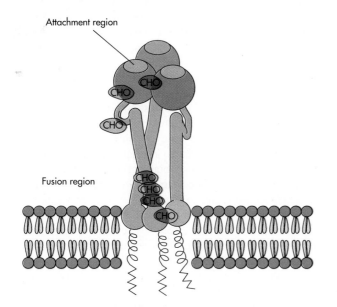

FIGURE 6-8 Diagram of the hemagglutinin glycoprotein trimer of influenza A virus, a representative spike protein. The region for attachment to the cellular receptor is exposed on the spike protein's surface. Under mild acidic conditions, the hemagglutinin changes conformation to expose a hydrophobic sequence at the "fusion region." *CHO,* N-linked carbohydrate attachment sites. (Modified from Schlesinger MJ, Schlesinger S: *Adv Virus Res* 33:1-44, 1987.)

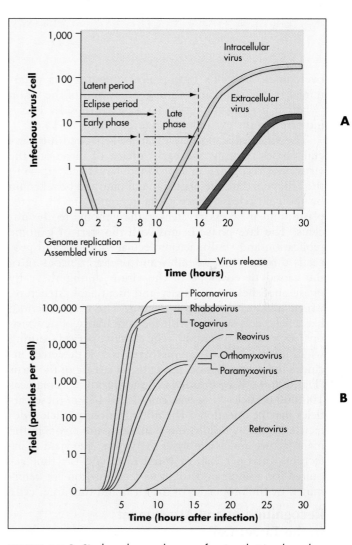

FIGURE 6-9 A, Single-cycle growth curve of a virus that is released on cell lysis. The different stages are defined by the presence or absence of visible viral components (eclipse period), infectious virus in the media (latent period), or macromolecular synthesis (early/late phases). **B,** Growth curve and burst size of representative viruses. (**B** modified from White DO, Fenner F: *Medical virology,* ed 3, New York, 1986, Academic.)

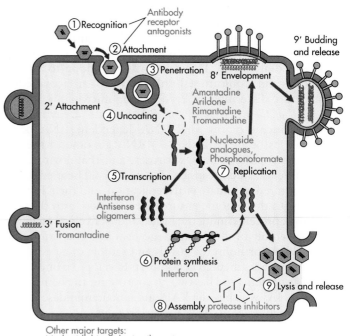

FIGURE 6-10 A general scheme of viral replication. Enveloped viruses have alternative means of entry *(3)*, assembly, and exit from the cell *(8′ and 9′).* The steps in viral replication susceptible to antiviral drugs are listed in magenta.

overcomes the cell's biochemical limitations is determined by the structure of the genome and of the virion (whether it is enveloped or has a naked capsid). This is indicated in the examples in Figures 6-12 to 6-14.

The viral replication cycle can be separated into several phases. During the **early phase** of infection, the virus must recognize an appropriate target cell; attach to the cell; penetrate the plasma membrane and be taken up by the cell; release (uncoat) its genome into the cytoplasm; and if necessary, deliver the genome to the nucleus. The **late phase** begins with the start of genome replication and viral macromolecular synthesis and proceeds through viral assembly and release. Uncoating of the capsid or envelope of the virion during the early phase abolishes its infectivity and identifiable structure, which initiates the **eclipse period.** The eclipse period, like a solar eclipse, ends with the appearance of new virions after virus assembly. The **latent period,** during which extracellular infectious virus is not detected, includes the eclipse period and ends on release of the virus (Figure 6-9). Each infected cell may produce as many as 100,000 particles; however, only 1% to 10% of these particles may be infectious. The noninfectious particles (defective particles) result from mutations and errors in the manufacture and assembly of the virion. The yield of infectious virus per cell, or **burst size,** and the time required for a single cycle of virus reproduction are determined by the properties of the virus and the target cell.

Recognition of and Attachment to the Target Cell

The binding of the **VAPs,** or structures on the surface of the virion capsid (Table 6-5), to **receptors on the cell** (Table 6-6) initially determines which cells can be infected by a virus. *The viral receptors on the cell may be proteins or carbohydrates.*

The viral attachment structure for a capsid virus may be part of the capsid or a protein that extends from the capsid. A canyon on the surface of rhinovirus 14, a pi-

cornavirus, serves as a "keyhole" for the insertion of a portion of the intercellular adhesion molecule (ICAM-1) from the cell surface. The fibers of the adenoviruses and the sigma 1 proteins of the reoviruses at the vertices of the capsid interact with receptors expressed on specific target cells.

The glycoproteins of enveloped viruses are the VAPs. The HA of influenza A virus binds to sialic acid expressed on many different cells and has a broad host range and tissue tropism. Similarly, the alpha togaviruses and the flaviviruses are able to bind to receptors expressed on cells of many animal species, including arthropods, reptiles, amphibians, birds, and mammals. This allows them to infect and to be spread by animals, mosquitoes, and other insects.

Viruses that bind to receptors expressed on specific cell types may be restricted to certain species (**host range**) (e.g., human, mouse) or specific cell types. The susceptible target cell defines the tissue **tropism** (e.g., neurotropic, lymphotropic). The Epstein-Barr virus, a herpesvirus, has a very limited host range and tropism because it binds to the C3d receptor (CR2) expressed on human B cells.

Penetration

Multiple interactions between the VAPs and the cellular receptors initiate the internalization of the virus into the cell. The mechanism of internalization depends on the virion structure and cell type. Most nonenveloped viruses enter the cell by receptor-mediated endocytosis

TABLE 6-5   Examples of VAPs

VIRUS FAMILY	VIRUS	VAP
Picornaviridae	Rhinovirus	VP1-VP2-VP3 complex
Adenoviridae	Adenovirus	Fiber protein
Reoviridae	Reovirus	Sigma 1
	Rotavirus	VP7
Togaviridae	Semliki Forest virus	E1-E2-E3 complex
Rhabdoviridae	Rabies virus	G Protein
Orthomyxoviridae	Influenza A virus	HA
Paramyxoviridae	Measles virus	HA
Herpesviridae	Epstein-Barr virus	gp350 and gp220
Retroviridae	Murine leukemia virus	gp70
	Human immunode-ficiency virus	gp120

gp, Glycoprotein.

TABLE 6-6   Examples of Viral Receptors

VIRUS	TARGET CELL	RECEPTOR*
Epstein-Barr virus	B cell	C3 complement receptor CR2 (CD21)
Human immuno-deficiency virus	Helper T cell	CD4 molecule and chemokine co-receptor
Rhinovirus	Epithelial cells	ICAM-1 (immunoglobulin superfamily protein)
Poliovirus	Epithelial cells	Immunoglobulin super-family protein
Rabies virus	Neuron	Acetylcholine receptor
Influenza A virus	Epithelial cells	Sialic acid
B19 parvovirus	Erythroid precursors	Erythrocyte P antigen (globoside)

ICAM-1, Intercellular adhesion molecule.
*Other receptors for these viruses may also exist.

or by viropexis. **Endocytosis** is a normal process used by the cell for the uptake of receptor-bound molecules such as hormones, low-density lipoproteins, and transferrin. Picornaviruses and papovaviruses may enter by **viropexis.** Hydrophobic structures of capsid proteins may be exposed after viral binding to the cells, and these structures help the virus slip through (direct penetration) the membrane.

Enveloped viruses fuse their membranes with cellular membranes to deliver the nucleocapsid or genome directly into the cytoplasm. *The optimum pH for fusion of an enveloped virus is a major determinant of whether penetration occurs at the cell surface at neutral pH or whether the virus must be internalized by endocytosis and fusion occurs in an endosome at acidic pH.* The fusion activity may be provided by the VAP or another protein. The HA of influenza A (Figure 6-6) binds to sialic acid receptors on the target cell. Under the mild acidic conditions of the endosome, the HA undergoes a dramatic conformational change to expose hydrophobic portions capable of promoting membrane fusion. Paramyxoviruses have a fusion protein that is active at neutral pH to promote virus-cell fusion. Paramyxoviruses can also promote cell-cell fusion to form multinucleated giant cells (**polykaryocytes** or **syncytia**). Some herpesviruses and retroviruses fuse with cells at a neutral pH and induce syncytia after replication.

Uncoating

Once internalized, the nucleocapsid must be delivered to the site of replication within the cell and the capsid or envelope removed. The genome of DNA viruses, except for poxviruses, must be delivered to the nucleus, whereas most RNA viruses remain in the cytoplasm. The uncoating process may be initiated by attachment to the receptor or promoted by the acidic environment or proteases found in an endosome or lysosome. Picornavirus capsids are weakened by the release of the VP4 capsid protein to allow uncoating. VP4 is released by the insertion of the receptor into the keyholelike canyon attachment site of the capsid. Enveloped viruses are uncoated on fusion with cell membranes. Fusion of the herpesvirus envelope with the membrane releases its nucleocapsid, which then "docks" with the nuclear membrane to deliver its DNA genome directly to the site of replication. The release of the influenza nucleocapsid from its matrix and envelope is facilitated by protons from inside the endosome, which passes through the ion pore formed by the influenza M2 matrix protein.

The reovirus and poxvirus are only partially uncoated on entry. The outer capsid of reovirus is removed, but the genome remains in an inner capsid, which contains the polymerases necessary for RNA synthesis. The initial uncoating of the poxviruses exposes a subviral particle to the cytoplasm, allowing synthesis of mRNA by virion-contained enzymes. An uncoating enzyme can then be synthesized to release the DNA-containing core into the cytoplasm.

Macromolecular Synthesis

Each virus must make mRNA and protein and generate an identical copy of its genome. *Transcription, translation, and replication of the genome are therefore probably the most important steps in viral multiplication.* Once the genome has been delivered to the cell, it is useless unless it can be transcribed into functional mRNAs capable of binding to ribosomes and being translated into proteins. The means by which each virus accomplishes these steps depends on the structure of the genome (Figure 6-11) and the site of replication.

The cellular machinery for transcription and mRNA processing is found in the nucleus. *Most DNA viruses use*

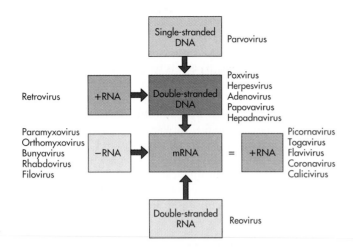

FIGURE 6-11 Strategies for production of mRNA. The arrows indicate the action of a viral or cellular polymerase. (Based on the Baltimore Schema; modified from *Bacterial Rev* 35:235-241, 1971.)

the cell's DNA-dependent RNA polymerase II and other enzymes to make mRNA. For example, eukaryotic mRNAs acquire a 3′ polyadenylated (poly A) tail and a 5′ methylated cap (for binding to the ribosome) and are processed to remove introns before being exported to the cytoplasm. Viruses that replicate in the cytoplasm must provide these functions or an alternative. Although poxviruses are DNA viruses, they replicate in the cytoplasm and therefore must encode enzymes for all these functions. *RNA viruses must encode the necessary enzymes for transcription and replication because the cell has no means of replicating RNA.* The mRNAs for RNA viruses are produced in the cytoplasm and may or may not acquire a 5′ cap or poly A tail.

The naked genome of DNA viruses (except poxviruses) and the positive-sense RNA viruses (except retroviruses) are *sufficient* for initiating replication on injection into a cell. These genomes can interact directly with host machinery to promote mRNA or protein synthesis or both.

DNA Viruses

The smaller the DNA virus, the more dependent the virus is on the host cell (Box 6-7). *The larger DNA viruses encode a DNA polymerase and proteins to enhance and control transcription and genome replication.* Viral DNA and mRNA synthesis can be enhanced by speeding up the growth of the cell or by increasing the number of DNA templates for transcription after the replication of the genome. A growing cell provides deoxyribonucleotides, polymerases, and other materials required for DNA virus replication. As a result, many DNA viruses encode proteins, which promote the growth of the host cell.

Transcription of the DNA virus genome (except for poxviruses) occurs in the nucleus using host cell polymerases and other enzymes for viral mRNA synthesis. Transcription of the viral genes is regulated by the inter-

---

BOX 6-7   **Properties of DNA Viruses**

Viral DNA resembles host DNA for transcription and replication.
DNA is not transient or labile.
  Viral genomes remain in the infected cell.
  Many DNA viruses establish persistent infections (e.g., latent, immortalizing).
DNA genomes reside in the nucleus (except in pox viruses).
Viral genes must interact with host transcriptional machinery (except in pox viruses).
  Viral gene transcription is temporarily regulated.
  Early genes encode DNA-binding proteins and enzymes.
  Late genes encode structural proteins.
DNA polymerases require a primer to replicate the viral genome.
The larger DNA viruses have more control over the replication of their genome.
  Parvovirus: requires cells undergoing DNA synthesis to replicate.
  Papovavirus: stimulates cell growth and DNA synthesis.
  Hepadnavirus: stimulates cell growth (?) and encodes its own polymerase.
  Adenovirus: stimulates cellular DNA synthesis and encodes its own polymerase.
  Herpesvirus: stimulates cell growth, encodes its own polymerase, and encodes enzymes to provide deoxyribonucleotides for DNA synthesis.
  Poxvirus: encodes its own polymerase and enzymes to provide deoxyribonucleotides for DNA synthesis, replication machinery, and transcription machinery.

---

action of specific *DNA-binding proteins* with *promoter and enhancer elements* in the viral genome. The viral promoter and enhancer elements are similar in sequence to those of the host cell to allow binding of the cell's transcriptional activation factors and DNA-dependent RNA polymerase. The tissue-specific DNA-binding proteins determine which viral mRNA is synthesized and whether the virus replicates. This is a factor in determining the **tissue tropism and host range** of the virus.

Different DNA and RNA viruses control the duration, sequence, and quantity of viral gene and protein synthesis in different ways. The more complex viruses encode their own transcriptional activators, which enhance or regulate the expression of viral genes. For example, the herpes simplex virus encodes many proteins that regulate the kinetics of viral gene expression, including the VMW 65 (alpha TIF protein, VP16). VMW 65 is carried in the virion, binds to the host cell transcription-activating complex (Oct-1), and enhances its ability to stimulate transcription of the immediate early genes of the virus.

In general, mRNA for nonstructural proteins is transcribed first. **Early gene products** (nonstructural proteins) are often DNA-binding proteins and enzymes, including viral encoded polymerases. These proteins are catalytic, and only a few are required. Replication of the genome usually initiates the transition to transcription of late gene products. **Late viral genes** encode structural proteins. Many copies of these proteins are required to package the virus but are generally not required before the genome is replicated. Newly replicated genomes also provide new templates that amplify late gene mRNA synthesis. Different DNA and RNA viruses control the time and amount of viral gene and protein synthesis in different ways.

Genes may be transcribed from either DNA strand of the genome and in opposite directions. For example, the early and late genes of the SV40 papovavirus are on opposite, nonoverlapping DNA strands. Viral genes may have introns requiring posttranscriptional processing of the mRNA by the cell's nuclear machinery (**splicing**). The late genes of papovaviruses and adenoviruses are initially transcribed as a large RNA from a single promoter and then processed to produce several different mRNAs after removal of different intervening sequences (introns).

Replication of viral DNA follows the same biochemical rules as for cellular DNA. Replication is initiated at a unique DNA sequence of the genome, called the **origin (ori)**. This is a site recognized by cellular or viral nuclear factors and the **DNA-dependent DNA polymerase.** Viral DNA synthesis is semiconservative, and viral and cellular DNA polymerases require a **primer** to initiate synthesis of the DNA chain. The parvoviruses have DNA sequences that are inverted and repeated to allow the DNA to fold back and hybridize with itself to provide a primer. Replication of the adenovirus genome is primed by deoxycytidine monophosphate attached to a terminal protein. A cellular enzyme (primase) synthesizes an RNA primer to start the replication of the papovavirus genome while the herpesviruses encode a primase.

Replication of the genome of the simple DNA viruses (e.g., parvoviruses, papovaviruses) uses the host DNA-dependent DNA polymerases, whereas the larger, more complex viruses (e.g., adenoviruses, herpesviruses, poxviruses) encode their own polymerases. Viral polymerases are usually faster but less precise than host cell polymerases, causing a higher mutation rate in viruses, as well as providing a target for antiviral drugs.

Hepadnavirus replication is unique in that a circular, positive-strand RNA intermediate is first synthesized by the cell's DNA-dependent RNA polymerase. An RNA-dependent DNA polymerase (reverse transcriptase) in the virion core makes a negative-strand DNA, and the RNA is degraded. Positive-strand DNA synthesis is initiated but stops when the genome and core are enveloped, yielding a partially double-stranded circular DNA genome.

Major limitations for replication of a DNA virus include availability of the DNA polymerase and deoxyribonucleotide substrates. Most cells in the resting phase

---

BOX 6-8   Properties of RNA Viruses

RNA is labile and transient.
Most RNA viruses replicate in the cytoplasm.
Cells cannot replicate RNA. RNA viruses must encode an RNA-dependent RNA polymerase.
The genome structure determines the mechanism of transcription and replication.
RNA viruses are prone to mutation.
The genome structure and polarity determine how viral mRNA is generated and proteins are processed.

Picornaviruses, Togaviruses, Flaviviruses, Caliciviruses, and Coronaviruses

(+) RNA genome resembles mRNA and is translated into a polyprotein, which is proteolyzed. A (−) RNA template is used for replication.

Orthomyxoviruses, Paramyxoviruses, Rhabdoviruses, Filoviruses, and Bunyaviruses

(−) RNA genome is a template for mRNA, which may also be the (+) RNA template for replication.

Reoviruses

(+/−) segmented RNA genome is a template for mRNA. (+) RNA may also be encapsulated to generate the (+/−) RNA and then more mRNA.

Retroviruses

(+) retrovirus RNA genome is converted into DNA, which is integrated into the host chromatin and transcribed as a cellular gene.

---

of growth are not undergoing DNA synthesis, and deoxythymidine pools are limited. The parvoviruses are the smallest DNA viruses and are very dependent on the host cell. They replicate only in growing cells such as erythroid precursor cells or fetal tissue. The larger DNA viruses are more independent. They may provide enzymes and other proteins that stimulate cell growth, and they may scavenge for deoxyribonucleotides (Box 6-7). The T antigen of SV40, the E7 of papillomavirus, and the E1a protein of adenovirus bind to and alter the function of growth-inhibitory DNA-binding proteins (p53 and the retinoblastoma gene product), which results in cell growth. Herpes simplex virus encodes scavenging enzymes such as deoxyribonuclease, ribonucleotide reductase, and thymidine kinase to generate the necessary deoxyribonucleotide substrates for replication of its genome.

RNA Viruses

Replication and transcription of RNA viruses are similar processes because the viral genomes are usually either an mRNA (positive-strand RNA) or a template for mRNA (negative-strand RNA) (Box 6-8). During replication

FIGURE 6-12 Replication of picornaviruses: a simple (+) RNA virus. *(1)*, Interaction of the picornaviruses with receptors on the cell surface defines the target cell and weakens the capsid. *(2)*, The genome is injected through the virion and across the cell membrane. *2'*, The virion is endocytosed, and then the genome is released. *(3)*, Alternatively, the genome is used as mRNA for protein synthesis. One large polyprotein is translated from the virion genome. *(4)*, Then the polyprotein is proteolytically cleaved into individual proteins, including an RNA-dependent RNA polymerase. *(5)*, The polymerase makes a (−) strand template from the genome and replicates the genome. A protein (VPg) is covalently attached to the 5' end of the viral genome. *(6)*, The structural proteins associate into the capsid structure, the genome is inserted, and the virions are released on cell lysis.

FIGURE 6-13 Replication of rhabdoviruses: a simple, enveloped (−) RNA virus. *(1)*, Rhabdoviruses bind to the cell surface and are *(2)* endocytosed. The envelope fuses with the endosome vesicle membrane to deliver the nucleocapsid to the cytoplasm. The virion must carry a polymerase, which *(3)* produces five individual mRNAs and a full-length (+) RNA template. *(4)*, Proteins are translated from the mRNAs, including one glycoprotein (G), which is cotranslationally glycosylated in the endoplasmic reticulum *(ER)*, processed in the Golgi apparatus, and delivered to the cell membrane. *(5)*, The genome is replicated from the (+) RNA template, and N, L, and NS proteins associate with the genome to form the nucleocapsid. *(6)*, The matrix protein associates with the G protein–modified membrane, which is followed by assembly of the nucleocapsid. *(7)*, The virus buds from the cell in a bullet-shaped virion.

and transcription, a double-stranded RNA replicative intermediate, a structure not normally found in uninfected cells, is formed.

The RNA virus genome must code for **RNA-dependent RNA polymerases (replicases** and **transcriptases)** because the cell has no means of replicating RNA. Because RNA is degraded relatively quickly, the RNA-dependent RNA polymerase must be provided or synthesized soon after uncoating to generate more viral RNA, or the infection will be aborted. Replication of the genome also provides new templates for production of more mRNA, which amplifies and accelerates virus replication.

The **positive-strand RNA virus** genomes of the picornaviruses, caliciviruses, coronaviruses, flaviviruses, and togaviruses act as mRNA, bind to ribosomes, and direct protein synthesis. The naked positive-strand RNA viral genome is sufficient to initiate infection by itself. After the virion encoded, RNA-dependent RNA poly-

merase is produced, a negative-strand RNA template is synthesized. The template can then be used to generate more mRNA and to replicate the genome. The negative-sense RNA template of the togaviruses is also used to produce a smaller RNA for the structural proteins (late genes). The mRNAs for these viruses are not capped at the 5' end, but the genome encodes a short poly A sequence. Transcription and replication of coronaviruses share many of these aspects but are more complex.

The **negative-strand RNA virus** genomes of the rhabdoviruses, orthomyxoviruses, paramyxoviruses, filoviruses, and bunyaviruses are the templates for production of mRNA. The negative-strand RNA genome is not infectious by itself, and *a polymerase must be carried into the cell with the genome* (associated with the genome as part of the nucleocapsid) to make mRNA and initiate viral protein synthesis. The mRNA or another positive-strand RNA species can then act as a template to generate more copies of the genome. Except for influenza viruses, transcription and replication of negative-strand RNA viruses occurs in the cytoplasm. The influenza transcriptase requires a primer to produce mRNA. It uses the 5′ ends of cellular mRNA in the nucleus as primers for its polymerase and in the process steals the 5′ cap from the cellular mRNA. The influenza genome is also replicated in the nucleus.

The reoviruses have a **segmented, double-stranded RNA** genome and undergo a more complex means of replication and transcription. The reovirus RNA polymerase is part of the inner capsid cores. mRNA units are transcribed from each of the 10 or more segments of the genome while they are still in the core. The negative strands of the genome segments are used as templates for mRNA in a manner similar to the negative-strand RNA viruses. The mRNA is released into the cytoplasm, where it directs protein synthesis or is sequestered into new cores. Reovirus-encoded enzymes contained in the inner capsid add the 5′ cap to viral mRNA. The mRNA does not have poly A. The positive-strand RNA in the cores acts as a template for negative-strand RNA, producing the progeny double-stranded RNA.

The arenaviruses have an **ambisense circular** genome with (+) sequences adjacent to (−) sequences. The early genes of the virus are transcribed from the negative-sense portion of the genome, and the late genes of the virus are transcribed from the full-length replicative intermediate.

Although the **retroviruses** have a positive-strand RNA genome, the virus provides no means for replication of the RNA in the cytoplasm. Instead, the retroviruses carry two copies of the genome, two tRNA molecules, and an RNA-dependent DNA polymerase (**reverse transcriptase**) in the virion. The tRNA is used as a primer for synthesis of a DNA copy (**cDNA**) of the genome. The cDNA is synthesized in the cytoplasm and then integrated into the host chromatin. The viral genome is then transcribed as a cellular gene. Promoters at the end of the integrated viral genome enhance the extent of their transcription. Full-length transcripts are used as new genomes, and individual mRNAs are generated by differential splicing of the RNA.

The most unusual mode of replication is reserved for the **delta virus.** The delta virus resembles a viroid. The genome is a circular, rod-shaped, single-stranded (+) RNA, which is extensively hybridized to itself. As the exception, the delta virus RNA genome is replicated by the host cell DNA-dependent RNA polymerase II in the nucleus. The genome forms an RNA structure called a *ribozyme,* which cleaves the RNA circle to produce a mRNA.

Viral Protein Synthesis

All viruses depend on the host-cell ribosomes, transfer RNA (tRNA), and mechanisms for posttranslational modification to produce their proteins. Unlike bacterial ribosomes, which can bind to a polycistronic mRNA and translate several gene sequences into separate proteins,

the eukaryotic ribosome binds to mRNA, makes a continuous protein, and then falls off the mRNA. Each virus deals with this limitation differently, depending on the structure of the genome. For example, the entire genome of a positive-strand RNA virus is read by the ribosome and translated into one giant **polyprotein.** The polyprotein is subsequently cleaved by cellular and viral proteases into functional proteins. DNA viruses, retroviruses, and most negative-strand RNA viruses transcribe mRNA for smaller polyproteins or individual proteins. The orthomyxovirus and reovirus genomes are segmented, and most of the segments code for single proteins for this reason.

Viruses use different tactics to promote preferential translation of their viral mRNA instead of cellular mRNA. In many cases the concentration of viral mRNA in the cell is so large that it occupies most of the ribosomes, preventing translation of cellular mRNA. Adenovirus infection blocks the egress of cellular mRNA from the nucleus. Herpes simplex virus and other viruses inhibit cellular macromolecular synthesis and induce degradation of the cell's DNA and mRNA. To promote selective translation of its mRNA, poliovirus inactivates the 200,000-dalton cap-binding protein of the ribosome with a viral-coded protease, preventing binding and translation of 5′ capped cellular mRNA. Togaviruses and many other viruses increase the permeability of the cell's membrane, which decreases the ribosomal affinity for most cellular mRNA. All these actions also contribute to the cytopathology of the virus infection. The pathogenic consequences of these actions are discussed further in Chapter 46.

Some viral proteins require **posttranslational modifications** such as phosphorylation, glycosylation, acylation, or sulfation. Protein phosphorylation is accomplished by cellular or viral protein kinases and is a means of modulating, activating, or inactivating proteins. Several herpesviruses and other viruses encode their own protein kinase. *Viral glycoproteins are synthesized on membrane-bound ribosomes and have the amino acid sequences to allow insertion into the rough endoplasmic reticulum and N-linked glycosylation.* The high-mannose precursor form of the glycoproteins progresses from the endoplasmic reticulum through the vesicular transport system of the cell and is processed through the Golgi apparatus. The sialic acid–containing mature glycoprotein is expressed on the plasma membrane of the cell unless the glycoprotein expresses protein sequences for retention in an intracellular organelle. The presence of the glycoproteins will determine where the virion will assemble. Other modifications, such as O-glycosylation, acylation, and sulfation of the proteins, can also occur during progression through the Golgi apparatus.

Assembly

Virion assembly is analogous to a three-dimensional interlocking puzzle that puts itself together in the box. The virion is built from small, easily manufactured parts that enclose the genome in a functional package. The site and mechanism of virion assembly in the cell depend on where genome replication occurs and whether the final structure is a naked capsid or an enveloped virus.

Assembly of the DNA viruses, other than poxviruses, occurs in the nucleus and requires transport of the virion proteins into the nucleus. These proteins must have the appropriate peptide signals for nuclear transport in addition to structural features. RNA virus and poxvirus assembly occurs in the cytoplasm.

Each part of the virion has recognition structures that allow the virus to form the appropriate protein-protein,

protein-nucleic acid, and (for enveloped viruses) protein-membrane interactions needed to assemble into the final structure. The assembly process begins when the necessary pieces are synthesized and the concentration of structural proteins in the cell is sufficient to thermodynamically drive the process, much like a crystallization reaction.

Assembly may be facilitated by scaffolding proteins or other proteins that are activated or release energy on proteolysis. For example, cleavage of the VP0 protein of poliovirus releases the VP4 peptide, which solidifies the capsid. For the human immunodeficiency virus and other retroviruses, polyproteins containing the protease, polymerase, and structural proteins accumulate at viral glycoprotein-modified membranes. The virion buds from the membrane, and the viral-encoded **protease** is activated within the virion and cleaves the polyprotein to produce the final, infectious nucleocapsid within the envelope. Herpesviruses and other capsid viruses also use a virion protease to finish the assembly of a nucleocapsid.

Capsid viruses may be assembled as empty structures (procapsids) to be filled with the genome (e.g., picornaviruses, herpesviruses), or they may be assembled around the genome. Nucleocapsids of the retroviruses, togaviruses, and the negative-strand RNA viruses assemble around the genome and are subsequently enclosed in an envelope.

Acquisition of an envelope occurs after association of the nucleocapsid with regions of host-cell membrane modified with viral glycoproteins. Matrix proteins for negative-strand RNA viruses line and promote the adhesion of nucleocapsids with the glycoprotein-modified membrane. As more interactions occur, the membrane surrounds the nucleocapsid, and the virus buds from the membrane.

The site of budding is determined by the type of genome and the protein sequence of the glycoproteins. Most RNA viruses bud from the plasma membrane, and the virus is released from the cell at the same time. The flaviviruses, coronaviruses, and bunyaviruses acquire their envelope by budding into the endoplasmic reticulum and Golgi membranes and may remain in these organelles. The herpes simplex virus nucleocapsid assembles in the nucleus and buds at the nuclear membrane. The enveloped herpesvirus is transported through the Golgi apparatus and is released by exocytosis or is released on cell lysis.

Assembly of a complete, functional influenza or reovirus virion requires accumulation of at least one copy of each gene segment. Although the influenza virus has only 8 genome segments, virions can randomly package 10 to 11 segments. Statistically, this yields approximately 1 complete set of genomes and functional virus per 20 defective viruses. Reovirus genomes are likely to assemble in a similar manner.

Errors are made during viral assembly. Empty virions and virions containing defective genomes are produced. As a result, the particle–to–infectious virus ratio,

FIGURE 6-14 Replication of herpes simplex virus, a complex enveloped DNA virus. The virus binds to specific receptors and fuses with the plasma membrane. The nucleocapsid then delivers the DNA genome to the nucleus. Transcription and translation occur in three phases: immediate early, early, and late. Immediate early proteins promote the takeover of the cell; early proteins consist of enzymes, including the DNA-dependent DNA polymerase; and the late proteins are structural proteins, including the viral capsid and glycoproteins. The genome is replicated before transcription of the late genes. Capsid proteins migrate into the nucleus, assemble into icosadeltahedral capsids and are filled with the DNA genome. The viral glycoproteins are inserted into the endoplasmic reticulum, and carbohydrate is attached. The glycoproteins diffuse to the contiguous nuclear envelope. The capsids filled with genomes bud through these modified membranes and are transferred to the Golgi apparatus; the glycoproteins are processed, and the virus is released by exocytosis. Alternatively, the virus may be released on cell lysis.

Labels in figure: Attachment and penetration by fusion; Immediate early Protein synthesis; Early Protein synthesis and genome replication; Late Protein synthesis (structural protein); Exocytosis and release; Assembly and release; Lysis and release; Nucleus; DNA genome; mRNA; Protein; DNA also called *particle–to–plaque-forming unit ratio,* is high, usually greater than 10 and during rapid viral replication can even be 10^4. Defective viruses can occupy the machinery required for normal virus replication to prevent (interfere with) virus production (**defective interfering particles**).

Release

Viruses can be released from cells after lysis of the cell, by exocytosis, or by budding from the plasma membrane. Naked capsid viruses are generally released after lysis of the cell. Release of some enveloped viruses occurs after budding from the plasma membrane. Lysis and plasma membrane budding are efficient means of release. Viruses that bud or acquire their membrane in the cytoplasm (e.g., flaviviruses, poxviruses) are released by exocytosis or cell lysis and are more cell associated. Viruses that bind to sialic acid receptors may also have a neuraminidase (e.g., orthomyxoviruses, certain paramyxoviruses). The neuraminidase removes potential sialic acid receptors on the glycoproteins of the virion and the host cell to prevent clumping and facilitate release.

Reinitiation of the Replication Cycle

The virus released to the extracellular medium is usually responsible for initiating new infections; however, **cell-cell fusion** or **vertical transmission** of the genome to daughter cells can also spread the infection. Some herpesviruses, retroviruses, and paramyxoviruses can induce cell-cell fusion to create multinucleated giant cells (syncytia). The retroviruses can transmit their integrated copy of the genome vertically to daughter cells on cell division.

VIRAL GENETICS

As with other genetic systems, mutations spontaneously occur in viral genomes, creating new virus strains with properties differing from the parental, or **wild-type, virus.** These variants can be identified by their nucleotide sequences, antigenic differences (serotypes), or differences in functional or structural properties. Most mutations have no effect or are detrimental to the virus. Mutations in essential genes inactivate the virus, but mutations in other genes can produce antiviral drug resistance or alter the antigenicity or pathogenicity of the virus.

Errors in copying the viral genome during virus replication produce many mutations. This is due to the **poor fidelity of the viral polymerase** and the rapid rate of DNA virus replication. In addition, **RNA viruses do not have a genetic error-checking mechanism.** As a result, the rates of mutation for DNA viruses are usually lower than for RNA viruses.

Mutants are identified by the changes induced by the mutation. Mutations in essential genes are termed **lethal mutations.** These mutants are difficult to isolate because the virus cannot replicate. A **deletion mutant** results

from the loss or selective removal of a portion of the genome and the function that it encodes. Other mutations may produce **plaque mutants,** which differ from the wild type in the size or appearance of the infected cell; **host range mutants,** which differ in the tissue type or species of target cell that can be infected; or **attenuated mutants,** which are variants that cause less serious infections in animals or humans. **Conditional mutants,** such as **temperature-sensitive (ts)** or **cold-sensitive mutants,** have a mutation in a gene for an essential protein that allows virus production only at certain temperatures. ts mutants generally grow well or relatively better at 30 to 35° C, whereas elevated temperatures of 38 to 40° C will inactivate the mutated, essential gene product and prevent virus production.

New virus strains can also arise by genetic interactions between viruses or between the virus and the cell (Figure 6-15). Intramolecular genetic exchange between viruses or the virus and the host is termed **recombination.** Recombination can occur readily between two related DNA viruses. For example, coinfection of a cell with the two closely related herpesviruses (herpes simplex virus types 1 and 2) yields intertypic recombinant strains. These new hybrid strains have genes from both types 1 and 2. Integration of retroviruses into host-cell chromatin is a form of recombination.

Viruses with segmented genomes (such as influenza viruses and reoviruses) form hybrid strains on infection of one cell with more than one virus strain. This process, termed **reassortment,** is analogous to picking 10 marbles out of a box containing 10 black and 10 white marbles. New strains of influenza A virus are created on

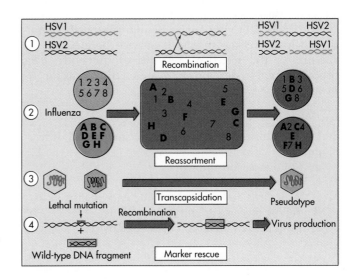

FIGURE 6-15 Genetic exchange between viral particles can give rise to new viral types, as illustrated. Representative viruses include the following: *1,* intertypic recombination of herpes simplex virus type 1 *(HSV1)* and type 2 *(HSV2); 2,* reassortment of two strains of influenza virus; *3,* rescue of a papovavirus defective in assembly by a complementary defective virus (transcapsidation); and *4,* marker rescue of a lethal or conditional mutation.

coinfection with a virus from different species (see Figure 56-5).

In some cases a defective viral strain can be rescued by the replication of another mutant, by the wild-type virus, or by a cell line bearing a replacement viral gene. The replication of the other virus provides the missing function required by the mutant (**complementation**), allowing replication to occur. Rescue of a lethal or conditional-lethal mutant with a defined genetic sequence, such as a restriction endonuclease DNA fragment, is called **marker rescue.** Marker rescue is used to map the genomes of viruses such as herpes simplex virus. Virus produced from cells infected with different virus strains may be **phenotypically mixed** and have the proteins of one strain but the genome of the other (**transcapsidation**). **Pseudotypes** are generated when transcapsidation occurs between different types of virus, but this is rare.

Individual virus strains or mutants are **selected** by their ability to use the host-cell machinery and to withstand the conditions of the body and the environment. Cellular properties that can act as selection pressures include the growth rate of the cell and tissue-specific expression of certain proteins required by the virus (e.g., enzymes, glycoproteins, transcription factors). The conditions of the body, its elevated temperature, natural and immune defenses, and tissue structure are also selection pressures for viruses. The viruses that cannot endure these conditions or evade the host defenses are eliminated. A small selective advantage in a mutant virus can shortly lead to its becoming the predominant viral strain. The high mutation rate of the human immunodeficiency virus promotes a switch in target-cell tropism from macrophage to T cell, the development of antiviral drug-resistant strains after treatment, and the generation of antigenic variants during a patient's course of infection.

The growth of virus under benign laboratory conditions allows weaker strains to survive because of the absence of the selective pressures of the body. This process is used to develop attenuated virus strains for use in vaccines.

QUESTIONS

1. What features of these viruses are similar and different?
   a. Poliovirus and rhinovirus
   b. Poliovirus and rotavirus
   c. Poliovirus and western equine encephalitis virus
   d. Yellow fever virus and dengue virus
   e. Epstein-Barr virus and cytomegalovirus

2. Match the characteristics from column A with the appropriate viral families in column B based on your knowledge of their physical and genome structure and its implications.

A	B
1. Is resistant to detergents	Picornaviruses
2. Is resistant to drying	Togaviruses
3. Replication in the nucleus	Orthomyxoviruses
4. Replication in the cytoplasm	Paramyxoviruses
5. Can be released from the cell without cell lysis	Rhabdoviruses
6. Provides a good target for antiviral drug action	Reoviruses
	Retroviruses
7. Undergoes reassortment on coinfection with two strains	Herpesviruses
8. Makes DNA from an RNA template	Papovaviruses
9. Uses a (+) RNA template to replicate the genome	Adenoviruses
	Poxviruses
10. Genome translated into a polyprotein	Hepadnaviruses

3. Based on structural considerations, which of the virus families listed in *2* should be able to endure fecal-oral transmission?
4. List the essential enzymes encoded by the virus families listed in *2.*
5. A mutant defective in the herpes simplex virus type 1 DNA polymerase gene replicates in the presence of herpes simplex virus type 2. The progeny virus contains the herpes simplex virus type 1 genome but is recognized by antibodies to herpes simplex virus type 2. Which genetic mechanisms may be occurring?
6. How are the early and late genes of the togaviruses, papovaviruses, and herpesviruses distinguished and how is the time of their expression regulated?
7. What are the consequences (no effect, decreased efficiency, or inhibition of replication) of a deletion mutation in the following viral enzymes?
   a. Epstein-Barr virus polymerase
   b. Herpes simplex virus thymidine kinase
   c. Human immunodeficiency virus reverse transcriptase
   d. Influenza B virus neuraminidase
   e. Rabies virus (rhabdovirus) G protein

Bibliography

Belshe RB, editor: *Textbook of human virology,* ed 2, St Louis, 1991, Mosby.
Fields BN, Knipe DM, Howley PM, editors: *Virology,* ed 3, New York, 1996, Lippincott-Raven.

Fungal Classification, Structure, and Replication

The branch of biology that deals with the study of fungi is called *mycology*. The systematic study of these organisms is approximately 150 years old; yet the practical manifestations of these organisms have been known since antiquity. In addition to their disease-producing potential in humans, fungi are directly or indirectly harmful in many other ways. They contribute to food spoilage, are the major cause of plant diseases, and destroy timber, textiles, and several synthetic materials. However, as saprobes, they share with bacteria (particularly organisms such as the *Streptomyces*) a role in the decay of complex plant and animal remains in the soil, breaking them down into simpler molecules to be absorbed by future generations of plants. Without this essential decay process the growth of plants, on which life depends, would eventually cease for lack of basic materials. Fungi are also specifically beneficial to humans. They are used in the production of antibiotics, organic acids, steroids, and products of fermentation, such as alcoholic beverages and soya sauce. The carbon dioxide produced by fungi makes dough rise in breadmaking, and the various ketones, aldehydes, and organic acids that result from the metabolic activities of fungi on milk curd and the juice of grapes provide the unique cheeses and wines we enjoy. Furthermore, fungi serve as scientific models to study genetics, biochemical processes, and relationships involving parasites and hosts.

Fungi are a diverse group of organisms that occupy many niches in the environment. In general they are free living and abundant in nature, with only a few in the normal flora of humans. Although tens of thousands of species have been described, fewer than 100 are routinely associated with human diseases. Unlike viruses, protozoan parasites, and some species of bacteria, fungi do not need to colonize or infect the tissues of humans or animals to preserve or perpetuate the species. With only two major exceptions (candidiasis and tinea versicolor), virtually all fungal infections originate from an exogenous source, either by inhalation or by traumatic implantation.

Fungi are **eukaryotic organisms.** Most important, they possess a nucleus enclosed by a nuclear membrane. Unlike plant cells and some bacteria, fungi do not contain chlorophyll and cannot synthesize macromolecules from carbon dioxide and energy derived from light rays. Therefore all fungi lead a heterotrophic existence in nature as **saprobes** (organisms that live on dead or decaying organic matter), **symbionts** (organisms that live together and in which the association is of mutual advantage), **commensals** (two organisms living in a close relationship in which one benefits by the relationship and the other neither benefits nor is harmed), or **parasites** (organisms that live on or within a host from which they derive benefits without making any useful contributions in return; in the case of pathogens the relationship is harmful to the host).

CLASSIFICATION

Conflicts often arise in considering relationships between certain fungi, and no universal consensus may be possible concerning the classification or even the nomenclature of a given organism. Differences of opinion occasionally arise, since one taxonomist may place greater emphasis on certain phenotypic features of an isolate than on criteria deemed more important by other individuals. Another difficulty is the conflict between those who group many organisms and those who prefer to emphasize minor phenotype differences and split them into many groups. The result of these conflicting opinions is the controversy that frequently arises over the proper names of individual fungi. As a practical matter, the use of multiple names for the same organism has created a great deal of confusion in the medical literature.

Organisms are classified for convenience of reference; thus the scheme of classification should reflect natural relationships between them. Biochemical, ultrastructural, molecular biological, and genetic studies support the concept that at least five kingdoms are necessary to accommodate all living things. These are the Monera (prokaryotes), Protista (protozoa), Fungi, Plantae, and Animalia. The Fungi kingdom is composed of two phyla (Table 7-1), the Zygomycota (organisms that produce a zygote during their sexual cycle) and the Dikaryomycota (organisms that have an extended state in which nuclei of different genotypes replicate autonomously in the same

TABLE 7-1	**Taxonomic Classification of the Fungi Kingdom**	
CLASSIFICATION	**SEXUAL CHARACTERISTICS**	**MEDICALLY IMPORTANT GENERA**
Phylum Zygomycota	Sexual reproduction occurs through fusion of two compatible gametangia to produce zygote. Asexual reproduction is characterized by production of sporangiospores.	Agents causing zygomycosis
Phylum Dikaryomycota	Dikaryotic life cycle includes extended dikaryotic phase after sexual conjugation; that is, haploid nuclei do not fuse immediately.	—
Subphylum Ascomycotina	Sexual reproduction occurs through fusion of two compatible nuclei to form diploid nucleus followed by meiosis to yield haploid progeny; entire process occurs within sac called *ascus*, and resultant spores are called *ascospores*.	Agents causing ringworm, histoplasmosis, and blastomycosis
Subphylum Basidiomycotina	Sexual reproduction takes place in sac called *basidium*, where two compatible nuclei fuse to form diploid nucleus, followed by meiosis to yield haploid progeny. These then mature on outer surface of basidium. Haploid progeny are called *basidiospores*.	Agent causing cryptococcosis
Form-class Deuteromycotina (Fungi imperfecti)	Sexual stage has not been observed in fungi classified in this category	*Candida, Trichosporon, Torulopsis, Pityrosporum, Epidermophyton, Coccidioides,* and *Paracoccidioides* species

protoplasm as a result of sexual conjugation). The phylum Dikaryomycota is divided into two subphyla, the Ascomycotina and the Basidiomycotina, which are defined according to the type of structure that forms and houses the haploid progeny. Those organisms for which a sexual phase has not been observed are classified in the form-class Deuteromycotina or Fungi imperfecti.

STRUCTURE

Fungi have structures typical of eukaryotic cells. Figure 7-1 illustrates a section of a model fungal cell with its component parts. In contrast with bacterial cells, fungal cells possess a complex cytosol that contains microvesicles, microtubules, ribosomes, mitochondria, Golgi apparatus, nuclei, a double-membraned endoplasmic reticulum, and other structures. The nuclei of fungi are enclosed by a membrane and contain virtually all of the cellular DNA. They have a true nucleolus rich in RNA. An interesting and unique property of this membrane is that during the mitotic cycle it persists throughout metaphase, in contrast to the nuclear membrane of plant and animal cells, which dissolves and then reforms after the chromosomes segregate to their centromeres.

Enclosing the complex cytosol is another membrane called the *plasmalemma* that is composed of glycoproteins, phospholipids, and ergosterol. The fact that fungi possess ergosterol in contrast to cholesterol, which is the major sterol found in tissues of mammals, is important because most antifungal strategies are based on the presence of ergosterol in fungal membranes. (Antifungal agents are discussed in Chapter 67.)

FIGURE 7-1 Diagram of the apical portion of a hyphal cell illustrating its component parts.

Unlike mammalian cells, fungi possess a multilayered rigid cell wall immediately exterior to the plasmalemma. The cell wall is structurally and biochemically complex, containing **chitin,** a homopolymer of beta-(1,4)-linked *N*-acetylglucosamine residues, as its structural foundation. Layered on the chitin are glucans, mannoproteins, and other complex polysaccharides in association with polypeptides. In filamentous fungi, the biosynthesis of chitin occurs at the growing tip. The synthesis of chitin is controlled by the activity of three chitin synthases. These enzymes exist in the cytosol in discrete membrane-bound packets called *chitosomes.* The active form of chitin synthase is found in the plasmalemma, and polymerization of chitin microfibrils occurs outside this membrane.

In addition to the cell wall, some fungi produce a capsular polysaccharide. This structure isolates the organism from its surrounding environment and at the same time is in direct communication with that environment; in the case of pathogens, this environment is host tissue. The cell wall and structures such as the capsular material determine virulence and play a role in eliciting host immune responses. (See Chapter 70 for a discussion of *Cryptococcus neoformans.*)

Most fungi respire aerobically but some have a limited capacity for anaerobiosis (fermentation), and others are strict anaerobes. Metabolically, they are heterotrophic and biochemically versatile, producing primary (e.g., citric acid, ethanol, glycerol) and secondary (e.g., penicillin, amanitins, aflatoxins) metabolites. The division time for these organisms is long (hours) compared with that of bacteria (minutes).

Fungi are gram positive, and the vegetative cells are not acid-fast. In histopathological sections, fungi can be stained by special procedures because of the glucans and other complex polysaccharides that make up the cell wall (methenamine-silver or periodic acid-Schiff staining methods).

Whereas the ability of fungi to cause disease in humans or animals appears to be accidental, most disease-producing fungi have developed characteristics that enable them to adapt to hostile tissue environments and grow. Fungi that colonize the cutaneous layers of the epidermis or invade hair and nails metabolize **keratin,** the tough, fibrous, insoluble protein that forms the principal matter of these tissues. Other fungi, such as *Histoplasma capsulatum, Blastomyces dermatitidis, Paracoccidioides brasiliensis,* and *Coccidioides immitis* have developed the capacity to overcome various host cellular defense mechanisms, can grow at the higher temperatures of the host (37° C) as well as the temperatures found in natural environments (around 25° C), and can survive in a lowered oxidation-reduction state (a situation found in damaged tissues).

Fungi can be divided into two basic morphological forms: yeast and hyphae. Their developmental histories encompass both vegetative and reproductive phases. These phases are frequently present simultaneously in growing cultures and may not be easily separated.

Yeasts are unicellular and reproduce asexually by processes termed *blastoconidia formation* (budding) (Figure 7-2, *A*) or fission (Figure 7-2, *B*).

Most fungi have branching, threadlike tubular filaments called *hyphae* (Figure 7-2, *C* to *F*) that elongate at their tips by a process called *apical extension.* These filamentous structures are either coenocytic (hollow and multinucleate) (Figure 7-2, *D*) or **septate** (divided by partitions) (Figure 7-2, *E* and *F*). The collective term for a mass of hyphae is **mycelium** (synonymous with **mold**). Hyphae that grow submerged or on the surface of a cul-

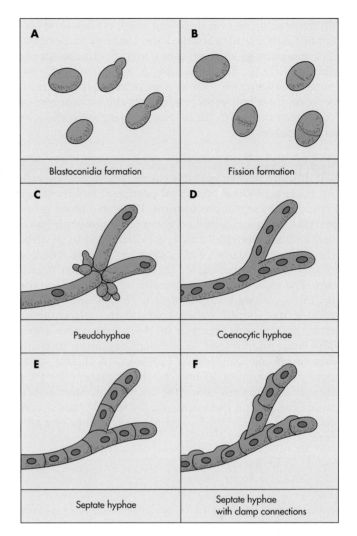

FIGURE 7-2 Fungal cell morphology. **A,** Yeast cells reproducing by blastocondia formation. **B,** Yeast cells dividing by fission. **C,** Pseudohyphal development. **D,** Coenocytic hyphae. **E,** Septate hyphae. **F,** Septate hyphae with clamp connections.

ture medium are called **vegetative hyphae** because they are responsible for absorbing nutrients. Those that project above the surface of the medium are called **aerial hyphae.** Aerial hyphae often produce specialized structures called *conidia* (i.e., asexual reproductive elements also called *propagules*) that are easily airborne and disseminated into the environment. The shape, size, and certain developmental features of conidia are useful to the mycologist in identifying the specific species. This is illustrated in Chapters 69 to 71.

The morphology of *Candida albicans,* part of the normal flora of the mouth, gastrointestinal tract, and membranes lining the mucosa of other cavities and tissues, is unique. In addition to being yeastlike or filamentous, this organism can assume a pseudohyphal morphology wherein the cells are elongated and linked like sausages (Figure 7-2, *C*). Pseudohyphal development is an exaggerated form of budding; the newly formed cells do not take on an oval shape and pinch off from the parent but rather remain attached and continue to elongate. The morphology of fungi is not fixed because some are dimorphic (e.g., *H. capsulatum, B. dermatitidis, C. immitis, P. brasiliensis*); that is, they can exist in a mycelial or yeast morphology depending on the environmental conditions of growth (in soil, on decaying vegetation, or in host tissues).

REPLICATION

All fungi reproduce by asexual processes, and most can reproduce by sexual mechanisms. If a sexual phase is observed for any fungal isolate, the terms **anamorph** (asexual) and **teleomorph** (sexual) are often used to describe the taxonomic status of the organism. This is reflected mostly in the nomenclature used to refer to that organism. For example, the anamorphic designation for the organism causing histoplasmosis is *Histoplasma capsulatum;* if the specific isolate exists in the teleomorphic state, the name is changed to *Ajellomyces capsulatum.* This convention is used for all fungal organisms to maintain taxonomic consistency. However, in clinical situations it is common to refer to the organisms by their asexual designations, since the anamorphic state is isolated from clinical specimens and the sexual phase occurs only under the extremely controlled conditions of a culture.

QUESTIONS

1. How do fungi differ from bacteria (size, nucleus, cytosol, cytosolic membrane, cell wall, physiology, staining properties, generation time)?
2. What is the basic difference between the cell membrane (plasmalemma) of fungal and mammalian cells?
3. How do yeasts differ from molds and what does the term *dimorphism* mean when it is applied to fungi?
4. What do the terms *anamorph* and *teleomorph* mean and of what importance are they?

Bibliography

Evans EGV, Gentles JC: *Essentials of medical mycology,* New York, 1985, Churchill Livingstone.

Gozalbo D et al: Critical steps in fungal cell wall synthesis: strategies for their inhibition, *Pharmacol Ther* 60:337-345, 1993.

Kreger-van Rij NJW, editor: *The yeasts: a taxonomic study,* ed 3, Amsterdam, 1984, Elsevier Science.

Margulis L, Schwartz KV: *Five kingdoms,* ed 2, New York, 1988, WH Freeman.

Moore-Landecker E: *Fundamentals of the fungi,* ed 3, Englewood Cliffs, NJ, 1990, Prentice-Hall.

Ruiz-Herrera J: *Fungal cell wall: structure, synthesis, and assembly,* Boca Raton, Fla, 1991, CRC.

CHAPTER 8

Parasitic Classification, Structure, and Replication

This chapter provides an introduction to parasite classification and physiology. This brief review is intended to enhance the reader's comprehension of the interrelationships among parasitic organisms, their epidemiology and transmission of disease, the specific disease processes involved, and the possibilities for prevention and control of maladies. We have deliberately attempted to simplify the taxonomy by using it to address the major divisions involved in medical parasitology: specifically, intestinal and urogenital protozoa, blood and tissue protozoa, nematodes, trematodes, and cestodes.

THE IMPORTANCE OF PARASITES

Medical parasitology is the study of invertebrate animals capable of causing disease in humans and other animals. Although parasitic diseases are frequently considered "tropical" and thus of little importance to physicians practicing in the more temperate, developed countries of the world, it is clear that the world has become a very small place and that physician knowledge of parasitic diseases is essential. The global impact of parasitic infections and the number of parasite-associated deaths is staggering and must be of concern to all health care workers (Table 8-1). Increasingly tourists, missionaries, Peace Corps volunteers, and others are visiting and working for extended periods of time in exotic, remote parts of the world. Thus they are at risk for parasitic and other infections that are rare in the United States and other developed countries. Another source of infected patients is the ever-increasing number of refugees from developing countries. Finally, the profound immunosuppression problems that accompany advances in medical therapy (e.g., organ transplantation), as well as those associated with persons infected with the human immunodeficiency virus (HIV), place a growing number of individuals at risk for developing infections caused by certain parasites. Given these considerations, clinicians and laboratory workers should be aware of the possibility of parasitic disease and should be trained in ordering, performing, and interpreting the appropriate laboratory tests to aid in the diagnosis and therapy.

CLASSIFICATION AND STRUCTURE

The parasites of humans are classified within the kingdom Animalia and are separated into two subkingdoms, Protozoa and Metazoa (Table 8-2). Parasite classification takes into account the morphology of intracytoplasmic structures, such as the nucleus, the type of locomotive organelles, and the mode of reproduction (Table 8-3). The Protozoa are animals in which all life functions occur in a single cell. The Metazoa are multicellular animals in which life functions occur in cellular structures organized as tissue and organ systems.

Protozoa

Protozoa are simple microorganisms that range in size from 2 to 100 μm. Their protoplasm is enclosed by a cell membrane and contains numerous organelles, including a membrane-bound nucleus, an endoplasmic reticulum, food-storage granules, and contractile and digestive vacuoles. The nucleus contains clumped or dispersed chromatin and a central karyosome. Organs of motility vary from simple cytoplasmic extrusions or pseudopods to more complex structures such as flagella or cilia. The subkingdom Protozoa comprises seven major subgroups or phyla, four of which are the concern of medical parasitology.

Sarcomastigophora

Phylum Sarcomastigophora consists of the amebae (subphylum Sarcodina) and the flagellates (subphylum Mastigophora). Locomotion of amebae is accomplished by the extrusion of pseudopodia ("false feet"), whereas flagellates move by the lashing of their whiplike flagella. The number and position of flagella vary a great deal in different species. In addition, specialized structures associated with the flagella may produce a characteristic morphological appearance that may be useful in species identification.

Ciliophora

Phylum Ciliophora consists of the ciliates, which include a variety of free-living and symbiotic species. Ciliate locomotion involves the coordinated movement of rows of

TABLE 8-1	Estimated Worldwide Prevalence of Parasitic Infections	
INFECTION	**NUMBER OF INFECTED**	**ANNUAL DEATHS***
Amebiasis	10% of world population	40,000-110,000
Malaria	400-490 million	2.2-2.5 million
African trypanosomiasis	100,000 new cases/yr	5000
American trypanosomiasis	24 million	60,000
Leishmaniasis	1.2 million	—
Schistosomiasis	>200 million	0.5-2 million
Opisthorchiasis	19 million	—
Paragonimiasis	3.2 million	—
Fasciolopsiasis	10 million	—
Filariasis	85-100 million	—
Onchocerciasis	>30 million	—
Dracunculiasis	10 million	—
Ascariasis	1 billion	1550†
Hookworm	900 million	—
Trichuriasis	500-800 million	—
Strongyloidiasis	35 million	—
Cestodiasis	65 million	—

Based on data from Sherris JC: *Medical microbiology: an introduction to infectious diseases,* ed 2, New York, 1990, Elsevier.
*Mortality data included where available.
†From intestinal obstruction.

TABLE 8-2	Medically Important Parasites (Kingdom, Animalia)	
SUBKINGDOM	**PHYLUM**	**ORGANISMS**
Protoza	Sarcomastigophora	Ameba, flagellates
	Ciliophora	Ciliates
	Apicomplexa	Sporozoa, Coccidia
	Microspora	Microsporidia
Metazoa	Nematoda	Roundworms
	Platyhelminthes	Flatworms
	Trematodes	Flukes
	Cestodes	Tapeworms
	Arthropoda	
	Chilopoda	Centipedes
	Pentastomida	Tongue worms
	Crustacea	Crabs, crayfish, shrimp, copepods
	Arachnida	Mites, ticks, spiders, scorpions
	Insecta	Mosquitoes, flies, lice, fleas, wasps, ants, beetles, moths, roaches, true bugs

Apicomplexa

Phylum Apicomplexa organisms are often referred to as *sporozoa* or *coccidia*. These unicellular organisms have a system of organelles at their apical end that produces substances to help the organism penetrate host cells and thus become an intracellular parasite.

Microspora

Phylum Microspora organisms were formerly classified with the Sporozoa. The Microspora are small intracellular parasites that differ significantly in structure from the Apicomplexa. These parasites are characterized by the structure of their spores, which have a complex tubular extrusion mechanism (polar tubule) used to inject the infective material (sporoplasm) into host cells.

Metazoa

The subkingdom Metazoa includes all animals that are not Protozoa. This text discusses two groups of organisms of major importance: the helminths ("worms") and the arthropods (crabs, insects, ticks, and the like).

Helminths

The helminths are complex, multicellular organisms that are elongated and bilaterally symmetrical. They are considerably larger than the protozoan parasites and generally are macroscopic, ranging in size from less than 1 mm to 1 m or more. The external surface of some worms is covered with a protective cuticle, which is acellular and may be smooth or possess ridges, spines, or tubercles. The protective covering of flatworms is known as a *tegument*. Frequently, helminths possess elaborate attach-

hairlike structures, or cilia. Cilia are structurally similar to flagella but are usually shorter and more numerous. Some ciliates are multinucleate. The only ciliate parasite of humans, *Balantidium coli,* contains two nuclei: a large macronucleus and a small micronucleus.

ment structures such as hooks, suckers, teeth, or plates. These structures are usually located anteriorly and may be useful in classifying and identifying the organisms (Table 8-3). Helminths typically have primitive nervous and excretory systems. Some have alimentary tracts; however, none has a circulatory system (Table 8-3). The helminths are separated into two phyla, the Nematoda and the Platyhelminthes.

Nematoda. Phylum Nematoda consists of the roundworms, which have cylindrical bodies. The sexes of roundworm are separate, and these organisms have a complete digestive system. The nematodes may be intestinal parasites or may infect the blood and tissue.

Platyhelminthes. Phylum Platyhelminthes consists of the flatworms, which have flattened bodies that are leaflike or resemble ribbon segments. Platyhelminthes can be further separated into trematodes and cestodes.

Trematodes, or **flukes,** have leaf-shaped bodies. Most are hermaphroditic, with male and female sex organs in a single body. Their digestive systems are incomplete and have only saclike tubes. Their life cycle is complex; snails serve as first intermediate hosts and other aquatic animals or plants as second intermediate hosts.

Cestodes, or **tapeworms,** have bodies composed of ribbons of proglottids, or segments. All are hermaphroditic, and all lack digestive systems, with nutrition being absorbed through the body walls. The life cycles of some cestodes are simple and direct, whereas those of others are complex and require one or more intermediate hosts.

Arthropods

Phylum Arthropoda is the largest group of animals in the kingdom Animalia. Arthropods are complex, multicellular organisms that may be involved directly in causing an invasive or a superficial (infestation) disease processes or indirectly as intermediate hosts and vectors of many infectious agents, including protozoan and metazoan parasites (Table 8-4). In addition, envenomization by biting and stinging arthropods can result in adverse reactions in humans that range from local allergic and hypersensitivity reactions to severe anaphylactic shock and death. There are five major classes of arthropods (Table 8-2).

Chilopoda. Class Chilopoda consists of terrestrial forms, such as centipedes. These organisms are of medical importance because of their poison claws, which may produce a painful "bite."

Pentastomida. The pentastomids, or tongue worms, are bloodsucking endoparasites of reptiles, birds, and mammals. Adult pentastomids are white and cylindrical or flattened parasites that possess two distinct body regions: an anterior cephalothorax and an abdomen. Humans may serve as intermediate hosts for these parasites.

Crustacea. Class Crustacea consists of familiar aquatic forms, such as crabs, crayfish, shrimp, and copepods. Several are involved as intermediate hosts in life cycles of various intestinal or blood and tissue helminths.

Arachnida. Class Arachnida consists of familiar terrestrial forms, such as mites, ticks, spiders, and scorpions.

These animals have no wings or antennae, like insects do, and adults have four pairs of legs, as opposed to three pairs for insects. Of medical importance are those serving as vectors for microbial diseases (mites and ticks) or as venomous animals that bite (spiders) or sting (scorpions).

Insecta. Class Insecta consists of familiar aquatic and terrestrial forms, such as mosquitoes, flies, midges, fleas, lice, bugs, wasps, and ants. Wings and antennae are present, and adult forms have three pairs of legs. Of medical importance are the many insects that serve as vectors for microbial diseases (mosquitoes, fleas, flies, lice, and bugs) or as venomous animals that sting (bees, wasps, and ants).

PHYSIOLOGY AND REPLICATION
Protozoa

The nutritional requirements of the parasitic protozoa are generally simple and require the assimilation of organic nutrients. The amebae, ameboflagellates, and certain other protozoa accomplish this assimilation by the rather primitive process of pinocytosis or phagocytosis of soluble or particulate matter (Table 8-3). The engulfed material is enclosed in digestive vacuoles. The flagellates and ciliates generally ingest food at a definitive site or structure, the peristome or cytostome. Other protozoan parasites, such as the intracellular microsporidia, assimilate nutrients by simple diffusion. The ingested food material may be retained in intracytoplasmic granules or invacuoles. The undigested particles and waste may be eliminated from the cell by extrusion of the material at the cell surface. Respiration in most parasitic protozoa is accomplished by facultatively anaerobic processes.

To ensure survival under harsh or unfavorable environmental conditions, many parasitic protozoa develop into a **cyst** form that is less metabolically active. This cyst is surrounded by a thick external cell wall capable of protecting the organism from otherwise lethal physical and chemical insults. The cyst form is an integral part of the life cycle of many protozoan parasites and facilitates the transmission of the organism from host to host in the external environment (Table 8-4). Parasites that cannot form cysts must rely on direct transmission from host to host or require an arthropod vector to complete their life cycles (Table 8-4).

In addition to cyst formation, many protozoan parasites have developed elaborate immunoevasive mechanisms that allow them to respond to attack by the host immune system by continuously changing their surface antigens, thus ensuring continued survival within the host. Reproduction among the protozoa is generally by simple binary fission (merogony), although the life cycle of some protozoa, such as the sporozoans, includes cycles of multiple fission (**schizogony**) alternating with a period of sexual reproduction (**sporogony or gametogony**).

TABLE 8-3   **Biological, Morphological, and Physiological Characteristics of Pathogenic Parasites**

ORGANISM CLASS	MORPHOLOGY	REPRODUCTION	ORGANELLES OF LOCOMOTION	RESPIRATION	NUTRITION
PROTOZOA					
Ameba	Unicellular; cyst and trophocyte forms	Binary fission	Pseudopods	Facultative anaerobe	Assimilation by pinocytosis or phagocytosis
Flagellates	Unicellular; cyst and trophozoite forms; possibly intracellular	Binary fission	Flagella	Facultative anaerobe	Simple diffusion or ingestion via cytostome, pinocytosis, or phagocytosis
Ciliates	Unicellular; cysts and trophozoite	Binary fission or conjugation	Cilia	Facultative anaerobe	Ingestion via cytostome, food vacuole
Coccidia	Unicellular, frequently intracellular; multiple forms, including trophozoites, sporozoites, cysts (oocysts), gametes	Schizogony and sporogony	None	Facultative anaerobe	Simple diffusion
Microsporidia	Obligate intracellular forms; small, simple cells and spores	Binary fission, schizogony and sporogony	None	Facultative anaerobe	Simple diffusion
HELMINTHS					
Nematodes	Multicellular; round, smooth, spindle shaped, tubular alimentary tract; possibility of teeth or plates for attachment	Separate sexes	No single organelle; active muscular motility	Adults: usually anaerobic, larvae: possibly aerobic	Ingestion or absorption of body fluids, tissue, or digestive contents
Trematodes	Multicellular; leaf shaped with oral and ventral suckers, blind alimentary tract	Hermaphroditic (*Schistosoma* group has separate sexes)	No single organelle; muscle-directed motility	Adults: usually anaerobic	Ingestion or absorption of body fluids, tissue, or digestive contents
Cestodes	Multicellular; head with segmented body (proglottids); lack of alimentary tract; head equipped with hood and/or suckers for attachment	Hermaphroditic	No single organelle; usually, attachment to mucosa, possible muscular motility (proglottids)	Adults: usually anaerobic	Absorption of nutrients from intestine
ARTHROPODS					
Chilopoda	Elongated; many legs; distinctive head and trunk; poison claws on first segment	Separate sexes	Legs	Aerobic	Carnivore
Pentastomida	Wormlike; cylindrical, or flattened; two distinct body regions; digestive and reproductive organs; lack of circulatory and respiratory systems	Separate sexes	Muscle-directed motility	Aerobic	Ingestion of body fluids and tissue
Crustacea	Hard external carapace; one pair of maxillae; five pairs of biramous legs	Separate sexes	Legs	Aerobic	Ingestion of body fluids and tissue, carnivorous
Arachnida	Body divided into cephalothorax and abdomen; eight legs and poisoning fangs	Separate sexes	Legs	Aerobic	Carnivore
Insecta	Body: head, thorax, and abdomen; one pair of antennae; three pairs of appendages, up to two pairs of wings	Separate sexes	Legs, wings	Aerobic	Ingestion of fluids and tissues

TABLE 8-4	Transmission and Distribution of Pathogenic Parasites		
ORGANISM	**INFECTIVE FORM**	**MECHANISM OF SPREAD**	**DISTRIBUTION**
Intestinal Protozoa			
Entamoeba histolytica	Cyst/trophozoite	Indirect (fecal-oral) Direct (venereal)	Worldwide
Giardia lamblia	Cyst	Fecal-oral route	Worldwide
Dientamoeba fragilis	Trophozoite	Fecal-oral route	Worldwide
Balantidium coli	Cyst	Fecal-oral route	Worldwide
Isospora belli	Oocyst	Fecal-oral route	Worldwide
Cryptosporidium species	Oocyst	Fecal-oral route Unknown	Worldwide
Enterocytozoon bieneusi	Spore	?Fecal-oral route	North America, Europe
Urogenital Protozoa			
Trichomonas vaginalis	Trophozoite	Direct (venereal) route	Worldwide
Blood and Tissue Protozoa			
Naegleria and Acantha- moeba species	Cyst/trophozoite	Direct inoculation, inhalation	Worldwide
Plasmodium species	Sporozoite	Anopheles mosquito	Tropical and subtropical areas
Babesia species	Pyriform body	Ixodes tick	North America, Europe
Toxoplasma gondii	Oocysts and tissue cysts	Fecal-oral route, carnivorism	Worldwide
Leishmania species	Promastigote	Phlebotomus sandfly	Tropical and subtropical areas
Trypanosoma cruzi	Trypomastigote	Reduviid bug	North, Central, and South America
Trypanosom brucei	Trypomastigote	Tsetse fly	Africa
Nematodes			
Enterobius vermicularis	Egg	Fecal-oral route	Worldwide
Ascaris lumbricoides	Egg	Fecal-oral route	Areas of poor sanitation
Toxocara species	Egg	Fecal-oral route	Worldwide
Trichuris trichiura	Egg	Fecal-oral route	Worldwide
Ancylostoma duodenale	Filariform lava	Direct skin penetration from contaminated soil	Tropical and subtropical areas
Necator americanus	Filariform larva	Direct skin penetration, autoinfection	Tropical and subtropical areas
Strongyloides stercoralis	Filariform larva	Direct skin penetration, autoinfection	Tropical and subtropical areas
Trichinella spiralis	Encysted larva in tissue	Carnivorism	Worldwide
Wuchereria bancrofti	Third-stage larva	Mosquito	Tropical and subtropical areas
Brugia malayi	Third-stage larva	Mosquito	Tropical and subtropical areas
Loa loa	Filariform larva	Chrysops fly	Africa
Mansonella speices	Third-stage larva	Biting midges or black flies	Africa, Central and South America
Onchocerca volvulus	Third-stage larva	Simulium black fly	Africa, Central and South America
Dracunculus medinensis	Third-stage larva	Ingestion of infected cyclops	Africa, Asia
Dirofilaria immitis	Third-stage larva	Mosquito	Japan, Australia, United States
Trematodes			
Fasciolopsis buski	Metacercaria	Ingestion of metacercaria encysted on aquatic plants	China, Southeast Asia, India

Continued.

| **TABLE 8-4** | **Transmission and Distribution of Pathogenic Parasites—cont'd** | | |

ORGANISM	INFECTIVE FORM	MECHANISM OF SPREAD	DISTRIBUTION
Fasciola hepatica	Metacercaria	Metacercaria on water plants	Worldwide
Opisthorchis (Clonorchis) sinensis	Metacercaria	Metacercaria encysted in freshwater fish	China, Japan, Korea, Vietnam
Paragonimus westermani	Metacercaria	Metacercaria encysted in freshwater crustaceans	Asia, Africa, India, Latin America
Schistosoma species	Cercaria	Direct penetration of skin by free-swimming cercaria	Africa, Asia, India, Latin America
Cestodes			
Taenia solium	Cysticercus, embryonated egg or proglottid	Ingestion of infected pork Ingestion of egg (cysticercosis)	Pork-eating countries: Africa, Southeast Asia China, Latin America
Taenia saginata	Cysticercus	Ingestion of cysticercus in meat	Worldwide
Diphyllobothrium latum	Sparganum	Ingestion of sparganum in fish	Worldwide
Echinococcus granulosus	Embryonated egg	Ingestion of eggs from infected canines	Sheep-raising countries: Europe, Asia, Africa, Australia, United States
Echinococcus multilocularis	Embryonated egg	Ingestion of eggs from infected animals, fecal-oral route	Canada, Northern United States, Central Europe
Hymenolepsis nana	Embryonated egg	Ingestion of eggs, fecal-oral route	Worldwide
Hymenolepsis diminuta	Cysticercus	Ingestion of infected beetle larvae in contaminated grain products	Worldwide
Dipylidium caninum	Cysticercoid	Ingestion of infected fleas	Worldwide

Metazoa

Helminths

The nutritional requirements of helminthic parasites are met by active ingestion of host tissue, fluids, or both, with resultant tissue destruction, or by more passive absorption of nutrients from the surrounding fluids and intestinal contents (Table 8-3). The muscular motility of many helminths expends considerable energy, and the worms rapidly metabolize carbohydrates. Nutrients are stored in the form of glycogen, the content of which is high in most helminths. Similar to respiration in protozoa, respiration in helminths is primarily anaerobic, although the larval forms may require oxygen.

A significant proportion of the energy requirement of helminths is dedicated to supporting the reproductive process. Many worms are quite prolific, producing as many as 200,000 offspring each day. In general, helminthic parasites are egg laying (**oviparous**), although a few species may bear live young (**viviparous**). The resulting larvae are always morphologically distinct from the adult parasites and must undergo several developmental stages or **molts** before attaining adulthood.

The major protective barrier for most helminths is the tough external layer (cuticle or tegument). Worms may also secrete enzymes that destroy host cells and neutralize immunological and cellular defense mechanisms. Similar to protozoan parasites, some helminths possess the ability to alter the antigenic properties of their external surfaces and thus evade the host immune response. This is accomplished in part by incorporating host antigens into their external cuticular layer. In this way the worm avoids immunological recognition, and in some diseases (e.g., schistosomiasis), it allows the parasite to survive within the host for decades.

Arthropods

Arthropods have segmented bodies, paired jointed appendages, and well-developed digestive and nervous systems. Sexes are separate. Respiration by aquatic forms is via gills and by terrestrial forms is via tubular body structures. All have a hard chitin covering as an exoskeleton.

SUMMARY

Physician awareness of parasitic diseases is undoubtedly more critical now than at any time in the history of medical practice. Physicians today must be prepared to answer questions from patients about protection from malaria and the risks of drinking water and eating fresh fruits and vegetables in remote areas where they may be traveling. With this knowledge of parasitic diseases, the physician can also evaluate signs, symptoms, and incubation periods in returning travelers and make a diagnosis and begin treatment for a patient with a possible parasitic disease. The risks of parasitic diseases in immunosuppressed individuals and those with acquired immunodeficiency syndrome must also be understood and taken into account.

Proper education regarding parasitic diseases in medical curricula cannot be overemphasized as a requirement for physicians whose practice includes travelers to foreign countries and refugee populations. Many of the important parasites responsible for human diseases are transmitted by arthropod vectors or are acquired by the consumption of contaminated food or water. The various modes of transmission and distribution of parasitic diseases are presented in appropriate detail in the following chapters; however, the data in Table 8-4 are provided as an outline.

QUESTIONS

1. How do protozoa adapt to harsh environmental conditions?
2. Which morphological form is important in the transmission of protozoa from host to host?
3. How do helminths, such as schistosomes, avoid the host immune response?
4. How do arthropods cause human disease?

Bibliography

Beaver PC, Jung RC, Cupp EW: *Clinical parasitology,* ed 9, Philadelphia, 1984, Lea & Febiger.

Brown HW, Neva FA: *Basic clinical parasitology,* ed 5, Norwalk, Conn, 1983, Appleton-Century-Crofts.

Howard BJ et al: *Clinical and pathogenic microbiology,* ed 2, St Louis, 1993, Mosby.

Markell EK, Voge M, John DT: *Medical parasitology,* ed 7, Philadelphia, 1992, WB Saunders.

Schmidt GD, Roberts LS: *Foundations of parasitology,* ed 4, St Louis, 1989, Mosby.

Sherris JC: *Medical microbiology: an introduction to infectious diseases,* ed 2, New York, 1990, Elsevier.

Microbial Flora in Health and Disease

9

Medical microbiology is the study of the interactions between animals (primarily humans) and microorganisms such as bacteria, viruses, fungi, and parasites. Although the primary interest is in diseases caused by these interactions, it must also be appreciated that microorganisms play a critical role in human survival. The normal population of endogenous organisms participates in the metabolism of food products, provides essential growth factors, protects against infections with highly virulent microorganisms, and stimulates the immune response. In the absence of these organisms, life as we know it would be impossible.

The microbial flora in and on the human body is in a continual state of flux determined by a variety of factors such as age, diet, hormonal state, health, sanitary conditions, and personal hygiene. Whereas the human fetus lives in a protected, sterile environment, the newborn is exposed to microbes from the mother and environment. The infant's skin is initially colonized, followed by the oropharynx, gastrointestinal tract, and other mucosal surfaces. Through the life of an individual, this microbial population continues to change. Changes in physical well-being can drastically disrupt the delicate balance that is maintained among the heterogeneous organisms coexisting within us. For example, hospitalization can lead to the replacement of normally avirulent organisms in the oropharynx with gram-negative bacilli (e.g., *Klebsiella* and *Pseudomonas* species) that can invade the lungs and cause pneumonia. Likewise, the growth of *Clostridium difficile* in the gastrointestinal tract is controlled by the indigenous bacteria present in the intestines. However, in the presence of antibiotics, the normal bacterial flora is eliminated, and *C. difficile* is able to proliferate and produce gastrointestinal disease. The mild form is referred to as *antibiotic-associated diarrhea*, whereas more severe forms include pseudomembranous colitis.

Exposure of an individual to an organism can lead to one of three outcomes. The organism can (1) transiently colonize the person, (2) permanently colonize the person, or (3) produce disease. It is important to understand the distinction between **colonization** and **disease.** (NOTE: The term **infection** has been used inappropriately as a synonym for both terms.) Organisms that colonize humans (whether for a short period [transient] or permanently) do not disrupt normal body functions. In contrast, disease occurs when the interaction between microbe and human leads to a pathological process characterized by damage to the human host. This process can result from microbial factors (e.g., damage to organs caused by the proliferation of the microbe or the production of toxins) or the host's immune response to the organism.

An understanding of medical microbiology requires knowledge not only of the different classes of microbes but also of their propensity for causing disease. Relatively few infections are caused by **strict pathogens** (i.e., organisms always associated with human disease). Some examples of strict pathogens and the diseases they cause include *Mycobacterium tuberculosis* (tuberculosis), *Neisseria gonorrhoeae* (gonorrhea), *Francisella tularensis* (tularemia), *Plasmodium* species (malaria), and rabies virus (rabies). Most infections are caused by **opportunistic pathogens**, organisms that are typically members of the patient's normal microbial flora (e.g., *Staphylococcus aureus, Escherichia coli, Candida albicans*). These organisms do not produce disease in their normal setting but establish disease when they are introduced into unprotected sites (e.g., bloodstream, tissues). The factors responsible for the virulence of strict and opportunistic pathogens are discussed in Chapters 19, 46, 66, and 72.

The microbial population that colonizes the human body is numerous and diverse. The most common organisms that form the commensal flora and their propensity to cause disease are summarized here.

RESPIRATORY TRACT AND HEAD
Mouth, Oropharynx, and Nasopharynx

The upper respiratory tract is colonized with numerous organisms, with 10 to 100 anaerobes for every aerobic bacteria (Box 9-1). The most common anaerobic bacteria are *Peptostreptococcus, Veillonella, Actinomyces,* and *Fusobacterium* species; the most common aerobic bacteria are *Streptococcus* and *Neisseria* species. The relative proportion of these organisms varies at different anatomical sites; for example, the microbial flora on the surface of a tooth is quite different from the flora in saliva or in the subgingival spaces. Most of the common organisms in the upper respiratory tract are relatively avirulent and are rarely associated with disease unless they are introduced into normally sterile sites (e.g., sinuses, middle ear, brain). Potentially pathogenic organisms can also be found in the upper airways, including group A *Streptococcus, Streptococcus pneumoniae, S. aureus, Neisseria meningitidis, Haemophilus influenzae, Moraxella catarrhalis,* and Enterobacteriaceae. Isolation of these organisms from an upper respiratory tract specimen does not define their pathogenicity. Their involvement with a disease process must be demonstrated to the exclusion of other pathogens. For example, with the exception of group A streptococci, these organisms are rarely responsible for pharyngitis, even though they can be isolated from patients with this disease.

Ear

The most common organism colonizing the outer ear is coagulase-negative *Staphylococcus*. Other organisms colonizing the skin have been isolated from this site, as well as potential pathogens such as *S. pneumoniae, Pseudomonas aeruginosa,* and the Enterobacteriaceae. The last group has also been associated with disease at this site.

Eye

The surface of the eye is colonized with coagulase-negative staphylococci as well as rare numbers of organisms found in the nasopharynx (e.g., *Haemophilus* species, *Neisseria* species, viridans streptococci). Disease is typically associated with *S. pneumoniae, S. aureus, H. influenzae, N. gonorrhoeae, Chlamydia trachomatis,* and *P. aeruginosa.*

Lower Respiratory Tract

The larynx, trachea, bronchioles, and lower airways are generally sterile, although transient colonization with secretions of the upper respiratory tract may occur after aspiration. Acute disease of the lower airway is usually caused by the more virulent bacteria present in the mouth (e.g., *S. pneumoniae, S. aureus, H. influenzae,* members of the family Enterobacteriaceae such as *Klebsiella*). Chronic aspiration may lead to a polymicrobial disease in which anaerobes are the predominant pathogens, particularly peptostreptococci and anaerobic gram-negative bacilli. Fungi such as *Candida* species can cause disease of the lower airway, but organisms must be demonstrated in tissue to exclude simple colonization. In contrast, the presence of the dimorphic fungi (e.g., *Histoplasma, Coccidioides,* and *Blastomyces* species) is diagnostic because colonization with these organisms does not occur.

GASTROINTESTINAL TRACT

The gastrointestinal tract is colonized with microbes at birth and remains the home for a diverse collection of organisms throughout the life of the host (Box 9-2). Although the opportunity for colonization with new organisms occurs daily with the ingestion of food and water, the population remains relatively constant unless exogenous factors such as antibiotic treatment disrupt the balanced flora.

Esophagus

Oropharyngeal bacteria and yeast, as well as the bacteria that colonize the stomach, can be isolated from the esophagus; however, most organisms are believed to be transient colonizers that do not establish permanent residence. Bacteria rarely cause disease of the esophagus (esophagitis); most infections are caused by *Candida* organisms and viruses such as herpes simplex virus and cytomegalovirus.

Stomach

Because the stomach contains hydrochloric acid and pepsinogen (secreted by the parietal and chief cells lining the gastric mucosa), the only organisms present are small numbers of acid-tolerant organisms such as the lactic

---

BOX 9-1   Most Common Microbes Colonizing the Respiratory Tract

Bacteria
  Actinomyces species
  Cardiobacterium species
  Corynebacterium species
  Eikenella species
  Enterobacteriaceae
  Eubacterium species
  Fusobacterium species
  Haemophilus species
  Kingella species
  Moraxella species
  Mycoplasma species
  Neisseria species
  Peptostreptococcus species
  Porphyromonas species
  Prevotella species
  Propionibacterium species
  Staphylococcus species
  Streptococcus species (groups A, C, F, and G)
  Streptococcus pneumoniae
  Streptococcus species (viridans group)
  Stomatococcus species
  Treponema species (not *T. pallidum*)
  Veillonella species
Fungi
  Candida species
Parasites
  Entamoeba gingivalis
  Trichomonas tenax

BOX 9-2 **Most Common Microbes Colonizing the Gastrointestinal Tract**

Bacteria
  Acinetobacter species
  Actinomyces species
  Bacteroides species
  Bifidobacterium species
  Clostridium species
  Corynebacterium species
  Eubacterium species
  Enterobacteriaceae
  Enterococcus species
  Fusobacterium species
  Helicobacter species
  Lactobacillus species
  Peptostreptococcus
    species
  Porphyromonas species
  Prevotella species
  Propionibacterium
    species
  Pseudomonas species

Bacteria—cont'd
  Staphylococcus species
  Streptococcus species
    (groups A, B, C, F,
    and G)
  Streptococcus bovis
  Streptococcus species
    (viridans group)
  Veillonella species
Fungi
  Candida species
Parasites
  Blastocystis species
  Chilomastix species
  Endolimax species
  Entamoeba coli
  Entamoeba hartmanni
  Entamoeba polecki
  Iodamoeba species
  Trichomonas hominis

acid-producing bacteria (*Lactobacillus* and *Streptococcus* species) and *Helicobacter pylori*. *H. pylori* is a cause of gastritis and ulcerative disease. The microbial population can dramatically change in numbers and diversity in patients receiving drugs that neutralize or reduce the production of gastric acids.

Small Intestine

In contrast with the anterior portion of the digestive tract, the small intestine is colonized with many different bacteria, fungi, and parasites. Most of these organisms are anaerobes, such as *Peptostreptococcus, Porphyromonas,* and *Prevotella* species. Common causes of gastroenteritis (e.g., *Salmonella* and *Campylobacter* species) can be present in small numbers as asymptomatic residents; however, their detection in the clinical laboratory generally indicates disease. If obstruction of the small intestine occurs, such as after abdominal surgery, then a condition called **blind loop syndrome** can occur. In this case, stasis of the intestinal contents leads to the colonization and proliferation of the organisms typically present in the large intestine, with a subsequent malabsorption syndrome.

Large Intestine

More microbes are present in the large intestine than anywhere else in the human body. It is estimated that more than 10^{11} bacteria per gram of feces can be found, with anaerobic bacteria in excess by 1000-fold. Various yeasts and nonpathogenic parasites can also establish residence in the large intestine. The most common bacteria

include *Bifidobacterium* species, *Eubacterium* species, *Bacteroides fragilis* group, *Enterococcus* species, and *E. coli*. *E. coli* is present in virtually all humans from birth until death. Although this organism represents less than 1% of the intestinal population, it is the most common aerobic organism responsible for intraabdominal infections. Likewise, *B. fragilis* is a minor member of the intestinal flora but the most common anaerobe responsible for intraabdominal disease. In contrast, *Eubacterium* and *Bifidobacterium* species are the most common bacteria but are rarely responsible for disease.

Antibiotic treatment can rapidly alter the population, causing the proliferation of antibiotic-resistant organisms such as enterococci, *Pseudomonas* species, and fungi. *C. difficile* can also grow rapidly in this situation, leading to disease ranging from diarrhea to pseudomembranous colitis. Exposure to other enteric pathogens, such as *Shigella* species, enterohemorrhagic *E. coli,* and *Entamoeba histolytica,* can also rapidly disrupt the colonic flora and produce significant intestinal disease.

GENITOURINARY SYSTEM

In general, the anterior urethra and vagina are the only anatomical areas of the genitourinary system permanently colonized with microbes (Box 9-3). Although the urinary bladder can be transiently colonized with bacteria migrating upstream from the urethra, these should be rapidly cleared by the bactericidal activity of the uroepithelial cells and the flushing action of voided urine. The other structures of the urinary system should be sterile except when disease or an anatomical abnormality is present. Likewise, the uterus should also remain free of organisms.

Anterior Urethra

The indigenous population of the urethra consists of a variety of organisms, with lactobacilli, streptococci, and coagulase-negative staphylococci the most numerous. These organisms are relatively avirulent and are rarely associated with human disease. In contrast, the urethra can be transiently colonized with fecal organisms such as *Enterococcus* species, Enterobacteriaceae, and *Candida* species—all of which can invade the urinary tract, multiply in urine, and lead to significant disease. Pathogens such as *N. gonorrhoeae* and *C. trachomatis* are common causes of urethritis and can persist as asymptomatic colonizers of the urethra. The isolation of these two organisms in clinical specimens should always be considered significant, regardless of the presence or absence of clinical symptoms.

Vagina

The microbial population of the vagina is more diverse and is dramatically influenced by hormonal factors. Newborn girls are colonized with lactobacilli at birth, and these bacteria predominate for approximately 6 weeks. After that time, the levels of maternal estrogen have declined, and the vaginal flora changes to include staphylo-

BOX 9-3   Most Common Microbes Colonizing the Genitourinary Tract

Bacteria
- *Actinomyces* species
- *Bacteroides* species
- *Bifidobacterium* species
- *Clostridium* species
- *Corynebacterium* species
- *Enterococcus* species
- Enterobacteriaceae
- *Eubacterium* species
- *Gardnerella* species
- *Haemophilus* species
- *Lactobacillus* species
- *Mobiluncus* species
- *Mycoplasma* species
- *Peptostreptococcus* species

Bacteria—cont'd
- *Porphyromonas* species
- *Prevotella* species
- *Propionibacterium* species
- *Staphylococcus* species
- *Streptococcus* species (group B)
- *Streptococcus* species (viridans group)
- *Treponema* species (not *T. pallidum*)
- *Ureaplasma* species

Fungi
- *Candida* species

BOX 9-4   Most Common Microbes Colonizing the Skin Surface

Bacteria
- *Acinetobacter* species
- *Aerococcus* species
- *Bacillus* species
- *Clostridium perfringens*
- *Corynebacterium* species
- *Micrococcus* species
- *Peptostreptococcus* species
- *Propionibacterium* species
- *Staphylococcus* species
- *Streptococcus* species (group A)

Fungi
- *Candida* species
- *Malassezia* species

cocci, streptococci, and Enterobacteriaceae. When estrogen production is initiated at puberty, the microbial flora again changes. Lactobacilli reemerge as the predominant organisms, and many other organisms are also isolated, including staphylococci (*S. aureus* less commonly than the coagulase-negative species), streptococci (including group B *Streptococcus*), *Enterococcus* species, *Gardnerella vaginalis*, *Mycoplasma* species and the related *Ureaplasma* species, Enterobacteriaceae, and a variety of anaerobic bacteria. *N. gonorrhoeae* is a common cause of vaginitis. In the absence of this organism, significant numbers of cases develop when the balance of vaginal bacteria is disrupted, resulting in decreases in the number of lactobacilli and increases in the number of *Mobiluncus* and *Gardnerella* organisms. *Trichomonas vaginalis*, *C. albicans*, and *Candida glabrata* are also important causes of vaginitis. Although herpes simplex virus and papillomavirus would not be considered normal flora of the genitourinary tract, these viruses can establish persistent infections.

Cervix

Although the cervix is not normally colonized with bacteria, *N. gonorrhoeae* and *C. trachomatis* are important causes of cervicitis. Actinomyces can also produce disease at this site.

SKIN

Although many organisms come into contact with the skin surface, this relatively hostile environment does not support the survival of most organisms (Box 9-4). Gram-positive bacteria (e.g., coagulase-negative *Staphylococcus* and less commonly *S. aureus*, corynebacteria, and propionibacteria) are the most common organisms found on the skin surface. *Clostridium perfringens* is isolated on the skin of approximately 20% of healthy individuals, and the fungi *Candida* and *Malassezia* are also found on skin surfaces, particularly in moist sites. Streptococci can transiently colonize the skin, but the volatile fatty acids produced by the anaerobe propionibacteria are toxic for these organisms. Gram-negative bacilli do not permanently colonize the skin surface (with the exception of *Acinetobacter* and a few other less common genera) because the skin is too dry.

QUESTIONS

1. What is the distinction between *colonization* and *disease*?
2. Give examples of strict pathogens and opportunistic pathogens.
3. What factors regulate the microbial populations of organism that colonize humans?

Bibliography

Balows A, Truper H: *The prokaryotes*, ed 2, New York, 1992, Springer-Verlag.

Isenberg H, D'Amato R: Indigenous and pathogenic microorganisms of humans. In Murray P et al, editors: *Manual of clinical microbiology*, ed 6, Washington, DC, 1995, American Society for Microbiology.

Murray P: Human microbiota. In Balows A et al: *Topley & Wilson's microbiology & microbial infections*, ed 9, London, 1997, Edward Arnold.

10

Sterilization, Disinfection, and Antisepsis

Medical microbiology involves the study of the pathogenesis and chemotherapy of infectious diseases, as well as the examination of how diseases can be prevented. An important aspect of the control of infections is an understanding of the principles of sterilization, disinfection, and antisepsis (Box 10-1).

STERILIZATION

Sterilization is the total destruction of all microbes, including the more resilient forms such as bacterial spores, mycobacteria, nonenveloped (nonlipid) viruses, and fungi (Figure 10-1). This can be accomplished using physical, gas vapor, or chemical sterilants (Table 10-1).

Physical sterilants such as **moist** and **dry heat** are the most common sterilizing methods used in hospitals and are indicated for most materials except those that are heat sensitive or consist of toxic or volatile chemicals. **Filtration** is useful for removing bacteria and fungi from air (with high-efficiency particulate air [HEPA] filters) or from solutions. These filters are unable to remove viruses and some small bacteria. Sterilization by **ultraviolet** or **ionizing** (e.g., microwave or gamma rays) **radiation** is also commonly used. The limitation of UV radiation is that direct exposure is required.

The gas vapor sterilant most commonly used is **ethylene oxide**. Although it is highly efficient, strict regulations limit its use because ethylene oxide is extremely toxic. Sterilization with **formaldehyde** gas is also limited because the chemical is carcinogenic. Its use is primarily restricted to sterilization of HEPA filters. **Hydrogen peroxide** vapors are effective sterilants because of the oxidizing nature of the gas. It is used for the sterilization of instruments. A variation is **plasma gas** sterilization, in which hydrogen peroxide is vaporized and then reactive free radicals are produced with either microwave-frequency or radiofrequency energy. Because this is an efficient sterilizing method that does not produce toxic byproducts, it is anticipated that plasma gas sterilization will replace many of the applications for ethylene oxide. One additional gas vapor sterilant is the use of **chlorine dioxide** gas, which denatures proteins by oxidation. Although further work with this method is required, the lack of toxicity also makes chlorine dioxide gas an attractive alternative to ethylene oxide sterilization.

Two chemical sterilants have also been used: **peracetic acid** and **glutaraldehyde**. Peracetic acid, an oxidizing agent, has excellent activity and the end products (i.e., acetic acid and oxygen) are nontoxic. In contrast, safety concerns exist with glutaraldehyde, and care must be used when handling this chemical.

DISINFECTION

Microbes are also destroyed by disinfection procedures, although more resilient organisms can survive. Unfortunately, the terms *disinfection* and *sterilization* are casually interchanged, which can result in some confusion. This occurs because disinfection processes have been categorized as high level, intermediate level, and low level. High-level disinfection can generally approach sterilization in effectiveness, whereas spore forms can survive intermediate-level disinfection, and many microbes can remain viable when exposed to low-level disinfection.

BOX 10-1   Definitions

Sterilization—Use of physical procedures or chemical agents to destroy all microbial forms, including bacterial spores.

Disinfection—Use of physical procedures or chemical agents to destroy most microbial forms; bacterial spores and other relatively resistant organisms (e.g., mycobacteria, viruses, fungi) may remain viable; disinfectants are subdivided into high-, intermediate-, and low-level agents.

Antisepsis—Use of chemical agents on skin or other living tissue to inhibit or eliminate microbes; no sporicidal action is implied.

Germicide—Chemical agent capable of killing microbes; spores may survive.

Sporicide—Germicide capable of killing bacterial spores.

Sanitation—Process by which microbial contamination on inanimate surfaces is reduced to a "safe" level.

Even the classification of disinfectants (Table 10-2) by their level of activity is misleading. The effectiveness of these procedures is influenced by the nature of the item to be disinfected, number and resilience of the contaminating organism or organisms, amount of organic material present (which can inactivate the disinfectant), type and concentration of disinfectant, and duration and temperature of exposure.

High-level disinfectants are used for items involved with invasive procedures that cannot withstand sterilization procedures (e.g., certain types of endoscopes, surgical instruments with plastic or other components that cannot be autoclaved). Disinfection of these and other items is most effective if treatment is preceded by cleaning the surface to remove organic matter. Examples of high-level disinfectants include treatment with moist heat and use of liquids such as **glutaraldehyde, hydrogen peroxide, peracetic acid, chlorine dioxide,** and other **chlorine compounds.**

Intermediate-level disinfectants (i.e., **alcohols, iodophor compounds, phenolic compounds**) are used to clean surfaces or instruments in which contamination with bacterial spores and other highly resilient organisms is unlikely. These have been referred to as *semicritical instruments* and *devices* and include flexible fiberoptic endoscopes, laryngoscopes, vaginal specula, anesthesia breathing circuits, and other items. **Low-level disinfectants** (i.e., **quaternary ammonium compounds**) are used to treat noncritical instruments and devices such as blood culture cuffs, electrocardiogram electrodes, and stethoscopes. Although these items come into contact with patients, they do not penetrate through mucosal surfaces or into sterile tissues.

The level of disinfectants used for environmental surfaces is determined by the relative risk these surfaces pose as a reservoir for pathogenic organisms. For example, a higher level of disinfectant should be used to clean the surface of instruments contaminated with blood than those surfaces that are "dirty," such as floors, sinks, and countertops. The exception to this rule is if a particular surface has been implicated in a nosocomial infection,

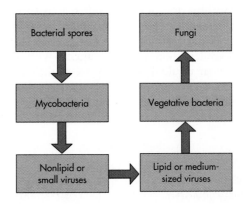

FIGURE 10-1 Microbes listed in decreasing order of resistance to germicidal chemicals. (Modified from Favero M, Bond W: Sterilization, disinfection, and antisepsis in the hospital. In Balows A et al, editors: *Manual of clinical microbiology,* ed 5, Washington, DC, 1991, American Society for Microbiology.)

TABLE 10-1	Methods of Sterilization
METHOD	**CONCENTRATION OR LEVEL**
PHYSICAL STERILANTS	
Steam under pressure	121° or 132° C for various time intervals
Dry heat	1 hr at 171° C; 2 hr at 160° C; 16 hr at 121° C
Filtration	0.22- to 0.45-μm pore size; HEPA filters
UV radiation	Variable exposure to 254-nm wavelength
Ionizing radiation	Variable exposure to microwave or gamma radiation
GAS VAPOR STERILANTS	
Ethylene oxide	450 to 1200 mg/L at 29° to 65° C for 2 to 5 hr
Formaldehyde vapor	2% to 5% at 60° to 80° C
Hydrogen peroxide vapor	30% at 55° to 60° C
Plasma gas	Highly ionized hydrogen peroxide gas
Chlorine dioxide gas	Variable
CHEMICAL STERILANTS	
Glutaraldehyde	2%
Peracetic acid	0.2%

TABLE 10-2	Methods of Disinfection	
METHOD	**CONCENTRATION (LEVEL OF ACTIVITY)**	
Heat		
Moist heat	75° to 100° C for 30 min (high)	
Liquid		
Glutaraldehyde	2% (high)	
Hydrogen peroxide	3% to 25% (high)	
Formaldehyde	3% to 8% (high/intermediate)	
Chlorine dioxide	Variable (high)	
Peracetic acid	Variable (high)	
Chlorine compounds	100 to 1000 ppm of free chlorine (high)	
Alcohol (ethyl, isopropyl)	70% to 95% (intermediate)	
Phenolic compounds	0.4% to 5.0% (intermediate/low)	
Iodophor compounds	30 to 50 ppm of free iodine/L (intermediate)	
Quaternary ammonium compounds	0.1% to 1.6% (low)	

such as a bathroom contaminated with *Clostridium difficile* (spore-forming anaerobic bacterium) or a sink contaminated with *Pseudomonas aeruginosa*. In these cases, a disinfectant with appropriate activity against the implicated pathogen should be selected.

ANTISEPSIS

Antiseptic agents (Table 10-3) are used to reduce the number of microbes on skin surfaces. These compounds are selected for their safety and efficacy. A summary of their germicidal properties is presented in Table 10-4. **Alcohols** have excellent activity against all groups of organisms except spores and are nontoxic, although they tend to dry the skin surface because of their removal of lipids. They also do not have residual activity and are inactivated by organic matter. Thus the surface of the skin should be cleaned before alcohol is applied. **Iodophors** are also excellent skin antiseptic agents with a range of activity similar to alcohols. They are slightly more toxic to the skin than alcohol, have limited residual activity, and are inactivated by organic matter. Iodophors and iodine preparations are frequently used with alcohols for disinfecting the skin surface. **Chlorhexidine** has broad antimicrobial activity, although it kills organisms at a much slower rate than alcohol. Its activity persists, although organic material and high pH levels decrease its effectiveness. The activity of **parachlorometaxylenol (PCMX)** is limited primarily to gram-positive bacteria. Because it is nontoxic and has residual activity, it has been used in handwashing products. **Triclosan** is active against bacteria but not other organisms. This is a common antiseptic agent in deodorant soaps.

MECHANISMS OF ACTION

The following section briefly reviews the mechanisms by which the most common sterilants, disinfectants, and antiseptics work.

Moist Heat

Attempts to sterilize items using boiling water are inefficient because only a relatively low temperature (100° C) can be maintained. Indeed, spore formation by a bacterium is commonly demonstrated by boiling a solution of organisms and then subculturing the solution. Vegetative organisms are killed by boiling, but the spores remain viable. If organisms grow on the subculture plate, the bacteria are capable of sporulating. In contrast, steam under pressure in an autoclave is a very effective form of sterilization; the higher temperature causes denaturation of microbial proteins. The rate of killing organisms during the autoclave process is rapid but is influenced by the temperature and duration of autoclaving, size of the autoclave, flow rate of the steam, density and size of the load, and placement of the load in the chamber. Care must be used to avoid creating air pockets, which inhibit

TABLE 10-3   Antiseptic Agents

ANTISEPTIC AGENT	CONCENTRATION
Alcohol (ethyl, isopropyl)	70% to 90%
Iodophors	1 to 2 mg of free iodine/L; 1% to 2% available iodine
Chlorhexidine	0.5% to 4%
Parachlorometaxylenol	0.5% to 3.75%
Triclosan	0.3% to 2%

TABLE 10-4   Germicidal Properties of Disinfectants and Antiseptic Agents

AGENT	BACTERIA	MYCOBACTERIA	BACTERIAL SPORES	FUNGI	VIRUSES
DISINFECTANTS					
Alcohol	+	+	−	+	+/−
Hydrogen peroxide	+	+	+	+	+
Formaldehyde	+	+	+	+	+
Phenolics	+	+	−	−	+
Chlorine	+	+	+/−	+/−	+
Iodophors	+	+/−	−	−	+/−
Glutaraldehyde	+	+	+	+	+
Quaternary ammonium compounds	+	−	−	−	+/−
ANTISEPTIC AGENTS					
Alcohol	+	+	−	+	+
Iodophors	+	+	−	+	+
Chlorhexidine	+	+	−	+/−	+
Parachlorometaxylenol	+/−	+/−	−	+	−
Triclosan	+	+/−	−	−	?

penetration of the steam into the load. In general, most autoclaves are operated at 121° to 132° C for 15 minutes or longer. The effectiveness of sterilization can be monitored by including commercial preparations of *Bacillus stearothermophilus* spores. An ampule of these spores is placed in the center of the load, removed at the end of the autoclave process, and incubated at 37° C. If the sterilization process was successful, the organisms fail to sporulate and do not grow.

Dry Heat

Hot air can also be used to sterilize items such as glassware. This is not as efficient as with moist air because diffusion and penetration of heat is slow, long sterilization periods and high temperatures are required, materials can be damaged by the oxidation process of this prolonged heating, and dry heat tends to stratify in the processing chamber. Sterilization requires processing for 1 hour at 171° C, 2 hours at 160° C, or 16 hours at 121° C. The effectiveness is monitored with spore tests using *Bacillus subtilis,* which is relatively resistant to killing by dry air (in contrast with *B. stearothermophilus*).

Ethylene Oxide

Ethylene oxide is a colorless gas, soluble in water and common organic solvents, that is used to sterilize heat-sensitive items. The sterilization process is relatively slow and influenced by the concentration of gas, relative humidity and moisture content of the item to be sterilized, exposure time, and temperature. The exposure time is reduced by 50% for each doubling of ethylene oxide concentration. Likewise, the activity of ethylene oxide approximately doubles with each temperature increase of 10° C. Sterilization with ethylene oxide is optimal in a relative humidity of approximately 30%, with decreased activity at higher or lower humidity. This is particularly problematic if the contaminated organisms are dried onto a surface or lyophilized. Ethylene oxide exerts its sporicidal activity through the alkylation of terminal hydroxyl, carboxyl, amino, and sulfhydryl groups. This process blocks the reactive groups required for many essential metabolic processes. Examples of other strong alkylating gases used as sterilants are formaldehyde and beta-propiolactone. Because ethylene oxide can damage viable tissues, the gas must be dissipated before the item can be used. This aeration period is generally 24 hours or longer. The effectiveness of sterilization is monitored with the *B. subtilis* spore test.

Aldehydes

As with ethylene oxide, the aldehydes exert their effect through alkylation. The two best known aldehydes are formaldehyde and glutaraldehyde, both of which can be used as sterilants or high-level disinfectants. Formaldehyde gas can be dissolved in water (called *formalin*) at a final concentration of 37%. Stabilizers such as methanol are added to formalin. Low concentrations of formalin are bacteriostatic (inhibit but do not kill organisms), whereas higher concentrations (e.g., 20%) can kill all organisms. This microbicidal activity can be enhanced by combining formaldehyde with alcohol (e.g., 20% formalin in 70% alcohol). Exposure of skin or mucous membranes to formaldehyde can be toxic. Glutaraldehyde is less toxic for viable tissues, but it can still cause burns on the skin or mucous membranes. Glutaraldehyde is more active at alkaline pH levels ("activated" by sodium hydroxide) but less stable. Glutaraldehyde is also inactivated by organic material, so items to be treated must first be cleaned.

Oxidizing Agents

Examples of oxidants include ozone, peracetic acid, and hydrogen peroxide, with the last used most commonly. Hydrogen peroxide effectively kills most bacteria at a concentration of 3% to 6% and kills all organisms, including spores, at higher concentrations (10% to 25%). The active oxidant form is not hydrogen peroxide but rather the free hydroxyl radical formed by the decomposition of hydrogen peroxide. Hydrogen peroxide is used to disinfect plastic implants, contact lenses, and surgical prostheses.

Halogens

Halogens, such as compounds containing iodine or chlorine, are extensively used as disinfectants. Iodine compounds are the most effective halogens available for disinfection. Iodine is a highly reactive element that precipitates proteins and oxidizes essential enzymes. It is microbicidal against virtually all organisms, including spore-forming bacteria and mycobacteria. Neither the concentration nor the pH of the iodine solution affect the microbicidal activity, although the efficiency of iodine solutions is increased in acid solutions because more free iodine is liberated. Iodine acts more rapidly than other halogen compounds or quaternary ammonium compounds. However, the activity of iodine can be reduced in the presence of some organic and inorganic compounds, including serum, feces, ascitic fluid, sputum, urine, sodium thiosulfate, and ammonia. Elemental iodine can be dissolved in aqueous potassium iodide or alcohol, or complexed with a carrier. The latter compound is referred to as an *iodophor* (*iodo,* "iodine"; *phor* "carrier"). Povidone iodine (iodine complexed with polyvinylpyrrolidone) is used most commonly, is relatively stable and nontoxic to tissues and metal surfaces, but is expensive compared with other iodine solutions.

Chlorine compounds are also used extensively as disinfectants. Aqueous solutions of chlorine are rapidly bactericidal, although their mechanisms of action are not defined. Three forms of chlorine may be present in water: elemental chlorine (Cl_2), which is a very strong oxidizing agent; hypochlorous acid ($HOCl$); and hypochlorite ion (OCl^-). Chlorine also combines with ammonia and other nitrogenous compounds to form chloramines or *N*-chloro compounds. Chlorine can exert its effect by the irreversible oxidation of SH groups of essential enzymes. Hypochlorites are believed to interact with cytoplasmic components to form toxic *N*-chloro compounds, which interfere with cellular metabolism. The efficacy of chlorine is inversely proportional to the pH, with greater activity observed at acid pH levels. This is consistent with greater activity associated with hypochlorous acid rather than hypochlorite ion concentration. The activity of chlorine compounds also increases with concentration (e.g., a twofold increase in concentration results in a 30% decrease in time required for killing) and temperature (e.g., a 50% to 65% reduction in killing time with a 10° C increase in temperature). Organic matter and alkaline detergents can reduce the effectiveness of chlorine compounds. These compounds demonstrate good germicidal activity, although spore-forming organisms are tenfold to 1000-fold more resistant to chlorine than vegetative bacteria.

Phenolic Compounds

Phenolic compounds (germicides) are rarely used as disinfectants. However, they are of historical interest because they were used as a comparative standard for assessing the activity of other germicidal compounds. The ratio of germicidal activity by a test compound to that by a specified concentration of phenol yielded the **phenol coefficient**. A value of 1 indicated equivalent activity, greater than 1 indicated activity less than phenol, and less than 1 indicated activity greater than phenol. These tests are limited by the fact that phenol is not sporicidal at room temperature (but is at temperatures approaching 100° C) and has poor activity against non-lipid–containing viruses. This is understandable because phenol is believed to act by disrupting lipid-containing membranes, resulting in leakage of cellular contents. Phenolic compounds are active against the normally resilient mycobacteria because the cell wall of these organisms has a very high concentration of lipids. Exposure of phenolics to alkaline compounds significantly reduces their activity, whereas halogenation of the phenolics enhances their activity. The introduction of aliphatic or aromatic groups into the nucleus of halogen phenols also increases their activity. Bisphenols are two phenol compounds linked together. The activity of these compounds can also be potentiated by halogenation. One example of a halogenated bis-phenol is hexachlorophene, an antiseptic with activity against gram-positive bacteria.

Quaternary Ammonium Compounds

Quaternary ammonium compounds consist of four organic groups covalently linked to nitrogen. The germicidal activity of these cationic compounds is determined by the nature of the organic groups, with the greatest activity observed with compounds with 8 to 18 carbon long groups. Examples of quaternary ammonium compounds include benzalkonium chloride and cetylpyridinium chloride. These compounds act by denaturing cell membranes to release the intracellular components. Quaternary ammonium compounds are bacteriostatic at low concentrations and bactericidal at high concentrations. However, organisms such as *Pseudomonas, Mycobacterium,* and the fungus *Trichophyton,* among others, are resistant to these compounds. Indeed, some *Pseudomonas* strains can grow readily in quaternary ammonium solutions. Many viruses and all bacterial spores are also resistant. Quaternary ammonium compounds are neutralized by ionic detergents, organic matter, and dilution.

Alcohols

The germicidal activity of alcohols increases with increasing chain length (maximum of 5 to 8 carbons). The two most commonly used alcohols are ethanol and isopropanol. These are rapidly bactericidal against vegetative bacteria, mycobacteria, some fungi, and lipid-containing viruses. Unfortunately, alcohols have no activity against bacterial spores and poor activity against some fungi and non-lipid–containing viruses. Activity is greater in the presence of water. Thus 70% alcohol is more active than 95% alcohol. Alcohol is a common disinfectant for skin surfaces and, when followed by treatment with an iodophor, is extremely effective for this purpose. Alcohols are also used to disinfect items such as thermometers.

QUESTIONS

1. Define the following terms and give three examples of each: *sterilization, disinfection,* and *antisepsis.*
2. Define the three levels of disinfection and give examples of each. When would each type of disinfectant be used?
3. What factors influence the effectiveness of sterilization with moist heat, dry heat, and ethylene oxide?
4. Give examples of each of the following disinfectants and their mode of action: iodine compounds, chlorine compounds, phenolic compounds, and quaternary ammonium compounds.

Bibliography

Block SS: Disinfection, sterilization, and preservation, ed 2, Philadelphia, 1977, Lea & Febiger.

Brody TM, Larner J, Minneman KP: *Human pharmacology: molecular to clinical,* ed 3, St Louis, 1998, Mosby.

Marsik F, Denys G: Sterilization, decontamination, and disinfection procedures for the microbiology laboratory. In Murray P et al, editors: *Manual of clinical microbiology,* ed 6, Washington, DC, 1995, American Society for Microbiology.

Rutala W: Antisepsis, disinfection, and sterilization in hospitals and related institutions. In Murray P et al, editors: *Manual of clinical microbiology,* ed 6, Washington, DC, 1995, American Society for Microbiology.

SECTION II

Basic Concepts in the Immune Response

Elements of Host Protective Responses

We live in a microbial world, and our bodies are constantly being exposed to bacteria, fungi, parasites, and viruses. Our bodies' defenses to this onslaught are similar to a military defense. The initial defense mechanisms are barriers, such as the skin, that prevent entry of the foreign agents. If these barriers are compromised or the agent gains entry in another way, the local militia (natural killer cells, neutrophils, macrophages) must quickly rally to the challenge and prevent expansion of the invasion. Finally, if this is not effective, a major campaign must be specifically directed against the invader (antibody and T cells) at whatever cost (immunopathogenesis). Similarly, knowledge of the characteristics (antigens) of the enemy before an attack allows a faster, more effective response (activation of memory B and T cells on rechallenge).

The different elements of the immune system interact and communicate with soluble molecules and by direct cell-to-cell interaction. These interactions provide the mechanisms for activation and control of the protective responses. Unfortunately, the protective responses to some infectious agents are insufficient; in other cases, the response to the challenge is excessive. In either case, disease occurs.

ACTIVATORS AND STIMULATORS OF IMMUNE FUNCTION

Immune cells communicate by direct cell-to-cell interactions (touch) and by the sensing of soluble molecules (similar to taste or smell), including proteins such as lymphokines, chemokines, and interferons and lipids such as steroids and prostaglandins. **Lymphokines** and **cytokines** are proteins produced by lymphoid and other cells that stimulate and regulate the immune response (Table 11-1 and Box 11-1). **Interferons** are low-molecular-weight proteins produced in response to viral infections (interferon-alpha and interferon-beta) or on activation of the immune response (interferon-gamma), which promote antiviral and antitumor responses and stimulate immune responses (see Chapter 14). The chemokines and other proteins (e.g., the C5a product of the complement cascade) are **chemotactic factors** that attract phagocytic and inflammatory cells to the site of infection. **Chemokines** are small proteins (~8000 daltons) that are associated with inflammatory responses. Neutrophils, basophils, monocytes, and T cells express receptors for specific chemokines.

CELLS OF THE IMMUNE RESPONSE

Immune responses are mediated by specific cells with defined functions. The characteristics of the most important cells of the immune system and their appearances are presented in Figure 11-1 and Table 11-2.

The white blood cells can be distinguished morphologically, by histological staining, by their immunological functions, and by intracellular and cell surface markers. The discovery of monoclonal antibodies has allowed the identification of cell surface markers, which distinguish subsets of the different types of cells. These markers have been defined within **clusters of differentiation** and the markers indicated by **"CD" numbers** (Table 11-3). Class II major histocompatibility complex (MHC) antigens (HLA-DR, HLA-DP, HLA-DQ) are expressed on B cells, macrophages, and a limited number of other cell types. In addition, these and all nucleated cells express class I MHC antigens (MHC I: HLA-A, HLA-B, HLA-C).

BOX 11-1 Major Lymphokine-Producing Cells

Macrophage—IL-1, TNF-alpha, TNF-beta, IL-6, IL-12, GM-CSF
CD4 TH1—IL-2, Interferon-gamma, TNF-beta, IL-3, GM-CSF, TNF-alpha
CD4 TH2—IL-4, IL-5, IL-6, IL-10, IL-3, IL-9, IL-13, GM-CSF, TNF-alpha

IL, Interleukin; *TNF*, tumor necrosis factor; *GM-CSF*, granulocyte-macrophage colony-stimulating factor.

Hematopoietic Cell Differentiation

Differentiation of a common progenitor cell, termed the *pluripotent stem cell*, gives rise to all blood cells. Differentiation begins during development of the fetus and continues throughout life. The **pluripotent stem cell** differentiates into stem cells for different lineages of blood cells, including the **lymphoid (T and B cell), myeloid, monocytic, erythrocytic,** and **megakaryoblastic** (source of platelets) lineages (Figure 11-1). The stem cells reside primarily in the bone marrow. Differentiation into the functional blood cells is triggered by specific cell surface interactions with the stromal cells of the

Text continued on p. 86

TABLE 11-1	Cytokines, Lymphokines, and Chemokines		
FACTOR	**SOURCE**	**MAJOR TARGET**	**FUNCTION**
Interferon-alpha, interferon-beta	Leukocytes, fibroblasts	Virally infected cells, tumor cells; NK cells	Induction of antiviral state; activation of NK cells, enhancement of cell-mediated immunity
Interferon-gamma	CD4 TH1 cells, NK cells	Macrophages,* T cells	Activation of macrophage, promotion of inflammation, promotion of TH1 and inhibition of TH2 responses
IL-1-alpha, IL-1-beta	Macrophage, fibroblasts, epithelial cells, endothelial cells	T cells, B cells, PMN leukocytes, tissue, CNS	Many actions: promotion of inflammatory and acute phase responses, fever, activation of T cells
TNF-alpha (cachectin)	Similar to IL-1	—	Similar to IL-1, antitumor and wasting (cachexia-weight loss) functions
TNF-beta	T cells	PMN leukocytes, tumors	Lymphotoxin: tumor killing, activation of PMN
Colony-stimulating factors (e.g., GM-CSF)	T cells, stromal cells	Stem cells	Growth and differentiation of specific cell types
IL-2	CD4 T cells (TH0, TH1)	T cells, B cells, NK cells	T- and B-cell **growth**
IL-3	CD4 T cells, keratinocytes	Stem cells	Differentiation
IL-4	CD4 (TH0, TH2), T cells	B and T cells	B-cell growth and differentiation; Ig production; TH2 responses
IL-5	CD4 TH2 cells	B cells, eosinophils	B-cell growth and differentiation, IgA and IgE production, eosinophil production, allergic responses
IL-6	Macrophages, T cells and B cells, fibroblasts, epithelial cells, endothelial cells	T cells and B cells, hepatocytes	Stimulation of acute-phase and inflammatory responses, fever, Ig secretion, B-cell growth and development
IL-7	Bone marrow, stroma	Precursor cells and stem cells	Growth of pre–B cell, thymocyte, T cell, and CTL
IL-10	CD4 TH2 cells	B cells, CD4 TH1 cells	B-cell growth, inhibition of TH1 response
IL-12	Macrophage	NK cells, CD4 TH1 cells	Activation
TGF-beta	CD4 TH3 cells	B cells	IgA production; immunosuppression of B, T, and NK cells and macrophages; promotion of oral tolerance, wound healing
Alpha-chemokines: C-X-C chemokines—two cysteines separated by one amino acid (IP-10; platelet factor 4; GRO alpha, beta-delta; IL-8)	Many cells	Neutrophils, T cells, macrophages	Chemotaxis, activation
Beta chemokines: C-C chemokines—two adjacent cysteines (MCP-1; MIP-1alpha; MIP-1beta, RANTES)	Many cells	T cells, macrophages, basophils	Chemotaxis, activation

NK, Natural killer; *IL,* interleukin; *PMN,* polymorphonuclear; *CNS,* central nervous system; *TNF,* tumor necrosis factor; *GM-CSF,* granulocyte-macrophage colony-stimulating factor; *Ig,* immunoglobulin; *CTL,* cytotoxic lymphocyte; *TGF,* transforming growth factor; *IP,* interferon-alpha protein; *MCP,* monocyte chemoattractant protein; *MIP,* macrophage inflammatory protein; *RANTES,* regulated on activation normal T expressed and secreted.
*Applies to one or more cells of the monocyte-macrophage lineage.

TABLE 11-2 **Cells of the Immune Response**

CELLS	CHARACTERISTICS	MARKERS	FUNCTIONS
NATURAL CYTOLYTIC CELLS			
Natural killer cells	Large granular lymphocytes	Fc receptors for antibody; CD16, CD56, CD57	Kill antibody-decorated cells and virus-infected or tumor cell (**no MHC restriction**)
PHAGOCYTIC CELLS			
Neutrophils (polymorphonuclear leukocytes)	Granulocytes with short life span, multilobed nucleus and granules, segmented band forms (more immature)	—	*Phagocytise* and kill *bacteria*
Eosinophils	Bilobed nucleus, heavily granulated cytoplasm	Staining with eosin	Are involved in parasite defense and allergic response
Macrophages	See below	—	—
ANTIGEN-PRESENTING CELLS (APCS)		**CLASS II MHC EXPRESSING CELLS**	**PRESENT ANTIGEN TO CD4 + T CELLS**
Monocytes*	Found in lymphocytes, blood, lungs, and other organs	Horseshoe-shaped nucleus, lysosomes, granules	Are *precursors to macrophage-lineage*, lymphokine release
Macrophages*	Possible residence in tissue, spleen, lymph nodes, and other organs; activated by interferon-gamma and TNF	Large, granular cells; Fc and C3 receptors	Initiate inflammatory and acute phase response; activated cells are antibacterial and have antiviral and antitumor activities
Langerhans' cells*	Presence in skin	—	Transport antigen to lymph nodes
Dendritic cells*	Alpha lymph nodes, tissue	—	Are efficient antigen presenter
Microglial cells*	CNS and brain	—	Produce cytokines
Kupffer's cells*	Presence in liver	—	Filter particles from blood (e.g., viruses)
B cells	See below	—	
ANTIGEN-RESPONSIVE CELLS			
T cells	Mature in thymus; large nucleus, small cytoplasm	CD2, CD3, T-cell receptor	Produce lymphokines
CD4 T cells	Helper/DTH cells; **activation** by APC through **class II MHC antigen presentation**	CD2, CD3, T-cell receptor, CD4	Produce IL-2, other lymphokines; stimulate T- and B-cell growth; promote B-cell differentiation (class-switching), antibody production
	TH1 subtype	IL-2, Ifn-gamma, LT production	Promote initial defenses (local), DTH, T killer cells
	TH2 subtype	IL-4, IL-5, IL-6, IL-10 production	Promote humoral responses
CD8 T killer cells	**Recognition** of antigen presented by **class I MHC antigens**	CD2, CD3, T-cell receptor, CD8	Kill viral, tumor, non-self (transplant) cells; secrete TH1 lymphokines
CD8 T cells (suppressor cells)	**Recognition** of antigen presented by **class I MHC antigens**	CD2, CD3, T-cell receptor, CD8	Suppress T- and B-cell response
ANTIBODY-PRODUCING CELLS			
B cells	Mature in Peyer's patches, bone marrow, bursal equivalent; large nucleus, small cytoplasm; activation by antigens and T-cell factors	Surface antibody, **class II MHC antigens**	Produce antibody and present antigen
Plasma cells	Small nucleus, large cytoplasm	—	Are terminally differentiated, antibody factories
OTHER CELLS			
Basophils/mast cells	Granulocytic	Fc receptors for IgE	Release histamine, provide allergic response, are antiparasitic

MHC, Major histocompatibility complex; *TNF*, tumor necrosis factor; *CNS*, central nervous system; *DTH*, delayed type hypersensitivity; *IL*, interleukin; *Ig*, immunoglobulin; *LPS*, lipopolysaccharide.
*Monocytes are macrophage lineage cells.

FIGURE 11-1 Morphology of cells involved in the immune response. Mononuclear cells include lymphocytes, monocytes, and macrophages. Polymorphonuclear leukocytes include neutrophils, eosinophils, basophils, and mast cells.

TABLE 11-3   Selected CD Markers of Importance

CD	IDENTITY/FUNCTION	T CELL	B CELL	NK	MONOCYTE	MACROPHAGE
CD2 (LFA-3R)	Erythrocyte receptor	**		■		
CD3	TCR subunit (gamma, delta, epsilon, zeta, eta); activation	**				
CD4	Class II MHC receptor	**			■	
CD5		■	■			
CD8	Class I MHC receptor	**		■		
CD11b (CR3)	C3b complement receptor 3 (alpha chain)		■	■	■	
CD11c (CR4)	Fibrinogen-binding receptor (alpha chain)				■	
CD14	LPS-binding protein receptor				■	
CD16 (Fc-gamma RIII)	Mediation of phagocytosis and ADCC			**		■
CD18	(Beta chain of CD11)	■	■	■	■	■
CD21 (CR2)	C3d complement receptor, EBV receptor		**			
CD25 (TAC)	IL-2 receptor (alpha chain)	*	*		*	
CD28	Receptor for B-7 costimulation	**	*			
CD32 (Fc-gamma RII)	Low-affinity receptor for immune complexes		■		■	**
CD35 (CR1)	Cb4 and C4b complement receptor		**			
CD40	Stimulation of B-cell		■		■	
CD40 L	Receptor for CD40	**				

Marker	Description
CD45 (LCA)	Leukocyte common antigen augments antigen signalling
CD45RA	
CD45RO	LCA isoform (memory cells)
CD56 (NKH1)	Adhesion molecule
CD57 (leu-7)	
CD64 (Fc-gamma RI)	High-affinity IgG receptor
CD70	CD27-ligand
CD80	B7: costimulation of T cells
ADHESION MOLECULES	
CD11a	LFA-1 (alpha chain)
CD29	VLA (beta chain)
VLA-1, VLA-2, VLA-3	Alpha integrins
VLA-4	Alpha$_4$ integrin homing receptor
CD50	ICAM-3
CD54	ICAM-1
CD58	LFA-3

Modified from Male D et al: *Advanced immunology*, ed 3, St Louis, 1996, Mosby.

R, Receptor; *LFA*, leukocyte function-associated antigen; *TCR*, T-cell antigen receptor; *MHC*, major histocompatibility complex; *LPS*, lipopolysaccharide; *IL*, interleukin; *LCA*, leukocyte common antigen; *VLA*, very late activation (antigen); *ICAM*, intracellular adhesion molecule.

This table shows the recognized CD markers of hemopoietic cells and their distribution. A filled rectangle or + means cell population present; a half-filled triangle is subpopulation. *, activated cells only; **, markers that identify or are critical to the cell type.

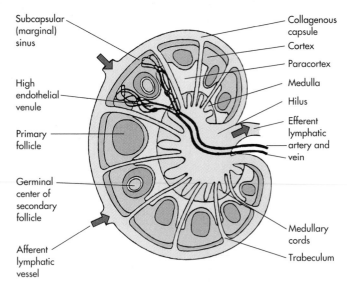

FIGURE 11-2 Thymus and bone marrow are primary lymphoid organs. They are sites of maturation for T and B cells, respectively. Cellular and humoral immune responses occur in the secondary (peripheral) lymphoid organs and tissues; effector and memory cells are generated here. The spleen responds predominantly to blood-borne antigens. Lymph nodes mount immune responses to antigens in intercellular fluid and in the lymph, absorbed either through the skin (superficial nodes) or from internal viscera (deep nodes). Tonsils, Peyer's patches, and other mucosa-associated lymphoid tissues (blue boxes) respond to antigens that have penetrated the surface mucosal barriers. (From Roitt I, Brostoff J, Male D: *Immunology,* ed 4, St Louis, 1996, Mosby.)

FIGURE 11-3 Beneath the collagenous capsule is the subcapsular sinus, which is lined with phagocytic cells. Lymphocytes and antigens from surrounding tissue spaces or adjacent nodes pass into the sinus via the afferent lymphatic system. The cortex contains aggregates of B cells (primary follicles), most of which are stimulated (secondary follicles) and have a site of active proliferation or germinal center. The paracortex contains mainly T cells, many of which are associated with the interdigitating cells (antigen-presenting cells.) Each lymph node has its own arterial and venous supply. Lymphocytes enter the node from the circulation through the specialized high endothelial venules in the paracortex. The medulla contains both T and B cells, as well as most of the lymph node plasma cells organized into cords of lymphoid tissue. Lymphocytes can leave the node only through the efferent lymphatic vessel. (From Roitt I, Brostoff J, Male D: *Immunology,* ed 4, St Louis, 1996, Mosby.)

marrow and specific lymphokines produced by these and other cells. **The thymus and the "bursal equivalent" in the Peyer's patches promote T- and B-cell development, respectively.** Helper T cells, macrophages, and other cells release lymphokines in response to infections and activation, which promote hematopoietic cell growth and terminal differentiation.

The bone marrow and thymus are considered **primary lymphoid organs** (Figure 11-2). These sites of initial lymphocyte differentiation are essential to the development of the immune system. **Secondary lymphoid organs** include the **lymph nodes, spleen,** and mucosa-associated lymphoid tissues **(MALT),** which also include gut-associated lymphoid tissue **(GALT)** (e.g., Peyer's patches) and bronchus-associated lymphoid tissue **(BALT)** (e.g., tonsils, appendix). These sites are where B and T cells reside and respond to antigenic challenges. Proliferation of the lymphocytes in response to infectious challenge causes these tissues to swell (swollen glands). The cells of the primary and secondary lymphoid organs express cell surface adhesion molecules **(addressins)** that

interact with **homing receptors** (cell adhesion molecules) expressed on B and T cells.

The spleen and lymph nodes are capsulated organs in which the macrophages and B and T cells reside in defined regions. Their location facilitates interactions that promote immune responses to antigen (Figure 11-3). The **lymph nodes** are kidney-shaped organs 2 to 10 mm in diameter that filter the fluid that passes from intercellular spaces into the lymphatic system and then through the lymph nodes. The lymph node consists of three layers. The cortex is the outer layer and contains mainly B cells and macrophages arranged in clusters called *follicles.* The paracortex contains dendritic cells that bring antigens from the tissues to be presented to the T cells to initiate immune responses. The medulla contains B and T cells and antibody-producing plasma cells. The **spleen** is a large organ that filters antigens from blood and removes aged blood cells and platelets (Figure 11-4). The spleen consists of two types of tissue: the white pulp and the red pulp. The white pulp consists of arterioles surrounded by lymphoid cells (periarteriolar lymphoid

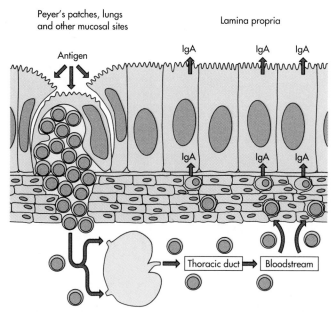

FIGURE 11-4 Organization of lymphoid tissue in the spleen. The white pulp contains germinal centers and is surrounded by the marginal zone, which contains numerous macrophages, antigen-presenting cells, slowly recirculating B cells, and natural killer cells. The red pulp contains venous sinuses separated by splenic cords. Blood enters the tissues via the trabecular arteries, which give rise to the many-branched central arteries. Some end in the white pulp, supplying the germinal centers and mantle zones, but most empty into or near the marginal zones. *PALS,* Periarteriolar lymphoid sheath. (From Roitt I, Brostoff J, Male D: *Immunology,* ed 4, St Louis, 1996, Mosby.)

FIGURE 11-5 Lymphoid cells stimulated with antigen in Peyer's patches (or the lungs or another mucosal site) migrate via the regional lymph nodes and thoracic duct into the bloodstream and then to the lamina propria of the gut and probably other mucosal surfaces. Thus lymphocytes stimulated at one mucosal surface may become distributed throughout the MALT system. IgA, Immunoglobulin A. (From Roitt I, Brostoff J, Male D: *Immunology,* ed 4, St Louis, 1996, Mosby.)

sheath) in which the T cells surround the central arteriole. B cells are organized into primary unstimulated or secondary stimulated follicles that have a germinal center. The germinal center contains memory cells, macrophages, and follicular dendritic cells. The red pulp is a storage site for blood cells and the site of turnover of aged platelets and erythrocytes. **MALT** contains less structured aggregates of lymphoid cells (Figure 11-5). For example, the **Peyer's patches** along the intestinal wall have special cells in the epithelium (M cells) that deliver antigens to the lymphocytes contained in defined regions (T [interfollicular] and B [germinal]).

POLYMORPHONUCLEAR LEUKOCYTES

Polymorphonuclear leukocytes (neutrophils) constitute 50% to 70% of circulating white blood cells (Figure 11-1) and are a primary **phagocytic defense** against bacterial infection. These short-lived cells circulate in the blood for 7 to 10 hours and then migrate into the tissue with a life span of an additional 3 days. Neutrophils are

11 to 14 μ in diameter, lack mitochondria, have a granulated cytoplasm with granules staining with both acidic and basic stains, and have a multilobed nucleus. Neutrophils leave the blood and concentrate at the site of infection in response to chemotactic factors. During infection, the number of neutrophils in the blood increases and includes precursor forms. These precursors are termed **band forms,** in contrast to the terminally differentiated and **segmented** neutrophil. This is sometimes termed *a left shift with an increase in bands vs. segs.* Neutrophils ingest bacteria by phagocytosis and expose the bacteria to antibacterial substances and enzymes contained in **primary (azurophilic)** and **secondary (specific) granules.** Azurophilic granules are reservoirs for enzymes such as myeloperoxidase, beta-glucuronidase, elastase, and cathepsin G. **Specific granules** serve as reservoirs for lysozyme and lactoferrin.

Eosinophils are heavily granulated cells (11 to 15 μ in diameter) with a bilobed nucleus and stain with the acid dye eosin Y. Eosinophils are also phagocytic, motile, and granulated. The granules contain acid phosphatase,

FIGURE 11-6 The mononuclear phagocyte system includes blood monocytes and phagocytes resident in tissues or fixed to the endothelial layer of blood capillaries. In the liver, these resident macrophages are known as *Kupffer's cells*, whereas in the kidney they are called the *intraglomerular mesangial cells*. Alveolar and serosal (e.g., peritoneal) macrophages are examples of "wandering" macrophages. Brain microglia are cells that enter the brain around the time of birth and differentiate into fixed cells. (From Roitt I, Brostoff J, Male D: *Immunology,* ed 4, St Louis, 1996, Mosby.)

peroxidase, and eosinophilic basic proteins. Eosinophils play a role in the defense against **parasitic infections**. The eosinophilic basic proteins are toxic to many parasites. **Basophils,** another type of granulocyte, are not phagocytic but release the contents of their granules during allergic responses (type 1 hypersensitivity).

MONONUCLEAR PHAGOCYTE SYSTEM

The mononuclear phagocyte system (previously called the *reticuloendothelial system*) includes **monocytes** (Figure 11-1) in the blood and cells derived from monocytes such as **macrophages, alveolar macrophages in the lungs, dendritic cells in tissue, Kupffer's cells in the liver, histiocytes in connective tissue, synovial A cells,** and **microglial cells in the brain** (Figure 11-6). Monocytes are 10 to 18 μ in diameter with a single-lobed, kidney bean–shaped nucleus and represent 3% to 8% of peripheral blood leukocytes. The different macrophages have different morphologies corresponding to their ultimate tissue location and function. Macrophages are long-lived cells that are phagocytic and contain mitochondria and lysosomes. **Macrophages**

have three basic functions: **phagocytosis, antigen presentation** to T cells to initiate specific immune responses, and **secretion of lymphokines** to activate and promote immune and inflammatory responses. Macrophages express cell surface receptors for the Fc portion of immunoglobulin G (IgG) **(Fc-gamma RI, Fc-gamma RII, Fc-gamma RIII)** and for the C3b product of the complement cascade **(CR1, CR3),** which facilitates the uptake of antigen, bacteria, or viruses coated with these proteins. Macrophages also express the **class II MHC antigen,** which allows these cells to present antigen to helper T cells to initiate the immune response. Macrophages secrete **interleukin-1, interleukin-6, and interleukin-12** and **tumor necrosis factor** in response to bacterial stimulation, which stimulates immune and inflammatory responses, including fever. A T-cell–derived lymphokine, **interferon-gamma,** activates macrophages. **Activated macrophages** have enhanced phagocytic, killing, and antigen-presenting capabilities. Specific cells of the macrophage lineage may not express one or more of the macrophage activities or cell surface markers; for example, Langerhans' cells lack phagocytic function.

TABLE 11-4   Comparison of B and T Cells

PROPERTY	T CELLS	B CELLS
Origin	Bone marrow	Bone marrow
Maturation	Thymus	Bursal equivalent: bone marrow, Peyer's patches
Functions	Helper: initiation and promotion of immune response	Antibody production
	DTH: Promotion and amplification of inflammatory response	Antibody presentation
	CTL: Class I MHC–restricted cytolysis	—
Protective response	Resolution of intracellular and fungal infections	Protection against rechallenge, block spread of agent in blood, opsonize, etc.
Products	Lymphokines,* interferon-gamma, growth factors, cytolytic substances (perforin, granzymes)*	IgM, IgD, IgA, or IgE
Distinguishing surface markers	CD2 (sheep red blood cell receptor), TCR, CD3, CD4 or CD8	Surface antibody, complement receptors, class II MHC antigens
Subsets	CD4 TH0: helper	B cells: antibody
	CD4 TH1: DTH	Plasma cell: antibody factories
	CD4 TH2: B-cell growth, differentiation class switching	
	CD4 TH3: Class switching-IgA	Memory cells: long-lived, anamnestic response
	CD8: cytotoxic T cells	
	CD8: suppressor cells	
	Memory cells: long-lived, anamnestic response	

DTH, Delayed type hypersensitivity; *CTL*, cytotoxic lymphocyte.
*Depending on subset.

LYMPHOCYTES

The lymphocytes are 6 to 10 μ in diameter, smaller than leukocytes. The two classes of lymphocytes, B and T cells, have a large nucleus and smaller, agranular cytoplasm. Although B and T cells are indistinguishable by morphological features, they can be distinguished by function and by surface markers (Table 11-4). The **large granular lymphocytes (LGLs)** are **natural killer (NK)** and **antibody-dependent killer (K) cells.** These cells contain cytoplasmic granules with cytolytic proteins.

The primary function of **B cells** is to **make antibody,** but they also internalize antigen, process the antigen, and present the antigen to T cells to initiate or enhance the immune response. B cells can be distinguished by the **cell surface presence of immunoglobulins, class II MHC molecules,** and receptors for the C3b and C3d products of the complement cascade **(CR1, CR2)** (Figure 11-7). The *B cell* name is derived from its site of differentiation in birds, the *b*ursa of Fabricius. In mammals, B-cell differentiation occurs in the fetal liver, fetal spleen, and bone marrow. B cells can develop into memory cells, which express the CD45RO cell surface marker, and circulate until activated by specific antigen. Activated B cells can terminally differentiate into **plasma cells.** Plasma cells are factories for antibody production with small nuclei and large cytoplasm.

T cells acquired their name because they develop in the **thymus.** T cells have three major functions in response to foreign antigen: They activate immune and in-

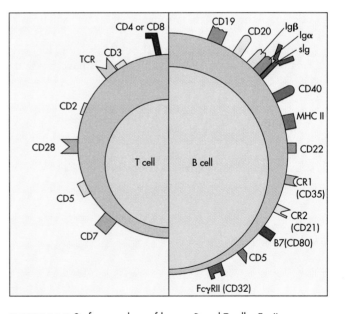

FIGURE 11-7 Surface markers of human B and T cells. *FcγII,* Fc-gamma RII.

flammatory responses by releasing lymphokines; they directly kill viral infected cells, foreign cells (e.g., tissue grafts), and tumors; and they control and suppress (when necessary) the immune response. T cells make up 60% to 80% of peripheral blood lymphocytes.

T cells were initially distinguished from B cells by their ability to bind and surround themselves (rosette) with sheep erythrocytes through the CD2 molecule. All T cells express an antigen-binding **T-cell receptor (TCR),** which resembles but differs from antibody, and **CD2 and CD3** associated proteins on their cell surface (Figure 11-7). T cells are divided into three major groups based on the type of TCR and the cell surface expression of two proteins, CD4 and CD8. Most lymphocytes express the **alpha beta (αβ) TCR. CD4-expressing T cells** include the **helper** and **delayed type hypersensitivity–inducing** (DTH-inducing) cells. These T cells produce and secrete lymphokines that stimulate and activate other immune responses. The CD4 T cells can be further divided into TH0, TH1, TH2, and TH3 subgroups. TH1 cells promote inflammatory and DTH responses, whereas TH2 cells promote antibody production. TH3 cells promote IgA production. The **CD8** T cells also release lymphokines but are better known for their ability to recognize and kill virally infected cells, foreign tissue transplants (nonself grafts), and tumor cells as **cytotoxic killer T cells.** CD8 T cells are also responsible for suppressing immune responses. T cells also produce memory cells that express CD45RO. Terminally differentiated CD4 and CD8 T cells express the class II MHC antigen. A small number of T cells express the **gamma delta (γδ) TCR** but do not express CD4 or CD8. These cells generally reside in tissue and are important for mucosal immunity.

Lymphoid cells that are not B or T cells (non-B/non-T or null cells) include LGLs. These cells have cytolytic activities and include the **NK** and **antibody-dependent cellular cytotoxicity (ADCC or K) cells.** They resemble the CD8 T cells in cytolytic function toward virally infected and tumor cells but differ in the mechanism for identifying the target cell.

QUESTIONS

1. A professor was teaching an introductory course and described the different immune cells with nicknames. Describe why the nicknames are appropriate or why they are not.
   a. Macrophage: Pac man (a computer game character that eats dots but eats bad guys when activated)
   b. T cells: Police department
   c. CD4 T cell: Desk sergeant/dispatch officer
   d. CD8 T cell: "Cop on the beat"/patrol officer
   e. B cell: Product design and building company
   f. Plasma cell: Factory
   g. Mast cell: Activable chemical warfare unit
   h. Neutrophil: Trash collector and disinfector

Bibliography

Immunology Today: Issues contain understandable reviews on current topics in immunology.
Male D et al: *Advanced immunology,* ed 3, St Louis, 1996, Mosby.
Roitt I, Brostoff J, Male D: *Immunology,* ed 4, St Louis, 1996, Mosby.

12

The Humoral Immune Response

The primary molecular component of the humoral immune response is antibody. Antibody molecules are synthesized by B and plasma cells in response to challenge by antigen. Antibodies provide protection from rechallenge by an infectious agent, block spread of the agent in the blood, and facilitate the elimination of a primary infection. To accomplish these tasks, an incredibly large repertoire of antibody molecules must be available to recognize the tremendous number of infectious agents and molecules that challenge our bodies. In addition to interacting specifically with foreign structures, antibody must interact with host systems and cells (e.g., complement, macrophages) to promote clearance of antigen and activation of subsequent immune responses (Box 12-1). Antibody molecules also serve as the cell surface receptors on the B cell to stimulate these antibody factories to grow and produce more antibody in response to antigenic challenge.

IMMUNOGENS, ANTIGENS, AND EPITOPES

Almost all of the proteins and carbohydrates associated with an infectious agent, whether a bacterium, fungus, virus, or parasite, are considered foreign to the human host and have the potential to induce an immune response. A protein or carbohydrate that challenges the immune system and that can initiate an immune response is called an **immunogen** (Box 12-2). Immunogens may contain more than one antigen (e.g., bacteria). An **antigen** is a molecule that is recognized by specific antibody or T cells. An **epitope (antigenic determinant)** is the actual molecular structure that interacts with a single antibody molecule. Within a protein, an epitope may be formed by a specific sequence **(linear epitope)** or a three-dimensional structure **(conformational epitope).** Antigens and immunogens usually contain several epitopes, each capable of binding to a different antibody molecule. As described later, a **monoclonal antibody** recognizes a single epitope.

Not all molecules are immunogens. In general, proteins are the best immunogens, carbohydrates are weaker immunogens, and lipids and nucleic acids are poor immunogens. The immunogen must be of sufficient size, and proteins must be degradable by phagocytes so that they can be presented to lymphocytes to initiate an immune response. **Haptens** (incomplete immunogens) cannot initiate but can be recognized by an immune response. Often, the hapten is too small to immunize an individual but can be recognized by antibody. Haptens can be made immunogenic by attachment to a **carrier** molecule, such as a protein. For example, dinitrophenol conjugated to bovine serum albumin is an immunogen for the dinitrophenol hapten.

During artificial immunization (e.g., vaccines), an **adjuvant** is used to enhance the response to antigen. Adjuvants usually prolong the presence of antigen in the tissue and activate or promote uptake of the immunogen by macrophages and lymphocytes. Most vaccines are precipitated onto alum to promote the slow release of antigen and the uptake by macrophages. Cells are stimulated and antigen is released slowly when emulsified in complete Freund's adjuvant (consisting of heat-killed mycobacteria in mineral oil). Newer, less toxic adjuvants being tested for use with human vaccines include liposomes (defined lipid complexes), bacterial cell wall components, molecular cages for antigen, and polymeric surfactants. Cholera toxin and *E. coli* lymphotoxin are potent adjuvants for secretory antibody (immunoglobulin A).

Some molecules will not elicit an immune response in an individual. During growth of the fetus, the body develops **immune tolerance** toward self-antigens as well as any foreign antigens that may be introduced before the maturation of the immune system. Later in life, toleration may occur under special conditions; for example, ingestion of high concentrations of bovine myelin can tolerize an individual to myelin. This has been proposed as a potential therapy for the autoimmunopathogenesis that causes multiple sclerosis.

The type of immune response initiated by an immunogen depends on its molecular structure. A primitive but rapid antibody response can be initiated toward *bacterial polysaccharides, peptidoglycan,* or *flagellin.* These molecules have a *large, repetitive structure,* which is sufficient to activate B cells to make antibody without the participation of T-cell help and are termed **thymus-independent antigens.** In these cases, the response is

FIGURE 12-1 Comparative structures of the immunoglobulin classes and subclasses in humans. IgA and IgM are held together in multimers by the J chain. IgA can acquire the secretory component for the traversal of epithelial cells.

BOX 12-1	**Antimicrobial Action of Antibodies**

Are opsonic: promote ingestion and killing by phagocytic cells (IgG)

Block attachment of toxins and virus

Neutralize toxins and virus

Agglutinate bacteria: may aid in clearing

Render motile organisms nonmotile

Combine with antigens on the microbial surface, activate the complement cascade, thus inducing an inflammatory response and bringing fresh phagocytes and serum Abs into the site

Combine with antigens on the microbial surface, activate the complement cascade, and form the membrane attack complex involving C5b to C9

BOX 12-2	**Definitions**

Immunogen—Substance capable of *eliciting* an immune response

Antigen—Substance *recognized* by immune response

Epitope—Molecular structure recognized by immune response

Hapten—Incomplete immunogen that cannot initiate response but that can be recognized by antibody

Carrier—Protein modified by hapten to elicit response

Adjuvant—Substance that promotes immune response to immunogen

T-independent antigens—Antigens with large, repetitive structures (e.g., bacterial, flagellin, lipopolysaccharide, polysaccharide)

T-dependent antigens—Antigens that must be presented to T and B cells for antibody production

---

limited to production of immunoglobulin M (IgM) antibody and fails to stimulate an anamnestic (memory) response. In most cases, B-cell production of antibody requires help, in the form of lymphokines, from T cells; therefore the antigen must be recognized and stimulate *both* T and B cells. Thymus-dependent antigens are usually proteins, stimulate all five classes of immunoglobulins, and elicit an anamnestic response. *The structure of the antigen, the amount of antigen, the route of administration of antigen, and other factors influence the type of immune response, including the types of antibody produced.* These factors influence the activation of different subclasses of helper T cells (TH1, TH2, and TH3) to pro-

duce different lymphokines, which promote the production of different types of antibody. For example, oral or nasal administration of a vaccine promotes the production of a secretory form of immunoglobulin A (sIgA) that would not be produced on intramuscular challenge.

IMMUNOGLOBULIN TYPES AND STRUCTURES

Immunoglobulins are subdivided into classes and subclasses based on the structure and antigenicity of their heavy chains. IgG, IgM, and IgA are the major antibody forms, whereas IgD and IgE comprise less than 1% of the

TABLE 12-1   Immunoglobulins

Ig	IgG	IgM	IgA	IgD	IgE
CD4 T helper subclass association	TH1, TH2	TH1 and T independent	TH2, TH3	—	TH2
Total Ig (%)	85	5-10	5-15	<1	<1
Molecular weight (kD)	154	900	160 (+ dimer)	185	190
H-chain class	Gamma	Mu	Alpha	Delta	Epsilon
Subclass	Gamma-1, gamma-2, gamma-3, gamma-4	—	Alpha-1, alpha-2	—	—
Serum half-life (days)	23	5	6	2-3	2-3
Principal site of action	Serum	Serum	Secretions	Receptor for B cells	Mast cells
Principal biological effect	Resistance: opsonin, secondary response	Resistance: precipitin, primary response	Resistance: prevention of movement across mucous membranes	B-cell activation	Anaphylaxis
Complement fixation	+	++++	−	−	−
Opsonin for macrophage, PMN	+				
Antibacterial lysis	+	+++	+	−	−
Crossing of placenta	+	−	−	−	−

PMN, Polymorphonuclear neutrophil (leukocyte); +/−, relative activity.

total immunoglobulins. Two immunoglobulin classes, IgA and IgG, are divided further into subclasses based on differences in the Fc portion. Four IgG subclasses are designated as IgG1 through IgG4 and two IgA subclasses (IgA1 and IgA2) (Figure 12-1).

Antibody molecules are Y-shaped molecules with two major structural regions that mediate the two major functions of the molecule (Figure 12-1 and Table 12-1). The **variable-region/antigen-combining site** must be able to identify and specifically interact with an epitope on an antigen. A large number of different antibody molecules, each with a different variable region, is produced in every individual to recognize the seemingly infinite number of different antigens in nature. The **Fc portion** (stem of the antibody Y) interacts with host systems and cells (e.g., complement, macrophages) to promote clearance of antigen and activation of subsequent immune responses. For IgG and IgA, the Fc portion interacts with other proteins to promote transfer across the placenta and the mucosa, respectively (Table 12-2).

For IgG and IgA, there is a flexible **hinge region** rich in proline and susceptible to cleavage by proteolytic enzymes. Digestion of IgG molecules with **papain** yields two **Fab** and one **Fc** fragment (Figure 12-2). Each Fab fragment has one antigen-binding site. By contrast, the Fc fragment has no antigen-binding site but is responsible for fixation of complement and attachment of the molecule to a cell surface immunoglobulin receptor. **Pepsin** cleaves the molecule, producing an **F(ab')2** fragment with two antigen-binding sites and a **pFc'** fragment.

The different types and parts of immunoglobulin can also be distinguished using antibodies directed against

TABLE 12-2   Fc Interactions with Immune Components

IMMUNE COMPONENT	INTERACTION	FUNCTION
Fc receptor	Macrophages	Opsonization
	PMNs	Opsonization
	T cells	Activation
	Cells responsible for antibody-dependent cellular cytotoxicity	Killing
	Mast cells for IgE	Allergic reactions, antiparasitic cellular
Complement	Complement system	Opsonization, killing (especially bacteria)

PMN, Polymorphonuclear neutrophils.

different portions of the molecule. **Isotypes (IgM, IgD, IgG, IgA, IgE)** are determined by antibodies directed against the Fc portion of the molecule. (*Iso is the same for each person.*) Allotypic differences occur for antibody molecules with the same isotype but contain protein sequences that differ from one person to another (in addition to the antigen-binding region). (*Every one ["Allo"] of them can't have the same IgG.*) The **idiotype** refers to the protein sequences in the variable region that gener-

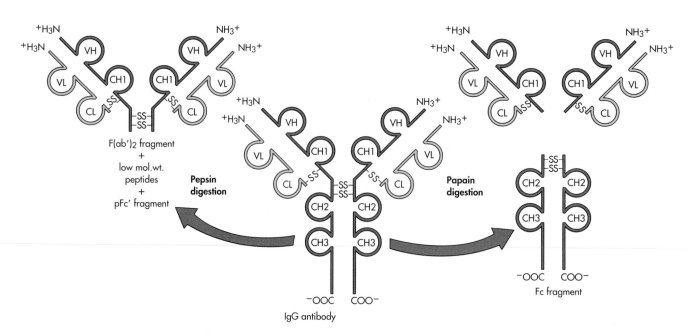

FIGURE 12-2 Proteolytic digestion of IgG. Pepsin treatment produces a dimeric F(ab')2 fragment. Pepsin treatment produces monovalent Fab fragments and an Fc fragment. The F(ab')2 and the Fab fragments bind antigen but lack a functional Fc region. *Blue,* heavy chain; *orange,* light chain.

ate the large number of antigen-binding regions. *(There are lots of different idiots.)*

On a molecular basis, each antibody molecule is made up of heavy and light chains encoded by separate genes. The basic immunoglobulin unit consists of two heavy (H) and two light (L) chains. IgM and IgA consist of multimers of this basic structure. The heavy and light chains of immunoglobulin are fastened together by interchain **disulfide bonds.** There are two types of **light chains—kappa and lambda**—that are present in all five immunoglobulin classes, although only one type is present in an individual molecule. Approximately 60% of human immunoglobulin molecules have kappa light chains, and 40% have lambda light chains. There are 5 types of **heavy chains, one for each type of antibody (IgM: mu, IgG: gamma, IgD: delta, IgA: alpha, IgE: epsilon).** Intrachain disulfide bonds define molecular **domains** within each chain. *Light chains have a variable and a constant domain. The heavy chains have a variable and three (IgG, IgA) or four (IgM, IgE) constant domains.* The variable domains on the heavy and light chains interact to form the antigen-binding site. The constant domains from each chain provide the molecular structure to the immunoglobulin and define the interaction of the antibody molecule with host systems and hence its ultimate function. The heavy chain of the different antibody molecules can also be synthesized with a membrane-spanning region to make the antibody an antigen-specific receptor for the B cell.

Immunoglobulin D

IgD, which has a molecular weight of 185 kD, comprises less than 1% of serum immunoglobulins. IgD exists primarily as **membrane IgD,** which serves with IgM as an antigen receptor on early B-cell membranes to help initiate antibody responses by activating B-cell growth.

Immunoglobulin M

IgM is the first antibody produced in response to antigenic challenge and can be produced in a T-independent manner. **IgM** comprises 5% to 10% of the total immunoglobulins in adults and has a half-life of 5 days. It is a pentameric molecule with five immunoglobulin units joined by disulfide bonds and the **J chain,** with a total molecular weight of 900 kD. Theoretically this immunoglobulin has 10 antigen-binding sites. IgM is the most efficient immunoglobulin for fixing (binding) complement. A single IgM pentamer can activate the classical complement pathway. Monomeric IgM is found with IgD on the B-cell surface, where it serves as the receptor for antigen. Because IgM is relatively large, it cannot spread from the blood into tissue. IgM is particularly important for immunity against polysaccharide antigens on the exterior of pathogenic microorganisms. It also promotes phagocytosis and promotes bacteriolysis through its complement-activation activity. IgM is also a major component of rheumatoid factors (autoantibodies).

Immunoglobulin G

IgG comprises approximately 85% of the immunoglobulins in adults. It has a molecular weight of 154 kD based on two L chains of 22,000 daltons each and two H chains of 55,000 daltons each. The four subclasses of IgG differ in structure (Figure 12-1), relative concentration, and function. The production of IgG requires T-cell help. IgG, as a class of antibody molecules, has the longest half-life (23 days) of the five immunoglobulin classes, crosses the placenta, and is the principal antibody in the anamnestic or booster response. IgG shows high avidity or binding capacity for antigens, fixes complement, stimulates chemotaxis, and acts as an opsonin to facilitate phagocytosis.

Immunoglobulin A

IgA comprises 5% to 15% of the serum immunoglobulins and has a half-life of 6 days. It has a molecular weight of 160 kD and a basic four-chain monomeric structure. However, it can occur as monomers, dimers, trimers, and multimers combined by the J chain (similar to IgM). In addition to serum IgA, a secretory or exocrine variety appears in body secretions and provides localized immunity. IgA production requires T-cell help and special mucosal stimulation to promote production of sIgA. **Adjuvants,** such as cholera toxin and attenuated salmonella bacteria, can promote an IgA response. **sIgA** acquires a **secretory component,** which promotes release through epithelial cells. sIgA (exocrine IgA) appears in colostrum, intestinal and respiratory secretions, saliva, tears, and other secretions. IgA-deficient individuals have an increased incidence of respiratory infections.

Immunoglobulin E

IgE constitutes less than 1% of the total immunoglobulins and has a half-life of approximately 2.5 days. Most IgE is bound to Fc receptors on mast cells, on which it serves as a receptor for allergens and parasite antigens. When sufficient antigen binds to the IgE on the mast cell, the mast cell releases histamine, prostaglandin, platelet-activating factor, and cytokines. IgE is important for protection against **parasitic infection** and is responsible for **anaphylactic hypersensitivity.**

IMMUNOGENETICS

The antibody response can recognize as many as 10^8 structures but can still specifically amplify and focus a response directed to a specific challenge. The mechanisms for generating this antibody repertoire and the different immunoglobulin subclasses are tied to the genetic events that accompany the development (differentiation) of the B cell (Figures 12-3 and 12-4).

Human chromosomes 2, 22, and 14 contain immunoglobulin genes for kappa, lambda, and H chains, respectively. The **germline form** of these genes consists of different and separate sets of genetic building blocks for the light (**V and J gene segments**) and heavy chains (**V, D, and J gene segments**), which are genetically recombined to produce the immunoglobulin variable regions and then associated with the constant-region **C** gene segments. For the kappa light chain, there are 300 V gene segments, 5 J gene segments, and 1 C gene segment. The number of lambda gene segments for V and J is more limited. For the heavy chain, there are 300 to 1000 V genes, 12 D (heavy-chain) genes, 5 (light-chain) or 6 (heavy-chain) J genes, but only 9 C genes (one for each class and subclass of antibody [mu; delta; gamma_3, gamma_1, gamma_2, and gamma_4; alpha_1 and alpha_2; and

FIGURE 12-3 Rearrangement of the germline genes to produce the human immunoglobulin kappa (κ) light chains. Genetic recombination juxtaposes one of the 100 V-region genes with a J-region gene and a C_k gene during differentiation into a pre–B cell. The remaining intervening sequences are removed by splicing the mRNA. *L,* Leader sequence.

FIGURE 12-4 Rearrangement of the germline genes to produce the human immunoglobulin heavy chains. A V-region gene (of 100 possible) combines with a D-region gene (of 12 possible) and a J-region gene (of 6 possible). Constant-region genes (corresponding to IgM $[\mu]$, IgD $[\delta]$, IgG $[\gamma]$, IgE $[\epsilon]$, and IgA $[\alpha]$) are attached to the VDJ region. *M,* Membrane-spanning segment.

epsilon]). In addition, gene segments for membrane-spanning peptides can be attached to the heavy-chain genes to allow the antibody molecule to insert into the B-cell membrane as an antigen-activation receptor.

Production of the final antibody molecule in the pre–B and B cell requires genetic recombination at the

DNA level and posttranscriptional processing at the RNA level. (Figure 12-5). Each of the V, D, and J segments is surrounded by DNA sequences that promote **directional recombination and the loss of the intervening DNA sequences.** Juxtaposition of randomly chosen V and J gene segments of the light chains and the V, D, and J gene segments of the heavy chains produce the variable region of the immunoglobulin chains. **Somatic mutation** of the immunoglobulin gene occurs later in activated B cells to increase the variability and the enormous number of possible coding sequences for the variable region. Attachment of the variable-region sequences (VDJ) to the beginning of the C gene segments by recombination produces a heavy-chain gene containing the mu; delta; gamma$_3$, gamma$_1$, gamma$_2$, and gamma$_4$; epsilon; and alpha$_1$ and alpha$_2$ sequences in the indicated order. In the **pre–B and immature B cells,** mRNAs are produced that contain the variable-region gene segments connected to the C gene sequences for mu and delta. Processing of the mRNA removes either

the mu or delta, as if it were an intron, to produce the final immunoglobulin. The pre-B cell expresses cytoplasmic IgM, whereas the B cell expresses cytoplasmic and cell surface IgM and cell surface IgD.

Class switching (IgM to IgG, IgE, or IgA) occurs in mature B cells in response to different lymphokines produced by TH1, TH2, or TH3 CD4 helper T cells. Genetic recombination juxtaposes the appropriate constant-region sequence with the variable-region sequences and in the process deletes the intervening C-region gene segments (Figure 12-5). Each of the C gene segments, except for delta, is preceded by a DNA sequence called the **switch site.** After the appropriate lymphokine signal, the switch in front of the mu sequence recombines with the switch in front of the gamma$_3$, gamma$_1$, gamma$_2$, or gamma$_4$; epsilon, or alpha$_1$, or alpha$_2$ sequences, creating a DNA loop that is subsequently removed. Processing of the RNA transcript yields the final mRNA for the immunoglobulin heavy-chain protein. For example, IgG1 production would result from the excision of DNA containing the C gene segments C mu, C delta, and C gamma$_3$ to attach the variable region to the gamma$_1$ C gene segment. *Class switching does not change the variable region.*

The final steps in B-cell differentiation to **memory cells** or **plasma cell** do not change the antibody gene. Memory cells are long-lived, antigen-responsive B cells expressing the CD45RO surface marker. Memory cells can be activated in response to antigen later in life to grow and produce specific antibody. Plasma cells are terminally differentiated B cells with a small nucleus but a large cytoplasm filled with endoplasmic reticulum. Plasma cells are antibody factories.

FIGURE 12-5 Differentiation of the B cell promotes genetic recombination and class switching. Switch regions in front of the constant-region genes (including IgG subclasses) allow recombination of the VDJ region with different heavy-chain constant-region genes, genetically removing the mu and other intervening genes. This produces the different heavy-chain genes. Splicing of mRNA produces the final IgM RNA.

ANTIBODY RESPONSE

An initial repertoire of IgM and IgD immunoglobulins is generated in pre–B cells by the genetic events previously described (Figure 12-6). Differentiation of the pre–B cell to the B cell is accompanied by the expression of cell surface IgM and IgD. Cell surface antibody associates with Ig-alpha (CD79a) and Ig-beta (CD79b) in the membrane. Binding of antigen initiates an activation signal. T-independent antigens cross-link sufficient numbers of surface antibody to promote B-cell growth and **clonal expansion** of the antigen-specific B cells. The activation signal is mediated by a cascade of protein tyrosine kinases, phospholipase C, and calcium fluxes that activate transcription and cell growth. The activation signal is amplified by other surface molecules, including the CR2 complement (C3d) receptor (CD21). Production of antibody to T-dependent antigens requires interaction of the B cell with the helper T cell through CD40 (on the B cell), CD40L (T cell), and lymphokines (interleukin-4 [IL-4], IL-5, IL-2, and interferon-gamma).

Clonal expansion of the antigen-specific B cells increases the number of antibody factories making the relevant antibody, which increases the strength of the antibody response. Activation of the B cells also promotes somatic mutation, increasing the diversity of antibody molecules directed at the specific antigen. The B-cell clones that express antibody with the strongest antigen binding are preferentially stimulated, selecting for a better antibody response.

Class switching is induced by the different combinations of lymphokines produced by helper T cells. TH1-helper responses (IL-2, interferon-gamma) promote production of IgM and IgG1, IgG2$_a$ subclasses. TH2-helper responses (IL-4, IL-10) promote production of IgM, IgG, IgE, and IgA. IgA production also requires

transforming growth factor–beta (TGF-beta), a TH3 response. TH2 cells also promote the development of memory cells. Terminal differentiation produces the plasma cell.

The primary antibody response is characterized by the initial production of IgM, and then as the response matures, IgG antibodies rapidly increase in concentration (Figure 12-7). IgM antibodies appear in the blood within 3 days to 2 weeks after exposure to a novel immunogen. The first antibodies that are produced react with residual antigen and therefore are rapidly cleared. However, after the initial lag phase, the antibody titer increases logarithmically to reach a plateau.

Reexposure to an immunogen induces a heightened antibody response (also termed **anamnestic response**). The antibodies develop more rapidly, last longer, and reach a higher titer. The **secondary** antibodies are principally of the IgG class, although IgM antibodies can also be detected in response to some infections.

During an immune response, antibodies are made against different epitopes of the foreign object, protein, or infectious agent. Specific antibody is a mixture of many different immunoglobulin molecules made by many different B cells **(polyclonal antibody),** each immunoglobulin molecule differing in the epitope that it recognizes and the strength of the interaction. Different antibody molecules are made and bind with different strengths (**avidity,** multivalent binding of antibody to antigen; **affinity,** monovalent binding to an epitope) for the same antigen and to different epitopes on the antigen.

Monoclonal antibodies are identical antibodies produced by a single clone of cells or by **myelomas** (cancers of plasma cells) or **hybridomas.** Hybridomas are cloned, laboratory-derived cells obtained by the fusion of antibody-producing spleen cells and a myeloma cell. In 1975, Kohler and Millstein developed the technique for producing monoclonal antibodies from B cell hybridomas. The hybridoma is immortal and produces a single

FIGURE 12-6 B-cell activation. Cross-linking of cell surface receptors activates lymphocytes. Lymphokines activate the growth and differentiation of B cells. *Ifnγ,* Interferon-gamma; *APC,* antigen-presenting cell.

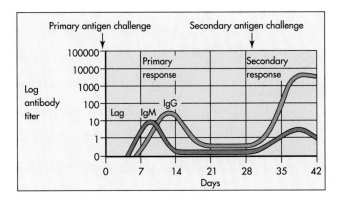

FIGURE 12-7 Time course of immune responses. The primary response occurs after a lag period. The IgM response is the earliest response. The secondary immune response (anamnestic response) reaches a higher titer, lasts longer, and consists predominantly of IgG.

(monoclonal) antibody. This technique has revolutionized the study of immunology because it allows the selection (cloning) of individual antibody-producing cells and their development into cellular factories for the production of large quantities of that antibody. Monoclonal antibodies have been commercially produced for both diagnostic reagents and therapeutic purposes.

COMPLEMENT

The complement system is an alarm and a weapon against infection, especially bacterial infection. The complement system is activated directly by bacteria and bacterial products **(alternate or properdin pathway),** by lectin binding to sugars on the bacterial cell surface **(mannan binding protein),** or by complexes of antibody and antigen **(classical pathway)** (Figure 12-8). Activation by either pathway initiates a **cascade of proteolytic events** that produce **chemotactic factors** to attract phagocytic and inflammatory cells to the site, **increase vascular permeability** to allow access to the site of infection, bind to the agent to promote their phago-

cytosis **(opsonization)** and elimination, and also **directly kill** the infecting agent. The two activation pathways of complement coalesce at a common junction point, the activation of the **C3 component**.

Alternate Pathway

The alternate pathway is activated directly by bacterial cell surfaces and their components, (e.g., endotoxin, microbial polysaccharides) as well as human IgA and other factors (Figure 12-9). This pathway can be activated before the establishment of an immune response to the infecting bacteria, since it does not depend on antibody activation and does not involve the early complement components (C1, C2, and C4). The initial activation of the alternate pathway is mediated by **properdin factor B** binding to C3b and then with properdin factor D, which splits factor B in the complex to yield the Bb active fragment that remains linked to C3b (activation unit). Inactive Ba is split from this complex, which leads to cleavage and activation of C3. The complement cascade continues in a manner analogous to the classical pathway, described later.

Classical Pathway

The classical complement cascade is initiated by binding to aggregates of antibody and antigen on the cell surface

FIGURE 12-8 The classic and alternate complement pathways. The goal of these pathways is activation of C3 and then C5. *MBP,* Mannan-binding protein; *MASP,* MBP-associated serine protease.

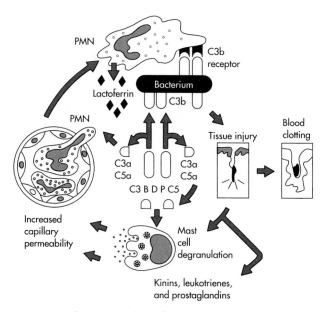

FIGURE 12-9 Alternative pathway for the activation of complement. Activation of the alternative complement pathway by bacterial cell surfaces produces C3b, which opsonizes the bacteria, and C5a, which is chemotactic for polymorphonuclear neutrophils *(PMNs)* and macrophages and triggers mast-cell degranulation. Other agents increase capillary blood flow and permeability.

or an immune complex. Aggregation of antibody (**IgG or IgM, not IgA or IgE**) changes the structure of the heavy chain to allow binding to complement (Figure 12-8).

The first complement component, designated *C1*, consists of a complex of three separate proteins designated *C1q*, *C1r*, and *C1s* (see Figure 12-8). One molecule each of C1q and C1s with two molecules of C1r compose the C1 complex or **recognition unit.** C1q facilitates binding of the recognition unit to cell surface antigen-antibody complexes. Activation of the classical complement cascade requires linkage of C1q to two IgG antibodies through their Fc regions. In contrast, one pentameric IgM molecule attached to a cell surface may interact with C1q to initiate the classical pathway. Binding of C1q activates C1r (referred to now as *C1r**) and in turn C1s (*C1s**). C1s* then cleaves C4 to C4a and C4b and C2 to C2a and C2b. The ability of a single recognition unit to split numerous C2 and C4 molecules represents an amplification mechanism in the complement cascade. The union of C4b and C2a produces **C4b2a,** which is known as **C3 convertase.** This complex binds to the cell membrane and cleaves C3 into C3a and C3b fragments. The C3 convertase amplifies the response by splitting many C3 molecules. The interaction of C3b with C4b2a bound to the cell membrane produces C4b3b2a, which is termed **C5 convertase.** This **activation unit** splits C5 into C5a and C5b fragments and represents yet another amplification step.

Lectin Pathway

The **mannan-binding protein (MBP)** (previously known as *RaRF*) is a large serum protein that binds to nonreduced mannose, fucose, and glucosamine on bacterial and other cell surfaces. MBP resembles and replaces the C1q component and on binding to bacterial surfaces activates the cleavage of **MBP-associated serine protease (MASP).** MASP cleaves the C4 and C2 components to produce the C3 convertase, the junction point of the complement cascade.

Biological Activities of Complement Components

Cleavage of the C3 and C5 components produces important factors that enhances clearance of the infectious agent, by promoting access to the infection site, and by attracting the cells that mediate of protective inflammatory reactions. **C3b** is an **opsonin,** which promotes the clearance of bacteria by binding directly to the cell membrane to make the cell more attractive to phagocytic cells such as neutrophils and macrophages, which have receptors for C3b. Complement fragments **C3a** and **C5a** also serve as powerful **anaphylatoxins** that stimulate **mast cells** to release **histamine,** which enhances *vascular per-*

meability and *smooth muscle contraction.* **C3a and C5a** also act as **attractants** (chemotactic factor) for neutrophils and macrophages. These cells also express receptors for C3b, are phagocytic, and promote inflammatory reactions.

Membrane Attack Complex

The terminal stage of the classical pathway involves creation of the **membrane attack complex (MAC),** which is also called the **lytic unit** (Figure 12-10). The five terminal complement proteins (C5 through C9) associate into a MAC on target-cell membranes to mediate injury. Initiation of MAC assembly begins with C5 cleavage into C5a and C5b fragments. A $(C5b,6,7,8)_1(C9)_n$ complex forms and drills a hole in the membrane, which leads to the hypotonic lysis of cells.

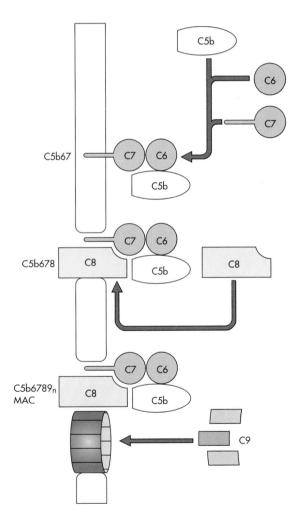

FIGURE 12-10 Cell lysis by complement. Activation of C5 initiates the molecular construction of an oil-well–like MAC.

QUESTIONS

What is wrong with each of these statements and why?

1. The laboratory tested a baby for IgM maternal antibodies.
2. An investigator attempted to use fluorescent-labeled F(ab')$_2$ fragments to locate class II MHC molecules on the cell surface of antigen-presenting cells without cross-linking (binding two molecules together) these cell surface molecules.
3. A patient is diagnosed as having been infected with a specific strain of influenza A (A/Bangkok/1/79/H3N2) based on the presence of antiinfluenza IgG in serum taken from the patient at the initial visit (within 2 days of symptoms).
4. A patient with a T-cell deficiency, unable to promote class switching of B cells, was also considered unable to use the complement systems.

5. Analysis of immunoglobulin genes from B cells taken from the patient described in *4* did not contain recombined VDJ variable-region gene sequences.
6. A patient was considered to have a B-cell deficiency because serum levels of IgE and IgD were undetectable despite proper concentrations of IgG and IgM.

Bibliography

Immunology Today: Issues contain understandable reviews on current topics in immunology.

Janeway CA, Travers P: *Immunobiology,* ed 2, New York, 1996, Garland.

Male D et al: *Advanced immunology,* ed 3, St Louis, 1996, Mosby.

Roitt I, Brostoff J, Male D: *Immunology,* ed 4, St Louis, 1996, Mosby.

Cellular Immune Responses

Cellular immune responses are mediated by mono-cyte-macrophage lineage cells, large granular lymphocytes (LGLs) (natural killer [NK] cells), and T cells. The **LGLs** provide early responses to infection, releasing lymphokines and killing virally infected and tumor (NK) cells and antibody-decorated cells (antibody-dependent cellular cytotoxicity [ADCC]). Cells of the **monocyte-macrophage** lineage bridge the gap between the innate and the antigen-specific protective responses as phagocytic, killer, cytokine-producing, and antigen-presenting cells. The **T cell** plays a central role in activating and controlling **(helping)** immune and inflammatory responses through the release of lymphokines. T cells are also very important for eliminating **(killing)** tumor cells and virally infected cells. T cells are morphologically similar to B cells but can be distinguished from B cells by specific cell surface antigenic markers. These include the antibody-like **T-cell receptor (TCR)** and its associated components **(CD3) (cluster of differentiation [CD])** and a receptor for sheep red blood cells **(CD2)**. These cells communicate through direct cell-to-cell interactions and with cytokines.

T-CELL DEVELOPMENT

T-cell precursors develop into T cells in the **thymus** (Figure 13-1). Contact with the thymic epithelium and hormones such as thymosin, thymulin, and thymopoietin II in the thymus promote extensive proliferation and differentiation of the individual's T-cell populations during fetal development. While in the thymus, genetic events generate numerous TCRs, each expressed on a different T-cell clone. T cells that react with the host (self-reactive) are forced into committing suicide (apoptosis), and the remaining T cells differentiate into the subpopulations of T cells.

The **helper T cells (CD4)** activate and control immune and inflammatory responses by the release of lymphokines (soluble messengers). Helper T cells interact with peptide antigens presented on **class II major histocompatibility (MHC) molecules** expressed on antigen-presenting cells (macrophages and B cells) (Figure 13-2). The vocabulary of lymphokines secreted by a spe-

cific CD4 T cell in response to antigenic challenge further distinguishes the CD4 T cell as a TH1 or a TH2 cell. TH1 cells promote inflammatory responses, especially important for controlling intracellular (mycobacterial and viral) and fungal infections, as well as certain types of antibody production. TH2 cells promote antibody and memory responses. A TH3 subtype has recently been described; it is involved in immunoglobulin A (IgA) production. The TH1 and TH2 responses are antagonistic.

Cytolytic and suppressor T cells (CD8) "patrol" the body for cells expressing virus or tumorlike abnormal proteins presented by the **class I MHC molecules**. Class I MHC molecules are found on all nucleated cells.

T-CELL CHARACTERISTICS

T cells were initially distinguished from B cells by their ability to bind sheep red blood cells and form rosettes. T cells are defined using antibodies that distinguish their cell surface molecules. The T-cell surface proteins include the TCR, the CD4 and CD8 coreceptors, accessory proteins that promote recognition and activation, lymphokine receptors, and adhesion proteins. These proteins determine the types of cell-to-cell interactions for the T cell and therefore the functions of the cell.

The **TCR complex** is a combination of the antigen recognition structure **(TCR)** and cell-activation machinery **(CD3)** (Figure 13-3). There are two types of T-cell antigen receptors, the TCR1, consisting of gamma and delta chains, and the TCR2, consisting of alpha and beta chains. T cells expressing TCR1 **(gamma/delta T cells)** are more primitive T cells, are generally restricted to mucosal epithelium and other tissue locations, and are important for stimulating mucosal immunity. TCR2 is expressed on most T cells **(alpha/beta T cells)**, and these cells are primarily responsible for antigen-activated immune responses.

As for the B cell, each T-cell clone recognizes and responds to a different antigen, as defined by its TCR. Each TCR molecule is made up of two different polypeptide chains. Like antibody, each TCR chain has a constant and a variable region. The repertoire of T-cell

FIGURE 13-1 Human T-cell development. T-cell markers are useful for the identification of the differentiation stages of the T cell and for characterizing T-cell leukemias and lymphomas. *Tdt,* Cytoplasmic terminal deoxynucleotide transferase.

FIGURE 13-2 MHC restriction and antigen presentation to T cells. *Left,* Antigenic peptides bound to class I MHC molecules are presented to the TCR on CD8+ killer/suppressor T cells. *Right,* Antigenic peptides bound to class II MHC molecules on the antigen-presenting cell *APC* (B cell or macrophage) are presented to CD4+ helper and delayed-type hypersensitivity T cells.

FIGURE 13-3 T-cell receptor. The TCR consists of different subunits. Antigen recognition occurs through the alpha/beta (α/β) or gamma/delta (γ/δ) subunits. The CD3 complex of gamma (γ), delta (δ), epsilon (ϵ), and zeta (ζ) subunits promotes T-cell activation. *V,* Variable region; *C,* constant region.

FIGURE 13-4 TCR and gene loci. Note the similarity to immunoglobulin genes.

antigen receptors is very large and can identify a tremendous number of antigenic specificities (estimated to be able to recognize 10^{15} separate epitopes). The genetic mechanisms for the development of this diversity are similar to those for antibody (Figure 13-4). The TCR gene is made up of multiple V, D, and J segments, similar to the antibody gene. Different V, D, and J segments recombine to form different TCR genes. Unlike the antibody genes, more than one D segment can be present in the TCR gene, which increases the potential for diversity. However, somatic mutation does not occur for the TCR gene.

The **CD3 complex** is found on all T cells and consists of the gamma, (epsilon)$_2$, epsilon, and (zeta)$_2$ polypeptide chains. The CD3 complex is the signal transduction unit for the TCR. **Tyrosine protein kinases** associate with the CD3 complex when antigen is bound to the TCR complex, promoting a cascade of protein phosphorylations and other events leading to activation of the T cell and production of interleukin-2 (IL-2) and its receptor (IL-2R).

The **CD4 and CD8** proteins are coreceptors for the TCR because they facilitate the interaction of the TCR with the antigen-presenting MHC molecule and can enhance the activation response. The **CD4** molecule is present on and identifies the helper or delayed type hypersensitivity (DTH) T cells. CD4 binds to class II MHC molecules on the surface of antigen-presenting cells. **CD8** is present on and identifies the killer or suppressor T cells. CD8 binds to class I MHC molecules on the surface of the target cell. Class I MHC molecules are expressed on all nucleated cells (see later section). The cytoplasmic tails of CD4 and CD8 associate with a protein tyrosine kinase (p56^{lck}), which enhances the TCR-induced activation of the cell on binding the antigen-presenting or target cell. CD4 or CD8 are found on alpha/beta T cells but not gamma/delta T cells.

Accessory molecules expressed on the T cell include several protein receptors on the cell surface that interact with proteins on antigen-presenting and target cells, leading to activation of the T cell, promoting tighter interactions between the cells, or facilitating the killing of the target cell. These accessory molecules include **CD45RA (native T cells) and CD45RO (memory T cells)**, a transmembrane protein tyrosine phosphatase; **CD28** and **CTLA-4** (on activated T cells), which binds to the **B7** protein on antigen-presenting cells to deliver a costimulation signal to the T cell; **CD5**, which is present on all T cells and promotes activation on binding to its ligand on B cells; and the **Fas ligand (FasL),** which initiates apoptosis in a target cell that expresses **Fas** on its cell surface.

Adhesion molecules tighten the interaction of the T cell with the antigen-presenting cell or target cell and may also promote activation. Adhesion molecules include **lymphocyte function antigen (LFA-1)**, which interacts with the **intracellular adhesion molecules (ICAM-1, ICAM-2, and ICAM-3)** on the target cell. **CD2** was originally identified by its ability to bind to sheep red blood cells **(erythrocyte receptor).** CD2 binds to LFA-3 on the target cell and promotes cell-to-cell adhesion and T cell activation. **Very late antigens (VLA-4 and VLA-5)** are expressed on activated cells later in the response and bind to fibronectin on target cells to enhance the interaction.

T cells express receptors for many lymphokines that activate and regulate T-cell function. The **lymphokine receptors** activate protein kinase cascades on binding of lymphokine to deliver their signal to the nucleus. IL-1 and IL-2 receptors are activation receptors. The **IL-2 receptor (IL-2R)** is composed of three subunits. Beta/gamma subunits are on most T cells (also NK cells) and have intermediate affinity for IL-2. The alpha subunit is synthesized in response to cell activation, forming high-affinity alpha/beta/gamma **IL-2R.** Binding of IL-2 to the IL-2R initiates a growth-stimulating signal to the T cell, which also promotes the production of more IL-2 and IL-2R. Other lymphokine receptors regulate the growth and lymphokine expression of the T cell.

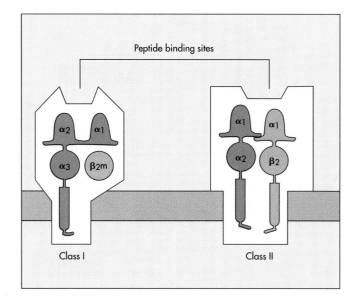

FIGURE 13-5 Structure of class I and II MHC molecules. The class I MHC molecules consist of two subunits: the heavy chain and beta-2-microglobulin. Class II MHC molecules consist of two subunits: alpha and beta.

ANTIGEN PRESENTATION TO T CELLS

Unlike cell surface immunoglobulin on B cells that sense ("taste" or "sniff") the presence of soluble foreign molecules that float past the cell, the TCR on the T cell must be presented with the relevant epitope, which is cleaved from the protein and cradled in a molecular holder on the surface of antigen-presenting cells for the T cell to "touch" and respond. **Class I and II MHC** molecules provide the molecular cradle for the peptide. The **CD8** molecule on cytolytic/suppressor T cells binds to and enhances the interaction with class I MHC molecules on target cells. This allows the T cell to sense the presence of self-antigenic and non-self-antigenic peptides. The **CD4** molecule on helper/DTH T cells binds to class II MHC molecules on antigen-presenting cells.

Class I MHC molecules are found on all nucleated cells and are the major determinate of "self." The class I MHC molecule, also known as **HLA** for human and H-2 for mouse, consists of two chains, a **variable heavy chain and a light chain (beta-2-microglobulin)** (Figure 13-5). Differences in the heavy chain of the HLA molecule between individuals *(allotypic differences)* elicit the T-cell response that prevents graft (tissue) transplantation. There are three separate HLA genes and proteins: **HLA-A, HLA-B,** and **HLA-C** (Figure 13-6). Each cell expresses a pair of different HLA-A, HLA-B, and HLA-C genes, one from each parent. The class I MHC molecule binds an antigenic peptide of nine amino acids in a cleft formed by the heavy chain. The class I MHC molecule presents antigenic peptides from within the cell **(endogenous)** to CD8-expressing T cells.

Class II MHC molecules are found *only on antigen-presenting cells*, cells that interact with CD4 T cells (e.g.,

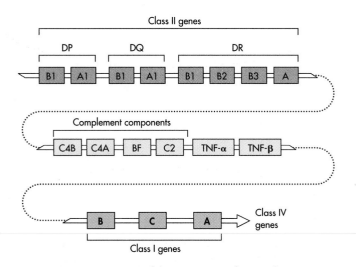

FIGURE 13-6 Genetic map of the MHC. Genes for complement components and tumor necrosis factor *(TNF)* are also within the MHC gene complex.

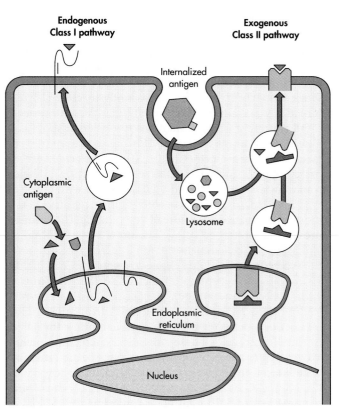

FIGURE 13-7 Antigen presentation by MHC molecules. *Endogenous* antigen (produced by the cell and analogous to cell trash) is proteolysed and transported into the endoplasmic reticulum. The peptide binds to a groove in the class I MHC molecule, allowing the complex to move to the cell surface for presentation to CD8+ T cells. *Exogenous* antigen (phagocytised) is degraded in lysosomes, transfers to endosomes containing the class II MHC molecules, binds to the class II MHC molecules, and is presented at the cell surface to CD4+ T cells.

macrophages, B cells). The class II MHC molecule (once known as *HLA-D*) is encoded by the **DP, DQ,** and **DR** loci. The class II MHC molecule is a dimer of alpha and beta subunits (Figure 13-5). The class II MHC molecule binds an antigenic peptide of 11 or more amino acids in a cleft formed by the alpha and beta subunits. The class II MHC molecule presents ingested **(exogenous)** antigenic peptides to CD4-expressing T cells.

Peptide Presentation by Class I and II MHC Molecules

Unlike antibodies that can recognize conformational epitopes, T-cell antigenic peptides must be linear epitopes. A T-cell antigen must be an 8 to 11 amino acid peptide that can bind to the molecular cleft of the class I or class II MHC molecule and still expose a T-cell epitope to the TCR. Because of these constraints, a protein may have only one or more T-cell antigenic peptides. The route of proteolysis producing the antigenic peptide differs for cells expressing "self" vs. "non-self" peptides **(endogenous route of antigen presentation)** to CD8 T cells in contrast to antigen-presenting cells, which present antigen to CD4 T cells **(exogenous route of antigen presentation)** (Figure 13-7).

Class I MHC molecules bind and present peptides from **endogenous** proteins—proteins synthesized within a cell. Class I MHC molecules present peptides, which are degraded from cellular proteins (trash) and then shuttled into the endoplasmic reticulum (ER). These peptides are often from nuclear proteins and glycoproteins. An antigenic peptide binds to the heavy chain of the class I MHC molecule as the class I MHC molecule is being assembled and is required for the class I MHC molecule to assemble properly, exit the ER, and proceed to the cell membrane. The peptide binding cleft of class I MHC molecule holds an 8 to 9 amino acid pep-

tide. During a **viral infection,** large quantities of viral proteins are produced and degraded into peptides, bound to class I MHC molecules and presented to CD8 T cells. **Transplanted cells** (grafts) express peptides on their MHC molecules that differ from the host and therefore may be recognized as foreign. **Tumor cells** often express peptides derived from abnormal or embryonic proteins, which may elicit responses in the host, since the host was not tolerized to these proteins.

Class II MHC molecules present peptides from exogenous proteins that were phagocytised and degraded in lysosomes by antigen-presenting cells, macrophages, or B cells. The class II MHC protein acquires its antigenic peptide as a result of a merging of the vesicular transport pathway (carrying newly synthesized class II MHC molecules) and the lysosomal degradation pathway (carrying phagocytised and proteolyzed proteins). The antigenic peptides displace a peptide attached in the ER and associate with the cleft formed in the class II MHC protein, and the complex is then delivered to the cell surface. The class II MHC peptide binding cleft holds an 11 to 12 amino acid peptide.

To analogize, all cells degrade their protein trash and then display it on the cell surface on class I MHC molecules. CD8 T cells policing the neighborhood are not alarmed by the normal, everyday peptide trash. A viral intruder would produce large amounts of viral peptide trash (e.g., beer cans, pizza boxes) displayed on class I MHC molecular garbage cans, which would alert the policing CD8 T cells. Antigen-presenting cells (macrophages and B cells) are similar to garbage collectors and gobble up the neighborhood trash, degrade it, display it on class II MHC molecules, and then move to a lymph node to present the antigenic peptides to the CD4 T cells in the "police station." Foreign antigens would alarm the CD4 T cells to release lymphokines and activate an immune response.

CD4 T-CELL ACTIVATION AND RESPONSE TO ANTIGEN

CD4 T helper cells are activated by the interaction of the TCR with antigenic peptide in the context of class II MHC molecules (Figure 13-8). The interaction is strengthened by CD4 binding to the class II MHC molecule and the linkage of adhesion proteins on the T cell and the antigen-presenting cell. The signal is transmitted to the nucleus through the CD3 complex by activation of phospholipase C, protein kinase C, intracellular calcium release, and specific protein kinase cascades. Several tyrosine protein kinase cascades are also activated by the CD3 complex. The result is the activation of specific transcription factors in the nucleus. However, a **costimulatory signal** is required to induce growth of the T cell as a fail-safe mechanism to ensure legitimate activation. Costimulatory signals are generated by the interaction of **CD28** or **CTLA-4** on the T cell, with the **B7-1** and **B7-2** molecules on the macrophage or B cell antigen-presenting cell, or by lymphokines binding to their receptors. Resting T cells require lymphokine signals (e.g., IL-1) to initiate growth of the cell. Partial activation (T-cell receptor interaction with MHC-peptide) without the IL-1 or CD28-B7 costimulation leads to **anergy** (unresponsiveness) or death of the T cell. This is a mechanism for eliminating self-reactive T cells in the developing thymus and development of **tolerance.** Proper activation of the helper T cell promotes production of IL-2 to activate other T cells and increases expression of IL-2 receptors on the cell surface, enhancing its own ability to bind and maintain activation by IL-2. Once activated, the IL-2 sustains the growth of the cell, and other lymphokines influence whether the T helper cell matures into a TH1 or a TH2 helper cell (see below).

TH1 and TH2 Cells

CD4 T cells are responsible for initiating DTH reactions and helping promote and enhance antibody responses. The CD4 T cells are divided into TH0, TH1, TH2, and a recently described TH3 class, depending on the lymphokines that they secrete and thus the responses that

FIGURE 13-8 The molecules involved in the interaction between T cells and antigen-presenting cells (*APC*). The various cytokines and their direction of action are also shown. Note that other cell surface molecules, as yet uncharacterized, may also be important in antigen presentation. *TNF*, Tumor necrosis factor; *GM-CSF*, granulocyte-macrophage colony stimulating factor; *IFN-α*, interferon-gamma; *ICAM-1*, intercellular adhesion molecule 1. (From Roitt I, Brostoff J, Male D: *Immunology*, ed 4, St Louis, 1996, Mosby.)

TABLE 13-1 Cytokines Produced by TH1, TH2, and TH0 Cells*

CYTOKINE	TH0	TH1	TH2
IFN-gamma	+	++	–
IL-2	+	++	–
TNF-beta (LT)	+	++	–
CHEMOKINES	+	+	–
GM-CSF	+	++	+
TNF-alpha	+	++	+
IL-3	+	++	++
IL-4	+	–	++
IL-5	+	–	++
IL-6		–	++
IL-10	+	–	++

IFN, Interferon; *TNF*, tumor necrosis factor; *GM-CSF*, granulocyte-macrophage colony-stimulating factor; +, minor product; ++, major product; –, no product

*The relative ability of TH0, TH1, and TH2 cells to produce different cytokines after activation. The cytokines that differentiate TH1 and TH2 cells are boxed.

they induce (Figure 13-9 and Table 13-1). TH0 cells produce IL-2, interferon-gamma (IFN-gamma), and IL-4. TH0 cells mature into either TH1 or TH2 cells, depending on the antigen, concentration of antigen, antigen-presenting cell, and lymphokine stimulation. Once activated, the TH1 and TH2 cells produce lymphokines that stimulate their own growth (autocrine) but inhibit the growth of the other type of CD4 T cell.

TH1 cells are more likely to be activated by large amounts of antigen, macrophage presentation of anti-

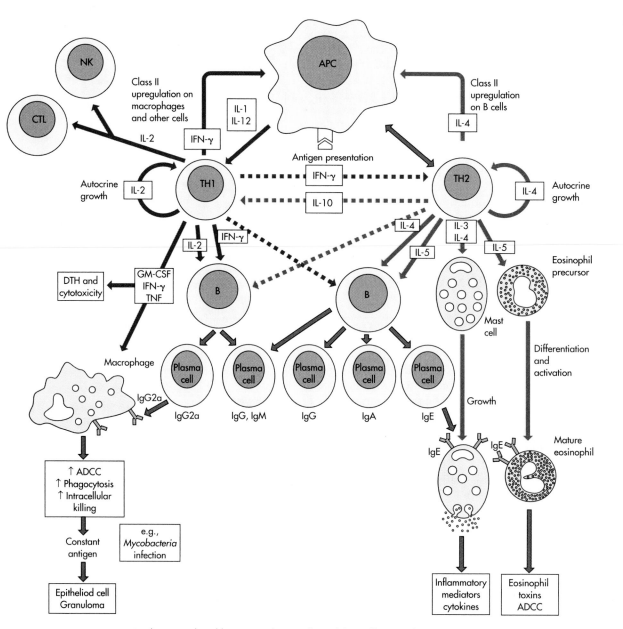

FIGURE 13-9 Cytokines produced by TH1 and TH2 cells and their effects on the immune system. TH1 responses are initiated by IL-12 and interferon-gamma and TH2 responses by IL-4. TH1 cells promote inflammation and the production of complement and macrophage-binding antibody *(solid blue lines)* and inhibit TH2 responses *(dotted blue lines)*. TH2 cells promote humoral response *(solid red lines)* and inhibit TH1 responses *(dotted red lines)*. *APC,* Antigen-presenting cell; *CTL,* cytotoxic T cell; *GM-CSF,* granulocyte-macrophage colony-stimulating factor; *TNF,* tumor necrosis factor; *DTH,* delayed-type hypersensitivity; *ADCC,* antibody-dependent cellular cytotoxicity.

gen, and secretion of **IL-2, IFN-gamma,** and **tumor necrosis factor-beta (TNF-beta) (lymphotoxin).** These lymphokines stimulate inflammatory responses and the production of IgM and specific subclasses of IgG. TH1 cells are stimulated by IL-2 and inhibited by IL-10. **TH2** cells are activated by B-cell, dendritic cell, or macrophage presentation of antigen and release **IL-4, IL-5, IL-6,** and **IL-10.** These lymphokines encourage antibody production and stimulate B-cell differentiation, resulting in immunoglobulin class switching and mem-

ory cell and plasma cell production. TH2 cells are stimulated by IL-4 and inhibited by IFN-gamma. Lymphokines and cytokines secreted by TH1 and TH2 cells include IL-3, TNF-alpha, granulocyte-macrophage colony-stimulating factor, and chemokines. **TH3** cells are characterized by their production of **TGF-beta,** which is important for promoting B-cell differentiation to produce IgA.

In summary, the TH1 response *(1 meaning first)* usually occurs first, often early in the infection, when antigen is abundant and is stimulated by macrophage presentation of antigen. The TH1 responses amplify local inflammatory reactions. The TH2 response *(2 meaning second)* results later, when antigen concentrations are lower and B cells expressing specific cell surface antibody can capture, process, and present the antigen. B-cell presentation of antigen to TH2 cells initiates an activation circuit, stimulating the growth and clonally expanding the helper T cells and B cells, which are specific for the same antigen. The TH2 response results in maturation of the immune response to the antigen and the development of antibody and memory cells for future protection. The inflammatory responses and complement-binding antibody stimulated by TH1 responses are important for eliminating intracellular infections (e.g., viruses, bacteria, and parasites) and fungi but are associated with autoimmune inflammatory diseases (e.g., multiple sclerosis, Crohn's disease, rheumatoid arthritis). Stimulation of TH2 responses against intracellular infections can exacerbate these infectious diseases by prematurely shutting off the TH1 responses but can modulate inflammatory and autoimmune diseases.

CD8 T CELLS

CD8 T cells include **cytotoxic T cells (CTLs) and suppressor cells.** CTLs are part of the **TH1 response** and are important for eliminating virally infected and tumor cells. CD8 T cells can also secrete TH1-like lymphokines. Less is known about suppressor cells.

The CTL response is initiated when CTL precursors are stimulated by binding of TCR and CD8 to the antigenic peptide on class I MHC molecules and a costimulatory signal from IL-2 or a CD28-B7 interaction (Figure 13-10). The activated CD8 T cells divide and differentiate into mature CTLs. The T cell and target cell are bound tightly together by interactions of the TCR with antigen-bearing class I MHC proteins and adhesion molecules on both cells (similar to a zipper). **Granules** containing toxic molecules, **granzymes** (esterases), and a pore-forming protein **(perforin)** move to the site of interaction and release their contents into the pocket formed between the T cell and target cell. Perforin generates holes in the target cell membrane to allow the granule contents to enter and destroy the target cell. T cells can also initiate **apoptosis** (programmed cell death) in target cells through the interaction of the **FasL** on the CTL with the **Fas** protein on the target cell surface. Apoptosis is characterized by degradation of the target cell DNA into discrete fragments of multiples of approximately 200 base pairs and disruption of internal membranes. Neurons and cells in the eye do not express the Fas protein (immune privileged) and cannot be killed by this mechanism. TH1 CD4 T cells also express FasL and can initiate apoptosis in target cells.

Suppressor T cells provide antigen-specific regulation of T helper cell function. Like CTLs, suppressor T cells are class I MHC restricted.

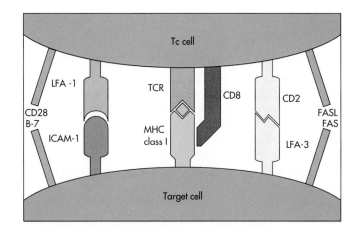

FIGURE 13-10 Interactions between CD8 CTL and target cells. The Fas-FasL interaction promotes apoptosis. *ICAM-1,* Intercellular adhesion molecule 1. (From Roitt I, Brostoff J, Male D: *Immunology,* ed 4, St Louis, 1996, Mosby.)

NATURAL KILLER CELLS

NK cells are an important part of the natural immune system. NK cells are often the first cellular response to a viral infection, are important for their antitumor activity, and amplify inflammatory reactions after bacterial infection. NK cells are also responsible for **ADCC,** in which they bind and kill antibody-coated cells.

NK cells are LGLs that share many characteristics with T cells. NK cells are stimulated by IFN-alpha and IFN-beta (produced early in response to a viral infection), TNF-alpha and IL-12 (produced by activated macrophages), and IL-2 (produced by CD4 T cells). The NK cells also express many of the same cell surface markers as T cells (e.g., CD2, CD7, IL-2R, **Fc receptor for IgG,** and **FasL**). Activated NK cells produce IFN-gamma, IL-1, and granulocyte-macrophage colony-stimulating factor on activation, which stimulate the macrophage. The granules in an NK cell contain **perforin** and **granzymes,** which are similar to the granules in a CD8 CTL. Unlike T cells, NK cells do not express TCR or CD3. NK cells neither recognize a specific antigen nor require presentation of antigen by MHC-restricted antigens. The NK system does not involve memory or require sensitization and cannot be enhanced by specific immunization.

The NK cell binds to carbohydrates and other cell surface proteins on target cells and kill the cell unless it receives an **inhibitory signal** on binding (killer-cell inhibitory receptors) to **HLA-C** or other MHC molecules. The proper expression of class I MHC on the cell surface is like a secret password that sends an inhibitory signal to prevent NK activation and killing of the target cell. Binding of the NK cell to antibody-coated target cells (ADCC) also initiates killing but without control by the inhibitory signal. The **killing mechanisms** are similar to those of CTLs, including **perforin** disruption of the target cell membrane, the toxic effects of the **granzymes,** and the **FasL-Fas** protein induction of apoptosis.

Lymphokine-Activated Killer Cells

Lymphokine-activated killer (LAK) cells are IL-2–activated effectors that are able to bind and kill many types of tumor and virally infected cells. Most LAK cell activity is derived from NK cells, but some T cells also become LAK cells.

CELLS OF THE MONOCYTE-MACROPHAGE LINEAGE

Monocytes are myeloid cells and develop from the same lineage as polymorphonuclear granulocytes. Macrophages and cells of the macrophage lineage (see Figure 11-6) develop from the monocyte and differ depending on their tissue location. Langerhans' cells (skin), follicular dendritic cells (lymph node and spleen), and interdigitating cells (lymph node and spleen) also develop from the monocyte and are nonphagocytic antigen-presenting cells.

The **surface markers** on monocyte-macrophages correspond to the cells' functions. These cells express receptors for opsonins (e.g., immunoglobulin Fc receptors [Fc-gamma RI, Fc-gamma RII, Fc-gamma RIII] and complement receptors [CR1, CR3]); lectins (specific sugar-binding proteins such as mannosyl-fucosyl receptors) and a receptor for the lipopolysaccharide-binding protein (CD14) to facilitate bacterial uptake; adhesion molecules (e.g., LFA-1) to promote cell-to-cell interactions; and the B7 and class II MHC proteins to allow antigen presentation to T cells.

Macrophages are activated to different functional levels by different stimuli. Ingestion of microbes promotes the release of IL-1, IL-12, and TNF, which initiate inflammatory reactions. Sufficient levels of TNF or IFN-gamma, produced by NK and CD4 TH1 cells, activate killing mechanisms in the macrophage (angry macrophage). The activated macrophage can kill phagocytised microbes and virus-infected and tumor cells. Continuous stimulation of macrophages by T cells, as in the case of an unresolved mycobacterial infection, pro-motes the fusion of macrophages into multinucleate giant cells and epithelioid cells that surround the infection and form a granuloma.

QUESTIONS

1. The following results were obtained on immunization with tetanus toxoid (TT) with or without cholera toxin (CT):

Vaccine	Antibody
TT	Serum IgG anti-TT
CT	Serum IgG, IgA, IgE anti-CT
	Secretory IgA anti-CT
TT + CT	Serum IgG, IgA, IgE anti-TT
	Secretory IgG anti-TT
	Serum IgG, IgA, IgE anti-CT
	Secretory IgA anti-CT

From these results, answer the following questions:
a. What effect did the CT have on the TT immunization?
b. Which subset of CD4 T cells was likely to be involved in each of the immunizations?
c. Which lymphokines were likely to be important in promoting the different immunization responses?

2. The importance of specific molecules can be determined by developing genetically deficient strains of mice (knock-out mice) and then testing the immune systems of these mice. Describe the immune functions that should be missing and the cell types that should be affected for the mice deficient in the following molecules:

a. Class I MHC   e. CD4
b. Class II MHC   f. B7-1 and B7-2
c. TCR gamma/delta   g. IFN-gamma
d. IL-2 receptor   h. IL-1

Bibliography

Immunology Today: Issues contain understandable reviews on current topics in immunology.
Male D et al: *Advanced immunology,* ed 3, St Louis, 1996, Mosby.
Roitt I, Brostoff J, Male D: *Immunology,* ed 4, St Louis, 1996, Mosby.

CHAPTER 14

Immune Responses to Infectious Agents

The previous chapters introduced the different components of host protection. This chapter describes how the different components interact to produce a protective response and the immunopathogenic consequences that may arise as a result of the response. The importance of any one of these protective responses becomes obvious when it is genetically deficient or blocked by chemotherapy, disease, or infection (e.g., acquired immunodeficiency syndrome [AIDS]).

We have three basic lines of protection against invasion by infectious agents: **natural barriers,** which restrict entry of the agent (e.g., skin, mucus, ciliated epithelium, gastric acid, bile); **innate antigen-nonspecific immune defenses,** which provide rapid, local responses to challenge by an invader (e.g., fever, interferon, neutrophils, macrophages, natural killer [NK] cells); and **antigen-specific immune responses,** which specifically target, attack, and eliminate the invaders that make it past the first two defenses (e.g., antibody, T cells). The importance of each of these different mechanisms for resolving an infection differs for different agents (Table 14-1). Phagocytic cells, the alternative pathway of complement and antibody, are most important for resolving bacterial infections, except for intracellular bacteria. Intracellular bacteria (i.e., mycobacteria) are inaccessible to antibody and therefore require **delayed type hypersensitivity (DTH)**–related T-cell and macrophage responses. Interferon, NK, and T-cell responses are most important for viral infections. Antibody also plays a role in antiviral immunity, especially in restricting the spread of virus by viremia. **DTH** responses are especially important for antifungal protection. Activated macrophage, T-cell, eosinophil, and immunoglobulin E (IgE)–mast cell responses are important for protection against parasitic infections. The protections initiated by **TH1-type immune responses** (interferon-gamma, cytolytic and inflammatory responses) are especially important for resolving infections by intracellular bacteria, viruses, fungi, and parasites. **TH2 responses** (humoral) are most important for resolving bacterial and parasitic infections and for the establishment of memory cells and production of secretory immunoglobulin A (IgA) for the protection of mucosal surfaces.

BARRIERS TO INFECTION

The **skin** and **mucous membranes** serve as barriers to most infectious agents (Figure 14-1 and Table 14-2), with few exceptions (e.g., papilloma virus, dermatophytes ["skin loving" fungi]). Free fatty acids produced in sebaceous glands and by organisms on the skin surface, lactic acid in perspiration, and the low pH and relatively dry environment of the skin all form unfavorable conditions for the survival of most organisms.

The mucosal epithelium covering the orifices of the body is protected by mucus secretions and cilia. For example, pulmonary airways are coated with mucus, which is continuously transported toward the mouth by ciliated epithelial cells. Large airborne particles get caught in the mucus, whereas small particles (0.05 to 3 μ, the size of viruses or bacteria) that reach the alveoli are phagocytised by macrophages and transported out of the air spaces. Cigarette smoke or other pollutants, as well as some bacteria and viruses (e.g., *Bordetella pertussis,* influenza virus), can interfere with this clearance mechanism by damaging the ciliated epithelial cells, thus rendering the patient susceptible to secondary bacterial pneumonia. Antimicrobial substances (lysozyme, lactoferrin, and secretory IgA) found in secretions at mucosal surfaces (e.g., tears, mucus, saliva) also provide protection. Lysozyme induces lysis of bacteria by cleaving the polysaccharide backbone of the peptidoglycan of gram-positive bacteria. Lactoferrin, an iron-binding protein, deprives microbes of the free iron they need for growth.

The **acidic environment of the stomach,** bladder, and kidneys and the **bile** of the intestines inactivate many viruses and bacteria. Urinary flow also limits the establishment of infection.

Body temperature and especially **fever** limit or prevent the growth of many microbes. In addition, the immune response is more efficient at elevated temperatures.

ANTIBACTERIAL RESPONSES

Figure 14-2 illustrates the progression of protective responses to a bacterial challenge. Protection is initiated on

TABLE 14-1 Antimicrobial Defenses for Infectious Agents

	BACTERIA	INTRACELLULAR BACTERIA	VIRUSES	FUNGI	PARASITES
Neutrophils	++	—	—	—	—
Macrophages	+	+	+	+	—
Complement	+	—	—	—	—
NK cells	—	—	+	—	—
CD4 TH1—DTH	—†	+	++	—	—
CD8—CTL	—	—	++	—	—
Antibody	++	+	+	+	++(IgE)*

++, Major component of the antimicrobial defense; −, possible role; +, important; *DTH*, delayed type hypersensitivity.
*Immunoglubulin E and mast cells are especially important for worm infections.
†DTH is important for intracellular infections.

BOX 14-1 Summary of Antibacterial Responses

COMPLEMENT

Alternative pathway activated by bacterial surfaces
Classical pathway activated later by antibody-antigen complexes
Production of chemotactic and anaphylotoxic proteins (C3a, C5a)
Opsonization of bacteria (C3b)
Promotion of killing of gram-negative bacteria

NEUTROPHILS

Important antibacterial phagocytic cell
Killing by oxygen-dependent and oxygen-independent mechanisms

MACROPHAGES

Important antibacterial phagocytic cell
Killing by oxygen-dependent and oxygen-independent mechanisms
Production of IL-1, IL-6, IL-12, TNF–alpha, TNF–beta, and Ifn-alpha
Activation of acute-phase and inflammatory responses
Presentation of antigen to CD4 T cell

T CELLS

TH1 CD4 responses important for intracellular bacterial infections
TH2 CD4 response important for all bacterial infections
CD8 T cytolytic T cells not very important

ANTIBODY

Binding to surface structures of bacteria (fimbriae, lipoteichoic acid, capsule)
Blocking of attachment
Opsonization of bacteria for phagocytosis
Promotion of complement action
Promotion of clearance of bacteria
Neutralization of toxins and toxic enzymes

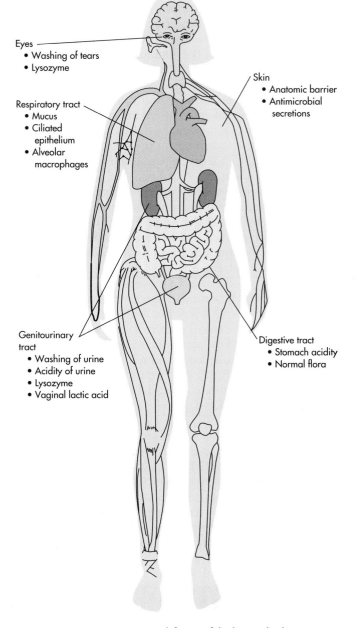

Eyes
• Washing of tears
• Lysozyme

Respiratory tract
• Mucus
• Ciliated epithelium
• Alveolar macrophages

Skin
• Anatomic barrier
• Antimicrobial secretions

Genitourinary tract
• Washing of urine
• Acidity of urine
• Lysozyme
• Vaginal lactic acid

Digestive tract
• Stomach acidity
• Normal flora

FIGURE 14-1 Barrier defenses of the human body.

TABLE 14-2	Nonspecific Humoral Defense Mechanisms	
FACTOR	**FUNCTION**	**SOURCE**
Lysozyme	Catalyses hydrolysis of bacterial peptidoglycan	Tears, saliva, nasal secretions, body fluids, lysosomal granules
Lactoferrin, transferrin	Bind iron and compete with microorganisms for it	Specific granules of PMNs
Lactoperoxidase	May be inhibitory to many microorganisms	Milk and saliva
Beta-lysin	Is effective mainly against gram-positive bacteria	Thrombocytes, normal serum
Chemotactic factors	Induce directed migration of PMNs, monocytes, and other cells	Bacterial substances, products of cell injury, denatured proteins, complement, and chemokines
Properdin	Activates complement in the absence of antibody-antigen complex	Normal plasma
Defensins	Block cell-transport activities	Polymorphonuclear granules

PMNs, Polymorphonuclear neutrophils.

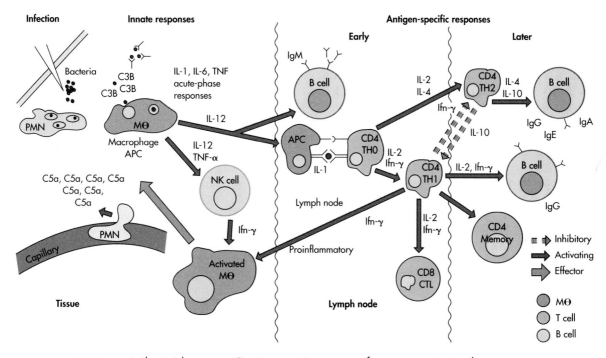

FIGURE 14-2 Antibacterial responses. First, innate antigen-nonspecific responses attract and promote PMN and macrophage responses. Antigen-presenting cells and antigen reach the lymph node to activate early immune responses (TH1 and IgM). Later, TH 2 mature antibody responses and memory cells are developed. *PMN*, Polymorphonuclear neutrophil; *IL*, interleukin; *TNF*, tumor necrosis factor; *Ifn*, interferon; *APC*, antigen-presenting cell.

activation of innate responses on a local basis and progresses to acute-phase and antigen-specific responses on a systemic scale. A summary of all antibacterial responses is presented in Box 14-1.

Acute inflammation is an early defense mechanism to contain an infection, prevent its spread from the initial focus, and signal subsequent specific immune responses. Inflammatory responses are beneficial but can also cause tissue damage and as a result contribute to the symptoms of disease. The three major events in acute inflammation

are (1) expansion of capillaries to increase blood flow (seen as blushing or a rash); (2) increased permeability of the microvasculature structure to allow escape of fluid, plasma proteins, and leukocytes from the circulation (source of edema); and (3) exit of leukocytes from the capillaries and accumulation at the site of injury.

Activation of Response

Bacterial components are excellent activators of the innate antigen-nonspecific protective responses (Box

BOX 14-2 **Bacterial Components that Activate Protective Responses**

Direct activation
  Lipopolysaccharide (endotoxin)
  Lipoteichoic acid
  Lipoarabinomannan
  Polyanions
  Formyl peptides (formyl-methionyl-leucyl-phenylalanine)
Chemotactic
  Peptidoglycan fragments
  Cell surface activation of alternative pathways of complement (C5a)

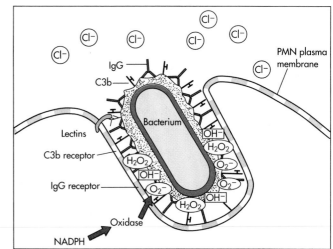

FIGURE 14-3 Killing of bacteria by a phagocyte. Bacteria are bound directly or are opsonized by mannose-binding protein, immunoglobulin G *(IgG)* and/or C3b, promoting their adherence and uptake by phagocytes. Bactericides and hydrogen peroxide are produced and released in response to bacterial adherence to kill the bacteria. *NADPH,* Reduced form of nicotinamide-adenine dinucleotide phosphate.

14-2). The peptidoglycan layer in bacterial cell walls (teichoic acid and peptidoglycan fragments of gram-positive bacteria) and lipopolysaccharide (LPS) in gram-negative bacterial cell walls can activate the **alternative complement pathway (properdin)** in the absence of antibody and with **mannose-binding protein** can activate the **classical complement pathway**. LPS (endotoxin) is a very strong activator of macrophages, B cells, and selected other cells (e.g., endothelial cells).

Activation of the **complement system** by the **alternative pathway** or via the mannose-binding protein (see Chapter 12) is a very early and important antibacterial defense. Complement activates inflammatory responses and can also directly kill gram-negative bacteria and, to a much lesser extent, gram-positive bacteria (the thick peptidoglycan of gram-positive bacteria shields the cell from lysis). Activation of the complement cascade by gram-positive or gram-negative bacteria provides **chemotactic factors (C5a)** to attract neutrophils and macrophages to the site of infection; **anaphylotoxins (C3a and C5a)** to stimulate mast cell release of histamine to increase vascular permeability, which allows access to the infection site; and **opsonins (C3b)**, which bind to bacteria and promote their phagocytosis. **Antibody (IgM or IgG)**, which is present later in an infection, enhances the complement response through activation of the classic **complement cascade**.

Kinins and clotting factors induced by tissue damage are also involved in inflammation (e.g., factor XII [Hageman factor], bradykinin, fibrinopeptides). These factors increase vascular permeability and are chemotactic for leukocytes. Products produced during arachidonic acid metabolism also affect inflammation. These products include **prostaglandins** and **leukotrienes,** which can mediate essentially every aspect of acute inflammation.

Phagocytosis

Polymorphonuclear neutrophils (PMNs), monocytes, and occasionally eosinophils are the first cells to appear in response to acute inflammation; they are followed later by macrophages. Chemotactic factors, including complement components (C5a) and bacterial products (e.g., formyl-methionyl-leucyl-phenylalanine [f-met-leu-phe]), are powerful chemoattractants for phagocytic cells.

Neutrophils provide a major antibacterial response. They are attracted to the site of infection and phagocytise and then kill the internalized bacteria. An increased number of neutrophils in the blood, body fluid (e.g., cerebrospinal fluid), or tissue indicates a bacterial infection. The mobilization of neutrophils is accompanied by a "left shift," an increase in the number of immature **band forms** released from the bone marrow (*left* refers to the beginning of a chart of neutrophil development).

Phagocytosis of bacteria by macrophages and neutrophils involves several steps, including attachment, internalization, and digestion. **Attachment** of the bacteria to the macrophage is mediated by **receptors for bacterial carbohydrates (lectins** [specific sugar-binding proteins]), **receptors for opsonins** (e.g., complement [C3b], mannose-binding protein receptors), fibronectin receptors (especially for *Staphylococcus aureus*), and Fc receptors for antibody. After attachment, the particle is surrounded by a portion of plasma membrane, which forms a phagocytic vacuole around the microbe. This vacuole fuses with the primary lysosomes (macrophages) or granules (PMNs) to allow inactivation and digestion of the vacuole contents. Phagocytic killing is oxygen dependent or oxygen independent, depending on the antimicrobial chemicals produced by the granules (Figure 14-3). Activation of macrophages is promoted

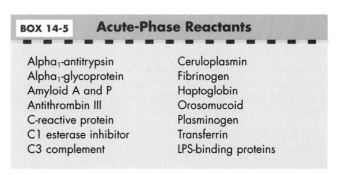

BOX 14-3	**Antibacterial Compounds of the Phagolysosome**

OXYGEN-DEPENDENT COMPOUNDS

Hydrogen peroxide: NADPH oxidase and NADH oxidase
Superoxide
Hydroxyl radicals (OH)
Activated halides (Cl⁻, I⁻, Br⁻): myeloperoxidase

OXYGEN-INDEPENDENT COMPOUNDS

Acids
Lysosome (degrades bacterial peptidoglycan)
Lactoferrin (chelates iron)
Defensins and other cationic proteins (damage membranes)
Proteases, elastase, cathepsin G

BOX 14-4	**Secreted Products of Macrophages with a Protective Effect on the Body**

Hematopoietic factors IL-6, IL-12, GM-CSF, G-CSF, M-CSF
Cytotoxic factors
Oxygen metabolites
  Hydrogen peroxide
  Superoxide anion
  Nitric oxide
Hydrolytic enzymes
  Collagenase
  Lipase
  Phosphatase
Endogenous pyrogen IL-1

Tumor necrosis factor
Interferon–alpha
Complement components
  C1 to C5
  Properdin
  Factors B, D, I, and H
Coagulation factors
Plasma proteins
Arachidonic acid metabolites
Prostaglandin
Thromboxane
Leukotrienes

---

by interferon-gamma (Ifn-gamma) (best), granulocyte-macrophage colony-stimulating factor (GM-CSF), tumor necrosis factor–alpha (TNF-alpha), and lymphotoxin (TNF–beta), which are produced earlier in the infection by NK cells or later by CD4 T cells. Activation of macrophages is required for macrophages to kill internalized microbes.

Oxygen-dependent killing is activated by a powerful oxidative burst that culminates in the formation of **hydrogen peroxide** and other antimicrobial substances (Box 14-3). The fusion of specific lysosomal granules and phagosomes permits the interaction of NADPH oxidase with cytochrome b. With the aid of quinone, this combination reduces oxygen to superoxide anion (O_2^-), which in the presence of a catalyst (e.g., superoxide dismutase) is converted to hydrogen peroxide. In the neutrophil, hydrogen peroxide with **myeloperoxidase** (released by primary granules during fusion to the phagolysosome) transforms chloride ions into **hypochlorous ions** that kill the microorganisms. **Nitric oxide** produced during this response has antimicrobial activity (as peroxynitrite [$N_2O_2^-$]) and is also a major second messenger molecule (like cyclic AMP), which enhances the inflammatory and other responses by activating guanylate cyclase.

The neutrophil can also mediate **oxygen-independent killing** on fusion of the phagosome with azurophil granules containing cationic proteins (e.g., cathepsin G) and specific granules containing lysozyme and lactoferrin. These proteins kill gram-negative bacteria by interrupting their cell membrane integrity, but they are far less effective against gram-positive bacteria, which are killed principally through the oxygen-dependent mechanism. The release of cytotoxins, cytokines, and other molecules (Box 14-4) can also injure endothelium and tissue.

BOX 14-5	**Acute-Phase Reactants**

Alpha₁-antitrypsin
Alpha₁-glycoprotein
Amyloid A and P
Antithrombin III
C-reactive protein
C1 esterase inhibitor
C3 complement

Ceruloplasmin
Fibrinogen
Haptoglobin
Orosomucoid
Plasminogen
Transferrin
LPS-binding proteins

Macrophages and **cells of the macrophage lineage** have several purposes in addition to the phagocytosis of bacteria and antigen (Figure 14-4). Macrophages trigger the **acute-phase response** by releasing interleukin-1 (IL-1), IL-6, tumor necrosis factor, and chemokines in response to LPS and the other bacterial cell wall components present during a bacterial challenge. Macrophages are also activated by tumor necrosis factor and IL-1 or interferon-gamma, which promote their passage into the affected tissue and activate oxygen-dependent killing. The macrophages also produce IL-12, which activates NK cells at the site of infection. NK cells can produce interferon-gamma to further activate macrophages.

Macrophages play a major role in the transition between the antigen-nonspecific and antigen-specific responses. Macrophages, especially dendritic cells, deliver the antigen to the lymph nodes for presentation to CD4 T cells and stimulate the T cells with IL-1.

The **acute-phase response** is triggered by inflammation, tissue injury, and release of IL-1, IL-6, tumor necrosis factor (produced by macrophages), prostaglandin E₁, and interferons associated with infection (Box 14-5). Acute-phase proteins that are produced

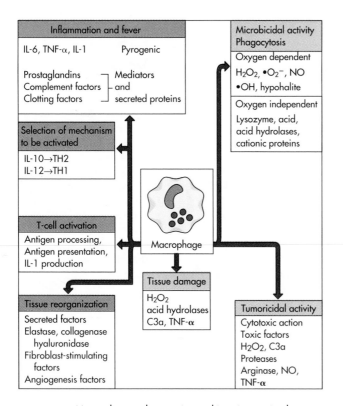

Inflammation and fever
IL-6, TNF-α, IL-1   Pyrogenic
Prostaglandins ⎤ Mediators
Complement factors ⎬ and
Clotting factors ⎦ secreted proteins

Microbicidal activity Phagocytosis
Oxygen dependent
H₂O₂, •O₂⁻, NO
•OH, hypohalite
Oxygen independent
Lysozyme, acid, acid hydrolases, cationic proteins

Selection of mechanism to be activated
IL-10→TH2
IL-12→TH1

T-cell activation
Antigen processing, Antigen presentation, IL-1 production

Macrophage

Tissue damage
H₂O₂ acid hydrolases C3a, TNF-α

Tissue reorganization
Secreted factors
Elastase, collagenase hyaluronidase
Fibroblast-stimulating factors
Angiogenesis factors

Tumoricidal activity
Cytotoxic action Toxic factors H₂O₂, C3a Proteases Arginase, NO, TNF-α

FIGURE 14-4 Macrophages phagocytise and inactivate microbes, present antigen, activate specific immunity, and promote inflammatory and acute-phase responses by releasing lymphokines. Activated macrophages can also kill tumor and other cells. *IL,* Interleukin; *TNF,* tumor necrosis factor. (From Roitt I, Brostoff J, Male D: *Immunology,* ed 4, St Louis, 1996, Mosby.)

and released into the serum include complement, coagulation proteins, LPS-binding proteins, transport proteins, protease inhibitors, and adherence proteins. **Fever** is triggered by IL-1, TNF–alpha, and interferon. IL-1 stimulation of the liver promotes production of C-reactive protein. C-reactive protein complexes with polysaccharides of numerous bacteria and fungi and activates the alternate complement pathway, which facilitates removal of these organisms from the body through increased phagocytosis. The acute-phase proteins *reinforce* the innate defenses against infection.

SPECIFIC IMMUNE RESPONSES TO BACTERIA

Ingestion of bacteria or bacterial antigens mobilizes the macrophages to move to the lymph nodes and interact with CD4 T cells (Figure 14-2). The initial interaction occurs with CD4 TH0 cells. Antigenic peptides (11+ amino acids) produced from phagocytised proteins (exogenous route) are bound to class II major histocompatibility complex (MHC) molecules and presented by the macrophage to the TH0 cells. The TH0 cells are activated by the interaction of its T-cell antigen receptor and CD4 with the antigenic peptide–class II MHC molecule complex in conjunction with the costimulatory

signals provided by the interaction of CD28 molecules on the T cells with the B7 molecule on the macrophage and by IL-1 and IL-12. The TH0 cells produce IL-2, interferon-gamma, and IL-4. Simultaneously, B cells expressing surface IgM and immunoglobulin D specific for the bacterial antigens are activated and produce IgM. Microbial cell wall polysaccharides, especially LPS, activate B cells and promote the specific IgM antibody responses. Swollen lymph nodes are an indication of lymphocyte activation in response to antigenic challenge.

Activated TH1 CD4 T cells promote and reinforce inflammatory responses (e.g., interferon-gamma activation of macrophage) and the class switching of B cells to produce complement-binding antibody (IgM, IgG). These are important for the early phases of an antibacterial response. TH1 responses are also *essential* for combating intracellular bacterial infections such as mycobacteria because these bacteria are protected from antibody. Interferon-gamma activates macrophage and other inflammatory processes (DTH) to kill the infected cell. Alternatively, the continuous stimulation induced by a chronic infection (e.g., tuberculosis) can promote fusion of macrophage to giant cells and epithelioid cells, forming a **granuloma** around the infection. **CD8 T cells** are not very important for antibacterial immunity.

CD4 TH2 T-cell responses occur later and are often initiated by the B-cell presentation of antigen. Binding of antigen to the cell surface antibody on B cells activates the B cell and also promotes uptake, processing of the antigen, and presentation of antigenic peptides on class II MHC molecules to the CD4 TH2 helper cell. The TH2 cell produces IL-4, IL-5, IL-6, and IL-10, which enhances IgG production and, depending on other factors, production of IgA or IgE. The TH2 response also promotes terminal differentiation of the B-cell to plasma-cell antibody factories or production of memory B cells.

Antibodies are the primary protection against extracellular bacteria and reinfection. Antibody is important for promoting complement activation, opsonizing the bacteria for phagocytosis, blocking bacterial adhesion, and neutralizing (inactivating) exotoxins (e.g., tetanospasmin, botulinum toxin) and other cytotoxic proteins produced by bacteria (e.g., degradative enzymes). Vaccine immunization with inactivated exotoxins (toxoids) is the primary means of protection against the potentially lethal effects of exotoxins.

IgM antibodies are produced early in the antibacterial response. IgM bound to bacteria activates the classic complement cascade, promoting both the direct killing of gram-negative bacteria and the inflammatory responses. The large size of IgM limits its ability to spread into the tissue. Later in the immune response, T-cell help promotes differentiation of the B-cell and immunoglobulin class switching to produce IgG. **IgG** antibodies are the predominant antibody, especially on rechallenge. IgG antibodies, except IgG4, fix complement and promote phagocytic uptake of the bacteria through Fc receptors on macrophages. The production of **IgA** requires TH2 and TH3 (transforming growth factor–beta) lymphokines. IgA is the primary secretory antibody and is important for protecting mucosal membranes. Secretory IgA contains the secretory component that promotes interaction and passage through mucosal epithelial cells. It neutralizes the binding of bacteria and their toxins.

Bacterial Immunopathogenesis

Activation of the inflammatory and acute-phase responses can initiate significant tissue and systemic damage. Acute inflammation promotes tissue damage and edema, and the responses to IL-1, IL-6, and tumor necrosis factor that are induced by endotoxin can lead to hemodynamic failure (see Chapter 19). Antibodies produced against bacterial antigens that share determinants with human proteins can initiate tissue destruction (e.g., antibodies produced in poststreptococcal glomerulonephritis and rheumatic fever). Nonspecific activation of CD4 T cells by **superantigens** (e.g., toxic shock syndrome toxin of *S. aureus*) promotes the production of large amounts of cytokines and eventually the death of the activated T cell. The sudden, massive release of cytokines can cause shock and severe tissue damage (e.g., toxic shock syndrome) (see Chapter 19).

Bacterial Evasion of Protective Responses

The mechanisms used by bacteria to evade host protective responses are discussed in Chapter 19 as virulence factors. These mechanisms include the inhibition of phagocytosis and intracellular killing in the phagocyte, inactivation of complement function, and intracellular growth (avoidance of antibody). Some microorganisms, including but not limited to mycobacteria (*Listeria* and *Brucella* species), survive and multiply within macrophages and use the macrophage as a protective reservoir or transport system to help spread the organisms throughout the body. However, activated macrophages can kill the intracellular pathogens.

SPECIFIC IMMUNE RESPONSES TO VIRUSES
Host Defenses Against Viral Infection

The immune response is the best and in most cases the only means of controlling a viral infection. The humoral and cellular immune responses are important for antiviral immunity. Unlike a bacterial infection, the ultimate goal of the antiviral immune response is to eliminate *both* the virus and the host cells harboring or replicating the virus. Interferon, NK cells, CD4 DTH responses, and CD8 cytotoxic killer cells are more important for viral infections than for bacterial infections. Failure to resolve the infection may lead to persistent or chronic infections or death.

Nonspecific Immune Defenses

Body temperature, fever, interferons, other cytokines, the mononuclear phagocyte system, and NK cells provide a local, rapid response to viral infection and also activate the specific immune defenses. Often, the nonspe-

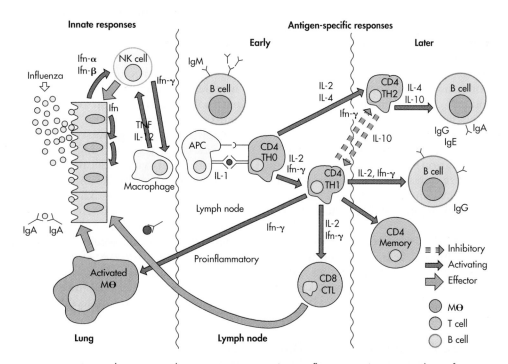

FIGURE 14-5 Antiviral responses. The response to a virus (e.g., influenza virus) initiates with interferon production and action and NK cells. Activation of antigen-specific immunity resembles the antibacterial response except that CD8 CTLs are important antiviral responses. *HLA,* Human leukocyte antigen; *Ifn,* interferon. *TNF,* tumor necrosis factor; *APC,* antigen-presenting cell.

TABLE 14-3	**Basic Properties of Human Interferons**		

| | **INTERFERON** | | |
PROPERTY	**ALPHA**	**BETA**	**GAMMA**
Previous designations	Leukocyte-IFN	Fibroblast-IFN	Immune IFN
	Type I	Type I	Type II
Genes	>20	1	1
Molecular weight (daltons)*			
Major subtypes	16,000-23,000	23,000	20,000-25,000
Cloned†	19,000	19,000	16,000
Glycosylation	No‡	Yes	Yes
pH 2 stability	Stable‡	Stable	Labile
Induction	Viruses	Viruses	Immune activation
Principal source	Epithelium, leukocytes	Fibroblast	Lymphocyte
Introns in gene	No	No	Yes
Homology with human IFN-alpha	100%	30%-50%	<10%

From White DO: *Antiviral chemotherapy, interferons and vaccines,* Basel, 1984, Karger; and Samuel CE: *Virol* 183:1-11, 1991.
IFN, Interferon.
*Molecular weight of monomeric form. Interferons often occur as polymers.
†Nonglycosylated form, as produced in bacteria by recombinant DNA technology.
‡Most subtypes, but not all.

cific defenses are sufficient to control a viral infection, thus preventing the occurrence of symptoms.

Viral infection can induce the release of cytokines (e.g., tumor necrosis factor, IL-1) and interferon from infected cells and macrophages. These soluble protein factors trigger local and systemic responses. Induction of fever and stimulation of the immune system are two of these systemic effects.

Body temperature and fever can limit the replication of or destabilize some viruses. Many viruses are less stable (e.g., herpes simplex virus) or cannot replicate (rhinoviruses) at 37° C or higher.

Cells of the **mononuclear phagocyte system** phagocytize the viral and cell debris from virus-infected cells. Macrophages in the liver (Kupffer's cells) and spleen rapidly filter many viruses from the blood. Antibody and complement bound to a virus facilitate its uptake by macrophages (**opsonization**). Macrophages also present antigen to T cells and release IL-1 and interferon to initiate the antigen-specific immune response. Activated macrophages can also distinguish and kill infected target cells.

NK cells are activated by interferon and specific lymphokines to kill virus-infected cells. Viral infection may reduce the expression of MHC antigens or alter the carbohydrates on cell surface proteins to provide cytolytic signals to the NK cell.

Interferon

Interferon was first described by Isaacs and Lindemann as a factor that "interferes" with the replication of many different viruses. Interferon is the body's *first* active defense against a viral infection, an "early warning system" at the local and systemic levels. In addition to activating a **target cell antiviral defense** to block viral replication, interferons also **activate the immune response** and **enhance T-cell recognition of the infected cell.** Interferon is a very important defense against infection but is also a cause of the **malaise, myalgia, chills,** and **fever (nonspecific influenza-like symptoms)** associated with many viral infections.

Interferon comprises a family of proteins that can be subdivided by several properties, including size, stability, cell of origin, and mode of action (Table 14-3). Interferon-alpha and interferon-beta share many properties, including structural homology and mode of action. **Interferon-alpha** is made by B cells, monocytes, and macrophages. **Interferon-beta** is made by fibroblasts and other cells in response to viral infection and other stimuli. **Interferon-gamma** is produced by activated T and NK cells later in the infection. Although interferon-gamma inhibits viral replication, its structure and mode of action differ from the other interferons. Interferon-gamma is also known as **macrophage activation factor** and is an integral component of the TH1 response.

One of the best inducers of interferon-alpha and interferon-beta production is double-stranded RNA, such as the replicative intermediates of RNA viruses (Box 14-6). One double-stranded RNA molecule per cell is sufficient to induce the production of interferon. Expression of the interferon gene is also induced when protein synthesis in the cell is reduced. This also decreases the concentration of a repressor protein of the interferon gene, which allows expression of the interferon gene. Nonviral interferon inducers include intracellular microorganisms (e.g., mycobacteria, fungi, and protozoa), immune stimulators or mitogens (e.g., endotoxins, phytohemagglutinin), double-stranded polynucleotides (e.g., poly I:C,

FIGURE 14-6 Induction of the antiviral state by interferon-alpha or interferon-beta. Interferon is produced in response to viral infection but does not affect the initially infected cell. The interferon binds to a cell surface receptor on other cells and induces production of antiviral enzymes (antiviral state). The infection and production of double-stranded RNA activates the antiviral activity.

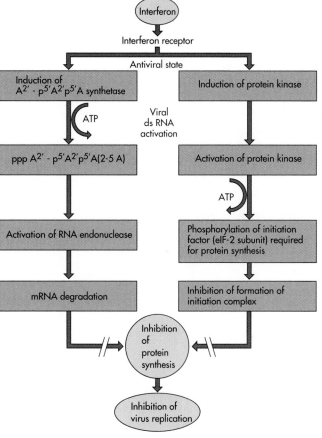

FIGURE 14-7 The two major routes for interferon inhibition of viral protein synthesis. One mechanism involves the induction of an unusual polymerase (2'-5' oligoadenylate synthetase *[2-5A]*) that is activated by double-stranded RNA. The activated enzyme synthesizes an unusual adenine trinucleotide with a 2', 5'-phosphodiester linkage. The trinucleotide activates an endonuclease that degrades mRNA. The other mechanism involves the induction of a protein kinase that inactivates the eIF-2 by phosphorylating one of the subunits to prevent initiation of protein synthesis. *ATP,* Adenosine triphosphate.

poly dA:dT), synthetic polyanion polymers (e.g., polysulfates, polyphosphates, and pyran), antibiotics (e.g., kanamycin, cycloheximide), and low-molecular-weight synthetic compounds (e.g., tilorone, acridine dyes).

Interferon-alpha and interferon-beta can be induced and released within hours of infection (Figure 14-6). The interferon binds to specific receptors on the neighboring cells and induces the production of antiviral proteins—**the antiviral state**. However, these antiviral proteins are not activated until they bind double-stranded RNA. The major antiviral effects of interferon are produced by two enzymes, 2'-5' oligoadenylate synthetase (an unusual polymerase) and a protein kinase specific for ribosomal initiating factor (eukaryotic initiation factor [eIF-2]). Viral infection of the cell and production of double-stranded RNA activate these enzymes and trigger a cascade of biochemical events that leads to the inhibition of protein synthesis, the degradation of messenger RNA (preferentially viral mRNA), and other activities. This process essentially puts the cellular factory "on strike" and prevents viral replication (Figure 14-7). It

---

BOX 14-6   Interferons

INDUCTION

Interferon production is stimulated by viral infection:
   Double-stranded RNA (e.g., RNA virus intermediate)
   Viral inhibition of cellular protein synthesis

MECHANIM OF ACTION

Release from an initial infected cell occurs.
Interferon binds to a specific cell surface receptor on another cell.
Interferon induces the "antiviral state": synthesis of protein kinase, 2'-5' oligoadenylate synthetase, and ribonuclease L.
Viral infection of the cell activates these enzymes.
Inhibition of viral and cellular protein synthesis occurs.

BOX 14-7   Activities of Interferons

ANTIVIRAL ACTIONS

Interferons initiate an antiviral state in cells.
Interferons block viral protein synthesis.
Interferons inhibit cell growth.

IMMUNOMODULATORY ACTIONS

Interferon-alpha and interferon-beta activate NK cells.
Interferon-alpha activates macrophages.
Interferon-gamma activates macrophages.
Interferons increase MHC antigen expression.
Interferons regulate the activities of T cells.

OTHER ACTIONS

Interferons regulate inflammatory processes.
Interferons regulate tumor growth.

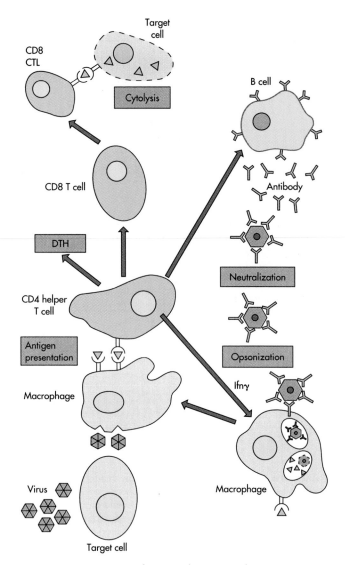

FIGURE 14-8 Antigen-specific antiviral immunity. The immune response is initiated by phagocytosis, proteolysis, and antigen presentation on macrophage lineage cells. Antigen-specific CD4 T cells are activated and release lymphokines, which activate DTH, cytolytic T cells, and B cells. Antibody binds to virus and neutralizes or opsonizes free virus. Macrophages phagocytise virus particles and restart the cycle. *Ifn*, Interferon.

must be stressed that interferon induces an antiviral state but does not directly block viral replication. The antiviral state lasts for 2 to 3 days, which may be sufficient for the cell to degrade and eliminate the virus without being killed.

Interferons stimulate cell-mediated immunity by activating effector cells and enhancing recognition of the virus-infected target cell. Interferons stimulate pre-NK cells to differentiate to NK cells to activate an *early, local,* natural defense against infection. Activation of macrophages by interferon-gamma promotes the production of more interferon, the secretion of other biological response modifiers, phagocytosis, recruitment, and inflammatory responses.

All interferon types stimulate the expression of class I MHC (human leukocyte antigen) and class II MHC antigens on the cell surface. Interferon-gamma increases the expression of class II MHC antigens on the macrophage to help promote antigen presentation to T cells. Interferon-alpha and interferon-beta increase the expression of class I MHC antigens, which enhances the cell's ability to present antigen, making the cell a better target for cytotoxic T cells (CTLs).

Interferon also has widespread regulatory effects on cell growth, protein synthesis, and the immune response (Box 14-7). All three interferon types block cell proliferation at appropriate doses.

Genetically engineered recombinant interferon is being used as an antiviral therapy for some viral infections (e.g., condyloma acuminata, hepatitis C). Effective treatment requires the use of the correct interferon subtype and its prompt delivery at the appropriate concentration. Interferons have also been used in clinical trials for the treatment of certain cancers. Interferon treatment is accompanied by influenza-like side effects such as chills, fever, and fatigue.

ANTIGEN-SPECIFIC IMMUNITY

Humoral and cell-mediated immunity play different roles in resolving viral infections. Humoral immunity (antibody) acts mainly on extracellular virions, whereas cell-mediated immunity (T cells) is directed at the virus-producing cell (Figure 14-8).

Humoral Immunity

Practically all viral proteins are foreign to the host and are immunogenic (capable of eliciting an antibody response). However, not all immunogens elicit protective immunity. *Protective humoral immunity is developed*

BOX 14-8   **Summary of Antiviral Responses**

INTERFERON

Interferon is induced by double-stranded RNA or inhibition of cellular protein synthesis.

Interferon initiates the antiviral state in surrounding cells.

Interferon blocks local viral replication.

Interferon initiates systemic antiviral responses.

NK CELLS

NK cells are activated by interferon-alpha and interferon-beta.

NK cells are activated by interferon-alpha and IL-12 and activate macrophages (interferon-gamma).

NK cells target and kill virus-infected cells (especially enveloped viruses).

MACROPHAGES (FAMILY OF CELLS)

Macrophages filter viral particles from blood.

Macrophages inactivate opsonized virus particles.

Macrophages present viral antigen to CD4 T cells.

T CELLS

T cells are essential for controlling enveloped and noncytolytic viral infections.

T cells recognize viral peptides presented by MHC molecules on cell surfaces.

T CELLS—cont'd

Antigenic viral peptides (linear epitopes) can come from any viral protein (e.g., glycoproteins, nucleoproteins).

TH1 CD4 responses are more important than TH2 responses.

CD8 cytotoxic T cells respond to viral peptide–class I MHC protein complexes on the cell surface.

TH2 CD4 responses are important for the maturation of antibody response.

TH2 CD4 responses may be detrimental if they prematurely limit the TH1 inflammatory and cytolytic responses.

ANTIBODY

Antibody neutralizes extracellular virus:

It blocks viral attachment proteins (glycoproteins, capsid proteins).

It destabilizes viral structure.

Antibody opsonizes virus for phagocytosis.

Antibody promotes killing of target cell by the complement cascade and antibody-dependent cellular cytotoxicity.

Antibody resolves lytic viral infections.

Antibody blocks viremic spread to target tissue.

IgM is an indicator of recent or current infection.

IgG is more effective than IgM.

Secretory IgA is important for protecting mucosal surfaces.

---

against the structural antigens located at the surface of the virus. These antigens include the viral capsid proteins of naked viruses and the glycoproteins of enveloped viruses. The best protective response is generated toward the viral proteins that interact with cell surface receptors (viral attachment proteins). An antibody response to other viral antigens may be useful for serological analysis of the viral infection (Box 14-8).

Antibody blocks the progression of disease by the **neutralization** and **opsonization** of cell-free virus. Antibody can neutralize the virus by binding to the viral attachment proteins, thus preventing their interaction with target cells, or by destabilizing the virus, thus initiating its degradation. Binding of antibody to the virus also opsonizes the virus, promoting its uptake and clearance by macrophages. Antibody recognition of infected cells can also promote antibody-dependent cellular cytotoxicity by NK cells.

The major antiviral role of antibody is to prevent the spread of extracellular virus to other cells, which is especially important in **preventing a viremia**. Antibody is most effective at **resolving cytolytic infections.** Resolution occurs because the virus kills the cell factory and the antibody eliminates the extracellular virus. Antibody is the primary defense initiated by vaccination.

T-Cell Immunity

T-cell–mediated immunity promotes antibody and inflammatory responses (CD4 helper and T cells) and kills infected cells (CD8 CTLs) (Box 14-8). **The CD4 TH1 response is generally more important than TH2 responses for controlling a viral infection, especially noncytolytic and enveloped viruses. CTLs (CD8)** kill infected cells and as a result eliminate the source of new virus. CTLs are activated by lymphokines produced by CD4 TH1 cells and kill cells expressing the appropriate complex of viral peptide with class I MHC protein. The peptides expressed on class I MHC antigens are obtained from viral proteins synthesized within the infected cell (endogenous route). CTL targets include peptides derived from viral proteins that may not elicit protective antibody (e.g., intracellular or internal virion proteins, nuclear proteins, improperly folded or processed proteins [cell trash]), in addition to viral glycoproteins. For example, the matrix and nucleoproteins of the influenza virus and the ICP4 (nuclear) protein of herpes simplex virus are targets for CTL lysis but do not elicit protective antibody.

Cell-mediated immunity is especially important for resolving infections by *syncytia-forming viruses,* which can spread from cell to cell without exposure to anti-

TABLE 14-4	Viral Evasion of Immune Responses

MECHANISM	VIRAL EXAMPLES	ACTION
HUMORAL RESPONSE		
Hidden from antibody	Herpesviruses, retroviruses	Latent infection
	Herpes simplex virus, varicella-zoster virus, paramyxoviruses, human immunodeficiency virus	Cell-to-cell infection (syncytia formation)
Antigenic variation	Lentiviruses (human immunodeficiency virus)	Genetic change after infection
	Influenza virus	Annual genetic changes
Secretion of blocking antigen	Hepatitis B virus	Hepatitis B surface antigen
Decay of complement	Herpes simplex virus	Glycoprotein C, which binds and promotes C3 decay
INTERFERON		
Block production	Hepatitis B virus	Inhibition of interferon transcription
	Epstein-Barr virus	IL-10 analogue (BRCA1) blocks interferon-gamma production
Block action	Adenovirus	Inhibits up-regulation of MHC expression VA1 RNA blocking double-stranded RNA activation of interferon-induced protein kinase
IMMUNE CELL FUNCTION		
Cytolysis of lymphocytes	Herpes simplex virus	Prevention of CD8 T-cell killing cells
Impairment of function	Human immunodeficiency virus	Kills CD4 T cells and alteration of macrophages
	Measles virus	Suppression of NK, T, and B cells
Immunosuppressive factors	Epstein-Barr virus	BCRF (similar to interleukin-10) suppression of THI CD4 helper T-cell responses
DECREASED ANTIGEN PRESENTATION		
Reduced human leukocyte antigen expression	Adenovirus 12	Inhibition of class I MHC transcription
		19-kD protein (E3 gene) binds class I MHC heavy chain, blocking translocation to surface
	Cytomegalovirus	H301 protein blocks surface expression of beta-2-microglobulin
INHIBITION OF INFLAMMATION		
—	Poxvirus, adenovirus	Blocking of action of IL-1 or tumor necrosis factor

PMNs, Polymorphonuclear neutrophils.

body (e.g., measles, herpes simplex, and varicella-zoster viruses), and *noncytolytic viruses* (e.g., hepatitis A and measles viruses) and for controlling *latent viruses* (herpes viruses and papillomaviruses).

IMMUNE RESPONSE TO VIRAL CHALLENGE
Primary Viral Challenge

The nonspecific immune responses are the earliest responses to viral challenge and are often sufficient to limit viral spread (Figure 14-5). The interferon produced in response to most viral infections initiates the protection of adjacent cells, enhances antigen presentation by increasing the expression of MHC antigens, and initiates the clearance of infected cells by activating NK cells and antigen-specific responses. Virus and viral components released from the infected cells are phagocytised by resident macrophages that mobilize and move to the lymph nodes. Macrophages in the liver and spleen are especially important for clearing virus from the bloodstream (**filters**). The macrophages degrade and process the viral antigens and express on their cell surface appropriate peptide fragments bound to class II MHC antigens. Macrophages also release IL-1, IL-6, and tumor necrosis factor to induce fever and promote helper T-cell activation.

Antiviral antigen-specific responses are similar to antibacterial antigen-specific responses except that the CD8 T cell plays a more important role. **IgM** is the first antiviral antibody produced, and its production indicates a primary infection. **IgG** and **IgA** are produced 2 to 3 days after IgM. Secretory IgA is made in response to a viral challenge through the natural openings of the body: the eyes, mouth, and respiratory and gastrointestinal systems. **CD8+ killer/suppressor T cells** are present at approximately the same time as serum IgG. CD8 T cells move to the site of infection and kill virus-infected cells. Recognition and binding to class I MHC viral peptide–expressing target cells promotes the release of perforin and granzymes to disrupt the cell membrane, whereas binding of the Fas ligand with Fas on the target cell promotes apoptosis of the target cell. Resolution of the infection occurs later, when sufficient antibody is available to neutralize all virus progeny or when cellular immunity has been able to reach and eliminate the infected cells. DTH and CTL responses are required for the resolution of most enveloped and noncytolytic viral infections. In many cases, IgG and CTLs in the blood are detected after viral replication has been controlled.

Secondary Viral Challenge

In any war it is easier to eliminate an enemy if its identity and origin are known and if establishment of its foothold can be prevented. Similarly, in the body, prior immunity allows rapid, specific mobilization of defenses to prevent disease symptoms, promote rapid clearance of the virus, and prevent viral access to the target tissue. As a result, most secondary viral challenges are asymptomatic. Antibody and memory B and T cells are present in an immune host to act on the viral infection and generate a more rapid and extensive anamnestic response. Secretory IgA provides an important defense to reinfection through the natural openings of the body but is produced only transiently. IgG antibody **prevents viremic spread** from the primary site of infection.

The nature of the immune response to a viral infection is determined by host, viral, and other factors. Host factors include genetic background, immune status, age, and the general health of the individual. Viral factors include viral strain, infectious dose, and route of entry. The time required to initiate immune protection, the extent of the response, the level of control of the infection, and the potential for **immunopathology** (see Chapter 46) resulting from the infection differ after a primary infection and a rechallenge.

Viral Mechanisms for Escaping the Immune Response

A major factor in the virulence of a virus is its ability to escape immune resolution. Viruses may escape immune resolution by evading detection, preventing activation, or blocking the delivery of the immune response. Specific examples are presented in Table 14-4. Some viruses even encode special proteins that suppress the immune response.

SPECIFIC IMMUNE RESPONSES TO FUNGI

The primary protective responses to fungal infection are promoted by **TH1-mediated inflammatory reactions.**

Patients deficient in these responses (e.g., patients with AIDS) are most susceptible to fungal infections. Macrophages activated by interferon-gamma are important for killing the fungi. Neutrophil production of cationic proteins may be important for some fungal infections (e.g., mucormycosis), and nitric oxide may be important for use against *Cryptococcus* and other fungi. Antibody, as an opsonin, may facilitate clearance of the fungi.

SPECIFIC IMMUNE RESPONSES TO PARASITES

It is difficult to generalize about the mechanisms of antiparasite immunity because there are many different parasites and different forms and tissue locations expressed during their life cycles (Table 14-5). In general, TH1 stimulation of **CD4, CD8 T-cell,** and **macrophage** responses is important for intracellular infections, and TH2 antibody responses are important for extracellular parasites in blood and fluids. **IgE** and **eosinophil** and **mast cell** action are especially important for eliminating worm (cestodes and nematodes) infections. Control of the infection may depend on which response is initiated in the host. For example, initiation of a TH2 response to *Leishmania* species is detrimental because it halts (IL-10 inhibition) the protective TH1 response. Parasites have developed sophisticated mechanisms for avoiding immune clearance and often establish chronic infections.

Extracellular parasites such as *Trypanosome cruzi*, *Toxoplasma gondii*, and *Leishmania* species are phagocytised by **macrophage. Antibody** may promote the uptake (opsonize) of the parasites. Killing of the parasites follows activation of the macrophage by **interferon-gamma** (produced by NK or CD4 TH1 cells) or **tumor necrosis factor–alpha** (produced by other macrophages) and induction of **oxygen-dependent killing mechanisms** (peroxide, superoxide, nitric oxide). In the absence of macrophage activation, the parasites may replicate in the macrophage. The observation that IL-4 and antibody production to *Leishmania* species correlated with the inhibition of protective inflammatory responses and poor outcome provided the basis for the discovery that TH1 and TH2 responses are separate and antagonistic.

Neutrophils act in a similar manner to macrophages: They phagocytize and kill extracellular parasites by oxygen-dependent and oxygen-independent mechanisms. **Eosinophils** localize near parasites, bind to IgG or IgE on the surface of larvae or worms (e.g., helminths, *Schistosoma mansonii*, *Trichinella spiralis*), degranulate by fusing their intracellular granules with the plasma membrane, and release the **major basic protein** into the intercellular space. The major basic protein is toxic to the parasite.

As indicated previously, **T-cell–dependent responses** are important for antiparasite responses. **CD4 TH1** production of **interferon-gamma** and activation of macro-

TABLE 14-5   **Examples of Antiparasitic Immune Responses**

PARASITE	HABITAT	MAIN HOST EFFECTOR MECHANISM	METHOD OF AVOIDANCE
Trypanosoma brucei	Bloodstream	Antibody + complement	Antigenic variation
Plasmodium species	Hepatocyte, blood cell	Antibody, cytokines	Intracellular, antigenic variation
Toxoplasma gondii	Macrophage	O_2 metabolites, NO, lysosomal enzymes	Inhibition of fusion with lysosomes
Trypanosoma cruzi	Many cells	O_2 metabolites, NO, lysosomal enzymes	Escape into cytoplasm, thus avoiding digestion in lysosome
Leishmania species	Macrophage	O_2 metabolites, NO, lysosomal enzymes	Impairment of O_2 burst and scavenging of products; avoidance of digestion
Trichinella spiralis	Gut, blood, muscle	Myeloid cells, antibody + complement	Encystment in muscle
Schistosoma mansoni	Skin, blood, lungs, portal vein	Myeloid cells, antibody + complement	Acquisition of host antigens, blockade by antibody; soluble antigens and immune complexes; antioxidants
Wuchereria bancrofti	Lymphatic system	Myeloid cells, antibody + complement	Thick extracellular cuticle; antioxidants

From Roitt I, Brostoff J, Male D: *Immunology*, ed 4, St Louis, 1996, Mosby.

*Antibody is most important for extracellular pathogens. Cell-mediated immunity (TH1 response) is most important for intracellular pathogens.

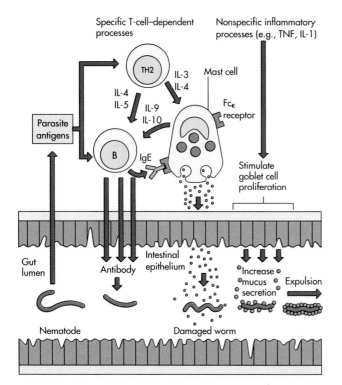

FIGURE 14-9 Elimination of nematodes from the gut. TH2 responses are important for stimulating the production of antibody. Antibody can damage the worm. IgE is associated with mast cells, the release of histamine, and toxic substances. Increased mucus secretion also promotes expulsion. *TNF*, Tumor necrosis factor. (From Roitt I, Brostoff J, Male D: *Immunology*, ed 4, St Louis, 1996, Mosby.)

phages are essential for protection against intracellular protozoa and the development of granulomas around *S. mansoni* eggs and worms in the liver. The granuloma, formed by layers of inflammatory cells, protects the liver from toxins produced by the eggs but also causes fibrosis. The development of fibrosis interrupts the venous blood supply to the liver, leading to hypertension and cirrhosis.

Cytokines produced by CD4 TH2 responses are very important for stimulating the production of IgE and the activation of mast cells (Figure 14-9). IgE bound to Fc receptors on mast cells targets the cell to antigens of the infecting parasite. In the lumen of the intestine, antigen binding and cross-linking of the IgE on the mast cell surface stimulates the release of histamine and substances toxic to the parasite and promotes mucus secretion to coat and promote expulsion of the worm.

IgG antibody also plays an important role in antiparasite immunity as an opsonin and by activating complement on the surface of the parasite.

Evasion of Immune Mechanisms by Parasites

Animal parasites have developed remarkable mechanisms for establishing chronic infections in the vertebrate host (Table 14-5). These mechanisms include intracellular growth, inactivation of phagocytic killing, release of blocking antigen (e.g. *Trypanosoma brucei, Plasmodium falciparum*), and development of cysts (e.g., protozoa: *Entamoeba histolytica*; helminths: *T. spiralis*) to limit access by the immune response. The African trypanosomes can reengineer the genes for their surface antigen (variable surface glycoprotein) and therefore change their antigenic appearance. Schistosomes can coat themselves with host antigens, including MHC molecules.

OTHER IMMUNE RESPONSES

Antitumor responses and rejection of tissue transplants are primarily mediated by T cells. CD8 cytolytic T cells recognize and kill tumors expressing peptides from embryological proteins, mutated proteins, or other proteins on class I MHC molecules (endogenous route of peptide presentation). IL-2 treatment in vitro generates **lymphokine-activated killer** and **NK cells** that target tumor cells, possibly a result of reductions in class I MHC molecules on the cell surface. Interferon-gamma–activated ("angry") macrophages can also distinguish and kill tumor cells.

Rejection of allografts used for organ transplants results from the expression of foreign peptides on foreign class I MHC antigens. In addition to host rejection of the transplanted tissue, cells from the donor of a blood transfusion or a tissue transplant can react against the new host in a **graft vs. host response.** An in vitro test of T-cell activation and growth in a graft vs. host–like response is the **mixed lymphocyte reaction.** Activation is usually measured by DNA synthesis (radioactive thymidine uptake).

IMMUNOPATHOGENESIS
Hypersensitivity Responses

Once activated, the immune response is sometimes difficult to control and causes tissue damage. Hypersensitivity reactions are responsible for many of the symptoms associated with microbial infections, especially viral infections. The four types of hypersensitivity responses are distinguished primarily by the mechanism of initiation and the time course.

Type I hypersensitivity is caused by **IgE** and is associated with allergic, atopic, and anaphylactic reactions (Figure 14-10). IgE binds to Fc receptors on mast cells and becomes the cell surface receptor for antigens **(allergens).** Cross-linking of the IgE triggers degranulation, releasing **chemoattractants** (cytokines, leukotrienes) to attract eosinophils, neutrophils, and mononuclear cells; **activators** (histamine, platelet-activating factor, tryptase, kininogenase) to promote vasodilatation and edema; and **spasmogens** (histamine, prostaglandin D_2, leukotrienes), to directly affect bronchial smooth muscle and promote mucus secretion. IgE allergic reactions are rapid-onset reactions. Desensitization (allergy shots) produces IgG to bind the allergen and prevent allergen binding to IgE.

Type II hypersensitivity is caused by antibody binding to cell surface molecules and the subsequent activation of cytolytic responses by the classic complement cascade or by cellular mechanisms (Figure 14-11). Examples of these reactions include myasthenia gravis

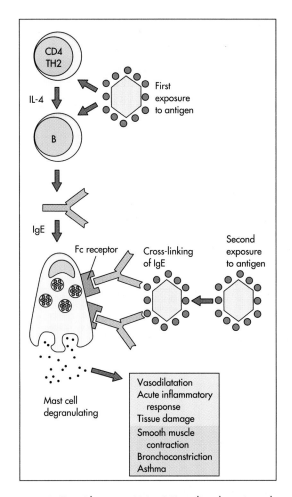

FIGURE 14-10 Type I hypersensitivity: IgE-mediated atopic and anaphylactic reactions. IgE produced in response to the initial challenge binds to Fc receptors on mast cells and basophils. Allergen binding to the cell surface IgE promotes the release of histamine and prostaglandins from granules to produce symptoms. Examples are hay fever, asthma, penicillin allergy, and reaction to bee stings.

because of antibodies to acetylcholine receptors on neurons, autoimmune hemolytic anemia, Goodpasture syndrome (lung and kidney basement membrane damage), and hemolytic disease of the newborn (blue babies) caused by the reaction of maternal antibody generated during the first pregnancy to Rh factors on fetal erythrocytes of a second baby (Rh incompatibility).

Type III hypersensitivity responses result from immune complexes and complement (Figure 14-12). In the presence of an abundance of soluble antigen in the bloodstream, large antigen-antibody complexes form, get trapped in capillaries (especially in the kidney), and then initiate the classic complement cascade. Activation of the complement cascade initiates inflammatory reactions. Immune complex disease may be caused by persistent infections (e.g., hepatitis B, malaria, staphylococcal infective endocarditis), autoimmunity (e.g., rheumatoid arthritis, systemic lupus erythematosus), or consistently inhaled antigen (e.g., mold, plant or animal antigens).

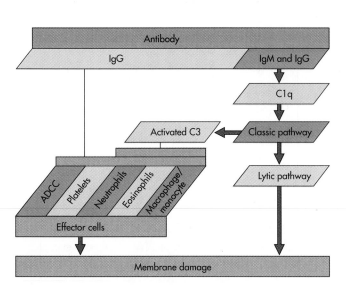

FIGURE 14-11 Type II hypersensitivity: mediated by antibody and complement. Complement activation promotes direct cell damage through the complement cascade and by the activation of effector cells. Examples are Goodpasture's syndrome, the response to Rh factor in newborns, and autoimmune endocrinopathies.

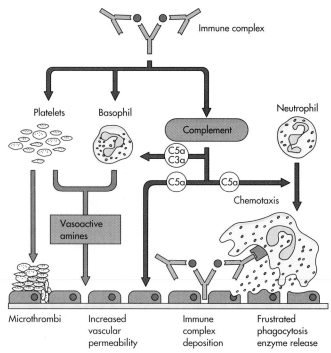

FIGURE 14-12 Type III hypersensitivity: immune complex deposition. Immune complexes can be trapped in the kidney and elsewhere in the body, can activate complement, and cause other damaging responses. Examples are serum sickness, nephritis associated with chronic hepatitis B infection, and Arthus reaction.

FIGURE 14-13 Type IV hypersensitivity: DTH mediated by CD4+ T cells (TH1). Activation of the CD4+ T cells releases lymphokines, including interferon-gamma, which promote inflammation. Examples are the tuberculin response (purified protein derivative test) and contact sensitivity to poison ivy and metals such as nickel. *APC*, Antigen-presenting cell; *TCR*, T-cell receptor.

TABLE 14-6		Important Characteristics of Four Types of DTH Reactions		
TYPE	**REACTION TIME**	**CLINICAL APPEARANCE**	**HISTOLOGICAL APPEARANCE**	**ANTIGEN**
Jones-Mote	24 hours	Skin swelling	Basophils, lymphocytes, mononuclear cells	Intradermal antigen: ovalbumin
Contact	48 hours	Eczema	Mononuclear cells, edema, raised epidermis	Epidermal: nickel, rubber, poison ivy
Tuberculin	48 hours	Local induration and swelling with or without fever	Mononuclear cells, lymphocytes and monocytes, reduced macrophages	Dermal: tuberculin, mycobacterial, and leishmanial
Granulomatous	4 weeks	Skin induration	Epithelioid cell granuloma, giant cells, macrophages, fibrosis with or without necrosis	Persistent antigen or antigen-antibody complexes in macrophages or "nonimmunological" (e.g., talcum powder)

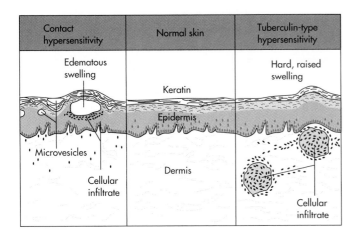

Contact hypersensitivity	Normal skin	Tuberculin-type hypersensitivity

FIGURE 14-14 Contact and tuberculin hypersensitivity responses. These type IV responses are cell-mediated but differ in the site of cell infiltration and in the symptoms. Contact hypersensitivity occurs in the epidermis and leads to the formation of blisters; tuberculin-type hypersensitivity occurs in the dermis and is characterized by swelling.

For example, hepatitis B infection produces large amounts of hepatitis B surface antigen, which may form immune complexes leading to glomerulonephritis. Type III hypersensitivity reactions can be induced in presensitized people by the intradermal injection of antigen to cause an **Arthus reaction,** a skin reaction characterized by redness and swelling. Serum sickness, extrinsic allergic alveolitis (a reaction to inhaled fungal antigen), and glomerulonephritis result from type III hypersensitivity reactions.

Type IV hypersensitivity responses are CD4 T-cell–induced DTH inflammatory responses (Figure 14-13 and Table 14-6). Although essential for the control of fungal infections and intracellular bacteria (e.g., mycobacteria), DTH is also responsible for **contact dermatitis** (e.g., cosmetics, nickel) and the response to poison ivy. Intradermal injection of **tuberculin** antigen (purified protein derivative) elicits firm swelling that is maximal 48 to 72 hours after injection and is indicative of prior exposure to *Mycobacterium tuberculosis* (Figure 14-14). **Granulomas** form in response to the intracellular growth of *M. tuberculosis*. These structures consist of an epithelioid (Langhans' cells) created from chronically activated macrophages, fused epithelioid cells (Giant cells) surrounded by lymphocytes, and fibrosis caused by the deposition of collagen from fibroblasts. Granulomatous hypersensitivity occurs with tuberculosis, leprosy, schistosomiasis, sarcoidosis, and Crohn's disease.

AUTOIMMUNE RESPONSES

Normally, a person is tolerized to self-antigens during the development of the immune system as a fetus and later in life by other mechanisms (e.g., oral tolerization). However, deregulation of the immune response may be initiated by cross-reactivity with microbial antigens (e.g.,

Group A streptococcal infection, rheumatic fever), polyclonal activation of lymphocytes induced by tumors or infection (e.g., malaria, Epstein-Barr virus infection), or a genetic predisposition caused by lack of tolerization to specific antigens.

Autoimmune reactions result from the presence of autoantibodies, activated T cells, and hypersensitivity reactions. People with certain MHC antigens are at higher risk to autoimmune responses (e.g., B27 and juvenile rheumatoid arthritis and ankylosing spondylitis). Many of these responses are associated with inflammatory TH1-type responses. Activation of TH2 responses to counteract the TH1 inflammation may provide a therapeutic approach for these diseases.

IMMUNODEFICIENCY

Immunodeficiency may result from genetic deficiencies, starvation, drug-induced immunosuppression (e.g., steroid treatment, cancer chemotherapy, chemotherapeutic suppression of tissue graft rejection), cancer (especially of immune cells), or disease (e.g., AIDS). Deficiencies in specific protective responses puts a patient at high risk for serious disease by infectious agents controlled by that response (Table 14-7). These "natural experiments" illustrate the importance of specific responses for controlling specific infections.

Hereditary Complement Deficiencies and Microbial Infection

Inherited deficiencies of C1q, C1r, C1s, C4, and C2 components are associated with defects in activation of the classic pathway that lead to increased susceptibility to **pyogenic** (pus-producing) staphylococcal and streptococcal infections (Figure 14-15). A deficiency of **C3** leads to a defect in activation of both the classic and alternative pathways, which also results in an increased incidence of pyogenic infections.

As expected, opsonization and phagocytosis are defective in some people (see the following section). **Defects of the properdin factors** impair activation of the alternative pathway, which also results in an increased susceptibility to pyogenic infections. Finally, **deficiencies of C5 through C9** are associated with defective cell killing, which increases the susceptibility to disseminated *Neisseria* infections.

Defects in Phagocyte Action

People with defective phagocytic function are more susceptible to bacterial infections but not to viral or protozoal infections (Figure 14-16). The clinical relevance of oxygen-dependent killing is illustrated by **chronic granulomatous disease** in children who have diminished cytochrome b and fail to form superoxide anions. Even though phagocytosis is normal, these children have an impaired ability to oxidize NADPH and destroy bacteria through the oxidative pathway. In patients with **Chédiak-Higashi syndrome,** the neutrophil granules fuse

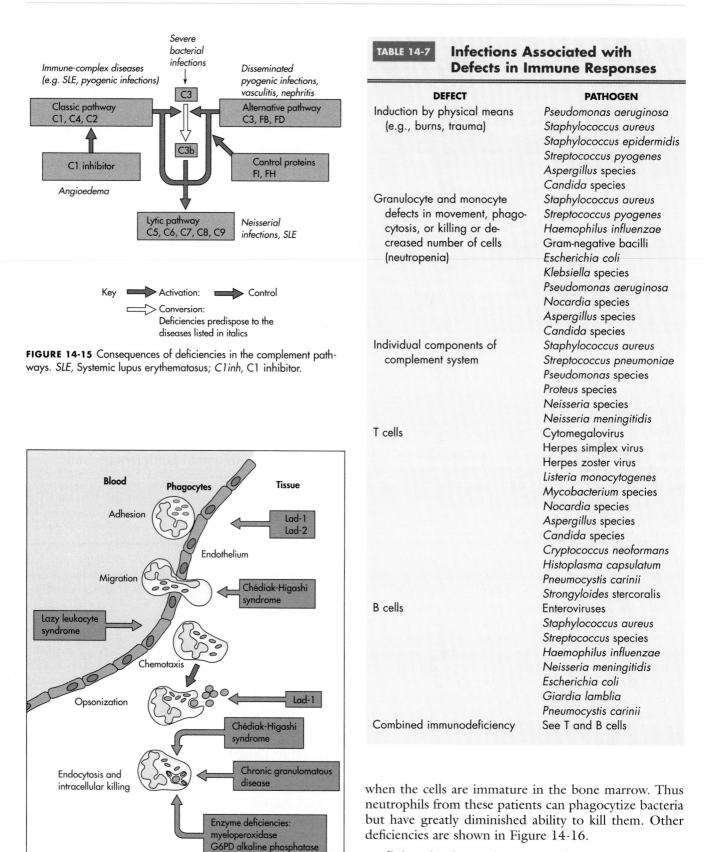

FIGURE 14-15 Consequences of deficiencies in the complement pathways. *SLE*, Systemic lupus erythematosus; *C1inh*, C1 inhibitor.

FIGURE 14-16 Consequences of phagocyte dysfunction. *G6PD*, Glucose-6-phosphate dehydrogenase. *Lad*, Leukocyte adhesion deficiency.

TABLE 14-7	Infections Associated with Defects in Immune Responses
DEFECT	**PATHOGEN**
Induction by physical means (e.g., burns, trauma)	Pseudomonas aeruginosa
	Staphylococcus aureus
	Staphylococcus epidermidis
	Streptococcus pyogenes
	Aspergillus species
	Candida species
Granulocyte and monocyte defects in movement, phagocytosis, or killing or decreased number of cells (neutropenia)	Staphylococcus aureus
	Streptococcus pyogenes
	Haemophilus influenzae
	Gram-negative bacilli
	Escherichia coli
	Klebsiella species
	Pseudomonas aeruginosa
	Nocardia species
	Aspergillus species
	Candida species
Individual components of complement system	Staphylococcus aureus
	Streptococcus pneumoniae
	Pseudomonas species
	Proteus species
	Neisseria species
	Neisseria meningitidis
T cells	Cytomegalovirus
	Herpes simplex virus
	Herpes zoster virus
	Listeria monocytogenes
	Mycobacterium species
	Nocardia species
	Aspergillus species
	Candida species
	Cryptococcus neoformans
	Histoplasma capsulatum
	Pneumocystis carinii
	Strongyloides stercoralis
B cells	Enteroviruses
	Staphylococcus aureus
	Streptococcus species
	Haemophilus influenzae
	Neisseria meningitidis
	Escherichia coli
	Giardia lamblia
	Pneumocystis carinii
Combined immunodeficiency	See T and B cells

when the cells are immature in the bone marrow. Thus neutrophils from these patients can phagocytize bacteria but have greatly diminished ability to kill them. Other deficiencies are shown in Figure 14-16.

Deficiencies in Antigen-Specific Immune Responses

People **deficient in T-cell function** are susceptible to **opportunistic infections** by viruses, especially en-

TABLE 14-8   Immunodeficiencies of Lymphocytes

CONDITION	T CELL NO.	T CELL FUNCTION	B CELL NO.	SERUM ANTIBODIES	INCIDENCE*
XLA, Bruton's syndrome	✓	✓	↓↓	IgG, IgA, IgM↓↓	Rare
X-SCID	↓↓	↓	✓	↓	Rare
XLP, Duncan's syndrome	✓	↓	✓	✓ or ↓	Rare
X-hyper IgM	✓	↓	✓	IgG↓↓, IgA↓↓, IgM↑	Rare
Wiskott-Aldrich syndrome	✓	↓	✓	IgA↑, IgE↑, IgM↓	Rare
ADA deficiency (SCID)	↓↓	↓↓	↓	↓	Very rare
PNP deficiency (SCID)	↓	↓	✓	✓	Very rare
HLA deficiency	✓	↓	✓	Poor Ag response	Very rare
Ataxia telangiectasia	↓	↓	✓	IgE↓, IgA↓, IgG2↓	Uncommon
DiGeorge syndrome	↓↓	↓	✓	✓	Very rare
IgA deficiency	✓	✓	✓	IgA↓	Common

From Brostoff J, Male DK: *Clinical immunology: an illustrated outline*, St Louis, 1994, Mosby.
XLA, X-linked agammaglobulinenia; *X-SCID*, X-linked severe combined immunodeficiency disease; *XLP*, X-linked lymphoproliferative (syndrome), *ADA*, adenosine deaminase; *PNP*, purine nucleoside phosphorylase; *HLA*, human leukocyte antigen; ✓, normal; ↑, increased; ↓, decreased or defective.
*Approximate incidence: Very rare $<10^{-6}$; rare 10^{-5}-10^{-6}. Uncommon 10^{-4}-10^{-5}; common 10^{-2}-10^{-3}.

veloped and noncytolytic viruses and viruses that establish latent or recurrent infections, intracellular bacteria, and fungi (Table 14-7). T-cell deficiencies can also prevent the maturation of B-cell antibody responses. T-cell deficiencies can arise from **genetic disorders** (e.g., X-linked immunodeficiency syndrome or Duncan's disease, DiGeorge syndrome) (Table 14-8), **infection (e.g., human immunodeficiency virus and AIDS), cancer chemotherapy, or immunosuppressive therapy for tissue transplantation.**

B-cell deficiencies may result in a complete lack of antibody production (hypogammaglobulinemia), inability to undergo class switching, or inability to produce specific subclasses of antibody. People deficient in antibody production are very susceptible to **bacterial infection.** IgA deficiency occurs in 1 of 700 Caucasians and results in an increased susceptibility to respiratory infections. A deficiency in IgG2 antibodies increases the risk to capsular bacterial infections, since this is the primary anticapsule response.

The immaturity of the immune system of **neonates** increases their susceptibility to infections by herpes viruses and other infections resolved by TH1-associated responses. Similarly, the less pronounced cell-mediated immune and inflammatory responses of **children** decrease the severity (in comparison to adults) of herpes (e.g., infectious mononucleosis, chickenpox) and hepatitis B infections but also increases the potential for the establishment of a chronic hepatitis B virus infection because of incomplete resolution.

QUESTIONS

1. Describe the types of immune responses that would be generated to the following different types of vaccines. Consider the route of processing and presentation of the antigens and the cells and lymphokines involved in generating the response.

a. Tetanus toxoid: intramuscular injection of formalin-fixed, heat-inactivated tetanus toxin protein.
b. Inactivated polio vaccine: intramuscular injection of chemically inactivated polio virus incapable of replication.
c. Live, attenuated measles vaccine: intramuscular injection of virus that replicates in cells and expresses antigen in cells and on cell surfaces.

2. Reproduce the table that follows and fill in the appropriate columns:

IMMUNODEFICIENCY DISEASE	IMMUNE DEFECT	SUSCEPTIBILITY TO SPECIFIC INFECTIONS
Chediak-Higashi syndrome		
Chronic granulomatous disease		
Complement C5 deficiency		
Complement C3 deficiency		
Complement C1 deficiency		
IgA deficiency		
X-linked agammaglobulinemia		
X-linked T-cell deficiency		
AIDS		
DiGeorge syndrome		
IgE deficiency		

Bibliography

Immunology Today: Issues contain understandable reviews on current topics in immunology.
Janeway CA, Travers P: *Immunobiology*, ed 2, New York, 1996, Garland.
Male D et al: *Advanced immunology*, ed 3, St Louis, 1996, Mosby.
Roitt I, Brostoff J, Male D: *Immunology*, ed 4, St Louis, 1996, Mosby.

15

Antimicrobial Vaccines

Antibodies produced in response to immunization or administered as therapy can prevent or lessen the serious symptoms of disease by **blocking the spread** of a bacterium, bacterial toxin, or virus to its target organ. Preventing an infection is better and cheaper than treating an infection. The immunization of a population, like personal immunity, stops the spread of the infectious agent by reducing the number of susceptible hosts **(herd immunity)**. Such immunization that has been done on a national and international level has succeeded in protecting the populace from the symptoms of pertussis, diphtheria, tetanus, and rabies; in controlling the spread of measles, mumps, and rubella; and in eliminating wild-type poliomyelitis in the Western Hemisphere and small-pox in the world. In conjunction with this immunization of the person and the populace, diseases can be prevented by limiting the exposure of healthy people to infected people **(quarantine)** and by eliminating the source (e.g., water purification) or means of spread (e.g., mosquito eradication) of the infectious agent. Smallpox is an example of an infection that was controlled by such means. As of 1977 it was eliminated through a successful World Health Organization (WHO) program combining vaccination and quarantine. However, vaccine-preventable diseases still occur where immunization programs are unavailable or too expensive (third-world countries) or neglected (e.g., the United States), as shown by the fact that measles causes 2 million deaths annually worldwide and outbreaks are becoming more frequent in the United States.

TYPES OF IMMUNIZATION

The injection of purified antibody or antibody-containing serum for the rapid, temporary protection or treatment of a person is termed *passive immunization.* Newborns receive natural passive immunity from maternal immunoglobulin that crosses the placenta or is present in the mother's milk.

Active immunization occurs when an immune response and immunological memory are stimulated in response to a challenge with an immunogen. Such immunization occurs after each exposure to an infectious agent **(natural immunization)** and through exposure to microbes or their antigens in **vaccines.** The term *vaccine* is derived from the vaccinia virus, a less virulent member of the poxvirus family that was used to immunize people against smallpox. Vaccines can be subdivided into two groups on the basis of whether they infect the person **(live vaccines** such as vaccinia) or whether they do not **(inactivated/subunit/killed vaccines)** (Figure 15-1). **DNA vaccines** represent a new potential means of immunization. In this approach, plasmid DNA is injected into muscle or skin, after which it expresses the gene for the immunogen.

Passive Immunization

Passive immunization may be used to prevent disease after a known exposure (e.g., needlestick injury with hepatitis B virus-contaminated blood), to ameliorate the symptoms of an ongoing disease, to protect immunosuppressed patients, or to block the action of bacterial toxins and prevent the diseases they cause (i.e., as therapy). Immune serum globulin preparations derived from seropositive humans or animals (e.g., horses) are available as prophylaxis for several bacterial and viral diseases (Table 15-1). Human serum globulin is prepared from pooled plasma and contains the normal repertoire of antibodies for an adult. Special high-titered immunoglobulin preparations are available for hepatitis B virus (HBIg), varicella zoster virus (VZIg), rabies (RIg), and tetanus (TIg). Human immunoglobulin is preferable to animal immunoglobulin, because of the attendant reduced risk of a hypersensitivity reaction (serum sickness).

Monoclonal antibody preparations are being developed for protection against various agents and diseases. Also being developed are monoclonal antibodies that can block the pathogenic mechanisms associated with infection, such as neutrophil adherence and septic shock.

Active Immunization

Inactivated Vaccines

Inactivated vaccines, rather than live vaccines, are used to confer protection against most bacteria and the viruses that may be too virulent or that can cause recurrent infection or be oncogenic. Inactivated vaccines can be produced through the chemical (e.g., formalin) or heat inactivation of bacteria, bacterial toxins, or viruses or through the purification of the components or subunits of the infectious agents.

These vaccines are usually administered with an **adjuvant,** such as alum, which boosts their immunogenicity. Better adjuvants are being developed that use bacterial cell wall components, synthetic polymers, or liposomes. The adjuvant also influences the type of immune response induced by the vaccine (TH1 or TH2). Attenuated forms of cholera toxin (CT) and *E. coli* lymphotoxin (LT) are being developed as potent adjuvants that promote secretory IgA production after intranasal or oral immunization.

Inactivated vaccines are generally safe, except in people who have allergic reactions to vaccine components. For example, many vaccines are produced in eggs, so these vaccines cannot be administered to people who are allergic to eggs. The immune response evoked by inactivated vaccines is predominantly a TH2 immune response and is more limited than that evoked by live vaccines. The immunity is not usually lifelong, may be limited to humoral and not cell-mediated immunity, does not elicit a local immunoglobulin A (IgA) response, requires booster shots, and requires a larger dose of an inactivated vaccine than of a live vaccine (Table 15-2).

There are three major types of inactivated bacterial vaccines: **toxoid** (inactivated toxins), **inactivated** (killed) bacteria, and **capsule or protein subunits** of the bacteria. The bacterial vaccines currently available are listed in Table 15-3. Most antibacterial vaccines protect against the pathogenic action of toxins.

Inactivated viral vaccines are available for **polio, hepatitis A, influenza, rabies,** and other viruses. The Salk polio (inactivated poliomyelitis vaccine or IPV) and the influenza vaccines are prepared by the formaldehyde inactivation of virions. The influenza vaccine is formulated annually and is a mixture of viruses predicted to threaten the population that particular year. In the past, a rabies vaccine was prepared by the formalin inactivation of infected rabbit neurons or duck embryos, but it is now prepared by the chemical inactivation of virions grown in human diploid tissue culture cells. Because of the slow course of rabies, the vaccine can be administered immediately after a person is exposed to the virus and still elicit a protective antibody response.

A **subunit vaccine** can be developed after identification of the bacterial or viral components that elicit a protective immune response. Either the immunogenic component is isolated from the bacterium, virus, or virus-infected cells by biochemical means or the vaccine is prepared through genetic engineering involving the expression of cloned viral genes in bacteria or eukaryotic cells. For example, the hepatitis B virus subunit vaccine was initially prepared from surface antigen obtained from human sera of chronic carriers of the virus, although it is no longer used in the United States. The vaccine is now purified from yeast bearing the gene for the antigen. The

antigen is purified, chemically treated, and absorbed onto alum to be used as a vaccine. **Vaccines against** *Haemophilus influenzae* **B,** *Neisseria meningitidis,* *Salmonella typhi,* **and** *Streptococcus pneumoniae* **are prepared from capsular polysaccharides.** Unfortu-

TABLE 15-1	**Immune Globulins Available for Postexposure Prophylaxis***
DISEASE	**SOURCE**
Hepatitis A	Human
Hepatitis B	Human†
Measles	Human
Rabies	Human†
Chickenpox, zoster	Human†
Tetanus	Human,† equine
Botulism	Equine
Diphtheria	Equine

*Immune globulins to other agents may also be available.
†Specific, high-titer antibody is available and is the preferred therapy.

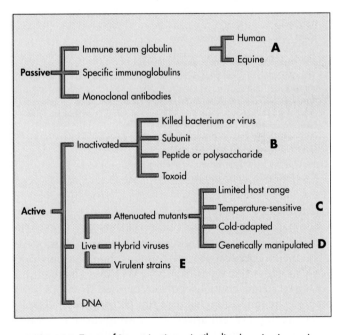

FIGURE 15-1 Types of immunizations. Antibodies (passive immunization) can be provided to block the action of an infectious agent, or an immune response can be elicited (active immunization) by natural infection or vaccination. The different forms of passive and active immunization are indicated. **A,** Equine antibodies can be used if human antibody is not available. **B,** Vaccine can consist of components purified from the infectious agent or can be developed through genetic engineering. **C,** Vaccine selected by passage in animals, embryonated eggs, or tissue culture cells. **D,** Deletion, insertion, reassortment, and other laboratory-derived mutants. **E,** Vaccine composed of a virus from a different species, which has a common antigen with the human virus.

TABLE 15-2	Advantages and Disadvantages of Live Versus Inactivated Vaccines	
PROPERTY	**LIVE**	**INACTIVATED**
Route of administration	Natural[a] or injection	Injection
Dose of virus, cost	Low	High
Number of doses	Single[b]	Multiple
Need for adjuvant	No	Yes[c]
Duration of immunity	Long term	Short term
Antibody response	IgG, IgA[d]	IgG
Cell-mediated immune response	Good	Poor
Heat lability in tropics	Yes[e]	No
Interference[f]	Occasional	None
Side effects	Occasional mild symptoms[g]	Occasional sore arm
Reversion to virulence	Rarely	None

From White DO, Fenner FJ: *Medical virology,* ed 3, New York, 1986, Academic.

[a]Oral or respiratory, in certain cases.

[b]A single booster may be required by law (yellow fever) or may be desirable (measles, rubella?) after about a decade.

[c]However, no satisfactory adjuvants other than alum are licensed for human use.

[d]IgA if delivered via the oral or respiratory route. Oral polio vaccine can prevent wild-type poliovirus from multiplying in the gut and thus facilitate near eradication of the virus from the community.

[e]Magnesium chloride and other stabilizers and maintenance of refrigeration or cold storage assist preservation.

[f]Interference from other viruses or diseases.

[g]Especially rubella and measles.

nately, polysaccharides are generally poor immunogens. The meningococcal vaccine contains the polysaccharides of four major serotypes (A/C/Y/W-135). The pneumococcal vaccine contains polysaccharides from 23 serotypes. The immunogenicity of the **H. influenzae B polysaccharide was enhanced by conjugation (chemical linkage) to a protein carrier** (e.g., diphtheria toxoid, *N. meningitidis* outer membrane protein, or *Corynebacterium diphtheriae* protein). The *H. influenzae* B polysaccharide-diphtheria toxoid carrier complex is approved for administration to infants. The other polysaccharide vaccines are less immunogenic and should only be administered to children older than 2 years.

Live Vaccines

Live vaccines are prepared with organisms limited in their ability to cause disease (**avirulent** or **attenuated**). Most live vaccines are used to protect people against vi-

ral diseases, especially infections caused by enveloped viruses, which require T-cell immune responses for the infection to resolve. Immunization with a live vaccine resembles the natural infection and elicits both humoral and cellular immunity. Initiation of the TH1 and TH2 immune responses generates an immunity that is generally long lived and, depending on the route of administration, can mimic the normal immune response to the infecting agent. However, there are two problems with live vaccines: (1) The vaccine virus may still be dangerous for immunosuppressed people or pregnant women who do not have the immunological resources for even a weakened virus infection to resolve, and (2) the vaccine may revert to a virulent viral form, a process that is rare.

Live bacterial vaccines include the orally administered live, attenuated *S. typhi* strain Ty2la vaccine for typhoid; the bacille Calmette-Guérin (BCG) vaccine for tuberculosis, which consists of an attenuated strain of *Mycobacterium bovis;* and an attenuated tularemia vaccine. A live vaccine may be required to elicit protection against infections such as these because both antibody- and cell-mediated immunity are important to confer protection against the intracellularly growing bacteria. The BCG vaccine is not routinely used in the United States because it causes people vaccinated with it to show a false-positive reaction to the purified protein derivative test, which is the screening test used to control tuberculosis in the United States.

Live virus vaccines consist of less virulent mutants (**attenuated**) of the wild-type virus, viruses from other species that share antigenic determinants, or genetically engineered viruses lacking virulence properties (Figure 15-1). Wild-type viruses are attenuated by growth in embryonated eggs or tissue culture cells at nonphysiological temperatures (32° to 34° C) and away from the selective pressures of the host immune response. These conditions select for or allow the growth of viral strains (mutants) that are less virulent because they grow poorly at 37° C (temperature-sensitive strains [e.g., measles vaccine] and cold-adapted strains), do not replicate well in any human cell (host-range mutants), or can replicate at a benign site but do not disseminate, bind, or replicate in the target tissue characteristically affected by the disease (e.g., polio vaccine replicates in the gastrointestinal tract but does not reach or infect the brain). Examples of attenuated live virus vaccines currently in use are listed in Table 15-4.

The first vaccine, that for smallpox, was developed by Jenner. The idea for the vaccine came to him when he noted that cowpox (vaccinia), a virulent virus from another species that shares antigenic determinants with smallpox, caused benign infections in humans but conferred protective immunity against smallpox. Similarly, the vaccine for the first tumor virus, Marek's disease virus of chickens, consists of the turkey herpesvirus. In addition, vaccines consisting of bovine or simian rotavirus have shown initial success in protecting infants against human rotavirus in clinical trials.

TABLE 15-3 **Bacterial Vaccines***

BACTERIA (DISEASE)	VACCINE COMPONENTS	INDICATIONS
Corynebacterium diphtheriae (diphtheria)	Toxoid	Children and adults
Clostridium tetani (tetanus)	Toxoid	Children and adults
Bordetella pertussis (pertussis)	Killed cell or cellular	Children
H. influenzae B (Hib; *Haemophilus* disease)	Capsule polysaccharide; capsule polysaccharide–protein conjugate	Children
N. meningitidis A and C (meningococcal disease)	Capsule polysaccharide	People at high risk (e.g., those with asplenia), travelers to epidemic areas (e.g., military personnel), children
S. pneumoniae (pneumococcal disease)	Capsule polysaccharide	People at high risk (e.g., those with asplenia)
Vibrio cholerae (cholera)	Killed cell	Travelers at risk to exposure
S. typhi (typhoid)	Killed cell, polysaccharide	Travelers at risk to exposure, household contacts, sewage workers
Bacillus anthracis (anthrax)	Killed cell	Handlers of imported fur
Yersinia pestis (plague)	Killed cell	Veterinarians, animal handlers
Francisella tularensis (tularemia)	Live attenuated	Animal handlers in endemic areas
Coxiella burnetii (Q fever)	Inactivated	Sheep handlers, laboratory personnel working with *C. burnetii*
Mycobacterium tuberculosis	Live attenuated bacille Calmette-Guérin (*M. bovis*)	Not recommended in United States

TABLE 15-4 **Viral Vaccines***

VIRUS	VACCINE COMPONENTS	INDICATIONS
Polio	Inactivated (IPV, Salk vaccine)	Children
	Attenuated (oral polio vaccine, Sabin vaccine)	Children
Measles	Attenuated	Children
Mumps	Attenuated	Children
Rubella	Attenuated	Children
Varicella zoster	Attenuated	Children
Influenza	Inactivated	Adults, especially medical personnel and the elderly
Hepatitis B	Subunit	Newborns, health care workers, high-risk groups (e.g., promiscuous people, intravenous drug users)
Hepatitis A	Inactivated	Children, child-care workers, travelers to endemic areas, Native Americans and Alaskans
Adenovirus	Attenuated	Military personnel
Yellow fever	Attenuated	Travelers at risk to exposure, military personnel
Rabies	Inactivated	Postexposure
		Preexposure: veterinarians, animal handlers
Smallpox	Vaccinia	No longer necessary
Japanese encephalitis	Inactivated	Travelers at risk to exposure
Eastern, Western, Russian spring-summer encephalitis viruses	Inactivated	Military personnel

* Listed in order of frequency of use.

Sabin developed the first live oral polio vaccine in the 1950s. The attenuated virus vaccine is obtained by multiple passage of the three types of poliovirus through monkey kidney tissue culture cells. At least 57 mutations are accumulated in the polio type 1 vaccine strain. When this vaccine is administered orally, IgA is secreted in the gut and immunoglobulin G (IgG) in the serum, which provides protection along the normal route of infection by the wild-type virus.

Live vaccines for measles, mumps, and rubella are often administered together (the MMR vaccine). Protection against these infections requires a potent cellular immune response, so the vaccine is administered at 2 years of age, late enough to prevent interference by maternal antibodies and to elicit a mature T-cell response. A killed measles vaccine proved to be a failure because it conferred an incomplete immunity that induced more serious symptoms (atypical measles) on challenge with wild-type measles virus than the symptoms associated with the natural infection. The initial live measles vaccine consisted of the Edmonston B strain, which was developed by Enders and colleagues. This virus was extensively passaged at 35° to 36° C through primary human kidney cells, human amnion cells, and chicken embryo cells. The currently used Moraten (United States) and Schwarz (other countries) vaccine strains of measles were obtained by further passage of the Edmonston B strain in chick embryos at 32° C. The mumps vaccine (Jeryl Lynn strain) and rubella vaccine (Wistar RA 27/3) viruses were also attenuated by extensive passage of the virus in cell culture. The varicella zoster vaccine uses the Oka strain, similarly requires a mature T-cell response, and is administered with the MMR vaccine.

Future Directions for Vaccination

Molecular biological techniques are being used to develop new vaccines. New live vaccines can be created by genetically engineering mutations that inactivate or delete a virulence gene instead of by randomly attenuating the virus by passage through tissue culture. Genes from infectious agents that cannot be properly attenuated can be inserted into safe viruses (e.g., vaccinia) to form **hybrid virus vaccines.** This approach holds the promise of allowing the development of a polyvalent vaccine to many agents in a single, safe, inexpensive, and relatively stable vector. On infection, the hybrid virus vaccine expresses and initiates an immune response to itself and the inserted antigens. The vaccinia virus vector system has been used in several experimental hybrid vaccines. Other vectors that have been considered include retroviruses, adenovirus, and herpes simplex virus.

Genetically engineered **subunit vaccines** are being developed by cloning genes encoding immunogenic proteins into bacterial and eukaryotic vectors. The greatest difficulty in the development of such vaccines is identifying the appropriate subunit or peptide immunogen that can elicit protective antibody and, ideally, T-cell responses. Once identified, the gene can be isolated, cloned, and expressed in bacteria or yeast cells, and then large quantities of these proteins can be produced. Genes for protective immunogens such as the surface antigen of hepatitis B, the gp120 of the human immunodeficiency virus (HIV), the hemagglutinin of influenza, the G antigen of rabies, and the gD antigen of herpes simplex virus have been cloned and grown in bacteria or eukaryotic cells for use or potential use as subunit vaccines.

Peptide subunit vaccines consist of specific epitopes of microbial proteins that elicit neutralizing antibody responses. To generate such a response, the peptide must contain sequences that allow it to be processed by an antigen-presenting cell, bind to an major histocompatibility complex antigen for presentation to T cells, and be recognized by helper T cells to facilitate antibody production. The immunogenicity of the peptide can be enhanced by its covalent attachment to a carrier protein. Better vaccines will be developed as the mechanisms of antigen presentation and T-cell receptor–specific antigens become better understood.

Antiidiotype antibodies are also being investigated as potential vaccines. Such antibodies recognize the variable region of a monoclonal antiviral antibody, which is like a cast of the viral epitope. The antiidiotype antibody resembles the original viral epitope, as if it were molded in the cast. Immunization with an antiidiotype antibody or the viral peptide would therefore elicit the production of similar antibodies.

DNA vaccines offer the exciting potential for immunization against infectious agents that require T-cell and antibody responses but that are not appropriate for use in live vaccines. These vaccines involve the cloning of the gene for a protein that elicits protective responses into a bacterial plasmid, which also allows the protein to be expressed in eukaryotic cells. The naked DNA is injected into the muscle or skin of the vaccine recipient, where the DNA is taken up by cells, the gene is expressed, and the protein is produced and presented to the immune response to elicit TH1 and TH2 responses. It is easier to develop a DNA vaccine than other types of vaccines.

With the advent of new technology it should be possible to develop vaccines against infectious agents such as *Streptococcus mutans* (to prevent tooth decay), the herpesviruses, HIV, and parasites such as *Plasmodium falciparum* (malaria) and *Leishmania*. In fact, it should be possible to produce a vaccine to almost any infectious agent once the appropriate protective immunogen is identified and its gene isolated.

IMMUNIZATION PROGRAMS

An effective vaccine program can save millions of dollars in health care costs. Such a program not only protects the person against infection and disease but also reduces the number of susceptible people in the population, thereby preventing the spread of the infectious agent

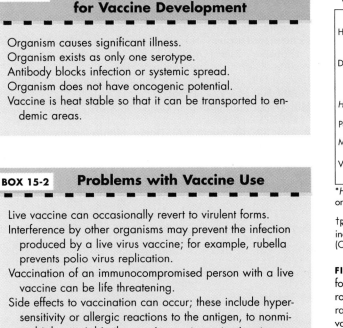

BOX 15-1   Properties of a Good Candidate for Vaccine Development

Organism causes significant illness.
Organism exists as only one serotype.
Antibody blocks infection or systemic spread.
Organism does not have oncogenic potential.
Vaccine is heat stable so that it can be transported to endemic areas.

BOX 15-2   Problems with Vaccine Use

Live vaccine can occasionally revert to virulent forms.
Interference by other organisms may prevent the infection produced by a live virus vaccine; for example, rubella prevents polio virus replication.
Vaccination of an immunocompromised person with a live vaccine can be life threatening.
Side effects to vaccination can occur; these include hypersensitivity or allergic reactions to the antigen, to nonmicrobial material in the vaccine, or to contaminants (e.g., eggs).
Vaccine development and liability insurance for the manufacturer are very expensive.
Organisms with many serotypes are difficult to control by vaccination.

*H. influenzae B (Hib) conjugate vaccine. Third dose may not be required depending on commercial source of vaccine.

†Recently, Centers for Disease Control and Prevention recommended two doses of inactivated polio vaccine (IPV) first, followed by two doses of oral polio vaccine (OPV) according to the schedule shown.

FIGURE 15-2 Recommended immunization schedule from the Centers for Disease Control and Prevention. Vaccines are listed under the ages routinely recommended for their administration. Bars indicate the range of acceptable ages for vaccination. For example, hepatitis B vaccine should be administered to children at 11 to 12 years of age who have not been previously vaccinated; varicella zoster virus vaccine should be administered to children who were not previously vaccinated and who lack a reliable history of chickenpox. *HB,* Hepatitis B; *DTP,* diphtheria and tetanus toxoids and whole-cell pertussis vaccines; *DTaP,* diphtheria and tetanus toxoids and acellular pertussis vaccines; *Td,* tetanus and diphtheria toxoids, absorbed, for adult use; *Var,* varicella zoster.

within the population. Although immunization may be the best means of protecting people against infection, vaccines cannot be developed for all infectious agents. One reason for this is that it is very time consuming and costly to develop vaccines. Considerations to weigh when choosing a candidate for a vaccine program are listed in Box 15-1.

Smallpox was eliminated by means of an effective vaccine program because the virus existed in only one serotype, symptoms were always present, and the vaccine was relatively benign and stable. However, its elimination came about only as the result of a concerted, cooperative effort on the part of the WHO and local health agencies worldwide. Rhinovirus is an example of a poor candidate for vaccine development because the viral disease is not serious and there are too many serotypes for vaccination to be successful. Practical aspects and problems with vaccine development are listed in Box 15-2.

From the standpoint of the individual, the ideal vaccine should elicit dependable, lifelong immunity to infection without producing serious side effects. Factors that influence the success of an immunization program include not only the composition of the vaccine, but also the timing, site, and conditions of its administration.

The recommended schedules of vaccinations for children are given in Figure 15-2. Infants are immunized with the diphtheria, tetanus, pertussis, and *H. influenzae* B conjugate inactivated vaccines as well as the inactivated or live oral polio vaccine. The inactivated hepatitis A vaccine can also be administered on this schedule or to adults at risk of infection. The live MMR vaccines are administered at 2 years of age, after the baby's immune response has matured and maternal antibodies have dissipated. Booster immunizations of inactivated vaccines and the live measles vaccine are required later in life. Adults should be immunized with vaccines for *S. pneumoniae* (pneumococcus), influenza, hepatitis B virus, and other diseases, depending on their jobs, the type of traveling they do, or other risk factors that make them particularly susceptible to specific infectious agents.

QUESTIONS

1. Why is an inactivated rather than a live vaccine used for the following immunizations: rabies, influenza, tetanus, hepatitis B virus, *H. influenzae* B, diphtheria, and pertussis?
2. Tetanus is treated with passive immunization and prevented by active immunization. Compare the nature and function of each of these therapies.

3. The inactivated polio vaccine is administered intramuscularly, whereas the live polio vaccine is administered as an oral vaccine. How does the course of the immune response and the immunoglobulins produced in response to each vaccine differ? What step in polio virus infection is blocked in a person vaccinated by each vaccine?

4. Why have large-scale vaccine programs not been developed for rhinovirus, herpes simplex virus, and respiratory syncytial virus?

5. Describe the public or personal health benefits that justify the development of the following major vaccine programs: measles, mumps, rubella, polio, smallpox, tetanus, and pertussis.

Bibliography

Centers for Disease Control: Update on adult immunization: recommendations of the Immunization Practices Advisory Committee, *MMWR* 40:RR-12, 1991.

Centers for Disease Control and Prevention: Immunization Information Page [Online]. (1997). Available: http://www.cdc.gov/diseases/immuni.html.

Conrad DA, Jensen HB: New and improved vaccines, *Postgrad Med* 100:113-127, 1996.

Hill DR: Immunizations, *Infect Dis Clin North Am* 6:291, 1992.

Plotkin SA, Mortimer EA: *Vaccines*, Philadelphia, 1988, WB Saunders.

SECTION

III

General Principles of Laboratory Diagnosis

CHAPTER 16

Microscopic Principles and Applications

The true complexity of our surroundings was unappreciated until microorganisms were revealed with the microscope. Indeed, the use of microscopy has helped define the relationships among a diversity of organisms, ranging from the smallest viruses consisting of a few proteins and minimal genetic information to multicellular parasites almost 10 meters long.

In general, microscopy is used in microbiology for two basic purposes: the initial detection of microbes and the preliminary or definitive identification of microbes. The microscopic examination of clinical specimens is used to detect bacterial cells, fungal elements, parasites (eggs, larvae, or adult forms), and viral inclusion bodies present in infected cells. Characteristic morphological properties of the microbe can be used for the preliminary identification of the organism, and for many fungi and parasites, microscopy is the definitive method for identifying the organism. The microscopic detection of organisms stained with antibodies labeled with fluorescent dyes has proved to be very useful for the specific identification of many viruses and bacteria. Five general microscopic methods have been used (Box 16-1).

MICROSCOPIC METHODS
Brightfield (Light) Microscopy

The basic components of light microscopes consist of a **light source** used to illuminate the specimen positioned on a stage, a **condenser** used to focus the light on the specimen, and two lens systems (**objective lens** and **ocular lens**) used to magnify the image of the specimen. In brightfield microscopy the specimen is visualized by transillumination, with light passing up through the condenser to the specimen. The image is then magnified first by the objective lens and then by the ocular lens. The total magnification of the image is the product of the magnifications of the objective and ocular lenses. Three different objective lenses are commonly used: low power ($\times 10$), which can be used to scan a specimen; high dry ($\times 40$), which is used to look for large microbes such as parasites and filamentous fungi; and oil immersion ($\times 100$), which is used to observe bacteria, yeasts (single-cell stage of fungi), and the morphological details of larger organisms and cells. Ocular lenses can further magnify the image (generally $\times 10$ to $\times 15$).

The limitation of brightfield microscopy is the resolution of the image (i.e., the ability to distinguish that two objects are separate and not one). The **resolving power** of a microscope is determined by the wavelength of light used to illuminate the subject and the angle of light entering the objective lens (referred to as the *numerical aperture*). The best brightfield microscopes have a resolving power of approximately 0.2 μm, which allows most bacteria but not viruses to be visualized. Although most bacteria and larger microorganisms can be seen with brightfield microscopy, the refractive indices of the organisms and background are similar. Thus organisms must be stained with a dye so that they can be observed, or an alternative method must be used.

Darkfield Microscopy

The same objective and ocular lenses used in brightfield microscopes are used in darkfield microscopes; however, a special condenser is used that prevents transmitted light from directly illuminating the specimen. Only oblique, scattered light reaches the specimen and passes into the lens systems, which causes the specimen to be brightly illuminated against a black background. The advantage of this method is that the resolving power of darkfield microscopy is significantly improved compared with that of brightfield microscopy (i.e., 0.02 μm versus 0.2 μm), which makes it possible for extremely thin bacteria such as *Treponema pallidum* (etiological agent of syphilis), *Borrelia burgdorferi* (Lyme disease), and *Leptospira* species (leptospirosis) to be detected. The disadvantage of this method is that because light passes around rather than through organisms, their internal structure cannot be studied.

Phase-Contrast Microscopy

Phase-contrast microscopy enables the internal details of microbes to be examined. In this form of microscopy, as parallel beams of light are passed through objects of different densities, the wavelength of one beam moves out of "phase" relative to the other beam of light (i.e., the beam moving through the more dense material is retarded more than the other beam). Through the use of annular rings in the condenser and the objective lens, the differences in phase are amplified so that in-phase light appears brighter than out-of-phase light. This creates a three-dimensional image of the organism or specimen, which permits more detailed analysis of the internal structures.

Fluorescent Microscopy

Some compounds called *fluorochromes* can absorb short-wavelength ultraviolet or ultrablue light and emit energy at a higher visible wavelength. Although some microorganisms show natural fluorescence (**autofluorescence**), fluorescent microscopy typically involves staining organisms with fluorescent dyes and then examining them with a specially designed fluorescent microscope. The microscope uses a high-pressure mercury, halogen, or xenon vapor lamp that emits a shorter wavelength of light than that emitted by traditional brightfield microscopes. A series of filters are used to block the heat generated from the lamp, eliminate infrared light, and select the appropriate wavelength for exciting the fluorochrome. The light emitted from the fluorochrome is then magnified through traditional objective and ocular lenses. Organisms and specimens stained with fluorochromes appear brightly illuminated against a black background, although the colors vary depending on the fluorochrome selected. The contrast between the organism and background is great enough that the specimen can be screened rapidly under low magnification and then the material examined under higher magnification once fluorescence is detected.

Electron Microscopy

Unlike other forms of microscopy, magnetic coils (rather than lenses) are used in electron microscopes to direct a beam of electrons from a tungsten filament through a specimen and onto a screen. Because a much shorter wavelength of light is used, magnification and resolution are dramatically improved. Individual viral particles (as opposed to viral inclusion bodies) can be seen only by electron microscopy. There are two types of electron microscopes: **transmission electron microscopes,** in which particles pass directly through the specimen, and **scanning electron microscopes,** in which particles pass

through the specimen at an angle and a three-dimensional picture is produced.

EXAMINATION METHODS

Clinical specimens or suspensions of microorganisms can be placed on a glass slide and examined under the microscope (i.e., direct examination of a wet mount). Although large organisms and cellular material can be seen using this method, analysis of the internal detail is frequently difficult. Phase-contrast microscopy can overcome some of these problems; alternatively, the specimen or organism can be stained by a variety of methods (Table 16-1).

Direct Examination

Direct examination methods are the simplest for preparing samples for microscopic examination. The sample can be suspended in water or saline (wet mount), mixed with alkali to dissolve background material (potassium hydroxide [KOH] method), or mixed with a combination of alkali and a contrasting dye (e.g., lactophenol cotton blue, iodine). The dyes nonspecifically stain the cellular material, increasing the contrast with the background, and permit examination of the detailed structures. A variation is the India ink method, in which the ink darkens the background rather than the cell. This method is used to detect capsules surrounding organisms such as the yeast *Cryptococcus* (the dye is excluded by the capsule, creating a clear halo around the yeast cell) and is a rapid method for the preliminary detection and identification of this important fungus.

Differential Stains

A variety of differential stains are used to stain specific organisms or components of cellular material. The Gram stain is the best known and most widely used stain and forms the basis for the phenotypic classification of bacteria. Yeasts can also be stained with this method (yeasts are gram-positive). The iron hematoxylin and trichrome stains are invaluable for the identification of protozoan parasites, and the Wright-Giemsa stain is used to identify blood parasites and other selected organisms. Stains such as methenamine silver and toluidine blue-O have largely been replaced by more sensitive or technically easier to use differential or fluorescent stains.

Acid-Fast Stains

At least three different acid-fast stains are used, each exploiting the fact that some organisms retain a primary stain even when exposed to strong decolorizing agents such as mixtures of acids and alcohols. The Ziehl-Neelsen is the oldest method used but requires heating the specimen during the staining procedure. Many laboratories have now replaced this method with either the cold acid-fast stain (Kinyoun method) or the fluorochrome stain (auramine-rhodamine method). The fluorochrome method is preferred, however, because a large area of the

BOX 16-1	*Microscopic Methods*

Brightfield (light) microscopy
Darkfield microscopy
Phase-contrast microscopy
Fluorescence microscopy
Electron microscopy

TABLE 16-1	Microscopic Preparations and Stains Used in the Clinical Microbiology Laboratory

STAINING METHOD	PRINCIPLE AND APPLICATIONS
DIRECT EXAMINATION	
Wet mount	Unstained preparation examined by brightfield, darkfield, or phase-contrast microscopy. Dyes used to examine gross morphology of organisms and specimens.
10% KOH	KOH used to dissolve proteinaceous material and facilitate detection of fungal elements, which are not affected by strong alkali solution. Dyes such as lactophenol cotton blue can be added to increase contrast between fungal elements and background.
India ink	Modification of KOH procedure in which ink is added as contrast material. Dyes primarily used to detect *Cryptococcus* species in cerebrospinal fluid and other body fluids. Polysaccharide capsule of *Cryptococcus* species excludes ink, creating halo around yeast cell.
Lugol's iodine	Iodine is added to wet preparations of parasitology specimens to enhance contrast of internal structures. Facilitates differentiation of ameba from host white blood cells.
DIFFERENTIAL STAINS	
Gram stain	Most commonly used stain in microbiology laboratory, forming basis for separating major groups of bacteria (e.g., gram-positive, gram-negative). After fixation of specimen to glass slide (by heating or alcohol treatment), specimen is exposed to crystal violet, and then iodine is added to form complex with primary dye. During decolorization with alcohol or acetone, complex is retained in gram-positive bacteria but lost in gram-negative organisms; counterstain safranin is retained by gram-negative organisms (hence their red color). Degree to which organism retains stain is function of organism, culture conditions, and staining skills of microscopist.
Iron hematoxylin stain	Used for detection and identification of fecal protozoa. Helminth eggs and larvae generally retain too much stain and are more easily identified with wet-mount preparation.
Methenamine silver stain	Generally performed in histology laboratories rather than microbiology laboratories. Used primarily for detection of fungal elements in tissues, although other organisms such as bacteria can be detected. Silver staining requires skill because nonspecific staining can render slide findings uninterpretable.
Toluidine blue-O stain	Used primarily for detection of *Pneumocystis* organisms in respiratory specimens. Cysts stain reddish blue to dark purple on light-blue background. Background staining is removed by sulfation reagent. Yeast cells stain and are difficult to differentiate from *Pneumocystis* cells. Trophozoites do not stain. Many laboratories have replaced it with specific fluorescent stains.
Trichrome stain	Alternative to iron hematoxylin for staining protozoa. Protozoa have bluish-green to purple cytoplasms with red or purplish-red nuclei and inclusion bodies; specimen background is green.
Wright-Giemsa stain	Used to detect blood parasites; viral and chlamydial inclusion bodies; and *Borrelia, Toxoplasma, Pneumocystis,* and *Rickettsia* species. Polychromatic stain that contains mixture of methylene blue, azure B, and eosin Y. Giemsa stain combines methylene blue and eosin. Eosin ions are negatively charged and stain basic components of cells to orange to pink, whereas other dyes stain acidic cell structures various shades of blue to purple. Protozoan trophozoites have red nucleus and grayish-blue cytoplasm; intracellular yeasts and inclusion bodies typically stain blue; rickettsiae, chlamydiae, and *Pneumocystis* species stain purple.
ACID-FAST STAINS	
Ziehl-Neelsen stain	Used to stain mycobacteria, as well as other acid-fast organisms. Organisms are stained with basic carbol fuchsin and resist decolorization with acid-alkali solutions. Background is counterstained with methylene blue. Organisms appear red against light-blue background. Uptake of carbol fuchsin requires heating specimen (hot acid-fast stain).
Kinyoun stain	Cold acid-fast stain (does not require heating). Same principle as Ziehl-Neelsen stain.
Auramine-rhodamine stain	Same principle as other acid-fast stains except that fluorescent dyes (auramine and rhodamine) are used for primary stain and potassium permanganate (strong oxidizing agent) is the counterstain and inactivates unbound fluorochrome dyes. Organisms fluoresce yellowish green against black background.

KOH, Potassium hydroxide.

| TABLE 16-1 | **Microscopic Preparations and Stains Used in the Clinical Microbiology Laboratory—cont'd** |

STAINING METHOD	PRINCIPLE AND APPLICATIONS
ACID-FAST STAINS—cont'd	
Modified acid-fast stain	Weak decolorizing agent is used with any of three acid-fast stains listed. Whereas mycobacteria are strongly acid-fast, other organisms stain more weakly (e.g., *Nocardia, Rhodococcus, Tsukamurella, Gordona, Cryptosporidium, Isospora, Sarcocystis,* and *Cyclospora* organisms). These organisms can be stained more efficiently by using weak decolorizing agent with acid-fast stains. Organisms that retain this stain are referred to as being *partially acid-fast.*
FLUORESCENT STAINS	
Acridine orange stain	Used for detection of bacteria and fungi in clinical specimens. Dye intercalates into nucleic acid (native and denatured). At neutral pH, bacteria, fungi, and cellular material stain reddish orange. At acid pH (4.0), bacteria and fungi remain reddish orange, but background material stains greenish yellow.
Auramine-rhodamine stain	Same as acid-fast stains.
Calcofluor white stain	Used to detect fungal elements and *Pneumocystis* species. Stain binds to cellulose and chitin in cell walls; clinician can mix dye with KOH. (Many laboratories have replaced traditional KOH stain with this stain.)
Direct fluorescent antibody stain	Antibodies (monoclonal or polyclonal) are complexed with fluorescent molecules. Specific binding to an organism is detected by presence of microbial fluorescence. Technique has proved useful for detecting or identifying many organisms (e.g., *Streptococcus pyogenes; Bordetella, Francisella, Legionella, Chlamydia, Cryptosporidium,* and *Giardia* species; influenza virus; herpes simplex virus). Test's sensitivity and specificity are determined by number of organisms present in test sample and quality of antibodies used in reagents.

specimen can be examined rapidly by simply searching for fluorescing organisms against a black background. Some organisms are "partially acid-fast," retaining the primary stain only when they are decolorized with a weakly acidic solution. This property is characteristic of a only a few organisms (Table 16-1), making it quite valuable for their preliminary identification.

Fluorescent Stains

The auramine-rhodamine acid-fast stain is a specific example of a fluorescent stain. Numerous other fluorescent dyes have also been used to stain specimens. For example, the acridine orange stain can be used to stain bacteria and fungi, and calcofluor white stains the chitin in fungal cell walls. Although the acridine orange stain is rather limited in its applications, the calcofluor white stain has rapidly replaced the potassium hydroxide stains. Another type of fluorescent stain is the examination of specimens with specific antibodies labeled with fluorescent dyes. The presence of fluorescing organisms is a rapid method for both the detection and identification of the organism.

QUESTIONS

1. Explain the principles underlying brightfield, darkfield, phase-contrast, fluorescent, and electron microscopy. Give one example in which each method would be used.
2. List three examples of direct microscopic examinations, differential stains, acid-fast stains, and fluorescent stains.

Bibliography

Chapin K: *Clinical microscopy.* In Murray P et al, editors: *Manual of clinical microbiology,* ed 6, Washington, DC, 1995, American Society for Microbiology.
Murray P: *ASM pocket guide to clinical microbiology,* Washington, DC, 1996, American Society for Microbiology.

Molecular Diagnosis

Like the evidence left at the scene of a crime, the DNA, RNA, or proteins of an infectious agent in a clinical sample can be used to help identify the agent. In many cases the agent can be detected and identified in this way even if it cannot be isolated or detected by immunological means. Many of the techniques discussed in this chapter were initially developed for the analysis of viruses, with new applications of the techniques being developed for the analysis of other types of infectious agents.

The advantages of molecular techniques are their sensitivity, specificity, and safety. From the standpoint of their safety, these techniques do not require isolation of the infectious agent and can be performed on chemically fixed (inactivated) samples or extracts. Because of their sensitivity, very dilute samples or DNA (e.g., viral DNA) can be detected in a tissue even if the agent is not replicating or producing other evidence of infection. The potential specificity of these techniques allows strains to be distinguished on the basis of differences in their genotype (i.e., mutants). This is especially useful for distinguishing antiviral drug-resistant strains, which may differ by a single nucleotide.

DETECTION OF VIRAL GENETIC MATERIAL
Electrophoretic Analysis of DNA and Restriction Fragment Length Polymorphism

The genome structure and genetic sequence are major distinguishing characteristics of the family, type, and strain of bacterium or virus. Specific strains of bacteria or viruses can be distinguished on the basis of their DNA or RNA or by the DNA fragments produced when the DNA is cleaved by specific restriction endonucleases. **Restriction endonucleases** are enzymes that recognize specific DNA sequences that have a palindromic structure; an example follows:

$\rightarrow$
G AATTC   EcoR1 recognition sequence
CTTAA G   and cleavage
$\leftarrow$

Restriction endonuclease recognition sequences differ in their sequence, length, and frequency of occur-

rence. As a result, different restriction endonucleases cleave the DNA of a sample in different places, yielding fragments of different lengths. The cleavage of different DNA samples with one restriction endonuclease can also yield fragments of many different lengths. The differences in the length of the DNA fragments among the different strains of a specific virus or bacterium produced on cleavage with one or more restriction endonucleases is termed **restriction fragment length polymorphism (RFLP).**

DNA or RNA of different sizes or structures can be distinguished by its electrophoretic mobility in an agarose or polyacrylamide gel. Different forms of the same DNA sequence and different lengths of DNA move through the mazelike structure of an agarose gel at different speeds, allowing their separation. The DNA can be visualized by staining with ethidium bromide. Smaller fragments (less than 20,000 base pairs), such as those from bacterial plasmids or from viruses, can be distinguished by normal electrophoretic methods. Larger fragments, such as those from whole bacteria, can be distinguished only by using a special electrophoretic technique called *pulsed-field gel electrophoresis.*

RFLP is useful, for example, for distinguishing different strains of herpes simplex virus (HSV). Comparison of the electrophoretic analysis of the restriction endonuclease cleavage patterns of DNA from different isolates can identify a pattern of virus transmission from one person to another or can distinguish HSV-1 from HSV-2. RFLP has also been used to show, for example, the spread of a strain of *Streptococcus* producing necrotizing fasciitis from a patient to other patients, an emergency medical technician, and the emergency room and attending physicians (Figure 17-1).

Genetic Probes

*DNA **probes** can be used like antibodies as sensitive and specific tools to detect, locate, and quantitate specific nucleic acid sequences in clinical specimens* (Figure 17-2). Because of the specificity and sensitivity of DNA probe techniques, individual species or strains of an infectious agent can be detected even if they are not growing or replicating.

140

DNA probes are chemically synthesized or obtained by cloning specific genomic fragments or an entire viral genome into bacterial vectors (plasmids, cosmids). DNA copies of RNA viruses are made with the retrovirus reverse transcriptase and then cloned into these vectors. After chemical or heat treatments to melt (separate) the DNA strands in the sample, the DNA probe is added and allowed to **hybridize** (bind) with the identical or nearly identical sequence in the sample. The **stringency** (the requirement for an exact sequence match) of the interaction can be varied so that related sequences can be detected or different strains (mutants) can be distinguished. The DNA probes are labeled with radioactive or chemically modified nucleotides (e.g., biotinylated uridine) so that they can be detected and quantitated. The use of a biotin-labeled DNA probe allows the use of a fluorescent- or enzyme-labeled avidin or streptavidin (a protein that binds tightly to biotin) molecule to detect viral nucleic acids in a cell in a way similar to the way in which indirect immunofluorescence or an enzyme immunoassay localizes an antigen.

The DNA probes can detect specific genetic sequences in fixed, permeabilized tissue biopsy specimens by **in situ hybridization.** The localization of cytomegalovirus-

(Figure 17-3) or papillomavirus-infected cells by in situ hybridization is preferable to an immunological means of doing so and is the only commercially available means of localizing papillomavirus. There are now many commercially available viral probes and kits for detecting viruses.

Specific nucleic acid sequences in extracts from a clinical sample can be detected by applying a small volume of the extract to a nitrocellulose filter (**dot blot**) and then probing the filter with labeled, specific viral DNA. Alternatively, the restriction endonuclease cleavage pattern separated electrophoretically can be transferred

FIGURE 17-1 RFLP distinction of DNA from bacterial strains separated by pulsed-field gel electrophoresis. Lanes *1* to *3* show Sma 1–digested DNA isolated from two family members suffering from necrotizing fasciitis and from their physician (pharyngitis). Lanes *4* to *6* are from unrelated *Streptococcus pyogenes* strains. (Courtesy Dr. Joe DiPersio, Akron, Ohio.)

FIGURE 17-2 DNA probe analysis of virus-infected cells. Such cells can be localized in histologically prepared tissue sections using DNA probes consisting of as few as nine nucleotides or bacterial plasmids containing the viral gene. A tagged DNA probe is added to the sample. In this case the DNA probe is labeled with biotin-modified thymidine, but radioactive agents can also be used. The sample is heated to denature the DNA and cooled to allow the probe to hybridize to the complementary sequence. Horseradish peroxidase–labeled avidin is added to bind to the biotin on the probe. The appropriate substrate is added to color the nuclei of virally infected cells. *b*, Biotin; *C*, cytosine; *G*, guanine; *A*, adenine.

FIGURE 17-3 In situ localization of cytomegalovirus (CMV) infection using a genetic probe. CMV infection of the renal tubules of a kidney is localized with a biotin-labeled, CMV-specific DNA probe and visualized by means of the horseradish peroxidase–conjugated avidin conversion of substrate, in a manner similar to enzyme immunoassay. (Courtesy Donna Zabel, Akron, Ohio.)

onto a nitrocellulose filter (**Southern blot**—DNA:DNA probe hybridization), and then the specific sequence can be identified by hybridization with a specific genetic probe and by its characteristic electrophoretic mobility. Electrophoretically separated RNA (**Northern blot**—RNA:DNA probe hybridization) blotted onto a nitrocellulose filter can be detected in a similar manner.

The **polymerase chain reaction** (PCR) can detect single copies of viral DNA and is one of the newest techniques of genetic analysis (Figure 17-4). In this technique, a sample is incubated with two short DNA oligomers that are complementary to the ends of a known genetic sequence of the viral DNA, a heat-stable DNA polymerase (*Taq* polymerase obtained from a thermophilic bacteria), nucleotides, and buffers. The oligomers hybridize to the appropriate sequence of DNA and act as primers for the polymerase, which copies that segment of the DNA. The sample is then heated to denature the DNA (separating the strands of the double helix) and cooled to allow hybridization of the primers to the new DNA. Each copy of DNA becomes a new template. The process is repeated many (20 to 40) times to amplify the original DNA sequence in an exponential manner. A target sequence can be amplified a million-fold in a few hours using this method. This technique is especially useful for detecting latent and integrated virus sequences, such as is the case for retroviruses, herpesviruses, papillomaviruses, and other papovaviruses.

The **RT-PCR** technique is a variation of the PCR, and it involves the use of the reverse transcriptase of retroviruses to convert viral RNA or messenger RNA to DNA before PCR amplification. In 1993, Hantavirus sequences were used as primers for RT-PCR to identify the agent causing an outbreak of hemorrhagic pulmonary disease in the Four Corners area of New Mexico. It showed the infectious agent to be a Hantavirus.

DETECTION OF PROTEINS

In some cases, viruses and other infectious agents can be detected on the basis of the finding of certain character-

FIGURE 17-4 PCR. This technique is a rapid means of amplifying a known sequence of DNA. A sample is mixed with a heat-stable DNA polymerase, excess deoxyribonucleotide triphosphates, and two DNA oligomers **(primers)**, which complement the ends of the target sequence to be amplified. The mixture is heated to denature the DNA and then cooled to allow binding of the primers to the target DNA and extension of the primers by the polymerase. The cycle is repeated 20 to 30 times. After the first cycle, only the sequence bracketed by the primers is amplified. In the **RT-PCR** technique, RNA can also be amplified after its conversion to DNA by reverse transcriptase. *A* and *B*, DNA oligomers used as primers; + and −, DNA strands. (Modified from Blair GE, Blair Zajdel ME: *Biochem Educ* 20:87-90, 1992.)

TABLE 17-1	Molecular Techniques		
TECHNIQUE	**PURPOSE**	**CLINICAL EXAMPLES**	
RFLP	Comparison of DNA	Molecular epidemiology, HSV-1 strains	
DNA electrophoresis	Comparison of DNA	Viral strain differences (up to 20,000 bases)	
Pulsed-field gel electrophoresis	Comparison of DNA (large pieces of DNA)	Streptococcal strain comparisons	
In situ hybridization	Detection and localization of DNA sequences in tissue	Detection of nonreplicating DNA virus (e.g., cytomegalovirus, human papillomavirus)	
Dot blot	Detection of DNA sequences in solution	Detection of viral DNA	
Southern blot	Detection and characterization of DNA sequences by size	Identification of specific viral strains	
Northern blot	Detection and characterization of RNA sequences by size	Identification of specific viral strains	
PCR	Amplification of very dilute DNA samples	Detection of DNA viruses	
RT-PCR	Amplification of very dilute RNA samples	Detection of RNA viruses	
SDS-PAGE	Separation of proteins by molecular weight	Molecular epidemiology of HSV	

istic enzymes or specific proteins. For example, the detection of reverse transcriptase in serum or cell culture indicates the presence of a retrovirus. The pattern of proteins from a virus or another agent after sodium dodecyl sulfate–polyacrylamide gel electrophoresis (**SDS-PAGE**) can also be used to identify and distinguish different strains of viruses or bacteria. In the SDS-PAGE technique, SDS binds to the backbone of the protein to generate a uniform peptide structure and protein length-to-charge ratio, such that the mobility of the protein in the gel is inversely related to the logarithm of its molecular weight. For example, the patterns of electrophoretically separated HSV proteins can be used to distinguish different types and strains of HSV-1 and HSV-2. Antibody can be used to identify specific proteins separated by SDS-PAGE using a **Western blot** technique (see Chapters 48 and 61). The molecular techniques used to identify infectious agents are summarized in Table 17-1.

Bibliography

Baron EJ, Peterson LR, Finegold SM: *Bailey and Scott's diagnostic microbiology,* ed 9, St Louis, 1994, Mosby.

DiPersio JR et al: Spread of serious disease-producing M3 clones of group A *Streptococcus* among family members and health care workers, *Clin Infect Dis* 22:490-495, 1996.

Murray PR: *ASM pocket guide to clinical microbiology,* Washington, DC, 1996, ASM.

Serological Diagnosis

Immunological techniques are used to detect, identify, and quantitate antigen in clinical samples as well as to evaluate the antibody response to infection and a person's history of exposure to infectious agents. The specificity of the antibody-antigen interaction and the sensitivity of many of the immunological techniques make them powerful laboratory tools (Table 18-1). In most cases the same technique can be used to evaluate a person's antigen and antibody status.

ANTIBODIES

Antibodies can be used as sensitive and specific tools to detect, identify, and quantitate the antigens from a virus, bacterium, fungus, or parasite. Specific antibodies may be obtained from convalescent patients (e.g., antiviral antibodies) or prepared in animals. These antibodies are **polyclonal,** heterogeneous antibody preparations that can recognize many epitopes on a single antigen. **Monoclonal** antibodies recognize individual epitopes on an antigen. Monoclonal antibodies for some antigens are commercially available, especially for lymphocyte cell surface antigens.

The development of monoclonal antibody technology revolutionized the science of immunology. For example, because of the specificity of these antibodies, lymphocyte subsets (e.g., CD4 and CD8 T cells) and lymphocyte cell surface antigens were identified. Monoclonal antibodies are the products of hybrid cells generated by the fusion and cloning of splenocytes from an immunized mouse and a myeloma cell line, which produces a hybridoma. The myeloma provides immortalization to the antibody-producing splenocytes. *Each hybridoma clone is a factory for one antibody molecule, yielding a monoclonal antibody that recognizes only one epitope.* In the near future, monoclonal antibodies will be prepared by genetic engineering. The advantages of monoclonal antibodies are that their specificity can be defined to a single epitope on an antigen and they can be prepared in industrial-sized tissue culture preparations. A major disadvantage of monoclonal antibodies is that they are often too specific, such that a monoclonal antibody specific for one epitope on a

viral antigen of one strain may not be able to detect different strains of the same virus.

METHODS OF DETECTION

Antibody-antigen complexes can be detected directly by precipitation techniques; by labeling the antibody with a radioactive, fluorescent, or enzyme probe; or indirectly by measuring an antibody-directed reaction such as complement fixation. *Most of the procedures for detecting and identifying antigen can also be used for serologically evaluating antibody levels.*

Precipitation and Immunodiffusion Techniques

Precipitation techniques are based on the ability of most antibody preparations to interact with more than one epitope on a protein or infectious agent and on the fact that each antibody molecule interacts with more than one antigen (e.g., immunoglobulin G [IgG] has two antigen-binding domains). Within a limited concentration range for both antigen and antibody, termed the **equivalence zone,** the antibody cross-links the antigen into a complex that is too large to stay in solution and therefore precipitates. The antigen-antibody complexes are soluble at concentration ratios of antigen to antibody that are above and below the equivalence concentration.

Various immunodiffusion techniques make use of the equivalence concept to determine the identity of an antigen or the presence of antibody. **Single radial immunodiffusion** can be used to detect and quantify an antigen. In this technique, antigen is placed into a well and allowed to diffuse into antibody-containing agar. The higher the concentration of antigen, the farther it diffuses before it reaches equivalence with the antibody in the agar and precipitates as a ring around the well. The **Ouchterlony immunodouble diffusion** technique is used to determine the relatedness of different antigens, as shown in Figure 18-1. In this technique, solutions of antibody and antigen are placed in separate wells cut into agar, and the antigen and antibody are allowed to diffuse toward each other to establish concentration gradients of

TABLE 18-1 **Selected Immunological Techniques**

TECHNIQUE	PURPOSE	CLINICAL EXAMPLES
Ouchterlony immunodouble diffusion	Detect and compare antigen and antibody	Fungal antigen and antibody
Immunofluorescence	Detection and localization of antigen	Viral antigen in biopsy (e.g., rabies, herpes simplex virus)
Enzyme immunoassay (EIA)	Same as immunofluorescence	Same as immunofluorescence
Immunofluorescence flow cytometry	Population analysis of antigen-positive cells	Immunophenotyping
Enzyme-linked immunosorbent assay (ELISA)	Quantitation of antigen and antibody	Viral antigen (rotavirus), viral antibody (anti-HIV)
Western blot	Detection of antigen-specific antibody	Confirmation of anti-HIV seropositivity
Radioimmunoassay (RIA)	Same as ELISA	Same as ELISA
Complement fixation	Quantitate specific antibody titer	Fungal, viral antibody
Hemagglutination inhibition	Antiviral antibody titer, serotype of virus strain	Seroconversion to current influenza strain, identification of influenza
Latex agglutination	Quantitation and detection of antigen and antibody	Rheumatoid factor, fungal antigens, streptococcal antigens

HIV, Human immunodeficiency virus.

FIGURE 18-1 Analysis of antigens and antibodies by immunoprecipitation. The precipitation of protein occurs at the equivalence point when multivalent antibody forms large complexes with antigen. **A,** Ouchterlony immunodouble diffusion. Antigen and antibody diffuse from wells, meet, and form a precipitin line. If *identical antigens* are used, the concentration of antigen between the wells is doubled, and precipitation does not occur in this region. If different antigens are used, two different precipitin lines are produced. If one sample shares antigen *(1/2)* but is not identical, then a single spur results for the complete antigen. **B,** Countercurrent electrophoresis. This technique is similar to the Ouchterlony method but is facilitated by electrophoresis. **C,** Single radial immunodiffusion. This technique involves the diffusion of antigen into an antibody-containing gel. Precipitin rings indicate an immune reaction, and the area of the ring is proportional to the concentration of antigen. **D,** Rocket electrophoresis. Antigens are first separated by electrophoresis, antibody is added to a trough, and then the diffusion of antibody and separated antigen produces an area of precipitation. **E,** Immunoelectrophoresis. Antigen is placed in a well and separated by electrophoresis. Antibody is then placed in the trough, and precipitin lines form as antigen and antibody diffuse toward each other.

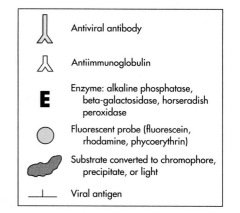

FIGURE 18-2 Immunofluorescence and EIAs for antigen localization in cells. Antigen can be detected by *direct* assay with antiviral antibody modified covalently with a fluorescent or enzyme probe or by *indirect* assay using antiviral antibody and chemically modified antiimmunoglobulin. The enzyme converts substrate to a precipitate, chromophore, or light.

FIGURE 18-3 Immunofluorescence localization of herpes simplex virus–infected nerve cells in a brain section from a patient with herpes encephalitis. (From Emond RT, Rowland HAK: *A color atlas of infectious diseases,* ed 2, London, 1987, Wolfe.)

each substance. A visible precipitin line occurs where the concentrations of antigen and antibody reach equivalence (Figure 18-1). On the basis of the pattern of the precipitin lines, this test can also be used to determine whether samples are identical, share some but not all epitopes (partial identity), or are distinct. This technique is used to detect fungal antigens (e.g., *Histoplasma* species, *Blastomyces* species, coccidioidomycoses). In other immunodiffusion techniques the antigen may be separated by electrophoresis in agar and then reacted with antibody (immunoelectrophoresis), it may be electrophoresed into agar that contains antibody (rocket electrophoresis), or antigen and antibody may be placed in separate wells and electrophoresed toward each other (countercurrent immunoelectrophoresis).

IMMUNOASSAYS FOR CELL-ASSOCIATED ANTIGEN (IMMUNOHISTOLOGY)

Antigens on the cell surface or within the cell can be detected by **immunofluorescence** and **enzyme immunoassay (EIA)**. In **direct immunofluorescence** a fluorescent molecule is covalently attached to the antibody (e.g., fluorescein isothiocyanate–labeled rabbit antiviral

antibody). In **indirect immunofluorescence** a fluorescent second antibody specific for the primary antibody (e.g., fluorescein isothiocyanate–labeled goat antirabbit antibody) is used to detect the primary antiviral antibody and locate the antigen (Figures 18-2 and 18-3). In **EIA** an enzyme such as horseradish peroxidase or alkaline phosphatase is conjugated to the antibody and converts a substrate into a chromophore to mark the antigen. These techniques are useful for the analysis of tissue biopsy specimens, blood cells, or tissue culture cells.

The **flow cytometer** can be used to analyze the immunofluorescence of cells in suspension and is especially useful for identifying and quantitating lymphocytes (immunophenotyping). Unlike an immunofluorescent microscope, a laser is used in the flow cytometer to excite

FIGURE 18-4 Flow cytometry. **A,** The flow cytometer evaluates individual cell parameters as the cells flow past a laser beam at rates of more than 5000 per minute. Cell size and granularity are determined by light scattering *(LS)*, and antigen expression is evaluated by immunofluorescence *(F)* using antibodies labeled with different fluorescent probes. **B** to **D,** T-cell analysis of a normal patient. **B,** Light-scatter analysis was used to define the lymphocytes *(Ly)*, monocytes *(Mo)*, and polymorphonuclear leukocytes *(PMN)*. **C,** The lymphocytes were analyzed for CD3 expression to identify T cells (presented in a histogram). **D,** The CD4- and CD8-positive cells were determined for the T cells. Each dot represents one T cell. (Data proved by Dr. Tom Alexander, Akron, Ohio.)

the fluorescent antibody attached to the cell and to determine the size of the cell by light-scattering measurements. The cells flow past the laser at rates of more than 5000 cells per minute, and analysis is performed electronically. The **fluorescence-activated cell sorter** is a

flow cytometer that can also isolate specific subpopulations of cells for tissue culture growth based on their size and immunofluorescence. The data obtained from a flow cytometer are usually presented in the form of a histogram, with the fluorescence intensity on the x-axis and the number of cells on the y-axis, or in the form of a dot plot in which more than one parameter is compared. The flow cytometer can perform a differential analysis of white blood cells and compare CD4 and CD8 T-cell populations simultaneously (Figure 18-4). Flow cytometry is also useful for analyzing cell growth after the fluorescent labeling of DNA and other fluorescent applications.

IMMUNOASSAYS FOR SOLUBLE ANTIGEN (IMMUNOHISTOCHEMISTRY)

The **enzyme-linked immunosorbent assay (ELISA)** uses antigen immobilized on a plastic surface, bead, or filter to capture and separate the specific antibody from other antibodies in a patient's serum (Figure 18-5). The affixed patient antibody is then detected by an antihuman antibody with a covalently linked enzyme (e.g., horseradish peroxidase, alkaline phosphatase, beta-galactosidase). It is quantitated spectrophotometrically by the intensity of the color produced in response to the enzyme conversion of an appropriate substrate. The actual concentration of antigen can be determined by comparison with standard antigen solutions. The many variations of ELISAs differ in the way in which they capture or detect antibody or antigen.

ELISAs can also be used to quantitate the soluble antigen in a patient's sample. In these assays, soluble antigen is captured and concentrated by an immobilized antibody and then detected with a different antibody labeled with the enzyme. An example of a commonly used ELISA is the home pregnancy test for the human chorionic gonadotropin hormone.

Western blot analysis is a variation of an ELISA. In this technique, viral proteins separated by electrophoresis according to their molecular weight or charge are transferred (blotted) onto a filter paper (e.g., nitrocellulose, nylon). When exposed to a patient's serum, the immobilized proteins capture virus-specific antibody and are visualized with an enzyme-conjugated antihuman antibody. This technique shows the proteins recognized by the patient serum. Western blot analysis is used to confirm ELISA results in patients suspected to be infected with the human immunodeficiency virus (HIV) (Figures 18-6 and 48-7).

In **radioimmunoassay (RIA),** radiolabeled (e.g., iodine-125) antibody or antigen is used to quantitate antigen-antibody complexes. RIA can be performed as a capture assay, as described previously for ELISA, or as a competition assay. In a competition assay, antibody in a patient's serum is quantitated by its ability to compete with and replace a laboratory-prepared radiolabeled antibody from antigen-antibody complexes. The antigen-antibody complexes are precipitated and separated from

A
Antibody detection

B
Antigen capture and detection

FIGURE 18-5 EIAs for quantitation of antibody or antigen. **A,** Antibody detection. *1,* Viral antigen obtained from infected cells, virions, or genetic engineering is affixed to a surface. *2,* Patient serum is added and allowed to bind to the antigen. Unbound antibody is washed away. *3,* Enzyme-conjugated antihuman antibody is added, and unbound antibody is washed away. *4,* Substrate is added and, *5,* converted into chromophore, precipitate, or light. **B,** Antigen capture and detection. *1,* Antiviral antibody is affixed to a surface. *2,* A specimen containing antigen is added, and unbound antigen is washed away. *3,* A second antiviral antibody is added to detect the captured antigen. *4,* Enzyme-conjugated antihuman antibody is added, washed, and followed by, *5,* substrate, which is, *6,* converted into chromophore, precipitate, or light.

Western blot

FIGURE 18-6 Western blot. Proteins are separated by sodium dodecyl sulfate–polyacrylamide gel electrophoresis *(SDS-PAGE),* electroblotted onto nitrocellulose *(NC)* paper, and incubated with antigen-specific or patient's antisera *(1°Ab)* and then enzyme-conjugated antihuman serum *(2°Ab).* Enzyme conversion of substrate identifies the antigen.

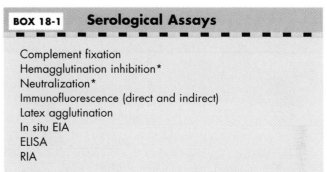

BOX 18-1   Serological Assays

Complement fixation
Hemagglutination inhibition*
Neutralization*
Immunofluorescence (direct and indirect)
Latex agglutination
In situ EIA
ELISA
RIA

*For detection of antibody or serotyping of virus.

free antibody, and the radioactivity is measured for both fractions. The amount of the patient's antibody is then quantitated from standard curves prepared using known quantities of competing antibody. The radioallergosorbent assay is a variation of an RIA capture assay in which radiolabeled antiimmunoglobulin E (IgE) is used to detect allergen-specific responses.

Complement fixation is a standard but technically difficult serological test (Box 18-1). In this test the patient's serum sample is reacted with laboratory-derived antigen and extra complement. Antibody-antigen complexes bind, activate, and fix (use up) the complement. The residual complement is then assayed by the lysis of red blood cells coated with antibody. Antibodies measured by this system generally develop slightly later in an illness than those measured by other techniques.

Antibody inhibition assays make use of the specificity of an antibody to prevent infection (**neutralization**) or other activity (**hemagglutination inhibition**) to identify the strain of the infecting agent, usually a virus, or to quantitate antibody responses to a specific strain of virus. For example, hemagglutination inhibition is used to distinguish different strains of influenza A. These tests are discussed further in Chapter 48.

Latex agglutination is a rapid, technically simple assay for detecting the antibody or soluble antigen. Virus-specific antibody causes latex particles coated with viral antigens to clump. Conversely, antibody-coated latex particles are used to detect soluble viral antigen. Passive hemagglutination makes use of antigen-modified erythrocytes as indicators instead of latex particles.

SEROLOGY

The humoral immune response provides a history of a patient's infections. Serology can be used to identify the infecting agent, evaluate the course of an infection, or determine the nature of the infection—whether it is a primary infection or a reinfection and whether it is acute or chronic. Serological data on an infection are provided by the antibody type and titer and the identity of the antigenic targets. Serological testing is used to identify viruses and other agents that are difficult to isolate and grow in the laboratory or that cause disease with slower courses (Box 18-2).

The relative antibody concentration is reported as a **titer.** A titer is the inverse of the greatest dilution, or lowest concentration (e.g., dilution of 1:64 = titer of 64), of a patient's serum that retains activity in the assays just described. The patient's specific IgG, immunoglobulin A (IgA), IgE, or immunoglobulin M (IgM) can be evaluated separately using a labeled second antihuman antibody specific for the antibody isotype by indirect immunofluorescence, latex agglutination, ELISA, or RIA.

Serology is used to determine the time course of an infection by determining whether **seroconversion** has occurred. Seroconversion occurs when antibody is produced in response to a primary infection. *Specific IgM antibody, found during the first 2 to 3 weeks of a primary infection, generally indicates a recent primary infection.* Seroconversion is indicated by the finding of *at least a fourfold increase in the antibody titer* between serum obtained during the acute phase of disease and that obtained at least 2 to 3 weeks later during the convalescent phase. Reinfection or recurrence later in life causes an anamnestic (secondary or booster) response. Antibody titers may remain high, however, in patients whose disease recurs frequently (e.g., herpesviruses).

Because of the inherent imprecision of serological assays based on twofold serial dilutions, it is necessary that there be a fourfold increase in the antibody titer between acute and convalescent sera for seroconversion to be confirmed. For example, samples with 512 units and 1023 units of antibody would both give a signal on a 512-fold dilution but not a 1024-fold dilution and would be reported as 512. On the other hand, samples with 1020 units and 1030 units are not significantly different but would be reported as titers of 512 and 1024, respectively.

BOX 18-2	**Viruses Diagnosed by Serology***

Epstein-Barr virus
Rubella virus
Hepatitis A, B, C, D, and E viruses
HIV
Human T-cell leukemia virus
Arboviruses (encephalitis viruses)

*Serological testing is also used to determine a person's immune status with regard to other viruses.

Serology can also be used to determine the stage of a slower or chronic infection (e.g., hepatitis B, infectious mononucleosis caused by Epstein-Barr virus) on the basis of the presence of antibody to specific antigens. The first antibodies to be detected are those directed against antigens most available to the immune system (e.g., on the virion, on infected-cell surfaces, secreted). Later in the infection, when cells have been lysed by the infecting virus or the cellular immune response, antibodies directed against the intracellular proteins and enzymes are detected.

QUESTIONS

Describe the diagnostic procedure or procedures (molecular or immunological) that would be appropriate for each of the following applications:

1. Determination of the apparent molecular weights of the HIV proteins.
2. Detection of human papillomavirus 16 (a nonreplicating virus) in a Papanicolaou (Pap) smear.
3. Detection of herpes simplex virus (a replicating virus) in a Pap smear.
4. Presence of *Histoplasma* fungal antigens in a patient's serum.
5. CD4 and CD8 T-cell concentrations in blood from a patient infected with HIV.
6. The presence of antibody and the titer of anti-HIV antibody.
7. Genetic differences between two herpes simplex viruses (DNA virus).
8. Genetic differences between two parainfluenza viruses (RNA virus).
9. Amount of rotavirus antigen in stool.
10. Detection and distinction of group A streptococci from other streptococci.

Bibliography

Baron EJ, Peterson LR, Finegold SM: *Bailey and Scott's diagnostic microbiology,* ed 9, St Louis, 1994, Mosby.
Murray PR: *ASM pocket guide to clinical microbiology,* Washington, DC, 1996, ASM.

SECTION ·················· IV

Bacteriology

CHAPTER 19

Mechanisms of Bacterial Pathogenesis

To a bacterium, the human body is a collection of environmental niches that provide the warmth, moisture, and food necessary for organisms to grow. The bacteria have acquired genetic traits that enable them to enter (invade) the environment, remain in a niche (adhere or colonize), gain access to food sources (degradative enzymes), and escape clearance by host immune and nonimmune protective responses (e.g., capsule). Unfortunately, many of the mechanisms that bacteria use to maintain their niche and the by-products of bacterial growth (e.g., acids, gas) are incompatible with the system of the human host. Many of these genetic traits are **virulence factors**, which enhance the ability of a bacterium to cause disease. Although most bacteria cause disease by directly destroying tissue, some release **toxins,** which are then disseminated by the blood to cause system-wide pathogenesis (Box 19-1).

Not all bacteria cause disease, but some always cause disease once infection occurs. The human body is colonized with numerous microbes **(normal flora),** many of which serve important functions for their hosts, such as aiding in the digestion of food, producing vitamins (e.g., vitamin K), and protecting the host from colonization with pathogenic microbes. Although many of these endogenous bacteria can cause disease, they normally reside in locations such as the gastrointestinal (GI) tract, skin, and upper respiratory tract, which are technically outside the body (Figure 19-1). Normal flora bacteria cause disease if they enter normally sterile sites of the body. **Virulent bacteria** have mechanisms that promote their growth in the host at the expense of the host's tissue or organ function. Symptoms result from the damage or loss of tissue or organ function or the development of host inflammatory responses. **Opportunistic bacteria** cause disease only in people with preexisting diseases or conditions that enhance their susceptibility. For example, *Pseudomonas aeruginosa* infect burn patients and the lungs of patients with cystic fibrosis.

The symptoms of a disease are determined by the function of the tissue affected, although systemic responses, produced by toxins, and immune responses may also occur. The seriousness of the symptoms depends on the importance of the organ affected and the extent of the damage caused by the infection. Infections of the central nervous system are always serious. In some cases the route of exposure and the target tissue for the pathogen or a toxin made by the pathogen determine the particular tissue affected. The **inoculum size** is also a major factor in determining whether disease occurs. However, this can vary from a relatively small inoculum (e.g., fewer than 200 *Shigella* for shigellosis) to a very large inoculum (e.g., 10^8 *Vibrio cholerae* or *Campylobacter* organisms for GI tract infections). Host factors also play a role in determining the potential for disease to be produced. For example, although a million or more *Salmonella* organisms are necessary for gastroenteritis to become established in a healthy person, only a few thousand organisms are necessary in a person whose gastric pH is neutral. The number of staphylococci necessary to produce a wound infection in a person with a foreign body (e.g., prosthesis, catheter, suture material) can also be dramatically reduced. Congenital defects, immunodeficiency states (see Chapter 14), and other disease-related conditions may also increase a person's susceptibility to infection.

ENTRY INTO THE HUMAN BODY

For infection to become established, bacteria must first gain entry into the body (Figure 19-1 and Table 19-1). Natural defense mechanisms and barriers, such as skin, mucus, ciliated epithelium, and secretions containing antibacterial substances (e.g., lysozyme), make it difficult for bacteria to gain entry into the body. However, these barriers are sometimes broken (e.g., a cut in the skin, a tumor or ulcer in the bowel), providing a portal of entry for the bacteria, or the bacteria may have the means to compromise the barrier and invade the body. On invasion, the bacteria can travel in the bloodstream to other sites in the body.

The skin has a thick, horny layer of dead cells that protects the body from infection. However, cuts in the skin, produced accidentally or surgically or kept open with catheters or other surgical appliances, provide a means for the bacteria to gain access to the susceptible tissue underneath. For example, *Staphylococcus aureus*

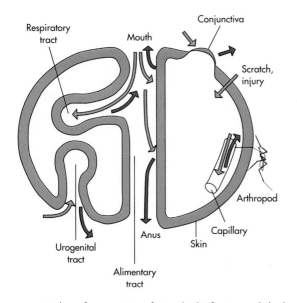

FIGURE 19-1 Body surfaces as sites of microbial infection and shedding. *Green arrows,* Infection; *purple arrows,* shedding. (Redrawn from Mims C et al: *Medical microbiology,* London, 1993, Mosby-Wolfe.)

TABLE 19-1	**Bacterial Port of Entry**
ROUTE	**EXAMPLES**
Ingestion	*Salmonella* species, *Shigella* species, *Yersinia enterocolitica,* enterotoxigenic *Escherichia coli, Vibrio* species, *Campylobacter* species, *Clostridium botulinum, Bacillus cereus, Listeria* species, *Brucella* species
Inhalation	*Mycobacterium* species, *Nocardia* species, *Mycoplasma pneumoniae, Legionella* species, *Bordetella, Chlamydia psittaci, Chlamydia pneumoniae*
Direct penetration	
Trauma	*Clostridium tetani*
Needlestick	*Staphylococcus aureus, Pseudomonas* species
Arthropod bite	*Rickettsia* species, *Ehrlichia* species, *Coxiella* species, *Francisella* species, *Borrelia* species, *Yersinia pestis*
Sexual transmission	*Neisseria gonorrhoeae, Chlamydia trachomatis, Treponema pallidum*
Transplacental	*Treponema pallidum*

BOX 19-1	**Bacterial Virulence Mechanisms**

Adherence
Invasion
By-products of growth (gas, acid)
Toxins
   Degradative enzymes
   A-B toxins
Endotoxin
Superantigen
Induction of excess inflammation
Evasion of phagocytic and immune clearance
Resistance to antibiotics

nize the GI tract, where they serve the beneficial function of producing the vitamin K that the body needs. These endogenous bacteria are normally benign and restricted to the body cavities that they colonize. However, these bacteria can enter normally sterile sites of the body, such as the peritoneum and the bloodstream, through a break in the normal barrier. An example of this is the patient whose colon tumor was detected through the identification of a septicemia (blood-borne infection) caused by enteric bacteria.

COLONIZATION, ADHESION, AND INVASION

As previously indicated, the GI tract is naturally colonized by benign and potentially beneficial bacteria. In some cases, environmental conditions determine the bacteria that can or will colonize a site. For example, *Legionella* grows in the lung but does not readily spread because it cannot tolerate high temperatures (>35° C). Colonization of sites that are normally sterile, such as the lung, implies the existence of a defect in a natural defense mechanism or a portal of entry. Patients with cystic fibrosis have such defects because of the reduction in their ciliary mucoepithelial function and altered mucosal secretions; as a result, they suffer from colonization by *S. aureus* and *P. aeruginosa.*

Bacteria may need to have specific mechanisms so that they can adhere to and colonize many different body surfaces (Table 19-2). If the bacteria can adhere to epithelial or endothelial cell linings of the bladder, intestine,

and *Staphylococcus epidermidis,* which are a part of the normal flora on skin, can enter the body through breaks in the skin and pose a major problem for people with indwelling catheters and intravenous lines.

The mouth, nose, respiratory tract, ears, eyes, urogenital tract, and anus are sites through which bacteria can enter the body. These natural openings in the skin and their associated body cavities are protected by natural defenses such as the mucus and ciliated epithelium that line the upper respiratory tract, the lysozyme and other antibacterial secretions in tears and mucus, and the acid and bile in the GI tract. However, many bacteria are unaffected or have the means to evade these defenses. For example, the outer membrane of the gram-negative bacteria makes these bacteria more resistant to lysozyme, acid, and bile. This enables the enterobacteria to colo-

TABLE 19-2   Examples of Bacterial Adherence Mechanisms

MICROBE	ADHESIN	RECEPTOR
Bacteria		
S. aureus	Lipoteichoic acid	Unknown
Staphylococcus species	Slime	Unknown
Streptococcus, group A	LTA-M protein complex	Unknown
Streptococcus, group B	Protein	N-Acetyl-glucosamine
Escherichia coli	Type 1 fimbriae	D-Mannose
	Colonization factor antigen I fimbriae	GM ganglioside
	P fimbriae	P blood group glycolipid
Other Enterobacteriaceae	Type 1 fimbriae	D-Mannose
Neisseria gonorrhoeae	Fimbriae	GD₁ ganglioside
Treponema pallidum	P₁, P₂, P₃	Fibronectin
Chlamydia species	Cell surface lectin	N-Acetyl-glucosamine
Mycoplasma pneumoniae	Protein P1	Sialic acid

LTA, Lipoteichoic acid.

and blood vessels, they cannot be washed away, which allows them to colonize the tissue. For example, natural bladder function eliminates any bacteria not affixed to the bladder wall. *Escherichia coli* and other bacteria have adhesins that bind to specific receptors on the tissue surface and this keeps them from being washed away. Many of these adhesin proteins are present at the tips of **fimbriae** (pili) and bind tightly to specific sugars on the target tissue. (This sugar-binding activity defines these proteins as lectins.) For example, most *E. coli* strains that cause pyelonephritis produce a fimbrial adhesin termed *P fimbriae*. This adhesin can bind to receptors for alpha-D-galactosyl-beta-D-galactoside (Gal-Gal), which is part of the P blood group antigen structure on human erythrocytes and uroepithelial cells. *Neisseria gonorrhoeae* pili are also important virulence factors; they bind to oligosaccharide receptors on epithelial cells. *Yersinia* organisms, *Bordetella pertussis*, and *Mycoplasma pneumoniae* express adhesin proteins that are not on fimbriae. *Streptococcus pyogenes* uses **lipoteichoic acid** and the F protein (binds to fibronectin) to bind to epithelial cells.

A special bacterial adaptation that facilitates colonization, especially of surgical appliances such as artificial valves or indwelling catheters, is a **biofilm** produced by the bacteria. Bacteria in biofilms are bound within a sticky web of polysaccharide that binds the cells together and to the surface. Dental plaque is an example of a biofilm. The biofilm matrix can also protect the bacteria from host defenses and antibiotics.

Although bacteria do not have mechanisms that enable them to cross skin, several bacteria can cross mucosal membranes and other tissue barriers to enter normally sterile sites and more susceptible tissue. These invasive bacteria either destroy the barrier or penetrate into the cells of the barrier. *Shigella* and *Salmonella* organisms bind to tissue and initiate its destruction so that they can then invade the host. Enteropathogenic *Yersinia* organisms produce an invasin protein that promotes the binding of the bacteria to cells, which in turn stimulates the cell to invaginate and take in the bacteria.

PATHOGENIC ACTIONS OF BACTERIA
Tissue Destruction

Although bacteria are part of the normal flora in many sites, their growth in normally sterile sites causes problems. **Bacterial growth,** especially fermentation, results in the production of acids, gas, and other by-products that are toxic to tissue. In addition, many bacteria release *degradative enzymes that break down tissue, thereby providing food for the growth of the organisms and promoting the spread of the bacteria,* especially if blood vessels are involved. For example, *Clostridium perfringens* are part of the normal flora of the GI tract but are also opportunistic pathogens that can establish infection in oxygen-depleted tissues and cause gas gangrene. These anaerobic bacteria produce enzymes (e.g., phospholipase C, collagenase, protease, hyaluronidase), several toxins, and acid and gas from bacterial metabolism, which destroys the tissue. Staphylococci produce many different enzymes that modify the tissue environment. These enzymes include hyaluronidase, fibrinolysin, and lipases. Streptococci also produce enzymes, including streptolysins S and O, hyaluronidase, and streptokinases; these enzymes facilitate the development of infection and its spread.

Toxins

Toxins are bacterial components that directly harm tissue or trigger destructive biological activities. Toxin and toxinlike activities are caused by cell wall components, degradative enzymes that cause lysis of cells, and specific receptor-binding proteins that initiate toxic reactions in a specific target tissue or initiate a systemic response (such as fever) by promoting the release of lymphokines. In many cases the toxin is completely responsible for causing the characteristic symptoms of the disease. For example, the **preformed toxin** present in food mediates the food poisoning caused by *S. aureus* and *Bacillus cereus* and the botulism caused by *Clostridium botulinum*. The food poisoning caused by preformed toxin occurs much sooner than other forms of gastroenteritis, however, because bacteria do not need to grow for the symptoms to occur. Because a toxin can be spread systemically through the bloodstream, symptoms may arise at a site distant from the site of infection, such as occurs in tetanus, which is caused by *Clostridium tetani*, or the toxin can be disseminated throughout the body, as occurs in the staphylococcal scalded skin syndrome.

Endotoxin and Other Cell Wall Components

The presence of bacterial cell wall components indicates infection. These components activate host protective responses. In some cases, the host response is excessive and may even be life threatening. On infection with gram-positive bacteria, peptidoglycan and its breakdown products, as well as teichoic and lipoteichoic acids, are released, and these stimulate toxinlike **pyrogenic responses.** The lipopolysaccharide produced by gram-negative bacteria is an even more powerful activator of inflammatory reactions, and its presence is like a multi-alarm warning to the body to activate the host's protective systems. *The lipid A portion of lipopolysaccharide is responsible for endotoxin activity.* It is important to appreciate that endotoxin is not the same as exotoxin and that only gram-negative bacteria make endotoxin.

Gram-negative bacteria release endotoxin during infection. Endotoxin binds to specific receptors on macrophages, B cells, and other cells and stimulates the production and release of **acute phase lymphokines,** such as interleukin-1, tumor necrosis factor–alpha, interleukin-6, and prostaglandins (Figure 19-2). Endotoxin also stimulates the growth (mitogenic) of B cells. At low concentrations, endotoxin stimulates the mounting of protective responses such as fever, vasodilatation, and the activation of the immune and inflammatory responses (Box 19-2). However, the endotoxin levels in the blood of patients with gram-negative bacterial sepsis (bacteria in the blood) can be very high, and the response to these can be overpowering, resulting in shock and possibly death. High concentrations of endotoxin activate the alternative pathway of complement and promote high fever, hypotension, shock produced by vasodilatation and capillary leakage, and disseminated intravascular coagulation stemming from the activation of the blood coagulation pathways. The high fever, pe-

techiae (skin lesions resulting from the capillary leakage), and potential symptoms of shock (resulting from increased vascular permeability) associated with *Neisseria meningitidis* infection can be related to the large amounts of endotoxin released during infection.

Exotoxins

Exotoxins are proteins produced by gram-positive or gram-negative bacteria and include **cytolytic enzymes** and **dimeric toxins with A and B subunits.** In many cases the toxin gene is encoded on a plasmid (tetanus toxin of *C. tetani*, LT and ST toxins of enterotoxigenic *E. coli*) or a lysogenic phage *(Corynebacterium diphtheriae* and *C. botulinum).* An example of a cytolytic toxin is the alpha toxin (phospholipase C) produced by *C. perfringens,* which enzymatically attacks sphingomyelin and other membrane phospholipids, resulting in cell lysis. The B portion of the A-B toxins that constitute the dimeric toxins binds to a specific cell surface receptor, and then the A subunit is transferred into the interior of the cell, where cell injury is induced. The tissues targeted by these toxins are very defined and limited (Figure 19-3 and Table 19-3). The functional properties of cytolytic and bipartite exotoxins are discussed in greater

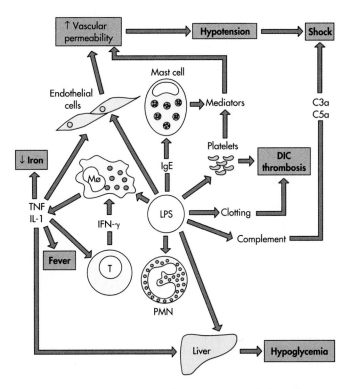

FIGURE 19-2 The many activities of lipopolysaccharide *(LPS).* This bacterial endotoxin activates almost every immune mechanism as well as the clotting pathway, which together make lipopolysaccharide one of the most powerful immune stimuli known. *DIC,* Disseminated intravascular coagulation; *IFN-γ* interferon-gamma; *IgE,* immunoglobulin E; *IL-1,* interleukin-1; *PMN,* polymorphonuclear neutrophil leukocytes; *TNF,* tumor necrosis factor. (Redrawn from Mims C et al: *Medical microbiology,* London, 1993, Mosby-Wolfe.)

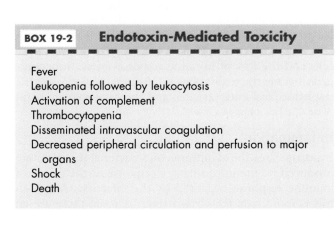

BOX 19-2   Endotoxin-Mediated Toxicity

Fever
Leukopenia followed by leukocytosis
Activation of complement
Thrombocytopenia
Disseminated intravascular coagulation
Decreased peripheral circulation and perfusion to major organs
Shock
Death

A   Inhibition of protein synthesis

B   Hyperactivation

C   Effects on nerve–muscle transmission

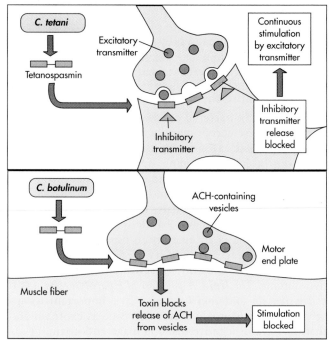

FIGURE 19-3 The mode of action of dimeric A-B exotoxins. The bacterial A-B toxins often consist of a two-chain molecule. The B chain promotes entry of the bacteria into cells, and the A chain has inhibitory activity against some vital function. *cAMP,* Cyclic adenosine monophosphate. ACH, Acetylcholine. (Redrawn from Mims C et al: *Medical microbiology,* London, 1993, Mosby-Wolfe.)

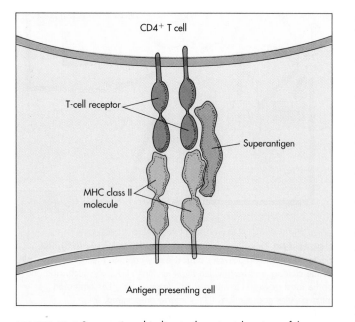

FIGURE 19-4 Superantigen binding to the external regions of the T-cell receptor and the class II major histocompatibility complex *(MHC)* molecules.

detail in the chapters dealing with the specific diseases involved.

Superantigens are also a special group of toxins (Figure 19-4). These are toxinlike molecules that activate T cells by binding to both the T-cell receptor and a class II major histocompatibility complex molecule on another cell without requiring antigen. This nonspecific means of activating T cells can trigger life-threatening autoimmune-like responses by stimulating the release of large amounts of interleukins, such as interleukin-1 and interleukin-2. This superantigen stimulation of T cells can also lead to death of specific T-cell receptor–expressing T cells and the loss of immune responsiveness. Superantigens include the toxic shock syndrome toxin of *S. aureus,* staphylococcal enterotoxins, and the erythrogenic toxin A or C of *S. pyogenes.*

Inflammation

In many cases the symptoms of a bacterial infection are produced by the inflammatory response or the excessive immune response triggered by the infection. Although this is more true for viruses than bacteria, these are an important cause of the symptoms in patients with infec-

TABLE 19-3   Properties of A-B Type Bacterial Toxins

TOXIN	ORGANISM	GENETIC CONTROL	SUBUNIT STRUCTURE	TARGET CELL RECEPTOR	BIOLOGICAL EFFECTS
Anthrax toxins	*Bacillus anthracis*	Plasmid	Three separate proteins (EF, LF, PA)	Unknown, probably glycoprotein	EF + PA: increase in target-cell cAMP level, localized edema; LF + PA: death of target cells and experimental animals
Bordetella adenylate cyclase toxin	*Bordetella* species	Chromosomal	A-B	Unknown, probably glycolipid	Increase in target cell cAMP level, modified cell function or cell death
Botulinum toxin	*C. botulinum*	Phage	A-B	Possibly ganglioside (GD_{1b})	Decrease in peripheral, presynaptic acetylcholine release, flaccid paralysis
Cholera toxin	*V. cholerae*	Chromosomal	A-5B	Ganglioside (GM_1)	Activation of adenylate cyclase, increase in cAMP level, secretory diarrhea
Diphtheria toxin	*C. diphtheriae*	Phage	A-B	Probably glycoprotein	Inhibition of protein synthesis, cell death
Heat-labile enterotoxins	*E. coli*	Plasmid	Similar or identical to cholera toxin		
Pertussis toxin	*B. pertussis*	Chromosomal	A-5B	Unknown, probably glycoprotein	Block of signal transduction mediated by target G proteins
Pseudomonas exotoxin A	*P. aeruginosa*	Chromosomal	A-B	Unknown, but different from diphtheria toxin	Similar or identical to diphtheria toxin
Shiga toxin	*Shigella dysenteriae*	Chromosomal	A-5B	Glycoprotein or glycolipid	Inhibition of protein synthesis, cell death
Shiga-like toxins	*Shigella* species, *E. coli*	Phage	Similar or identical to Shiga toxin		
Tetanus toxin	*C. tetani*	Plasmid	A-B	Ganglioside (GT_1) and/or GD_{1b}	Decrease in neurotransmitter release from inhibitory neurons, spastic paralysis

Based on data from Mandell G, Douglas G, Bennett J: *Principles and practice of infectious disease,* ed 3, New York, 1990, Churchill Livingstone.
cAMP, Cyclic adenosine monophosphate.

tions caused by *Chlamydia,* treponemes (syphilis), and *Borrelia* (Lyme disease). In addition, the sequelae of streptococcal infections such as rheumatic fever result from the effects of the antibodies to the bacterial M protein, which cross-react with and initiate damage to the heart. Poststreptococcal glomerulonephritis results from the formation of immune complexes deposited in the glomeruli of the kidney.

MECHANISMS FOR ESCAPING HOST DEFENSES

Logically, the longer bacteria remain in a host, the more time they have to cause damage. Therefore bacteria that can evade or incapacitate the host defenses have a greater potential for causing disease. Bacteria have developed ways to avoid being recognized and killed by phagocytic cells and to inactivate or evade the complement system and antibody, and some bacteria can hide from immune responses by growing intracellularly (Box 19-3).

*The **capsule** is one of the most important virulence factors* (Box 19-4). These slime layers function by shielding the bacteria from immune and phagocytic responses. Capsules are usually made of polysaccharides, which are usually poor immunogens. The *S. pyogenes* capsule, for example, is made of hyaluronic acid, which mimics human connective tissue, thereby masking the bacteria and keeping it from being recognized by the immune system. The capsule also acts like a slimy football jersey, in that it is hard to grasp and tears away when grabbed by a phagocyte. The capsule also protects a bacteria from the environment of a phagolysosome within the macrophage or leukocyte. Mutants of normally encapsulated bacteria that lose the ability to make a capsule also lose their virulence; examples of such bacteria are *Streptococcus pneumoniae* and *N. meningitidis*.

Bacteria can circumvent phagocytic killing in a variety of ways. They can produce enzymes capable of lysing phagocytic cells (e.g., the streptolysin produced by *S. pyogenes* or the alpha toxin produced by *C. perfringens*). They can inhibit phagocytosis (e.g., the effect of the **capsule** surrounding and the **M protein** produced by *S. pyogenes*) or block intracellular killing. Bacteria have also developed mechanisms to protect them from intracellular killing. These include their ability to prevent phagolysosome fusion, to resist being killed by bactericidal lysosomal enzymes or substances, and to exit the phagosome

TABLE 19-4   Methods That Circumvent Phagocytic Killing

METHOD	EXAMPLE
Inhibition of phagolysosome infusion	*Legionella* species, *Mycobacterium tuberculosis*, *Chlamydia* species
Resistance to lysosomal enzymes	*Salmonella typhimurium*, *Coxiella* species, *Ehrlichia* species, *Mycobacterium leprae*, *Leishmania* species
Adaptation to cytoplasmic replication	*Listeria* species, *Francisella* species, *Rickettsia* species

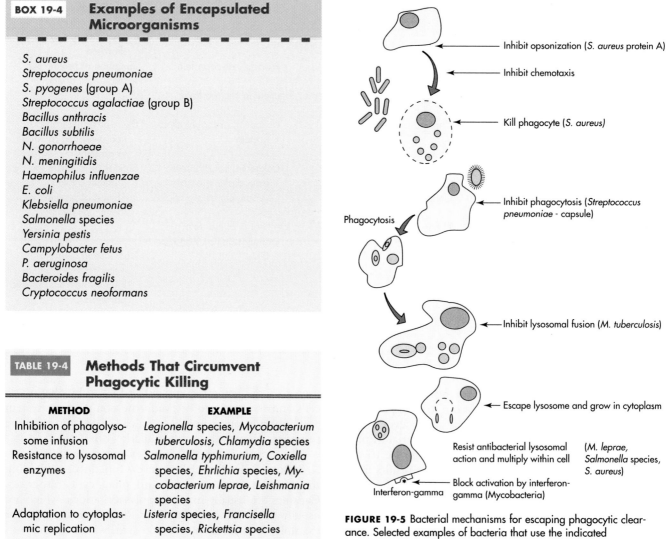

FIGURE 19-5 Bacterial mechanisms for escaping phagocytic clearance. Selected examples of bacteria that use the indicated antiphagocytic mechanisms are given.

into the host cytoplasm before being exposed to lysosomal enzymes (Table 19-4 and Figure 19-5). Staphylococci can also produce catalase, an enzyme that makes the myeloperoxidase system less effective. Many of the bacteria that are internalized but survive phagocytosis use the cell as a place to grow and a means of being disseminated throughout the body.

Other important host defenses subverted by bacteria include the **alternate pathway of complement** and **antibody.** Bacteria evade complement action by masking themselves and by inhibiting activation of the cascade. The long O antigen of lipopolysaccharide prevents the complement from gaining access to the membrane and protects gram-negative bacteria from damage. Immunoglobulin A antibody is inactivated by an immunoglobulin A–specific protease made by *N. gonorrhoeae. S. aureus* makes an immunoglobulin G–binding protein, protein A, which masks the bacteria and thereby prevents antibody action.

S. aureus can also escape host defenses by walling off the site of infection. *S. aureus* can produce **coagulase,** an enzyme that promotes the conversion of fibrin to fibrinogen to produce a clotlike barrier; this feature distinguishes *S. aureus* from *S. epidermidis. Mycobacterium tuberculosis* is able to survive in a host by promoting the development of a granuloma, within which viable bacteria may reside for the life of the infected person. The bacteria may resume growth if there is a decline in the immune status of the person.

SUMMARY

The primary virulence factors of bacteria are adhesins, invasins, degradative enzymes, toxins, the capsule, and mechanisms for escaping elimination by host defenses. Disease produced by some bacteria results from the action of only one virulence mechanism. For example, *C. diphtheria* has only one virulence mechanism: diphtheria toxin. Other bacteria express many virulence factors. *S. aureus* is an example of such a bacterium; it expresses adhesins, degradative enzymes, toxins, catalase, and coagulase, which are responsible for producing a spectrum of diseases. In addition, different strains within a bacterial species may express different virulence mechanisms. For example, the symptoms and sequelae of gastroenteritis (diarrhea) caused by *E. coli* may include invasion and bloody stools, cholera-like watery stools, and even severe hemorrhagic disease, depending on the specific infecting strain.

QUESTIONS

1. Name three routes by which exogenous pathogens can infect a person. List five examples of organisms that use each route.
2. How are microbes able to resist immunological clearance? Give at least one specific example of each mechanism.
3. What are the two general types of exotoxins? List examples of each type.

Bibliography

Gorbach S et al: *Infectious diseases,* Philadelphia, 1992, WB Saunders.

Mandell GJ et al: *Mandell, Douglas and Bennett's principles and practice of infectious diseases,* ed 4, New York, 1995, Churchill Livingstone.

McGee J et al: *Oxford textbook of pathology,* vol 1, Oxford, 1992, Oxford University Press.

Antibacterial Agents

This chapter will provide an overview of the mechanisms of action and antibacterial spectrum of the most commonly used antibiotics as well as a description of the common mechanisms of bacterial resistance. The terminology appropriate for this discussion is summarized in Box 20-1.

The year 1935 was an important one for the chemotherapy of systemic bacterial infections. Although antiseptics had been applied topically to prevent the growth of microorganisms, systemic bacterial infections had not as yet responded to any existing agents. In this year the red azo dye protosil was shown to protect mice against systemic streptococcal infection and to be curative in patients suffering from such infections. It was soon found that protosil was cleaved in the body to release *p*-aminobenzene sulfonamide, or sulfanilamide, which was subsequently shown to have antibacterial activity. These observations regarding the first "sulfa" drug ushered in a new era in medicine. Compounds (antibiotics) produced by microorganisms were eventually discovered to inhibit the growth of other microorganisms. For example, Fleming first noted that the mold *Penicillium* prevented the multiplication of staphylococci. A concentrate from a culture of this mold was prepared, and the remarkable activity and lack of toxicity of the first antibiotic, penicillin, were demonstrated. Streptomycin and the tetracyclines were developed in the 1940s and 1950s, followed rapidly by the development of additional aminoglycosides, semisynthetic penicillins, cephalosporins, quinolones, and other antimicrobials. All these antibacterial agents greatly increased the range of infectious diseases that could be prevented or cured.

Despite the rapidity with which new chemotherapeutic agents are introduced, bacteria have shown a remarkable ability to develop resistance to these agents. Thus antibiotic therapy will not be the predicted magical cure for all infections; rather it is only one weapon, albeit an important one, against infectious diseases. It is also important to recognize that because resistance to antibiotics is frequently not predictable, physicians must rely on their clinical experience for the initial selection of empirical therapy. Guidelines for the management of infections caused by specific organisms are discussed in the relevant chapters of this text.

The results of in vitro antimicrobial susceptibility testing are valuable for selecting chemotherapeutic agents active against the infecting organism. Extensive work has been performed in an effort to standardize the testing methods and improve the clinical predictive value of the results. Despite these efforts, the in vitro tests are simply a measurement of the effect of the antibiotic against the organism. The selection of an antibiotic and the patient's outcome are influenced by a variety of interrelated factors, including the pharmacokinetic properties of the antibiotic, drug toxicity, and the patient's general medical status.

The basic mechanisms and sites of antibiotic activity are summarized in Table 20-1 and Figure 20-1, respectively.

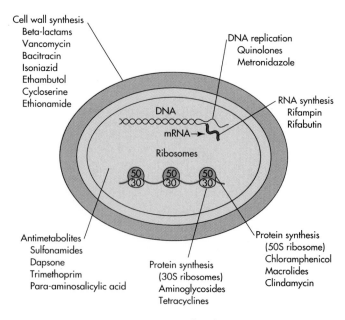

FIGURE 20-1 Basic sites of antibiotic activity.

BOX 20-1   **Terminology**

Antibacterial spectrum—Range of activity of an antimicrobial against bacteria. A **broad-spectrum** antibacterial drug can inhibit a wide variety of gram-positive and gram-negative bacteria, whereas a **narrow-spectrum** drug is active only against a limited variety of bacteria.

Bacteriostatic activity—The level of antimicrobial activity that inhibits the growth of an organism. This is determined in vitro by testing a standardized concentration of organisms against a series of antimicrobial dilutions. The lowest concentration that inhibits the growth of the organism is referred to as the **minimum inhibitory concentration (MIC).**

Bactericidal activity—The level of antimicrobial activity that kills the test organism. This is determined in vitro by exposing a standardized concentration of organisms to a series of antimicrobial dilutions. The lowest concentration that kills 99.9% of the population is referred to as the **minimum bactericidal concentration (MBC).**

Antibiotic combinations—Combinations of antibiotics that may be used (1) to broaden the antibacterial spectrum for empiric therapy or the treatment of polymicrobial infections, (2) to prevent the emergence of resistant organisms during therapy, and (3) to achieve a synergistic killing effect.

Antibiotic synergism—Combinations of two antibiotics that have enhanced bactericidal activity when tested together compared with the activity of each antibiotic.

Antibiotic antagonism—Combination of antibiotics in which the activity of one antibiotic interferes with the activity of the other (e.g., the sum of the activity is less than the activity of the individual drugs).

Beta-lactamase—An enzyme that hydrolyzes the beta-lactam ring in the beta-lactam class of antibiotics, thus inactivating the antibiotic. The enzymes specific for penicillins and cephalosporins are the **penicillinases** and **cephalosporinases,** respectively.

TABLE 20-1   Basic Mechanisms of Antibiotic Action

ANTIBIOTIC	ACTION
INHIBITION OF CELL WALL SYNTHESIS	
Penicillin	Binds PBPs and enzymes responsible for peptidoglycan synthesis
Cephalosporin	Binds PBPs and enzymes responsible for peptidoglycan synthesis
Cephamycin	Binds PBPs and enzymes responsible for peptidoglycan synthesis
Carbapenem	Binds PBPs and enzymes responsible for peptidoglycan synthesis
Monobactam	Binds PBPs and enzymes responsible for peptidoglycan synthesis
Beta-lactamase inhibitor/beta-lactam	Binds beta-lactamase and prevents enzymatic inactivation of beta-lactam
Vancomycin	Disrupts cross-linkage of peptidoglycan layers
Bacitracin	Disrupts movement of peptidoglycan precursors
Isoniazid	Disrupts mycolic acid synthesis
Ethionamide	Disrupts mycolic acid synthesis
Ethambutol	Disrupts arabinogalactan synthesis
Cycloserine	Disrupts cross-linkage of peptidoglycan layers
INHIBITION OF PROTEIN SYNTHESIS	
Aminoglycoside	Binds 30S ribosomal proteins
Tetracycline	Prevents polypeptide elongation at 30S ribosome
Macrolide	Prevents polypeptide elongation at 50S ribosome
Clindamycin	Prevents polypeptide elongation at 50S ribosome
ALTERATION OF CELL MEMBRANES	
Polymyxin	Disrupts bacterial cytoplasmic membrane
Bacitracin	Disrupts bacterial cytoplasmic membrane
INHIBITION OF NUCLEIC ACID SYNTHESIS	
Quinolone	Binds alpha subunit of DNA gyrase
Rifampin	Prevents transcription by binding DNA-dependent RNA polymerase
Rifabutin	Prevents transcription by binding DNA-dependent RNA polymerase
Metronidazole	Disrupts bacteria DNA (is cytotoxic compound)
ANTIMETABOLITE	
Sulfonamides	Inhibit dihydropteroate synthase and disrupt folic acid synthesis
Dapsone	Inhibits dihydropteroate synthase
Trimethoprim	Inhibits dihydrofolate reductase and disrupts folic acid synthesis

PBPs, Penicillin-binding proteins.

INHIBITION OF CELL WALL SYNTHESIS

By far the most common mechanism of antibiotic activity is interference with bacterial cell wall synthesis. Most of the cell wall–active antibiotics are classified as beta-lactam antibiotics (e.g., penicillins, cephalosporins, cephamycins, carbapenems, monobactams, beta-lactamase inhibitors), so named because they share a common beta-lactam ring structure (Figure 20-2). Other antibiotics that interfere with construction of the bacterial cell wall include vancomycin, bacitracin, and the antimycobacterial agents isoniazid, ethambutol, cycloserine, and ethionamide.

Beta-Lactam Antibiotics

The major structural component of bacterial cell walls is the peptidoglycan layer. The basic structure is a chain of 10 to 65 disaccharide residues consisting of alternating molecules of N-acetylglucosamine and N-acetylmuramic acid. Attached to the latter sugar is a pentapeptide composed of L-alanine, D-glutamic acid, either meso-diaminopimelic acid (DAP) or L-lysine, D-alanine, and D-alanine. Individual chains are covalently cross-linked with a pentaglycine bridge between DAP or L-lysine on one chain and D-alanine on the adjacent chain. The building of the pentapeptides and pentaglycine bridges is catalyzed by specific enzymes (e.g., transpeptidases, transglycosylases, carboxypeptidases, endopeptidases). These regulatory enzymes are also called **penicillin-binding proteins (PBPs)** because they can be bound by beta-lactam antibiotics. When growing bacteria are exposed to these antibiotics, the antibiotic binds to the PBPs in the bacterial cytoplasmic membrane, thereby inhibiting synthesis of the cell wall peptidoglycan layer and causing the release of autolytic enzymes that degrade the preformed cell wall, resulting in bacterial cell death. Thus the beta-lactam antibiotics generally act as bactericidal agents.

Bacteria can develop resistance to beta-lactam antibiotics by three mechanisms: (1) Prevention of the interaction between the antibiotic and the target PBP, (2) failure of the antibiotic to bind to the PBP, and (3) hydrolysis of the antibiotic by beta-lactamases (Figure

FIGURE 20-2 General structures of beta-lactam antibiotics. Additional variations are possible at some of the non–R group positions. For example, the cephamycins and cephalosporins differ by replacing the sulfur molecule at the 5 position with oxygen. The arrow points to the bond that is broken during beta-lactamase–catalyzed hydrolysis. (Modified from Brody TM et al, editors: *Human pharmacology: molecular to clinical*, ed 4, St Louis, 1994, Mosby.)

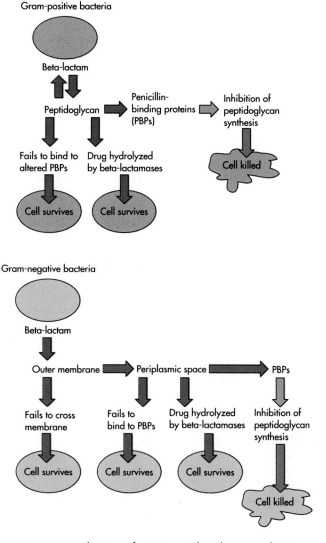

FIGURE 20-3 Mechanisms of resistance to beta-lactam antibiotics. (Modified from Brody TM et al, editors: *Human pharmacology: molecular to clinical*, ed 4, St Louis, 1994, Mosby.)

20-3). The first mechanism of resistance is seen only in gram-negative bacteria (particularly *Pseudomonas* species) because they have an outer membrane that overlies the peptidoglycan layer. Penetration of beta-lactam antibiotics into gram-negative bacilli requires transit through the outer membrane pores. Changes in the proteins that form the walls of the pores can alter the size or charge of these channels and result in the exclusion of the antibiotic. Bacteria can also acquire a modified PBP that fails to bind to beta-lactam antibiotics but will contribute to the synthesis of the peptidoglycan layer. The modified PBP can either originate from a mutation in the PBP gene (e.g., *Streptococcus pneumoniae* resistant to penicillins) or through the acquisition of a new PBP (e.g., *Escherichia coli* PBP introduced into *Staphylococcus aureus* confers resistance to oxacillin). Finally, bacteria can produce **beta-lactamases** that inactivate the beta-lactam antibiotics. More than 200 different beta-lactamases have been described. Some are specific for penicillins (i.e., penicillinases) and cephalosporins (i.e., cephalosporinases), whereas others have a broad range of activity and are capable of inactivating most beta-lactam antibiotics. This latter group of beta-lactamases **(extended-spectrum beta-lactamases [ESBLs])** is particularly troublesome because they are commonly encoded on plasmids and can be transferred from organism to organism. This has severely limited the use of beta-lactam antibiotics in some hospitals.

Penicillins

Penicillin compounds are highly effective antibiotics with an extremely low toxicity. The basic compound is an organic acid with a beta-lactam ring obtained from culture of the mold *Penicillium chrysogenum* (Figure 20-2). If the mold is grown by a fermentation process, large amounts of a key intermediate, 6-aminopenicillinacic acid (the beta-lactam ring is fused with a thiazolidine ring), are produced. The biochemical substitution of this intermediate yields derivatives that have decreased acid lability and increased absorption in the gastrointestinal tract, resistance to destruction by penicillinase, or a broader spectrum of activity that includes gram-negative bacteria (Box 20-2).

Penicillin G is incompletely absorbed because it is inactivated by gastric acid. Thus it is used mainly as an intravenous drug for the treatment of infections caused by the limited number of susceptible organisms. Penicillin V is more resistant to acid and is the preferred oral form for the treatment of susceptible bacteria. Penicillinase-resistant penicillins such as methicillin and oxacillin are used to treat infections caused by susceptible staphylococci. Ampicillin was the first penicillin active against gram-negative bacilli, although the spectrum of activity was limited primarily to *Escherichia* and *Proteus* species. However, other penicillins (e.g., carbenicillin, ticarcillin, piperacillin) that have been developed are effective against a broad spectrum of gram-negative bacteria,

---

BOX 20-2   Penicillins

NATURAL PENICILLINS

Benzylpenicillin (penicillin G)
Phenoxymethyl penicillin (penicillin V)

PENICILLINASE-RESISTANT PENICILLINS

Nafcillin	Cloxacillin
Methicillin	Dicloxacillin
Oxacillin	

EXTENDED-SPECTRUM PENICILLINS

Aminopenicillins (ampicillin, amoxicillin)
Carboxypenicillins (carbenicillin, ticarcillin)
Ureidopenicillins (mezlocillin, piperacillin)

---

including *Klebsiella*, *Enterobacter*, and *Pseudomonas* species.

Cephalosporins and Cephamycins

The cephalosporins are beta-lactam antibiotics derived from 7-aminocephalosporanic acid (the beta-lactam ring is fused with a dihydrothiazine ring), which was originally isolated from the mold *Cephalosporium* (Figure 20-2). The cephamycins are closely related to the cephalosporins, except that they contain oxygen in place of sulfur in the dihydrothiazine ring, rendering them more stable to beta-lactamase hydrolysis. The cephalosporins and cephamycins have the same mechanism of action as the penicillins but have a wider antibacterial spectrum, are resistant to many beta-lactamases, and have improved pharmacokinetic properties.

Biochemical modifications in the basic antibiotic molecule resulted in the development of antibiotics with improved activity and pharmacokinetic properties. The activity of narrow-spectrum, first-generation antibiotics is primarily restricted to *Escherichia* species, *Klebsiella* species, *Proteus* species, and oxacillin-susceptible gram-positive cocci (Box 20-3). Many of the expanded-spectrum, second-generation antibiotics are also active against *Haemophilus influenzae*, *Enterobacter* species, *Citrobacter* species, *Serratia* species, and some anaerobes such as *Bacteroides fragilis*. The broad-spectrum, third-generation antibiotics are active against most Enterobacteriaceae and *Pseudomonas aeruginosa*. Unfortunately, gram-negative bacteria have rapidly developed resistance to cephalosporins and cephamycins (primarily as the result of beta-lactamase production), which has significantly compromised the use of all these agents.

Other Beta-Lactam Antibiotics

Other classes of beta-lactam antibiotics include the carbapenems such as imipenem, monobactams, and the combination of a beta-lactam antibiotic with a beta-

BOX 20-3	**Selected Examples of Cephalosporins and Cephamycins**

NARROW-SPECTRUM (FIRST-GENERATION) AGENTS

Cephalexin	Cephapirin
Cephalothin	Cephradine
Cefazolin	

EXTENDED-SPECTRUM (SECOND-GENERATION) AGENTS

Cefaclor	Cefuroxime
Cefamandole	Cefotetan
Cefonicid	Cefoxitin

BROAD-SPECTRUM (THIRD-GENERATION) AGENTS

Cefepime	Cefotaxime
Cefixime	Ceftazidime

BOX 20-4	**Other Beta-Lactam Antibiotics**

Carbapenem
  Imipenem
  Meropenem
Monobactam
  Aztreonam
Beta-lactamase inhibitor/beta-lactam
  Clavulanic acid/amoxicillin
  Clavulanic acid/ticarcillin
  Sulbactam/ampicillin
  Tazobactam/piperacillin

lactamase inhibitor (Box 20-4). The **carbapenems** are broad-spectrum antibiotics that are active against virtually all groups of organisms, with only a few exceptions (e.g., resistance has been reported for all oxacillin-resistant staphylococci and selected Enterobacteriaceae, *Pseudomonas* species, and other gram-negative bacilli). In contrast, the **monobactams** are narrow-spectrum antibiotics that are active only against aerobic, gram-negative bacteria. Finally, the **beta-lactamase inhibitors** (e.g., clavulanic acid, sulbactam, tazobactam) are relatively inactive by themselves but are combined with some penicillins (e.g., ampicillin, amoxicillin, ticarcillin, piperacillin) to treat infections caused by beta-lactamase–producing bacteria. The inhibitors irreversibly bind and inactivate susceptible bacterial beta-lactamases (although not all are bound by these inhibitors), permitting the companion drug to enter the cell and disrupt bacterial cell wall synthesis.

Vancomycin

Vancomycin, originally obtained from *Streptomyces orientalis,* is a complex glycopeptide that disrupts cell wall synthesis in growing gram-positive bacteria. Vancomycin interacts with the D-alanine–D-alanine termini of the pentapeptide side chains, which interferes sterically with the formation of the bridges between the peptidoglycan chains. Vancomycin is used for the management of infections caused by oxacillin-resistant staphylococci, *Clostridium difficile,* and other gram-positive bacteria resistant to beta-lactam antibiotics. Vancomycin is inactive against gram-negative bacteria because the molecule is too large to pass through the outer membrane and reach the peptidoglycan target site. In addition, some organisms are intrinsically resistant to vancomycin (e.g., *Leuconostoc, Lactobacillus, Pediococcus,* and *Erysipelothrix* species) because the pentapeptide terminates in D-alanine–D-lactate, which does not bind vancomycin. In-

trinsic resistance is also found in some species of enterococci that contain a D-alanine–D-serine terminus (i.e., *Enterococcus gallinarum, E. casseliflavus*). Finally, some species of enterococci (particularly *E. faecium* and *E. faecalis*) have acquired resistance to vancomycin. The genes for this resistance, which is also related to changes in the pentapeptide terminus, are carried on plasmids and have seriously compromised the usefulness of vancomycin for the treatment of enterococcal infections.

Bacitracin

Bacitracin, which was isolated from *Bacillus licheniformis,* is a mixture of polypeptides used in topically applied products (e.g., creams, ointments, sprays) for the treatment of skin infections caused by gram-positive bacteria. Bacitracin inhibits cell wall synthesis by interfering with dephosphorylation of the lipid carrier responsible for moving the peptidoglycan precursors through the cytoplasmic membrane to the cell wall. It may also damage the bacterial cytoplasmic membrane and inhibit RNA transcription. Resistance to the antibiotic is most likely due to failure of the antibiotic to penetrate into the bacterial cell.

Isoniazid, Ethionamide, Ethambutol, and Cycloserine

Isoniazid, ethionamide, ethambutol, and cycloserine are cell wall–active antibiotics used for the treatment of mycobacterial infections. Isoniazid (isonicotinic acid hydrazide [INH]) is bactericidal against actively replicating mycobacteria. Although the exact mechanism of action is unknown, the synthesis of mycolic acid is affected (the desaturation of the long-chain fatty acids and the elongation of fatty acids are disrupted). Ethionamide, a derivative of INH, also blocks mycolic acid synthesis. Ethambutol interferes with the synthesis of arabinogalactan in the cell wall, and cycloserine inhibits two enzymes, D-alanine–D-alanine synthetase and alanine racemase, that catalyze cell wall synthesis. Resistance to these four antibiotics results primarily from reduced drug uptake into the bacterial cell or alteration of the target sites.

INHIBITION OF PROTEIN SYNTHESIS

The primary action of the agents in the second largest class of antibiotics is the inhibition of protein synthesis (Table 20-1).

Aminoglycosides

The aminoglycoside antibiotics consist of amino sugars linked through glycosidic bonds to an aminocyclitol ring (Box 20-5). Streptomycin, neomycin, kanamycin, and tobramycin were originally isolated from *Streptomyces* species, and gentamicin and sisomicin were isolated from *Micromonospora* species. Amikacin and netilmicin are synthetic derivatives of kanamycin and sisomicin, respectively. These antibiotics exert their effort by passing through the bacterial outer membrane (in gram-negative bacteria), cell wall, and cytoplasmic membrane to the cytoplasm, where they inhibit bacterial protein synthesis by irreversibly binding to the 30S ribosomal proteins. This attachment to the ribosomes has two effects: production of aberrant proteins as the result of misreading of the messenger RNA (mRNA), and interruption of protein synthesis by causing the premature release of the ribosome from mRNA.

The aminoglycosides are bactericidal because of their ability to bind irreversibly to ribosomes and are commonly used to treat serious infections caused by many gram-negative bacilli and some gram-positive organisms. Streptococci and anaerobes are resistant to aminoglycosides. The most commonly used antibiotics in this class are gentamicin and tobramycin, both of which have a broad spectrum of activity. Netilmicin is reported to be less ototoxic than gentamicin or tobramycin, but netilmicin also has less antibacterial activity. All three aminoglycosides are used to treat systemic infections caused by susceptible gram-negative bacteria, including the Enterobacteriaceae and *Pseudomonas* species. Amikacin is frequently used to treat infections caused by gram-negative bacteria that are resistant to other aminoglycosides, and streptomycin has been used for the treatment of tuberculosis, tularemia, and streptomococcal or enterococcal endocarditis (in combination with a penicillin). Although kanamycin was one of the first aminoglycosides with a broad activity against gram-negative bacteria, it is now rarely used because it is inactive against *Pseudomonas* species.

Resistance to the antibacterial action of aminoglycosides can develop in one of three ways: mutation of the ribosome binding site, decreased uptake of the antibiotic into the bacterial cell, or enzymatic modification of the antibiotic. Resistance caused by alteration of the bacterial ribosome is relatively uncommon, except in members

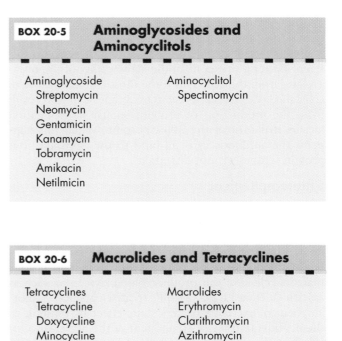

BOX 20-5 Aminoglycosides and Aminocyclitols

Aminoglycoside	Aminocyclitol
Streptomycin	Spectinomycin
Neomycin	
Gentamicin	
Kanamycin	
Tobramycin	
Amikacin	
Netilmicin	

BOX 20-6 Macrolides and Tetracyclines

Tetracyclines	Macrolides
Tetracycline	Erythromycin
Doxycycline	Clarithromycin
Minocycline	Azithromycin
	Spiramycin

of the genus *Enterococcus*. Because these important gram-positive cocci can be killed only with the synergistic combination of an aminoglycoside with a cell-wall antibiotic, this resistance is clinically significant. Resistance caused by inhibited transport of the antibiotic into the bacterial cell is occasionally observed with *Pseudomonas* but more commonly seen with anaerobic bacteria. This is because the uptake of aminoglycoside by the cell is oxygen dependent. Enzymatic phosphorylation, adenylation, and acetylation of the amino and hydroxyl groups of the aminoglycosides are the most common mechanisms of resistance. The differences in the antibacterial activity among the aminoglycosides are determined by their relative susceptibility to these enzymes.

Tetracyclines

The tetracylines are broad-spectrum, bacteriostatic antibiotics that inhibit protein synthesis in bacteria by blocking the binding of aminoacyl–transfer RNA (tRNA) to the 30S ribosome–mRNA complex (Box 20-6). Tetracyclines are effective in the treatment of infections caused by *Chlamydia, Mycoplasma, Rickettsia,* and other selected gram-positive and gram-negative bacteria. All tetracyclines have a similar spectrum of activity, with the primary difference among the antibiotics in their pharmacokinetic properties. Resistance to the tetracyclines can stem from decreased penetration of the antibiotic into the bacterial cell, active efflux of the antibiotic out of the cell, or the protection of the 30S ribosome. Mutations in the chromosomal gene encoding the outer membrane porin protein, OmpF, can lead to low-level resistance to the tetracyclines, as well as other antibiotics (e.g., beta-lactams, quinolones, chloramphenicol).

Researchers have identified a variety of genes in different bacteria that control the active efflux of the tetracyclines from the cell. This is the most common cause of resistance. Resistance to the tetracyclines can also result from the production of proteins similar to elongation factors that protect the 30S ribosome. When this happens, the antibiotic can still bind to the ribosome, but protein synthesis is not disrupted.

Chloramphenicol

Chloramphenicol has a broad antibacterial spectrum similar to that of tetracycline but is the drug of choice only for the treatment of typhoid fever. The reason for its limited use is that besides interfering with bacterial protein synthesis, it disrupts protein synthesis in human bone marrow cells and can produce blood dyscrasias such as aplastic anemia (1 per 24,000 treated patients). Chloramphenicol exerts its bacteriostatic effect by binding to the peptidyl transferase component of the 50S ribosomal subunit, thus blocking peptide elongation. Resistance to chloramphenicol is observed in bacteria producing plasmid-encoded chloramphenicol acetyltransferase, which catalyzes the acetylation of the 3-hydroxy group of chloramphenicol. The product is incapable of binding to the 50S subunit. Less commonly, chromosomal mutations alter the outer membrane porin proteins, causing the gram-negative bacilli to be less permeable.

Macrolides

Erythromycin, derived from *Streptomyces erythreus,* is the model macrolide antibiotic. The basic structure of this class of antibiotics is a macrocyclic lactone ring bound to two sugars, desosamine and cladinose. Modification of the macrolide structure has led to the development of newer agents, including azithromycin and clarithromycin (Box 20-6). Macrolides are bacteriostatic antibiotics with a broad spectrum of activity. They have been used to treat pulmonary infections caused by *Mycoplasma, Legionella,* and *Chlamydia* species, as well as infections caused by *Campylobacter* species and gram-positive bacteria in patients allergic to penicillin. Azithromycin and clarithromycin have also been used to treat infections caused by mycobacteria (e.g., *Mycobacterium avium* complex). Macrolides exert their effect by their reversible binding to the 50S ribosome, which blocks polypeptide elongation. Resistance to the macrolides stems from the methylation of the 23S ribosomal RNA, which prevents binding by the antibiotic. Destruction of the lactone ring by an erythromycin esterase or the active efflux of the antibiotic from the bacterial cell can also be the source of resistance.

Clindamycin

Clindamycin is a derivative of lincomycin, which was originally isolated from *Streptomyces lincolnensis.* Like chloramphenicol and the macrolides, clindamycin blocks protein elongation by binding to the 50S ribosome. It inhibits peptidyl transferase by interfering with the binding of the amino acid–acyl-tRNA complex. Clindamycin is active against staphylococci and anaerobic gram-negative bacilli but generally inactive against aerobic gram-negative bacteria. Methylation of the 23S ribosomal RNA is the source of bacterial resistance. Because both erythromycin and clindamycin can induce this enzymatic resistance (also plasmid mediated), cross-resistance between these two classes of antibiotics is observed.

ALTERATION OF CELL MEMBRANES

Another mechanism by which antibiotics exert their action is by altering the bacterial cell membranes (Table 20-2). The polymyxin class of antibiotics is an important example of agents that have this effect. These antibiotics, which were isolated from *Bacillus polymyxa,* consist of cationic, branched cyclic decapeptides that destroy the cytoplasmic membranes of susceptible bacteria. Members of this class of antibiotics include polymyxin B and polymyxin E (colistin). These antibiotics are active against gram-negative bacteria, particularly *Pseudomonas* organisms. However, because these antibiotics are capable of causing serious nephrotoxicity, their use has been limited chiefly to the external treatment of localized infections such as external otitis, eye infections, and skin infections caused by sensitive organisms. The detergent-like activity of the polymyxins is prevented when the antibiotic is unable to penetrate through the outer membrane of gram-negative bacilli to the inner cytoplasmic membrane. Bacitracin can also disrupt bacterial cytoplasmic membranes.

INHIBITION OF NUCLEIC ACID SYNTHESIS
Quinolones

The quinolones are synthetic chemotherapeutic agents that inhibit bacterial DNA gyrases or topoisomerases, which are required to supercoil strands of bacterial DNA into the bacterial cell (Box 20-7). Nalidixic acid was used to treat urinary tract infections caused by a variety of gram-negative bacteria, but resistance to the drug developed rapidly, causing it to fall out of use. This drug has now been replaced by newer, more active quinolones such as ciprofloxacin. These antibiotics have excellent

BOX 20-7	Quinolones
Nalidixic acid	Levofloxacin
Norfloxacin	Lomefloxacin
Ciprofloxacin	Sparfloxacin
Ofloxacin	

activity against gram-positive and gram-negative bacteria, although resistance can develop rapidly in *Pseudomonas* organisms, oxacillin-resistant staphylococci, and enterococci.

DNA gyrase consists of two alpha and two beta subunits, with the quinolones binding to the alpha subunits. Alteration of this subunit is the principal mechanism of bacterial resistance, although decreased drug uptake has also been observed. Decreased uptake stems from changes in porin proteins on the bacterial surface. Both resistance mechanisms are chromosomally mediated.

Rifampin and Rifabutin

Rifampin, a semisynthetic derivative of rifamycin B produced by *Streptomyces mediterranei*, binds to DNA-dependent RNA polymerase, and inhibits the initiation of RNA synthesis. Rifampin is bactericidal for *Mycobacterium tuberculosis* and is very active against aerobic gram-positive cocci, including staphylococci and streptococci.

Because resistance can develop rapidly, rifampin is usually combined with one or more other effective antibiotics. Rifampin resistance in gram-positive bacteria results from a mutation in the chromosomal gene that codes for the beta subunit of RNA polymerase. Gram-negative bacteria are resistant intrinsically to rifampin as the result of decreased uptake of the hydrophobic antibiotic. Rifabutin, a derivative of rifamycin, has a similar mode of activity and spectrum of activity. It is particularly active against *M. avium*.

Metronidazole

Metronidazole was originally introduced as an oral agent for the treatment of *Trichomonas* vaginitis. However, it was also found to be effective in the treatment of amebiasis, giardiasis, and serious anaerobic bacterial infections (including those caused by *B. fragilis*). Metronidazole has no significant activity against aerobic or facultatively anaerobic bacteria. The antimicrobial properties of metronidazole stem from the reduction of its nitro group by bacterial nitroreductase, thereby producing cytotoxic compounds that disrupt the host DNA. Resistance results from either decreased uptake of the antibiotic or elimination of the cytotoxic compounds before they can interact with host DNA.

ANTIMETABOLITES

The sulfonamides are antimetabolites that compete with *p*-aminobenzoic acid, thereby preventing the synthesis of the folic acid required by certain microorganisms (Figure 20-4). Because mammalian organisms do not synthesize folic acid (required as a vitamin), sulfonamides do not interfere with mammalian cell metabolism. Trimethoprim is another antimetabolite that interferes with folic acid metabolism by inhibiting dihydrofolate reductase, thereby preventing the conversion of dihydrofolate to

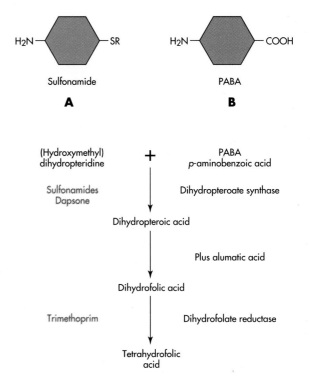

FIGURE 20-4 Antimetabolic activity or competitive antagonism. **A,** Sulfonamides, which resemble *p*-aminobenzoic acid, and dapsone competitively inhibit dihydropterate synthase. **B,** Trimethoprim inhibits the enzymatic action of dihydrofolate reductase. Both of these actions cause interference with the synthesis of folic acid, which is required by bacteria.

tetrahydrofolate. This blocks the formation of thymidine, some purines, methionine, and glycine. Trimethoprim is commonly combined with sulfamethoxazole to produce a synergistic combination active at two steps in the synthesis of folic acid. Dapsone and *p*-aminosalicylic acid are also antifolates that have proved to be useful for treating mycobacterial infections.

Sulfonamides are effective against a broad range of gram-positive and gram-negative organisms, such as *Nocardia, Chlamydia,* and some protozoa. Short-acting sulfonamides such as sulfisoxazole are among the drugs of choice for the treatment of acute urinary tract infections caused by susceptible bacteria such as *E. coli.* Trimethoprim-sulfamethoxazole is effective against a large variety of gram-positive and gram-negative microorganisms and is the drug of choice for the treatment of acute and chronic urinary tract infections. The combination is also effective in the treatment of infections caused by *Pneumocystis carinii,* bacterial infections of the lower respiratory tract, otitis media, and uncomplicated gonorrhea.

Resistance to these antibiotics can stem from a variety of mechanisms. Bacteria such as *Pseudomonas* are resistant as the result of permeability barriers. A decreased affinity of dihydrofolate reductase can be the source of trimethoprim resistance. In addition, bacteria that use exogenous thymidine (e.g., enterococci) are also intrinsically resistant.

OTHER ANTIBIOTICS

Clofazimine is a lipophilic antibiotic that binds to mycobacterial DNA. It is highly active against *M. tuberculosis,* is a first-line drug for the treatment of *Mycobacterium leprae* infections, and has been recommended as a secondary antibiotic for the treatment of infections caused by other mycobacterial species.

Pyrazinamide (PZA) is active against *M. tuberculosis* at a low pH, such as that found in phagolysosomes. The active form of this antibiotic is pyrazinoic acid, produced when PZA is hydrolyzed in the liver. The mechanism by which PZA exerts its effect is unknown.

QUESTIONS

1. Describe the mode of action of the following antibiotics: penicillin, vancomycin, isoniazid, gentamicin, tetracycline, erythromycin, polymyxin, ciprofloxacin, and sulfamethoxazole.
2. What three mechanisms of resistance are observed with by beta-lactam antibiotics? What is the mechanism responsible for oxacillin resistance in *Staphylococcus* species? Imipenem resistance in *Pseudomonas* species? Penicillin resistance in *S. pneumoniae?*
3. By what three mechanisms have organisms developed resistance to aminoglycosides?
4. What mechanism is responsible for resistance to the quinolones?
5. How do trimethoprim and the sulfonamides differ in their mode of action?

Bibliography

Kucers A, Bennett NM: *The use of antibiotics: a comprehensive review with clinical emphasis,* ed 4, Philadelphia, 1989, Lippincott.

Mandell GL, Bennett JE, Dolin R: *Principles and practice of infectious diseases,* ed 4, New York, 1995, Churchill Livingstone.

Murray P et al: *Manual of clinical microbiology,* ed 6, Washington, DC, 1995, American Society for Microbiology.

CHAPTER 21

Laboratory Diagnosis of Bacterial Diseases

Microbiology differs from all other specialties in clinical pathology in that the objective of many of the tests is to isolate viable organisms. This means that the proper specimen must be collected, delivered expeditiously to the laboratory in the appropriate transport system, and inoculated onto media that will support the growth of the most likely pathogens. Care must also be taken to keep the specimen from being contaminated with clinically insignificant organisms that are present in the environment or that colonize the patient's mucosal surfaces. Collection of the proper specimen and its rapid delivery to the clinical laboratory are primarily the responsibility of the patient's physician, whereas the appropriate transport system and culture methods are selected by the clinical microbiologist. However, these responsibilities are not mutually exclusive in that the microbiologist should be prepared to instruct the physician about the most appropriate specimen to collect if a particular diagnosis is suspected and the physician must provide the microbiologist with information about the clinical diagnosis so that the right culture media and growth conditions are selected. The chapters that follow provide information about the selection of culture media for specific pathogens. The reference texts listed in the bibliography also give information on this topic. The primary focus of this chapter, however, is to provide guidelines for the proper collection and transport of different specimens (summarized in Table 21-1) as well as general information about the laboratory processing of specimens. Whenever an unusual or fastidious pathogen is suspected (e.g., *Bordetella pertussis*, *Francisella tularensis*), the laboratory should be notified so that the appropriate transport system and culture media can be obtained.

BLOOD

The culture of blood is one of the most important procedures performed in the clinical microbiology laboratory. The success of this test is directly related to the methods used to collect the blood sample. The single most important factor that determines the success of a blood culture is the volume of blood processed. Specifically, there is a 40% increase in the rate of cultures positive for organisms if 20 ml rather than 10 ml of blood is cultured because more than half of all septic patients have fewer than one organism per milliliter of blood. Therefore approximately 20 ml of blood should be collected from an adult for each blood culture and proportionally smaller volumes should be collected from children and neonates. Because many hospitalized patients are susceptible to infections with organisms colonizing their skin, careful disinfection of the patient's skin with alcohol followed by 2% iodine is important.

Bacteremia and *fungemia* are defined as the presence of bacteria and fungi, respectively, in the bloodstream, and these infections are referred to collectively as **septicemia**. Clinical studies have shown that septicemia can be continuous or intermittent. **Continuous septicemia** occurs primarily in patients with intravascular infections (e.g., endocarditis, septic thrombophlebitis, intravascular catheter infections) or with overwhelming sepsis (e.g., septic shock). **Intermittent septicemia** occurs in patients with other infections in which the focus of the infection is at a distal site (e.g., lungs, urinary tract, soft tissue). The timing of blood collection is not important for patients with continuous septicemias, but it is critical for patients with intermittent septicemias. In addition, because clinical signs of sepsis (e.g., fever, chills, hypotension) are a response to the release of endotoxins or exotoxins from the organisms, these signs may occur as long as 1 hour after the organisms have been cleared from the bloodstream. Thus the worst time to collect blood samples for culture is when the patient develops a fever. Two to three blood samples should be collected at random times during a 24-hour period; it is not necessary to collect any additional samples, even in patients receiving antibiotics.

Most blood samples are inoculated into bottles filled with enriched nutrient broths. This should be done when the sample is collected. To ensure the maximal recovery of important organisms, two bottles of media should be inoculated for each culture. When these inoculated bottles of broth are received in the laboratory, they are incubated at 37° C and inspected at regular intervals for evidence of microbial growth. When growth is detected, the broths are subcultured to isolate the or-

	TRANSPORT SYSTEM	SPECIMEN VOLUME	OTHER CONSIDERATIONS
...cter-	Blood culture bottle with nutrient medium	Adults: 20 ml/culture Children: 5-10 ml/culture Neonates: 1-2 ml/culture	Skin should be disinfected with 70% alcohol followed by 2% iodine; 2-3 cultures collected every 24 hr unless patient is in septic shock or antibiotics will be started immediately; blood collections should be separated by 30-60 min; blood is divided equally into two bottles of nutrient media.
Blood—intracellular bacteria (e.g. *Brucella, Francisella, Neisseria* species)	Same as routine blood cultures; lysis-centrifugation system	Same as routine blood cultures	Considerations are same as those of routine blood cultures; release of intracellular bacteria may improve organism's recovery; *Neisseria* species is inhibited by some anticoagulants (sodium polyanethoesulfonate).
Blood—*Leptospira* species	Sterile heparinized tube	1-5 ml	Specimen is useful only during the first week of illness; afterward, urine should be cultured.
Cerebrospinal fluid	Sterile screw-capped tube	Bacterial culture: 1-5 ml Mycobacterial culture: as large a volume as possible	Specimen must be collected aseptically and delivered immediately to laboratory; it should not be exposed to heat or refrigeration.
Other normally sterile fluids (e..g, abdominal, chest, synovial, pericardial)	Small volume: sterile screw-capped tube; large volume: blood culture bottle with nutrient medium	As large a volume as possible (Pathogens can be present in small numbers.)	Specimens are collected with needle and syringe; swab is not used because quantity of collected specimen is inadequate; air should not be injected into culture bottle because it will inhibit growth of anaerobes.
Catheter	Sterile screw-capped tube or specimen cup	N/A	The entry site should be disinfected with alcohol; catheter should be aseptically removed on receipt of specimen in laboratory; catheter is rolled across blood agar plate and then discarded.
Respiratory—throat	Swab immersed in transport medium	N/A	Area of inflammation is swabbed; exudate is collected if present; contact with saliva should be avoided because it can inhibit recovery of group A streptococci.
Respiratory—epiglottis	Collection of blood for culture	Same as blood culture	Swabbing the epiglottis can precipitate complete airway closure; blood cultures should be collected for specific diagnosis.
Respiratory—sinuses	Sterile anaerobic tube or vial	1-5 ml	Specimens must be collected with needle and syringe; culture of nasopharynx or oropharynx has no value; specimen should be cultured for aerobic and anaerobic bacteria.
Respiratory—lower airways	Sterile screw-capped bottle; anaerobic tube or vial only for specimens collected by avoiding upper tract flora	1-2 ml	Expectorated sputum; if possible, patient rinses mouth with water before collection of the specimen; patient should cough deeply and expectorate lower airway secretions directly into sterile cup; collector should avoid contamination with saliva. Bronchoscopy specimen: anesthetics can inhibit growth of bacteria, so specimens should be processed immediately; if "protected" bronchoscope is used, anaerobic cultures can be performed. Transtracheal aspirate or direct lung aspirate: specimens can be processed for aerobic and anaerobic bacteria.

N/A, Not applicable.

| TABLE 21-1 | Specimen Collection for Bacterial Pathogens—cont'd |

SPECIMEN	TRANSPORT SYSTEM	SPECIMEN VOLUME	OTHER CONSIDERATIONS
Ear	Capped, needleless syringe; sterile screw-capped tube	Whatever volume is collected	Specimen should be aspirated with needle and syringe; culture of external ear has no predictive value for otitis media.
Eye	Inoculate plates at bedside (seal and transport to lab immediately)	Whatever volume can be collected	For infections on surface of eye, specimens are collected with swab or by corneal scrapings; for deep-seated infections, aspiration of aqueous or vitreous fluid is performed; all specimens should be inoculated onto appropriate media at collection; delays will result in significant loss of organisms.
Exudates (transudates, drainage, ulcers)	Swab immersed in transport medium; aspirate in sterile screw-capped tube	Bacteria: 1-5 ml Mycobacteria: 3-5 ml	Contamination with surface material should be avoided; specimens are generally unsuitable for anaerobic culture.
Wounds (abscess, pus)	Aspirate in sterile screw-capped tube or sterile anaerobic tube or vial	1-5 ml of pus	Specimens should be collected with sterile needle and syringe; curette is used to collect specimen at base of wound; swabbed specimens should be avoided.
Tissues	Sterile screw-capped tube; sterile anaerobic tube or vial	Representative sample from center and border of lesion	Specimen should be aseptically placed into appropriate sterile container; adequate quantity of specimen must be collected to recover small numbers of organisms.
Urine—midstream	Sterile urine container	Bacteria: 1 ml Mycobacteria: ≥10 ml	Contamination of specimen with bacteria from the urethra or vagina should be avoided; first portion of the voided specimen is discarded; organisms can grow rapidly in urine, so specimens must be transported immediately to laboratory, held in bacteriostatic preservative, or refrigerated.
Urine—catheterized	Sterile urine container	Bacteria: 1 ml Mycobacteria: ≥10 ml	Catheterization is not recommended for routine cultures (risk of inducing infection); first portion of collected specimen is contaminated with urethral bacteria, so it should be discarded (similar to midstream voided specimen); specimen must be transported rapidly to laboratory.
Urine—suprapubic aspirate	Sterile anaerobic tube or vial	Bacteria 1 ml Mycobacteria: ≥10 ml	This is invasive specimen, so urethral bacteria are avoided; it is only valid method available for collecting specimens for anaerobic culture; also useful for collection of specimens from children or adults unable to void uncontaminated specimens.
Genitals	Specially designed swabs for *Neisseria gonorrhoeae* and *Chlamydia* probes	N/A	Area of inflammation or exudate should be sampled; endocervix (not vagina) and urethra should be cultured for optimal detection.
Feces (stool)	Sterile screw-capped container	N/A	Rapid transport to laboratory is necessary to prevent production of acid (bactericidal for some enteric pathogens) by normal fecal bacteria; it is unsuitable for anaerobic culture; because large number of different media will be inoculated, swab should not be used for specimen collection.

ganism for identification and antimicrobial susceptibility testing. Most clinically significant isolates are detected within the first 2 days of incubation; however, all cultures should be incubated for a minimum of 5 to 7 days. More prolonged incubation is generally unnecessary, except for fastidious organisms. Because few organisms are typically present in the blood of a septic patient, it is not worthwhile to stain samples of blood (e.g., Gram stain) for microscopic analysis.

CEREBROSPINAL FLUID

Bacterial meningitis is a serious disease that is associated with high morbidity and mortality if the etiological diagnosis is delayed. Because some common pathogens that cause bacterial meningitis are labile (e.g., *Neisseria meningitidis, Streptococcus pneumoniae*), specimens of cerebrospinal fluid (CSF) should be processed immediately after they are collected. Under no circumstance should the specimen be refrigerated or heated. The patient's skin is disinfected with alcohol and iodine before lumbar puncture, and the CSF is collected into sterile screw-capped tubes. On receipt of the specimen in the microbiology laboratory, it is concentrated by centrifugation, and the sediment is used to inoculate bacteriological media and prepare a Gram stain. Other stains are used if fungal (potassium hydroxide or KOH stain) or mycobacterial (acid-fast stain) infections are suspected. The laboratory technician should notify the physician immediately if the culture is positive for organisms.

OTHER NORMALLY STERILE FLUIDS

A variety of other normally sterile fluids may be collected for bacteriological culture, including abdominal (peritoneal), chest (pleural), synovial, and pericardial fluids. If a large volume of fluid can be collected by percutaneous aspiration (e.g., abdominal or chest fluids), it should be inoculated into blood culture bottles containing nutrient media. A small portion should also be sent to the laboratory in a sterile tube so that appropriately stained specimens (e.g., Gram, KOH, acidfast) can be prepared. A large variety of organisms may be responsible for causing infections at these sites, including polymicrobial mixtures of aerobic and anaerobic organisms. For this reason, biological staining is useful for identifying the organisms responsible for the infection. If only small quantities of fluid are collected, the specimen can be inoculated directly onto agar media. Because relatively few organisms may be in the sample (as a result of the dilution of organisms or microbial elimination by the host immune response), it is important to culture as large a volume of fluid as possible. Because anaerobes may also be present in the sample (particularly samples obtained from patients with intraabdominal or pulmonary infections), the specimen should not be exposed to oxygen.

UPPER RESPIRATORY TRACT SPECIMENS

Group A streptococci cause most bacterial infections of the pharynx. Other bacteria that can cause pharyngitis include *Corynebacterium diphtheriae, B. pertussis, Neisseria gonorrhoeae, Chlamydia* species, and *Mycoplasma pneumoniae*. These bacteria, however, are relatively uncommon, and special techniques must be used to isolate them. Other potentially pathogenic bacteria, such as *Staphylococcus aureus, S. pneumoniae, Haemophilus influenzae*, Enterobacteriaceae, and *Pseudomonas* species may be present in the oropharynx, but they rarely cause pharyngitis.

A Dacron or calcium alginate swab should be used to collect pharyngeal specimens. The tonsillar areas, posterior pharynx, and any exudate or ulcerative area should be sampled. Contamination of the specimen with saliva should be avoided because bacteria in saliva can overgrow or inhibit the growth of group A streptococci. If a pseudomembrane is present (e.g., as with *C. diphtheriae* infections), a portion should be dislodged and submitted for culture. Group A streptococci and *C. diphtheriae* are very resistant to drying, so special precautions are not required for transport of the specimen to the laboratory. In contrast, specimens collected for the recovery of *B. pertussis* and *N. gonorrhoeae* should be inoculated onto culture media immediately after they are collected and before they are sent to the laboratory. Specimens obtained for the isolation of *Chlamydia* species and *M. pneumoniae* should be transported in a special transport medium.

Group A streptococci can be detected directly in the clinical specimen through the use of immunoassays for the group-specific antigen. Although these tests are very specific, they are insensitive and cannot be used to reliably exclude the diagnosis of group A streptococcal pharyngitis.

Other upper respiratory tract infections can involve the epiglottis and sinuses. Complete airway obstruction can be precipitated by attempts to culture the epiglottis (particularly in children). Thus these cultures should never be performed. The specific diagnosis of a sinus infection requires the direct aspiration of the sinus, appropriate anaerobic transport of the specimen to the laboratory (using a system that avoids exposing anaerobes to oxygen and drying), and prompt processing. Culture of the nasopharynx or pharynx is not useful and should not be performed. *S. pneumoniae, H. influenzae, Moraxella catarrhalis, S. aureus*, and anaerobes are the most common pathogens that cause sinusitis.

LOWER RESPIRATORY TRACT SPECIMENS

A variety of techniques can be used to collect lower respiratory tract specimens; these include expectoration, induction with saline, bronchoscopy and bronchial alveolar lavage, transtracheal aspiration (rarely used today), and direct aspiration through the chest wall. Because upper airway bacteria may contaminate expectorated and induced sputa, the specimen should be inspected microscopically to assess the magnitude of oral contamination and the value of processing the specimen. Specimens containing many squamous epithelial cells and no predominant bacteria in association with leukocytes should not be submitted for culture. The presence of squamous epithelial cells indicates that the specimen has been contaminated with saliva. Such contamination can be avoided by obtaining the specimen using a protected bronchoscope, transtracheal aspiration, or direct lung aspiration. These invasive procedures must be used to collect uncontaminated specimens from patients with anaerobic lung infections. Most lower respiratory tract pathogens grow within 2 to 3 days, although it may take additional time for the bacterium to be isolated and identified. If infection with a mycobacterium such as *Mycobacterium tuberculosis* is suspected, the laboratory should be notified so that special culture techniques and acid-fast stains can be used.

EAR AND EYE

Tympanocentesis (the aspiration of fluid from the middle ear) is required to make the specific diagnosis of a middle ear infection. However, this is unnecessary in most patients because the most common pathogens that cause these infections (*S. pneumoniae, H. influenzae,* and *M. catarrhalis*) can be treated empirically. Outer ear infections are typically caused by *Pseudomonas aeruginosa* ("swimmer's ear") or *S. aureus*. The proper specimen to be obtained for culture is a scraping of the involved area of the ear.

Collection of specimens for the diagnosis of ocular infections is difficult because the sample obtained is generally very small and relatively few organisms may be present. Samples of the eye surface should be collected by a swab before topical anesthetics are applied, followed by corneal scrapings whenever necessary. The eye must be directly aspirated to collect intraocular specimens. The culture media should be inoculated when the specimens are collected and before they are sent to the laboratory. Although most common ocular pathogens grow rapidly (e.g., *S. aureus, S. pneumoniae, H. influenzae, P. aeruginosa, Bacillus cereus*), some may require prolonged incubation (e.g., coagulase-negative staphylococci) or the use of specialized culture media (*N. gonorrhoeae, Chlamydia trachomatis*).

WOUNDS, ABSCESSES, AND TISSUES

Open, draining wounds can frequently be colonized with potentially pathogenic organisms unrelated to the specific infectious process. Therefore it is important to collect samples from deep in the wound after the surface has been cleaned. Whenever possible, a swab should be

avoided because it is difficult to obtain a representative sample without contamination with organisms colonizing the surface. Likewise, aspirates from a closed abscess should be collected from both the center and the wall of the abscess. Simply collecting pus from an abscess is generally nonproductive because most organisms actively replicate at the base of the abscess rather than in the center. Drainage from soft tissue infections can be collected by aspiration. If fluctuance is not obtained, a small quantity of saline can be infused into the tissue and then withdrawn for culture. Saline containing a bactericidal preservative should not be used.

Tissues should be obtained from representative portions of the infectious process, with multiple samples collected whenever possible. The tissue specimen should be transported in a sterile screw-capped container, and sterile saline should be added to prevent drying if a small sample (e.g., biopsy specimen) is collected. A sample of tissue should also be submitted for histological examination. Because collection of tissue specimens requires invasive procedures, every effort should be made to collect the proper specimen and ensure that it is cultured for all clinically significant organisms that may be responsible for the infection. This requires close communication between the physician and microbiologist.

URINE

Urine is one of the most frequently submitted specimens for culture. Because potentially pathogenic bacteria colonize the urethra, the first portion of urine collected by voiding or catheterization should be discarded. Urinary tract pathogens can also grow in urine, so there should be no delay in the transport of specimens to the laboratory. If the specimen cannot be cultured immediately, it should be refrigerated or placed in a bacteriostatic urine preservative. Once the specimen is received in the laboratory, 1 to 10 μl is inoculated onto each culture medium (generally one nonselective agar medium and one selective medium). This is done so that the number of organisms in the urine can be quantitated, which is useful for assessing the significance of an isolate, although small numbers of organisms in a patient with pyuria can be clinically significant. Numerous urine screening procedures (e.g., biochemical tests, microscopy stains) have been developed and are used widely; however, these procedures cannot be recommended because they are invariably insensitive in detecting a clinically significant, low-grade bacteriuria.

GENITAL SPECIMENS

Despite the variety of bacteria associated with sexually transmitted diseases, most laboratories concentrate on detecting *N. gonorrhoeae* and *C. trachomatis*. Traditionally this was done by inoculating the specimen onto media selective for these organisms. However, this is a slow process, taking 2 or more days for a positive culture to be obtained and more time for isolates to be identified definitively. Culture was also found to be insensitive because both organisms are extremely labile and die rapidly during transit under less than optimal conditions. For these reasons, researchers have developed nonculture methods, including direct immunofluorescent staining and antigen-directed immunoassays for *Chlamydia* species, as well as commercial molecular probes and molecular amplification procedures (e.g., amplification by the polymerase chain reaction, ligase chain reaction, and other methods) for both organisms. The direct staining methods and immunoassays have proved to be relatively insensitive, particularly in identifying asymptomatic carriers of *Chlamydia* organisms. However, the probes are both sensitive and specific and have rapidly replaced all other methods of detection.

The other major bacterium that causes sexually transmitted diseases is *Treponema pallidum*, the etiological agent of syphilis. This organism cannot be cultured in the clinical laboratory, so the diagnosis is made using microscopy or serology. Material from lesions must be examined using darkfield microscopy because the organism is too thin to be detected using brightfield microscopy. In addition, the organism dies rapidly when exposed to air and drying conditions, so the microscopic examination must be performed at the time the specimen is collected. The serological diagnosis of syphilis is discussed in Chapter 41.

FECAL SPECIMENS

A large variety of bacteria can cause gastrointestinal infections. For these bacteria to be recovered in culture, an adequate stool sample must be collected (generally not a problem in a patient with diarrhea), transported to the laboratory in a manner that ensures the viability of the infecting organisms, and inoculated onto the appropriate selective media. Rectal swabs should not be submitted because a variety of selective media must be inoculated for the various possible pathogens to be recovered. The quantity of feces collected on a swab would be inadequate.

Stool specimens should be collected in a clean pan and then transferred into a tightly sealed waterproof container. The specimens should be transported promptly to the laboratory to prevent acidic changes in the stool (caused by bacterial metabolism), which are toxic for organisms such as *Shigella*. If a delay is anticipated, the feces should be mixed with a preservative such as phosphate buffer mixed with glycerol or Cary-Blair transport medium (if *Campylobacter* infection is suspected). In general, however, rapid transport of the specimen to the laboratory is always superior to the use of any transport medium.

It is important to notify the laboratory if a particular enteric pathogen is suspected because this will help the laboratory select the appropriate culture medium. For example, although *Vibrio* species can grow on the common media used for the culture of stool specimens, the use of media selective for *Vibrio* facilitates the rapid isolation and identification of this organism. In addition, some organisms are not routinely isolated by the laboratory procedures (e.g., enterotoxigenic *Escherichia coli*), whereas others would not be expected to be in a stool sample because their disease is caused by toxin production in the food and not by growth of the organism in the gastrointestinal tract (e.g., *S. aureus*). The microbiologist should be able to select the appropriate test (e.g., culture, toxin assay) if the specific pathogen is indicated. *Clostridium difficile* is a significant cause of antibiotic-associated gastrointestinal disease. Although the organism can be cultured from stool specimens if they are promptly delivered to the laboratory, the most specific way to diagnose the infection is by detecting the *C. difficile* toxin in fecal extracts; the toxin is responsible for the disease.

Because many bacteria, both pathogenic and nonpathogenic, are present in fecal specimens, it frequently takes at least 3 days for the enteric pathogen to be isolated and identified. For this reason, stool cultures are used to confirm the clinical diagnosis, and therapy, if indicated, should not be delayed pending the culture results. Indeed, antimicrobial susceptibility testing is usually not performed with most enteric pathogens.

QUESTIONS

1. What is the most important factor that influences the recovery of microorganisms in blood collected from septic patients?
2. Which organisms are important causes of bacterial pharyngitis?
3. What criteria should be used to assess the quality of a lower respiratory tract specimen?
4. What methods are used to detect the three most common bacteria that cause sexually transmitted diseases?

Bibliography

Baron EJ, Peterson L, Finegold SM: *Bailey and Scott's diagnostic microbiology,* ed 9, St Louis, 1995, Mosby.

Mandell G, Bennett JE, Dolin R: *Principles and practice of infectious diseases,* ed 4, New York, 1995, Churchill Livingstone.

Murray PR et al: *Manual of clinical microbiology,* ed 6, Washington, DC, 1995, American Society for Microbiology.

22

Staphylococcus and Related Organisms

The gram-positive cocci are a heterogeneous collection of approximately 16 genera that colonize humans. Features that they have in common are their spherical shape, their Gram stain reaction, and an absence of endospores. The catalase-positive genera *(Staphylococcus, Micrococcus,* and *Stomatococcus)* are discussed in this chapter, the catalase-negative genera *(Streptococcus, Enterococcus,* and related organisms) are discussed in the next two chapters, and the anaerobic gram-positive cocci *(Peptostreptococcus)* are discussed in Chapter 36.

The name *Staphylococcus* is derived from the Greek term *staphylé,* meaning "a bunch of grapes." This name refers to the fact that the cells of these gram-positive cocci grow in a pattern resembling a cluster of grapes, although organisms in clinical material may appear as single cells, pairs, or short chains (Figure 22-1). Staphylococci are 0.5 to 1 μm in diameter, nonmotile, facultatively anaerobic, and catalase positive, and they are able to grow in a medium containing 10% sodium chloride and at a temperature of 18° to 40° C. The organisms are present on the skin and mucous membranes of humans, as well as the skin and mucous membranes of other mammals and birds. The genus currently comprises 32 species, 16 of which are found on humans (Table 22-1). *Staphylococcus* is an important pathogen in humans that can cause a wide spectrum of diseases, including life-threatening systemic maladies, cutaneous infections, opportunistic infections, and urinary tract disease (Table 22-2). The species most commonly associated with human diseases are *S. aureus* (the most virulent and best-known member of the genus), *S. epidermidis, S. saprophyticus, S. haemolyticus, S. lugdunensis,* and *S. schleiferi. S. aureus* colonies are golden as the result of the carotenoid pigments that form during their growth, hence the species name. It is also the only species found in humans that produces the enzyme coagulase; thus all other species are commonly referred to as **coagulase-negative staphylococci.**

Nine species of *Micrococcus* have been described, eight of which colonize humans, primarily on the surface of the skin. The cocci are 0.5 to 2.0 μm in diameter and arranged as single cells, pairs, or irregular clusters. The organisms grow only aerobically, and the colonies commonly are yellow or red. Although micrococci may be found in patients with opportunistic infections, their isolation in clinical specimens almost invariably represents a clinically insignificant contamination with skin flora.

Stomatococcus mucilaginosus, the only species in this genus, is a commensal organism that resides in the oropharynx and upper respiratory tract. Cells are 1.0 to 1.5 μm in diameter and are usually arranged in clusters. The organism is facultatively anaerobic, unable to grow in the presence of 5% salt, and weakly positive for catalase. Colonies have a prominent mucoid capsule, which makes them adhere to culture media, the body surfaces, and foreign material (e.g., catheters, shunts, prosthetic valves and joints). In recent years, this organism has been reported to be the cause of an increasing number of opportunistic infections in immunocompromised patients. The most common clinical manifestations of *S. mucilaginosus* infection are endocarditis, septicemia, and catheter-related infections.

The remainder of this chapter will concentrate on a description of *Staphylococcus* and its role in human disease.

PHYSIOLOGY AND STRUCTURE

The structure of the staphylococcal cell wall is illustrated in Figure 22-2.

Capsule

A loose-fitting, polysaccharide layer (slime layer) is only occasionally found on staphylococci cultured in vitro, but it is believed to be more commonly present in vivo. This capsule protects the bacteria by inhibiting the chemotaxis and phagocytosis of the organisms by polymorphonuclear leukocytes, as well as by inhibiting the proliferation of mononuclear cells after mitogen exposure. It also facilitates the adherence of bacteria to catheters and other synthetic material (e.g., grafts, shunts, prosthetic valves and joints) (Figure 22-3). This property is particularly important for the survival of relatively avirulent coagulase-negative staphylococci.

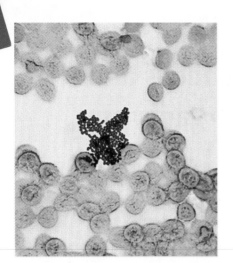

FIGURE 22-1 Gram stain of *Staphylococcus aureus*.

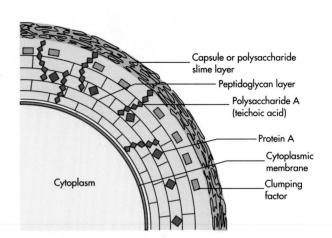

FIGURE 22-2 Structure of staphylococcal cell wall.

TABLE 22-1	Human Colonization and Disease Caused by *Staphylococcus, Micrococcus,* and *Stomatococcus* Species		
SPECIES	**HUMAN COLONIZATION**	**HUMAN DISEASE**	
Staphylococcus species			
S. aureus	Common	Common	
S. epidermidis	Common	Common	
S. saprophyticus	Common	Common	
S. haemolyticus	Common	Uncommon	
S. lugdunensis	Common	Uncommon	
S. schleiferi	Common	Uncommon	
S. saccharolyticus	Common	Rare	
S. warneri	Common	Rare	
S. hominis	Common	Rare	
S. auricularis	Common	Rare	
S. xylosus	Common	Rare	
S. simulans	Common	Rare	
S. capitis	Common	Rare	
S. cohnii	Common	Rare	
S. caprae	Uncommon	Rare	
S. pasteuri	Uncommon	Rare	
Micrococcus species			
M. luteus	Common	Rare	
M. varians	Common	Rare	
M. agilis	Uncommon	Rare	
M. kristinae	Uncommon	Rare	
M. lylae	Uncommon	Rare	
M. nishinomiyaensis	Uncommon	Rare	
M. roseus	Uncommon	Rare	
M. sedentarius	Uncommon	Rare	
Stomatococcus mucilaginosus	Common	Uncommon	

TABLE 22-2	*Staphylococcus, Micrococcus,* and *Stomatococcus* Species and Their Diseases
ORGANISM	**DISEASES**
Staphylococcus aureus	Toxin mediated (scalded skin syndrome, toxic shock syndrome, food poisoning)
	Cutaneous (impetigo, folliculitis, furuncles, carbuncles, wound infections)
	Other (bacteremia, endocarditis, pneumonia, empyema, osteomyelitis, septic arthritis)
Coagulase-negative *Staphylococcus* species	Opportunistic infections (bacteremia, endocarditis, catheter and shunt infections, prosthetic joint infections)
	Urinary tract infection
Micrococcus species	Opportunistic infections (bacteremia, peritonitis, shunt infections)
Stomatococcus species	Opportunistic infections (bacteremia, endocarditis, catheter and shunt infections, peritonitis)

FIGURE 22-3 Slime-producing *Staphylococcus epidermidis* on the surface of an intravascular catheter. (From Rupp ME, Archer GL: *Clin Infect Dis* 19:231, 1994.)

Peptidoglycan

The peptidoglycan layer, composed of peptide cross-linked glycan chains, is the major structural component of the staphylococcal cell wall. The glycan chains are built with 10 to 12 alternating subunits of *N*-acetylmuramic acid and *N*-acetylglucosamine. Tetrapeptide side chains are attached to the *N*-acetylmuramic acid subunits, and the glycan chains are then cross-linked with diagonal peptide bridges that form between the tetrapeptide side chains. For example, the glycan chains in *S. aureus* are cross-linked with pentaglycine bridges that are attached to L-lysine in one tetrapeptide chain and to D-alanine in an adjacent chain. Unlike gram-negative bacteria, the peptidoglycan layer in gram-positive organisms consists of many cross-linked layers, which makes the cell wall more rigid. The peptidoglycan layer stimulates the production of endogenous pyrogens, activates the production of interleukin-1 from monocytes, attracts polymorphonuclear leukocytes (a process responsible for abscess formation), and can activate complement.

Protein A

The surface of most *S. aureus* strains (but not the coagulase-negative staphylococci) is uniformly coated with protein A. This protein is covalently linked to the peptidoglycan layer and has a unique affinity for binding to the Fc receptor of IgG1, IgG2, and IgG4, thus effectively preventing the antibody-mediated immune clearance of the organism. Extracellular protein A can also bind antibodies, thereby forming immune complexes with the subsequent consumption of the complement.

The presence of protein A has been exploited in some serological tests, in which protein A-coated *S. aureus* is used as a nonspecific carrier of antibodies directed against other antigens.

Teichoic Acids

Teichoic acids are species-specific, phosphate-containing polymers that are bound covalently to the peptidoglycan layer or through lipophilic linkage to the cytoplasmic membrane (lipoteichoic acids). Ribitol teichoic acid with *N*-acetylglucosamine residues (polysaccharide A) is present in *S. aureus,* and glycerol teichoic acid with glucosyl residues (polysaccharide B) is present in *S. epidermidis.* Teichoic acids mediate the attachment of staphylococci to mucosal surfaces through their specific binding to fibronectin. Although the teichoic acids are poor immunogens, a specific antibody response is stimulated when they are bound to peptidoglycan. The monitoring of this antibody response has been used to detect systemic staphylococcal disease.

Clumping Factor

The outer surface of most strains of *S. aureus* contains clumping factor, or **bound coagulase.** This protein binds fibrinogen, converts it to insoluble fibrin, and can cause the staphylococci to clump or aggregate.

Cytoplasmic Membrane

The cytoplasmic membrane is made up of a complex of proteins, lipids, and a small amount of carbohydrates. It serves as an osmotic barrier for the cell and provides an anchorage for the cellular biosynthetic and respiratory enzymes.

PATHOGENESIS AND IMMUNITY
Staphylococcal Toxins

S. aureus produces many virulence factors (Table 22-3), including at least five cytolytic or membrane-damaging toxins (alpha, beta, delta, gamma, and leukocidin), as well as exfoliative toxin, toxic shock syndrome toxin-1 (TSST-1), and five enterotoxins (A to E). The cytolytic toxins have also been described as *hemolysins,* but this is a misnomer because the activities of the first four toxins are not restricted solely to red blood cells and leukocidin is unable to lyse erythrocytes. The cytotoxins can lyse neutrophils, resulting in the release of the lysosomal enzymes that subsequently damage the surrounding tissues.

Exfoliative toxin, TSST-1, and the enterotoxins belong to a class of polypeptides known as **superantigens.** These toxins bind to class II major histocompatibility complex molecules on macrophages, which in turn interact with the beta-subunit of specific T-cell receptors, leading to the proliferation of the T cells and the release of cytokine. The systemic effects of these diseases result from this process.

Alpha Toxin

Alpha toxin, which is encoded on both the bacterial chromosome and a plasmid, disrupts the smooth muscle in blood vessels and is toxic to many types of cells, including erythrocytes, leukocytes, hepatocytes, platelets,

TABLE 22-3	*Staphylococcal* Virulence Factors	
VIRULENCE FACTORS	**BIOLOGIC EFFECTS**
STRUCTURAL COMPONENTS	
Capsule	Inhibits chemotaxis and phagocytosis
	Facilitates adherence to foreign bodies
Peptidoglycan	Provides osmotic stability
	Stimulates production of endogenous pyrogen (endotoxin-like activity)
	Leukocyte chemoattractant (abscess formation)
	Inhibits phagocytosis
Protein A	Inhibits antibody-mediated clearance by binding IgG1, IgG2, and IgG4 Fc receptors
	Leukocyte chemoattractant
	Anticomplementary
Teichoic acid	Regulates cationic concentration at cell membrane
	Binds to fibronectin
Cytoplasmic membrane	Osmotic barrier
	Regulates transport into and out of cell
	Site of biosynthetic and respiratory enzymes
TOXINS	
Cytotoxins (alpha, beta, delta, gamma, leukocidin)	Toxic for many cells, including leukocytes, erythrocytes, macrophages, platelets, and fibroblasts
Exfoliative toxin	Disrupts vascular smooth muscle
	Stimulates T cells to release cytokines (superantigens)
Toxic shock syndrome toxin-1	Splits desmosomes in stratum granulosum layer of epidermis
Enterotoxins (A to E)	Superantigen (stimulates T cells to release cytokines)
	Superantigen (stimulates mast cells)
	Increases intestinal peristalsis and fluid loss
	Central nervous system effect manifested by nausea and vomiting
ENZYMES	
Coagulase	
	Converts fibrinogen to fibrin
Catalase	Protects *S. aureus* from phagocytosis
Hyaluronidase	Converts hydrogen peroxide to water and oxygen
	Hydrolyzes hyaluronic acids in connective tissue, promoting the spread of staphylococci in tissue
Fibrinolysin	Dissolves fibrin clots
Lipases	Hydrolyzes lipids
Nucleases	Hydrolyzes DNA
Penicillinase	Hydrolyzes penicillins

and cultivated cells (e.g., human diploid fibroblasts, HeLa cells, Ehrlich ascites carcinoma cells). It appears to mediate cytolysis by inserting into hydrophobic regions of the cell membrane, which in turn leads to the disruption of membrane integrity. Alpha toxin is believed to be an important mediator of tissue damage in staphylococcal disease and causes necrosis when injected subcutaneously.

Beta Toxin

Beta toxin, also called **sphingomyelinase C,** is a heat-labile protein that is toxic to a variety of cells, including erythrocytes, leukocytes, macrophages, and fibroblasts. This enzyme catalyzes the hydrolysis of membrane phospholipids in susceptible cells, with the amount of lysis proportional to the concentration of sphingomyelin exposed on the cell surface. Beta toxin, together with alpha toxin, is believed to be responsible for the tissue destruction and abscess formation characteristic of staphylococcal diseases and for the ability of *S. aureus* to proliferate in the presence of a vigorous inflammatory response.

Delta Toxin

Delta toxin is a large, thermostable, hydrophobic, heterogeneous protein that has a wide spectrum of cytolytic activity, a property consistent with the belief that it disrupts cellular membranes by means of a detergent-like action.

Gamma Toxin

Gamma toxin is able to lyse human, sheep, and rabbit erythrocytes as well as human lymphoblastic cells. Although two separate proteins are required for the toxin to be activated, the mode of action is not defined.

Leukocidin

Leukocidin has two components, neither of which alone has appreciable activity against the leukocyte membrane. However, in combination the two molecules facilitate structural changes in the cell membrane, pore formation, and increased permeability to cations. Bacteria that produce leukocidin are more resistant to phagocytosis.

Exfoliative Toxin

Staphylococcal scalded skin syndrome (SSSS) a spectrum of diseases characterized by exfoliative dermatitis, is mediated by exfoliative toxin, also known as **exfoliatin** and **epidermolytic toxin.** Two distinct forms of exfoliative toxin (A and B) have been identified (Table 22-4), and either can produce disease. Ultrastructural studies have shown that exposure to the toxins, which are serine proteases, is followed by the splitting of the intercellular bridges (desmosomes) in the stratum granulosum epidermis. The toxins are not associated with cytolysis or inflammation, so neither staphylococci nor leukocytes are typically seen in the involved layer of the epidermis. After exposure of the epidermis to the toxin, protective neutralizing antibodies develop, leading to resolution of the toxic process. SSSS is seen mostly in young children and only rarely in older children and adults. Its rarity in the last two age groups may result from the presence of protective antibodies or an insensitivity of the adult epidermis to the toxin.

Toxic Shock Syndrome Toxin-1

Toxic shock syndrome (TSS) is characterized by fever, hypotension, and rash followed by desquamation and the involvement of multiple organ systems. It is toxin mediated. Toxic shock syndrome toxin-1 (**TSST-1**), formerly called *pyrogenic exotoxin C* and *enterotoxin F,* is an exotoxin secreted during the growth of some strains of *S. aureus* and can reproduce most of the clinical manifestations of TSS in an experimental rabbit model (rash and desquamation are not seen). TSST-1 has not been found in staphylococcal isolates from all patients with TSS, but most of these isolates not producing TSST-1 are reported to produce enterotoxin B. The role of this second toxin in TSS has not been adequately defined. Coagulase-negative staphylococci can also produce TSS.

Enterotoxins

Five serologically distinct staphylococcal enterotoxins (A through E) have been identified. The enterotoxins are resistant to hydrolysis by gastric and jejunal enzymes and are stable to heating at 100° C for 30 minutes. Thus once a food product has been contaminated with enterotoxin-producing staphylococci and the toxins have been produced, reheating the food will not be protective. These toxins are produced by *S. aureus* and *S. epidermidis,* with 30% to 50% of all *S. aureus* strains producing an enterotoxin. Enterotoxin A is most commonly associated with disease. Enterotoxins C and D are found in contaminated milk products, and enterotoxin B causes staphylococcal pseudomembranous enterocolitis. The precise mechanism of toxin activity is not understood because a satisfactory animal model is not available, but possibly the toxins bind and activate mast cells. Like the exfoliative toxin and TSST-1, the enterotoxins are strong inducers of the formation of cytokine such as interleukin-1. They also stimulate intestinal peristalsis and have a central nervous system effect, as manifested by the

TABLE 22-4	**Characteristics of Exfoliative Toxins**	
PROPERITES	**EXFOLIATIVE TOXIN A**	**EXFOLIATIVE TOXIN B**
Size	24,000 daltons	24,000 daltons
Temperature tolerance	Stable (100° C, 20 min)	Labile (60° C, 30 min)
EDTA treatment	Inactivated	No effect
DNA	Chromosomal	Plasmid

nausea and intense vomiting that occur in patients with this gastrointestinal disease.

Staphylococcal Enzymes
Coagulase

S. aureus strains possess two forms of coagulase: bound (also called *clumping factor*) and free. Coagulase bound to the staphylococcal cell wall can directly convert fibrinogen to insoluble fibrin and cause the staphylococci to clump. The cell-free coagulase accomplishes the same result by reacting with a globulin plasma factor (coagulase-reacting factor) to form staphylothrombin, a thrombinlike factor. This factor catalyzes the conversion of fibrinogen to insoluble fibrin. Coagulase is used as a marker for the virulence of *S. aureus*. The role of coagulase in the pathogenesis of disease is speculative, but coagulase may cause the formation of a fibrin layer around a staphylococcal abscess, thus localizing the infection and protecting the organisms from phagocytosis.

Catalase

All staphylococci produce catalase, which catalyzes the conversion of toxic hydrogen peroxide to water and oxygen. Hydrogen peroxide can accumulate during bacterial metabolism or after phagocytosis.

Hyaluronidase

Hyaluronidase hydrolyzes hyaluronic acids, the acidic mucopolysaccharides present in the acellular matrix of connective tissue. This enzyme facilitates the spread of *S. aureus* in tissues. More than 90% of *S. aureus* strains produce this enzyme.

Fibrinolysin

Fibrinolysin, also called **staphylokinase,** is produced by virtually all *S. aureus* strains and can dissolve fibrin clots. Staphylokinase is distinct from the fibrinolytic enzymes produced by streptococci.

Lipases

All strains of *S. aureus* and more than 30% of the strains of coagulase-negative *Staphylococcus* produce several different lipases. As their name implies, these enzymes hydrolyze lipids, an essential function to ensure the survival of staphylococci in the sebaceous areas of the body. It is believed that these enzymes must be present for staphylococci to invade cutaneous and subcutaneous tissues and for superficial skin infections (e.g., furuncles [boils], carbuncles) to develop.

Nuclease

A thermostable nuclease is another marker for *S. aureus*. The role of this enzyme in the pathogenesis of infection is unknown.

Penicillinase

More than 90% of staphylococcal isolates were susceptible to penicillin in 1941, the year the antibiotic was first used clinically. However, resistance to penicillin quickly developed, primarily because the organisms could produce penicillinase (beta-lactamase). The widespread distribution of this enzyme was ensured by its presence on transmissible plasmids.

EPIDEMIOLOGY

Staphylococci are ubiquitous. Virtually all people have coagulase-negative staphylococci on their skin, and transient colonization of moist skin folds with *S. aureus* is common (Boxes 22-1 and 22-2). *S. aureus* and coagulase-negative staphylococci are also found in the oropharynx, gastrointestinal tract, and urogenital tract. Colonization of the umbilical stump, skin, and perineal area of neonates with *S. aureus* is common. Short-term or persistent carriage in older children and adults is more common in the anterior nasopharynx. Adherence of the organism to the mucosal epithelium is regulated by fibronectin receptors for staphylococcal teichoic acids. Approximately 15% of normal healthy adults are persistent nasopharyngeal carriers of *S. aureus*, with a higher incidence reported for hospitalized patients, medical personnel, people with eczematous skin diseases, and people who regularly use needles, either illicitly (e.g., drug abusers) or for medical reasons (e.g., insulin-dependent diabetics, patients receiving allergy injections, those undergoing hemodialysis).

Because staphylococci are found on the skin and in the nasopharynx, shedding of the bacteria is common and is responsible for many hospital-acquired infections. Staphylococci are susceptible to high temperatures, as well as to disinfectants and antiseptic solutions. However, the organisms can survive on dry surfaces for long periods. The organisms can be transferred to a susceptible person either through direct contact or through contact with fomites (e.g., contaminated clothing, bed linens). Therefore medical personnel must use proper handwashing techniques to prevent the transfer of staphylococci from themselves to patients or among patients.

CLINICAL SYNDROMES
Staphylococcus aureus

S. aureus causes disease through the production of toxin or through the direct invasion and destruction of tissue. The clinical manifestations of some staphylococcal diseases almost exclusively are the result of toxin activity (e.g., SSSS, TSS, and staphylococcal food poisoning), whereas other diseases result from the proliferation of the organisms, leading to abscess formation and tissue destruction (e.g., cutaneous infections, endocarditis, pneumonia, empyema, osteomyelitis, septic arthritis) (Figure 22-4). In the presence of a foreign body (e.g., splinter, catheter, shunt, prosthetic valve or joint), significantly fewer staphylococci are necessary to establish disease. Likewise, patients with congenital diseases associated with an impaired chemotactic or phagocytic

BOX 22-1 Summary of *Staphylococcus aureus* Infections

BACTERIAL FACTORS

Diseases—see Table 22-2.

Virulence factors—see Table 22-3.

Common on skin and in oropharynx and gastrointestinal and urogenital tracts.

Lysozyme in tears and saliva, and human leukocytes, monocytes, and macrophages, forms a natural barrier to *S. aureus* infection.

Organisms can survive on dry surfaces for long periods.

TRANSMISSION

Person to person through direct contact or through contact with fomites (contaminated clothing, bed linens).

Food poisoning: ingestion of food or dairy products (e.g., processed meats, custards, potato salad, ice cream) contaminated with organisms producing heat-stable enterotoxin.

Pneumonia: aspiration of oral secretions.

Bacteremia: hematogenous spread from a localized infection (e.g., cutaneous) to distal sites (e.g., heart [endocarditis], bone [osteomyelitis], joints [septic arthritis]).

WHO IS AT RISK?

Hospitalized patients who have sustained trauma or undergone surgical procedures, particularly when a foreign body (e.g., suture, catheter, prosthesis) is present.

People taking antibiotics that suppress the normal flora.

Scalded skin syndrome: infants and young children.

Toxic shock syndrome: menstruating women and children or adults with localized staphylococcal infection.

Impetigo: young children.

WHO IS AT RISK?—cont'd

Bacteremia and endocarditis: hospitalized patients with contaminated intravascular catheters, those who use intravenous needles, and those with localized staphylococcal infections.

Pneumonia: children, hospitalized patients, elderly patients, and patients with compromised pulmonary function or an antecedent viral respiratory infections (e.g., influenza).

Septic arthritis: hematogenous spread from infected focus or secondary infection resulting from trauma.

GEOGRAPHY/SEASON

Ubiquitous and worldwide.

Food poisoning is more common in summer and during late-year holidays.

MODES OF CONTROL

Most strains are resistant to penicillins; beta-lactamase–resistant penicillins (e.g., oxacillin, methicillin) are used.

Vancomycin is drug of choice for strains resistant to beta-lactam antibiotics.

For bacteremia and endocarditis, prompt treatment is essential to prevent secondary foci of infection.

For toxic shock syndrome, the focus of infection must be eradicated.

Treatment is symptomatic for food poisoning. People with cutaneous staphylococcal infection should avoid food preparation.

Proper cleansing of wounds and use of disinfectant help prevent infection.

For medical personnel, thorough handwashing and covering of exposed skin help prevent infection.

BOX 22-2 Summary of Coagulase-Negative Staphylococcal Infections

BACTERIAL FACTORS

Diseases—see Table 22-2.

Virulence factors—see Table 22-3.

Coagulase-negative staphylococci are common on the skin, in the oropharynx, and in the gastrointestinal and urogenital tracts.

Organisms can survive on dry surfaces for long periods.

TRANSMISSION

Bacteremia: introduced through a contaminated catheter.

Endocarditis: infection of previously damaged or artificial heart valve.

Prosthesis infection: introduced at surgery or by bacteremia.

WHO IS AT RISK?

Hospitalized patients with catheters, shunts, prostheses, or damaged heart valves.

GEOGRAPHY/SEASON

Ubiquitous and worldwide.

No seasonal incidence.

MODES OF CONTROL

Most strains are resistant to penicillin and other beta-lactam antibiotics.

Vancomycin is the drug of choice for strains resistant to beta-lactam antibiotics.

For endocarditis, prompt treatment is essential.

Maintenance of sterile intravascular lines helps prevent infection.

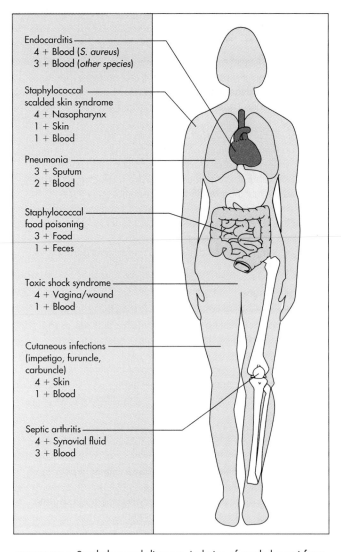

FIGURE 22-4 Staphylococcal diseases. Isolation of staphylococci from sites of infection. *1+*, Less than 10% positive cultures; *2+*, 10% to 50% positive cultures; *3+*, 50% to 90% positive cultures; *4+*, more than 90% positive cultures.

FIGURE 22-5 Staphylococcal scalded skin syndrome. (From Emond RT, Rowland HAK: *A color atlas of infectious diseases*, London, 1987, Wolfe.)

response (e.g., Job-Buckley syndrome, Wiskott-Aldrich syndrome, chronic granulomatous disease) are more susceptible to staphylococcal diseases.

Staphylococcal Scalded Skin Syndrome

In 1878 Gottfried Ritter von Rittershain described 297 infants younger than 1 month who had bullous exfoliative dermatitis. The disease he described, now called *Ritter's disease* or *staphylococcal scalded skin syndrome*, is characterized by the abrupt onset of a localized perioral erythema (redness and inflammation around the mouth) that covers the entire body within 2 days. Slight pressure displaces the skin (a positive Nikolsky's sign), and large bullae or cutaneous blisters form soon thereafter and are followed by desquamation of the epithelium (Figure 22-5). The blisters contain clear fluid but no organisms or leukocytes, a finding consistent with the fact that the disease is caused by the bacterial toxin. The epithelium becomes intact again within 7 to 10 days, when protective antibodies appear. Scarring does not occur because only the top layer of epidermis is sloughed. The mortality rate is low; when death does occur, it results from a secondary bacterial infection of the denuded skin areas.

Bullous impetigo is a localized form of SSSS. Specific strains of toxin-producing *S. aureus* (e.g., phage type 71) are associated with the formation of superficial skin blisters (Figure 22-6). Unlike patients with the disseminated manifestations of SSSS, patients with bullous impetigo have localized blisters that are culture positive. The erythema does not extend beyond the borders of the blister, and Nikolsky's sign is not present. The disease primarily occurs in infants and young children and is highly communicable.

Toxic Shock Syndrome

The first outbreak of TSS occurred in 1928 in Australia, where the disease developed in 21 children, 12 of whom died after an injection with an *S. aureus*–contaminated vaccine. Fifty years later, Todd observed what he called *toxic shock syndrome* in seven children with systemic disease, and the first reports of TSS in menstruating women were published in the summer of 1980. This was followed by a dramatic increase in the incidence of TSS, particularly in women. Subsequently, it was discovered that TSST-1–producing strains of *S. aureus* could multiply rapidly in hyperabsorbent tampons and release toxin. After the recall of these tampons, the incidence of disease, particularly in menstruating women, rapidly decreased.

FIGURE 22-6 Bullous impetigo, a localized form of staphylococcal scalded skin syndrome. (From Emond RT, Rowland HAK: *A color atlas of infectious diseases*, London, 1987, Wolfe.)

FIGURE 22-7 Toxic shock syndrome. Fatal infection with cutaneous and soft tissue involvement noted in photograph.

The disease is initiated with the localized growth of toxin-producing strains of *S. aureus* in the vagina or a wound, followed by release of the toxin into the bloodstream. Clinical manifestations start abruptly and include fever, hypotension, and a diffuse macular erythematous rash. Multiple organ systems (gastrointestinal, musculature, renal, hepatic, hematological, central nervous) are also involved, and the entire skin, including the palms and soles, desquamates (Figure 22-7). The initially high fatality rate has been decreased as the etiology and epidemiology of this disease have become better understood. However, unless the patient is specifically treated with an effective antibiotic, the risk of recurrent disease is as high as 65%.

Staphylococcal Food Poisoning

Staphylococcal food poisoning, one of the most common food-borne illnesses, is an intoxication rather than infection. Disease is due to toxin-contaminated food rather than a direct effect of the organisms. The most common infected foods are processed meats such as ham and salted pork, custard-filled pastries, potato salad, and ice cream. Growth of *S. aureus* in salted meats is consistent with the ability of this organism to replicate selectively in nutrient media supplemented with as much as 10% to 15% sodium chloride. Unlike many other forms of food poisoning in which an animal reservoir is important, staphylococcal food poisoning results from contamination of the food by a human carrier. Although contamination can be prevented by not allowing people with an obvious staphylococcal skin infection to prepare food, approximately half of the carriers are asymptomatic; col-

onization most commonly occurs in the nasopharynx. After the staphylococci have been introduced into the food, the food must remain at room temperature or warmer for the organisms to grow and release the toxin. Subsequent heating of the food will kill the bacteria but not inactivate the heat-stable toxin. Furthermore, the contaminated food will not appear or taste tainted.

After ingestion of contaminated food the onset of disease is abrupt and rapid, with a mean incubation period of 4 hours, which is consistent with a disease mediated by preformed toxin. Further toxin is not produced by ingested staphylococci, so the disease has a rapid course, with symptoms generally lasting less than 24 hours. Staphylococcal food poisoning is characterized by severe vomiting, diarrhea, and abdominal pain or nausea. Sweating and headache may occur, but fever is not seen. The diarrhea is watery and nonbloody, and dehydration may result from a considerable fluid loss.

The toxin-producing organisms can be cultured from the contaminated food if the organisms are not killed during food preparation. The enterotoxins are heat stable, so any contaminated food can be tested for toxins at a public health facility (these tests are not performed in most hospital laboratories).

Treatment is for the relief of the abdominal cramping and diarrhea and for the replacement of fluids. Antibiotic therapy is not indicated because as already noted, the disease is not mediated by the toxin produced in situ. Neutralizing antibodies to the toxin can be protective. However, a second episode of staphylococcal food poisoning can occur with a serologically distinct enterotoxin.

FIGURE 22-8 Pustular impetigo. Note the vesicles at different stages of development, including pus-filled vesicles on an erythematous base and dry, crusted lesions. (From Emond RT, Rowland HAK: *A color atlas of infectious diseases*, London, 1987, Wolfe.)

Certain strains of *S. aureus* can also cause enterocolitis, which is manifested clinically by profuse watery diarrhea, fever, and dehydration. Enterocolitis occurs primarily in patients who have received broad-spectrum antibiotics, which suppress the normal colonic flora and permit the growth of *S. aureus*. The diagnosis of staphylococcal enterocolitis can be confirmed only after other, more common causes of infection have been excluded (e.g., *Clostridium difficile* colitis). Abundant staphylococci are typically present in the stool of affected patients, and the normal gram-negative flora are absent. Fecal leukocytes are observed, and white plaques with ulceration are seen on the colonic mucosa.

Cutaneous Infections

Localized, pyogenic staphylococcal infections include impetigo, folliculitis, furuncles, and carbuncles. **Impetigo,** a superficial infection affecting mostly young children, occurs primarily on the face and limbs. Initially a small macule (flattened red spot) is seen, and then a pus-filled vesicle (pustule) on an erythematous base develops. Crusting occurs after the pustule ruptures. Multiple vesicles at different stages of development are common due to the secondary spread of the infection to adjacent skin sites (Figure 22-8). Impetigo is usually caused by *S. aureus*, although group A streptococci, either alone or with *S. aureus*, are responsible for 20% of cases.

Folliculitis is a pyogenic infection in the hair follicles. The base of the follicle is raised and reddened, and there is a small collection of pus beneath the epidermal surface. If this occurs at the base of the eyelid, it is called a **stye**. **Furuncles** (boils), an extension of folliculitis, are large,

painful, raised nodules with an underlying collection of dead and necrotic tissue. These can drain spontaneously or with a surgical incision.

Carbuncles occur when furuncles coalesce and extend to the deeper subcutaneous tissue. Multiple sinus tracts are usually present. Unlike patients with folliculitis and furuncles, patients with carbuncles have chills and fevers, indicating the systemic spread of staphylococci. Thus bacteremia with secondary spread to other tissues is common in patients with carbuncles.

Staphylococcal wound infections can also occur in patients after a surgical procedure or after trauma, with organisms colonizing the skin introduced into the wound. The staphylococci are not able to establish an infection in an immunocompetent person unless a foreign body is present in the wound (e.g., stitches, a splinter, dirt). Infections are characterized by edema, erythema, pain, and an accumulation of purulent material. The infection can be easily managed if the wound is reopened, the foreign matter removed, and the purulent material removed. If signs such as fever and malaise are observed or if the wound does not clear in response to localized management, antibiotic therapy directed against *S. aureus* is indicated.

Bacteremia and Endocarditis

S. aureus is a common cause of bacteremia. Although bacteremias caused by most other organisms originate from an identifiable focus of infection, such as an infection of the lungs, urinary tract, or gastrointestinal tract, the initial foci of infection in approximately one third of patients with *S. aureus* bacteremias are not known. Most likely the infection spreads to the bloodstream from an innocuous-appearing skin infection. More than half of the cases of *S. aureus* bacteremia are acquired in the hospital after a surgical procedure or result from the continued use of a contaminated intravascular catheter. *S. aureus* bacteremias, particularly prolonged episodes, are associated with dissemination to other body sites, including the heart.

Acute endocarditis caused by *S. aureus* is a serious disease, with a mortality rate approaching 50%. Although patients with *S. aureus* endocarditis may initially have nonspecific influenza-like symptoms, their condition can deteriorate rapidly and include disruption of cardiac output and peripheral evidence of septic embolization (Figure 22-9). Unless appropriate medical and surgical intervention is instituted immediately, the patient's prognosis is poor. An exception to this is *S. aureus* endocarditis in parenteral drug abusers, whose disease normally involves the right side of the heart (tricuspid valve) rather than the left. The initial symptoms may be mild, but fever, chills, and pleuritic chest pain caused by pulmonary emboli are generally present. Clinical cure of the endocarditis is the rule, although it is common for complications to occur as the result of secondary spread of the infection to other organs.

FIGURE 22-9 Septic embolization, caused by occlusion of capillaries with microcolonies of staphylococci, is common in bacteremic patients, particularly patients with endocarditis. (From Emond RT, Rowland HAK: *A color atlas of infectious diseases*, London, 1987, Wolfe.)

Pneumonia and Empyema

S. aureus respiratory disease can develop after the aspiration of oral secretions or from the hematogenous spread of the organism from a distant site. Aspiration pneumonia is primarily seen in the very young, the aged, and patients with cystic fibrosis, influenza, chronic obstructive pulmonary disease, and bronchiectasis. The clinical and radiographic presentations of the pneumonia are not unique. Radiographic examination reveals the presence of patchy infiltrates with consolidation or abscesses, the latter consistent with the organism's ability to secrete cytotoxic toxins and enzymes and form localized abscesses. Hematogenous pneumonia is common in patients with bacteremia or endocarditis.

Empyema occurs in 10% of patients with pneumonia, and *S. aureus* is responsible for one third of all cases. Because the organism can become consolidated in loculated areas, drainage of the purulent material is sometimes difficult.

Osteomyelitis and Septic Arthritis

S. aureus osteomyelitis can result from the hematogenous dissemination to bone, or it can be a secondary infection resulting from trauma or the extension of disease from an adjacent area. Hematogenous spread in children generally results from a cutaneous staphylococcal infection and usually involves the metaphyseal area of long bones, a highly vascularized area of bony growth. This infection is characterized by the sudden onset of localized pain over the involved bone and by high fever. Blood cultures are positive in about half of cases.

The hematogenous osteomyelitis that is seen in adults commonly occurs in the form of vertebral osteomyelitis and rarely in the form of an infection of the long bones. Intense back pain with fever is the initial symptom. Radiographic evidence of osteomyelitis in children and adults is not seen until 2 to 3 weeks after the initial symptoms appear. **Brodie's abscess** is a sequestered focus of staphylococcal osteomyelitis that arises in the metaphyseal area of a long bone and occurs only in adults. The staphylococcal osteomyelitis that occurs after trauma or a surgical procedure is generally accompanied by inflammation and purulent drainage from the wound or the sinus tract overlying the infected bone. With appropriate antibiotic therapy and surgery, the cure rate for staphylococcal osteomyelitis is excellent.

S. aureus is the primary cause of septic arthritis in young children and in adults who are receiving intraarticular injections or who have mechanically abnormal joints. *S. aureus* is replaced by *Neisseria gonorrhoeae* as the most common cause of septic arthritis in sexually active persons. Staphylococcal arthritis is characterized by a painful, erythematous joint, with purulent material obtained on aspiration. Infection is usually demonstrated in the large joints (e.g., shoulder, knee, hip, elbow). The prognosis in children is excellent, but in adults, it depends on the nature of the underlying disease as well as the occurrence of any secondary infectious complications.

Staphylococcus epidermidis and Other Coagulase-Negative Staphylococci
Endocarditis

S. epidermidis and the related coagulase-negative staphylococci can infect native and prosthetic heart valves. Infections of native valves are believed to result from the inoculation of organisms onto a damaged heart valve (e.g., a congenital malformation, damage resulting from rheumatic heart disease). This form of staphylococcal endocarditis is relatively rare and is more commonly caused by streptococci.

In contrast, staphylococci are a major cause of endocarditis of artificial valves. The organisms are introduced at the time of valve replacement, and the infection characteristically has an indolent course, with clinical signs and symptoms not developing for as long as 1 year after the procedure. Although the heart valve can be infected, more commonly the infection occurs at the site where the valve is sewn to the heart tissue. Thus infection with abscess formation can lead to separation of the valve at the suture line and mechanical heart failure. Because of the nature and site of infection, septic embolization and persistent bacteremia are less common in patients with staphylococcal prosthetic valve endocarditis than in those with other forms of endocarditis. The prognosis is guarded in patients who have this infection, and prompt medical and surgical management is critical.

Catheter and Shunt Infections

From 20% to 65% of all infections of prosthetic devices, catheters, and shunts are caused by coagulase-negative staphylococci. These infections have become a major medical problem as the result of the increased use of long-dwelling catheters for the feeding and medical management of critically ill patients. Because the coagulase-negative staphylococci can produce a polysaccharide slime that can bond them to catheters and shunts and protect them from antibiotics and inflammatory cells, they are particularly well adapted to causing these infections. Infections of cerebrospinal fluid shunts can lead to meningitis. A persistent bacteremia is generally observed in patients with such shunts because the organisms have continual access to the bloodstream. Immune complex-mediated glomerulonephritis occurs in patients with long-standing disease.

Prosthetic Joint Infections

Infections of artificial joints, particularly the hip, can be caused by coagulase-negative staphylococci. The patient usually only experiences localized pain and mechanical failure of the joint. Systemic signs such as fever and leukocytosis are not prominent, and blood culture findings do usually not contribute to the diagnostic process. Treatment consists of joint replacement and antimicrobial therapy. The risk of reinfection of the new joint is considerably increased in such patients.

Staphylococcus saprophyticus

S. saprophyticus has a predilection for causing urinary tract infections in young, sexually active women and is rarely responsible for infections in other patients. It is also infrequently found as an asymptomatic colonizer of the urinary tract. Infected women usually have dysuria (pain on urination), pyuria (pus in urine), and numerous organisms in the urine. Typically, patients respond rapidly to antibiotics, and reinfection is uncommon.

LABORATORY DIAGNOSIS
Microscopy

Staphylococci are gram-positive cocci that form clusters when grown on agar media but commonly appear as single cells or small groups of organisms in clinical specimens. The successful detection of organisms in a clinical specimen depends on the type of the infection (e.g., abscess, bacteremia, impetigo) and the quality of the material submitted for analysis. To obtain abscess material, the clinician scrapes the base of the abscess with a swab or curette; an abundance of organisms should be observed in Gram stain specimens. Aspirated pus consists primarily of necrotic material with relatively few organisms, so such specimens should not be collected. Few organisms are generally present in the blood of bacteremic patients (an average of less than 1 organism per milliliter of blood), so Gram stain blood specimens are typically unrewarding. Staphylococci are seen in the nasopharynx

of patients with SSSS and in the vagina of patients with TSS, but these organisms cannot be differentiated from the staphylococci that normally colonize these sites. Many staphylococci are implicated in documented outbreaks of staphylococcal food poisoning, but organisms are generally not found in fecal specimens collected from ill patients.

Culture

Clinical specimens should be inoculated onto nutritionally enriched agar media supplemented with sheep blood. If there is a mixture of organisms in the specimen (e.g., wound or respiratory specimen), *S. aureus* can be selectively isolated on agar media supplemented with 7.5% sodium chloride, which inhibits the growth of most other organisms, and mannitol, which is fermented by *S. aureus* but not most other staphylococci. Staphylococci grow rapidly on nonselective media, both aerobically and anaerobically, with large, smooth colonies seen within 24 hours. As noted earlier, *S. aureus* colonies are commonly golden, particularly when the cultures are incubated at room temperature. Almost all isolates of *S. aureus* and relatively few strains of coagulase-negative staphylococci grown on sheep blood agar show hemolysis; the hemolysis is caused by cytotoxins produced by the organisms.

Serology

Attempts to detect staphylococcal structural antigens in blood or clinical specimens have generally been unsuccessful. However, antibodies to cell wall teichoic acids are present in many patients with long-standing *S. aureus* infections. Antibodies develop within 2 weeks of the onset of disease and are detected in most patients with staphylococcal endocarditis. This test is less reliable, however, in the detection of antibodies in patients with staphylococcal osteomyelitis or wound infections because the focus of infection is sequestered in these settings and the organisms frequently do not stimulate a humoral immune response. The finding of elevated antibody titers in a bacteremic patient indicates the need for a prolonged course of antimicrobial therapy. However, the importance of negative serological findings must be carefully weighed because the test is relatively insensitive. Antibody titers are measured by immunodiffusion tests.

Identification

Relatively simple biochemical tests (e.g., positive reactions for coagulase, clumping factor, heat-stable nuclease, alkaline phosphatase, and mannitol fermentation) can be used to differentiate *S. aureus* from the other staphylococci. However, differentiation of the coagulase-negative staphylococci is more complex and is not routinely done in most clinical laboratories.

Antibiotic susceptibility patterns (antibiograms), biochemical profiles (biotyping), susceptibility to bacteriophages (phage typing), and nucleic acid analysis can be used for the intraspecies characterization of isolates for epidemiological purposes. Although the first two procedures can be performed in most laboratories and the results are reproducible if the tests are performed carefully, phage typing and nucleic acid analysis are performed at fewer laboratories. Phage typing differentiates among staphylococcal strains by their pattern of susceptibility to lysis by an international collection of specific bacteriophages. This testing is done only by research laboratories. The analysis of plasmid and genomic DNA by pulsed-field gel electrophoresis or similar techniques has rapidly evolved to be the most sensitive way to characterize isolates at the species and subspecies level. These methods are currently used in many research and clinical laboratories.

FIGURE 22-10 Penicillin-binding protein profiles of methicillin-resistant *Staphylococcus aureus* (6-1, 108-1, 123-1) and methicillin-susceptible revertant strains (6-1-4, 108-1-1, 123-1-2). Note that penicillin-binding protein 2' is present in all methicillin-resistant strains and absent in all methicillin-susceptible strains. (Based on data from Utsui Y, Yokota T: *Antimicrob Agents Chemother* 28:397-403, 1985.)

TREATMENT, PREVENTION, AND CONTROL

Staphylococci quickly developed drug resistance after penicillin was introduced, and today less than 10% of the strains are susceptible to this antibiotic. This resistance is mediated by penicillinase (beta-lactamase), which hydrolyzes the beta-lactam ring of penicillin. The genetic information encoding the production of this enzyme is carried on transmissible plasmids, which facilitated the rapid dissemination of resistance among staphylococci.

Because of the problems with penicillin-resistant staphylococci, semisynthetic penicillins resistant to beta-lactamase hydrolysis (e.g., methicillin, nafcillin, oxacillin, dicloxacillin) were developed. Unfortunately, the staphylococci developed resistance to these antibiotics as well. Currently, 30% to 50% of the strains of *S. aureus* and most of the coagulase-negative staphylococci are resistant to these newer penicillins. Resistance occurs as the result of alterations in the antibiotic target sites (i.e., penicillin-binding proteins) in the cell wall, which prevent the antibiotics from binding to the bacteria (Figure 22-10). This phenomenon is chromosomally mediated. It is sometimes difficult for laboratories to detect resistance to the semisynthetic penicillins because resistance is preferentially expressed at low temperatures (30° C) in vitro. Some strains of staphylococci, called *hyper–beta-lactamase producers,* also produce large quantities of beta-lactamases that can hydrolyze penicillin as well as oxacillin and the related antibiotics. These strains do not appear to be clinically resistant to oxacillin and related beta-lactam antibiotics; however, they can be mistaken in the laboratory for resistant strains that are producing penicillin-binding protein 2' (PBP2').

Despite the tendency of staphylococci to develop resistance to antibiotics, virtually all strains are uniformly susceptible to vancomycin. This is the antibiotic of choice in the treatment of disease caused by staphylococci resistant to beta-lactam antibiotics.

Staphylococci are ubiquitous organisms present on the skin and mucous membranes, and their introduction through breaks in the skin is frequently unavoidable. However, the number of organisms required to establish an infection (infectious dose) is generally large unless a foreign body is present in the wound (e.g., dirt, a splinter, stitches). Proper cleansing of the wound and the application of an appropriate disinfectant (e.g., germicidal soap, iodine solution, hexachlorophene) will prevent most infections in healthy people.

The spread of staphylococci from person to person is more difficult to prevent. An example of this is surgical wound infections, which can be caused by relatively few organisms because of the foreign bodies and devitalized tissue present. Although it is unrealistic to sterilize the operating room personnel and environment, the risk of contamination during an operative procedure can be minimized through proper hand-washing and the covering of exposed skin surfaces. The spread of methicillin-resistant organisms can also be difficult to control because asymptomatic nasopharyngeal carriage is the most frequent source of these organisms. However, some success in this regard has been achieved through the use of chemoprophylaxis consisting of vancomycin and rifampin.

CASE STUDY AND QUESTIONS

An 18-year-old man fell on his knee while playing basketball. The knee was painful, but the overlying skin was unbroken. The next day the knee was swollen and remained painful, so he was taken to the local emergency room. Clear fluid was aspirated from the knee, and the physician prescribed symptomatic treatment. Two days later the swelling returned, the pain increased, and erythema developed over the knee. Because the patient also felt systemically ill and had an oral temperature of 38.8° C, he returned to the emergency room. Aspiration of the knee yielded cloudy fluid, and cultures of the fluid and blood were positive for *S. aureus*.

1. Name two possible sources of this organism.
2. Staphylococci cause a variety of diseases, including SSSS, TSS, food poisoning, cutaneous infections, and endocarditis. How do the clinical symptoms of these diseases differ from the infection in this patient? Which of these diseases are intoxications?
3. What toxins have been implicated in staphylococcal diseases? Which staphylococcal enzymes have been proposed as virulence factors?
4. Which structures in the staphylococcal cell and which toxins protect the bacterium from phagocytosis?
5. What is the role of *S. epidermidis* in infections associated with prosthetic devices? What virulence property helps establish these infections? What infection is caused by *S. saprophyticus*? What population is most susceptible to this infection?

Bibliography

Committee on Toxic Shock Syndrome: The toxic shock syndrome: a conference held 20-22 November 1981, sponsored by the Institute of Medicine, National Academy of Sciences, *Ann Intern Med* 96(6 Pt 2):831-996, 1982.

Holmberg SD, Blake PA: Staphylococcal food poisoning in the United States: new facts and old misconceptions, *JAMA* 251:487-489, 1984.

Hovelius B, Mardh PA: *Staphylococcus saprophyticus* as a common cause of urinary tract infections, *Rev Infect Dis* 6:328-337, 1984.

Kloos WE, Bannerman TL: Update on clinical significance of coagulase-negative staphylococci, *Clin Microbiol Rev* 7:117-140, 1994.

Mandell GL: *Principles and practice of infectious diseases*, ed 4, New York, 1995, Wiley.

McWhinney PHM et al: *Stomatococcus mucilaginosus:* an emerging pathogen in neutropenic patients, *Clin Infect Dis* 14:641-646, 1992.

Mulligan ME et al: Methicillin-resistant *Staphylococcus aureus:* a consensus review of the microbiology, pathogenesis, and epidemiology with implications for prevention and management, *Am J Med* 94:313-323, 1993.

Murray PR et al: *Manual of clinical microbiology*, ed 6, Washington, DC, 1995, American Society of Microbiology.

Rogolsky M: Nonenteric toxins of *Staphylococcus aureus*, *Microbiol Rev* 43:320-360, 1979.

Rupp ME, Archer GL: Coagulase-negative staphylococci: pathogens associated with medical progress, *Clin Infect Dis* 19:231-245, 1994.

Sheagren JN: *Staphylococcus aureus*: the persistent pathogen, *N Engl J Med* 310:1368-1373, 1437-1442, 1984.

Streptococcus

The genus *Streptococcus* is a diverse collection of gram-positive cocci typically arranged in pairs or chains. Most species are facultative anaerobes, but some may be able to grow only in atmospheric conditions ranging from strictly anaerobic to capnophilic (i.e., growth dependent on carbon dioxide). Their nutritional requirements are complex, necessitating the use of blood- or serum-enriched media for isolation. Carbohydrates are fermented, resulting in the production of lactic acid, and unlike *Staphylococcus* species, the organisms are catalase negative.

The role of streptococci in human disease was appreciated very early (Box 23-1). However, the differentiation of species within the genus is complicated because at least three different schemes are still used to classify the organisms: serological properties (Lancefield groupings A through H, K through V); hemolytic patterns (complete [beta] hemolysis, incomplete [alpha] hemolysis, and no [gamma] hemolysis); and biochemical (physiological) properties. The serological classification scheme was developed by Lancefield in 1933 for differentiating beta-hemolytic strains. Most beta-hemolytic strains and some alpha-hemolytic and nonhemolytic strains possess group-specific antigens, most of which are cell wall carbohydrates. These antigens can be readily detected by immunological assays and have been useful for the rapid identification of many streptococcal pathogens. However, not all streptococci possess these group-specific cell wall antigens. For example, organisms such as *S. pneumoniae* and the numerous species of alpha-hemolytic and nonhemolytic streptococci (collectively termed the *viridans group of streptococci*) must be identified by their physiological properties. Unfortunately the classification schemes are not mutually exclusive (Table 23-1). For example, *S. anginosus* strains may be nontypeable (viridans group) or may react with the antisera for groups C, F, and G. Likewise, *S. agalactiae* (group B) is usually beta-hemolytic but may also be alpha-hemolytic or nonhemolytic.

GROUP A *STREPTOCOCCUS*

Group A *Streptococcus,* also called *S. pyogenes,* is an important cause of a variety of suppurative and nonsuppurative diseases (Box 23-1). Although they are the most common cause of bacterial pharyngitis, these organisms have become notorious in recent years because of their tendency to cause dramatic, life-threatening diseases. Indeed, reports of these "flesh-eating" bacteria have flooded both the scientific literature and the tabloid press.

Physiology and Structure

Group A streptococci are 0.5 to 1.0 μm spherical cocci that form short chains in clinical specimens and longer chains when grown in liquid media (Figure 23-1). Growth is optimal on enriched blood agar media but is inhibited if the medium contains a high concentration of glucose. After 24 hours of incubation, 1- to 2-mm white colonies with a large zone of beta-hemolysis are observed. Encapsulated strains may appear mucoid on freshly prepared media but wrinkled on dry media. Nonencapsulated colonies are smaller and glossy.

The antigenic structure of group A streptococci has been extensively studied. The basic structural framework of the cell wall is the peptidoglycan layer, which is similar in composition to that found in other gram-positive bacteria. Within the cell wall are the group- and type-specific antigens of group A streptococci.

Group-Specific Carbohydrate

Group-specific carbohydrate, which constitutes approximately 10% of the dry weight of the cell, is a dimer of *N*-acetylglucosamine and rhamnose. This antigen is used to classify group A streptococci and distinguish them from other streptococcal groups.

Type-Specific Proteins

The **M protein** is a major type-specific protein associated with virulent streptococci. This protein consists of two polypeptide chains complexed in an alpha helix. The carboxy terminus is anchored in the cell wall and cytoplasmic membrane, and the amino terminus is exposed above the cell surface. The carboxy end is highly conserved and shared among all M serotypes, whereas the amino end is responsible for the antigenic diversity of the more than 80 M serotypes. A secondary type-specific protein that is a useful epidemiological marker is the **T protein** (trypsin-resistant protein). The structural function of this protein is unknown.

Other Cell Surface Proteins

Other important proteins that have been described include the M-like proteins and F protein. The **M-like proteins** are structurally similar to the M proteins, with their carboxy termini anchored in the cell wall and their amino end exposed at the cell surface. The **F protein** is named for the fact that it binds fibronectin, a host cell protein.

Capsule

The outermost layer of the cell is the **capsule**, which is composed of hyaluronic acid identical to that found in connective tissue. For this reason the capsule is nonimmunogenic and protects bacteria from phagocytosis.

Pathogenesis and Immunity

The virulence of group A streptococci is determined by a variety of structural molecules and elaborated toxins and enzymes (Table 23-2). Although the precise role each plays in pathogenesis is often not well defined, it is likely that M protein, M-like proteins, and F protein are important in the establishment of infection and that the observed clinical manifestations can be directly attributed to effects of substances such as the pyrogenic exotoxins and streptolysins.

Capsule

The nonimmunogenic hyaluronic acid capsule protects the cells against phagocytosis.

M Protein

M protein is the main structural component protecting the streptococci from phagocytosis. M protein preferen-

---

BOX 23-1   Streptococci and Their Diseases

S. PYOGENES (GROUP A)

Pharyngitis, scarlet fever, pyoderma, erysipelas, cellulitis, necrotizing fasciitis, streptococcal toxic shock syndrome, bacteremia, rheumatic fever, glomerulonephritis

S. AGALACTIAE (GROUP B)

Neonatal infections (meningitis, pneumonia, bacteremia), urinary tract infections, amnionitis, endometritis, wound infections, pneumonia, bacteremia

OTHER BETA-HEMOLYTIC STREPTOCOCCI

Pharyngitis, abscess formation, bacteremia

S. PNEUMONIAE

Pneumonia, sinusitis, otitis media, meningitis, bacteremia

VIRIDANS GROUP STREPTOCOCCI

Bacteremia, endocarditis, abscess formation, dental caries

FIGURE 23-1 Gram stain of group A *Streptococcus*.

TABLE 23-1   Classification of Common Streptococcal Pathogens

SEROLOGICAL CLASSIFICATION	BIOCHEMICAL CLASSIFICATION	HEMOLYTIC PATTERNS
A	S. pyogenes	Beta
B	S. agalactiae	Beta, occasionally alpha or nonhemolytic
C	S. anginosus, S. equisimilis	Beta, occasionally alpha or nonhemolytic
D	S. bovis	Alpha, nonhemolytic; occasionally beta
F	S. anginosus	Beta
G	S. anginosus	Beta
—	S. pneumoniae	Alpha
Viridans group	S. mutans group, S. salivarius group, S. sanguis group, S. mitis group, S. milleri group	Alpha, nonhemolytic

tially binds the serum beta-globulin factor H, which is a regulatory protein for the alternative complement pathway. Complement component C3b mediates opsonization, and factor H destablizes C3b. Thus the C3b that binds to the cell surface in the region of the M protein is degraded by factor H.

Specific M serotypes are associated with rheumatic heart disease and glomerulonephritis. One explanation for this finding is that it represents autoimmune disease. In support of this hypothesis, amino acid sequence homology has been demonstrated in these serotypes with sequences in cardiac tropomyosin, cardiac muscle sarcolemma, and glomerular basement membrane antigens.

M-Like Proteins

Although the significance of the M-like proteins in causing virulence remains to be defined, it is known that they can bind the Fc portion of IgG and IgA, thereby essentially coating the bacterial cell with host antigens. These proteins can also bind alpha$_2$-macroglobulin, a protease inhibitor that can theoretically protect the bacteria from the proteases that are released by phagocytic cells.

F Protein

F protein has a receptor for fibronectin, a matrix protein on eukaryotic cells, and may be the major adhesin for bacterial attachment to the epithelial cells of the pharynx and skin.

Pyrogenic Exotoxins

The streptococcal pyrogenic exotoxins (Spe), originally called **erythrogenic toxins,** are produced by lysogenic strains of streptococci and are similar to the toxin produced in *Corynebacterium diphtheriae*. Three immunologically distinct, heat-labile toxins (SpeA, SpeB, and SpeC) have been described in group A streptococci and in rare strains of groups C and G streptococci. These toxins act as superantigens, interacting with both macrophages and helper T cells with the release of IL-1, IL-2, and IL-6; tumor necrosis factor–alpha; and interferon-gamma. These cytokines mediate a variety of important effects, including the shock and the organ failure characteristically seen in patients who have severe streptococcal disease. The toxins are also responsible for causing the rash observed in patients with scarlet fever, although it is unclear whether this results from the direct effect of the toxin on the capillary bed or, more likely, whether it is secondary to a hypersensitivity reaction. Exotoxin A has been found in more than half of the group A streptococcal strains that are responsible for causing severe streptococcal toxic shock disease. Although this toxin is important in the pathogenesis of this disease, other factors are also important.

Streptolysins S and O

Streptolysin S is an oxygen-stable, nonimmunogenic, cell-bound hemolysin that can lyse erythrocytes, leukocytes, and platelets. Streptolysin S can also stimulate the release of lysosomal contents after engulfment, with subsequent death of the phagocytic cell. Streptolysin O is inactivated reversibly by oxygen and irreversibly by cholesterol.

Unlike streptolysin S, antibodies are readily formed against streptolysin O and are useful for documenting recent group A streptococcal infection (**ASO test**). This hemolysin cross-reacts with similar oxygen-labile toxins produced by *S. pneumoniae* and *Clostridium* species. Streptolysin O can also kill leukocytes by lysing their cytoplasmic granules, with the subsequent release of hydrolytic enzymes.

Streptokinases

At least two forms of streptokinase (A and B) have been described. These enzymes can lyse blood clots and may be responsible for causing the rapid spread of group A streptococci in infected tissues.

TABLE 23-2	**Group A *Streptococcus* Virulence Factors**
VIRULENCE FACTOR	**BIOLOGICAL EFFECT**
Capsule	Nonimmunogenic; antiphagocytic
M protein	Antiphagocytic; degrades C3b
M-like proteins	Binds IgM, and IgG and alpha$_2$-macroglobulin (protease inhibitor)
F protein	Mediates adherence to epithelial cells
Pyrogenic exotoxins	Mediates pyrogenicity, enhancement of delayed hypersensitivity and susceptibility to endotoxin, cytotoxicity, nonspecific mitogenicity for T cells, immunosuppression of B-cell function, and production of scarlatiniform rash
Streptolysin S	Lyses leukocytes, platelets, and erythrocytes; stimulates release of lysosomal enzymes; nonimmunogenic
Streptolysin O	Lyses leukocytes, platelets, and erythrocytes; stimulates release of lysosomal enzymes; immunogenic
Streptokinase	Lyses blood clots; facilitates spread of bacteria in tissues
DNase	Depolymerizes cell-free DNA in purulent material
C5a peptidase	Degrades C5a

DNase, Deoxyribonuclease.

BOX 23-2   Summary of Group A Streptococcal Infections

BACTERIAL FACTORS

Transient colonization of oropharynx is common; disease occurs when strains establish infection of pharynx or skin before specific antibodies develop or competitive organisms proliferate.
Diseases—see Box 23-1.
Virulence factors—see Table 23-2.

TRANSMISSION

Person to person by respiratory droplets (pharyngitis) or through breaks in skin after direct contact with infected person, fomite, or arthropod vector.
Rheumatic fever: nonsuppurative complication of upper respiratory tract infections with group A streptococci.
Acute glomerulonephritis: nonsuppurative complication of upper respiratory tract or cutaneous infection with group A streptococci.

WHO IS AT RISK?

Pharyngitis: children 5 to 15 years old at greatest risk.
Streptococcal toxic shock syndrome: patients with extensive soft tissue infections and bacteremia.
Pyoderma: children 2 to 5 years old who have poor personal hygiene.
Erysipelas and cellulitis: young children and older adults with preexisting respiratory tract or skin infections caused by group A streptococci.
Bacteremia: patients with deep soft tissue infections or involvement of internal organs (e.g., pneumonia).
Rheumatic fever: children with severe streptococcal disease.
Pharyngitis-associated glomerulonephritis: school-age children.
Pyoderma-associated glomerulonephritis: preschool-age children.

GEOGRAPHY/SEASON

Pharyngitis and rheumatic fever are more common in autumn and winter.
Pyoderma is more common in warm, moist environments and during summer.
Pharyngitis-associated glomerulonephritis is more common in temperate and cold climates and during winter and spring.
Pyoderma-associated glomerulonephritis is more common in hot or tropical climates and during late summer and early autumn.

MODES OF CONTROL

Penicillin is drug of choice. Erythromycin or oral cephalosporin is used for patients allergic to penicillin; antistaphylococcal antibiotics are given for mixed infections.
Oropharyngeal carriage occurring after treatment can be retreated; treatment is not indicated for prolonged asymptomatic carriage because antibiotics disrupt normal protective flora.
Starting antibiotic therapy within 10 days in patients with pharyngitis prevents rheumatic fever.
For rheumatic fever, antibiotic prophylaxis prevents recurrences; prophylaxis is required before procedures (e.g., dental) that can induce bacteremias leading to endocarditis.
For glomerulonephritis, no specific antibiotic treatment or prophylaxis is indicated.

Deoxyribonuclease

Four immunologically distinct deoxyribonucleases (DNases A to D) have been identified. These enzymes are not cytolytic but can depolymerize free DNA present in pus. This reduces the viscosity of the abscess material and facilitates spread of the organisms. Antibodies developed against DNase B are an important marker of cutaneous group A streptococcal infections.

C5a Peptidase

Complement component C5a mediates inflammation by recruiting and activating phagocytic cells. **C5a peptidase** disrupts this by degrading C5a.

Other Enzymes

Other enzymes, including hyaluronidase ("spreading factor") and diphosphopyridine nucleotidase (DPNase), have been described. Their role in pathogenesis is unknown.

Epidemiology

Group A streptococci commonly colonize the oropharynx of healthy children and young adults (Box 23-2). Although the incidence of carriage is reported to be 15% to 20%, these figures are misleading. Highly selective culture techniques are necessary to detect small numbers of organisms in oropharyngeal secretions. Colonization with group A streptococci is transient, regulated by the person's ability to mount specific immunity to the M protein of the colonizing strain, and the presence of any competitive organisms in the oropharynx. Bacteria such as the alpha-hemolytic and nonhemolytic streptococci are able to produce antibiotic-like substances called **bacteriocins**, which suppress the growth of group A streptococci.

In general, group A streptococcal disease is caused by recently acquired strains that can establish an infection of the pharynx or skin before specific antibodies are produced or competitive organisms are able to proliferate.

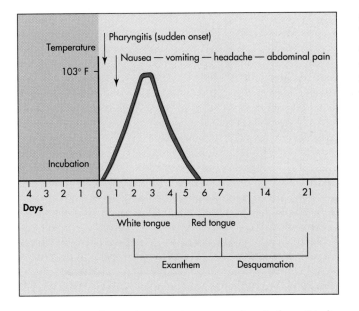

FIGURE 23-2 Evolution of signs and symptoms of scarlet fever. (Modified from Habif TP: *Clinical dermatology: a color guide to diagnosis and therapy,* St Louis, 1985, Mosby.)

Group A streptococci are the major cause of bacterial pharyngitis, with group C and G organisms occasionally involved. This is primarily a disease of children between the ages of 5 to 15 years, but infants and adults are also susceptible. The pathogen is spread person to person through respiratory droplets. Crowding, such as in classrooms and day-care facilities, increases the opportunity for the organism to spread. Soft tissue infections (i.e., pyoderma, erysipelas, cellulitis, fasciitis) are typically preceded by initial skin colonization with group A streptococci, after which the organisms are introduced into the superficial or deep tissues through a break in the skin.

Clinical Syndromes

Suppurative Streptococcal Disease

Pharyngitis. Pharyngitis generally develops 2 to 4 days after exposure to the pathogen, with an abrupt onset of sore throat, fever, malaise, and headache. The posterior pharynx can appear erythematous with an exudate, and cervical lymphadenopathy can be prominent. Despite these clinical signs and symptoms, differentiating streptococcal pharyngitis from viral pharyngitis is difficult. For example, only about 50% of patients with "strep throat" have pharyngeal or tonsillar exudates. Likewise, most young children with exudative pharyngitis have viral disease. The specific diagnosis can be made only by bacteriological or serological tests.

Scarlet fever is a complication of streptococcal pharyngitis (Figure 23-2) and occurs when the infecting strain is lysogenized by a temperate bacteriophage that stimulates production of a pyrogenic exotoxin. Within 1 to 2 days after the initial clinical symptoms of pharyngitis develop, a diffuse erythematous rash initially appears

on the upper chest and then spreads to the extremities. The area around the mouth is generally spared (circumoral pallor), as are the palms and soles. A yellowish white coating initially covers the tongue and is later shed, revealing a red, raw surface beneath ("strawberry tongue"). The rash, which blanches when pressed, is best seen on the abdomen and in skin folds (Pastia's lines). The rash disappears over the next 5 to 7 days and is followed by desquamation.

Suppurative complications of streptococcal pharyngitis have become rare since the advent of antimicrobial therapy. However, abscesses of the peritonsillar and retropharyngeal areas are seen, as well as disseminated infections to the brain, heart, bones, and joints.

Pyoderma. Pyoderma (impetigo) is a confined, purulent *(pyo)* infection of the skin *(derma)* that primarily affects exposed areas (i.e., face, arms, legs). Infection begins when the skin is colonized with group A streptococci after direct contact with an infected person or a fomite, after which the organism is introduced into the subcutaneous tissues through a break in the skin (e.g., scratch, insect bite). Initially, vesicles develop and then become pustules (pus-filled vesicles), which then rupture and crust over. The regional lymph nodes can become enlarged, but the systemic signs of infection (e.g., fever, sepsis, involvement of other organs) are uncommon. Secondary spread of the infection caused by scratching is typical. Pyoderma is seen primarily in young children (2 to 5 years of age) with poor personal hygiene and occurs primarily during the warm, moist summer months. Although group A streptococci are responsible for most streptococcal skin infections, groups C and G have also been implicated. *Staphylococcus aureus* is frequently present in the lesions. The strains of streptococci that cause skin infections are different from those that cause pharyngitis, although pyoderma serotypes can colonize the pharynx and establish a persistent carriage state.

Erysipelas. Erysipelas (*erythros,* "red"; *pella,* "skin") is an acute infection of the skin. Patients experience local pain and inflammation (erythema, warmth), lymph node enlargement, and systemic signs (chills, fever, leukocytosis). The involved skin area is typically raised and distinctly differentiated from the uninvolved skin (Figure 23-3). Erysipelas occurs most commonly in young children or older adults, historically on the face but now more commonly on the legs, and usually is preceded by respiratory tract or skin infections with group A streptococci (less frequently with group C or G streptococci).

Cellulitis. Unlike erysipelas, cellulitis typically involves the deeper subcutaneous tissues, and the distinction between infected and noninfected skin is not as clearly separated. Like erysipelas, local inflammation and systemic signs are observed. Precise identification of the offending organism is necessary because many different microbes can cause cellulitis.

Necrotizing fasciitis. Necrotizing fasciitis, an infection that occurs deep in the subcutaneous tissue, is

FIGURE 23-3 Acute stage of erysipelas of the leg. Note the erythema in the involved area and bullae formation. (From Emond RTD, Rowland HAK: *A colour atlas of infectious diseases*, ed 2, London, 1989, Wolfe.)

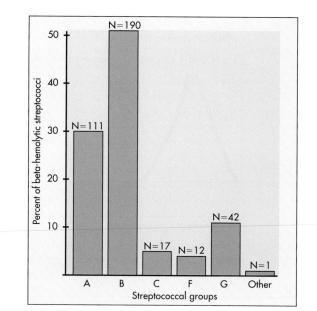

FIGURE 23-4 Distribution of streptococcal groups in bacteremic adults admitted to Barnes Hospital in St. Louis from 1986 to 1995. A total of 373 patients with beta-hemolytic streptococcal bacteremia was seen during this period.

characterized by an extensive destruction of muscle and fat that spreads along the fascial planes. The organism (referred to by the news media as *flesh-eating bacteria*) is introduced into the tissue through a break in the skin (e.g., minor cut or trauma, vesicular viral infection, burn, surgery). Initially there is evidence of cellulitis, after which bullae form and gangrene and systemic symptoms develop. Systemic toxicity, multiorgan failure, and death (mortality exceeds 50%) are the hallmarks of this disease; thus prompt therapy is necessary to prevent them. Unlike cellulitis, which can be treated with antibiotic therapy alone, fasciitis must be treated aggressively with the surgical debridement of nonviable tissue.

Streptococcal toxic shock syndrome. Although the incidence of severe group A streptococcal disease declined steadily after the advent of antibiotics, this trend changed dramatically in the late 1980s, when infections characterized by multisystem toxicity were reported. Most patients initially experience soft tissue inflammation at the site of the infection and pain, as well as nonspecific symptoms such as fever, chills, malaise, nausea, vomiting, and diarrhea. The pain intensifies as the disease progresses to shock and organ failure (e.g., kidney, lungs, liver, heart)—features similar to those of staphylococcal toxic shock syndrome. However, patients with streptococcal disease are bacteremic, and most have necrotizing fasciitis. Although people of all age groups are susceptible to streptococcal toxic shock syndrome, patients with certain conditions are at increased risk, such as those with human immunodeficiency virus infection, cancer, diabetes mellitus, heart or pulmonary dis-

ease, and Varicella virus infection, as well as intravenous drug abusers and those who abuse alcohol. The group A streptococci responsible for causing this syndrome differ from the strains causing pharyngitis, in that most are M serotypes 1, 3, 12, or 28 and some have prominent mucopolysaccharide hyaluronic acid capsules (mucoid strains). The production of pyrogenic exotoxins, particularly exotoxin A, is also a prominent feature of these organisms.

Other suppurative diseases. Group A streptococci have been associated with a variety of other suppurative infections, including puerperal sepsis, lymphangitis, and pneumonia. Although these infections are seen occasionally, they became less common after the introduction of antibiotic therapy.

Bacteremia. Group A streptococci are the second most common beta-hemolytic streptococci isolated in blood cultures (Figure 23-4). Patients with localized infections such as pharyngitis, pyoderma, and erysipelas are rarely bacteremic; however, the blood cultures in most patients with necrotizing fasciitis or toxic shock syndrome are positive for the organism. The mortality in this population of patients approaches 40%.

Nonsuppurative Streptococcal Disease

Rheumatic fever. Rheumatic fever is a nonsuppurative complication of group A streptococcal disease. It is characterized by inflammatory changes involving the heart, joints, blood vessels, and subcutaneous tissues. Chronic, progressive damage to the heart valves may occur. The incidence of rheumatic fever has decreased from

(Table 23-3). Diagnosis is determined on the basis of the clinical presentation and the finding of evidence of a recent group A streptococcal infection. Young patients generally have an uneventful recovery, but the long-term prognosis for adults is unclear. Progressive, irreversible loss of renal function has been observed in adults.

Laboratory Diagnosis

Microscopy

Gram stain of samples of affected tissue can be used to make a rapid, preliminary diagnosis of group A streptococcal soft issue infections or pyoderma. Because streptococci do not normally colonize the skin surface, the finding of gram-positive cocci in pairs and chains in association with leukocytes is important. In contrast, streptococci are part of the normal oropharyngeal flora, so their presence in a respiratory specimen from a patient with pharyngitis has poor predictive value.

Antigen Detection

A variety of immunological tests that react with the group-specific carbohydrate in the bacterial cell wall can be used to detect group A streptococci directly in throat swabs. The antigen is extracted by treating the specimen with nitrous acid for 5 minutes. The extract is then neutralized and mixed with specific antibodies that are immobilized on a filter membrane (enzyme immunoassay [EIA]) or bound to latex particles. The development of a positive indicator in the EIA or the agglutination of the latex particles represents a positive result. Although these assays are very specific, the sensitivity of the tests is low (probably no better than 75% to 80%), so all negative results must be confirmed by culture. Nonrespiratory specimens can not be used in direct antigen tests because the sensitivity of the tests is low.

Culture

Despite the difficulty of collecting throat swab specimens from children, specimens must be obtained from the posterior oropharynx (e.g., tonsils). Fewer group A streptococci are present in the anterior areas of the mouth and the mouth (particularly saliva) is colonized with bacteria that inhibit the growth of group A streptococci. Therefore contamination of even a properly collected specimen may obscure or suppress the growth of group A streptococci. The recovery of group A streptococci from skin infections is not a problem. The crusted top of the lesion is raised, and the purulent material and base of the lesion are cultured. An abundance of group A streptococci should be recovered. Cultures should not be obtained from open, draining skin pustules because they might be superinfected with staphylococci.

As discussed previously, streptococci have fastidious growth requirements. Antibiotics (e.g., trimethoprim-sulfamethoxazole) can be added to blood agar plates to suppress the growth of oral bacterial flora. Although these selective plates have proved very useful, the growth of group A streptococci on the plates is delayed, and

---

TABLE 23-3	Epidemiological Features of Acute Streptococcal Glomerulonephritis	
FEATURE	**PHARYNGITIS ASSOCIATED**	**PYODERMA ASSOCIATED**
Seasonal occurrence	Winter and spring	Late summer and early autumn
Geographical distribution	Temperate and cold climates	Hot and tropical climates
Age	School-age children	Preschool-age children
Familial occurrence	Common	Common
Attack rate after infection with nephritogenic strain	10%-15%	10%-15%
Carrier state	Pharynx (common)	Skin (rare)
Serological types	Limited to pharynx	Limited to skin
Antistreptolysin O response	Common	Uncommon
Anti-DNase B response	Common	Common

---

a peak of more than 10,000 cases per year reported 30 years ago to 112 cases reported in 1994 (the last year of mandatory reporting). The disease is caused by specific M serotypes of group A streptococci (e.g., M18, M3, and to a lesser extent, M5). Rheumatic fever is associated with streptococcal pharyngitis but not cutaneous streptococcal infections. As would be expected, the epidemiological characteristics of the disease mimic those of streptococcal pharyngitis: it is most common in young school-age children, with no male or female predilection, and occurs primarily during the fall or winter. As many as one third of patients have an asymptomatic or mild infection with group A streptococci before rheumatic fever develops. Streptococcal infection recurs if antibiotic prophylaxis is not used. The risk for recurrence decreases with time.

Because no specific diagnostic test can identify patients with rheumatic fever, the diagnosis is made on the basis of clinical findings. In making the diagnosis, it is critical to document evidence of recent group A streptococcal disease by culture results, antigen detection, or serological findings.

Acute glomerulonephritis. The second nonsuppurative complication of streptococcal disease is acute glomerulonephritis, which is characterized by acute inflammation of the renal glomeruli with edema, hypertension, hematuria, and proteinuria. Specific nephritogenic strains of group A streptococci are associated with this disease. The pharyngeal and pyodermal strains differ. The epidemiological characteristics of the disease are similar to those of the initial streptococcal infection prolonged incubation must be used (2 to 3 days). It is also unclear what atmosphere of incubation should be used. Because virtually all group A streptococci produce streptolysin S, cultures can be incubated in air. They should not be incubated in air supplemented with carbon dioxide, however, because such an environment favors the growth of inhibitory bacteria.

Identification

Group A streptococci historically were identified by their susceptibility to bacitracin (Table 23-4). A disk saturated with bacitracin is placed onto a plate inoculated with group A streptococci, and after overnight incubation, strains inhibited by bacitracin are considered group A streptococci. Group A streptococci are now definitively identified by demonstrating the group-specific carbohydrate, a technique that was not routinely practical until the introduction of direct antigen detection tests.

Antibody Detection

Patients with group A streptococcal disease produce antibodies to many specific enzymes. Although antibodies against the M protein are produced and are important for maintaining immunity, these antibodies appear late in the clinical course of the disease and are type specific. In contrast, the measurement of antibodies against streptolysin O (the ASO test) is useful for confirming rheumatic fever or acute glomerulonephritis resulting from a recent streptococcal infection. These antibodies appear 3 to 4 weeks after the initial exposure to the organism and persist. An elevated ASO titer is not observed in patients with streptococcal pyoderma, however; it is thought that the streptolysin O is inactivated by lipids present on the skin. The production of other antibodies against streptococcal enzymes, particularly DNase B, has been documented in patients with streptococcal pyoderma and pharyngitis. The anti-DNase B test should be performed if streptococcal glomerulonephritis is suspected.

Treatment, Prevention, and Control

Group A streptococci are very sensitive to penicillin. Erythromycin or an oral cephalosporin can be used in patients with a history of penicillin allergy. However, this therapy is ineffective in patients with mixed infections that include *S. aureus*. Treatment in this case should include oxacillin or vancomycin. Drainage and aggressive surgical debridement must be promptly initiated in patients with serious soft tissue infections.

Persistent oropharyngeal carriage of group A streptococci can occur after a complete course of therapy. This may stem from poor compliance with the prescribed course of therapy, reinfection with a new strain, or persistent carriage in a sequestered focus. Because antibiotic resistance has not been observed in such patients, they can be given an additional course of treatment. If carriage persists, retreatment is not indicated because prolonged antibiotic therapy can disrupt normal bacterial flora. Antibiotic therapy in patients with pharyngitis speeds the relief of symptoms and, if initiated within 10 days of the initial clinical disease, prevents rheumatic fever. Antibiotic therapy does not appear to influence the progression to acute glomerulonephritis.

Patients with a history of rheumatic fever require long-term antibiotic prophylaxis to prevent recurrence of the disease. Because damage to the heart valve predisposes these patients to endocarditis, they also require antibiotic prophylaxis before they undergo procedures that can induce transient bacteremias (e.g., dental procedures). Specific antibiotic therapy does not alter the course of acute glomerulonephritis, however, and prophylactic therapy is not indicated because recurrent disease is not observed in these patients.

GROUP B *STREPTOCOCCUS*

Group B *Streptococcus*, or *S. agalactiae*, was initially recognized as a cause of puerperal sepsis. Although the organism is still associated with this disease, it has become more notorious as an important cause of septicemia, pneumonia, and meningitis in newborn children, as well as serious disease in adults (Box 23-1).

Physiology and Structure

Group B streptococci are gram-positive cocci (0.6 to 1.2 μm) that form short chains in clinical specimens and

TABLE 23-4   Presumptive Identification of Streptococci

ORGANISM	SUSCEPTIBILITY BACITRACIN	SUSCEPTIBILITY OPTOCHIN	CAMP	HYDROLYSIS OF HIPPURATE	HYDROLYSIS OF ESCULIN	GROWTH IN BILE	GROWTH IN 6.5% NaCl	LYSIS BY BILE
Beta-hemolytic streptococci								
Group A	S	R	−	−	−	−	−	−
Group B	R*	R	+	+	−	−	+*	−
Groups C, F, G	R	R	−	−	−	−	−	−
Viridans group	R*	R	−	−	−*	−*	−	−
S. pneumoniae	R	S	−	−	−	−	−	+

NaCl, Sodium chloride; S, susceptible; R, resistant; −, negative; +, positive.
*Test variations can be seen.

longer chains in culture. They grow well on nutritionally enriched medium as buttery-appearing colonies larger than group A streptococci colonies. The colonies are surrounded by a narrow zone of beta-hemolysis. Rare strains are nonhemolytic or alpha-hemolytic.

These streptococci have group-specific cell wall polysaccharide antigen (composed of rhamnose, *N*-acetylglucosamine, and galactose), type-specific capsular polysaccharides (Ia, Ib, and II to VI), and the surface protein, **antigen c.** Nine immunologically distinct serotypes have been described: Ia, Ia/c, Ib/c, II, IIc, III, IV, V, and VI. These serotypes are important epidemiological markers.

Pathogenesis and Immunity

Antibodies developed against the type-specific capsular antigens in group B streptococci are protective, which partly explains the predilection of this organism for neonates. Infants who do not have the type-specific maternal antibodies are at increased risk for infection. Bactericidal activity for group B streptococci also requires complement. As a result, there is a greater likelihood of systemic spread of the organism in colonized infants with low complement levels.

Group B streptococci produce several enzymes, including DNases, hyaluronidase, neuraminidase, proteases, hippurase, and hemolysins. Although these enzymes are useful for identifying the organism, their role in the pathogenesis of infection is unknown.

Epidemiology

Group B streptococci colonize the lower gastrointestinal tract and the genitourinary tract (Box 23-3). Transient vaginal carriage has been observed in 10% to 30% of pregnant women, but the incidence of the finding depends on the time during the gestation period when the sampling is done and the culture techniques used. A similar incidence has been observed in nonpregnant women. Approximately 60% of infants born to colonized mothers become colonized with their mother's organism. The likelihood of colonization at birth is increased if the mother is heavily colonized, but neonatal disease is not more common in these infants. This finding emphasizes that the maternal immune status is more important than exposure to the bacteria in the colonization of infants with the organism. Other risk factors for neonatal colonization include premature delivery, prolonged membrane rupture, and intrapartum fever. Approximately 1% to 2% of colonized mothers give birth to infants who subsequently develop systemic disease. The most common serotypes isolated in pregnant and nonpregnant adults are Ia, Ia/c, III, and V. These are also the serotypes most commonly associated with neonatal disease.

Infection with subsequent development of infection in the neonate can occur in utero, at birth, or during the first few months of life. Infections in infants younger than 7 days of age are called **early onset disease**; those occurring from 1 week to 3 months of life are generally considered **late-onset disease.** Neonatal disease occurs in approximately 3 per 1000 live births, but early onset disease is 3 times more frequent than late-onset disease (Figure 23-5). In 1990, 7600 episodes of neonatal disease were documented, and there were 310 (4.1%) deaths from the disease.

There are proportionally more group B streptococcal infections in adults than in neonates, but the overall in-

---

BOX 23-3	Summary of Group B Streptococcal Infections

BACTERIAL FACTORS

Neonatal disease can occur in utero, at birth, or during the first few months of life.
Diseases—see Box 23-1.

TRANSMISSION

Early onset neonatal disease: transfer from mother by means of colonized birth canal, premature rupture of membranes, prolonged labor, preterm birth, or disseminated maternal group B streptococcal disease.
Late-onset neonatal disease: person to person through contact with infected infant or mother.
Postpartum sepsis: spread of organisms colonizing vagina to surgical incision site or uterus.
Other adult diseases: spread from gastrointestinal or genitourinary tract.

WHO IS AT RISK?

Neonates, particularly those without type-specific maternal antibodies and with low complement levels.

WHO IS AT RISK—cont'd

Pregnant women.
Men and nonpregnant women with diabetes mellitus, cancer, or alcoholism.

GEOGRAPHY/SEASON

Ubiquitous.
No seasonal incidence.

MODES OF CONTROL

Penicillin G is drug of choice; combination of penicillin and aminoglycoside is used in patients with serious infections.
Vancomycin is used for patients allergic to penicillin.
For high-risk babies, antibiotic therapy and passive immunization by transfusion with blood containing type-specific antibodies are performed.

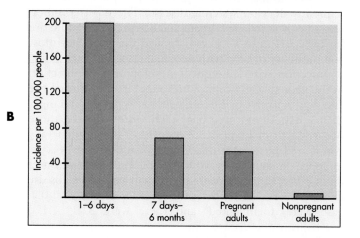

FIGURE 23-5 Incidence of invasive group B streptococcal disease in metropolitan Atlanta in 1992 and 1993. **A,** Percentage distribution of 279 cases of invasive disease. No disease was observed in residents 6 months to 15 years of age. **B,** Calculated incidence per 100,000 neonates or adults. (Based on data from Blumberg HM et al: *J Infect Dis* 173:365-373, 1996.)

cidence is higher in neonates (Figure 23-5). The risk of disease is greater in pregnant women than in men and nonpregnant women. Urinary tract infections, amnionitis, endometritis, and wound infections are the most common manifestations in pregnant women. Infections in men and nonpregnant women are primarily skin and soft tissue infections, bacteremia, urosepsis, and pneumonia. Group B streptococci are the most common beta-hemolytic streptococci isolated in blood cultures (Figure 23-4). Conditions that predispose to the development of adult disease include diabetes mellitus, cancer, and alcoholism.

Clinical Syndromes

Early Onset Neonatal Disease

Clinical symptoms of group B streptococcal disease acquired in utero or at birth generally develop during the first week of life. Early onset disease, which is character-

ized by bacteremia, pneumonia, or meningitis, is indistinguishable from sepsis caused by other organisms. The mortality rate has decreased to less than 5% as a result of rapid diagnosis and better supportive care; however, 15% to 30% of infants surviving meningitis have neurological sequelae, including blindness, deafness, and severe mental retardation.

Late-Onset Neonatal Disease

Disease in older infants is acquired from an exogenous source (e.g., mother, another infant). The predominant manifestation is bacteremia with meningitis, which again resembles disease caused by other bacteria. Although the survival rate is high, neurological complications are common in children with meningitis.

Infections in Pregnant Women

Urinary tract infections frequently occur in women during and immediately after pregnancy. Because childbearing women are generally in good health, the prognosis is excellent for those who receive appropriate therapy. Secondary complications of bacteremia, such as endocarditis, meningitis, or osteomyelitis, are rare.

Infections in Men and Nonpregnant Women

Men and nonpregnant women with group B streptococcal infections are generally older than the pregnant women who acquire the infection, and they have debilitating underlying conditions. For this reason, mortality is higher in this population (i.e., between 15% and 32%).

Laboratory Diagnosis

Antigen Detection

Direct detection of the organism with antibodies prepared against the group-specific carbohydrate is useful for the rapid detection of group B streptococcal disease in neonates. A variety of methods are used, including staphylococcal coagglutination, latex agglutination, and EIAs. Unfortunately, the direct antigen test is too insensitive to be used to screen mothers and predict which newborns are at increased risk for acquiring neonatal disease; thus it should not be used to replace culture.

Culture

Group B streptococci readily grow on a nutritionally enriched medium, producing large colonies after 24 hours of incubation. Beta-hemolysis may be difficult to detect or absent, which poses a problem in the detection of the organism in mixed cultures. Thus a selective broth medium, with antibiotics added to suppress the growth of other organisms, should be used to detect group B streptococcal carriage in pregnant women.

Identification

A preliminary identification of an isolate can be made by demonstration of a positive CAMP test (Figure 23-6) or

FIGURE 23-6 CAMP reaction with group B streptococci. Group B streptococci produce a diffusible, heat-stable protein (CAMP factor) that enhances beta-hemolysis of *S. aureus*. *S. aureus* produces sphingomyelinase C, which can bind to erythrocyte membranes. When exposed to the group B CAMP factor, the cells undergo hemolysis. (From Howard BJ: *Clinical and pathogenic microbiology*, St Louis, 1987, Mosby.)

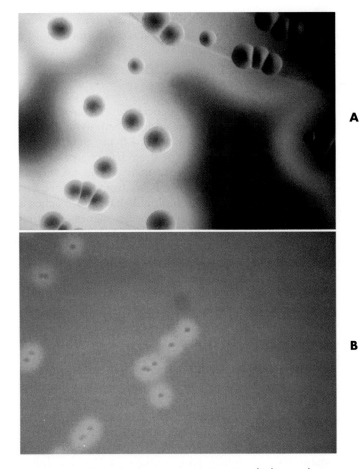

FIGURE 23-7 Group C streptococcus. **A,** *S. equisimilis,* large-colony species. **B,** *S. anginosus,* small-colony species.

by the hydrolysis of hippurate. Group B streptococci are definitively identified by the demonstration of the group-specific carbohydrate.

Treatment, Prevention, and Control

Group B streptococci are generally susceptible to penicillin G, which is the drug of choice. However, the minimum inhibitory concentration (MIC) needed to inhibit the organism is approximately 10 times greater than that needed to inhibit group A streptococci. In addition, **tolerance** to penicillin (the ability of the antibiotic to inhibit but not kill the organism) has been reported. For these reasons, a combination of penicillin and an aminoglycoside is frequently used in the management of serious infections. Vancomycin is an alternative therapy for patients allergic to penicillin. Resistance to erythromycin and tetracycline has been observed.

In an effort to prevent neonatal disease, intrapartum penicillin should be administered to the mother if group B streptococcal infection develops during pregnancy, if she has previously given birth to an infant with invasive group B disease, or if risk factors for the disease are present at birth (i.e., intrapartum temperature of at least 38° C, membrane rupture at least 18 hours before delivery, or a vaginal or rectal culture positive for organisms at 35 to 37 weeks' gestation).

Passive immunization of high-risk babies by transfusion with blood containing type-specific antibodies has reduced the morbidity and mortality associated with group B streptococcal disease; however, the therapy is not readily available. Efforts to eliminate this disease are directed to detection and immunization of women of childbearing age who have no protective antibodies.

OTHER BETA-HEMOLYTIC STREPTOCOCCI

Although 18 other groups of beta-hemolytic streptococci have been described, the most commonly isolated strains belong to groups C, F, and G. The two species of group C streptococci associated with human disease are *S. equisimilis* and *S. anginosus*. *S. equisimilis* produce large colonies with a large zone of beta-hemolysis on blood agar media (Figure 23-7, *A*), a behavior similar to that of group A streptococci. Like group A streptococci, *S. equisimilis* cause pharyngitis, which is sometimes complicated by acute glomerulonephritis but never rheumatic fever. *S. anginosus* produce smaller colonies (requiring 2 days of incubation) and a narrow zone of beta-hemolysis (Figure 23-7, *B*). This species is primarily associated with abscess formation and not pharyngitis.

S. anginosus is also a prominent member of groups F and G. That is, strains belonging to this species can possess polysaccharide antigens for groups C, F, or G. All group F streptococci and the "small colony" variants of group G are considered to be *S. anginosus*. Like group C streptococci, these organisms colonize the oropharynx, gastrointestinal tract, and genitourinary tract and produce human disease in which abscess formation is a prominent feature.

VIRIDANS STREPTOCOCCI

The viridans group of streptococci are a heterogeneous collection of alpha-hemolytic and nonhemolytic streptococci. Their group name is derived from *viridis* (Latin for "green") because many of these bacteria produce a green pigment on blood agar media. The taxonomic nomenclature for these species is confusing because European and American microbiologists have not reached a consensus on it. Thus different species names are often used interchangeably in the literature. At least 15 species have been identified in the United States, and they are classified into five subgroups. The precise classification of these bacteria can be problematic and is beyond the scope of this text. Although most isolates of viridans streptococci do not possess a group-specific carbohydrate, their reactivity with some groups of carbohydrates has been reported.

Like most other streptococci, these species are nutritionally fastidious, requiring complex media supplemented with blood products and frequently an incubation atmosphere augmented with 5% to 10% carbon dioxide. Some strains are "nutritionally deficient" in that they can grow only in the presence of exogenously supplied pyridoxal, the active form of vitamin B₆. These organisms can usually grow initially in blood cultures but cannot grow when subcultured unless pyridoxal-supplemented media are used. These strains have been recently been reclassified into a new genus *Abiotrophia* with two species recognized (*A. adiacens* and *A. defectiva*).

The viridans streptococci are isolated in the oropharynx, gastrointestinal tract, and genitourinary tract. Although these organisms can cause a variety of infections, they are most frequently associated with dental caries, subacute endocarditis, and suppurative intraabdominal infections. They adhere to tooth enamel or previously damaged heart valves, probably because of the insoluble dextran that they produce from glucose. This is the case for *S. mutans* and *S. sanguis*. Nongroupable *S. anginosus* is classified into the *S. milleri* group and is responsible for causing pyogenic infections.

Most strains of viridans streptococci are highly susceptible to penicillin, with MICs of less than 0.1 μg/ml, although moderately resistant streptococci (penicillin MIC of 0.2 to 0.5 μg/ml) have been observed in as many as 10% of species. Infections with these isolates can generally be treated with a combination of penicillin and an aminoglycoside. High-level resistance, resulting from an alteration in the penicillin-binding proteins, is rare. Tolerance to the killing activity of penicillin has also been reported, but the clinical significance of this is controversial.

STREPTOCOCCUS PNEUMONIAE

S. pneumoniae was isolated independently by Pasteur and Steinberg more than a hundred years ago. Since that time research with this organism has led to an increased understanding of molecular genetics, antibiotic resistance, and vaccine-related immunoprophylaxis. Unfortunately, pneumococcal disease is still a leading cause of morbidity and mortality.

Physiology and Structure

The pneumococcus is an encapsulated, gram-positive coccus. The cells are 0.5 to 1.2 μm in diameter, oval or lancet shaped, and arranged in pairs or short chains (Figure 23-8). Older cultures decolorize readily and appear gram-negative. Colonial morphology varies. Colonies of encapsulated strains are generally large (1 to 3 mm in diameter on blood agar; smaller on chocolatized or heated blood agar), round, mucoid, and unpigmented; colonies of nonencapsulated strains are smaller and appear flat. All colonies undergo autolysis with aging; the central portion of the colony dissolves, leaving a dimpled appearance. Colonies are alpha-hemolytic on blood agar if incubated aerobically and may be beta-hemolytic if grown anaerobically.

The organism has fastidious nutritional requirements and can grow only on enriched media (e.g., tryptic soy agar or brain-heart infusion agar) supplemented with blood products. *S. pneumoniae* can ferment several carbohydrates, with lactic acid the primary metabolic byproduct. *S. pneumoniae* grows poorly in media with high glucose concentrations because lactic acid rapidly reaches toxic levels. Like all streptococci, the organism lacks catalase. Unless an exogenous source of catalase is provided (e.g., from blood), the accumulation of hydrogen peroxide inhibits the growth of *S. pneumoniae*, as observed on chocolatized blood agar.

FIGURE 23-8 Gram stain of *S. pneumoniae*.

Virulent strains of *S. pneumoniae* are covered with a complex polysaccharide capsule. The capsular polysaccharides have been used for the serological classification of strains, with 90 serotypes that are currently recognized. Purified capsular material from the most commonly isolated serotypes are used in a polyvalent vaccine.

The peptidoglycan layer of the cell wall of the pneumococcus is typical of gram-positive cocci and consists of alternating subunits of *N*-acetylglucosamine and *N*-acetylmuramic acid cross-linked by peptide bridges. The other major component of the cell wall is teichoic acid rich in galactosamine, phosphate, and choline. The choline is unique to the cell wall of *S. pneumoniae* and plays an important regulatory role in cell wall hydrolysis. Choline must be present for activity of the pneumococcal autolysin, amidase, during cell division. Two forms of teichoic acid exist in the pneumococcal cell wall: one exposed on the cell surface and a similar form covalently bound to the plasma membrane lipids. The exposed teichoic acid (also called **C substance**) is species specific and unrelated to the group-specific carbohydrates observed by Lancefield in beta-hemolytic streptococci. The C substance precipitates a serum globulin fraction (**C-reactive protein [CRP]**) in the presence of calcium. CRP is present in low concentrations in healthy people but in elevated concentrations in patients with acute inflammatory diseases. The lipoteichoic acid in the membrane can cross-react with the Forssman surface antigens on mammalian cells.

Pathogenesis and Immunity

Despite the fact that this organism has been extensively studied, much remains to be learned about the pathogenesis of pneumococcal disease. The disease manifestations are caused primarily by the host response to infection rather than the production of organism-specific toxic factors. However, an understanding of how *S. pneumoniae* colonizes the oropharynx, spreads into normally sterile tissues, stimulates a localized inflammatory response, and evades being killed by phagocytic cells is crucial (Table 23-5).

Colonization and Migration

S. pneumoniae is a human pathogen that colonizes the oropharynx and then, in specific situations, is able to spread to the lungs, paranasal sinuses, or middle ear. It can also be transported in the bloodstream to distal sites such as the brain. The initial colonization of the oropharynx is mediated by the binding of the bacteria to epithelial cells by means of a poorly defined **protein adhesin**. Subsequent migration of the organism to the lower respiratory tract can be prevented if the bacteria are enveloped in mucus and removed from the airways by the action of ciliated epithelial cells. The bacteria can counteract this by producing **secretory IgA** (sIgA) **protease** and **pneumolysin**. sIgA traps bacteria in mucin by attaching itself to the bacteria at the antigen-binding site

and to mucin at the Fc region. The bacterial protease prevents this interaction. Pneumolysin, a cytotoxin similar to the streptolysin O in *S. pyogenes,* binds cholesterol in the host cell membrane and creates pores. This activity can destroy the ciliated epithelial cells.

Tissue Destruction

A pathognomonic characteristic of pneumococcal infections is the mobilization of inflammatory cells to the focus of infection. This is mediated by pneumococcal **teichoic acid, peptidoglycan fragments**, and **pneumolysin**. Teichoic acid and the peptidoglycan fragments activate the alternative complement pathway, producing C5a, which mediates the inflammatory process. Pneumolysin activates the classic complement pathway, resulting in the production of C3a and C5a. In turn, cytokines such as IL-1 and TNF–alpha are produced by the activated leukocytes, leading to the further migration of inflammatory cells to the site of infection, fever, tissue damage, and other characteristic signs of pneumococcal infection. The production of **hydrogen peroxide** by *S. pneumoniae* can also lead to tissue damage caused by reactive oxygen intermediates. Finally, **phosphorylcholine** present in the bacterial cell wall can bind to receptors for platelet-activating factor that is expressed on the surface of endothelial cells, leukocytes, platelets, and tissue cells such as those in the lungs and meninges. By binding

TABLE 23-5 *Streptococcus pneumoniae* **Virulence Factors**

VIRULENCE FACTOR	BIOLOGICAL EFFECT
COLONIZATION AND MIGRATION	
Protein adhesin	Binds to epithelial cells
Secretory IgA protease	Disrupts secretory IgA-mediated clearance
Pneumolysin	Possibly destroys ciliated epithelial cells
TISSUE DESTRUCTION	
Teichoic acid	Activates alternative C pathway
Peptidoglycan fragments	Activates alternative C pathway
Pneumolysin	Activates classic complement pathway
Hydrogen peroxide	Allows reactive oxygen intermediates to cause damage
Phosphorylchorine	Binds phosphodiesterase-activating factor, allowing bacteria to enter host cells
PHAGOCYTIC SURVIVAL	
Capsule	Antiphagocytic
Pneumolysin	Suppresses phagocytic oxidative burst

BOX 23-4   Summary of *S. pneumoniae* Infections

BACTERIAL FACTORS

Diseases—see Box 23-1.
Virulence factors—see Table 23-5.

TRANSMISSION

Endogenous spread from colonized nasopharynx or oropharynx to distal site: lungs, sinuses, ears, blood, meninges.
Person to person through infectious droplets (rare).

WHO IS AT RISK?

Persons with antecedent viral respiratory tract disease or other conditions that interfere with bacterial clearance from respiratory tract.
Children and the elderly.
People with hematological disorder (malignancy, sickle cell disease).

WHO IS AT RISK—cont'd

People with asplenia.
Renal transplant recipients.

GEOGRAPHY/SEASON

Ubiquitous.
Disease more common in cool months.

MODES OF CONTROL

Penicillin is drug of choice; cephalosporins, erythromycin, chloramphenicol are used for patients allergic to penicillin.
Penicillin resistance is increasingly common.
Immunization with 23-valent vaccine prevents infection.

---

these receptors, the bacteria can enter the cells, which protects them from opsonization and phagocytosis, and pass into sequestered areas such as blood and the central nervous system. This activity facilitates the spread of disease.

Phagocytic Survival

S. pneumoniae survives phagocytosis because of the antiphagocytic protection afforded by its **capsule** and the pneumolysin-mediated suppression of the phagocytic cell oxidative burst, which is required for intracellular killing. The virulence of *S. pneumoniae* is a direct result of this capsule. Encapsulated (smooth) strains can cause disease in humans and experimental animals, whereas nonencapsulated (rough) strains are avirulent. Antibodies directed against the type-specific capsular polysaccharides protect against disease caused by immunologically related strains. The capsular polysaccharides are soluble and have been called **specific soluble substances**. Free polysaccharides can protect viable organisms from phagocytosis by binding with opsonic antibodies.

Epidemiology

S. pneumoniae is a common inhabitant of the throat and nasopharynx of healthy people (Box 23-4). A 5% to 75% incidence of such carriage has been reported, but the incidence is significantly affected by the methods used to detect the organism and the population studied. Colonization is more common in children than in adults, with *S. pneumoniae* initially detected at about 6 months of age. Subsequently, the child is transiently colonized with other serotypes of the organism. The duration of carriage decreases with each successive serotype carried, in part because of the development of serotype-specific immunity. Although new serotypes are acquired throughout the year, the incidence of carriage and associated dis-

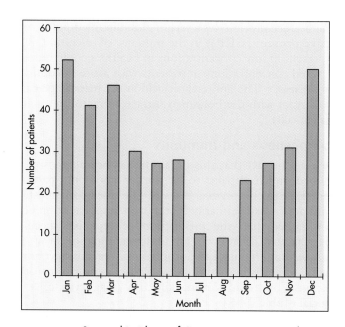

FIGURE 23-9 Seasonal incidence of *S. pneumoniae* invasive disease. Cumulative monthly incidence of invasive disease at Barnes Hospital in St. Louis from 1980 to 1995.

ease is highest during the cool months (Figure 23-9). The strains of pneumococci that cause disease are the same as the ones associated with carriage. When infection occurs, generally the patient acquires a new serotype rather than one associated with prolonged carriage.

Pneumococcal disease occurs when organisms colonizing the nasopharynx and oropharynx spread to distal loci, such as the lungs (pneumonia), paranasal sinuses (sinusitis), ears (otitis media), and meninges (meningitis). Bacteremia, with subsequent spread of the disease to other body sites, can occur with all of these infections.

S. pneumoniae is a common cause of bacterial pneumonia (an estimated 500,000 cases annually in the United States), meningitis (6000 cases annually), otitis media, sinusitis, and bacteremia (55,000 cases annually). The incidence of disease is highest in children and the elderly, populations with low levels of protective antibodies directed against the pneumococcal capsular polysaccharides.

Pneumonia occurs when the endogenous oral organisms are aspirated. Although strains can be transferred by airborne droplets from one person to another in a closed population, epidemics are rare. Disease occurs when the natural defense mechanisms (epiglottal reflex, trapping of bacteria by the mucus-producing cells lining the bronchus, removal of organisms by the ciliated respiratory epithelium and cough reflex) are circumvented, permitting organisms colonizing the oropharynx to gain access to the lower airways. Pneumococcal disease is most commonly associated with an antecedent viral respiratory disease such as influenza or measles or with other conditions that interfere with bacterial clearance, such as chronic pulmonary disease, alcoholism, congestive heart failure, diabetes mellitus, and chronic renal disease.

Clinical Syndromes

Pneumonia

Pneumococcal pneumonia develops when the bacteria multiply in the alveolar spaces. After aspiration, the bacteria grow rapidly in the nutrient-rich edema fluid. Erythrocytes, leaking from congested capillaries, accumulate in the alveoli. After this, first the neutrophils and then the alveolar macrophages migrate, and the organisms are phagocytosed and destroyed. The onset of the clinical manifestations of pneumococcal pneumonia is abrupt and includes a severe shaking chill and sustained fever of 39° to 41° C. The patient commonly has symptoms of a viral respiratory tract infection 1 to 3 days before the onset. Most patients have a productive cough with blood-tinged sputum, and they commonly have chest pain (pleurisy). Because the disease is associated with aspiration, it is generally localized in the lower lobes of the lungs (hence the name **lobar pneumonia**). However, children and the elderly can have a more generalized bronchopneumonia. Patients usually recover rapidly after the initiation of appropriate antimicrobial therapy, with complete radiologic resolution in 2 to 3 weeks. The overall mortality rate is 5%, although this is influenced by the serotype of the organism and the age and underlying disease of the patient. The mortality rate is considerably higher in patients with disease caused by *S. pneumoniae* type 3 as well as in elderly patients and patients with documented bacteremia. Patients with splenic dysfunction or splenectomy can also have severe pneumococcal disease, caused by decreased bacterial clearance from the bloodstream and the defective production of early antibodies.

Abscesses do not commonly form in patients with pneumococcal pneumonia, except in those with specific serotypes (e.g., serotype 3). Pleural effusions are seen in approximately 25% of patients with pneumococcal pneumonia, and empyema (purulent effusion) is a rare complication.

Sinusitis and Otitis Media

S. pneumoniae is a common cause of acute infections of the paranasal sinuses and ear. The disease is usually preceded by a viral infection of the upper respiratory tract, after which polymorphonuclear leukocytes infiltrate and obstruct the sinuses and ear canal. Middle ear infection (otitis media) is primarily seen in young children, but bacterial sinusitis can occur in patients of all ages.

Meningitis

S. pneumoniae can spread into the central nervous system after bacteremia, infections of the ear or sinuses, or head trauma that causes a communication between the subarachnoid space and the nasopharynx. Bacterial meningitis can occur in patients of all ages but is primarily a pediatric disease. Although pneumococcal meningitis is relatively uncommon in neonates, *S. pneumoniae* is now a leading cause of disease in children and adults. Mortality and severe neurological deficits are from 4 to 20 times more common in patients with meningitis caused by *S. pneumoniae* than in those with meningitis caused by other organisms.

Bacteremia

Bacteremia occurs in 25% to 30% of patients with pneumococcal pneumonia and in more than 80% of patients with meningitis. In contrast, bacteria are generally not present in the bloodstream of patients with sinusitis or otitis media. Endocarditis can occur in patients with normal or previously damaged heart valves. Destruction of valve tissue is common.

Laboratory Diagnosis

Microscopic Examination

Gram stain of sputum specimens is a rapid way to diagnose pneumococcal disease. The organisms characteristically appear as lancet-shaped diplococci surrounded by an unstained capsule; however, they may also appear to be gram negative because they tend not to stain well (particularly older cultures). In addition, their morphology may be distorted in a patient receiving antibiotic therapy. Gram stain consistent with *S. pneumoniae* can be confirmed with the **quellung** reaction (German for "swelling"). In this test, polyvalent anticapsular antibodies are mixed with the bacteria, and then the mixture is examined microscopically. An increased refractiveness around the bacteria is a positive reaction for *S. pneumoniae*.

Antigen Detection

Soluble pneumococcal capsular polysaccharide can be rapidly detected in infected body fluids by immunological assays such as counterimmunoelectrophoresis (CIE) and latex agglutination. The tests are very sensitive (able to detect 50 ng of antigen) and specific, although serotypes 7 and 14 are not detected by routine CIE procedures. The antigen detected in cerebrospinal fluid and serum is identical to the purified capsular polysaccharide; however, the antigen is degraded before it is excreted into the urine and has only a partial immunological identity.

Culture

Sputum specimens should be inoculated onto an enriched nutrient medium supplemented with blood. *S. pneumoniae* is recovered in the sputum cultures from only half of the patients who have pneumonia because the organism has fastidious nutritional requirements and is rapidly overgrown by contaminating oral bacteria. A selective medium such as blood agar with 5 μg/ml of gentamicin has been used with some success to isolate the organism from sputum specimens, but it takes some technical skill to distinguish *S. pneumoniae* from the other alpha-hemolytic streptococci that are frequently present in the specimen. For the organism responsible for sinusitis or otitis to be diagnosed definitively, an aspirate must be obtained from the infected focus. It is not difficult to isolate *S. pneumoniae* from specimens of cerebrospinal fluid unless antibiotic therapy has been initiated before the specimen is collected. Culture findings are negative in as many as half of infected patients who have received even a single dose of antibiotics.

Identification

Isolates of *S. pneumoniae* are rapidly lysed when the autolysins are activated after exposure to bile. The organism can be identified presumptively by placing a drop of bile on an isolated colony. Most colonies of *S. pneumoniae* are solubilized within a few minutes, whereas other alpha-hemolytic streptococci remain unchanged. This test can also be performed by adding bile to a broth culture of *S. pneumoniae*, which causes the organisms to be rapidly lysed and the broth to clear. *S. pneumoniae* can also be identified by its susceptibility to optochin (ethylhydrocupreine dihydrochloride). The isolate is streaked onto a blood agar plate, and a disk saturated with optochin is placed in the middle of the inoculum. A zone of inhibited bacterial growth is seen around the disk after overnight incubation. Additional biochemical, serological, or molecular diagnostic tests can be performed for a definitive identification.

Treatment, Prevention, and Control

Before the advent of antibiotics, specific treatment was guided by the passive infusion of type-specific capsular antibodies. These opsonizing antibodies enhanced polymorphonuclear leukocyte–mediated phagocytosis and the killing of bacteria. However, this immunotherapy was discontinued once antimicrobial therapy became available. Penicillin rapidly became the treatment of choice for pneumococcal disease. Alternative effective agents for patients allergic to penicillin have included the cephalosporins, erythromycin, and chloramphenicol (for meningitis). Resistance to tetracycline is well documented. In 1977, isolates of *S. pneumoniae* resistant to multiple antibiotics, including penicillin, were reported by researchers in South Africa. Until recently, high-level resistance to penicillin (MIC of at least 2 μg/ml) was relatively uncommon, and only 5% of all strains of *S. pneumoniae* isolated in the United States were considered to be moderately resistant (MIC of 0.1 to 1.0 μg/ml). However, this has changed dramatically in recent years: Resistance to penicillin has been observed for as many as a third of the strains isolated in the United States and in a higher number of those isolated in other countries. Increased resistance to penicillins is associated with a decreased affinity of the antibiotic for the penicillin-binding proteins present in the bacterial cell wall.

Efforts to prevent or control the disease have focused on the development of effective anticapsular vaccine. The current vaccine contains 23 different capsular polysaccharides. Approximately 94% of all strains isolated from infected patients either are included in the vaccine or are serologically related to the vaccine serotypes. Longitudinal studies have shown that the serotypes of *S. pneumoniae* associated with disease have not been influenced by the use of the vaccine. The vaccine is immunogenic in normal adults, and the immunity is long lived. However, the vaccine is not as effective in some patients at risk for pneumococcal disease; these include patients with asplenia, sickle cell disease, hematological malignancy, and human immunodeficiency virus infection; patients who have undergone renal transplant; young children; and the elderly.

CASE STUDY AND QUESTIONS

A 62-year-old man with a history of chronic obstructive pulmonary disease (COPD) came to the emergency room because of a fever of 40° C, chills, nausea, vomiting, and hypotension. The patient also produced tenacious, yellowish sputum, which had increased in quantity over the preceding 3 days. The patient had a respiratory rate of 18 breaths/min, and his blood pressure was 94/52 mm Hg. Chest x-ray examination showed extensive infiltrates in the left lower lung that involved both the lower lobe and the lingula. Multiple blood cultures and culture of the sputum yielded *S. pneumoniae*. The isolate was susceptible to cefazolin, vancomycin, and erythromycin but resistant to penicillin.

1. What predisposing condition made this patient more susceptible to pneumonia and bacteremia caused by *S. pneumoniae*? What other populations of patients are susceptible to these infections? What other infections are caused by this organism, and what populations are most susceptible?

2. What is the mechanism most likely responsible for this isolate's resistance to penicillin?

3. What are the major virulence factors of *S. pneumoniae,* group A *Streptococcus,* and group B *Streptococcus*? What infections are caused by group A and B streptococci and in what patient populations?

4. Group A streptococci can cause streptococcal toxic shock syndrome. Compare the pathogenesis of this disease with that produced by staphylococci.

5. What two nonsuppurative diseases can develop after localized group A streptococcal disease? Which serological tests can be used to confirm the clinical diagnosis of each nonsuppurative disease?

Bibliography

Bisno AL, Stevens DL: Streptococcal infections of skin and soft tissues, *N Engl J Med* 334:240-245, 1996.

Blumberg HM et al: Invasive group B streptococcal disease: the emergence of serotype V, *J Infect Dis* 173:365-373, 1996.

Breiman RF et al: Emergence of drug-resistant pneumococcal infections in the United States, *JAMA* 271:1831-1835, 1994.

Bruyn GAW et al: Mechanisms of host defense against infection with *Streptococcus pneumoniae, Clin Infect Dis* 14:251-262, 1992.

Centers for Disease Control and Prevention: Prevention of perinatal group B streptococcal disease: a public health perspective, *MMWR* 45(RR-7):1-14, 1996.

Fiorentino M: The return of rheumatic fever, *Clin Microbiol Newsletter* 18:25-29, 1996.

Holm SE: Invasive group A *Streptococcus* infections, *N Engl J Med* 335:590-591, 1996 (editorial).

Jackson LA et al: Risk factors for group B streptococcal disease in adults, *Ann Intern Med* 123:415-420, 1995.

Johnson DR et al: Epidemiologic analysis of group A streptococcal serotypes associated with severe systemic infections, rheumatic fever, or uncomplicated pharyngitis, *J Infect Dis* 166:374-382, 1992.

Katz AR, Morens DM: Severe streptococcal infections in historical perspective, *Clin Infect Dis* 14:298-307, 1992.

Musher DM: Infections caused by *Streptococcus pneumoniae:* clinical spectrum, pathogenesis, immunity, and treatment, *Clin Infect Dis* 14:801-809, 1992.

Salyers AA, Whitt DD: *Bacterial pathogenesis: a molecular approach,* Washington DC, 1994, ASM.

Stevens DL: Streptococcal toxic shock syndrome: spectrum of disease, pathogenesis, and new concepts in treatment, *Emerging Infect Dis* 1:69-78, 1995.

Enterococcus and Other Gram-Positive Cocci

Twelve genera of catalase-negative, gram-positive cocci are recognized as human pathogens (Table 24-1). *Streptococcus* (see Chapter 23) and *Enterococcus* are the most frequently isolated genera and the ones most commonly responsible for human disease. *Aerococcus, Leuconostoc, Pediococcus,* and *Alloiococcus* can also cause important, albeit uncommon, human disease (Table 24-2). The other genera of cocci are rarely recovered in clinical specimens or associated with human disease and will not be considered further.

ENTEROCOCCUS

The enterococci ("enteric cocci") were previously classified as group D streptococci because they possess the group D cell wall antigen (glycerol teichoic acid associated with the cytoplasmic membrane). Despite this observation, it was recognized that these organisms were distinct from other group D streptococci (referred to as *nonenterococcal group D streptococci* [e.g., *S. bovis*]). The enterococcal and nonenterococcal groups were originally differentiated by their physiological properties and then by nucleic acid analysis. In 1984 the enterococci were reclassified into the new genus *Enterococcus,* and there are currently 18 species in this genus. The most commonly isolated, clinically important species are *E. faecalis* ("pertaining to feces") and *E. faecium* ("of feces").

Physiology and Structure

The enterococci are gram-positive cocci typically arranged in pairs and short chains (Figure 24-1). The microscopic morphology of these isolates frequently cannot be differentiated from that of *Streptococcus pneumoniae.* The cocci are facultatively anaerobic and grow optimally at 35° C, although most isolates can grow from 10° to 45° C. They grow readily on blood agar media, with large, white colonies appearing after 24 hours of incubation; the colonies are typically nonhemolytic but can be alpha-hemolytic or beta-hemolytic. The enterococci grow in the presence of 6.5% NaCl, tolerate 40% bile salts, and can hydrolyze esculin. These basic properties can be used to distinguish enterococci from other catalase-negative, gram-positive cocci. Selected pheno-

typic tests (e.g., fermentation reactions, hydrolysis of pyrrolidonyl-beta-naphthylamide [PYR], motility, pigment production) are required to further differentiate the enterococcal species.

Pathogenesis and Immunity

Enterococci are commensal organisms that have a limited potential for causing disease. These bacteria do not possess a single potent toxin or hydrolytic enzyme, such as those produced by other microorganisms, and generally cannot avoid being engulfed and killed by phagocytic cells. However, a combination of virulence factors makes it possible for enterococci to cause serious disease (Table 24-3). For example, protein and carbohydrate factors regulate the colonization of the human intestine and vagina. These factors permit the organisms to bind to epithelial cells. Enterococci can also produce protein bacteriocins that inhibit competitive bacteria, and they possess multiple genes that encode resistance and regulate the survival of the organisms in the presence of empirical antibiotic therapy.

Epidemiology

As their name implies, enterococci are enteric bacteria, which are commonly recovered in feces collected from humans as well as a variety of animals. Many *E. faecalis* organisms are found in the large intestine (e.g., 10^7 organisms per gram of feces) and in the genitourinary tract. The distribution of *E. faecium* is similar to that of *E. faecalis,* but the organisms are found less frequently. The prevalence of the many other enterococcal species is unknown, although they are believed to colonize the intestines in small numbers. Enterococci are not commonly isolated from the respiratory tract or from the skin. Most human infections with enterococci originate from the patient's bowel flora, although the organisms can also be transferred from patient to patient or acquired through the consumption of contaminated food or water.

Clinical Syndrome

Despite the paucity of virulence factors, enterococci are well respected for their ability to cause life-threatening infections. Indeed, they have been one of the most feared nosocomial pathogens in the 1990s because many strains are completely resistant to all conventional antibiotics. Enterococci are the fourth leading cause of nosocomial infections, responsible for 10% of all these infections. The urinary tract and bloodstream are the most commonly involved sites. Enterococcal infections are particularly common in patients with urinary or intravascular catheters and in patients who have been hospitalized for prolonged periods and have received broad-spectrum antibiotics. Although enterococci are frequently associated with intraabdominal abscesses (because of their colonization of the intestines) and wound infections, the importance of these isolates is less clear because the infections are generally polymicrobial.

Laboratory Diagnosis

Enterococci grow readily on nonselective media such as blood agar or chocolate agar. Despite the fact that enterococci may resemble *S. pneumoniae* on Gram-stained specimens, the organisms can be readily differentiated on the basis of simple biochemical reactions (e.g., enterococci are resistant to optochin, do not dissolve when exposed to bile, and hydrolyze PYR). Phenotypic (e.g., pigment production, motility) and biochemical tests are

FIGURE 24-1 Gram-stained specimen showing *E. faecalis.*

TABLE 24-2	Catalase-Negative, Gram-Positive Cocci and Their Diseases*	
ORGANISM	**DISEASES**
Enterococcus	Urinary tract infections, bacteremia, endocarditis, wound infections
Aerococcus	Opportunistic infections (endocarditis, bacteremia), urinary tract infections
Leuconostoc	Opportunistic infections (bacteremia, dialysis infections), wound infections
Pediococcus	Opportunistic infections (bacteremia)
Alloiococcus	Chronic otitis media

*Streptococcal diseases are discussed in Chapter 23; all other catalase-negative, gram-positive cocci not listed here are rare opportunistic pathogens.

TABLE 24-1	Human Colonization and Disease Caused by Catalase-Negative, Gram-Positive Cocci	
GENUS	**HUMAN COLONIZATION**	**HUMAN DISEASE**
Streptococcus	Common	Common
Enterococcus	Common	Common
Aerococcus	Uncommon	Uncommon
Leuconostoc	Rare	Uncommon
Pediococcus	Rare	Uncommon
Alloiococcus	Rare	Rare
Gemella	Rare	Rare
Globicatella	Rare	Rare
Helcococcus	Rare	Rare
Lactococcus	Rare	Rare
Tetragenococcus	Rare	Rare
Vagococcus	Rare	Rare

TABLE 24-3	Enterococcal Virulence Factors	
VIRULENCE FACTOR	**BIOLOGICAL EFFECT**
COLONIZATION FACTORS	
Aggregation substance	Hairlike protein embedded in cytoplasmic membrane that facilitates plasmid exchange and binding to epithelial cells
Carbohydrate adhesins	Present in individual bacterium in multiple types; mediate binding to host cells
SECRETED FACTORS	
Cytolysin	Protein bacteriocin that inhibits growth of gram-positive bacteria (facilitates colonization); induces local tissue damage
Pheromone	Chemoattractant for neutrophils that may regulate inflammatory reaction
Gelatinase	Hydrolyzes gelatin, collagen, hemoglobin, and other small peptides
Antibiotic resistance	Resistant to aminoglycosides, beta-lactams, and vancomycin

necessary to differentiate among *E. faecalis, E. faecium,* and the other *Enterococcus* species, but this topic is beyond the scope of this text.

Treatment, Prevention, and Control

Antimicrobial therapy for enterococcal infections is complicated because most antibiotics are not bactericidal at clinically relevant concentrations. Therapy has traditionally consisted of the synergistic combination of an aminoglycoside and a cell wall–active antibiotic (e.g., ampicillin, vancomycin). However, resistance to aminoglycosides, ampicillin, penicillin, and vancomycin has become a major problem. Typically, more than 25% of enterococci are resistant to the aminoglycosides; more than 50% of some species (e.g., *E. faecium*) are resistant to ampicillin, and many medical centers report that more than 20% of enterococci are resistant to vancomycin. This resistance of these strains to aminoglycosides and vancomycin is particularly troublesome because it is mediated by plasmids and can be transferred to other bacteria.

It is difficult to prevent and control enterococcal infections. Infections typically develop in patients who are hospitalized for a long time and treated with broad-spectrum antibiotics for other infections. Careful restriction of antibiotic therapy and the implementation of appropriate infection-control practices (e.g., isolation of infected patients, use of gowns and gloves when in contact with patients) can reduce the risk of colonization with these bacteria.

OTHER CATALASE-NEGATIVE GRAM-POSITIVE COCCI

Other catalase-negative, gram-positive cocci or coccobacilli associated with human disease include *Aerococcus, Alloiococcus, Leuconostoc,* and *Pediococcus.* All are relatively avirulent, opportunistic pathogens that are rarely isolated in clinical specimens. *Aerococcus* ('air coccus') is typically an airborne organism that can contaminate the patient's skin or the specimen at the time it is collected or processed in the laboratory. As its name implies, *Alloiococcus otitidis* is an opportunistic organism that causes persistent middle ear infections. The epidemiology of infections caused by *Leuconostoc* and *Pediococcus* is less well understood, although they are likely part of the normal microbial flora of humans. These organisms are capable of causing opportunistic infections in patients with immunological defects and patients receiving antibiotic therapy. *Leuconostoc* and *Pediococcus* are particularly important because they are typically resistant to vancomycin, an antibiotic commonly used to treat infections with gram-positive cocci. It is difficult to identify most isolates precisely, and such identification is generally done only in reference laboratories.

CASE STUDY AND QUESTIONS

A 72-year-old man was admitted to the hospital because of a fever that had risen as high as 40° C, myalgias, and respiratory complaints. The clinical diagnosis of influenza was confirmed by the laboratory isolation of influenza virus from respiratory secretions. His hospitalization was complicated by the development of pneumonia caused by oxacillin-resistant *Staphylococcus aureus,* which was treated with a 2-week course of vancomycin. Declining pulmonary function necessitated the use of a ventilator, which led to the development of a secondary infection with *Klebsiella pneumoniae.* Ceftazidime (a cephalosporin) and gentamicin were added to the patient's treatment. After 4 weeks of hospitalization, the patient became septic. *E. faecium* resistant to vancomycin, gentamicin, and ampicillin was cultured from three blood specimens.

1. What predisposing conditions made this patient more susceptible to infection with *E. faecium*?
2. What is the most likely source of this organism?
3. What factors contribute to the virulence of enterococci?

Bibliography

Edmond MB et al: Vancomycin-resistant *Enterococcus faecium* bacteremia: risk factors for infection, *Clin Infect Dis* 20:1126-1133, 1995.

Handwerger S et al: Infection due to *Leuconostoc* species: six cases and review, *Rev Infect Dis* 12:602-610, 1990.

Jett BD et al: Virulence of enterococci, *Clin Microbiol Rev* 7:462-478, 1994.

Mandell GL et al: *Principles and practice of infectious diseases,* ed 4, New York, 1995, John Wiley & Sons.

Moellering RC: Emergence of *Enterococcus* as a significant pathogen, *Clin Infect Dis* 14:1173-1178, 1992.

Murray BE: ß-Lactamase–producing enterococci, *Antimicrob Agents Chemother* 36:2355-2359, 1992.

Patterson JE, Zervos MJ: High-level gentamicin resistance in *Enterococcus:* microbiology, genetic basis, and epidemiology, *Rev Infect Dis* 12:644-652, 1990.

Ruoff KL: The "new" catalase-negative, gram-positive cocci. *Clin Microbiol Newsletter* 16:153-159, 1994.

Shay DK et al: Epidemiology and mortality risk of vancomycin-resistant enterococcal bloodstream infections, *J Infect Dis* 172:993-1000, 1995.

25

Bacillus

The endospore-forming bacteria are classified in the family Bacillaceae. The two clinically important genera are *Bacillus* and *Clostridium* (see Chapter 37). Currently, 51 species are in the genus *Bacillus;* however, only one is a strict pathogen *(B. anthracis),* and relatively few species have been associated with human disease (Table 25-1). In addition to forming spores, all *Bacillus* species are aerobic or facultatively anaerobic, gram-positive or gram-variable bacilli (Figure 25-1), and most are motile and catalase positive. These organisms are saprophytes in nature and are found in soil worldwide. Their ability to form spores allows them to survive in soil for years without the need to replicate.

BACILLUS ANTHRACIS
Physiology and Structure

Bacillus anthracis (Greek, *anthracis,* "charcoal carbuncle") is a large (1 × 3 to 5 μm) organism arranged as single or paired bacilli in clinical specimens and as long, serpentine chains and clumps in culture. Although spores are readily observed in 2- or 3-day-old cultures, they are not seen in clinical specimens. A prominent polypeptide **capsule** (consisting of glutamic acid) is observed in clinical specimens but is not produced in vitro unless special growth conditions are used. In addition to the capsule, *B. anthracis* has a polysaccharide cell wall antigen and a toxin. **Anthrax toxin** consists of three antigenically distinct, heat-labile components: protective antigen, lethal factor, and edema factor. Although none of the components is active alone, the combination of protective antigen and either of the other two components has toxic properties.

Pathogenesis

The two major factors responsible for the virulence of *B. anthracis* are presence of the capsule and toxin production. The capsule is antiphagocytic, and antibodies directed against the capsule are not protective. Only one type of capsule has been identified, presumably because it is composed of only glutamic acid. The combination of anthrax toxin–protective antigen and the edema factor has been observed to cause edema in an-

imals in experiments, and the combination of this antigen with the lethal factor causes death. Anthrax toxin also inhibits phagocytosis and blocks leukocyte oxidative activity.

Epidemiology

Anthrax is primarily a herbivore disease; humans are infected through exposure to contaminated animals or animal products (Box 25-1). The disease is a serious problem in countries where animal vaccination is not practiced or is impractical (e.g., disease established in African wildlife). In contrast, anthrax is rarely seen in the United States; only five cases were reported between 1981 and 1996.

Human disease is acquired by one of three routes: inoculation, inhalation, or ingestion. Approximately 95% of anthrax infections result from the inoculation of *Bacillus* spores through exposed skin, either from contaminated soil or infected animal products such as hides, goat hair, or wool. Inhalation anthrax, also called **woolsorters' disease,** results from the inhalation of *B. anthracis* spores during the processing of goat hair. Ingestion anthrax is very rare in humans, but ingestion is a common route of infection in herbivores. The organism is not highly contagious, and person-to-person transmission does not occur.

Clinical Syndromes

Typically, **cutaneous anthrax** starts with the development of a painless papule at the site of inoculation that rapidly progresses to an ulcer surrounded by vesicles and then to a necrotic eschar. Systemic signs, as well as massive edema caused by the anthrax toxin, can develop. The mortality rate in patients with untreated cutaneous anthrax is 20%.

Inhalation anthrax may initially mimic a viral respiratory illness and then rapidly progress to diffuse pulmonary involvement leading to respiratory failure. The mortality rate is high even in appropriately treated patients because the disease is usually not suspected until the course is irreversible.

Gastrointestinal anthrax is a very rare human disease with varied clinical presentations. Mesenteric ade-

TABLE 25-1	*Bacillus* Species and Their Diseases
ORGANISM	**DISEASE**
B. anthracis	Anthrax (cutaneous, inhalation, gastrointestinal)
B. cereus	Gastroenteritis (emetic, diarrheal), ocular infections, catheter-related sepsis, opportunistic infections
B. circulans	Opportunistic infections
B. licheniformis	Opportunistic infections
B. subtilis	Opportunistic infections

FIGURE 25-1 *B. cereus.* Spores appear as clear areas within the individual bacilli.

BOX 25-1	**Summary of *Bacillus anthracis* Infections**

BACTERIAL FACTORS

Spores can survive in soil for years.
Virulence factors include polypeptide capsule and anthrax toxin (lethal factor, edema factor, and protective antigen).

TRANSMISSION

Inoculation (most common).
Inhalation (rare in humans, more common in herbivores).
Ingestion (rare).

WHO IS AT RISK?

People in endemic areas in contact with infected animals or contaminated soil.
People who work with animal materials (hides, fur, wool, hair) imported from endemic areas.

GEOGRAPHY/SEASON

Prevalent in impoverished areas where vaccination is not practiced.
No seasonal incidence.

MODES OF CONTROL

Penicillin is drug of choice; erythromycin or chloramphenicol is administered for patients allergic to penicillin.
Vaccination of animal herds and people in endemic areas is performed.
Disposal of animals that die of anthrax should occur.

nopathy, hemorrhage, and ascites have all been observed in affected individuals and are associated with a high mortality rate.

Laboratory Diagnosis

B. anthracis can be readily detected by the microscopic examination and culture of material from cutaneous papules or ulcers. Large gram-positive bacilli without spores are seen in the tissue. *B. anthracis* can grow on nonselective laboratory media. The colonies are non-hemolytic, rapidly growing, and adherent. The absence of hemolysis, the sticky consistency of the colonies, and the microscopic appearance of serpentine chains of bacilli ("medusa head") are characteristics of *B. anthracis* that can be used to distinguish them from other *Bacillus* species. Selected biochemical tests must be done and the organism shown to be nonmotile to identify *B. anthracis* definitively. Serological tests can also detect antibodies to the lethal and edema factors; however, antibiotic therapy frequently causes false-negative results.

Treatment, Prevention, and Control

Penicillin is the antibiotic of choice for the treatment of anthrax, although erythromycin or chloramphenicol is used for patients allergic to penicillin. The control of human disease requires the control of animal disease. This involves the vaccination of animal herds in endemic regions and the burning or burial of animals that die of anthrax. The vaccination of animals is an effective control measure. It has also been used to protect humans who live in areas where the disease is endemic and who work with animal hides, furs, bone meal, wool, and hair imported from countries with endemic anthrax. Complete eradication of anthrax is unlikely because the spores of the organism can exist for many years in soil.

BACILLUS CEREUS AND OTHER BACILLUS SPECIES

Bacillus species other than *B. anthracis* are primarily opportunistic pathogens that have relatively low capac-

TABLE 25-2 *Bacillus cereus* Food Poisoning		
	EMETIC FORM	**DIARRHEAL FORM**
Implicated	Rice	Meat, vegetables food
Incubation period	<6 hours (mean, 2 hours)	>6 hours (mean, 9 hours)
Symptoms	Vomiting, nausea, abdominal cramps	Diarrhea, nausea, abdominal cramps
Duration	8-10 hours (mean, 9 hours)	20-36 hours (mean, 24 hours)
Enterotoxin	Heat stable	Heat labile

ities for virulence. Although most of these species have been found to cause disease, *B. cereus* (Greek, *cereus*, "wax colored") is clearly the most important pathogen, with gastroenteritis, ocular infections, and intravenous catheter-related sepsis the diseases most commonly observed.

Pathogenesis

Gastroenteritis caused by *B. cereus* is mediated by one of two enterotoxins (Table 25-2). The heat-stable enterotoxin causes the **emetic form** of the disease, and the heat-labile enterotoxin causes the **diarrheal form** of the disease. The heat-labile enterotoxin is similar to the enterotoxin produced by *Escherichia coli* and *Vibrio cholera;* each stimulates the adenylate cyclase–cyclic adenosine monophosphate system in intestinal epithelial cells and can be assayed by measuring the fluid that accumulates in rabbit ileal loops inoculated with the toxin. The mechanism of action of the heat-stable enterotoxin is unknown.

The pathogenesis of *B. cereus* ocular infections is also incompletely defined. At least three toxins have been implicated: necrotic toxin (a heat-labile enterotoxin), **cereolysin** (a potent hemolysin named after the species), and **phospholipase C** (a potent lecithinase). It is likely that the rapid destruction of the eye that is characteristic of such *B. cereus* infections results from the interaction of these toxins and other unidentified factors.

Bacillus species can colonize skin transiently and be recovered as an insignificant contaminant in blood cultures. However, in the presence of an intravascular foreign body, these organisms can be responsible for causing persistent bacteremia and signs of sepsis (i.e., fever, chills, hypotension, shock).

Epidemiology

B. cereus, B. subtilis, and other *Bacillus* species are ubiquitous organisms, present in virtually all environments (Box 25-2). Isolation of bacteria from clinical specimens in the absence of characteristic disease usually represents insignificant contamination.

BOX 25-2 Summary of *Bacillus cereus* Infections

BACTERIAL FACTORS

Spores can survive in soil.
Virulence factors include enterotoxins (heat stable, heat labile), cereolysin, and phospholipase C.

TRANSMISSION

Ingestion (food poisoning).
Penetration into eye or systemic spread during bacteremia.
Infection of intravenous catheter.

WHO IS AT RISK?

People who eat contaminated foods (e.g., rice, meat, vegetables, sauces).
Patients with penetrating eye injury.
Patients with intravascular foreign bodies (e.g., catheters).

GEOGRAPHY/SEASON

Ubiquitous.
No seasonal incidence.

MODES OF CONTROL

Foods should be refrigerated after cooking.
Vancomycin, ciprofloxacin, and gentamicin are administered.

Clinical Syndromes

As mentioned previously, *B. cereus* is responsible for causing two forms of food poisoning: vomiting disease (emetic form) and diarrheal disease (diarrheal form). The emetic form results from the consumption of contaminated rice. Most bacilli are killed during the initial cooking of the rice, but the heat-resistant spores survive. If the cooked rice is not refrigerated, the spores germinate, and the bacilli can multiply rapidly. The heat-stable enterotoxin that is released is not destroyed when the rice is reheated. After ingestion of the enterotoxin and a 1- to 6-hour incubation period, a disease of short duration (less than 24 hours) develops. Symptoms consist of vomiting, nausea, and abdominal cramps. Fever and diarrhea are generally absent. *B. subtilis* can produce a similar disease.

The diarrheal form of *B. cereus* food poisoning results from the consumption of contaminated meat, vegetables, or sauces. There is a longer incubation period, during which the organism produces the heat-labile enterotoxin, and then the diarrhea, nausea, and abdominal cramps develop. This form of disease generally lasts 1 day or longer. *B. licheniformis* can also produce diarrheal disease.

B. cereus ocular infections usually occur after traumatic, penetrating injuries, but infections in intravenous drug abusers have also been documented. The organisms in patients with traumatic injuries can originate from contaminated soil on the object penetrating the eye, or the organism may be directly inoculated onto the eye surface. *Bacillus* panophthalmitis is a rapidly progressive disease that almost universally ends in the complete loss of light perception within 48 hours of the injury.

Other infections with *B. cereus*, *B. subtilis*, and other *Bacillus* species include intravenous catheter and central nervous system shunt infections and endocarditis (most commonly in drug abusers), as well as pneumonitis, bacteremia, and meningitis in severely immunosuppressed patients.

Laboratory Diagnosis

Like *B. anthracis*, other *Bacillus* species can be readily grown in the laboratory. For confirmation of the existence of food-borne disease, the implicated food (e.g., rice, meat, vegetables) should be cultured. Isolation of the organism from the patient should not be attempted because fecal colonization is common. The heat-labile enterotoxin can be detected using an animal model (e.g., rabbit ileal loop); however, the heat-stable emetic toxin can be detected only when the organism is grown on media prepared from rice (consistent with the fact that rice is the food most commonly contaminated with this organism). *Bacillus* organisms grow rapidly and are readily detected in specimens collected from infected eyes, intravenous culture sites, and other locations.

Treatment, Prevention, and Control

Because of the short and uncomplicated course of *B. cereus* gastroenteritis, symptomatic treatment is adequate. The treatment of other *Bacillus* infections is complicated by the fact that they have a rapid and progressive course and a high incidence of multidrug resistance (*B. cereus* is resistant to penicillins and cephalosporins). Vancomycin, ciprofloxacin, and gentamicin can be used. Food poisoning can be prevented by the proper refrigeration of food before serving and after cooking.

CASE STUDY AND QUESTIONS

A family of three ate dinner at a local restaurant. Two hours after eating, severe abdominal cramps, nausea, and vomiting developed in all three. They went to a local emergency room, where they were found to have normal blood pressures, no fever, and normal white blood cell counts and differential tests. They were treated symptomatically for food poisoning and sent home. Within 24 hours the symptoms subsided in all three.

1. Describe the two forms of *Bacillus* food poisoning. Which form do these patients have?
2. What is the most likely food responsible for this disease? Why was the onset of symptoms so rapid and the duration so short?
3. This organism can also cause eye infections. What risk factors are associated with these infections?
4. *B. anthracis* is responsible for three clinical forms of anthrax. Name them, the route of acquisition, and the prognosis.
5. What are two major virulence factors of *B. anthracis*?

Bibliography

Davey RT Jr, Tauber WB: Posttraumatic endophthalmitis: the emerging role of *Bacillus cereus* infection, *Rev Infect Dis* 9:110-123, 1987.

Drobniewski FA: *Bacillus cereus* and related species, *Clin Microbiol Rev* 6:324-338, 1993.

Ihde DC, Armstrong D: Clinical spectrum of infection due to *Bacillus* species, *Am J Med* 55:839-845, 1973.

Shamsuddin D et al: *Bacillus cereus* panophthalmitis: source of the organisms, *Rev Infect Dis* 4:97-103, 1982.

Terranova W, Blake PA: *Bacillus cereus* food poisoning, *N Engl J Med* 298:143-144, 1978.

Tuazon CU et al: Serious infections from *Bacillus* spp, *JAMA* 241:1137-1140, 1979.

Van Ness GB: Ecology of anthrax, *Science* 172:103-109, 1971.

Corynebacterium

Non-spore-forming, gram-positive bacilli can be subdivided into two large groups on the basis of their cell shape and the guanine plus cytosine content of their DNA. It has been proposed that the group of bacteria with an irregular shape and high guanine plus cytosine content should be placed in a new family, *Mycobacteriaceae*. Included in this family are *Corynebacterium*, *Nocardia* (see Chapter 39), *Rhodococcus* (see Chapter 39), and *Mycobacterium* (see Chapter 40).

Corynebacterium (Greek, *koryne*, "club"; *bakterion*, "small rod," referring to the fact that an individual organism is a small, club-shaped rod) is a large, heterogeneous collection of species that have a cell wall with arabinose, galactose, meso-diaminopimelic acid, and short-chain mycolic acids. Gram stains of these bacteria reveal short chains (V or Y configurations) or clumps resembling Chinese "letters" (Figure 26-1). Metachromatic granules within the cells may be seen with special stains. Corynebacteria are aerobic or facultatively anaerobic and generally grow slowly on enriched media. The organisms are nonmotile and catalase positive and ferment carbohydrates, producing lactic acid. Specific biochemical tests can identify the more than 20 species that colonize humans and can cause disease.

Corynebacteria are ubiquitous in plants and animals, and they normally colonize the skin, upper respiratory tract, gastrointestinal tract, and urogenital tract of humans. Although all species of corynebacteria can function as opportunistic pathogens, a few are commonly associated with disease (Table 26-1). The most famous of these is *C. diphtheriae*, the etiological agent of diphtheria (Greek, *diphthera*, "leathery skin," referring to the pseudomembrane that initially forms on the pharynx).

CORYNEBACTERIUM DIPHTHERIAE
Physiology and Structure

C. diphtheriae is an irregularly staining, pleomorphic bacillus (0.3 to 0.8 × 1.0 to 8.0 μm), with metachromatic granules observed in bacilli stained with methylene blue. After overnight incubation, 1- to 3-mm colonies are observed on blood agar medium. More selective, differential media can be used to recover this pathogen from specimens in which other organisms are present.

Pathogenesis and Immunity

C. diphtheriae is a classic model of bacterial virulence. The toxicity observed in diphtheria is directly attributed to an exotoxin secreted by the bacteria at the focus of infection. The organism does not need to enter the bloodstream to produce the systemic signs of disease.

The "tox" gene that codes for the exotoxin is introduced into strains of *C. diphtheriae* by a lysogenic bacteriophage (beta-phage). Two processing steps are necessary for the active gene product to be secreted: (1) proteolytic cleavage of the leader sequence from the "tox" protein during secretion from the bacterial cell and (2) cleavage of the toxin molecule into two polypeptides (A and B) that remain attached by a disulfide bond. This 58,300-Da protein is an example of the classic **A-B exotoxin**.

Three functional regions exist on the toxin molecule: a **receptor-binding region** and a **translocation region** on the B subunit and a **catalytic region** on the A toxin. The receptor for the toxin is the **heparin-binding epidermal growth factor**, which is present on the surface of many eukaryotic cells, particularly heart and nerve cells. This explains the cardiac and neurological symptoms observed in patients with severe diphtheria. After the toxin becomes attached to the host cell, it is engulfed in an endocytic vesicle. The A subunit is released into the host cell cytoplasm, an event mediated by the B subunit translocation region. The A subunit then catalyzes adenosine diphosphate–ribosylation of elongation factor 2 (EF-2), a factor required for the movement of nascent peptide chains on ribosomes. Because the turnover of EF-2 is very slow and only about one molecule per ribosome is present in a cell, it has been estimated that one exotoxin molecule can inactivate the entire EF-2 content in a cell, completely terminating host cell protein synthesis.

Epidemiology

Diphtheria is distributed worldwide in poor urban areas where there is crowding and the protective level of

FIGURE 26-1 Gram-stained specimen showing *Corynebacterium* species.

TABLE 26-1	*Corynebacterium* Species Commonly Associated with Human Disease
ORGANISM	**DISEASES**
C. diphtheriae	Diphtheria (respiratory, cutaneous)
C. jeikeium (group JK)	Septicemia, soft tissue infections, other opportunistic infections in immunocompromised patients
C. urealyticum (group D2)	Urinary tract infections, including pyelonephritis and alkaline-encrusted cystitis; opportunistic infections
C. minutissimum	Erythrasma, opportunistic infections
C. xerosis	Opportunistic infections
C. pseudodiphtheriticum	Endocarditis; opportunistic infections
C. striatum	Opportunistic infections

vaccine-induced immunity is low. *C. diphtheriae* is maintained in the population by asymptomatic carriage in the oropharynx or on the skin of immune people (after either exposure to *C. diphtheriae* or immunization). It is transmitted from person to person by respiratory droplets or skin contact (Box 26-1). Humans are the only known reservoir for this organism.

Diphtheria has become uncommon in the United States as the result of an active immunization program, as shown by the fact that more than 200,000 cases were reported in 1921 but fewer than 5 cases per year have been reported since 1980. Diphtheria is primarily a pediatric disease, but the highest incidence has shifted toward older age groups in areas where there are active immunization programs for children. Skin infection with toxigenic *C. diphtheriae* (cutaneous diphtheria) also occurs but is not a reportable disease in the United States, so the incidence is unknown.

Clinical Syndromes

The clinical presentation of diphtheria is determined by the site of infection, the immune status of the patient, and the virulence of the organism. Exposure to *C. diphtheriae* can result in asymptomatic colonization in fully immune people, mild respiratory disease in partially immune patients, or a fulminant, sometimes fatal disease in nonimmune patients.

Respiratory Diphtheria

The symptoms of diphtheria involving the respiratory tract develop after a 2- to 6-day incubation period. Organisms multiply locally on epithelial cells in the pharynx or adjacent surfaces and initially cause localized damage as the result of exotoxin activity. The onset is sudden, with malaise, sore throat, exudative pharyngitis, and a low-grade fever. The exudate evolves into a thick pseudomembrane composed of bacteria, lymphocytes, plasma cells, fibrin, and dead cells that can cover the tonsils, uvula, and palate and extend up into the nasopharynx or down into the larynx. The pseudomembrane firmly adheres to the respiratory tissue and is difficult to dislodge without making the underlying tissue bleed (unique to diphtheria). As the patient recovers after the approximately 1-week course of the disease, the membrane dislodges and is expectorated. Complications in patients with severe disease include breathing obstruction, cardiac arrhythmia, and coma. It can also cause death.

Cutaneous Diphtheria

Cutaneous diphtheria is acquired by skin contact with other infected persons. The organism colonizes the skin and gains entry into the subcutaneous tissue through breaks in the skin. A papule develops first and then evolves into a chronic nonhealing ulcer, sometimes covered with a grayish membrane. Systemic signs of disease can occur, a result of the effects of the exotoxin.

Laboratory Diagnosis

The initial treatment of a patient with diphtheria is instituted on the basis of the clinical diagnosis, not laboratory results, because definitive results are not available for at least 1 week.

Microscopy

The results from microscopic examination of clinical material are unreliable. Metachromatic granules in *C. diphtheriae* stained with methylene blue have been described, but this appearance is not specific to this or-

BACTERIAL FACTORS

Diseases include respiratory and cutaneous diphtheria.
Virulence factor is diphtheria exotoxin.

TRANSMISSION

Person to person by inhalation or skin contact.
Asymptomatic carriage maintains bacteria in population.
Humans are only known reservoir.

WHO IS AT RISK?

Unvaccinated people.
People in crowded, urban areas.
Children or adults with waning immunity.

GEOGRAPHY/SEASON

Worldwide, where vaccination programs are not maintained.
Respiratory diphtheria is rare in United States; incidence of cutaneous diphtheria is unknown but probably low.
No seasonal incidence.

MODES OF CONTROL

Diphtheria antitoxin neutralizes exotoxin.
Penicillin or erythromycin eliminates organism.
Active immunization with diphtheria toxoid should be provided during childhood (DPT vaccine); then booster shots should be given every 10 years.
Antimicrobial prophylaxis should be provided for people who have come in close contact with patients who have diphtheria.

ganism, and interpretation of the smear requires technical expertise.

Culture

Specimens for the recovery of *C. diphtheriae* should be collected from both the nasopharynx and throat and inoculated onto nonselective media, as well as media developed specifically for this organism (e.g., cysteine-tellurite agar, serum tellurite agar, Löffler's medium). *C. diphtheriae* has a characteristic gray-to-black color on tellurite agar, and the microscopic morphology is best seen on Löffler's medium. *C. diphtheriae* has been described as having three colonial morphologies on cysteine-tellurite agar: **gravis, intermedius,** and **mitis.** Gravis colonies are large, irregular, and gray; intermedius colonies are small, flat, and gray; and mitis colonies are small, round, convex, and black. Although these morphologies were initially correlated with the severity of illness, the distinctions are not now considered valid. However, they are useful for the epidemiological classification of isolates. The precise identification of *C. diphtheriae* is determined by the results from specific biochemical tests.

Toxigenicity Testing

All isolates of *C. diphtheriae* should be tested for the production of exotoxin. This can be done by an in vitro immunodiffusion assay (**Elek test**), a tissue culture neutralization assay using specific antitoxin, or an in vivo neutralization assay using guinea pigs injected subcutaneously with the patient's isolate.

Treatment, Prevention, and Control

The most important aspect of the treatment for diphtheria is the early administration of diphtheria antitoxin to specifically neutralize the exotoxin before it is bound by the host cell. Once the toxin is internalized by the cell, cell death is inevitable. Antibiotic therapy with penicillin or erythromycin is also used to eliminate *C. diphtheriae* and terminate toxin production. Bed rest, isolation to prevent secondary spread, and maintenance of an open airway in patients with respiratory diphtheria are all important.

Symptomatic diphtheria can be prevented by actively immunizing people with diphtheria toxoid during childhood and with booster doses every 10 years throughout life. The nontoxic, immunogenic toxoid is prepared by formalin treatment of the toxin. Initially, children are given monthly injections of this preparation with pertussis and tetanus antigens (**DPT vaccine**) for 3 months, after which they receive regular booster injections.

Immunity to diphtheria can be determined by measuring the neutralizing antibodies in a person (**Schick test**). This is done by injecting diphtheria toxin intradermally. No skin reaction is observed if neutralizing antibodies are present; localized edema with necrosis occurs if neutralizing antibodies are absent, indicating that the patient is susceptible to diphtheria.

People coming in close contact with patients with documented diphtheria are at risk for acquiring the disease. Nasopharyngeal cultures should be collected from all close contacts and antimicrobial prophylaxis with penicillin or erythromycin started immediately. Contacts who have not completed the series of diphtheria immunizations or who have not received a booster dose within the previous 5 years should receive a booster dose of toxoid. People exposed to cutaneous diphtheria should be managed in the same manner as those exposed to respiratory diphtheria. If the respiratory or cutaneous infection is caused by a nontoxigenic strain, then it is unnecessary to institute prophylaxis in contacts.

OTHER *CORYNEBACTERIUM* SPECIES

Other corynebacteria are part of the indigenous human flora (e.g., *C. jeikeium, C. urealyticum, C. minutissimum, C. xerosis, C. pseudodiphtheriticum, C. striatum*). With only a few exceptions, disease caused by these organisms is relatively rare.

C. jeikeium is a well-recognized opportunistic pathogen in immunocompromised patients, particularly those with hematological disorders and intravascular catheters. Carriage of this organism is uncommon in healthy people, but the skin of as many as 40% of hospitalized patients can be colonized regardless of their immunological state. Predisposing conditions for disease include prolonged hospitalization, granulocytopenia, prior or concurrent antimicrobial therapy, and chemotherapy, as well as a mucocutaneous portal of entry. This organism is very resistant to antibiotics, so antibiotic therapy during hospitalization may foster colonization of the skin. The organism can then gain access through an intravenous catheter and establish disease in the immunologically compromised patient.

C. urealyticum is uncommonly isolated from healthy people; however, this rare but important pathogen can infect the urinary tract. As the name implies, *C. urealyticum,* a strong urease producer, can produce enough urease to make the urine alkaline, which can lead to the formation of struvite calculi or stones. Other urinary tract pathogens may also produce large amounts of urease, which leads to renal stone formation. These include *Staphylococcus saprophyticus, Klebsiella pneumoniae,* and *Proteus mirabilis.* Risk factors associated with *C. urealyticum* infections include immunosuppression, underlying genitourinary disorders, an antecedent urological procedure, and prior antibiotic therapy.

C. minutissimum colonizes the skin of healthy people and has been associated with **erythrasma,** a superficial infection of the skin involving the formation of pruritic macular patches. This typically occurs in the genital area.

Numerous other *Corynebacterium* species have been associated with opportunistic infections. These bacteria are commonly present on the skin and mucosal surfaces, so their isolation in a clinical specimen may represent an important finding or may simply represent contamination of the specimen.

Treatment of *Corynebacterium* infections can be problematic. *C. jeikeium* and *C. urealyticum* are typically resistant to most antibiotics, so most patients require vancomycin. The other species tend to be more susceptible to antibiotics, but in vitro testing may be required to effect a cure.

CASE STUDY AND QUESTIONS

A 78-year-old man with a history of hypertension was admitted to the hospital because of a severe headache of 4 hours' duration. Evidence of subarachnoid hemorrhage and hydrocephalus was found, and the patient required the placement of a left subdural-to-atrial shunt. Fever developed 1 week after the operation. *C. jeikeium* was isolated from blood cultures and a subsequent culture of fluid collected from the shunt.

1. What risk factors are associated with infections with *C. jeikeium? C. urealyticum? C. diphtheriae?*
2. What antibiotic therapy could be given for infections with each of these organisms?
3. What additional therapy would be administered to a patient suspected of having a *C. diphtheriae* infection?
4. Explain the synthesis and mode of action of the diphtheria exotoxin.

Bibliography

Coyle MB, Lipsky BA: Coryneform bacteria in infectious diseases: clinical and laboratory aspects, *Clin Microbiol Rev* 3:227-246, 1990.

George MJ: Clinical significance and characterization of *Corynebacterium* species, *Clin Microbiol Newsletter* 17:177-180, 1995.

Lipsky BA et al: Infections caused by nondiphtheria corynebacteria, *Rev Infect Dis* 4:1220-1235, 1982.

Pascual C et al: Phylogenetic analysis of the genus *Corynebacterium* based on 16S rRNA gene sequences, *Intl J Syst Bacteriol* 45:724-728, 1995.

Salyers AA, Whitt DD: *Bacterial pathogenesis: a molecular approach,* Washington, DC, 1994, ASM.

Soriano F et al: Urinary tract infection caused by *Corynebacterium* group D2: report of 82 cases and review, *Rev Infect Dis* 12:1019-1034, 1990.

CHAPTER 27

Listeria, Erysipelothrix, and Other Gram-Positive Bacilli

A variety of aerobic, gram-positive bacilli that morphologically resemble *Corynebacterium* organisms colonize humans. Whereas most of these genera are clinically insignificant, some are associated with disease. The following four are discussed in this chapter: *Listeria*, *Erysipelothrix*, *Arcanobacterium*, and *Gardnerella*. The isolation of *Listeria* and *Erysipelothrix* organisms in clinical specimens is always an important finding. *Arcanobacterium* colonizes the oropharynx and skin of people but is almost always associated with disease. *Gardnerella*, which is commonly isolated in genital specimens, plays a poorly defined role in the pathogenesis of bacterial vaginosis (vaginitis).

LISTERIA

The genus *Listeria* consists of six species, with *L. monocytogenes* responsible for causing human disease. *L. monocytogenes* is a gram-positive, non-spore-forming, facultatively anaerobic bacillus capable of causing meningitis and bacteremia. These small coccobacilli (0.4 × 0.5 to 2 μm) can microscopically resemble corynebacteria or gram-positive diplococci (e.g., *Streptococcus pneumoniae*, *Enterococcus*) (Figure 27-1). The organisms are motile at room temperature, exhibiting a characteristic tumbling motion, but not at 37° C. This differential characteristic is useful for their preliminary identification. Although *Listeria* organisms are widely distributed in nature, human disease is uncommon and restricted to several well-defined populations: neonates and the elderly, pregnant women, and immunocompromised patients, particularly those with defective cell-mediated immunity.

Pathogenesis and Immunity

L. monocytogenes is a facultative intracellular pathogen that can grow in macrophages, epithelial cells, and cultured fibroblasts. All virulent strains produce a hemolysin, **listeriolysin O**, that is genetically related to streptolysin O and pneumolysin. This hemolysin is required for the bacterium to be released after phagocytosis and intracellular growth (Figure 27-2). No other virulence factors have been identified. As a result, the intracellular survival and spread of the bacilli are critically important.

Phagocytosis of the bacteria by activated macrophages leads to bacterial death, most likely because the oxidative metabolites of the macrophages inactivate the oxygen-labile hemolysin. In the absence of effective cellular immunity, *Listeria* can produce overwhelming infections.

Epidemiology

L. monocytogenes is isolated from soil, water, vegetation, and a variety of mammals, birds, fish, insects, and other animals (Box 27-1). Asymptomatic carriage, as well as disease, is well documented in humans and other mammals. Although the incidence of human carriage is unknown, fecal carriage is estimated to occur in 1% to 5% of healthy people. Recent studies have shown that there are 12.7 cases of invasive human disease per 100,000 live births and 7.4 cases per million population. However, the incidence of disease in patients with acquired immunodeficiency syndrome (AIDS) is more than 100-fold greater. Meningitis in renal transplant patients and in adults with cancer is frequently caused by *Listeria*, and it is the fourth most common cause of community-acquired bacterial meningitis.

Human listeriosis is a sporadic disease seen throughout the year, but the incidence peaks in the warmer months. Focal epidemics have been associated with the consumption of contaminated milk, soft cheese, undercooked meat (e.g., turkey franks, cold cuts), unwashed raw vegetables, and cabbage. Recent studies show that most cases of sporadic listeriosis are also foodborne. In fact, the mortality rate of symptomatic *Listeria* infections (20% to 30%) is higher than that of almost all other foodborne diseases. *Listeria* organisms can grow in a wide pH range as well as in cold temperatures—an attribute that has been exploited for the selective isolation of this organism (**"cold enrichment"**). Thus the refrigeration of contaminated food products permits the slow multiplication of the organisms to an infectious dose.

Clinical Disease
Neonatal Disease

Two forms of neonatal disease have been described: **early onset disease,** acquired transplacentally in utero, and **late-onset disease,** acquired at or soon after birth.

FIGURE 27-1 Gram-stain preparation showing *Listeria monocytogenes*.

Early onset disease, also called **granulomatosis infantiseptica,** is a devastating disease associated with a high mortality rate unless it is promptly treated. The disease is characterized by the formation of disseminated abscesses and granulomas in multiple organs. Late-onset disease occurs 2 to 3 weeks after birth in the form of meningitis or meningoencephalitis with septicemia. The clinical signs and symptoms are not unique; thus other causes of neonatal central nervous system disease, such as group B streptococcal disease, must be excluded.

Disease in Healthy Adults

Most infections in healthy adults are asymptomatic or occur in the form of a mild influenza-like illness. Gastrointestinal symptoms develop in some patients. In contrast, illness in patients with compromised immune sys-

FIGURE 27-2 *Listeria* is an intracellular pathogen. After binding to specific receptors on the surface of epithelial cells or macrophages and inducing phagocytosis, the bacillus moves into the cell in an endosome. Before this vesicle fuses with lysosomes and the bacterium is killed by the lysosomal enzymes, the endosome membrane is dissolved by listeriolysin O. A halo of actin filaments then surrounds the organism that after bacterial replication, is oriented into a tail and pushes the bacteria to the macrophage surface. A pseudopod extension then forms and facilitates transfer into another cell. *Listeria* produces two other hemolysins (phospholipase C enzymes) that lyse host cell membranes and can facilitate cell-to-cell spread. This process protects *Listeria* from exposure to antibodies and other extracellular bactericidal factors. (Redrawn from Tilney LG, Portnoy DA: *J Cell Biol* 109:1597-1608, 1989.)

BOX 27-1 **Summary of *Listeria* Infections**

BACTERIAL FACTORS

Organism can grow in macrophages and epithelial cells.
Organism can replicate at 4° to 8° C (in refrigerated foods).
Asymptomatic carriage occurs in healthy people.
Virulent strains produce hemolysins (listeriolysin O, phospholipase C).

TRANSMISSION

Ingestion of contaminated food.
Transplacental spread from bacteremic mother to fetus.

WHO IS AT RISK?

Neonates.
Elderly.
Pregnant women.
Patients with defective cell-mediated immunity.

GEOGRAPHY/SEASON

Worldwide.
Sporadic cases; incidence peaks in warmer months.
Epidemics have occurred.

MODES OF CONTROL

Penicillin or ampicillin, alone or in combination with gentamicin, is given.
People at high risk should avoid eating raw or partially cooked foods of animal origin, soft cheese, and unwashed raw vegetables.

tems (e.g., the aged; pregnant women; patients with AIDS, diabetes, and cancer) is more severe.

Meningitis in Adults

Meningitis is the most common form of *Listeria* infection in adults. Although the clinical signs and symptoms of meningitis caused by this organism are not specific, *Listeria* should always be suspected in organ transplant patients, patients with cancer, or pregnant women in whom meningitis develops.

Primary Bacteremia

Bacteremic patients may have an unremarkable history of chills and fever (commonly observed in pregnant women) or a more acute presentation with high-grade fever and hypotension. Only severely immunocompromised patients and the infants of septic pregnant women appear to be at risk of death.

Laboratory Diagnosis

Microscopy

Gram-stained preparations of cerebrospinal fluid typically show no *Listeria* organisms because such organisms are generally present in concentrations 100 to 1000 times less than those observed with other bacteria that cause meningitis. Intracellular and extracellular gram-positive coccobacilli are seen in a preparation that stains positively for the organism. Care must be taken in interpreting the Gram-stained preparation, however, because the organism can resemble *Corynebacterium, S. pneumoniae, Enterococcus,* or if the preparation is overdecolorized, *Haemophilus.*

Culture

Listeria organisms grow on most conventional laboratory media, with small, round colonies observed on agar media after incubation for 1 to 2 days. It may be necessary to use selective media and cold enrichment to detect *Listeria* in specimens contaminated with rapidly growing bacteria. Beta-hemolysis on sheep blood agar media can serve to distinguish *Listeria* from morphologically similar bacteria; however, the hemolysis is generally weak and may not be observed initially. The characteristic motility of the organisms in a liquid medium or semisolid agar is also helpful for the preliminary identification of *Listeria.* All gram-positive bacilli isolated from blood and cerebrospinal fluid should be identified to distinguish between *Corynebacterium* (presumably contaminants) and *Listeria.*

Identification

Selected biochemical and serological tests are used to definitively identify the pathogen. A total of 13 serotypes have been described, with 1/2a, 1/2b, and 4b responsible for most infections in neonates and adults. Serotyping is generally not useful in epidemiological investigations because relatively few serotypes are isolated from humans with disease. The molecular characterization of isolates is required in this instance.

Treatment, Prevention, and Control

Penicillin or ampicillin, either alone or with gentamicin, is the treatment of choice for infections with *L. monocytogenes.* Erythromycin can be used in patients allergic to penicillin, but resistance to trimethoprim and the tetracyclines has been observed. Because *Listeria* organisms are ubiquitous and most infections are sporadic, prevention and control are difficult. However, high-risk people (e.g., pregnant women, immunocompromised people, the elderly) should avoid eating raw or partially cooked foods of animal origin, soft cheeses, and unwashed raw vegetables. A vaccine is not available, and prophylactic antibiotic therapy for high-risk patients has not been evaluated.

ERYSIPELOTHRIX
Physiology and Structure

E. rhusiopathiae (Greek, "hair of erysipelas"; "of red disease"), the sole member of the genus, is a gram-positive, non-spore-forming, facultatively anaerobic bacillus that is distributed worldwide in wild and domestic animals. The bacilli are slender (0.2 to 0.4 × 0.8 to 2.5 μm) and sometimes pleomorphic, with a tendency to form filaments as long as 60 μm ("hairlike"). They may decolorize readily and appear gram negative. The organisms are microaerophilic, preferring a reduced oxygen atmosphere and supplemented carbon dioxide. Small, grayish, alpha-hemolytic colonies are observed after 2 to 3 days of incubation. Animal disease—particularly in swine—is widely recognized, but human disease is uncommon.

Pathogenesis

Little is known about specific virulence factors in *Erysipelothrix* organisms. Disease in swine has been associated with hyaluronidase and neuraminidase production. However, because this organism is an uncommon human pathogen, similar studies in humans have not been performed.

Epidemiology

Erysipelothrix is a ubiquitous organism that is distributed worldwide in many wild and domestic animals, including mammals, birds, and fish (Box 27-2). **Erysipeloid** is an occupational disease in humans: Butchers, meat processors, farmers, poultry workers, fish handlers, and veterinarians are at greatest risk. People working with swine and fish are especially at risk. Cutaneous infections typically develop after the organism is inoculated subcutaneously through an abrasion or puncture wound during the handling of contaminated animal products or soil. The incidence of human disease is unknown because it is not a reportable disease.

Clinical Syndromes

Three forms of human infection with *E. rhusiopathiae* have been described: a localized skin infection (**erysipeloid**), a generalized cutaneous form, and a septicemic form. Erysipeloid is an inflammatory skin lesion that develops at the site of trauma after a 1- to 4-day incubation period. The lesion, most commonly present on the fingers or hands, is violaceous and has a raised edge. It slowly spreads peripherally as the discoloration in the central area fades. The painful lesion is pruritic, and the patient experiences a burning or throbbing sensation. Suppuration is uncommon, which distinguishes erysipeloid from streptococcal erysipelas. The resolution can be spontaneous but can be hastened with appropriate antibiotic therapy.

The diffuse cutaneous infection is rare. It is often associated with systemic manifestations, but blood cultures are negative for the organism.

The septicemic form of *Erysipelothrix* infections is also uncommon, but when present, it is frequently associated with endocarditis. *Erysipelothrix* endocarditis may have an acute onset but is usually subacute. Involvement of previously undamaged heart valves (particularly the aortic valve) is common.

Laboratory Diagnosis

The bacilli are located only in the deep tissue of the lesion. Thus full-thickness biopsy specimens or deep aspirates must be collected from the margin of the lesion.

Microscopic studies and the culture of specimens collected from the surface invariably demonstrate the absence of organisms. *E. rhusiopathiae* is not fastidious and grows on most conventional laboratory media. The absence of motility and catalase production distinguishes this organism from *Listeria* species. Biochemical testing definitively identifies the organism.

Treatment, Prevention, and Control

Erysipelothrix is susceptible to penicillin, which is the antibiotic of choice. Cephalosporins, erythromycin, and clindamycin are also active in vitro, but the organism is resistant to the sulfonamides, aminoglycosides, and vancomycin. Infections in people at an increased occupational risk are prevented by use of gloves and other appropriate coverings on exposed skin. Vaccination is used to control disease in swine.

ARCANOBACTERIUM

Arcanobacterium haemolyticus (Latin, "secretive hemolytic bacterium") is a small, pleomorphic, gram-positive bacillus that was formerly classified in the genus *Corynebacterium*. Arcanobacteria colonize humans and are responsible for pharyngitis with or without a scarlet fever–like rash, as well as cutaneous infections. The erythematous, maculopapular rash is seen in more than half of patients. The incidence of pharyngitis caused by *A. haemolyticus* is unknown but is estimated to be between 5% and 13% of the incidence of the pharyngitis caused by *S. pyogenes*. *Arcanobacterius* infections occur in older patients, but the pharyngitis caused by this organism and *S. pyogenes* cannot be distinguished clinically. This does not pose a therapeutic problem, however, because *Arcanobacterium* organisms are susceptible to penicillin, erythromycin, clindamycin, and tetracycline.

The pathogenesis of these infections is not completely understood. Arcanobacteria produce at least two toxins, phospholipase D and hemolysin, and the enzyme neuraminidase. The phospholipase D is similar to that found in *C. pseudotuberculosis*, although it is antigenically distinct.

It is difficult to detect the organism in culture (as implied by the name). *A. haemolyticus* grows slowly and is only weakly hemolytic on sheep blood agar. Growth and hemolysis are better on agar medium supplemented with human or rabbit blood, but these media are rarely used in clinical laboratories. It is necessary to perform definitive biochemical tests to distinguish this organism from *Streptococcus* and *Corynebacterium* organisms.

GARDNERELLA

G. vaginalis (named after H.L. Gardner) morphologically resembles a gram-negative bacillus but has the cell wall structure of a gram-positive organism. *G. vaginalis* is pleomorphic (averaging 0.5 × 1.5 μm) and nonmotile and does not form spores or possess a capsule. The organism is facultatively anaerobic and grows slowly, requiring a carbon dioxide–enriched atmosphere.

G. vaginalis is part of the normal vaginal flora in almost 70% of healthy women. The number of *Gardnerella* and various obligate anaerobes (primarily *Bacteroides* species, *Mobiluncus* species, and *Peptostreptococcus* species) significantly increases in women with bacterial vaginosis (nonspecific vaginitis). However, the pathogenic role of *G. vaginalis* in this disease is incompletely defined. Most investigators now believe that the presence of *Gardnerella* organisms is a useful marker for bacterial vaginosis but that the organism is not responsible for the disease. Metronidazole, which is active against both *Gardnerella* and the anaerobes, is used to treat this infection.

The simple isolation of *Gardnerella* from vaginal secretions has little diagnostic significance because the organism is frequently recovered in healthy women. The diagnostic test for bacterial vaginosis is microscopic examination of vaginal secretions. The clinical diagnosis is supported by the finding of **"clue cells,"** which are epithelial cells covered with gram-positive or gram-variable bacilli (resembling *G. vaginalis*) and small, curved, gram-negative bacilli (resembling *Mobiluncus*). The presumptive identification of *Gardnerella* is based on the findings yielded by the Gram-stained preparation, the colonial morphologies, and a negative catalase reaction.

CASE STUDY AND QUESTIONS

A 35-year-old man was hospitalized because of headache, fever, and confusion. He received a kidney transplant 7 months before, after which he was maintained on immunosuppressive drugs to prevent organ rejection. Physical examination of the patient revealed a temperature of 39° C and obtundation. Analysis of cerebrospinal fluid disclosed a white blood cell count of 36 cells/mm³ (96% polymorphonuclear leukocytes), a glucose concentration of 40 mg/dl, and a protein concentration of 172 mg/dl. A Gram-stained preparation of cerebrospinal fluid was negative for organisms, but cultures of blood and cerebrospinal fluid revealed gram-positive coccobacilli.

1. What is the most likely cause of this patient's meningitis? What is the significance of his immunosuppression?
2. What are potential sources of this organism? What other people would be at increased risk for infection?
3. List the most important gram-positive bacilli discussed in this chapter and the diseases that they cause.
4. What is the epidemiology of infections caused by *E. rhusiopathiae* and *A. haemolyticum?*

Bibliography

Catlin BW: *Gardnerella vaginalis:* characteristics, clinical considerations, and controversies, *Clin Microbiol Rev* 5:213-237, 1992.

Gorby GL, Peacock JE Jr: *Erysipelothrix rhusiopathiae* endocarditis: microbiologic, epidemiologic, and clinical features of an occupational disease, *Rev Infect Dis* 10:317-325, 1988.

Jones EM, MacGowan AP: Antimicrobial chemotherapy of human infection due to *Listeria monocytogenes, Eur J Clin Microbiol Infect Dis* 14:165-175, 1995.

Jurado RL et al: Increased risk of meningitis and bacteremia due to *Listeria monocytogenes* in patients with human immunodeficiency virus infection, *Clin Infect Dis* 17:224-227, 1993.

Pinner RW et al: Role of foods in sporadic listeriosis. II. Microbiologic and epidemiologic investigation, *JAMA* 267:2046-2050, 1992.

Reboli AC, Farrar WE: The genus *Erysipelothrix.* In Ballows A et al, editors: *The prokaryotes,* New York, 1992, Springer-Verlag.

Salyers AA, Whitt DD: *Listeria monocytogenes.* In Salyers AA, Whitt DD, editors: *Bacterial pathogenesis: a molecular approach,* Washington, DC, 1994, ASM.

Schuchat A et al: Role of foods in sporadic listeriosis. I. Case-control study of dietary risk factors, *JAMA* 267:2041-2045, 1992.

Tilney LG, Portnoy DA: Actin filaments and the growth, movement, and spread of the intracellular bacterial parasite, *Listeria monocytogenes, J Cell Biol* 109:1597-1608, 1989.

CHAPTER 28

Neisseria

The genus *Neisseria* (named after A.L.S. Neisser, who originally described the organism responsible for gonorrhea) consists of 10 species. Two species, *N. gonorrhoeae* and *N. meningitidis*, are strictly human pathogens, and the remaining species are commonly present on mucosal surfaces of the oropharynx and nasopharynx and occasionally colonize the anogenital mucosal membranes. Members of the genus are aerobic, gram-negative cocci typically arranged in pairs (diplococci) with adjacent sides flattened together (resembling coffee beans) (Figure 28-1). The bacteria are not motile and do not form endospores. Pathogenic strains are usually encapsulated. All species are oxidase positive, and most produce catalase—properties that combined with the Gram-stain morphology, allow for a rapid, presumptive identification of a clinical isolate. Carbohydrates are used oxidatively (not fermentatively). Although diseases caused by *N. gonorrhoeae* and *N. meningitidis* are well known, the other *Neisseria* species have limited virulence and generally produce disease only in compromised patients (Table 28-1).

NEISSERIA GONORRHOEAE

Infection with *N. gonorrhoeae* has been recognized for centuries. Despite effective antibiotic therapy, it is still one of the most common sexually transmitted diseases in the United States.

Physiology and Structure

N. gonorrhoeae is a fastidious organism; it requires complex media to grow and is adversely affected by drying and fatty acids. Although this makes recovery of the organism from clinical specimens difficult, it is nevertheless easy for the organism to be transmitted from person to person. The structure of *N. gonorrhoeae* is well known; however, the names of the cell wall components and different colony types have recently been changed, which can cause confusion. The cell wall is typically gram-negative, with the thin peptidoglycan layer sandwiched between the inner cytoplasmic membrane and the outer membrane. The outer surface is covered with a loosely associated **capsule.**

The surface of the bacteria can be covered with pili, which are composed of **pilin proteins.** Expression of the pili is controlled by the *pil* gene complex, with phase shifts observed between the presence and the absence of pili (phase variation). Pilin proteins have a conserved region at the amino terminal end and highly variable regions at the exposed carboxy terminus. The lack of immunity to reinfection with *N. gonorrhoeae* partially results from the antigenic variation among the pilin proteins, as well as the phase variation in pilin expression, and this complicates attempts to develop effective vaccines.

Three other prominent families of proteins are present in the outer membrane. The **Por proteins** (formerly protein I) are porin proteins that form pores or channels in the outer membrane. An antigenic variation in these proteins is exploited for the serotype classification of *N. gonorrhoeae*. **Opa proteins** (opacity proteins; formerly protein II) are a family of membrane proteins that mediate binding to epithelial cells. Multiple alleles of these proteins can be expressed by an individual isolate. The third group of proteins in the outer membrane are the **Rmp proteins** (reduction-modifiable proteins; formerly protein III), which are closely associated with the Por proteins.

Iron is essential for the growth and metabolism of gonococci. Three proteins mediate the acquisition of iron. Two of them, **Tbp1** and **Tbp2**, form a receptor for binding transferrin; the third, **Lbp**, is a lactoferrin-binding protein. The mechanism by which these receptor proteins remove iron from transferrin and lactoferrin is unknown.

The last major antigen in the cell wall is lipooligosaccharide (**LOS**). This is composed of lipid A and a core oligosaccharide similar to gram-negative lipopolysaccharide (LPS). However, LOS does not have the antigenically diverse, strain-specific O polysaccharide antigens found in LPS.

Other proteins associated with the gonococci are a **protease** and **beta-lactamase.** The protease is capable of cleaving IgA, and the beta-lactamase hydrolytically destroys penicillin.

Pathogenesis and Immunity

Gonococci attach to mucosal cells, penetrate into the cells and multiply, and then pass through the cells into the subepithelial space, where infection is established. The presence of pili is important for the initial attachment (Table 28-2): Nonpiliated cells are avirulent. After the initial attachment, Opa protein directs first a tighter association with the host cell surface and then the migration of bacteria into the epithelial cell. Researchers believe that the Por protein protects the phagocytosed bacteria from intracellular killing by inhibiting phagolysosome fusion. The gonococcal LOS stimulates the inflammatory response and release of TNF–alpha, which causes most of the symptoms associated with gonococcal disease. IgG$_3$ is the predominant IgG antibody formed in response to gonococcal infection. Although the antibody response to Por is minimal, serum antibodies to pilin, Opa protein, and LOS are readily detected. Antibodies to LOS can activate complement, releasing C5a, which has a chemotactic effect on neutrophils. However, IgG and secretory IgA1 antibodies directed against Rmp protein can block this bactericidal antibody response. People with inherited complement deficiencies are at considerably greater risk for systemic disease.

Epidemiology

Gonorrhea occurs only in humans; it has no other known reservoir (Box 28-1). Although the incidence of disease has decreased since 1975 (Figure 28-2), more than 400,000 cases are reported annually in the United States. Even this large number is an underestimation of the true incidence of disease because the diagnosis and reporting of gonococcal infections are incomplete. The peak incidence of the disease is in adolescents, with one third of all infections occurring in this age group.

N. *gonorrhoeae* is transmitted primarily by sexual contact. Women have a 50% risk of acquiring the infection as the result of a single exposure to an infected man, whereas men have a risk of approximately 20% as the result of a single exposure to an infected woman. The risk

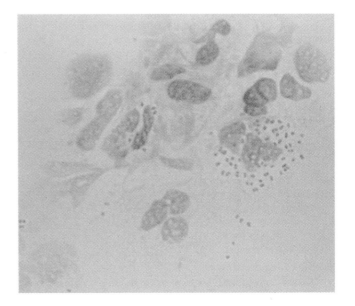

FIGURE 28-1 *N. gonorrhoeae* in urethral exudate. Note the spatial arrangement of the pairs of cocci with sides pressed together. This is characteristic of this genus.

TABLE 28-1	*Neisseria* **Species and Their Diseases**
ORGANISM	**DISEASE**
N. gonorrhoeae	Urethritis, cervicitis, salpingitis, pelvic inflammatory disease, proctitis, bacteremia, arthritis, conjunctivitis, pharyngitis
N. meningitidis	Meningitis, meningoencephalitis, bacteremia, pneumonia, arthritis, urethritis
Other *Neisseria* species	Opportunistic infections

TABLE 28-2	**Virulence Factors in *N. gonorrhoeae***
VIRULENCE FACTOR	**BIOLOGICAL EFFECT**
Capsule	Antiphagocytic
Pilin	Protein that mediates initial attachment to human cells, including epithelium of vagina, fallopian tube, and buccal cavity
Por (protein I)	Porin protein—promotes intracellular survival by preventing phagolysosome fusion in neutrophils
Opa (protein II)	Opacity protein—mediates firm attachment to epithelial cells and invasion into cells
Rmp (protein III)	Reduction-modifiable protein—protects other surface antigens (Por protein, LOS) from bactericidal antibodies
Tbp1, Tbp2	Two transferrin-binding proteins—mediate acquisition of iron for bacterial metabolism
Lbp	Lactoferrin-binding protein—mediates acquisition of iron for bacterial metabolism
LOS	Lipooligosaccharide—has endotoxin activity
IgA$_1$ protease	Destroys IgA$_1$ (role in virulence is unknown)
Beta-lactamase	Hydrolyzes beta-lactam ring in penicillin

BOX 28-1	*Summary of N. gonorrhoeae Infections*

BACTERIAL FACTORS

Diseases—see Table 28-1.
Virulence factors—see Table 28-2.

TRANSMISSION

Primarily by sexual contact.
Asymptomatic carriage major reservoir.

WHO IS AT RISK?

Humans are only natural hosts.
Patients with multiple sexual encounters.
Patients with late complement deficiencies.

GEOGRAPHY/SEASON

Worldwide distribution.
Disease corresponds to sexual activity.

MODES OF CONTROL

Ceftriaxone, cefixime, or ciprofloxacin can be administered in uncomplicated cases; penicillin should be avoided because resistance is common.
Doxycycline or azithromycin should be added for infections complicated by *Chlamydia*.
For neonates, prophylaxis with 1% silver nitrate; ophthalmia neonatorum is treated with ceftriaxone.
Prevention includes patient education, use of condoms or spermicides with nonoxynol 9 (only partially effective), and aggressive follow-up of sexual partners of infected patients.
Effective vaccines are not available.

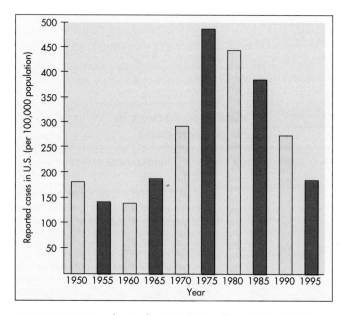

FIGURE 28-2 Gonorrhea in the United States from 1950 to 1995. (Data from *MMWR* Annual Summary, 1995.)

of infection increases as the person has more sexual encounters with infected partners.

The major reservoir for gonococci is the asymptomatically infected person. Determining a true incidence of asymptomatic infection is difficult. Although disease is more commonly diagnosed in men than in women, asymptomatic carriage is more common in women than in men. As many as half of all infected women have mild or asymptomatic infections, whereas most men are initially symptomatic. The symptoms generally clear within a few weeks in people with untreated disease, and asymptomatic carriage may then become established. The site of infection also determines whether carriage occurs, with rectal and pharyngeal infections more commonly asymptomatic than genital infections.

Clinical Syndromes

Genital infection in men is primarily restricted to the urethra. A purulent urethral discharge and dysuria develop after a 2- to 5-day incubation period. Approximately 95% of all infected men have acute symptoms. Although complications are rare, epididymitis, prostatitis, and periurethral abscesses can occur.

The primary site of infection in women is the cervix because the bacteria infect the endocervical columnar epithelial cells. The organism cannot infect the squamous epithelial cells that line the vagina of postpubescent women. Symptomatic patients commonly experience vaginal discharge, dysuria, and abdominal pain. Ascending genital infection, including salpingitis, tuboovarian abscesses, and pelvic inflammatory disease are observed in 10% to 20% of women. Disseminated infections with septicemia and infection of skin and joints occur in 1% to 3% of infected women and in a much lower percentage of infected men. The increased proportion of disseminated infections in women is caused by the numerous untreated asymptomatic infections in this population. The clinical manifestations of disseminated disease include fever; migratory arthralgias; suppurative arthritis in the wrists, knees, and ankles; and a pustular rash on an erythematous base over the extremities but not on the head and trunk. *N. gonorrhoeae* is a leading cause of purulent arthritis in adults.

Other diseases associated with *N. gonorrhoeae* include perihepatitis (**Fitz-Hugh–Curtis syndrome**); purulent conjunctivitis, particularly in newborns infected during vaginal delivery (**ophthalmia neonatorum**); anorectal gonorrhea in homosexual men; and pharyngitis.

Laboratory Diagnosis

Microscopy

Gram stain is very sensitive (greater than 90%) and specific (98%) in detecting gonococcal infection in men with purulent urethritis (Figure 28-1). However, its sensitivity in detecting infection in asymptomatic men is 60% or less. The test is also relatively insensitive in detecting gonococcal cervicitis in both symptomatic and asymptomatic women, although a positive result is considered reliable when an experienced microscopist sees gram-negative diplococci within polymorphonuclear leukocytes. Thus Gram stain can be reliably used to diagnose infections in men with purulent urethritis, but all negative results in women and asymptomatic men must be confirmed by culture. Gram stain is also useful for the early diagnosis of purulent arthritis but is insensitive for the detection of *N. gonorrhoeae* in patients with skin lesions, anorectal infections, or pharyngitis. Commensal *Neisseria* organisms in the oropharynx and morphologically similar bacteria in the gastrointestinal tract compromise the specificity of the stain for these specimens.

Culture

N. gonorrhoeae can be readily isolated from genital specimens if care is taken in collecting and processing the specimens (Figure 28-3). Because other commensal organisms normally colonize mucosal surfaces, all genital, rectal, and pharyngeal specimens must be inoculated onto both selective media (e.g., modified Thayer-Martin medium) and nonselective media (e.g., chocolate blood agar). Selective media suppress the growth of contaminating organisms. However, a nonselective medium should also be used because some gonococcal strains are inhibited by the vancomycin present in most selective media. The organisms are also inhibited by the fatty acids and trace metals present in the peptone hydrolysates and agar in other common laboratory media (e.g., blood agar, nutrient agar). The gonococci die rapidly if specimens are allowed to dry. Therefore drying, as well as cold temperatures, should be avoided by inoculating the specimen directly onto prewarmed media at the time of collection.

The endocervix must be properly exposed to ensure that an adequate specimen is collected. Although the endocervix is the most common site of infection in women, the rectal specimen may be the only one positive for gonococci in women who have asymptomatic infections, as well as in homosexual and bisexual men. Blood cultures are generally positive for gonococci only during the first week of the infection in patients with disseminated disease. In addition, special handling of blood specimens is required to ensure the adequate recovery of gonococci because supplements present in the blood culture media can be toxic to *Neisseria* organisms. Cultures of specimens from infected joints are positive for the organism if they are collected at the time the arthritis develops, but skin cultures are generally unrewarding.

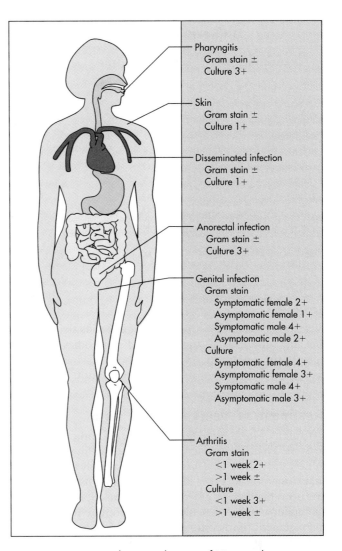

FIGURE 28-3 Laboratory detection of *N. gonorrhoeae*.

Identification

N. gonorrhoeae is preliminarily identified on the basis of the isolation of oxidase-positive, gram-negative diplococci that grow on chocolate blood agar or on media that are selective for pathogenic *Neisseria* species. Definitive identification is guided by the detection of acid produced from glucose but not from other sugars (Table 28-3).

Genetic Probes

Commercial probes specific for the nucleic acids of *N. gonorrhoeae* have been developed for the direct detection of bacteria in clinical specimens. Tests using these probes are sensitive, specific, and rapid (results are available in 2 to 4 hours). Combination assays for both *N. gonorrhoeae* and *Chlamydia* organisms are also available. In many laboratories, culture for these two pathogens has been replaced with probe assays. The primary problem with this approach is that antibiotic resistance cannot be monitored.

TABLE 28-3	Differential Characteristics of Commonly Isolated *Neisseria* Species					
CHARACTERISTIC	**N. GONORRHOEAE**	**N. MENINGITIDIS**	**N. LACTAMICA**	**N. SICCA**	**N. MUCOSA**	**N. FLAVESCENS**
Growth on:						
MTM, ML (35° C)	+	+	+	0	0	0
CHOC, BA (22° C)	0	0	V	+	+	+
Nutrient agar (35° C)	0	V	+	+	+	+
Acid from:						
Glucose	+	+	+	+	+	0
Maltose	0	+	+	+	+	0
Lactose	0	0	+	0	0	0
Sucrose	0	0	0	+	+	0
Fructose	0	0	0	+	+	0
Nitrate reduction	0	0	0	0	+	0

MTM, Modified Thayer-Martin agar; *ML,* Martin-Lewis agar; *CHOC,* chocolate agar; *BA,* blood agar; *V,* variable growth.

Serology

Researchers have developed serological tests that can detect the gonococcal antigens and antibodies directed against the organism. However, these tests are neither sensitive nor specific, and their use cannot be recommended.

Treatment, Prevention, and Control

Penicillin is no longer the antibiotic of choice for three reasons. First, the concentration of penicillin required to inhibit growth of *N. gonorrhoeae* has steadily increased so that doses considerably higher than those used originally are now needed to effect clinical cure. Specifically, the therapeutic dose of penicillin G recommended for the management of uncomplicated gonorrhea has risen from 200,000 units prescribed in 1945, to 4.8 million units required currently. Second, penicillin resistance mediated by enzymatic hydrolysis of the beta-lactam ring was initially reported from Southeast Asia and now is seen worldwide. The first case of beta-lactamase–producing *N. gonorrhoeae* observed in the United States was reported in 1976. During the next 4 years, relatively few new cases were detected, and most were related to imported cases. However, since 1980, the number of resistant strains has risen rapidly, and the increase is not attributable to foreign travel. This increase should continue because the resistance gene is encoded on a transmissible plasmid. Finally, strains of penicillin-resistant *N. gonorrhoeae* that do not produce beta-lactamase have also been isolated. This chromosomally mediated resistance is not limited only to penicillin but extends to tetracyclines, erythromycin, and aminoglycosides and results from changes on the cell surface that keep the antibiotic from penetrating into the gonococcal cell. Because the incidence of penicillin resistance is now high (>10% of all strains), the Centers for Disease Control and Prevention now recommends that ceftriaxone, cefixime, or a fluoroquinolone be used as the initial therapy for cases of uncomplicated gonorrhea and that these agents be given in combination with doxycy-

cline or azithromycin in the management of dual infections with *Chlamydia.*

Immunity to infections with *N. gonorrhoeae* is poorly understood. Antibodies can be detected to pili antigens, as well as to the Por proteins and LOS. However, multiple infections are common in sexually promiscuous people. This lack of protective immunity is explained in part by the antigenic diversity of gonococcal strains. The variable region at the carboxy terminus of the pilin protein is the immunodominant portion of the molecule. Antibodies developed against this region protect against reinfection with a homologous strain, but cross-protection against heterologous strains is incomplete. This also explains the ineffectiveness of vaccines developed against pilin proteins.

Chemoprophylaxis is also ineffective, except in the protection of newborns against gonococcal eye infections (ophthalmia neonatorum), in which 1% silver nitrate, 1% tetracycline, or 0.5% erythromycin eye ointments are routinely used. Prophylactic use of penicillin to prevent genital disease is ineffective and may select for resistant strains.

Major efforts to stem the epidemic of gonorrhea encompass education, aggressive detection, and follow-up screening of sexual contacts. It is important to realize that gonorrhea is not an insignificant disease. Chronic infections can lead to sterility, and asymptomatic infections perpetuate the reservoir of disease and lead to a higher incidence of disseminated infections.

NEISSERIA MENINGITIDIS

A paradox surrounds *N. meningitidis.* This encapsulated, gram-negative diplococci commonly colonizes the nasopharynx of healthy people. However, it is also the second most common cause of community-acquired meningitis in adults, and the swift progression from good health to life-threatening disease can cause fear and panic in a community unlike almost any other disease.

Physiology and Structure

The meningococci form transparent, nonpigmented, nonhemolytic colonies on chocolate blood agar, and their growth is enhanced in a moist atmosphere with 5% carbon dioxide. Isolates with large polysaccharide capsules appear as mucoid colonies. Meningococci are oxidase positive and are differentiated from other *Neisseria* species by the production of acid from the breakdown of glucose and maltose but not of sucrose or lactose (Table 28-3).

N. meningitidis is subdivided into serogroups and serotypes. Thirteen serogroups, with antigenic differences in their polysaccharide capsule, have been described. Serogroups A, B, C, X, Y, and W135 are most commonly associated with meningococcal disease. The serotype classification of isolates is based on differences in the proteins in the outer membrane and in the oligosaccharide component of LOS. Serotype classification has proved useful for epidemiological classification and for the characterization of virulent strains (certain LOS-based serotypes are more commonly associated with invasive disease); however, molecular analysis has replaced serological analysis in epidemiological investigations. All group A meningococci have the same outer membrane proteins and belong to a single serotype, whereas the meningococci in groups B and C belong to multiple serotypes. The membrane proteins and serotype classification are shared by these two serogroups.

Pathogenesis and Immunity

The outcome in a person exposed to *N. meningitidis* depends on four factors: (1) whether the bacteria are able to colonize the nasopharynx (mediated by pili), (2) whether specific group- and serotype-specific antibodies are present, (3) whether systemic spread occurs without antibody-mediated phagocytosis (protection afforded by polysaccharide capsule), and (4) whether toxic effects (mediated by the LOS endotoxin) are expressed.

Experiments with nasopharyngeal tissue organ cultures have shown that meningococci attach selectively to specific receptors for meningococcal pili on nonciliated columnar cells of the nasopharynx (Figure 28-4). Meningococci without pili are less able to bind to these cells.

Previous colonization with *N. meningitidis* provides protective immunity. However, progressive disease can occur in the absence of specific antibodies. Infants younger than 1 year are more susceptible to disease because of the decline in the level of maternal antibodies. Likewise, epidemic spread of disease results from the introduction of a new, virulent strain into a immunologically naive population. Bactericidal activity also requires the existence of complement. Patients with deficiencies in C5, C6, C7, or C8 of the complement system are estimated to be at a 6000-fold increased risk for meningococcal disease. Although immunity is primarily mediated by the humoral immune response, lymphocyte responsiveness to meningococcal antigens is markedly depressed in patients with acute disease.

FIGURE 28-4 Scanning electron micrograph showing attachment of *N. meningitidis* by pili to the microvilli of nonciliated cells but not to ciliated cells in the nasopharynx. (From Stephens DS et al: *J Infect Dis* 148:369-376, 1983.)

Like *N. gonorrhoeae*, meningococci are internalized into phagocytic vacuoles, able to avoid intracellular death, replicate, and then migrate to the subepithelial spaces. The antiphagocytic properties of the polysaccharide capsule protect *N. meningitidis* from phagocytic destruction.

The diffuse vascular damage associated with meningococcal infections (e.g., endothelial damage, inflammation of vessel walls, thrombosis, disseminated intravascular coagulation) is largely attributed to the action of the LOS endotoxin present in the outer membrane. *N. meningitidis* produces excess membrane fragments that are released into the extracellular space. This continuous hyperproduction of endotoxin may cause the severe endotoxic reaction seen in patients with meningococcal disease.

Epidemiology

Endemic meningococcal disease occurs worldwide, and epidemics are common in developing countries (Box 28-2). Pandemics of disease have been uncommon in developed countries since World War II. Approximately 90% of the cases of meningococcal disease are caused by serogroups A, B, or C, with B responsible for causing most cases of endemic disease in the United States. *N. meningitidis* is transmitted by respiratory droplets among people in prolonged close contact, such as family members living in the same household and soldiers living

BACTERIAL FACTORS

Diseases—see Table 28-1.

Specific receptors for meningococcal pili allow colonization of nasopharynx.

Polysaccharide capsule protects bacteria from antibody-mediated phagocytosis.

Bacteria can survive intracellular killing in the absence of humoral immunity.

Endotoxin mediates most clinical manifestations.

TRANSMISSION

Person to person by aerosolization of respiratory tract secretions.

WHO IS AT RISK?

Humans are the only natural hosts.

Children younger than 5 years (highest incidence).

Patients with late complement deficiencies.

WHO IS AT RISK?—cont'd

Close contacts of infected people (e.g., family members, day-care contacts, military personnel).

GEOGRAPHY/SEASON

Worldwide incidence, although epidemics are more common in developing countries.

Disease is more common in dry months.

MODES OF CONTROL

Breast-feeding infants have passive immunity (first 6 months).

Treatment is with penicillin (drug of choice), chloramphenicol, ceftriaxone, and cefotaxime.

Chemoprophylaxis for contacts is with rifampin or sulfadiazine (if susceptible).

For immunoprophylaxis, vaccination is an adjunct to chemoprophylaxis; it is used only for serogroups A, C, Y, and W135; no effective vaccine is available for serogroup B.

FIGURE 28-5 Incidence of meningococcal disease by age group in the United States from 1989 to 1991. (From Jackson LA, Wenger JD: *MMWR* 42:21-30, 1993.)

together in military barracks. Classmates in schools and hospital employees are not considered close contacts and are not at significantly increased risk of acquiring the disease unless they are in direct contact with the respiratory secretions of an infected person.

Humans are the only natural carriers for *N. meningitidis*. Studies of the asymptomatic carriage of *N. meningitidis* have shown that there is a tremendous variation in its prevalence, of less than 1% to almost 40%. The oral and nasopharyngeal carriage rates are highest for school-age children and young adults and higher in lower socioeconomic populations (caused by person-to-person spread in crowded areas) and do not vary with the seasons even though disease is most common during the dry season. Carriage is typically transient, with clearance occurring after specific antibodies develop. Endemic disease is most common in children younger than 5 years, particularly infants (Figure 28-5). People who are older and who live in closed populations (e.g., military barracks, prisons) are prone to infection during epidemics.

During the first months of life, maternal bactericidal antibodies in the infant are protective. However, children become susceptible to infection as this passive immunity wanes and before acquired immunity develops. Acquired immunity develops in asymptomatically colonized persons, with bactericidal antibodies detectable within 2 weeks of colonization. Cross-reacting antibodies can form and provide immunity to *N. meningitidis*. These can be antibodies to antigenically related strains of meningococci or to bacteria of other genera (e.g., *Escherichia coli* serotype K1 cross-reacts with group B *N. meningitidis*). Most meningococcal strains acquired during carriage are typeable.

Clinical Syndromes
Meningitis

A total of 2886 cases of meningococcal disease (approximately 1 case per 100,000 population) were reported in the United States in 1994. Most of these infections were meningitis. The disease usually begins abruptly with headache, meningeal signs, and fever. However, very young children may have only nonspecific signs such as fever and vomiting. Mortality approaches 100% in untreated patients but is less than 10% in patients in whom

FIGURE 28-6 Skin lesions in patient with meningococcemia. Note that the petechial lesions have coalesced and formed hemorrhagic bullae.

FIGURE 28-7 Gram stain of cerebrospinal fluid showing *N. meningitidis.*

appropriate antibiotic therapy is promptly instituted. The incidence of neurological sequelae is low, with hearing deficits and arthritis most commonly reported.

Meningococcemia

Septicemia (meningococcemia) with or without meningitis is a life-threatening disease. Thrombosis of small blood vessels and multiorgan involvement are the characteristic clinical features. Small petechial skin lesions on the trunk and lower extremities are common and may coalesce to form larger hemorrhagic lesions (Figure 28-6). Overwhelming disseminated intravascular coagulation with shock, together with the bilateral destruction of the adrenal glands **(Waterhouse-Friderichsen syndrome)**, may ensue.

A milder, chronic septicemia has also been observed. Bacteremia can persist for days or weeks, and the only signs of infection are a low-grade fever, arthritis, and petechial skin lesions. The response to antibiotic therapy in these patients is generally excellent.

Other Syndromes

Additional infections caused by *N. meningitidis* include pneumonia, arthritis, and urethritis. Meningococcal pneumonia is usually preceded by a respiratory tract infection. Symptoms include cough, chest pain, rales, fever, and chills. Evidence of pharyngitis is observed in most affected patients. The prognosis in these patients is good.

Laboratory Diagnosis

It is important to identify *N. meningitidis* infection definitively so that specific therapy can be initiated in the patient and prophylaxis can be started for the contacts,

when indicated. The most useful specimens for the detection of meningococci are blood and cerebrospinal fluid (CSF). Although the organism is present in the blood of most patients with systemic disease, additives in the blood culture broths can be toxic for *Neisseria* organisms and inhibit or delay bacterial growth. The laboratory should be notified if meningococcal disease is suspected so that alternative blood-culturing methods can be used. It is relatively easy to detect and grow the organism from the CSF of untreated patients because of the abundance of organisms in the fluid (i.e., more than 10^7 organisms per milliliter of fluid are normally found). However, the viability of organisms can be adversely affected in patients previously treated with antibiotics.

Because the bacterial count in CSF is high, the gram-negative diplococci are readily seen with polymorphonuclear leukocytes in Gram stain (Figure 28-7). Counter-immunoelectrophoresis or the agglutination of latex particles coated with specific antibodies can also be used to detect soluble polysaccharide antigen. However, the usefulness of these tests is limited because serogroup B *N. meningitidis* is relatively nonimmunogenic and does not react with the test reagents.

Treatment, Prevention, and Control

Antibiotic therapy and supportive management for the complications of meningococcal disease have significantly reduced the mortality associated with the disease. Sulfonamides were the basis for the initial therapeutic successes; however, widespread resistance to the agents has now negated their effectiveness. Penicillin is currently the antibiotic of choice, but resistance to it is also becoming more common. High-level resistance (MIC ≥ 2 μg/ml) mediated by beta-lactamase is very rare. Moderate resistance (MIC of 0.1 to 1.0 µg/ml) caused by the genetic alteration of penicillin-binding proteins is reported with increasing frequency, with approximately 4% to 5% of isolates in the United States resistant by this mechanism. Because penicillin therapy remains effective against most of these isolates, the clinical significance of low-level resistance is unknown. Chloramphenicol or broad-spectrum cephalosporins can be used as an alternative to penicillin.

Eradication of the pool of healthy carriers is unlikely. Because of this, efforts have been concentrated on the prophylactic treatment of people exposed to diseased patients and on the enhancement of immunity to the serogroups most commonly associated with disease. As just noted, sulfonamides were used for prophylaxis, but now they are no longer considered reliable. In addition, penicillin is ineffective in eliminating the carrier state. Minocycline and rifampin have been used effectively for antibiotic-mediated chemoprophylaxis; however, toxic effects have been associated with minocycline, and rifampin-resistant *N. meningitidis* can arise during treatment. At present, prophylaxis with a sulfonamide is recommended for people exposed to susceptible strains, with rifampin used for those with sulfonamide-resistant strains.

Vaccines directed against the group-specific capsular polysaccharides have been developed for antibody-mediated immunoprophylaxis. A polyvalent vaccine effective against groups A, C, Y, and W135, which can be administered to children older than 2 years of age, has been developed. However, the vaccine cannot be administered to high-risk children in younger age groups. Moreover, the group B polysaccharide is a weak immunogen and cannot induce a protective antibody response. Thus immunity to group B *N. meningitidis* must develop naturally after exposure to cross-reacting antigens. Vaccination with a suspension containing a serogroup can be used for control of an outbreak of disease, for travelers to hyperendemic areas, or for people at increased risk for disease (e.g., patients with complement deficiency).

OTHER *NEISSERIA* SPECIES

Neisseria species such as *N. sicca* and *N. mucosa* are commensal organisms in the oropharynx. These organisms have been implicated in isolated cases of meningitis, osteomyelitis, and endocarditis, as well as bronchopulmonary infections, acute otitis media, and acute sinusitis. The true incidence of respiratory tract infections caused by these organisms is not known because most specimens are contaminated with oral secretions. However, the observation of many gram-negative diplococci associated with inflammatory cells in a well-collected respiratory specimen would support the etiologic role of these organisms. Most isolates of *N. sicca* and *N. mucosa* are susceptible to penicillin, although low-level resistance caused by altered penicillin-binding protein (i.e., PBP2) has been observed.

CASE STUDY AND QUESTIONS

A 22-year-old female school teacher was brought to the emergency room after a 2-day history of headache and fever. On the day of admission the woman failed to come to school. When the woman's mother went to her apartment, she found her daughter in bed, confused and highly agitated. The patient was comatose when she arrived in the emergency room. Purpuric skin lesions were present on her trunk and arms. Analysis of her CSF revealed the presence of 380 cells/mm^3 (93% polymorphonuclear leukocytes), a protein concentration of 220 mg/dl, and a glucose concentration of 32 mg/dl. Gram stain of CSF showed many gram-negative diplococci, and the same organism was isolated from blood and CSF. The patient died despite prompt initiation of therapy with penicillin.

1. What is the most likely organism responsible for this fulminant disease? What is the most likely source of this organism?
2. Chemoprophylaxis should be administered to which people? What are the criteria for administering chemoprophylaxis?
3. What other diseases are caused by this organism?
4. What virulence factors have been associated with *N. gonorrhoeae*?
5. What measures should be used to control infections with *N. gonorrhoeae*?

Bibliography

Campos J et al: Genetic diversity of penicillin-resistant *Neisseria meningitidis, J Infect Dis* 166:173-177, 1992.

DeVoe IW: The meningococcus and mechanisms of pathogenicity, *Microbiol Rev* 46:162-190, 1982.

Feldman HA: The meningococcus: a twenty year perspective, *Rev Infect Dis* 8:288-294, 1986.

Hook EW, Holmes KK: Gonococcal infections, *Ann Intern Med* 102:229-243, 1985.

Jackson LA et al: Prevalence of *Neisseria meningitidis* relatively resistant to penicillin in the United States: 1991, *J Infect Dis* 169:438-441, 1994.

Moran JS, Levine WC: Drugs of choice for the treatment of uncomplicated gonococcal infections, *Clin Infect Dis* 20:S47-S65, 1995.

Morris SA et al: Perspectives on pathogenic *Neisseriae, Clin Microbiol Rev* 2(suppl):1-149, 1989.

Salyers AA, Whitt DD: *Bacterial pathogenesis: a molecular approach*, Washington, DC, 1994, ASM.

Stephens DS et al: Interaction of *Neisseria meningitidis* with human nasopharyngeal mucosa: attachment and entry into columnar epithelial cells, *J Infect Dis* 148:369-376, 1983.

Enterobacteriaceae

The family Enterobacteriaceae is the largest, most heterogeneous collection of medically important gram-negative bacilli. A total of 30 genera and more than 120 species have been described. These genera have been classified based on biochemical properties, antigenic structure, and nucleic acid hybridization and sequencing. Despite the complexity of this family, more than 95% of the medically important isolates belong to only 10 genera and constitute fewer than 25 species (Box 29-1).

Enterobacteriaceae are ubiquitous organisms that are found worldwide in soil, water, and vegetation and are part of the normal intestinal flora of most animals, including humans. These bacteria cause a variety of human diseases, including 30% to 35% of all septicemias, more than 70% of urinary tract infections, and many intestinal infections. Some species (e.g., *Salmonella* and *Shigella* species, *Yersinia pestis*) are always associated with disease in humans, whereas others (e.g., *Escherichia coli*, *Klebsiella pneumoniae*, *Proteus mirabilis*) are members of the normal commensal flora that can cause opportunistic infections. Infections can originate from an animal reservoir (e.g., most *Salmonella* species, *Yersinia* species), from a human carrier (e.g., *Shigella* species, *S. typhi*), or through the endogenous spread of organisms in a susceptible patient (e.g., *Escherichia* species) and can involve virtually all body sites (Figure 29-1).

PHYSIOLOGY AND STRUCTURE

Members of this family are moderately sized (0.3 to 1.0 × 1.0 to 6.0 μm), gram-negative bacilli (Figure 29-2). They are either nonmotile or motile with peritrichous flagella and do not form spores. All members can grow rapidly aerobically and anaerobically (facultative anaerobes) on a variety of nonselective (e.g., blood agar) and selective (e.g., MacConkey agar) media. The Enterobacteriaceae have simple nutritional requirements, ferment glucose, reduce nitrate, and are catalase positive and oxidase negative. The absence of cytochrome oxidase activity is an important characteristic because it can be measured rapidly and is used to distinguish Enterobacteriaceae from many other fermentative and nonfermentative gram-negative bacilli.

Morphological characteristics of the cultures on differential selective media have been used to identify members of the family Enterobacteriaceae. For example, the ability to ferment lactose has been used to differentiate lactose-fermenting strains (e.g., *Escherichia*, *Klebsiella*, *Enterobacter*, *Citrobacter*, and *Serratia* species) from strains that do not ferment lactose (e.g., *Proteus*, *Salmonella*, *Shigella*, *Yersinia* species). Resistance to bile salts in some selective media exhibited by the enteric pathogens *Shigella* and *Salmonella* has also been used to separate these bacteria from commensal organisms present in the gastrointestinal tract. Some members of the family have prominent capsules (e.g., *Klebsiella*), whereas other strains are surrounded by a loose-fitting, diffusible slime layer.

The heat-stable lipopolysaccharide (LPS) is the major cell wall antigen and consists of three components: the somatic O polysaccharide, a core polysaccharide common to all Enterobacteriaceae (common antigen), and lipid A (Figure 29-3). The serological classification of the Enterobacteriaceae is based on three major groups of antigens: somatic O polysaccharides, capsular K antigens (either protein or polysaccharide), and the flagellar H proteins. Specific O antigens are present in each genus, although cross-reactions between closely related genera are common (e.g., *Salmonella* with *Citrobacter*; *Escherichia* with *Shigella*). The antigens are detected by agglutination with specific antibodies. The heat-labile K antigens may interfere with detection of the O antigens. This is circumvented by boiling the organism, which removes the K antigens. Different genera both within and outside the family Enterobacteriaceae possess K antigens; for example, *E. coli* K1 cross-reacts with *Neisseria meningitidis* and *Haemophilus influenzae*, and *Klebsiella pneumoniae* cross-reacts with *Streptococcus pneumoniae*. The H antigens are heat-labile, flagellar proteins. They can be absent from a cell or undergo antigenic variation and be present in two phases.

PATHOGENESIS AND IMMUNITY

Numerous virulence factors have been identified in the members of the family Enterobacteriaceae. Some are common to all genera, and others are unique to specific virulent strains (Box 29-2).

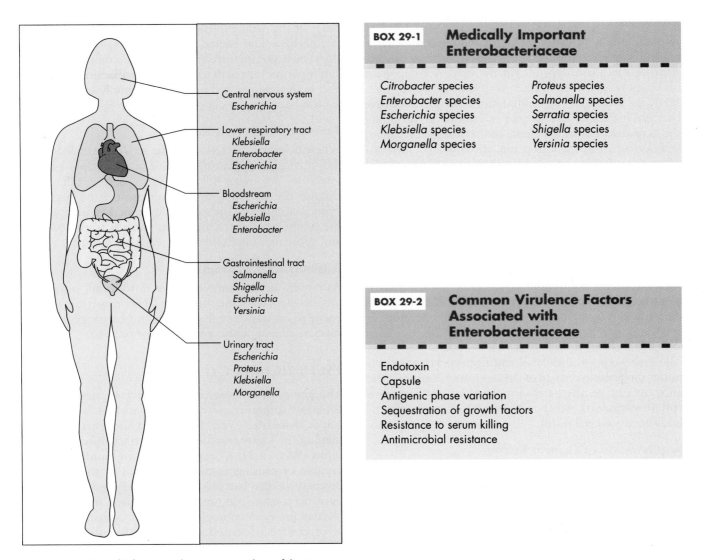

FIGURE 29-1 Sites of infections with common members of the Enterobacteriaceae listed in order of prevalence.

FIGURE 29-2 Gram stain of *K. pneumoniae.*

FIGURE 29-3 Antigenic structure of Enterobacteriaceae.

Endotoxin

Endotoxin is a virulence factor shared among all aerobic and some anaerobic gram-negative bacteria. The activity of this toxin depends on the lipid A component of lipopolysaccharide, which is released at cell lysis. Many of the systemic manifestations of gram-negative bacterial infections are initiated by endotoxin, including the activation of complement, the release of cytokines, leukocytosis, thrombocytopenia, disseminated intravascular coagulation, fever, decreased peripheral circulation, shock, and death.

Capsule

Encapsulated Enterobacteriaceae are protected from phagocytosis by the hydrophilic capsular antigens, which repel the hydrophobic phagocytic cell surface. These antigens interfere with the binding of antibodies to the bacteria and are poor immunogens or activators of complement. However, the protective role of the capsule is diminished if specific anticapsular antibodies develop.

Antigenic Phase Variation

The expression of capsular K and flagellar H antigens is under the genetic control of the organism. Each of these antigens can be alternately expressed or not expressed **(phase variation),** which can protect bacteria from antibody-mediated cell death.

Sequestration of Growth Factors

In contrast with the nutrients provided to the organisms in enriched media, the bacteria must become nutritional scavengers when growing in vivo. Iron is an important growth factor required by bacteria, but it is bound in heme proteins (e.g., hemoglobin, myoglobin) or in iron-chelating proteins (e.g., transferrin, lactoferrin). The bacteria counteract this by producing their own competitive iron-chelating compounds—the siderophores **enterobactin** and **aerobactin.** Iron can also be released from host cells by hemolysins produced by the bacteria.

Resistance to Serum Killing

Whereas many bacteria can be rapidly cleared from blood, virulent organisms capable of producing systemic infections are frequently resistant to serum killing. Although the bacterial capsule can protect the organism from serum killing, other poorly defined factors prevent the binding of complement components to the bacteria and subsequent complement-mediated clearance.

Antimicrobial Resistance

As rapidly as new antibiotics are introduced, organisms can develop resistance to them. This resistance can be encoded on transferable plasmids and exchanged among species, genera, and even families of bacteria.

ESCHERICHIA COLI

The genus *Escherichia* consists of five species; *E. coli* is the most common and clinically important. This organism is associated with a variety of diseases, including meningitis, gastroenteritis, urinary tract infections, and sepsis (Box 29-3). As expected, the multitude of strains capable of causing disease is reflected in the antigenic diversity of the bacteria. Many O, H, and K antigens have been described, and these are used to classify the isolates for epidemiological purposes. Specific antigenic serotypes are associated with increased virulence.

BOX 29-3 **Summary of *E. coli* Infections**

BACTERIAL FACTORS

Diseases—septicemia, urinary tract infections, neonatal meningitis, gastroenteritis.
Virulence factors—see Boxes 29-2 and 29-4.

TRANSMISSION

Present in soil, water, and vegetation and part of normal gastrointestinal tract flora.
Endogenous spread in susceptible patients (nosocomial infection).
Exogenous infections spread by ingestion of contaminated food or water.

WHO IS AT RISK?

Septicemia: patients with *E. coli* infections at other sites (e.g., urinary tract, abdomen).
Urinary tract infections: pregnant or sexually active women, men with prostatic hypertrophy, and patients with urinary catheters.

WHO IS AT RISK?—cont'd

Neonates colonized with *E. coli* K1.
Travelers to countries with poor hygienic standards (gastroenteritis).
People who consume undercooked hamburgers or unpasteurized milk or fruit juice.

GEOGRAPHY/SEASON

Worldwide (particularly in countries with substandard sanitation).
No seasonal incidence.

MODES OF CONTROL

Treatment with antibiotics showing in vitro activity.
Appropriate infection-control practices in hospitals.
Maintenance of high hygienic standards.

Pathogenesis and Immunity

E. coli possesses a broad range of virulence factors. In addition to the general factors possessed by all members of the family Enterobacteriaceae, *Escherichia* strains responsible for diseases such as gastroenteritis and urinary tract infections possess specialized virulence factors. Two general categories are adhesins and exotoxins (Box 29-4).

Adhesins

E. coli is able to remain in the gastrointestinal tract or urinary tract because they are able to adhere to the cells lining these tracts and to avoid being eliminated by intestinal motility or the flushing action of voided urine. Strains of *E. coli* possess numerous highly specialized adhesins. These include **type 1 pili** and colonization factor antigens (**CFA/I** and **CFA/II**) in enterotoxigenic *E. coli*; **GVVPQ fimbriae** in enteroaggregative *E. coli*; **bundle-forming pili** (Bfp) and **intimin** in enteroaggregative *E. coli*; and **P pili**, afimbrial adhesins (**AFAI** and **AFAIII**), and **Dr** adhesins in uropathogenic *E. coli*.

Exotoxins

E. coli also produces a diverse spectrum of exotoxins. Enterotoxigenic *E. coli* produces heat-stable toxins (**STa** and **STb**) and heat-labile toxins (**LT-I** and **LT-II**). Enterohemorrhagic *E. coli* produce Shiga-like toxins (**SLT-I** and **SLT-II**). Enteroaggregative *E. coli* has been observed to produce a heat-stable toxin, and hemolysins (**HlyA**) are considered important in uropathogenic *E. coli*. The precise mechanisms by which these toxins function are described in the following sections.

Epidemiology

Large numbers of *E. coli* are present in the gastrointestinal tract and the bacteria frequently found to be the cause of sepsis, neonatal meningitis, infections of the urinary tract, and gastroenteritis. For example, *E. coli* is the most common gram-negative bacilli isolated from septic patients (Figure 29-4), is responsible for causing more than 80% of all community-acquired urinary tract infections and most hospital-acquired infections, and is a prominent cause of gastroenteritis in developing countries. Most infections (with the exception of neonatal meningitis and gastroenteritis) are endogenous. That is, the person's normal microbial flora is able to establish infection when the host's defenses are compromised.

Clinical Syndromes

Septicemia

Typically, septicemia caused by gram-negative bacilli such as *E. coli* originates from infections in the urinary or gastrointestinal tract (e.g., an intraabdominal infection caused by intestinal perforation). The mortality associated with *E. coli* septicemia is influenced by the source of infection and the underlying disease of the patient, with a significantly higher incidence of death in immunocompromised patients and in those with intraabdominal infections.

Urinary Tract Infections

Most gram-negative bacilli that produce urinary tract infections originate in the colon, contaminate the urethra, ascend into the bladder, and may migrate to the kidney or prostate (an ascending infection as opposed to an infection caused by the hematogenous spread of the organism to the urinary tract). Although most strains of *E. coli* can produce urinary tract infections, disease is most common with certain specific serotypes. These bacteria are particularly virulent because of their ability to produce adhesins (primarily **P pili, AFAI, AFAIII,** and **Dr**), which bind to cells lining the bladder and upper urinary tract (preventing the elimination of the bacteria in voided urine), and hemolysin **HlyA**, which lyses erythrocytes and other cell types (leading to cytokine release and stimulation of an inflammatory response).

Neonatal Meningitis

E. coli with group B streptococci are the most common cause of neonatal meningitis; 75% of these strains possess the K1 capsular antigen. Although it is common for infants to be colonized with *E. coli* at birth, disease in infants is relatively infrequent.

BOX 29-4	**Specialized Virulence Factors Associated with *E. coli***

ADHESINS	EXOTOXINS
Type 1 pili	STa, STb
CFA/I, CFA/II	LT-I, LT-II
GVVPQ fimbriae	SLT-I, SLT-II
Bfp	Enteroaggregative heat-stable toxin
Intimin	
P pili	HlyA
AFAI, AFAIII	
Dr adhesin	

FIGURE 29-4 Incidence of Enterobacteriaceae associated with bacteremia. (Data courtesy Barnes-Jewish Hospital, St. Louis.)

Pie chart: 45% Escherichia, 22% Klebsiella, 20% Enterobacter, 4% Proteus, 4% Serratia, 2% Citrobacter, 3% Other.

TABLE 29-1   Gastroenteritis Caused by *Escherichia coli*

SITE OF ACTION	DISEASE	PATHOGENESIS
ENTEROTOXIGENIC *E. COLI* (ETEC)		
Small intestine	Traveler's diarrhea; infant diarrhea in under-developed countries; watery diarrhea, vomiting, cramps, nausea, low-grade fever	Plasmid-mediated heat-stable and/or heat-labile enterotoxins that stimulate hyper-secretion of fluids and electrolytes
ENTEROINVASIVE *E. COLI* (EIEC)		
Large intestine	Disease in underdeveloped countries; fever, cramping, watery diarrhea followed by development of dysentery with scant, bloody stools	Plasmid-mediated invasion and destruction of epithelial cells lining colon
ENTEROPATHOGENIC *E. COLI* (EPEC)		
Small intestine	Infant diarrhea with fever, nausea, vomiting, nonbloody stools	Plasmid-mediated adherence and destruction of epithelial cells
ENTEROHEMORRHAGIC *E. COLI* (EHEC)		
Large intestine	Hemorrhagic colitis with severe abdominal cramps, initial watery diarrhea, followed by grossly bloody diarrhea; little or no fever; hemolytic uremic syndrome	Mediation by cytotoxic shiga-like toxins (SLT-I, SLT-II), which disrupt protein synthesis; toxins encoded by lysogenic bacteriophages
ENTEROAGGREGATIVE *E. COLI* (EAggEC)		
Small intestine	Infant diarrhea in underdeveloped countries; persistent watery diarrhea with vomiting, dehydration, and low grade fever	Plasmid-mediated aggregative adherence that prevents fluid absorption

Gastroenteritis

The strains of *E. coli* that cause gastroenteritis are subdivided into five groups: enterotoxigenic, enteroinvasive, enteropathogenic, enterohemorrhagic, and enteroaggregative (Table 29-1). Gastroenteritis produced by **enterotoxigenic *E. coli* (ETEC)** is mediated by heat-labile (**LT-I,** and **LT-II**) and heat-stabile (**STa** and **STb**) enterotoxins. LT-1 is antigenically similar to the toxin produced by *Vibrio cholerae* in that it consists of one A subunit and five B subunits. The B subunits bind to the same receptor as cholera toxin (G_{M1} gangliosides) and allow entry of the A subunit into the target cell. The A subunit adenosine diphosphate–ribosylates a membrane protein (G_s), which regulates adenylate cyclase. The net effect of this interaction is an increase in cyclic adenosine monophosphate (cAMP) levels with activation of sodium, chloride, potassium bicarbonate, and water out of the cell into the intestinal lumen (e.g., watery diarrhea). In a similar fashion, STa binds to guanylate cyclase, leading to an increase in the level of cyclic guanosine monophosphate and subsequent hypersecretion of fluids. LT-II and STb are produced by strains of *E. coli* isolated from animals but not from humans. Genes for LT-I and STa are present on a transferable plasmid, which can also carry the genes for the adhesins **CFA/I** and **CFA/II.** The receptors for these colonization factors are glycoproteins.

Secretory diarrhea caused by ETEC develops after a 1- to 2-day incubation period and persists for an average of 3 to 4 days. The symptoms—cramps, nausea, vomiting, and watery diarrhea—are similar to those of cholera but are milder. Neither histological changes of the intestinal mucosa nor inflammation is observed. Disease mediated by heat-labile toxin is indistinguishable from that mediated by heat-stable toxin. Toxin production is not associated with specific serotypes, so tissue cultures or animal model assays for toxin activity must be performed for toxigenic strains to be detected. Nucleic acid probes have also been used to detect the toxin genes. Disease caused by these pathogenic *E. coli* is rarely observed in the United States.

Enteroinvasive *E. coli* (EIEC) invade and destroy the colonic epithelium, producing a disease characterized by fever and cramps, with blood and leukocytes in stool specimens. Specific O serotypes of *E. coli* produce disease; however, the serological analysis of isolates cannot identify invasive strains reliably. These organisms must have a large plasmid (**pINV**) for them to be able to invade epithelial cells, although chromosomal genes are also necessary for disease to develop. This disease is primarily seen in developing countries.

Enteropathogenic *E. coli* (EPEC) are considered an important cause of pediatric diarrhea in impoverished countries. Although specific O serotypes have been associated with outbreaks of EPEC diarrhea in nurseries, the serotyping of the *E. coli* isolated in random or endemic disease is discouraged except in epidemiological investigations. Disease occurs because the organism adheres to the enterocyte plasma membrane and cause destruction (effacement) of the adjacent microvilli. Thus these strains have also been called **enteroadherent *E. coli*.** Attachment and destruction of the cellular architecture proceed in three stages: loose attachment mediated by Bfp; stimulation of intracellular calcium level; and finally, rearrangement of intracellular actin, leading to the destruction of the microvilli. The intimate bacteria–host cell contact required for the final stage is mediated by an outer membrane protein, **intimin.** Bfp is plasmid mediated (EPEC adherence factor, or EAF plasmid), and intimin is encoded on the *E. coli* attachment-effacement (*eae*) gene located on the bacterial chromosome. The diarrhea likely results from the loss of the absorptive properties of the infected cells; a toxin has not been found.

Enterohemorrhagic *E. coli* (EHEC) are the most common strains producing disease in developed countries, with an estimated 20,000 cases occurring annually in the United States. The ingestion of fewer than 100 bacilli can produce disease. The severity of the disease caused by EHEC ranges from mild, uncomplicated diarrhea to hemorrhagic colitis with severe abdominal pain, bloody diarrhea, and little or no fever. **Hemolytic uremic syndrome** (acute renal failure, thrombocytopenia, and microangiopathic hemolytic anemia) is also associated with this organism. It is a complication in 10% of children younger than 10 years. Disease is most common in the warm months, with the greatest incidence in children younger than 5 years. Most cases of epidemic and endemic disease have been attributed to the consumption of undercooked ground beef or other beef products, as well as unpasteurized milk or fruit juices (e.g., cider made from apples contaminated with feces from cattle).

Initially a nonbloody diarrhea develops in patients after the bacilli become attached to the epithelium of the terminal ileum, cecum, and colon (mediated by intimin). Subsequent elaboration of toxins (called *verotoxin*, *Shiga toxin*, or *Shiga-like toxin*) mediates bloody diarrhea and increased abdominal pain. At least two toxins have been recognized (referred to here as **SLT-I** and **SLT-II**). SLT-I is identical to the Shiga toxin produced by *S. dysenteriae*, except for one amino acid; SLT-II has 60% homology. Both toxins are encoded by lysogenic bacteriophages. Both have five B subunits and one A subunit, with the B subunit binding to a specific glycolipid on the host cell (globotriaosylceramide). After the A subunit is internalized, it is cleaved into two molecules, and the A_1 fragment binds to the 28S ribosomal ribonucleic acid (rRNA) and disrupts protein synthesis. Hemolytic uremic syndrome has been preferentially associated with the production of SLT-II, which has been shown to destroy renal endothelial cells selectively. More than 50 serotypes of EHEC have been isolated; however, most are serotype O157:H7.

Enteroaggregative *E. coli* (EAggEC) have been implicated as a cause of persistent, watery diarrhea with vomiting and dehydration in infants in developing countries. The bacteria are characterized by their D-mannose–resistant aggregative adherence pattern. Expression of the aggregative pattern is mediated by a thin pili (GVVPQ fimbriae) present on a plasmid. A toxin and hemolysin have also been described, but their role in disease is undefined. Adherence of the bacteria to the intestinal mucosa does not provoke histological changes.

SALMONELLA

The taxonomic classification of the genus *Salmonella* is problematic, with more than 2000 unique serotypes described. Careful analysis of DNA homology has revealed that the genus consists of a single species subdivided into seven subgroups. Although the single species designation *S. enterica* has been recommended, this taxonomically correct approach has not been widely adopted. Most authorities continue to use the conventional approach of designating the serotype epithet as the species name.

Pathogenesis and Immunity

Although much is known about the genetic relationship of *Salmonella* strains, epidemiology of infections, and clinical manifestations of disease, relatively little is known about the role of specific virulence factors. After ingestion and passage through the stomach, *Salmonella* organisms are able to invade and replicate in the cells lining the lumen of the terminal portion of the small intestine. The adherence of the bacteria to the microvilli on the cell surface stimulates the rearrangement of actin (**ruffling**), with subsequent engulfment of the bacteria within endocytic vesicles. The bacteria remain in the vesicles and replicate until the cell is lysed. Chromosomal **invasin** (*inv*) genes mediate the attachment and penetration of the bacteria into the cells; however, the precise products of this gene complex have not been characterized. *Salmonella* species are also protected from stomach acids and the acid pH of the phagosome by an **acid tolerance response** (*ATR*) gene. Catalase and superoxide dismutase are other factors that protect the bacteria from intracellular killing. The inflammatory response confines the infection to the gastrointestinal tract, mediates the release of prostaglandins, and stimulates cAMP and active fluid secretion.

Epidemiology

Salmonella organismss are found in virtually all animals, including poultry, reptiles, livestock, rodents, domestic animals, birds, and humans (Box 29-5). Animal-to-animal spread and the use of *Salmonella*-contaminated animal feeds maintain an animal reservoir. Serotypes such as *S. typhi* and *S. paratyphi* are highly adapted to humans and do not cause disease in nonhuman hosts. Other *Salmonella* strains (e.g., *S. choleraesuis*) are adapted to animals and, when they infect humans, can cause severe disease. Finally, many strains have no host specificity and cause disease in both human and nonhuman hosts.

Most infections result from the ingestion of contaminated food products and, in children, from direct fecal-oral spread. The incidence of disease is greatest in children younger than 5 years and adults older than 60 years, who are infected during the summer and autumn months when contaminated foods are consumed at outdoor social gatherings. The most common sources of human infections are poultry, eggs, dairy products, and foods prepared on contaminated work surfaces (e.g., cutting boards where uncooked poultry was prepared). Approximately 50,000 cases of *Salmonella* infections are reported annually in the United States, although this probably represents only 10% of all human infections (Figure 29-5).

S. typhi infection occurs when food or water contaminated by infected food handlers is ingested. There is no animal reservoir. Approximately 400 to 500 *S. typhi* infections occur annually in the United States, with most acquired during foreign travel.

Although people are frequently exposed to *Salmonella* organisms, a large inoculum (10^6 to 10^8 bacteria) is required for symptomatic disease to develop. This can happen if the organism multiplies to a high density, such as in improperly stored, contaminated food products. The infectious dose is reduced for people at increased risk for disease because of age, immunosuppression or underlying disease (leukemia, lymphoma, sickle cell disease), or reduced gastric acidity.

Clinical Syndromes

Four forms of *Salmonella* infection exist: enteritis, septicemia, enteric fever, and asymptomatic colonization.

Enteritis

Enteritis is the most common form of salmonellosis. Symptoms generally appear 6 to 48 hours after the consumption of contaminated food or water, with the initial presentation of nausea, vomiting, and nonbloody diarrhea. Fever, abdominal cramps, myalgias, and headache are also common. Colonic involvement can be demonstrated in the acute form of the disease. Symptoms can persist from 2 days to 1 week before spontaneous resolution.

Septicemia

All *Salmonella* species can cause bacteremia, although infections with *S. choleraesuis*, *S. paratyphi*, and *S. typhi* more frequently lead to a bacteremic phase. The risk for *Salmonella* bacteremia is increased in pediatric and geriatric patients as well as in patients with acquired immunodeficiency syndrome. The clinical presentation of *Salmonella* bacteremia is like that of other gram-negative bacteremias; however, localized suppurative infections such as osteomyelitis, endocarditis, and arthritis can occur in as many as 10% of patients.

Enteric Fever

S. typhi produce a febrile illness called *typhoid fever*. A mild form of this disease, referred to as *paratyphoid fever*, is produced by *S. paratyphi A, S. schottmuelleri* (formerly *S. paratyphi B*), and *S. hirschfeldii* (formerly *S. paratyphi C*). In contrast to other *Salmonella* infections, the bacteria responsible for enteric fever pass through the cells lining the intestines and are engulfed by macrophages. They replicate after being transported to the liver, spleen, and bone marrow.

BOX 29-5   Summary of *Salmonella* Infections

BACTERIAL FACTORS

Diseases—enteritis, septicemia, enteric fever.

Virulence factors—ability to invade and replicate in enterocytes; protection from acid-mediated killing by *ATR* gene product; produce catalase and superoxide dismutase.

Animals are main reservoir for human disease, except for infection with bacteria responsible for typhoid and paratyphoid fevers (human reservoir).

Asymptomatic carriage with *S. typhi* and less commonly with other species.

TRANSMISSION

Ingestion of contaminated food products (e.g., poultry, eggs, dairy products).

Direct fecal-oral spread in children.

Person-to-person spread with contaminated food or water (typhoid or paratyphoid fevers).

WHO IS AT RISK?

Anyone who consumes foods contaminated with large numbers of salmonellae is at risk, particularly children younger than 5 years and adults older than 60 years, patients with reduced gastric acid levels, and immunocompromised patients (especially patients with acquired immunodeficiency syndrome).

Foreign travelers to areas where hygienic practices are substandard and people exposed to *S. typhi* carriers.

GEOGRAPHY/SEASON

Worldwide.

More common in summer and autumn months.

MODES OF CONTROL

Symptomatic treatment rather than antibiotics to prevent prolongation of carriage.

Proper preparation and refrigeration of foods.

Improved hygiene.

Ten to fourteen days after ingestion of the bacilli, patients experience gradually increasing fever with nonspecific complaints of headache, myalgias, malaise, and anorexia. These symptoms persist for a week or more and are followed by gastrointestinal symptoms. This cycle corresponds to an initial bacteremic phase and is followed by colonization of the gallbladder and then reinfection of the intestines.

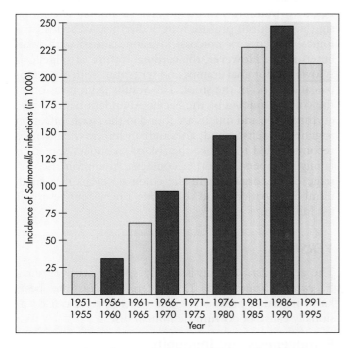

FIGURE 29-5 Annual reported incidence of *Salmonella* infections (excluding typhoid fever) in the United States from 1951 to 1995. (Redrawn from *MMWR* 44:74-79, 1995.)

Asymptomatic Carriage

The species of *Salmonella* responsible for causing typhoid and paratyphoid fevers are maintained by human carriage. Chronic carriage for more than 1 year after symptomatic disease will develop in 1% to 5% of patients, with the gallbladder the reservoir in most patients. Chronic carriage with other species of *Salmonella* occurs in less than 1% of patients and does not represent an important source of human infection.

SHIGELLA
Epidemiology

Unlike the genus *Salmonella*, the taxonomic classification of *Shigella* is quite simple (Box 29-6). Four species consisting of more than 45 O antigen–based serotypes have been described: *S. dysenteriae, S. flexneri, S. boydii,* and *S. sonnei. S. sonnei* is the most common cause of shigellosis in the industrial world, and *S. flexneri* is the most common in underdeveloped countries. More than 30,000 *Shigella* infections were reported in the United States in 1995 (Figure 29-6); however, this is a vast underestimate of the true incidence of infection. Shigellosis is primarily a pediatric disease, with more than half of all infections occurring in children between 1 and 10 years of age. Endemic disease in adults is common in male homosexuals and household contacts of infected children. Epidemic outbreaks of disease occur in day-care centers, nurseries, and custodial institutions. Shigellosis is transmitted by the fecal-oral route, primarily by people with contaminated hands and less commonly in water or food. Because as few as 200 bacilli can establish disease, shigellosis spreads rapidly in communities where sanitary standards and the level of personal hygiene are low.

BOX 29-6   **Summary of *Shigella* Infections**

BACTERIAL FACTORS

Disease—gastroenteritis (shigellosis).

Virulence factors—genes encode adherence, invasion, and intracellular replication in cells lining colon; Shiga toxin disrupts protein synthesis.

TRANSMISSION

Human carriage with spread by person-to-person contact; primarily transmitted by fecal-oral route by people with contaminated hands.

Consumption of contaminated food or water (less important means of transmission).

WHO IS AT RISK?

Anyone exposed to carrier, particularly young children or those in day-care centers, nurseries, and custodial institutions.

WHO IS AT RISK?—cont'd

Male homosexuals.

Communities with poor sanitation and hygienic practices.

GEOGRAPHY/SEASON

Worldwide.

No seasonal incidence.

MODES OF CONTROL

Antibiotic therapy is used to decrease number of organisms and duration of carriage in symptomatic patients (reducing person-to-person spread).

Institution of infection-control practices: handwashing and proper disposal of soiled linens.

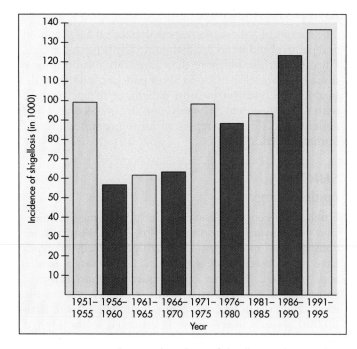

FIGURE 29-6 Annual reported incidence of shigellosis in the United States from 1951 to 1995. (Redrawn from *MMWR* 44:74-79, 1995.)

Pathogenesis and Immunity

Shigella organisms cause disease by invading and replicating in cells lining the colonic mucosa. Structural genes mediate the adherence of the organisms to the cells, as well as their invasion, intracellular replication, and cell-to-cell spread. These genes are carried on a large virulence plasmid but are regulated by chromosomal genes. Thus the presence of the plasmid does not ensure functional gene activity.

Shigella species appear unable to attach to differentiated mucosal cells; rather, they first attach to and invade the **M (microfold) cells** located in Peyer's patches. These cells typically transport foreign antigens to the underlying macrophages for clearance. However, *Shigella* species are able to lyse the phagocytic vacuole and replicate in the host cell cytoplasm (unlike *Salmonella* that replicate in the vacuole). With the rearrangement of actin filaments in the host cells, the bacteria are propelled through the cytoplasm to adjacent cells, where cell-to-cell passage occurs. In this way *Shigella* organisms are protected from immune-mediated clearance. Bacteremia with *Shigella* species is uncommon because bacteria that do spread to the bloodstream are rapidly engulfed and killed by macrophages.

S. dysenteriae produce an exotoxin, **Shiga toxin.** Like the toxin produced by EHEC, the Shiga toxin has one A subunit and five B subunits. The B subunits bind to a host cell glycolipid (Gb3) and facilitate transfer of the A subunit into the cell. The A subunit cleaves the 28S rRNA in the 60S ribosomal subunit. This prevents binding of aminoacyl–transfer RNA and disrupts protein syn-

thesis. The primary manifestation of toxin activity is endothelial damage. Renal damage results in the hemolytic uremic syndrome (as occurs in EHEC).

Clinical Syndromes

Shigellosis is characterized by abdominal cramps, diarrhea, fever, and bloody stools. The clinical signs and symptoms of shigellosis appear 1 to 3 days after bacilli are ingested. The bacilli colonize the small intestine and begin to multiply within the first 12 hours. The initial sign of infection, profuse watery diarrhea without histological evidence of mucosal invasion, is mediated by an enterotoxin. However, the cardinal feature of shigellosis is lower abdominal cramps and tenesmus, with abundant pus and blood in the stool. This results from invasion of the colonic mucosa by the bacilli. Abundant neutrophils, erythrocytes, and mucus are found in the stool. Infection is generally self-limited, although antibiotic treatment is recommended to reduce the risk of secondary spread to family members and other contacts. Asymptomatic carriage of the organism in the colon develops in a small number of patients and represents a persistent reservoir for infection.

YERSINIA

The genus *Yersinia* consists of 11 species, with *Y. pestis*, *Y. enterocolitica*, and *Y. pseudotuberculosis* the best-known human pathogens. The other species can occasionally cause opportunistic human disease.

Pathogenesis and Immunity

Y. pestis is a highly virulent pathogen that causes systemic disease with a high mortality rate; *Y. enterocolitica* and *Y. pseudotuberculosis* are primarily enteric pathogens that are rarely isolated from the bloodstream. *Y. pestis* can be introduced directly into the patient's blood by an infected flea. The organism is adapted to survive and replicate in nonactivated macrophages. *Y. enterocolitica* and *Y. pseudotuberculosis* are acquired through the ingestion of contaminated food or water and establish their infections by invading M cells in Peyer's patches. In contrast to *Shigella* infections, *Yersinia* organisms do not replicate in the M cells but rather pass through to the underlying tissue, are engulfed by macrophages, carried to the mesenteric lymph nodes, and replicate. These bacteria cannot survive in neutrophils, so infections are typically limited to the intestines and lymphoid tissues.

All three species of *Yersinia* have a plasmid that carries virulence genes for adherence (*Yersinia* **adherence gene [*yadA*]**), multifunctional *Yersinia* **outer membrane protein (*yop*) genes,** and regulatory (**low calcium response [*lcr*]**) genes. The 11 *yop* genes have cytotoxic activity, inhibit the migration and engulfment of phagocytes, and inhibit platelet aggregation. The *lcr* gene mediates the supply of calcium to the organism, which is believed to be important for the organism's intracellular

BOX 29-7   Summary of *Yersinia* Infections

BACTERIAL FACTORS

Diseases—*Y. pestis:* bubonic plague, pneumonic plague; *Y. enterocolitica:* enterocolitis, transfusion-related septicemia; *Y. pseudotuberculosis:* enterocolitis.

Virulence factors—factors common to *Yersinia:* genes for adherence, cytotoxic activity, inhibition of phagocytic migration and engulfment, and inhibition of platelet aggregation. Factors common to *Y. pestis:* antiphagocytic protein capsule that can degrade complement components, thereby preventing opsonization and phagocytic migration; can degrade fibrin clots; and is resistant to serum killing.

TRANSMISSION

Y. pestis: spread from mammalian reservoir (rats, squirrels, rabbits, domestic animals) by flea bites or contact with contaminated animal tissues.

Other *Yersinia* species: ingestion of contaminated food products, infusion of contaminated blood products.

WHO IS AT RISK?

Y. pestis: people in communities with poor hygienic conditions and with endemic plague; people exposed to infected animals.

WHO IS AT RISK?—cont'd

Other *Yersinia* organisms: people who eat contaminated food or receive contaminated blood products.

GEOGRAPHY/SEASON

Y. pestis primarily affects people living in Asia and Africa; however, it is distributed worldwide, including the southwestern United States; disease occurs cyclically as the reservoir population increases and decreases. Incidence of disease in the human population increases as infected animals die.

Other *Yersiniae* species: infections occur worldwide but primarily in cold climates.

MODES OF CONTROL

Y. pestis—control of rodent vector and improved hygiene; vaccination; chemoprophylaxis.

Other *Yersiniae* organisms: proper food preparation and storage.

---

survival. *Y. pestis* also has two additional plasmids, which encode virulence genes: **fraction 1 (Fra 1)** gene, which codes for an antiphagocytic protein capsule, and **plasminogen activator (*Pla*)** gene, which degrades complement components C3b and C5a, preventing opsonization and phagocytic migration, respectively. The *Pla* gene also degrades fibrin clots, permitting *Y. pestis* to spread rapidly. Other virulence factors specifically associated with *Y. pestis* include serum resistance and the ability of the organism to absorb organic iron as a result of a siderophore-independent mechanism.

Epidemiology

All *Yersinia* infections are zoonotic, with humans the accidental hosts. There are two forms of *Y. pestis* infection: **urban plague**, with rats as the natural reservoirs, and **sylvatic plague**, with infections in squirrels, rabbits, field rats, and domestic cats. Pigs, rodents, livestock, and rabbits are the natural reservoirs for *Y. enterocolitica*, whereas rodents, wild animals, and game birds are the natural reservoirs for *Y. pseudotuberculosis*.

One of the most devastating diseases in history was caused by *Y. pestis* (Box 29-7). Epidemics of the plague were recorded in the Old Testament. The first of three major pandemics (urban plague) started in 541 AD and continued through the end of the eighth century, with an estimated 40 million deaths caused by this bacterium. The second pandemic started in the 1320s and within 5

years resulted in more than 25 million deaths in Europe alone (30% of the population). The third pandemic began in China in the 1860s and spread to Africa, Europe, and the Americas. Epidemic and sporadic cases of the disease continue to this day. From 1950 through 1995, almost 400 cases of plague were reported in the United States (Figure 29-7), with disease (sylvatic plague) primarily in the western United States.

Urban plague is maintained in rat populations and spread among rats or between rats and humans by infected fleas. Fleas become infected during a blood meal from a bacteremic rat. After the bacteria replicate in the flea gut, the organisms can be transferred to another rodent or to humans. Urban plague has been eliminated from most communities by the effective control of rats and better hygiene. In contrast, sylvatic plague is difficult or impossible to eliminate because the mammalian reservoirs and flea vectors are widespread. *Y. pestis* produces a fatal infection in the animal reservoir. Thus cyclic patterns of human disease occur as the opportunity for contact with the reservoir population increases or decreases. Infections can also be acquired through the ingestion of contaminated animals or handling of contaminated animal tissues. Although the organism is highly infectious, human-to-human spread is uncommon unless the patient has pulmonary involvement.

Y. enterocolitica is a common cause of enterocolitis in Scandinavian and other European countries, as well as in

FIGURE 29-7 Annual reported incidence of *Y. pestis* infections in the United States from 1955 to 1995. (Redrawn from *MMWR* 44:74-79, 1995.)

the colder areas of North America. Most studies show that infections are more common during the cold months. Virulence with this organisms is associated with specific serotypes. The most common serotypes found in Europe, Africa, Japan, and Canada are O3 and O9, and O8 has been identified in the United States. *Y. pseudotuberculosis* is a relatively uncommon cause of human disease.

Clinical Syndromes

The two clinical manifestations of *Y. pestis* infection are bubonic plague and pneumonic plague. **Bubonic plague** is characterized by an incubation period of no more than 7 days after a person has been bitten by an infected flea. Patients have a high fever and a painful bubo (inflammatory swelling of the lymph nodes) in the groin or axilla. Bacteremia develops rapidly if patients are not treated, and as many as 75% die. The incubation period (2 to 3 days) is shorter in patients with **pneumonic plague.** Initially, these patients experience fever and malaise, with pulmonary signs developing within 1 day. The patients are highly infectious, with person-to-person spread by aerosols. The mortality rate in untreated patients with pneumonic plague exceeds 90%.

Approximately two thirds of all *Y. enterocolitica* infections are enterocolitis, as the name implies. The gastroenteritis is characterized by diarrhea, fever, and abdominal pain that last for as long as 1 to 2 weeks, although a chronic form of the disease can develop and persist for months. Disease involves the terminal ileum, and if the mesenteric lymph nodes become enlarged, the disease can mimic acute appendicitis. *Yersinia* infections are most common in children, with pseudoappendicitis posing a particular problem in this age group. *Y. pseudotuberculosis* can also produce a disease with the clinical features. Other manifestations seen in adults include septicemia, arthritis, intraabdominal abscess, hepatitis, and osteomyelitis.

In 1987, *Y. enterocolitica* was first reported to cause blood transfusion–related bacteremia and endotoxic shock. Because *Yersinia* organisms can grow at 4° C, this organism can multiply to toxic concentrations in nutritionally rich blood products that are contaminated and refrigerated for at least 3 weeks. There is no reliable method for detecting contaminated blood products. Use of products stored for a shorter time would probably eliminate the problem because the organisms would not be able to multiply to toxic levels. However, this is not practical given the current shortage of blood products.

OTHER ENTEROBACTERIACEAE
Klebsiella

Members of the genus *Klebsiella* have a prominent capsule that is responsible for the mucoid appearance of isolated colonies and the enhanced virulence of the organisms in vivo. The most commonly isolated member of this genus is *K. pneumoniae*, which can cause community-acquired primary lobar pneumonia. Alcoholics and people with compromised pulmonary function are at increased risk for pneumonia because of their inability to clear aspirated oral secretions from the lower respiratory tract. Pneumonia caused by *Klebsiella* species frequently involves the necrotic destruction of alveolar spaces, cavity formation, and the production of blood-tinged sputum. These bacteria also cause wound, soft tissue, and urinary tract infections.

Proteus

Infection of the urinary tract with *P. mirabilis* is the most common disease produced by this genus. *Proteus* strains produce large quantities of urease, which splits urea into carbon dioxide and ammonia. This raises the urine pH and facilitates the formation of renal stones. The increased alkalinity of the urine is also toxic to the uroepithelium. Despite the serological diversity of these organisms, infection has not been associated with any specific serotype. Furthermore, in contrast to *E. coli*, the pili on the *Proteus* organism may decrease its virulence by enhancing phagocytosis of the bacilli.

Enterobacter, Citrobacter, Morganella, and Serratia

Primary infections in immunocompetent patients are rarely caused by *Enterobacter*, *Citrobacter*, *Morganella*, or *Serratia* organisms. They are more commonly the cause of hospital-acquired infections in immunocompromised patients. Antibiotic therapy can be ineffective because these organisms are frequently resistant to multiple antibiotics. This is a particularly serious problem with *Enterobacter* species.

LABORATORY DIAGNOSIS
Culture

Members of the family *Enterobacteriaceae* grow readily on culture media. Specimens of normally sterile material such as spinal fluid or tissue collected at surgery can be inoculated onto nonselective blood agar media. Selective media (e.g., MacConkey agar, eosin–methylene blue agar [EMB]) are used for the culture of specimens normally contaminated with other organisms (e.g., sputum, feces). By using these selective differential agars, lactose-fermenting Enterobacteriaceae can be separated from nonfermentative strains, thereby providing information that can be used to guide empirical antimicrobial therapy. Highly selective or organism-specific media are useful for the recovery of organisms such as *Salmonella* and *Shigella* in stool specimens, where an abundance of normal flora can obscure the presence of important pathogens.

It is difficult to recover *Y. enterocolitica* because this organism grows slowly at traditional incubation temperatures and prefers cooler temperatures, where it is more active metabolically. Clinical laboratories have exploited this property, however, by mixing the fecal specimen with saline and then storing the specimen at 4° C for 2 weeks or more before subculturing it to agar media. This **cold enrichment** permits the growth of yersiniae but inhibits or kills other organisms in the specimen. Although use of cold enrichment method does not aid in the initial management of a patient with *Yersinia* gastroenteritis, it has helped elucidate the role of this organism in chronic intestinal disease.

Biochemical Identification

There are many diverse species in the family Enterobacteriaceae. The references listed at the end of this chapter provide additional information about biochemical identification. Biochemical test systems have become increasingly sophisticated, and now virtually all members of the family can be identified accurately in 4 to 24 hours with one of several commercially available identification systems.

Serological Classification

Serological testing is very useful for determining the clinical significance of an isolate (e.g., serotyping specific pathogenic strains such as *E. coli* O157:H7 or *Y. enterocolitica* O8) and for classifying isolates for epidemiological purposes. However, the usefulness of this procedure is limited by cross-reactions with antigenically related Enterobacteriaceae organisms as well as with organisms from other families.

TREATMENT, PREVENTION, AND CONTROL

Antibiotic therapy for infections with Enterobacteriaceae must be guided by in vitro susceptibility test results and clinical experience. Whereas some organisms such as *E. coli* and *P. mirabilis* are susceptible to many antibiotics, others can be highly resistant. Furthermore, susceptible organisms exposed to subtherapeutic concentrations of antibiotics in a hospital setting can rapidly develop resistance. In general, antibiotic resistance is more common in hospital-acquired infections than in community-acquired infections. Antibiotic therapy is not rec-

ommended for some infections. For example, symptomatic relief, but not antibiotic treatment, is usually recommended for patients with *Salmonella* gastroenteritis because antibiotics can prolong the fecal carriage of this organism.

It is difficult to prevent infections with Enterobacteriaceae because these organisms are a major part of the endogenous microbial population. However, some risk factors for the infections should be avoided. These include the unrestricted use of antibiotics that can select for resistant bacteria, the performance of procedures that traumatize mucosal barriers without prophylactic antibiotic coverage, and the use of urinary catheters. Unfortunately, many of these factors are present in patients at greatest risk for infection (e.g., immunocompromised patients confined to the hospital for extensive periods).

Exogenous infection with Enterobacteriaceae is theoretically easier to control. For example, the source of infections with organisms such as *Salmonella* is well defined. However, these bacteria are ubiquitous in poultry and eggs. Unless care is taken in the preparation and refrigeration of such foods, little can be done to control these infections. *Shigella* organisms are predominantly transmitted in young children, but it is difficult to interrupt the fecal-hand-mouth transmission responsible for spreading the infection in this population. Outbreaks of these infections can be effectively prevented and controlled only through the education of the people and the introduction of appropriate infection-control procedures (e.g., handwashing, proper disposal of soiled diapers and linens) in the settings where these infections typically occur.

Vaccination with formalin-killed *Y. pestis* has proved effective for people at high risk. Chemoprophylaxis with tetracycline has also proved useful for people in close contact with a patient with pneumonic plague. The administration of live, attenuated *S. typhi* vaccines has led to a 50% reduction in the incidence of typhoid fever in populations in which the incidence of endemic disease is high. However, this protection is short lived. Inactivated whole-cell vaccines, as well as vaccination with purified Vi antigen (the polysaccharide capsular antigen of *S. typhi* associated with virulence), are also protective.

CASE STUDY AND QUESTIONS

A 25-year-old, previously healthy woman came to the emergency room for the evaluation of bloody diarrhea and diffuse abdominal pain of 24 hours' duration. She complained of nausea and had vomited twice. She denied a history of inflammatory bowel disease, previous diarrhea, or contact with other people with diarrhea. The symptoms began 24 hours after she ate an undercooked hamburger at a local fast-food restaurant. Rectal examination revealed watery stool with gross blood. Sigmoidoscopy showed diffuse mucosal erythema and petechiae with a modest exudation but no ulceration or pseudomembranes. Cultures for *Salmonella*, *Shigella*, and *Yersinia* organisms and the examination for enteric parasites were negative.

1. Which two species of Enterobacteriaceae have been associated with hemorrhagic colitis? What virulence factor mediates this disease?
2. *Escherichia, Salmonella, Shigella,* and *Yersinia* organisms can all invade cells lining the intestines. What are the similarities and differences in the pathogenesis of the diseases caused by these bacteria?
3. What are the four forms of *Salmonella* infection?
4. Differentiate between disease caused by *S. typhi* and that caused by *S. sonnei*.
5. Describe the epidemiology of *Y. pestis* infections.

Bibliography

Brubaker RR: Factors promoting acute and chronic diseases caused by yersiniae, *Clin Microbiol Rev* 4:309-324, 1991.

Butler T: *Yersinia* infections: centennial of the discovery of the plague bacillus, *Clin Infect Dis* 19:655-663, 1994.

Cover TL, Aber RC: *Yersinia enterocolitica, N Engl J Med* 321:16-24, 1989.

Duplaix N: Fleas: the lethal leapers, *Natl Geograph* pp 672-694, May 1988.

Farmer JJ: *Enterobacteriaceae: introduction and identification.* In Murray PR et al, editors: *Manual of clinical microbiology,* ed 6, Washington, DC, 1995, American Society for Microbiology.

Gilchrist MJ: *Enterobacteriaceae: opportunistic pathogens and other genera.* In Murray PR et al, editors: *Manual of clinical microbiology,* ed 6, Washington, DC, 1995, American Society for Microbiology.

Gray LD: Escherichia, Salmonella, Shigella, *and* Yersinia. In Murray PR et al, editors: *Manual of clinical microbiology,* ed 6, Washington, DC, 1995, American Society for Microbiology.

Holt JG et al: *Bergey's manual of determinative bacteriology,* ed 9, Baltimore, 1994, Williams & Wilkins.

Johnson JR: Virulence factors in *Escherichia coli* urinary tract infection, *Clin Microbiol Rev* 4:80-128, 1991.

Kaye SA, Obrig T: Pathogenesis of *E. coli* hemolytic uremic syndrome, *Clin Microbiol Newsletter* 18:49-51, 1996.

Miller VL et al, editors: *Molecular genetics of bacterial pathogenesis,* Washington, DC, 1994, American Society for Microbiology.

Moulder JW: Comparative biology of intracellular parasitism, *Microbiol Rev* 49:298-337, 1985.

Reisner BS: Plague: past and present, *Clin Microbiol Newsletter* 18:153-155, 1996.

Salyers AA, Whitt DD: *Bacterial pathogenesis: a molecular approach,* Washington, DC, 1994, American Society for Microbiology.

Sansonetti PJ: Molecular and cellular biology of *Shigella flexneri* invasiveness: from cell assay systems to shigellosis, *Curr Topics Microbiol Immunol* 180:1-19, 1992.

Su C, Brandt LJ: *Escherichia coli* O157:H7 infection in humans, *Ann Intern Med* 123:698-714, 1995.

Tarr PI: *Escherichia coli* O157:H7: clinical, diagnostic, and epidemiological aspects of human infection, *Clin Infect Dis* 20:1-10, 1995.

CHAPTER······· 30

Vibrio, Aeromonas, and Plesiomonas

The second major group of gram-negative, facultatively anaerobic (i.e., growing aerobically and anaerobically), fermentative bacilli are the genera *Vibrio, Aeromonas,* and *Plesiomonas.* These organisms are distinguished from the Enterobacteriaceae by a positive oxidase reaction and the presence of polar flagella. They were at one time classified together in the family Vibrionaceae, in part because of their similar physiological properties and in part because they are primarily found in water and are well known for their ability to produce gastrointestinal disease. However, molecular biology techniques have established that these genera are only distantly related and belong in three separate families: Vibrionaceae, Aeromonadaceae, and Plesiomonadaceae. Despite this taxonomic reorganization, it is appropriate to consider these bacteria together because their epidemiology and range of diseases are similar.

VIBRIO

The genus *Vibrio* is composed of more than 34 species of curve-shaped bacilli. A total of 11 species have been implicated in human infections (Table 30-1), with *V. cholerae, V. parahaemolyticus,* and *V. vulnificus* the most prominent.

Physiology and Structure

Vibrio species can grow on a variety of simple media within a broad temperature range (from 18° to 37° C). *V. cholerae* can grow in the absence of salt; other species that are pathogenic in humans require salt (halophilic). *V. cholerae,* the etiological agent of cholera, is the best-known member of the genus; the disease was first documented more than 2000 years ago. Members of the species are subdivided on the basis of their somatic O antigens, with 139 described to date. *V. cholerae* O1 and O139 are responsible for causing classic cholera, which can occur in epidemics or pandemics. Other strains of *V. cholerae* can also cause human disease but not in epidemics. *V. cholerae* O1 can be subdivided into two biotypes (*el tor* and *cholerae*). These groups are important for the epidemiological classification of isolates. *V. parahaemolyticus* can also be subdivided on the basis of differences in the somatic O antigens.

Pathogenesis and Immunity

Multiple chromosomal genes involved in the virulence of *V. cholerae* O1 have been characterized (Table 30-2). These include genes for the two subunits of cholera toxin (*ctx*A and *ctx*B), the toxin coregulated pilus (*tcp*) gene complex, accessory colonization factor (*acf*) genes, the hemagglutination-protease (*hap*) gene, the zona occludens toxin (*zot*) gene, and the accessory cholera enterotoxin (*ace*) gene. Regulatory genes control the expression of these genes. Clearly, the best studied and most important of these virulence factors is **cholera toxin.** This toxin is a complex A-B toxin that binds to specific receptors in the small intestine, enters the mucosal cells, and effects a series of reactions that result in the rapid secretion of sodium, potassium, and bicarbonate into the intestinal lumen (Figure 30-1). Severely infected patients can lose as much as 1 L of fluid per hour during the height of the disease. Such a tremendous loss of fluid would normally flush the organisms out of the gastrointestinal tract; however, *V. cholerae* are able to adhere to the mucosal cell layer by the pili encoded by the *tcp* gene complex and the *acf* genes that code for an adhesin. Nonadherent strains are unable to establish infection. The release of bacteria from cells (e.g., after cell death) is mediated by the enzymatic activity of the *hap* gene product. The precise role of the *zot* toxin and *ace* toxin in disease remains undefined. Unlike other non-O1 serotypes, *V. cholerae* O139 possesses the same virulence complex possessed by the O1 strains. Thus the ability of the O139 strains to adhere to the intestinal mucosa and produce cholera toxin is the reason for these strains being as virulent as O1 strains.

The means by which other *Vibrio* species cause disease are less clearly understood, although a variety of potential virulence factors have been identified (Table 30-3). Most virulent strains of *V. parahaemolyticus* produce a heat-stable hemolysin (**Kanagawa-positive** strains) that is cytotoxic and cardiotoxic in experimental animals. Virulent vibrios can also adhere to and invade the intestinal tissue (unlike *V. cholerae,* which is considered an adherent but noninvasive pathogen).

Epidemiology

Vibrio species, including *V. cholerae,* grow naturally in estuarine and marine environments worldwide. All *Vibrio*

245

TABLE 30-1 *Vibrio* Species Associated with Human Disease

SPECIES	SOURCE OF INFECTION	CLINICAL DISEASE
V. cholerae*	Water, food	Gastroenteritis
V. parahaemolyticus	Shellfish, seawater	Gastroenteritis, wound infection, bacteremia
V. vulnificus	Shellfish, seawater	Bacteremia, wound infection, cellulitis
V. alginolyticus	Seawater	Wound infection, external otitis
V. hollisae	Shellfish	Gastroenteritis, wound infection, bacteremia
V. fluvialis	Seafood	Gastroenteritis, wound infection, bacteremia
V. damsela	Seawater	Wound infection
V. furnissii†	Unknown	Gastroenteritis
V. metschnikovii†	Unknown	Bacteremia
V. cincinnatiensis†	Unknown	Bacteremia, meningitis
V. carchariae†	Seawater	Wound (shark bite)

*V. mimicus, believed to be an atypical strain of V. cholerae, is included here.
†Isolates rarely associated with human infection.

The complete toxin binding to the GM1-ganglioside receptor on the cell membrane via the binding subunits (B).

The active portion (A₁) of the A subunit enters the cell and activates adenyl cyclase.

This activity results in accumulation of cyclic adenosine 3', 5' mono phosphate (cAMP) along the cell membrane.

The cAMP causes the active secretion of sodium (Na⁺), chloride (Cl⁻), potassium (K⁺), bicarbonate (HCO₃⁻), and water (H₂O) out of the cell into the intestinal lumen.

FIGURE 30-1 Mechanism of action of cholera toxin.

TABLE 30-2 Virulence Factors of *V. cholerae* O1 and O139

VIRULENCE FACTOR	BIOLOGICAL EFFECT
Cholera toxin	Hypersecretion of electrolytes and water
Coregulated pilus	Adherence to mucosal cells
Accessory colonization factor	Adhesin
Hemagglutination-protease (mucinase)	Releases bacteria from mucosal cells
Zona occludens toxin	Exotoxin
Accessory cholera enterotoxin	Exotoxin
Flagellum	Motility
Siderophores	Iron sequestration

TABLE 30-3 Virulence Factors of Other Species

ORGANISM	VIRULENCE FACTORS
V. parahaemolyticus	Cytotoxin, hemolysin, adhesin, mucinase
V. vulnificus	Serum resistance, antiphagocytic polysaccharides, cytolysins, collagenase, protease, siderophore
V. alginolyticus	Collagenase
V. hollisae	Heat-stable and heat-labile enterotoxin, hemolysin
V. damsela	Cytolysin

species appear able to survive and replicate in contaminated waters with increased salinity and at temperatures of 10° to 30° C. Pathogenic vibrios can also flourish in waters with chitinous shellfish, hence the association between *Vibrio* infections and the consumption of shellfish. Asymptomatically infected humans can also be an important reservoir for this organism in areas where *V. cholerae* disease is endemic.

Seven major pandemics of cholera have occurred since 1817, resulting in thousands of deaths and major socioeconomic changes. Sporadic disease and epidemics occurred before this time, but worldwide spread of the disease became possible only with intercontinental travel resulting from increased commerce and wars. The seventh pandemic, which was caused by *V. cholerae* O1 biotype *el tor*, began in Asia in 1961 and spread to Africa, Europe, and Oceania in the 1970s and 1980s. In 1991 the pandemic strain spread to Peru and subsequently has caused disease in most countries in South and Central America, as well as in the United States and Canada (Figure 30-2). By June 1995 more than 1 million cases and 10,000 deaths resulting from the disease had been reported in the Americas. A new epidemic strain emerged in 1992 in India and has rapidly spread across Asia. The strain, **V. cholerae O139 Bengal,** is the first non-O1 strain capable of causing epidemic disease; it produces disease in adults who were ill with the O1 strain (showing that no protective immunity is conferred) and appears destined to be responsible for causing the next pandemic.

Cholera is spread by contaminated water and food. Direct person-to-person spread is unusual, because a high inoculum (e.g., 10^8 organisms) is required to establish infection in a person with normal gastric acidity. The infectious dose in a person with achlorhydria or hypochlorhydria can be reduced to 10^3 to 10^5 organisms. Cholera is usually seen in communities with poor sanitation. Indeed, one benefit from the cholera pandemics was recognition of the role of contaminated water in the spread of disease and the need to improve community sanitation systems so that the disease could be controlled.

Infections caused by *V. parahaemolyticus, V. vulnificus,* and other pathogenic vibrios result from the consumption of improperly cooked seafood, particularly oysters, or exposure to contaminated seawater. Gastroenteritis caused by vibrios occurs throughout the year because oysters are typically contaminated with abundant organisms year-round. In contrast, septicemia and wound infections with *Vibrio* occur during the warm months when the number of organisms in seawater is high.

Clinical Syndromes

Vibrio cholerae

Infection with *V. cholerae* O1 can range from asymptomatic colonization or a mild diarrheal disease to severe, rapidly fatal diarrhea (Box 30-1). The clinical manifesta-

FIGURE 30-2 Spread of pandemic *V. cholerae* O1 *el tor* in the Americas from 1991 to 1994. (From Tauxe RV et al: *Emerging Infect Dis* 1:141-146, 1995.)

tions of cholera begin an average of 2 to 3 days after ingestion of the bacilli, with the abrupt onset of watery diarrhea and vomiting. As more fluid is lost, the feces-streaked stool specimens become colorless and odorless, free of protein, and speckled with mucus flecks (**rice-water stools**). The resulting severe fluid and electrolyte loss can lead to dehydration, metabolic acidosis (bicarbonate loss), and hypokalemia and hypovolemic shock (potassium loss), with cardiac arrhythmia and renal failure. The mortality rate is 60% in untreated patients but less than 1% in patients promptly treated to replace lost fluids and electrolytes. Cholera can resolve spontaneously after a few days of symptoms. Disease caused by *V. cholerae* O139 appears to be worse than disease caused by *V. cholerae* O1, with a higher incidence of severe dehydration and death. Gastroenteritis caused by other serotypes of *V. cholerae* is milder and not associated with epidemics.

Vibrio parahaemolyticus

The severity of gastroenteritis caused by *V. parahaemolyticus* can range from a self-limiting diarrhea to a mild cholera-like illness. In general the disease develops

BOX 30-1   Summary of *V. cholerae* Infections

BACTERIAL FACTORS

Disease—cholera.

Virulence factors—see Table 30-2.

Two biotypes: *V. cholerae* O1 biotype *cholerae* causes more severe disease than biotype *el tor*.

139 O antigens have been characterized; only strains with O1 or O139 can produce cholera toxin and cause pandemic disease.

TRANSMISSION

Bacteria can grow in estuarine and marine environment, particularly one with chitinous shellfish.

Asymptomatic human carriers serve as sources for the contamination of water or food.

Disease caused by the ingestion of large numbers of organisms in contaminated water or food.

Infectious inoculum less in patients whose gastric acidity is reduced.

WHO IS AT RISK?

People living in communities with poor sanitation.

People who consume raw shellfish, particularly oysters.

GEOGRAPHY/SEASON

Contaminated estuarine and marine waters.

V. cholerae gastroenteritis is not typically seasonal, but bacterial levels increase in contaminated waters during the warm months. The incidence of wound infections and septicemia caused by other vibrios increases during warm months.

MODES OF CONTROL

Fluid and electrolyte replacement is crucial.

Antibiotic therapy reduces the bacterial burden and exotoxin production; doxycycline (adults), trimethoprim-sulfamethoxazole (children), or furazolidone (pregnant women) is administered.

Improved hygiene is critical for control.

Killed cholera vaccine is of limited value for preventing O1 infections and of no value for preventing O139 infections.

---

after a 5- to 72-hour incubation period (mean, 24 hours) with an explosive, watery diarrhea. No gross blood or mucus is found in stool specimens except in very severe cases. Headache, abdominal cramps, nausea, vomiting, and low-grade fever may persist for 72 hours or more. The patient usually experiences an uneventful recovery. Wound infections with this organism can occur in people exposed to contaminated seawater.

Vibrio vulnificus

V. vulnificus is a particularly virulent species of *Vibrio* responsible for rapidly progressive wound infections after exposure to contaminated seawater and for septicemia after consumption of contaminated raw oysters. The wound infections are characterized by initial swelling, erythema, and pain followed by the development of vesicles or bullae and eventual tissue necrosis. Patients usually experience systemic signs of fever and chills. The mortality in patients with *V. vulnificus* septicemia can be as high as 50% unless antimicrobial therapy is started rapidly. Infections are most severe in patients with hepatic disease, hematopoietic disease, or chronic renal failure and in those receiving immunosuppressive drugs.

Other *Vibrio* Species

V. alginolyticus can cause infection in superficial wounds exposed to contaminated seawater. Infections of the ear, eye, and gastrointestinal tract have also been reported rarely. *V. hollisae*, *V. fluvialis*, *V. furnissii*, and *V. damsela* are responsible for causing gastroenteritis, wound infec-

tions, and bacteremia. Single cases of infections with *V. metschnikovii* (bacteremia), *V. cincinnatiensis* (meningitis), and *V. carchariae* (wound infection) have been documented.

Laboratory Diagnosis

Microscopy

Vibrio species are small (0.5×1.5 to $3 \mu m$), curved, gram-negative bacilli. The organisms are rarely seen in Gram-stained stool or wound specimens; however, an experienced observer using darkfield microscopy may be able to detect the characteristic motile bacilli.

Culture

Vibrio organisms survive poorly in an acidic or dry environment. Specimens must be collected early in the disease and cultured promptly onto media. If culturing is delayed, the specimen should be mixed in a Cary-Blair transport medium and refrigerated. Vibrios survive poorly in buffered glycerol-saline, the transport medium used for most enteric pathogens.

Vibrios grow on most media used in clinical laboratories for stool cultures, including blood agar and MacConkey agar. Special selective agar for vibrios (e.g., thiosulfate citrate bile salts sucrose agar), as well as an enrichment broth (e.g., alkaline peptone broth; pH, 8.6), can also be used. Isolates are identified with selective biochemical tests and serotyped using polyvalent antisera. In tests done to identify halophilic vibrios, the media must be supplemented with 1% sodium chloride.

Treatment, Prevention, and Control

Patients with cholera must be promptly treated with fluid and electrolyte replacement before the resultant massive fluid loss leads to hypovolemic shock. Antibiotic therapy, although of secondary value, can reduce exotoxin production and more rapidly eliminate the organism. Doxycycline or tetracycline is the drug of choice for adults, furazolidone is used for pregnant women, and trimethoprim-sulfamethoxazole is used for children. *V. cholerae* has been reported to be resistant to trimethoprim-sulfamethoxazole. *V. parahaemolyticus* gastroenteritis is usually a self-limited disease, although antibiotic therapy can be used in addition to fluid and electrolyte therapy in patients with severe infections. *V. vulnificus* wound infections and septicemia must be promptly treated with antibiotic therapy. Tetracycline is the most effective drug in vivo, although some success has been reported for the aminoglycosides.

Because vibrios are free living in estuarine and marine reservoirs and the incidence of human carriage of *V. cholerae* can range from 1% to 20% in previously infected patients, it is unlikely that the reservoir for this organism will be eradicated. Only improved sanitation can lead to effective control of the disease. This involves adequate sewage management, the use of purification systems to eliminate contamination of the water supply, and the implementation of appropriate steps to prevent contamination of food.

Although there is a killed cholera vaccine for O1 strains, the protection is short lived. Currently the vaccine is not recommended for people traveling to areas with endemic disease. There is no vaccine for the O139 strains. Tetracycline prophylaxis has also been used to reduce the risk of infection in people traveling to areas where the disease is endemic but has not prevented the spread of cholera. Because the infectious dose of *V. cholerae* is high, antibiotic prophylaxis is generally unnecessary in people who use appropriate hygiene.

AEROMONAS

Aeromonas is a gram-negative, facultative anaerobic bacillus that morphologically resembles members of the Enterobacteriaceae. A total of 11 species of *Aeromonas* have been described, including 9 associated with human disease; *A. hydrophila, A. caviae,* and *A. veronii* biovar *sobria* are most commonly isolated. The organisms are ubiquitous in fresh and brackish water, and infections typically occur after the ingestion of contaminated water or food. The asymptomatic gastrointestinal carriage of this organism is less than 3%, with a peak in carriage and disease during the warm months.

Although numerous potential virulence factors (e.g., endotoxin, hemolysins, enterotoxin, proteases, siderophores, adherence factors) have been identified, their precise role is unknown. *Aeromonas* species cause opportunistic systemic disease in immunocompromised patients (particularly those with hepatobiliary disease or an

TABLE 30-4	**Characteristics of *Aeromonas* and *Plesiomonas* Gastroenteritis**	
EPIDEMIOLOGICAL AND CLINICAL FEATURES	**AEROMONAS**	**PLESIOMONAS**
Natural habitat	Fresh or brackish water	Fresh or brackish water
Source of infection	Contaminated water or food	Contaminated water or food; contact with amphibians or reptiles
Clinical presentation		
Diarrhea	Present	Present
Vomiting	Present	Present
Abdominal cramps	Present	Present
Fever	Absent	Absent
Blood/leukocytes in stool	Absent	Present
Pathogenesis	Enterotoxin (?)	Invasive

underlying malignancy), diarrheal disease in otherwise healthy people, and wound infections (Table 30-4). Gastrointestinal disease in children is usually an acute, severe illness, whereas adults tend to have chronic diarrhea. Severe gastroenteritis resembles shigellosis in that blood and leukocytes are present in the stool of affected patients.

Acute diarrheal disease is self-limited, and only supportive care is indicated in such patients. Antimicrobial therapy is necessary in patients with chronic diarrheal disease or systemic infection. *Aeromonas* organisms are resistant to penicillins, most cephalosporins, and erythromycin; only gentamicin, trimethoprim-sulfamethoxazole, and chloramphenicol are consistently active.

PLESIOMONAS

The genus *Plesiomonas* consists of facultative anaerobic, gram-negative bacilli that are oxidase positive, have multiple polar flagella, and are differentiated from *Aeromonas* organisms by selected biochemical reactions. Only one species has been described, *P. shigelloides,* which is taxonomically related to *Proteus* species and serologically related to *Shigella sonnei.* The organism is found in freshwater and estuarine waters and is acquired through contact with fresh water, the consumption of seafood, or exposure to amphibians or reptiles.

As with *Aeromonas,* the absence of an animal model has prevented researchers from defining the pathogenic mechanisms of *Plesiomonas* disease. The primary disease caused by *P. shigelloides* is a self-limiting gastroenteritis (secretory, colitis, or chronic form), with the onset of disease occurring 48 hours after exposure to the organism. A variety of uncommon extraintestinal infections have also been described. Asymptomatic carriage is rare.

The organism is susceptible to chloramphenicol, cephalosporins, imipenem, trimethoprim-sulfamethoxazole, and fluoroquinolones. The organism is not susceptible to ampicillin, carbenicillin, erythromycin, and many aminoglycosides.

CASE STUDY AND QUESTIONS

A 57-year-old man was hospitalized in New York City with a 2-day history of severe, watery diarrhea. The illness began 1 day after he had returned from Ecuador. The patient was dehydrated and suffering from an electrolyte imbalance (acidosis, hypokalemia). The patient made an uneventful recovery after fluid and electrolyte replacement was instituted to compensate for the losses resulting from the watery diarrhea. Stool cultures were positive for *V. cholerae*.

1. What are the characteristic clinical signs of cholera?
2. What is the most important virulence factor in this disease? What other virulence factors have been described? What are the modes of their action?
3. How did this patient acquire this infection? How does this differ from the acquisition of infections caused by *V. parahaemolyticus* or *V. vulnificus*?
4. How can cholera be controlled in areas where infection is endemic?

Bibliography

Albert MJ: *Vibrio cholerae* O139 Bengal, *J Clin Microbiol* 32:2345-2349, 1994.

Besser RE et al: Diagnosis and treatment of cholera in the United States: are we prepared? *JAMA* 272:1203-1205, 1994.

Calia KE: *Vibrio cholerae* O139: an emerging pathogen, *Clin Microbiol Newsletter* 18:17-22, 1996.

Clark RB, Janda JM: *Plesiomonas* and human disease, *Clin Microbiol Newsletter* 13:49-52, 1991.

Hlady WG, Klontz KC: The epidemiology of *Vibrio* infections in Florida, 1981-1993, *J Infect Dis* 173:1176-1183, 1996.

Holmberg SD, Farmer JJ III: *Aeromonas hydrophila* and *Plesiomonas shigelloides* as causes of intestinal infections, *Rev Infect Dis* 6:633-639, 1984.

Janda JM: Recent advances in the study of the taxonomy, pathogenicity, and infectious syndromes associated with the genus *Aeromonas*, *Clin Microbiol Rev* 4:397-410, 1991.

Janda JM et al: *Aeromonas* species in septicemia: laboratory characteristics and clinical observations, *Clin Infect Dis* 19:77-83, 1994.

Ko W-C, Chuang Y-C: *Aeromonas* bacteremia: review of 59 episodes, *Clin Infect Dis* 20:1298-1304, 1995.

Lacey SW: Cholera: calamitous past, ominous future, *Clin Infect Dis* 20:1409-1419, 1995.

Lang DR, Guerrant RL: Summary of the 29th United States–Japan Joint Conference on Cholera and Related Diarrheal Diseases, *J Infect Dis* 171:8-12, 1995.

Mahon BE et al: Reported cholera in the United States, 1992-1994: a reflection of global changes in cholera epidemiology, *JAMA* 276:307-312, 1996.

Salyers AA, Whitt DD: *Bacterial pathogenesis: a molecular approach*, Washington, DC, 1991, ASM.

Tauxe RV et al: Epidemic cholera in the new world: translating field epidemiology into new prevention strategies, *Emerging Infect Dis* 1:141-146, 1995.

Wachsmuth LK et al, editors: Vibrio cholerae *and cholera: molecular to global perspectives*, Washington DC, 1994, ASM.

Waldor MK, Mekalanos JJ: Emergence of a new cholera pandemic: molecular analysis of virulence determinants in *Vibrio cholerae* O139 and development of a live vaccine prototype, *J Infect Dis* 170:278-283, 1994.

31

Campylobacter and Helicobacter

The classification of *Campylobacter* and *Helicobacter* has undergone many changes since the bacteria were first isolated at the beginning of this century. However, molecular biology techniques (e.g., sequence analysis of 16S rRNA genes), characterization of cell wall proteins and lipids, serological characterization, and analysis of biochemical properties have been used to resolve much of the taxonomic confusion. These genera, with *Arcobacter, Wolinella,* and *Flexispira,* belong to the same rRNA superfamily (Box 31-1), which consists of spiral, gram-negative bacilli with a low DNA–guanosine plus cytosine base ratio, an inability to ferment or oxidize carbohydrates (in contrast with the bacteria discussed in Chapters 29 and 30), and microaerophilic growth requirements (i.e., growth only in the presence of a reduced oxygen level). *Campylobacter* and *Arcobacter* are grouped into the family Campylobacteriaceae; *Helicobacter, Wolinella,* and *Flexispira* are grouped into an unnamed family. Because *Campylobacter* and *Helicobacter* species are the most commonly isolated and clinically important members of this superfamily, they are the only genera discussed in this chapter.

CAMPYLOBACTER

The genus *Campylobacter,* from the Greek word *kampylos* for "curved," consists of comma-shaped, gram-negative bacilli (Figure 31-1) that are oxidase and catalase positive and motile by means of a polar flagellum. A total of 15 species and 6 subspecies are now recognized; 12 of the species are associated with human disease (Table 31-1). Diseases caused by campylobacters are primarily gastroenteritis and septicemia. *C. jejuni* is the most common cause of bacterial gastroenteritis in the United States, and *C. coli* is responsible for 2% to 5% of the cases of *Campylobacter* gastroenteritis. The latter is a more common cause of gastroenteritis in underdeveloped countries. A variety of other species are rare causes of gastroenteritis or systemic infections. Unlike other species, *C. fetus* is most commonly responsible for causing systemic infections such as bacteremia, septic thrombophlebitis, arthritis, septic abortion, and meningitis.

Physiology and Structure

Campylobacter organisms have a typical gram-negative cell wall structure. The major antigen of the genus is the lipopolysaccharide of the outer membrane. In addition, the different somatic O polysaccharide antigens and the heat-labile capsular and flagellar antigens have been used for the epidemiological classification of clinical isolates.

Recognition of the role of campylobacters in gastrointestinal disease was delayed because the organisms grow best in an atmosphere of reduced oxygen (5% to 7%, microaerophilic) and increased carbon dioxide (5% to 10%). In addition, *C. jejuni* grow better at 42° C than at 37° C. These properties have now been exploited for the selective isolation of pathogenic campylobacters in stool specimens. The small size of the organisms (0.3 to 0.6 μm in diameter) has also been used to recover the bacteria by filtering stool specimens. Campylobacters pass through 0.45-μm filters, whereas other bacteria are retained.

Pathogenesis and Immunity

The major factors determining whether disease develops are the infectious dose of the organisms and the level of a person's immunity. Disease is more likely to develop in patients exposed to a large number of organisms or, for example, in those who lack gastric acids. People in a population of high endemic disease develop measurable levels of specific serum and secretory antibodies and have less severe disease. Patients with hypogammaglobulinemia have prolonged, severe disease with *C. jejuni.*

The pathogenesis of *C. jejuni* gastrointestinal disease is not completely understood. The mucosal surfaces of the jejunum (as implied by the name), ileum, and colon are damaged in the disease. On gross examination the mucosal surface appears edematous and bloody. Histologically the mucosal surface is ulcerated, with crypt abscesses in the epithelial glands and infiltration of the lamina propria with neutrophils, mononuclear cells, and eosinophils. This inflammatory process is consistent with invasion of the organisms into the intestinal tissue. Enterotoxins, cytopathic toxins, and endotoxic activity have been detected in *C. jejuni* isolates. However, the precise

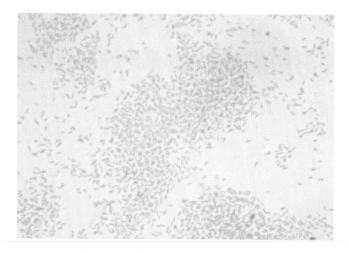

FIGURE 31-1 Gram stain showing *Campylobacter* organisms. Note the curved bacilli.

BOX 31-1   Members of Superfamily Vi of Class Proteobacteria

Campylobacter—15 species, 6 subspecies
Arcobacter—4 species
Helicobacter—17 species
Wolinella—1 species
Flexispira—1 species

roles of these factors in disease have not been defined. For example, strains lacking enterotoxin activity are still fully virulent. An adhesin that mediates the attachment of the organisms to the mucosal layer has been described. Strains without the adhesin, as well as nonmotile strains, are avirulent.

C. fetus has a propensity to spread from the gastrointestinal tract to the bloodstream and distal foci. This is particularly common in debilitated and immunocompromised patients, such as those with liver disease, diabetes mellitus, chronic alcoholism, or malignancies. In vitro studies have shown that *C. fetus* is resistant to complement- and antibody-mediated serum killing, whereas *C. jejuni* is killed rapidly. *C. fetus* is covered with a capsulelike protein (**S protein**) that prevents complement-mediated killing in serum (inhibition of C3b binding to the bacteria). *C. fetus* loses its virulence in an animal model if this protein layer is removed.

Specific serum and secretory antibodies that provide strain-specific immunity typically develop in patients who have been exposed to campylobacters. Although patients may be recolonized with the bacteria, disease is uncommon.

Epidemiology

Campylobacter infections are zoonotic, with a variety of animals serving as reservoirs (Table 31-1). Humans acquire the infections from the consumption of contaminated food, milk, or water; contaminated poultry is responsible for more than half of the *Campylobac-*

TABLE 31-1   *Campylobacter* Species Associated with Human Disease

SPECIES	RESERVOIR HOST	HUMAN DISEASE	FREQUENCY
C. jejuni subsp. jejuni	Poultry, pigs, bulls, dogs, cats, birds, mink, rabbits, insects	Gastroenteritis, septicemia, meningitis, spontaneous abortion, proctitis, Guillain-Barré syndrome	Common
C. jejuni subsp. doylei	Humans	Gastroenteritis, gastritis, septicemia	Uncommon
C. coli	Pigs, poultry, bulls, sheep, birds	Gastroenteritis, septicemia, gastroenteritis, spontaneous abortion, meningitis	Uncommon
C. fetus subsp. fetus	Cattle, sheep	Septicemia, gastroenteritis, spontaneous abortion, meningitis	Uncommon
C. fetus subsp. venerealis	Cattle	Septicemia	Uncommon
C. hyointestinalis subsp. hyointestinalis	Pigs, cattle, hamsters, deer	Gastroenteritis	Rare
C. concisus	Humans	Periodontal disease, gastroenteritis	Rare
C. sputorum subspecies sputorum	Humans, cattle, pigs	Abscesses, gastroenteritis	Rare
C. curvus	Humans	Periodontal disease, gastroenteritis	Rare
C. rectus	Humans	Periodontal disease	Rare
C. showae	Humans	Periodontal disease	Rare
C. gracilis	Humans	Periodontal disease, empyema, abscesses	Rare
C. upsaliensis	Dogs, cats	Gastroenteritis, septicemia, abscesses	Rare
C. lari	Poultry, birds, dogs, cats, monkeys, horses, seals	Gastroenteritis, septicemia	Rare

Based on data from On SLW: *Clin Microbiol Rev* 9:405-422, 1996.

ter infections in developed countries. Food products that neutralize gastric acids (e.g., milk) effectively reduce the infectious dose. Fecal-oral transmission from person to person may also occur, but it is uncommon for the disease to be transmitted by food handlers (Box 31-2).

The actual incidence of *Campylobacter* infections is unknown because disease is not reported to public health officials. However, more than 2 million *C. jejuni* infections may occur annually, and such infections are more common than *Salmonella* and *Shigella* infections combined (Figure 31-2). Disease is most common in the warm months but occurs throughout the year. The peak incidence of disease is in young adults. In underdeveloped countries, symptomatic disease occurs in young children, and persistent, asymptomatic carriage is observed in adults.

C. fetus infections are relatively uncommon, with fewer than 250 cases reported annually. Unlike *C. jejuni*, *C. fetus* infects immunocompromised, elderly people.

Clinical Syndromes

C. jejuni infections are seen most commonly as acute enteritis with diarrhea, malaise, fever, and abdominal pain. Affected patients can have 10 or more bowel movements per day during the peak of disease, and stools may be grossly bloody. The disease is generally self-limiting, although symptoms may last for 1 week or longer. The range of clinical manifestations can include colitis, acute abdominal pain, and bacteremia. In the most common presentation of *C. fetus* infection, the patient initially experiences gastroenteritis followed by septicemia with dissemination to multiple organs.

Laboratory Diagnosis

Microscopy

C. jejuni are thin (0.3 μm) and cannot be easily seen in Gram-stained specimens. When observed, the organisms appear as small, curved bacilli. The organism, with its characteristic darting motility, can be detected by dark-field or phase-contrast microscopy in freshly collected stool specimens; however, this is rarely done.

Culture

C. jejuni went unrecognized for many years because isolation requires growth in a microaerophilic atmosphere

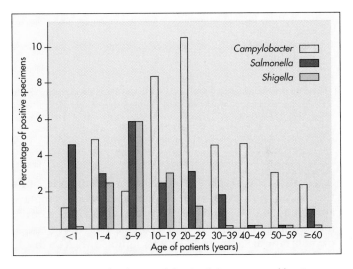

FIGURE 31-2 Age distribution of diarrheal disease caused by *Campylobacter*, *Salmonella*, and *Shigella* organisms.

BOX 31-2   **Summary of *Campylobacter* Infections**

BACTERIAL FACTORS

Diseases—gastroenteritis (primarily *C. jejuni*, *C. coli*), septicemia (primarily *C. fetus*).

Virulence factors—Factors that regulate adhesion, motility, and invasion into intestinal mucosa are poorly defined for *C. jejuni* and *C. coli*; S protein in *C. fetus* inhibits C3b binding and subsequent complement-mediated phagocytosis and killing.

TRANSMISSION

Zoonotic infection.

Animals with asymptomatic carriage: important reservoir of infection for humans.

Ingestion of contaminated food (especially poultry), milk, or water.

WHO IS AT RISK?

People who ingest undercooked poultry, unpasteurized milk, contaminated water, and uncooked foods prepared on surfaces where poultry was prepared.

WHO IS AT RISK?—cont'd

People who receive high infectious dose, except for patients with reduced gastric acid levels.

C. fetus infections primarily in immunocompromised elderly patients.

GEOGRAPHY/SEASON

Worldwide.

More common in warm months.

MODES OF CONTROL

For gastroenteritis, infection is self-limited and is managed by fluid and electrolyte replacement.

Severe gastroenteritis and septicemia are treated with erythromycin (drug of choice), tetracyclines, aminoglycosides, chloramphenicol, quinolones, or clindamycin.

Gastroenteritis is prevented by proper preparation of food and consumption of pasteurized milk; prevention of contaminated water supplies also controls infection.

| TABLE 31-2 | Phenotypic Properties of *Campylobacter* and *Helicobacter* Species |

CHARACTERISTICS	C. JEJUNI	C. COLI	C. FETUS	H. PYLORI	H. CINAEDI	H. FENNELLIAE
Oxidase	+	+	+	+	+	+
Catalase	+	+	+	+	+	+
Nitrate reduction	+	+	+	−	+	−
Urease	−	−	−	+	−	−
Hydrolysis of						
Hippurate	+	−	−	−	−	−
Indoxyl acetate	+	+	−	−	−	+
Growth at						
25° C	−	−	+	−	−	−
37° C	+	+	+	+	+	+
42° C	+	+	−	−	−	−
Growth in 1% glycine	+	+	+	−	+	+
Susceptibility to						
Nalidixic acid	S	S	V	R	S	S
Cephalothin	R	R	S	S	I	S

Based on data from Murray P et al, editors: *Manual of clinical microbiology*, ed 6, Washington DC, 1995, American Society for Microbiology.

+, Positive reaction; −, negative reaction; *S*, susceptible; *V*, variable reaction; *R*, resistant; *I*, intermediate.

(e.g., 5% to 7% oxygen, 5% to 10% carbon dioxide, and the balance nitrogen), at an elevated incubation temperature (e.g., 42° C), and on selective media. The selective media must contain blood or charcoal to remove toxic oxygen radicals and antibiotics to inhibit the growth of contaminating organisms. Campylobacters are slow-growing organisms, usually requiring incubation for 48 to 72 hours or longer. *C. fetus* is not thermophilic and cannot grow at 42° C. However, a microaerophilic atmosphere is still required for isolation.

Identification

Preliminary identification of isolates is based on growth under selective conditions, typical microscopic morphology, and detection of oxidase and catalase activity. Definitively identification of all isolates is guided by the reactions summarized in Table 31-2.

Treatment, Prevention, and Control

Campylobacter gastroenteritis is typically a self-limited infection managed by the replacement of lost fluids and electrolytes. Antibiotic therapy may be used in patients with severe infections or septicemia. Campylobacters are susceptible to a wide variety of antibiotics, including erythromycin, tetracyclines, aminoglycosides, chloramphenicol, quinolones, and clindamycin. Most isolates are resistant to penicillins, cephalosporins, and sulfonamide antibiotics. Erythromycin is the antibiotic of choice for the treatment of enteritis (tetracycline or quinolones are secondary antibiotics); systemic infections are treated with aminoglycosides.

Campylobacter gastroenteritis is prevented by the proper preparation of food, particularly poultry; the con-

sumption of pasteurized milk; and the implementation of safeguards to prevent the contamination of water supplies. It is unlikely that *Campylobacter* carriage in animal reservoirs such as chickens and turkeys will be eliminated.

HELICOBACTER

In 1983 spiral-shaped, gram-negative bacilli resembling campylobacters were found in patients with type B gastritis. The organisms were originally classified as *Campylobacter* but were subsequently reclassified as a new genus, *Helicobacter*. The bacteria, *H. pylori*, have now been shown to cause gastritis and peptic ulcers and are associated with gastric adenocarcinoma (Table 31-3). Helicobacters have been isolated from the stomachs of many other mammals (e.g., monkeys, dogs, cats, cheetahs, ferrets, mice, rats). The intestinal tract is also colonized by helicobacters, including *H. cinaedi* and *H. fennelliae*, which have been isolated from homosexual men with proctitis, proctocolitis, or enteritis.

Physiology and Structure

Helicobacter species are characterized by sequence analysis of their 16S rRNA genes; their cellular fatty acids; the presence of multiple polar, sheathed flagella; and selected biochemical tests (e.g., positive oxidase and catalase reactions, negative hippurate hydrolysis). Currently, 17 species have been characterized, but this taxonomy is rapidly changing. Helicobacters have a spiral shape in young cultures but assume coccoid forms in older cultures (Figure 31-3).

H. pylori is highly motile (corkscrew motility) and produce an abundance of urease. Urease production is a

TABLE 31-3 *Helicobacter* Species Associated with Human Disease

SPECIES	RESERVOIR HOST	HUMAN DISEASE	FREQUENCY
H. pylori	Humans, primates, pigs	Gastritis, peptic ulcers, gastric adenocarcinoma	Common
H. cinaedi	Humans, hamsters	Gastroenteritis, septicemia, proctocolitis, cellulitis	Uncommon
H. fennelliae	Humans	Gastroenteritis, septicemia, proctocolitis	Uncommon
H. canis	Dogs	Gastroenteritis	Rare
H. pullorum	Poultry	Gastroenteritis	Rare
H. strain "Mainz"	Humans	Septic arthritis	Rare
H. rappini	Humans, sheep, mice	Gastroenteritis	Rare
H. heilmanii	Humans	Gastritis	Rare

Based on data from On SL: *Clin Microbiol Rev* 9:405-422, 1996.

TABLE 31-4 Virulence Factors of *H. pylori*

VIRULENCE FACTOR	FUNCTION
Urease	Neutralizes gastric acids; stimulates monocytes and neutrophil chemotaxis
Acid-inhibitory protein	Induces hypochlorhydria during acute infection by blocking acid secretion from parietal cells
Flagella	Allows penetration into gastric mucous layer and protection from acid environment
Adhesins	Mediate binding to host cells (Examples of adhesins are hemagglutinins, sialic acid binding adhesin, Lewis blood group adhesin.)
Mucinase	Degrades gastric mucus
Superoxide dismutase	Prevents phagocytic killing by neutralizing oxygen metabolites
Catalase	Prevents phagocytic killing by neutralizing peroxides
Vacuolating cytotoxin	Induces vacuolation in epithelial cells; stimulates neutrophil migration into mucosa

consistent finding in *Helicobacter* species that colonize the stomach but is not seen in species found in the intestines.

Pathogenesis and Immunity

H. pylori possesses numerous potential virulence factors (Table 31-4). Initial colonization is facilitated by blockage of acid production of bacterial acid-inhibitory protein and neutralization of gastric acids by the ammonia produced from bacaterial urease activity. The actively motile helicobacters can then pass through the gastric mucus and adhere to the epithelial cells. Localized tissue damage is mediated by urease by-products, mucinase, and the activity of the vacuolating cytotoxin that induces epithelial cell damage and, together with urease and bacterial lipopolysaccharide, stimulates the inflammatory response. *H. pylori* is protected from phagocytosis and intracellular killing by production of superoxide dismutase and catalase. *H. pylori* also produces hemolysins, phospholipases, and alcohol dehydrogenase, but their role in disease is undefined.

Epidemiology

Serological studies performed in the United States have documented that the incidence of *H. pylori* infection in healthy people is relatively low during childhood but increases to approximately 45% in older adults (Box 31-3).

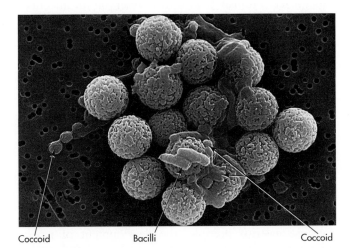

Coccoid   Bacilli   Coccoid

FIGURE 31-3 Scanning electron micrograph of *H. pylori* in a 7-day culture. Bacilli and coccoid forms *(arrows)* are bound to paramagnetic beads used in immunomagnetic separation. (Courtesy Dr. L. Engstrand, Uppsala, Sweden.)

However, considerable variations exist in the prevalence among different populations. For example, infection appears earlier in people in a low socioeconomic class and in developing nations. *H. pylori* is identified in 70% to 100% of patients with gastritis, gastric ulcers, and duo-

---

BOX 31-3   **Summary of *H. pylori* Infections**

BACTERIAL FACTORS

Diseases—gastritis, peptic ulcers, gastric adenocarcinoma (*H. pylori*); gastroenteritis, proctocolitis, septicemia, cellulitis (*H. cinaedi* and *H. fennelliae*).
Virulence factors—see Table 31-4.

TRANSMISSION

Not clearly defined, although person-to-person spread is most likely.
Humans are primary reservoir.

WHO IS AT RISK?

Older adults (incidence increases with age).
Infection appears earlier in people living in developing countries and in low socioeconomic populations.
Homosexual males are at increased risk for infections with *H. cinaedi* and *H. fennelliae*.

GEOGRAPHY/SEASON

Ubiquitous and worldwide.
No seasonal incidence.

MODES OF CONTROL

Treatment of *H. pylori* infection involves combination therapy. Current combination of agents recommended are omeprazole (reduces acid production and gives symptomatic relief) with one or more antibiotics (e.g., clarithromycin, amoxicillin, metronidazole). Bismuth can also be added.
It is difficult to prevent and control the disease because the organism is ubiquitous.

---

denal ulcers but is infrequently isolated from patients without histological evidence of gastritis. No animal reservoir has been identified definitively (although domestic cats were implicated in one study), and infection through the consumption of contaminated food or water has not been demonstrated. Although the mechanism of transmission is not known, family clustering has been recognized. Humans are the main reservoir for infection, which is probably spread person to person.

Clinical Syndromes

Clinical evidence is now overwhelming that *H. pylori* is the etiological agent in virtually all cases of type B gastritis. This evidence includes virtually a 100% association between gastritis and infection with the bacterium, experimental infection produced in both animals and humans, and histological resolution of the pathological changes when specific therapy is used to eradicate the organism. It is now generally accepted that *H. pylori* is the cause of most gastric and duodenal ulcers, with elimination of the organism leading to healing of the ulcers and a significant reduction in the incidence of recurrence. Because gastritis precedes the development of gastric adenocarcinomas, extensive epidemiological and experimental studies are underway to determine the role of *H. pylori* in the pathogenesis of this malignancy.

H. cinaedi and *H. fennelliae* can cause gastroenteritis and proctocolitis with septicemia in homosexual men. *H. cinaedi* also causes recurrent cellulitis with fever and bacteremia in immunocompromised patients.

Laboratory Diagnosis
Histopathology

H. pylori is detected by histological examination of gastric biopsies. Although the organism can be seen in hematoxylin-eosin or Gram-stained specimens, the Warthin-Starry silver stain is the most sensitive.

Urease Test

The urease test is the most rapid way to detect *H. pylori*. Urease activity can be measured directly in the clinical specimen or after an organism has been isolated. The abundance of urease produced by the organism permits detection of the alkaline by-product within 1 to 2 hours.

Culture

The organism can grow only in a microaerophilic atmosphere on enriched medium supplemented with blood, hemin, or charcoal. The supplementation of the medium protects the bacteria from oxygen free radicals, hydrogen peroxide, and fatty acids. Specimens should not be inoculated onto media used for the recovery of *Campylobacter* because these media are too inhibitory. Culture is insensitive unless multiple biopsy specimens from the gastric mucosa are processed.

Identification

Preliminary identification of isolates is based on their growth characteristics under selective conditions, typical microscopic morphological findings, and detection of oxidase, catalase, and urease activity. Definitive identification of *H. pylori* and related bacteria is guided by the reactions summarized in Table 31-2.

Serology

As already indicated, infection with *H. pylori* stimulates a humoral immune reaction that persists as the result of continuous exposure to the bacteria. Because the antibody titers persist for many years, the test cannot be used to discriminate between past and current infection. Furthermore, the titer of antibodies measured does not correlate with the severity of the disease or the response to therapy. However, the tests are useful for documenting exposure to the bacteria, either for epidemiological studies or for the initial evaluation of a symptomatic patient.

Treatment, Prevention, and Control

Numerous antibiotic regimens have been evaluated. Use of a single antibiotic or an antibiotic combined with bismuth is ineffective. The greatest success in curing gastritis or peptic ulcer disease has been accomplished with the combination of a proton pump inhibitor (e.g., omeprazole) and one or more antibiotics (e.g., clarithromycin, amoxicillin, metronidazole). Bismuth can also be added. At this time, the most efficacious treatment for *H. pylori* disease has not been determined. *H. cinaedi* and *H. fennelliae* are resistant to erythromycin but susceptible to ampicillin and gentamicin.

CASE STUDY AND QUESTIONS

A mother and her 4-year-old son came to the local emergency room with a 1-day history of diarrhea and abdominal cramping. Both patients had low-grade fevers, and the child had gross blood in the stool specimen. The symptoms developed 18 hours after a dinner of mixed green salad, chicken, corn, bread, and apple pie. Culture of blood samples was negative for organisms, but *C. jejuni* was isolated from stool specimens of both the mother and child.

1. What is the most likely food responsible for these infections? What measures should be used to prevent these infections?

2. What campylobacters are commonly found in blood specimens?
3. What diseases have been associated with *H. pylori*?
4. How do *H. pylori* survive the acidic environment of the stomach and produce disease?

Bibliography

Blaser MJ: *Helicobacter pylori:* its role in disease, *Clin Infect Dis* 15:386-393, 1992.

Blaser MJ, Pei Z: Pathogenesis of *Campylobacter fetus* infections: critical role of high molecular weight S-layer proteins in virulence, *J Infect Dis* 167:372-377, 1993.

Cardarelli-Leite P et al: Rapid identification of *Campylobacter* species by RFLP analysis of a PCR-amplified fragment of the gene coding for 16S rRNA, *J Clin Microbiol* 34:62-67, 1996.

Cover TL, Blaser MJ: *Helicobacter pylori* infection: a paradigm for chronic mucosal inflammation: pathogenesis and implications for eradication and prevention, *Adv Intern Med* 41:85-117, 1996.

Hunt R, editor: Proceedings of a symposium. *Helicobacter pylori*: from theory to practice, *Am J Med* 100:1-64, 1996.

NIH Consensus Development Panel: *Helicobacter pylori* in peptic ulcer disease, *JAMA* 272:65-69, 1994.

On SLW: Identification methods for campylobacters, helicobacters, and related organisms, *Clin Microbiol Rev* 9:405-422, 1996.

Soll A: Medical treatment of peptic ulcer disease: practice guidelines, *JAMA* 275:622-629, 1996.

Staat MA et al: A population-based serologic survey of *Helicobacter pylori* infection in children and adolescents in the United States, *J Infect Dis* 174:1120-1123, 1996.

Ursing JB et al: Proposal of minimal standards for describing new species of the family Campylobacteriaceae, *Intl J Syst Bacteriol* 44:842-845, 1994.

Van Enk R: Serologic diagnosis of *Helicobacter pylori* infection, *Clin Microbiol Newsletter* 18:89-92, 1996.

CHAPTER ···········

32

Pseudomonas and Related Organisms

Clinically important aerobic, gram-negative bacilli can be artificially classified into four general groups: (1) facultatively anaerobic and microaerophilic bacilli (i.e., bacilli discussed in Chapters 29 to 31), (2) aerobic nonfermenters (i.e., Pseudomonadaceae), (3) *Haemophilus* and related genera, and (4) unusual bacilli. Of the bacilli isolated in clinical specimens, 70% to 80% are members of the first group, 10% to 15% are in the second group, 10% to 15% are haemophilic bacilli, and fewer than 1% are classified into the unusual bacilli group. The focus of this chapter is *Pseudomonas* and related nonfermentative, gram-negative bacilli, whereas *Haemophilus* and the unusual bacilli are discussed in Chapters 33 to 35.

Pseudomonas and related bacilli are a complex mixture of opportunistic pathogens of plants, animals, and humans. To complicate the understanding of these organisms, the taxonomic classification has undergone numerous changes during the past decade. A partial listing of clinically important nonfermentative organisms is summarized in Box 32-1. Despite the many genera, only a few are isolated commonly. *P. aeruginosa, Burkholderia cepacia, Stenotrophomonas maltophilia, Acinetobacter baumannii,* and *Moraxella catarrhalis* constitute more than 75% of all isolates.

PSEUDOMONAS

Pseudomonads are ubiquitous organisms found in soil, decaying organic matter, vegetation, and water. They are also found throughout the hospital environment in moist reservoirs such as food, cut flowers, sinks, toilets, floor mops, respiratory therapy and dialysis equipment, and even disinfectant solutions. It is uncommon for carriage to persist in humans as part of the normal microbial flora unless the person is hospitalized or is an ambulatory, immunocompromised host. The broad environmental distribution of pseudomonads is made possible by their simple growth requirements. Many organic compounds can be used as a source of carbon and nitrogen, and some strains can even grow in distilled water by using trace nutrients. *Pseudomonas* organisms also possess many structural factors and toxins that enhance

their virulence, as well as render them resistant to most commonly used antibiotics. Indeed, it is surprising that these organisms are not more common pathogens, considering their ubiquitous presence, ability to grow in virtually any environment, virulence properties, and broad-based antimicrobial resistance. Instead, *Pseudomonas* infections are primarily opportunistic (i.e., restricted to patients with compromised host defenses). This illustrates the importance of the host's ability to prevent colonization and invasion with pseudomonads.

Physiology and Structure

Pseudomonads are straight or slightly curved gram-negative bacilli (0.5 to 1.0 × 1.5 to 5.0 μm) and motile by means of polar flagella. The organisms are nonfermentative and use relatively few carbohydrates (e.g., glucose, ribose, gluconate) during oxidative metabolism. Oxygen is the terminal electron acceptor, and the presence of cytochrome oxidase in *Pseudomonas* organisms is used to differentiate them from the Enterobacteriaceae. Although these organisms are defined as obligate aerobes, they can grow anaerobically, using nitrate as an alternate electron acceptor. Some strains appear mucoid because of the abundance of a polysaccharide capsule; these strains are particularly common in patients with cystic fibrosis. Some pseudomonads produce diffusible pigments (e.g., pyocyanin [blue], fluorescein [yellow], pyorubin [red-brown]). The genus consists of many different species subdivided by their biochemical and genetic differences; however, *P. aeruginosa* is the most common clinically significant pseudomonad and the species that will be emphasized here.

Pathogenesis and Immunity

P. aeruginosa has several virulence factors, including structural components, toxins, and enzymes (Table 32-1). Defining the role that each factor plays in disease is difficult, and most experts in this field believe virulence is multifactorial.

Adhesins

Adherence of *P. aeruginosa* to host cells is mediated by pili and nonpilus adhesins. Pili are important for binding to epithelial cells and are similar in structure to the pili found in *Neisseria gonorrhoeae*. *P. aeruginosa* also produces neuraminidase that removes sialic acid residues from the pili receptor, thereby enhancing adherence of the bacteria to the epithelial cells. Although these have not been well characterized, nonpilus adhesins on the bacterial surface are also important for the attachment of *P. aeruginosa* to host cells.

Polysaccharide Capsule

P. aeruginosa produce a mucoid alginate layer that protects the organism from phagocytosis. This polysaccharide layer can also anchor the bacteria to cell surfaces, particularly in patients with cystic fibrosis or other chronic respiratory diseases who are predisposed to colonization with mucoid strains of *P. aeruginosa*. The production of alginate is under complex regulation. In experimental animals, this feature is rapidly lost during in vitro growth and is regained after infection.

Endotoxin

Lipopolysaccharide endotoxin is a major cell wall antigen in *P. aeruginosa*, as it is in other gram-negative bacilli. The lipid A component of endotoxin mediates the various biological effects of the sepsis syndrome.

Exotoxin A

Exotoxin A is one of the most important virulence factors produced by pathogenic strains of *P. aeruginosa*. This toxin blocks protein synthesis in eukaryotic cells in a manner similar to diphtheria toxin. However, these toxins are structurally and immunologically different, and exotoxin A is less potent than diphtheria toxin. This toxin most likely mediates the tissue damage that occurs in burn wound infections and chronic pulmonary infections.

Exoenzyme S

Exoenzyme S is an extracellular toxin produced by one third of the clinical isolates of *P. aeruginosa*. It inhibits protein synthesis. Exotoxin A and exoenzyme S are adenosine diphosphate–ribosyltransferases, but they are distinguished from each other by the heat stability of exoenzyme S. Although this protein does not appear to mediate tissue damage, it may interfere with phagocytic killing.

Elastase

Two enzymes (LasA [serine protease] and LasB [zinc metalloprotease]) act synergistically to degrade elastin, resulting in the lung parenchymal damage and hemorrhagic lesions (**ecthyma gangrenosum**) associated with disseminated *P. aeruginosa* infections. These enzymes can also degrade complement components and inhibitors of leukocyte proteases, which leads to further tissue damage in acute infections. Chronic *Pseudomonas* infections are characterized by the formation of antibodies to LasA and LasB, with the deposition of immune complexes in the infected tissues.

Phospholipase C

Phospholipase C breaks down lipids and lecithin, facilitating tissue destruction. The exact role of this enzyme in infections of the respiratory and urinary tracts is unclear, although an important association between hemolysin production and disease has been recognized.

Pyocyanin

The blue pigment, pyocyanin, produced by *P. aeruginosa* catalyzes the production of superoxide and hydrogen peroxide, toxic forms of oxygen. In the presence of **pyochelin** (an iron-binding siderophore), the more toxic

---

BOX 32-1   **Clinically Important Nonfermentative Gram-Negative Bacilli**

Achromobacter species	*Flavobacterium* species
Acinetobacter species	*Moraxella* species
Agrobacterium species	*Ochrobactrum* species
Alcaligenes species	*Oligella* species
Burkholderia species	*Pseudomonas* species
Chryseomonas species	*Skewanella* species
Comamonas species	*Sphingomonas* species
Eikenella species	*Stenotrophomonas* species
Flavimonas species	*Weeksella* species

TABLE 32-1   **Virulence Factors Associated with *P. aeruginosa***

VIRULENCE FACTORS	BIOLOGICAL EFFECTS
Adhesins	Mediate attachment to host epithelial cells (pili and nonpilus adhesins), enhance pili adherence (bacterial production of neuraminidase)
Alginate production	Forms mucoid layer that protects bacteria from phagocytosis and facilitates adherence to host cells
Exotoxin A	Inhibits host protein synthesis; produces tissue damage
Exoenzyme S	Inhibits host protein synthesis; interferes with phagocytic killing
Elastolytic activity	Degrades elastin, with direct damage to lung tissue and vessels (elastolytic enzymes)
Phospholipase C	Mediates tissue damage
Pyocyanin	Mediates tissue damage through production of toxic oxygen radicals (i.e., hydrogen peroxide, superoxide, hydroxyl radicals)
Antibiotic resistance	Complicates antimicrobial therapy

BOX 32-2   Summary of *P. aeruginosa* Infections

BACTERIAL FACTORS

Diseases—infections of the respiratory tract, burn wounds, urinary tract, ear, and eye; bacteremia and endocarditis; gastroenteritis.

Virulence factors—see Table 32-1.

Growth in virtually any environment with minimal nutritional requirements and tolerance to a wide range of temperatures.

TRANSMISSION

Ubiquitous opportunistic pathogen of plants, animals, and humans.

Found throughout hospitals in moist reservoirs (respiratory and dialysis equipment, sinks, toilets, flowers).

Persistent carriage is uncommon in immunocompetent people but common in hospitalized patients. Risk factors: prior treatment with broad-spectrum antibiotics, respiratory therapy, prolonged hospitalization, and compromised immune function.

WHO IS AT RISK?

Opportunistic pathogen of immunocompromised patients, patients with chronic pulmonary disease (e.g., cystic fibrosis), and patients with compromised defense mechanisms (e.g., burn wounds, trauma to eye).

WHO IS AT RISK?—cont'd

Patients exposed to contaminated water (e.g., hot tubs, whirlpools, pools).

Diabetic or elderly patients (malignant external otitis).

Intravenous drug users.

GEOGRAPHY/SEASON

Worldwide.

No seasonal incidence.

MODES OF CONTROL

Combined use of effective antibiotics (e.g., aminoglycoside and beta-lactam antibiotics) is effective. Monotherapy is generally ineffective and selective for resistant strains.

Hyperimmune globulin and granulocyte transfusions may be beneficial in selected infections in immunocompromised patients.

Hospital infection-control efforts should concentrate on preventing contamination of sterile medical equipment and nosocomial infections.

Unnecessary use of broad-spectrum antibiotics, which select for resistant organisms such as *P. aeruginosa*.

---

hydroxyl radical is produced, which can mediate tissue damage.

Antibiotic Resistance

P. aeruginosa is inherently resistant to many antibiotics and can mutate to even more resistant strains during therapy. Although numerous resistance mechanisms have been identified, the mutation of porin proteins constitutes the major mechanism of resistance. Penetration of antibiotics into the pseudomonad cell is primarily through pores in the outer membrane. If the proteins forming the walls of these pores are altered to restrict flow through the channels, then resistance to many classes of antibiotics can develop.

Epidemiology

Pseudomonads are opportunistic pathogens present in a variety of environments (Box 32-2). The ability to isolate these organisms from moist surfaces may be limited only by the interest in searching for the organism. Pseudomonads have minimal nutritional requirements, can tolerate a wide range of temperatures (4° to 42° C), and are resistant to many antibiotics and disinfectants. Indeed, the recovery of *Pseudomonas* organisms from an environmental source (e.g., hospital sink or floor) means very little unless there is epidemiological evidence that the contaminated site is a reservoir for in-

fection. Furthermore, isolation of pseudomonads from a hospitalized patient is worrisome but does not normally justify therapeutic intervention unless there is evidence of disease. The recovery of *Pseudomonas* organisms, particularly species other than *P. aeruginosa*, from a clinical specimen may also result from environmental contamination of the specimen during collection or laboratory processing. Because these organisms are opportunistic pathogens, the significance of an isolate must be measured by assessing the clinical presentation of the patient.

Clinical Syndromes

Pulmonary Infections

P. aeruginosa infections of the lower respiratory tract can range in severity from colonization or a benign tracheobronchitis to severe necrotizing bronchopneumonia. Colonization is seen in patients with cystic fibrosis, other chronic lung diseases, or neutropenia. *Pseudomonas* pulmonary infection in patients with cystic fibrosis has been associated with exacerbation of the underlying disease, as well as invasive disease in the pulmonary parenchyma. Mucoid strains are commonly associated with these patients and are difficult to eradicate with antibiotic therapy. Neutropenic and other immunocompromised patients are frequently exposed to *Pseudomonas* organisms through exposure to contaminated respiratory therapy equipment. Invasive disease in this population is characterized by a diffuse, typically bilateral bronchopneumonia with microabscess formation and tissue necrosis.

Primary Skin Infections

P. aeruginosa can cause a variety of skin infections. The most recognized are infections of burn wounds. *P. aeruginosa* colonization of a burn wound, followed by localized vascular damage and tissue necrosis and ultimately bacteremia, is common in patients with severe burns. The moist surface of the burn and the lack of a neutrophilic response to tissue invasion predispose patients to such infections. The application of topical creams and wound management have had only limited success in controlling *Pseudomonas* colonization in these patients.

Folliculitis is another common infection caused by *Pseudomonas* species and results from immersion in contaminated water (e.g., hot tubs, whirlpools, swimming pools). Secondary infections with *Pseudomonas* organisms also occur in patients with acne and people who depilate their legs. Finally *P. aeruginosa* can cause nail infections in patients whose hands are frequently exposed to water.

Urinary Tract Infections

Infection of the urinary tract is seen primarily in patients with chronic indwelling urinary catheters. Typically these patients are treated with multiple courses of antibiotics that tend to select for the more resistant strains of *Pseudomonas* species.

Ear Infections

External otitis is most frequently caused by *P. aeruginosa*, with swimming (**swimmer's ear**) an important risk factor. This localized infection can be managed with topical antibiotics and drying agents. **Malignant external otitis** is a more virulent form of disease seen primarily in diabetics and elderly patients. It can invade the underlying tissues, damage the cranial nerves and bones, and be life threatening. Aggressive antimicrobial and surgical intervention is required for patients with the latter disease. *P. aeruginosa* is also associated with chronic otitis media.

Eye Infections

Infections of the eye occur after initial trauma to the cornea (e.g., abrasion from contact lens, scratch on the eye surface) and then exposure to *P. aeruginosa* in contaminated water. Corneal ulcers develop and can progress to eye-threatening disease unless prompt treatment is instituted.

Bacteremia and Endocarditis

Bacteremia caused by *P. aeruginosa* is clinically indistinguishable from that caused by other gram-negative infections, although the mortality rate in affected patients is higher. This higher mortality rate is due in part to the predilection of this organism for immunocompromised patients and in part to the inherent virulence of *Pseudomonas* organisms. Bacteremia occurs most often in patients with neutropenia, diabetes mellitus, extensive burns, and hematological malignancies. Most *Pseudomonas* bacteremias originate from infections of the lower respiratory tract, urinary tract, and skin and soft tissue (particularly burn wound infections). Although seen in a minority of patients, characteristic skin lesions (**ecthyma gangrenosum**) may develop. The lesions present as erythematous vesicles that become hemorrhagic, necrotic, and ulcerated. Microscopic examination of the lesion shows abundant organisms, vascular destruction (which explains the hemorrhagic nature of the lesions), and an absence of neutrophils, as would be expected in neutropenic patients.

Pseudomonas endocarditis is most commonly observed in intravenous drug abusers. These patients acquire the infection from the use of drug paraphernalia contaminated with the waterborne organisms. The tricuspid valve is often involved, and the infection is associated with a chronic course but with a more favorable prognosis than that in patients with infections of the aortic or mitral valve.

Other Infections

P. aeruginosa is also the cause of a variety of other infections, including those localized in the gastrointestinal tract, central nervous system, and musculoskeletal system. The underlying conditions required for most pseudomonad infections are the presence of the organism in a moist reservoir and the circumvention or elimination of host defenses (e.g., cutaneous trauma, elimination of normal microbial flora as a result of imprudent use of antibiotics, neutropenia).

OTHER PSEUDOMONADS

All *Pseudomonas* species can cause opportunistic infections in immunocompromised patients. Most true infections with these organisms have been localized to the respiratory tract in patients with underlying pulmonary disease or to the urinary tract in patients after instrumentation or catheterization. The clinical significance of an isolate is often difficult to assess because specific signs and symptoms of disease may be absent and the organism may be an insignificant waterborne contaminant.

Laboratory Diagnosis
Culture

Because pseudomonads have simple nutritional requirements, they grow easily on common isolation media such as blood or MacConkey agar. Aerobic incubation is required (unless nitrate is available), so growth in broth is generally confined to the broth-air interface.

Identification

The colonial morphology (e.g., colony size, hemolytic activity, pigmentation, odor) combined with the results of selected rapid biochemical tests (e.g., positive oxidase reaction) for the preliminary identification of these isolates. For example, *P. aeruginosa* grows rapidly and has flat colonies with a spreading border, a green pigmentation caused by the production of the blue pyocyanin and the yellow fluorescein, and a characteristic sweet, grapelike odor.

Although it is relatively easy to identify *P. aeruginosa* definitively, it may take an extensive battery of physiological tests to identify other pseudomonads. Biochemical profiles, antibiotic susceptibility patterns, susceptibility to bacteriophages (phage typing), production of pyocins, serological typing, and the molecular characterization of DNA or ribosomal RNA are used for the specific classification of isolates for epidemiological purposes. Although clinical laboratories often classify these organisms by their biochemical or susceptibility patterns, these are the least discriminatory methods. Phage typing, pyocin typing, and serotyping have all been used successfully but are performed only in reference laboratories. Nucleic acid analysis has rapidly become the most sensitive and practical epidemiological tool for clinical laboratories.

Treatment, Prevention, and Control

The antimicrobial therapy for *Pseudomonas* infections is frustrating because the infected patient with compromised host defenses cannot augment the antibiotic activity and pseudomonads are typically resistant to most antibiotics (Table 32-2). Even susceptible organisms can become resistant during therapy by inducing the formation of antibiotic-inactivating enzymes (e.g., betalactamases) or through the transfer of plasmid-mediated resistance from a resistant organism to a susceptible one. Furthermore, some groups of antibiotics, such as the aminoglycosides, are ineffective at certain sites of infection (poor activity in the acidic environment of an abscess). A combination of aminoglycoside and beta-lactam antibiotics, which have documented activity against the isolate, are generally required for therapy to be successful in patients with serious infections. The administration of hyperimmune globulin and granulocyte transfusions to augment compromised immune function may be beneficial in selected patients who have *Pseudomonas* infections.

Attempts to eliminate *Pseudomonas* organisms from the hospital are practically useless, given the ubiquitous presence of the organism in water supplies. Effective infection-control practices should concentrate on preventing the contamination of sterile equipment such as respiratory therapy and dialysis machines and the cross-contamination of patients by medical personnel. The inappropriate use of broad-spectrum antibiotics should also be avoided because such use can suppress the normal microbial flora and permit the overgrowth of resistant pseudomonads.

BURKHOLDERIA

Five species formerly classified as *Pseudomonas* have been reclassified as members of the genus *Burkholderia* (Table 32-3). *B. cepacia* and *B. pseudomallei* are important human pathogens, *B. pickettii* is an opportunistic pathogen, and *B. gladioli* and *B. mallei* do not cause human disease.

Like *P. aeruginosa*, *B. cepacia* can colonize a variety of moist environmental surfaces and is commonly associated with nosocomial infections. Infections caused by this organism include respiratory tract infections in patients with cystic fibrosis or chronic granulomatous disease; urinary tract infections in catheterized patients; septicemia, particularly in patients with contaminated intravascular catheters; and other opportunistic infections. With the exception of pulmonary infections, *B. cepacia* has a relatively low level of virulence, and infections with the organism do not commonly result in death. *B. cepacia* is susceptible to trimethoprim-

TABLE 32-2	Mechanisms of Antibiotic Resistance in *P. aeruginosa*
ANTIBIOTIC	**RESISTANCE MECHANISMS**
Beta-lactams (penicillins, cephalosporins, carbapenems)	Beta-lactamase hydrolysis, decreased permeability, altered binding proteins
Aminoglycosides	Enzymatic hydrolysis by acetylation, adenylation, or phosphorylation; decreased permeability; altered ribosomal target
Chloramphenicol	Enzymatic hydrolysis by acetyltransferase; decreased permeability
Fluoroquinolones	Altered target (DNA gyrase); decreased permeability

TABLE 32-3	*Burkholderia* Species and Associated Diseases
SPECIES	**DISEASES**
B. cepacia	Respiratory tract infections (particularly in patients with cystic fibrosis), urinary tract infections, septic arthritis, peritonitis, septicemia, opportunistic infections
B. pseudomallei	Melioidosis
B. pickettii	Opportunistic infection
B. gladioli	Colonization of respiratory tracts of patients with cystic fibrosis
B. mallei	Glanders in livestock

sulfamethoxazole. Although the organism appears to be susceptible in vitro to piperacillin, to broad-spectrum cephalosporins, and to ciprofloxacin, the clinical response is generally poor.

B. pseudomallei is a saprophyte found in soil, water, and vegetation. It has a worldwide distribution but is particularly prevalent in Southeast Asia, India, Africa, and Australia. The organism causes opportunistic infections; however, these infections (**melioidosis**) can occur in previously healthy people as an acute suppurative infection or a chronic pulmonary infection. The disease can occur from a few days to many years after exposure. Thus although *B. pseudomallei* is rarely isolated in people living in the Western hemisphere, latent disease can occur in people who have been in endemic areas.

Melioidosis has protean manifestations. Most people exposed to *B. pseudomallei* remain asymptomatic. However, a localized suppurative infection develops in some exposed cutaneously, and this is accompanied by regional lymphadenitis, fever, and malaise. This form of disease can resolve without incident or rapidly progress to overwhelming sepsis. The third form of infection is pulmonary disease, which may range in severity from a mild bronchitis to necrotizing pneumonia. Cavitation can develop if appropriate antimicrobial therapy is not instituted. Isolation of *B. pseudomallei* for diagnostic purposes should be approached carefully because the organism is highly infectious. The combination of trimethoprim-sulfamethoxazole and a broad-spectrum cephalosporin is recommended for the treatment of systemic infections.

STENOTROPHOMONAS MALTOPHILIA

S. maltophilia is one of the most commonly isolated nonfermentative, gram-negative bacilli. This organism was originally classified in the genus *Pseudomonas* and then more recently in the genus *Xanthomonas*. Despite the confusion created by these taxonomic changes, the clinical importance of this opportunistic pathogen is well known. It is responsible for causing infections in debilitated patients with impaired host-defense mechanisms, and because *S. maltophilia* is resistant to most commonly used beta-lactam and aminoglycoside antibiotics, patients receiving long-term antibiotic therapy are particularly at risk for acquiring infections with this organism.

The spectrum of nosocomial infections with *S. maltophilia* is broad and includes bacteremia, pneumonia, meningitis, wound infections, and urinary tract infections. Hospital epidemics with this organism have been traced to contaminated disinfectant solutions, respiratory therapy or monitoring equipment, and ice machines.

Antimicrobial therapy is complicated because the organism is resistant to many commonly used drugs. Trimethoprim-sulfamethoxazole is the most active against the organism; good activity is also seen with chloramphenicol and ceftazidime.

ACINETOBACTER

The genus *Acinetobacter* has also undergone taxonomic reorganization. Currently, 17 species are recognized, with *A. baumannii*, *A. lwoffii*, and *A. haemolyticus* the species most commonly isolated. Acinetobacters are recovered in nature and in the hospital. They survive on moist surfaces, including respiratory therapy equipment, and on dry surfaces such as the human skin, which is unusual for gram-negative bacilli. These bacteria are also part of the normal oropharyngeal flora of a small number of healthy people and can proliferate to large numbers during hospitalization.

Acinetobacters are opportunistic pathogens that cause infections in the respiratory tract, urinary tract, and wounds; they also cause septicemia. Treatment of *Acinetobacter* infections is problematic because these organisms, particularly *A. baumannii*, are often resistant to antibiotics. Specific therapy must be guided by in vitro susceptibility tests, but empirical therapy for serious infections should consist of a beta-lactam antibiotic (e.g., ceftazidime, imipenem) and an aminoglycoside.

MORAXELLA

Like other genera discussed in this chapter, the genus *Moraxella* has been reorganized on the basis of nucleic acid analysis. Although the species classified in the genus continue to change, *M. nonliquefaciens* remains the most frequently isolated species because it colonizes the upper respiratory tract and skin surface, and *M. catarrhalis* remains the most important pathogen. *M. catarrhalis* is a common cause of bronchitis and bronchopneumonia (in elderly patients with chronic pulmonary disease), sinusitis, and otitis. The last two infections occur most frequently in previously healthy people. Most isolates produce beta-lactamases and are penicillin resistant; however, these bacteria are uniformly susceptible to cephalosporins, erythromycin, tetracycline, trimethoprim-sulfamethoxazole, and the combination of penicillins with a beta-lactamase inhibitor (e.g., clavulanic acid).

CASE STUDY AND QUESTIONS

A 63-year-old man had been hospitalized for 21 days for the management of newly diagnosed leukemia. During this time, a urinary tract infection with *Escherichia coli* developed, and the patient was treated for 14 days with broad-spectrum antibiotics. On hospital day 21, fever and shaking chills developed. Within 24 hours the patient became hypotensive, and ecthymic skin lesions appeared. Despite aggressive therapy with antibiotics, the patient died. Multiple blood cultures were positive for *P. aeruginosa*.

1. What factors placed this man at increased risk for infection with *P. aeruginosa*?

2. What virulence factors possessed by the organism make it a particularly serious pathogen? What is the biological effect of these factors?

3. What antibiotics can be used to treat *P. aeruginosa* infections? Why is this organism resistant to many antibiotics?

4. What diseases are caused by *B. cepacia*? *S. maltophilia*? *A. baumannii*? *M. catarrhalis*? What antibiotics can be used to treat these infections?

Bibliography

Dance DAB: Melioidosis: the tip of the iceberg, *Clin Microbiol Rev* 4:52-60, 1991.

Gustafson TL et al: *Pseudomonas* folliculitis: an outbreak and review, *Rev Infect Dis* 5:1-8, 1983.

Krueger K, Barbieri J: The family of bacterial ADP-ribosylating exotoxins, *Clin Microbiol Rev* 8:34-47, 1995.

Mendelson M et al: *Pseudomonas aeruginosa* bacteremia in patients with AIDS, *Clin Infect Dis* 18:886-895, 1994.

Muder R et al: Bacteremia due to *Stenotrophomonas (Xanthomonas) maltophilia*: a prospective, multicenter study of 91 episodes, *Clin Infect Dis* 22:508-512, 1996.

Robin T, Janda JM: *Pseudo-, Xantho-, Stenotrophomonas maltophilia*: an emerging pathogen in search of a genus, *Clin Microbiol Newsletter*, 18:9-13, 1996.

Rossau R et al: Taxonomy of Moraxellaceae fam. nov.: a new bacterial family to accommodate the genera *Moraxella, Acinetobacter,* and *Psychrobacter* and related organisms, *Int J Syst Bacteriol* 41:310-319, 1991.

Sadoff JC, Sanford JP: Symposium on *Pseudomonas aeruginosa* infections, *Rev Infect Dis* 5(suppl):833-1004, 1983.

Salyers AA, Whitt DD: *Bacterial pathogenesis: a molecular approach*, Washington, DC, 1994, ASM.

Vartivarian SE et al: Mucocutaneous and soft tissue infections caused by *Xanthomonas maltophilia*: a new spectrum, *Ann Intern Med* 121:969-973, 1994.

Wick MJ et al: Structure, function, and regulation of *Pseudomonas aeruginosa* exotoxin A, *Annu Rev Microbiol* 44:335-363, 1990.

Bordetella, Francisella, and Brucella

Numerous gram-negative bacilli are classified together as genera of uncertain affiliation. Three clinically important genera in this group are *Bordetella*, *Francisella*, and *Brucella* (Table 33-1).

BORDETELLA

Bordetella organisms are extremely small (0.2 to 0.5 × 1 μm), strictly aerobic, nonfermentative, gram-negative coccobacilli. Three species have been associated with human disease: *B. pertussis* (Latin for "severe cough") the agent responsible for **pertussis** or **whooping cough**; *B. parapertussis* (Latin for "like pertussis"), responsible for a milder form of pertussis; and *B. bronchiseptica*, responsible for respiratory disease in dogs, swine, laboratory animals, and occasionally humans.

Physiology and Structure

Bordetella species are differentiated on the basis of their growth characteristics, biochemical reactivity, and antigenic properties (Table 33-2). Despite these phenotypic differences, genetic studies have shown that they are closely related or identical species, differing only in the expression of virulence genes. However, at this time the species have not been reclassified and are considered as distinct here.

B. pertussis does not grow on common laboratory media; these organisms require media supplemented with charcoal, starch, blood, or albumin to absorb the toxic substances present in agar. Nicotinamide is also required for growth. The organism is nonmotile and oxidizes amino acids but does not ferment carbohydrates. The other *Bordetella* species are less fastidious and can grow on blood and MacConkey agars. *Bordetella* species possess a genus-specific O antigen and strain-specific, heat-labile K antigens. The K antigens are used for differentiating isolates in epidemiological investigations.

Pathogenesis and Immunity

Infection with *B. pertussis* and the development of whooping cough require exposure to the organism, bacterial attachment to the ciliated epithelial cells of the bronchial tree, proliferation of the bacteria, and production of localized tissue damage and systemic toxicity. Attachment of the organisms to ciliated epithelial cells is mediated primarily by two bacterial adhesins: **filamentous hemagglutinin** and **pertussis toxin** (Table 33-3). The filamentous hemagglutinin binds to sulfated glycolipids on the membranes of ciliated respiratory cells. This adhesin also binds to CR3, a glycoprotein receptor on the surface of polymorphonuclear leukocytes. This interaction initiates the phagocytic uptake of the bacteria. The intracellular survival of *B. pertussis* may protect the bacteria from humoral antibodies and permit persistent carriage. Pertussis toxin consists of a toxic subunit (S1) and five binding subunits (S2 to S5; two S4 subunits are present in each toxin molecule). The S2 subunit binds to lactosylceramide, a glycolipid present on ciliated respiratory cells. The S3 subunit binds to receptors on phagocytic cells, which leads to an increase in CR3 on the cell surface, further bacterial attachment mediated by the filamentous hemagglutinin, and subsequent bacterial phagocytosis. Two other adhesins have been identified in *B. pertussis*: **pili** and **pertactin,** the latter a protein on the surface of the bacteria. Although both proteins mediate the binding to cultured mammalian cells, their role in the attachment to ciliated cells in vivo is unknown.

B. pertussis produces several toxins that mediate the localized and systemic manifestations of disease. The S1 portion of pertussis toxin has adenosine diphosphate–ribosylating activity for the membrane surface **G_i protein** (a guanosine triphosphate–hydrolyzing protein), which regulates adenylate cyclase activity. This causes the cyclic adenosine monophosphate (cAMP) levels to be unregulated, resulting in increased respiratory secretions and mucus production characteristic of the paroxysmal stage of pertussis.

Adenylate cyclase toxin, the second major toxin produced by *B. pertussis,* is activated by intracellular calmodulin and catalyzes the conversion of endogenous adenosine triphosphate to cAMP in eukaryotic cells (the same as pertussis toxin does). Adenylate cyclase toxin also inhibits leukocyte chemotaxis, phagocytosis, and killing. This toxin may be important for the initial protection of the bacteria during the early stages of disease.

TABLE 33-1 Human Pathogens

GENUS	SPECIES	DISEASE
Bordetella	pertussis	Pertussis
	parapertussis	Pertussis
	bronchiseptica	Bronchopulmonary disease
Francisella	tularensis	Tularemia
Brucella	melitensis	Brucellosis
	abortus	Brucellosis
	suis	Brucellosis
	canis	Brucellosis

TABLE 33-2 Differential Characteristics of Bordetella Species

CHARACTERISTICS	B. PER-TUSSIS	B. PARA-PERTUSSIS	B. BRON-CHISEPTICA
Oxidase	+	−	+
Urease	−	+	+
Motility	−	−	+
Browning on Mueller-Hinton agar	−	+	−
Growth on			
Sheep blood agar	−	+	+
MacConkey agar	−	+	+

Modified from Murray P et al: *Manual of clinical microbiology*, ed 6, Washington, DC, 1995, American Society for Microbiology.

Dermonecrotic toxin is a heat-labile toxin that at low doses causes vasoconstriction of peripheral blood vessels in an animal model; this is accompanied by localized ischemia, the movement of leukocytes to extravascular spaces, and hemorrhage. The toxin probably is responsible for the localized tissue destruction seen in pertussis, although further work is necessary to confirm this. At high doses, this toxin causes fatal reactions in an experimental mouse model.

Tracheal cytotoxin is a low-molecular-weight cell wall peptidoglycan monomer that has a specific affinity for ciliated epithelial cells. At low concentrations, it causes ciliostasis (inhibition of cilia movement), and at the higher concentrations produced later in the infection, it causes the extrusion of ciliated cells. Tracheal cytotoxin specifically interferes with DNA synthesis, thereby impairing the regeneration of damaged cells. This process disrupts the normal clearance mechanisms in the respiratory tree and leads to the characteristic cough associated with pertussis. The toxin also stimulates the release of the cytokine IL-1, which leads to fever.

B. pertussis produces two distinct **lipopolysaccharides,** one with lipid A and the other with lipid X. Both lipopolysaccharide molecules can activate the alternate complement pathway and stimulate cytokine release. Their role in the disease process is unknown.

Epidemiology

Although the incidence of pertussis, with its associated morbidity and mortality, was reduced considerably after the introduction of effective vaccines in 1949, the disease is still endemic worldwide and affects more than 60 million people annually. Between 2000 and 6000 new

TABLE 33-3 Virulence Factors Associated with *B. pertussis*

VIRULENCE FACTOR	BIOLOGICAL EFFECT
ADHESINS	
Filamentous hemagglutinin	Binds to sulfated glycolipids on ciliated cell membranes; binds to CR3 on surface of polymorphonuclear leukocytes and initiates phagocytosis.
Pertussis toxin	S2 subunit binds to glycolipid on surface of ciliated respiratory cells; S3 subunit binds to ganglioside on surface of phagocytic cells.
Pili	Binds to mammalian cells. (Role in disease is unknown.)
Pertactin	Binds to mammalian cells. (Role in disease is unknown.)
TOXINS	
Pertussis toxin	S1 subunit ADP-ribosylates host cell G_i protein, causing deregulation of host cell adenylate cyclase; toxin inhibits phagocytic killing and monocyte migration.
Adenylate cyclase toxin	Increases intracellular level of adenylate cyclase and inhibits phagocytic killing and monocyte migration.
Dermonecrotic toxin	Causes dose-dependent skin lesions or fatal reactions in experimental animal model. (Role in disease is unknown.)
Tracheal cytotoxin	A peptidoglycan fragment that kills ciliated respiratory cells and stimulates the release of interleukin-1 (fever).
Lipopolysaccharide	Two distinct lipopolysaccharide molecules with either lipid A or lipid X; activates alternate complement pathway and stimulates cytokine release. (Role in disease is unknown.)

cases are reported each year in the United States (Figure 33-1), but this is certainly an underestimation of the true incidence of disease. *B. pertussis* has no animal or environmental reservoir, so it must spread from patients with clinically apparent pertussis or with subclinical infections (Box 33-1). In theory, vaccination could eliminate *B. pertussis* in the same manner that the smallpox and polio viruses have been eradicated. Unfortunately, the vaccine has not been widely accepted because of fears concern-

ing vaccine-related toxicity. In addition, immunity produced by either natural infection or vaccination is not lifelong. For this reason the incidence of pertussis in the adult population has increased (Figure 33-2). In particular, there have been several reports of a large number of adults with coughs persisting for at least 2 weeks who have serological evidence of recent *B. pertussis* infection. Thus pertussis is seen in nonimmune infants and young children and in adults with waning immunity.

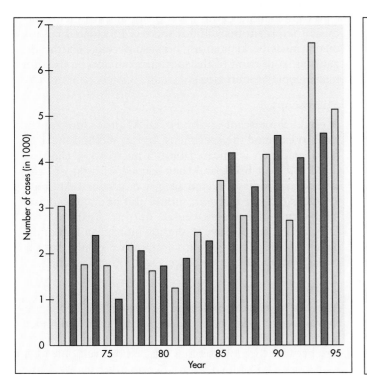

FIGURE 33-1 Incidence of pertussis in the United States from 1971 to 1995. (From *MMWR* 44:525-529, 1995.)

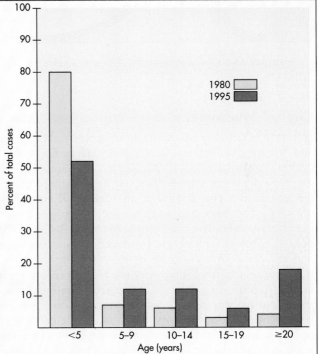

FIGURE 33-2 Age distribution for pertussis infections reported during 1980 and 1994.

BOX 33-1   **Summary of *B. pertussis* Infections**

BACTERIAL FACTORS

Disease—pertussis (whooping cough).
Virulence factors—see Table 33-3.

TRANSMISSION

Person-to-person spread through inhalation of infectious aerosols.
No animal or environmental reservoir.

WHO IS AT RISK?

Nonvaccinated or inadequately vaccinated children.
Adults with waning immunity, who are exposed to symptomatic patients.

GEOGRAPHY/SEASON

Worldwide.
No seasonal incidence.

MODES OF CONTROL

Treatment is primarily supportive.
Erythromycin can reduce infectivity.
Whole-cell and multivalent, acellular vaccines are generally effective; they are administered with vaccines for diphtheria and tetanus.

	Incubation	Catarrhal	Paroxysmal	Convalescent
Duration	7–10 days	1–2 weeks	2–4 weeks	3–4 weeks (or longer)
Symptoms	None	Rhinorrhea, malaise, fever, sneezing, anorexia	Repetitive cough with whoops, vomiting, leukocytosis	Diminished paroxysmal cough, development of secondary complications (pneumonia, seizures, encephalopathy)
Bacterial culture				

FIGURE 33-3 Clinical presentation of *B. pertussis* disease.

Clinical Syndromes

Infection is initiated when infectious aerosols are inhaled and the bacteria become attached to and proliferate on ciliated epithelial cells. After a 7- to 10-day incubation, the typical patient experiences the first of three stages (Figure 33-3). The first stage, the **catarrhal stage,** resembles a common cold, with serous rhinorrhea, sneezing, malaise, anorexia, and low-grade fever. Because the peak number of bacteria are produced during this stage and the cause of the disease is not yet recognized, patients in the catarrhal stage pose the highest risk to their contacts. After 1 to 2 weeks the **paroxysmal stage** begins. During this time, ciliated epithelial cells are extruded from the respiratory tract, and the clearance of mucus is impaired. This stage is characterized by the classic whooping cough paroxysms (i.e., a series of repetitive coughs followed by an inspiratory whoop). Mucus production in the respiratory tract is common and is partially responsible for causing airway restriction. The paroxysms are frequently terminated with vomiting and exhaustion. A marked lymphocytosis is also prominent during this stage. Affected patients may experience as many as 40 to 50 paroxysms daily during the height of the illness. After 2 to 4 weeks the disease enters the **convalescent stage;** at this time the paroxysms diminish in number and severity, but secondary complications can occur. This classic presentation of pertussis may not be seen in patients with partial immunity. Such patients may have a history of a chronic persistent cough with or without vomiting.

Laboratory Diagnosis

Specimen Collection and Transport

B. pertussis are extremely sensitive to drying and do not survive unless care is taken during the collection and transport of the specimen to the laboratory. The optimal diagnostic specimen is a nasopharyngeal aspirate. The yield from specimens obtained by oropharyngeal swabs is lower than that from nasopharyngeal aspirates, and synthetic fiber swabs (e.g., calcium alginate or Dacron) must be used. Cotton swabs should not be used because they contain fatty acids, which are toxic to *B. pertussis.*

The most important factors affecting the recovery of *Bordetella* organisms are the speed with which the specimen is cultured and the quality of the culture media. The specimen must be either directly inoculated onto freshly prepared isolation media (e.g., charcoal-horse blood agar, Bordet-Gengou medium) at the patient's bedside or placed in a suitable transport medium (e.g., Regan-Lowe transport medium). Specimens cannot be delivered to the laboratory in traditional transport media, because the organisms will not survive. Inoculated culture media must be kept moist because drying kills the organisms. A portion of the specimen can also be used for microscopic examination.

Microscopy

A direct fluorescent antibody (DFA) procedure can be used to examine the specimens. In this method the aspirated specimen is smeared onto a microscopic slide, air dried and heat fixed, and then stained with fluorescein-labeled antibodies directed against *B. pertussis.* Antibodies against *B. parapertussis* should also be used to detect mild forms of pertussis caused by this organism. The DFA results are positive in slightly more than half of the patients with pertussis, but false-positive results can occur as a result of cross-reactions with other bacteria.

Culture

After the inoculated media are received in the laboratory, they are incubated in air at 35° C and in a humidified chamber. Prolonged incubation (e.g., 7 days) is necessary because the tiny colonies can be observed only after 3 or more days of incubation. Because the quality of the media dramatically affects the success of culture, laboratories that infrequently culture specimens for *Bordetella* should arrange for the state public health department to process these specimens.

Identification

B. pertussis are identified by their characteristic microscopic and colonial morphology on selective media and their reactivity with a specific antiserum (either in an agglutination reaction or with the reagents used in the DFA test). The reactions summarized in Table 33-2 can be used to differentiate *B. pertussis* from *B. parapertussis.*

Serology

It is difficult to interpret the results of serological tests because microscopy and culture techniques are relatively insensitive standards by which to evaluate these results. Most investigators recommend using multiple tests (e.g., measure IgG and IgA antibodies against filamentous hemagglutinin and IgG antibodies against pertussis toxin). A significant rise in antibody titer between acute and convalescent serum or an initially high titer is consistant with a recent infection.

Treatment, Prevention, and Control

The treatment for pertussis is primarily supportive, with nursing supervision during the paroxysmal and convalescent stages of the illness. Antibiotics do not ameliorate the clinical course; in fact, convalescence depends on the rapidity and degree to which the layer of ciliated epithelial cells regenerates. Erythromycin is effective in eradicating the organisms and can reduce the duration of infectivity; however, this has limited value because the illness is usually unrecognized during peak of contagiousness.

Whole-cell, inactivated vaccines have been available for almost 50 years. In the United States, they are commonly administered with vaccines for diphtheria and tetanus (DPT vaccine) and are considered 80% to 85% effective in eliminating symptomatic pertussis. However, concern about the associated complications has limited the acceptance of the current whole-cell vaccine in some countries. Multivalent, acellular pertussis vaccines have been developed; these vaccines use components believed to evoke protective immunity, such as filamentous hemagglutinin, pertussis toxin, fimbriae agglutinins, and pertactin. Numerous clinical trials have shown that these vaccines confer a protective immunity at least equivalent to that conferred by whole-cell vaccines, and these vaccines are associated with a lower incidence of side effects. On the basis of these results, it has been recommended that multivalent, acellular vaccines should replace the older vaccines.

Because pertussis is highly contagious in a susceptible population and unrecognized infections in family members of a symptomatic patient can maintain disease in a community, erythromycin has been used for prophylaxis in select instances.

OTHER *BORDETELLA* SPECIES

B. parapertussis is responsible for causing 10% to 20% of the cases of mild pertussis seen annually in the United States. *B. bronchiseptica* causes respiratory disease primarily in animals but has been associated with human respiratory tract colonization and bronchopulmonary disease. Both organisms can be readily isolated on conventional laboratory media, and unlike *B. pertussis,* both have easily recognizable metabolic properties.

FRANCISELLA TULARENSIS

F. tularensis is the causative agent of **tularemia** (also called *glandular fever, rabbit fever, tick fever,* and *deer fly fever*) in animals and humans. The taxonomic classification of the organism is derived from Edward Francis, who demonstrated the association between rodent disease in Tulare County, California, and human disease (hence the genus and species name).

Physiology and Structure

F. tularensis is a very small (0.2×0.2 to 0.7μm), faintly staining, gram-negative coccobacillus. The organism is

		BIOVAR
CHARACTERISTIC	**BIOVAR *TULARENSIS***	**PALAEARCTICA**
Name	Jellison A; nearctica	Jellison B
Geographical distribution	North America	Europe, Asia, the Americas
Biochemical properties		
Glycerol fermentation	Positive	Negative
Citrulline-ureidase	Positive	Negative
Source of infection	Ticks, rabbits	Contaminated water or rodents
Human disease	Severe	Mild

TABLE 33-4   Differentiation Between *Francisella tularensis* biovar *tularensis* and biovar *palaearctica*

nonmotile and nonpiliated, is surrounded with a thin lipid capsule, and has fastidious growth requirements. Like *Bordetella,* this organism is strictly aerobic and requires enriched media and incubation for a minimum of 3 days.

Pathogenesis and Immunity

F. tularensis is an intracellular parasite that can survive for prolonged periods in macrophages of the reticuloendothelial system because the organism inhibits phagosome-lysosome fusion. Pathogenic strains possess an antiphagocytic capsule, and loss of the capsule is associated with decreased virulence (Box 33-2). Like all gram-negative bacilli, this organism has endotoxin, but it is considerably less active than the endotoxin found in other gram-negative bacilli (e.g., *Escherichia coli*).

Epidemiology

Although *F. tularensis* has a worldwide distribution, the prevalence of the two biochemical varieties (biovars *tularensis* and *palaearctica*) is somewhat restricted (Table 33-4). The organism is found in many wild mammals, domestic animals, birds, fish, and blood-sucking arthropods, as well as in contaminated water. The most common reservoirs of *F. tularensis* in the United States are rabbits, ticks, and muskrats. Human tularemia is acquired most often from the bite of an infected arthropod or from contact with an infected animal or domestic pet (e.g., cat) that has caught an infected animal (e.g., rabbit). However, disease can also be acquired from the consumption of contaminated meat or water or from the inhalation of an infectious aerosol (most commonly in a laboratory or during the dressing of an infected animal). Infection with *F. tularensis* requires as few as 10 organisms when exposure is by an arthropod bite or contami-

BOX 33-2   Summary of *F. tularensis* Infections

BACTERIAL FACTORS

Disease—tularemia: ulceroglandular, oculoglandular, glandular, typhoidal, oropharyngeal, pneumonic, gastrointestinal.

Virulence factors—intracellular pathogen resistant to killing in serum and by phagocytes; antiphagocytic capsule.

TRANSMISSION

Bite from infected insect (e.g., tick, biting fly, mosquito [uncommon in United States]).

Contact with infected animal (e.g., skinning, dressing, eating animal).

Inhalation of infectious aerosol.

WHO IS AT RISK?

Hunters.

People exposed to ticks or other infected insects.

Laboratory personnel.

GEOGRAPHY/SEASON

Worldwide.

Most infections in the United States occur in Arkansas, Missouri, and Oklahoma.

GEOGRAPHY/SEASON—cont'd

Most infections acquired by men occur during the summer (exposed to infected insects) or fall (hunting exposure).

MODES OF CONTROL

1 to 2 weeks of therapy with streptomycin or gentamicin.

Avoid exposure to infected animals (i.e., do not handle animals with uncovered hands) or ticks (use insect repellents and cover exposed skin).

Cook all meats thoroughly before consumption and treat water.

Laboratory personnel should wear gloves and perform all work in a biohazard hood.

Live attenuated vaccine can be used for people at significant risk for exposure.

Prophylactic antibiotics are not recommended, except for laboratory personnel with a significant exposure history.

FIGURE 33-4 Incidence of tularemia in the United States from 1971 to 1994. (From *MMWR* 44[53]:74-79, 1995.)

nation of unbroken skin, 50 organisms when inhaled, and 10^8 organisms when ingested.

The reported incidence of disease is low (Figure 33-4). Approximately 100 cases are reported in the United States each year; however, the actual number of infections is likely to be much higher because tularemia is frequently unsuspected and is difficult to confirm by laboratory tests. The disease is most common in Arkansas, Missouri, and Oklahoma. Most of the infections occur during the summer (when exposure to infected ticks is greatest) and the winter (when hunters are exposed to infected rabbits). People at greatest risk for infection are hunters, those exposed to ticks, and laboratory personnel. In areas where the organism is endemic, it is said that if a rabbit is moving so slowly that it can be shot by a hunter or caught by a pet, the rabbit could be infected.

Clinical Syndromes

The symptoms of tularemia develop abruptly after a 3- to 5-day incubation period and include fever, chills, malaise, and fatigue. *F. tularensis* disease is classified clinically on the basis of the site of the infection and the presence of skin ulcers and lymphadenopathy. Thus tularemia can be subdivided into several different forms: ulceroglandular, oculoglandular, glandular, typhoidal, oropharyngeal, pneumonic, and gastrointestinal.

The **ulceroglandular** form is the most common. A skin lesion, which starts as a painful papule in the area of the enlarged lymph node, develops at the site of an insect bite. The papule then ulcerates and has a necrotic center and raised border. Localized lymphadenopathy is also present.

Oculoglandular tularemia is a specialized form of the disease and results from direct contamination of the eye. The organism can be introduced into the eyes, for example, by contaminated fingers or through exposure to water or aerosols. Affected patients have a painful conjunctivitis and regional lymphadenopathy.

Patients with **glandular** tularemia initially have a painful adenopathy without the overlying ulcer. **Typhoidal** tularemia is a systemic illness characterized by sepsis with multiorgan involvement. This is the most difficult form to recognize and is associated with the highest mortality. **Oropharyngeal** and **gastrointestinal** tularemia results from the ingestion of contaminated meat or water. The **pneumonic** form results from the inhalation of infectious aerosols.

Laboratory Diagnosis
Specimen Collection

The collection and processing of specimens for the isolation of *F. tularensis* is extremely hazardous for both the physician and the laboratory worker. The organism, by virtue of its small size, can penetrate through the skin and mucous membranes during collection of the sample or be inhaled if aerosols are produced. Even though tularemia is rare, it is commonly reported as a laboratory-acquired infection. Gloves should be worn during collection of the specimen (e.g., aspiration of an ulcer or lymph node), and all processing should be performed in a biohazard hood.

Microscopy

The detection of *F. tularensis* in Gram-stained aspirates from infected nodes or ulcers is almost always unsuccessful because the organism is extremely small and stains faintly. A more sensitive and specific approach is direct staining of the clinical specimen with fluorescein-labeled antibodies directed against the organism.

Culture

It is stated that *F. tularensis* cannot be isolated on common laboratory media because the organism requires sulfhydryl-containing substances (e.g., cysteine) for it to grow. However, *F. tularensis* can grow on the chocolate blood agar plates used in most laboratories because these plates are supplemented with cysteine. Thus it is usually not necessary for a laboratory to use specialized media such as cysteine blood agar or glucose cysteine agar to grow most isolates. If infection with *F. tularensis* is suspected, the laboratory should be notified. *F. tularensis* grows slowly and may be overlooked if the cultures are not incubated for a prolonged period. Blood cultures are generally negative for the organism, but cultures of sputum and aspirates of lymph nodes or draining sinuses are usually positive.

Identification

F. tularensis are weakly catalase positive and oxidase negative. The results of most conventional biochemical tests are negative, so identification is confirmed by demonstrating the bacteria's reactivity with specific antiserum.

Serology

Tularemia is diagnosed in most patients by the finding of a fourfold or greater increase in the titer of antibodies during the illness or a single titer of 160 or greater. However, antibodies (including IgG, IgM, and IgA) can persist for many years, making it difficult to differentiate between past and current disease. Antibodies directed against *Brucella* can also cross-react with *Francisella*. Therefore the diagnosis of tularemia should not be based solely on serological tests.

Treatment, Prevention, and Control

Streptomycin is the antibiotic of choice for the treatment of all forms of tularemia. Gentamicin is an acceptable alternative, but there has been less clinical experience with this drug. *F. tularensis* strains produce beta-lactamase, which renders penicillins and cephalosporins ineffective. Tetracycline and chloramphenicol have been used to treat infections; however, these bacteriostatic antibiotics are associated with an unacceptably high rate of relapse. The mortality rate is less than 1% in patients treated promptly with appropriate antibiotics.

To prevent infection, people should avoid the reservoirs and vectors of infection (e.g., rabbits, ticks, biting insects), but this is often difficult. At a minimum, people should not handle ill-appearing rabbits and should wear gloves when skinning and eviscerating animals. Because the organism is present in the arthropod's feces and not saliva, the tick must feed for a prolonged time before the infection is transmitted. Therefore prompt removal of the tick can prevent infection. The wearing of protective clothing and use of insect repellents reduces the risk of exposure.

Live, attenuated vaccines are not completely effective in preventing disease but can lessen the severity of the disease. These are recommended for people at a significantly increased risk of exposure to the organism. Inactivated vaccines are not protective because they do not elicit protective, cellular immunity.

BRUCELLA

The genus *Brucella* consists of six species, four of which cause human **brucellosis**: *B. abortus, B. melitensis, B. suis,* and *B. canis.* However, nucleic acid hybridization studies have shown that only one species of *Brucella* actually exists *(B. melitensis);* the other species are considered closely related biological variants (biovars). Because the nomenclature for this genus is well established, however, the species designations for the individual groups are retained here. *Brucella* is closely related to *Bartonella* (see Chapter 35).

Brucellosis has a number of names based on the original microbiologists who isolated and described the organisms (Sir David Bruce and Bernhard Bang [**Bang's disease**]), its clinical presentation (**undulant fever**), and the sites of recognized outbreaks (e.g., Malta fever, Mediterranean remittent fever, rock fever of Gibraltar, county fever of Constantinople, fever of Crete).

Physiology and Structure

The individual species are distinguished by their reservoir host, growth properties, and biochemical reactivities, as well as by the fatty acid composition of their cell walls. *Brucella* are small (0.5×0.6 to 1.5 μm), nonmotile, nonencapsulated, gram-negative coccobacilli. The organism grows slowly on culture (taking a week or more), is strictly aerobic with some strains requiring supplemental carbon dioxide for growth, and does not ferment carbohydrates. Human isolates are catalase and oxidase positive, reduce nitrate, and have variable urease activity. *B. abortus, B. melitensis,* and *B. suis* have two surface antigens in common: A and M antigens. *B. abortus* has the highest concentration of **A antigen,** and *B. melitensis* has the highest concentration of **M antigen.** *B. canis* is antigenically distinct. Some characteristics of the four species that cause human disease are summarized in Table 33-5.

Pathogenesis and Immunity

Like *Francisella, Brucella* is an intracellular parasite of the reticuloendothelial system. After the initial exposure, the organisms are phagocytosed by macrophages and monocytes and then are carried to the spleen, liver, bone marrow, lymph nodes, and kidneys. Granulomas form in these organs, and destructive changes in these and other tissues occur in patients with advanced disease. These organisms are able to survive intracellularly because they can inhibit polymorphonuclear leukocyte degranulation, and their survival in cells can be prolonged unless specific cellular immunity develops. *B. melitensis* is the species most able to resist the bactericidal effect of serum and phagocytic killing, consistent with the increased virulence of this species.

Epidemiology

Brucella infections have a worldwide distribution, with more than 500,000 documented cases reported annually. However, the incidence of disease in the United States is much lower (119 reported infections in 1994 [Figure 33-5]), with approximately 1 reported case per 2 million

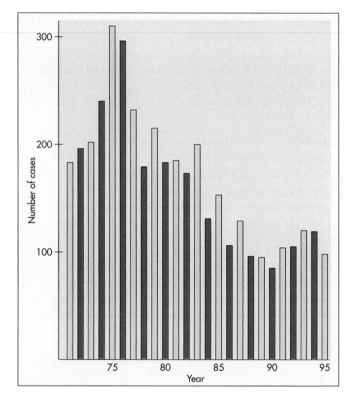

FIGURE 33-5 Incidence of brucellosis in the United States from 1971 to 1995. (From *MMWR* 44:525-529,1995.)

| TABLE 33-5 | **Characteristics of Human Brucellosis** |

| | | | GROWTH ON DYES | | |
SPECIES	ANIMAL RESERVOIR	CO₂ REQUIRED	BASIC FUCHSIN	THIONIN	CLINICAL DISEASE
B. melitensis	Goats, sheep	−	+	+	Severe, acute disease with complications (common)
B. abortus	Cattle	+	+	−	Mild disease with suppurative complications (uncommon)
B. suis	Swine	−	±	+	Suppurative, destructive disease with chronic manifestations
B. canis	Dogs	−	−	+	Mild disease with suppurative complications (uncommon)

people. The disease is rare in the United States because disease in the animal reservoir is well controlled.

Brucella causes mild or asymptomatic disease in the natural host: *B abortus* infects cattle; *B. melitensis,* goats and sheep; *B. suis,* swine; and *B. canis,* dogs, foxes, and coyotes (Box 33-3). The organism has a predilection for infecting organs rich in erythritol, a sugar metabolized by many *Brucella* strains in preference to glucose. Animal (but not human) tissues, including breast, uterus, placenta, and epididymis, are rich in erythritol. Thus the organisms localize in these tissues in nonhuman reservoirs and can cause sterility, abortions, or asymptomatic carriage. Human disease in the United States results primarily from the consumption of contaminated, unpasteurized milk and other dairy products. California and Texas are the areas in the United States where the highest number of cases are reported, and most of these infections occur in Hispanics from Mexico or visitors to that country. Laboratory personnel are also at significant risk for infection through direct contact or inhalation of the organism. Disease in the animal population in the United States has been effectively eliminated through the destruction of infected animals and the vaccination of disease-free animals, so infections in veterinarians, slaughterhouse workers, and farmers is now much less common than it was before 1980.

Clinical Syndromes

The disease spectrum of brucellosis depends on the infecting organism. *B. abortus* and *B. canis* tend to produce mild disease with rare suppurative complications. In contrast, *B. suis* causes the formation of destructive lesions and has a prolonged course. *B. melitensis,* the most common cause of brucellosis, also causes severe disease with a high incidence of serious complications because the organisms can survive in phagocytic cells and multiply to high concentrations.

Acute disease develops in approximately half of the patients infected with *Brucella,* with symptoms first appearing up to 2 months after exposure. Initial symptoms are nonspecific and consist of malaise, chills, sweats, fatigue, weakness, myalgias, weight loss, arthralgias, and nonproductive cough. Almost all patients have a fever, and this can be intermittent in untreated patients, hence the name *undulant fever.* Patients with advanced disease can have gastrointestinal tract symptoms (70% of patients), osteolytic lesions or joint effusions (20% to 60%), respiratory tract symptoms (25%), and less commonly, cutaneous, neurological, or cardiovascular manifestations. Chronic infections can also develop in inadequately treated patients.

Laboratory Diagnosis
Specimen Collection
Multiple blood samples should be collected for culture and serological testing. Bone marrow cultures, as well as cultures of infected tissues, may also be useful. To ensure safe handling of the specimen, the laboratory should be notified if brucellosis is suspected.

Microscopy
Brucella organisms are readily stained using conventional techniques, but their intracellular location and small size make them difficult to detect in clinical specimens.

BOX 33-3	**Summary of *Brucella* Infections**

BACTERIAL FACTORS

Disease—brucellosis (Bang's disease, undulant fever).
Virulence factors—intracellular pathogen that is resistant to killing in serum and by phagocytes.

TRANSMISSION

Zoonotic infection: animal reservoirs are goats and sheep (*B. melitensis*), cattle (*B. abortus*), swine (*B. suis*), and dogs (*B. canis*).
Ingestion of contaminated, unpasteurized milk or dairy products. Direct contact with infected animals or inhalation of infectious aerosols.

WHO IS AT RISK?

People who consume unpasteurized dairy products.
People in direct contact with infected animals (e.g., veterinarians, meat handlers, farmers).
Laboratory personnel.

GEOGRAPHY/SEASON

Worldwide; in the United States, it is most common in California and Texas (Hispanic population).
No seasonal incidence.

MODES OF CONTROL

Treatment for 3 to 6 weeks with doxycycline either alone or with rifampin or gentamicin for patients older than 8 years; doxycycline is replaced with trimethoprim-sulfamethoxazole for children younger than 8 years or for pregnant women.
The disease is controlled by eradication of the disease in the animal reservoir through vaccination and the serological monitoring of the animals for evidence of disease; the pasteurization of dairy products; the use of proper safety techniques in clinical laboratories working with this organism.

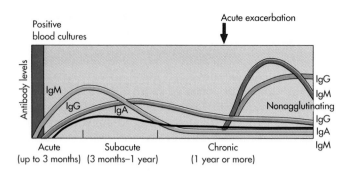

FIGURE 33-6 Antibody responses in untreated brucellosis. (From Mandell G et al: *Principles and practice of infectious diseases*, ed 2, New York, 1985, Churchill Livingstone.)

Culture

Brucella are slow-growing organisms during primary isolation. Isolates can grow on most enriched blood agars and occasionally on MacConkey agar; however, incubation for 3 or more days may be required. It can take as long as 4 to 6 weeks for the organisms to grow in blood cultures, although they grow faster if the blood culture is transferred to agar media (e.g., in biphasic cultures). *B. abortus*, but not other species, must be incubated in a carbon dioxide–enriched atmosphere.

Identification

An isolate can be preliminarily identified as *Brucella* by its microscopic and colonial morphology, positive oxidase reaction, and reactivity with antibodies directed against *Brucella*. Species are differentiated on the basis of their biochemical reactivity, growth in the presence of the dyes thionin and basic fuchsin (Table 33-5), and agglutination in specific antisera. However, most laboratories in the United States refer isolates to reference centers because they infrequently isolate these bacteria and cannot identify the specific species.

Serology

Subclinical brucellosis and many cases of acute and chronic diseases are identified by a specific antibody response in the infected patient. Antibodies are detected in virtually all patients; initially there is an IgM response, after which both IgG and IgA antibodies are produced (Figure 33-6). Antibodies can persist for many months or years, so a significant increase in the antibody titer is required to provide definitive serological evidence of current disease. A presumptive diagnosis can be made if there is a fourfold increase in the titer or a single titer is greater than or equal to 80. High antibody titers (160 or more) are noted in 5% to 10% of the population living in endemic areas, so serological tests should be used to confirm the clinical diagnosis of brucellosis and not to form the basis of the diagnosis. The antigen used in the *Brucella* agglutination test is from *B. abortus*. Antibodies directed against *B. melitensis* or *B. suis* cross-react with this antigen; however, there is no cross-reactivity with *B. canis*. The specific *B. canis* antigen must be used to diagnose infections with this organism. Antibodies directed against other genera of bacteria are also reported to cross-react with the *B. abortus* antigen.

Treatment, Prevention, and Control

Tetracyclines, with doxycycline the preferred agent, are generally active against most strains of *Brucella;* however, this is a bacteriostatic drug, so relapse is common after an initially successful response. The combination of doxycycline with rifampin or gentamicin has proved effective and has a low incidence of relapse. Because the tetracyclines are toxic for young children and fetuses, doxycycline should be replaced with trimethoprim-sulfamethoxazole for pregnant women and children younger than 8 years. Treatment must be continued for 6 weeks or longer for it to be successful. Relapse of disease is due to inadequate therapy and not the development of antibiotic resistance.

Control of human brucellosis is accomplished through control of the disease in livestock, as demonstrated in the United States. This requires the systematic identification (by serological testing) and elimination of infected herds and animal vaccination. The avoidance of unpasteurized dairy products, the observance of appropriate safety procedures in the clinical laboratory, and the wearing of protective clothing by abattoir workers are further ways to prevent brucellosis. Although the attenuated *B. abortus* vaccine has been used successfully to prevent infection in animal herds, it cannot be used in humans because it produces symptomatic disease.

CASE STUDY AND QUESTIONS

A 5-year-old girl was brought to the local public health clinic because of a severe, intractable cough. During the previous 10 days she had a persistent cold that had become worse. The cough developed the previous day and was so severe that it was frequently followed by vomiting. The child appeared exhausted from the coughing episodes. A blood cell count showed a marked leukocytosis with a predominance of lymphocytes. The examining physician suspected that the child has pertussis.

1. What laboratory tests can be performed to confirm the physician's clinical diagnosis? What specimens should be collected, and how should they be submitted to the laboratory?
2. What virulence factors are produced by *B. pertussis* and what are their biological effects?
3. What is the natural progression and prognosis for this disease? How can it be prevented? What are the differences between whole-cell and acellular vaccines?
4. Describe the epidemiology of *F. tularensis* infections. How is the clinical diagnosis confirmed in the laboratory?
5. Describe the epidemiology of the brucellosis.

Bibliography

Capellan J, Fong I: Tularemia from a cat bite: case report and review of feline-associated tularemia, *Clin Infect Dis* 16:472-475, 1993.

Chomel B et al: Changing trends in the epidemiology of human brucellosis in California from 1973 to 1992: a shift toward foodborne transmission, *J Infect Dis* 170:1216-1223, 1994.

Edwards K, Decker M: Acellular pertussis vaccines for infants, *N Engl J Med* 334:391-392, 1996 (editorial).

Hoppe J: Update on epidemiology, diagnosis, and treatment of pertussis, *Eur J Clin Microbiol Infect Dis* 15:189-193, 1996.

Nennig M et al: Prevalence and incidence of adult pertussis in an urban population, *JAMA* 275:1672-1674, 1996.

Pertussis: United States, January 1992-June 1995, *MMWR* 44:525-529, 1995.

Salyers A, Whitt D: *Bacterial pathogenesis: a molecular approach,* Washington, DC, 1994, ASM.

Vancanneyt M et al: Differentiation of *Bordetella pertussis, B. parapertussis,* and *B. bronchiseptica* by whole-cell protein electrophoresis and fatty acid analysis, *Int J Syst Bacteriol* 45:843-847, 1995.

Woolfrey BF, Moody JA: Human infections associated with *Bordetella bronchiseptica, Clin Microbiol Rev* 4:243-255, 1991.

Wright S et al: Pertussis infection in adults with persistent cough, *JAMA* 273:1044-1046, 1996.

Young EJ, Corbel MJ: *Brucellosis: clinical and laboratory aspects,* Boca Raton, Fla, 1989, CRC.

Pasteurellaceae

The family Pasteurellaceae consists of three genera: *Haemophilus*, *Actinobacillus*, and *Pasteurella*, with *Haemophilus* the most common human pathogen (Table 34-1). Although these genera are clearly related to each other, the taxonomic classification of the individual species is controversial. For example, it has been proposed that *Haemophilus* and *Pasteurella* species should be placed in the genus *Pasteurella*. Because the classification is unsettled, the traditional nomenclature has been maintained in this chapter.

The members of the family Pasteurellaceae are small (0.2 × 0.3 to 2.0 µm), gram-negative, non-spore-forming, nonmotile, and aerobic or facultative anaerobic bacilli. Most have fastidious growth needs, requiring enriched media for isolation.

HAEMOPHILUS

Haemophilus organisms are small, sometimes pleomorphic, gram-negative bacilli (Figure 34-1). They are obligate parasites present on the mucous membranes of humans and certain species of animal. *H. influenzae* is the species most commonly associated with disease. Although less frequently isolated, *H. ducreyi* is well recognized as the etiological agent of the sexually transmitted disease, **soft chancre** or **chancroid**. *H. aphrophilus* is a rare but important cause of endocarditis, and the other members of the genus primarily cause opportunistic infections.

Physiology and Structure

Most species of *Haemophilus* (from the Greek words for "blood loving") require media supplemented with growth-stimulating factors, specifically **X factor** (hematin), **V factor** (nicotinamide adenine dinucleotide [NAD]), or both factors. Although both factors are present in blood-enriched media, the blood must be gently heated to release the factors and destroy the inhibitors of V factor. For this reason, heated blood ("chocolate") agar is used for the in vitro isolation of *Haemophilus*.

The cell wall structure of *Haemophilus* is typical of other gram-negative bacilli. Lipopolysaccharide endotoxin activity is present in the cell wall, and strain-specific and species-specific proteins are found in the outer membrane. Analysis of these strain-specific proteins has been valuable in epidemiological investigations. The surface of many, but not all, strains of *H. influenzae* is covered with a polysaccharide capsule, and six antigenic serotypes (a through f) have been identified. Before the introduction of vaccines directed against *H. influenzae* type b antigen, this serotype was responsible for causing more than 95% of all invasive *Haemophilus* infections. After the introduction of the vaccines, serotypes a and f, as well as nonencapsulated *H. influenzae*, emerged as important pathogens. Other species of *Haemophilus* do not have capsules.

In addition to the serological differentiation of *H. influenzae*, the species is subdivided into nine biotypes (I to VIII and *aegyptius*) on the basis of three biochemical reactions: indole production, urease activity, and ornithine decarboxylase activity. Although biotype *aegyptius* and *H. influenzae* biotype III have identical biochemical profiles, they can be distinguished by the nature of the clinical disease, their in vitro growth properties, and the outer membrane protein profiles. *H. influenzae* biotype *aegyptius* is important because it causes purulent conjunctivitis and a systemic disease called *Brazilian purpuric fever*.

Pathogenesis and Immunity

Haemophilus species, particularly *H. parainfluenzae* and nonencapsulated *H. influenzae*, colonize the upper respiratory tract in virtually all people within the first few months of life. These organisms can spread locally and cause disease in the ears (otitis media), sinuses (sinusitis), and lower respiratory tract (bronchitis, pneumonia). Disseminated disease, however, is relatively uncommon. In contrast, encapsulated *H. influenzae* (particularly serogroup b) is uncommon in the upper respiratory tract or is present in only very small numbers but has been a common cause of disease in children (i.e., meningitis, epiglottitis, cellulitis). Pili and nonpilus adhesins are believed to mediate the colonization of the oropharynx with *H. influenzae*. Cell wall components of the bacteria (e.g., lipopolysaccharide and a low-molecular-weight glycopeptide) impair ciliary function, which leads to damage of the respiratory epithelium. The bacteria can then be translocated across both epithelial and endothelial cells and enter the bloodstream. In the absence of specific opsonic antibodies directed against the polysaccharide capsule, high-grade bacteremia can develop, with dissemination to the meninges or other distal foci.

The major virulence factor in *H. influenzae* type b is the antiphagocytic polysaccharide capsule, which contains ribose, ribitol, and phosphate (commonly referred to as *polyribitol phosphate* [**PRP**]). Antibodies directed against the capsule greatly stimulate bacterial phagocytosis and complement-mediated bactericidal activity. These antibodies develop as a result of natural infection, vaccination with purified PRP, or the passive transfer of maternal antibodies. The severity of systemic disease is inversely related to the rate of clearance of bacteria from the bloodstream. The risk of meningitis and epiglottitis is significantly greater in patients with no anti-PRP antibodies, with depletion of complement, or after splenectomy. The lipopolysaccharide lipid A component induces meningeal inflammation in an animal model and may be responsible for initiating this response in humans. IgA1–specific proteases are produced by *H. influenzae* (both encapsulated and nonencapsulated strains) and may facilitate colonization of the organisms on mucosal surfaces.

Epidemiology

Haemophilus species are present in almost all individuals. Most of the isolates are nonencapsulated *H. influenzae*, with encapsulated strains detectable only when highly selective culture methods are used. Although *H. influenzae* type b is the most common serotype that causes systemic disease, it is rarely isolated in healthy children (a fact that emphasizes the virulence of this bacterium). *H. parainfluenzae* constitutes 10% of the bacterial flora in saliva, and the other species are associated with dental plaque and periodontal disease.

Haemophilus species can also be isolated in the gastrointestinal and genitourinary tracts but typically in relatively low numbers.

The epidemiology of *Haemophilus* disease has changed dramatically in the past decade (Box 34-1). The incidence of invasive *Haemophilus* disease increased gradually up to the late 1980's, with an estimated 15,000 cases reported annually. Two thirds of the infections were meningitis, and most occurred in children younger than 1 year. The primary risk factor for invasive *Haemophilus* disease is the absence of protective antibodies directed against the polysaccharide capsule. The first vaccines for *H. influenzae* type b were not protective for children younger than 18 months of age (the population at greatest risk for disease) because there is a natural delay in the maturation of the immune response to polysaccharide antigens. However, vaccines containing purified PRP antigens conjugated to protein carriers were found to elicit a protective antibody response in infants 2 months of age and older. Since the introduction of conjugated vaccines in December 1987, there has been a 95% reduction in the incidence of systemic disease in children younger than 5 years old (Figure 34-2). Most of the *H. influenzae* type b infections now occur in non-immune children (incomplete vaccination or a poor response to the vaccine) and in elderly adults with waning immunity. In addition, invasive *H. influenzae* disease caused by other serotypes of encapsulated bacteria (particularly serotypes a and f) and by nonencapsulated strains has now become proportionally more common than that caused by serotype b.

The epidemiology of disease caused by nonencapsulated *H. influenzae* and other *Haemophilus* species is distinct. Because it is common for people to be colonized with these species, invasive disease is relatively uncommon. Ear and sinus infections caused by these organisms are primarily pediatric diseases but can occur in adults. Pulmonary disease most commonly affects the elderly, particularly those with a history of underlying obstruc-

TABLE 34-1	***Haemophilus* Species Associated with Human Disease**
SPECIES	**PRIMARY DISEASES**
H. influenzae	Pneumonia, sinusitis, otitis, conjunctivitis, meningitis, epiglottitis, cellulitis, bacteremia
H. ducreyi	Chancroid
H. aphrophilus	Endocarditis, opportunistic infections
H. parainfluenzae	Bacteremia, endocarditis, opportunistic infections
H. haemolyticus	Opportunistic infections
H. parahaemolyticus	Opportunistic infections
H. paraphrophilus	Opportunistic infections

FIGURE 34-1 Gram stain of *H. influenzae*.

BOX 34-1   Summary of *Haemophilus* Infections

BACTERIAL FACTORS

Diseases—see Table 34-1; biotype *aegypticus* is responsible for purulent conjunctivitis and Brazilian purpuric fever.

Virulence factors—Type b polysaccharide capsule inhibits complement-mediated phagocytosis; pili, and nonpilus adhesins mediate attachment to epithelial cells; lipopolysaccharide and glycopeptide impair cilia and damage epithelial surface.

Type b strains are now being rapidly replaced with types a and f strains, as well as nonencapsulated strains.

TRANSMISSION

Endogenous spread from upper respiratory tract directly to sinuses, ear, and lower respiratory tract. Bacteremia relatively uncommon except in pulmonary disease.

WHO IS AT RISK?

Patients with systemic infections, especially nonimmunized children or elderly people with waning immunity (particularly obstructive pulmonary disease).

Patients with depleted complement or after splenectomy.

GEOGRAPHY/SEASON

Worldwide.

No seasonal incidence.

H. ducreyi causes genital ulcers in people living in Africa and Asia; this occurs less commonly in the populations of Europe and North America.

MODES OF CONTROL

Severe infection should be treated with beta-lactamase—resistant cephalosporin with good CSF penetration (e.g., ceftriaxone) or chloramphenicol.

For mild infection, ampicillin (if susceptible), trimethoprim-sulfamethoxazole, or active cephalosporin is used.

Active immunization with purified capsular PRP conjugated to protein carrier is best prevention against *H. influenzae* type b.

Passive immunization with hyperimmune globulins active against *H. influenzae* type b is of some use in protecting high-risk children exposed to organism.

Rifampin prophylaxis is useful in eliminating carriage of *H. influenzae* type b in children at high risk for disease.

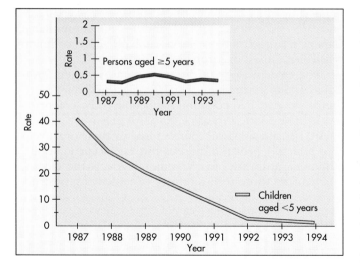

FIGURE 34-2 The rate of *H. influenzae* disease per 100,000 patients has dramatically decreased in children younger than 5 years but has remained relatively constant in older children. (From *MMWR* 44:546, 1995.)

tive pulmonary disease or conditions predisposing to aspiration (e.g., alcoholism, altered mental state).

H. ducreyi is an important cause of genital ulcers (chancroid) in Africa and Asia but is less common in Europe and North America. The incidence of disease in the United States is cyclic, with a peak incidence of more than 5000 cases reported in 1988, decreasing to less than 700 cases in 1995. Despite this favorable trend, the

Centers for Disease Control and Prevention has documented that the disease is significantly underreported, so the true incidence is unknown.

Clinical Syndromes

The clinical syndromes seen in patients with *H. influenzae* infections are represented in Figure 34-3. The diseases caused by all *Haemophilus* species are described in the following sections.

Meningitis

As mentioned already, *H. influenzae* type b was the most common cause of pediatric meningitis, but this changed rapidly once the conjugated vaccines became widely used. Disease in nonimmune patients results from the bacteremic spread of the organisms from the nasopharynx and cannot be differentiated clinically from other causes of bacterial meningitis. The intial presentation is a 1- to 3-day history of mild upper respiratory disease, after which the typical signs and symptoms of meningitis appear. Mortality is less than 10% in patients who receive prompt therapy, and carefully designed studies have also documented a low incidence of serious neurological sequelae (in contrast with the 50% incidence of severe residual damage in children seen in initial studies).

Epiglottitis

Epiglottitis, characterized by cellulitis and the swelling of the supraglottic tissues, represents a life-threatening emergency. Although epiglottitis is a pediatric disease, the peak incidence of this disease during the prevaccine era was primarily in children 2 to 4 years of age; this is in contrast with the incidence of meningitis, which peaked in children 3 to 18 months of age. Children with epiglottitis have pharyngitis, fever, and difficulty breathing, which can rapidly progress to complete obstruction of the airway and death. Since the introduction of the vaccine, the incidence of this disease has also decreased dramatically in children and remains relatively rare in adults.

Cellulitis

As with meningitis and epiglottitis, cellulitis is another pediatric disease that has largely been eliminated by vaccination. When it is observed, patients have fever and cellulitis characterized by the development of reddish-blue patches on the cheeks or periorbital areas. The diagnosis is strongly suggested by the typical clinical presentation, cellulitis proximal to the oral mucosa, and lack of documented vaccination in the child.

Arthritis

Before the advent of conjugated vaccines, the most common form of arthritis in children younger than 2 years of age was an infection of single large joints secondary to the bacteremic spread of *H. influenzae* type b. Disease does occur in older children and adults, but it is very uncommon and generally affects immunocompromised patients and patients with previously damaged joints.

Otitis, Sinusitis, and Lower Respiratory Tract Disease

Nonencapsulated strains of *H. influenzae* are opportunistic pathogens that can cause infections of the upper and lower airways. Most studies have shown that *H. influenzae* and *Streptococcus pneumoniae* are the two most common causes of acute and chronic otitis and sinusitis. Primary pneumonia is uncommon in children and adults who have normal pulmonary function. However, these organisms commonly colonize patients who have chronic pulmonary disease and frequently are associated with exacerbations of bronchitis as well as frank pneumonia.

Conjunctivitis and Brazilian Purpuric Fever

Epidemic, as well as endemic, conjunctivitis can be caused by *H. influenzae* biotype *aegyptius*. A specific strain of this organism has also been found to cause Brazilian purpuric fever, a fulminant pediatric disease characterized by an initial conjunctivitis followed a few days later by the acute onset of fever, vomiting, and abdominal pain. In untreated patients, petechiae, purpura, and shock, culminating in death, rapidly ensue. The pathogenesis of Brazilian purpuric fever and the specific virulence characteristics of the pathogen are poorly understood.

Chancroid

Chancroid is a sexually transmitted disease that is most commonly diagnosed in men, presumably because

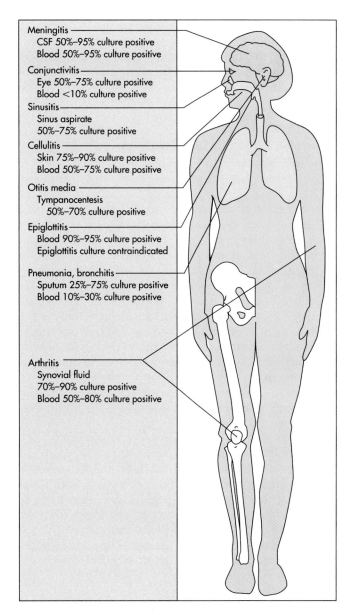

FIGURE 34-3 Infections caused by *H. influenzae*. With the advent of the conjugated vaccine, most infections in adults involve areas contiguous with the oropharynx (i.e., lower respiratory tract, sinuses, ears). Serious systemic infections (e.g., meningitis, epiglottitis) can occur in nonimmune patients. *CSF,* Cerebospinal fluid.

women can have asymptomatic or inapparent disease. Approximately 5 to 7 days after exposure, a tender papule with an erythematous base develops on the genitalia or perianal area. The lesion then ulcerates and becomes painful, and inguinal lymphadenopathy is frequently present. Other causes of genital ulcers, such as syphilis and herpes simplex disease, must be excluded.

Other Infections

Other species of *Haemophilus* can cause opportunistic infections, such as otitis media, conjunctivitis, sinusitis, meningitis, and dental abscesses. Some species, such as

H. aphrophilus, can spread from the mouth to the blood-stream and then infect a previously damaged heart valve, leading to the development of subacute endocarditis. This disease is particularly difficult to diagnose by laboratory testing because organisms cultured from blood grow slowly.

Laboratory Diagnosis

Specimen Collection and Transport

It is necessary to obtain samples of cerebrospinal fluid (CSF) and blood to diagnose *Haemophilus* meningitis. Because there are approximately 10^7 bacteria per milliliter of CSF in patients with untreated meningitis, 1 to 2 ml of fluid is generally adequate for microscopy, culture, and antigen-detection tests. Blood should also be cultured for the diagnosis of epiglottitis, cellulitis, arthritis, or pneumonia. These cultures are less useful, however, for the diagnosis of localized upper respiratory tract diseases (e.g., sinusitis, otitis). Culture of material obtained by direct needle aspiration is necessary for definitive microbiological confirmation of these diseases. Specimens should not be collected from the posterior pharynx in patients with suspected epiglottitis because the procedure may stimulate coughing and completely obstruct the airway. Specimens for the detection of *H. ducreyi* should be collected with a moistened swab from the base or margin of the ulcer.

Microscopy

If microscopy is performed carefully, the detection of *Haemophilus* species in clinical specimens is both sensitive and specific. Small gram-negative coccobacilli can be detected in more than 80% of CSF specimens from patients with untreated *Haemophilus* meningitis. The microscopic examination of Gram-stained specimens is also useful for the rapid diagnosis of arthritis and lower respiratory tract disease.

Culture

It is relatively easy to isolate *H. influenzae* from clinical specimens inoculated onto media supplemented with growth factors. Chocolate agar or Levinthal agar is used in most laboratories. However, if chocolate agar is overheated during preparation, V factor is destroyed, and *Haemophilus* species requiring this growth factor will not grow; thus each preparation of medium must be tested before use. The bacteria appear as 1- to 2-mm, smooth, opaque colonies after 24 hours of incubation. They can also be detected growing around colonies of *Staphylococcus aureus* on unheated blood agar (**satellite phenomenon**). The staphylococci provide the requisite growth factors by lysing the erythrocytes in the medium and releasing intracellular V factor. The colonies of *H. influenzae* in these cultures are much smaller than they are on chocolate agar, however, because the V factor inhibitors are not inactivated.

The growth of *Haemophilus* in blood cultures is generally delayed because most commercially prepared blood culture broths are not supplemented with optimum concentrations of X and V factors. Furthermore, the growth factors are released only when the blood cells lyse, but inhibitors of V factor present in the medium can delay recovery of the bacteria. Isolates of *H. influenzae* frequently grow better in anaerobically incubated blood cultures because under these conditions the organisms do not require X factor for growth.

H. influenzae biotype *aegyptius* and *H. ducreyi* are fastidious and require specialized growth conditions. Biotype *aegyptius* grows best on chocolate agar supplemented with 1% IsoVitaleX, with growth detected after incubation in a carbon dioxide atmosphere for 2 to 4 days. The recovery of *H. ducreyi* in culture is relatively insensitive (less than 85% of cultures yield organisms under optimal conditions) but reportedly best on GC agar supplemented with 1% to 2% hemoglobin, 5% fetal bovine serum, 10% CVA enrichment, and vancomycin (3 µg/ml). Cultures should be incubated at 33° C in 5% to 10% carbon dioxide for 7 days or more.

Antigen Detection

The immunological detection of *H. influenzae* antigen, specifically the PRP capsule, is a rapid and sensitive way to diagnose *H. influenzae* type b disease. PRP can be detected by particle agglutination, which can detect less than 1 ng/ml of PRP. In this test, antibody-coated latex particles are mixed with the clinical specimen; agglutination occurs if PRP is present. Antigen can be detected in CSF and urine (in which the antigen is eliminated intact). This test detects only disease caused by *H. influenzae* type b. Other capsular serotypes and nonencapsulated strains will not give a positive reaction.

Identification

H. influenzae is readily identified by demonstrating a requirement for both X and V factors and the specific biochemical properties summarized in Table 34-2. Further subgrouping of *H. influenzae* can be done by biotyping, electrophoretic characterization of the membrane protein antigens, and analysis of the strain-specific nucleic acid sequences.

Treatment, Prevention, and Control

Patients with systemic *H. influenzae* infections require prompt antimicrobial therapy because the mortality rate in patients with meningitis or epiglottitis approaches 100%. Serious infections are treated with broad-spectrum cephalosporins. Less severe infections, such as sinusitis and otitis, can be treated with ampicillin (if susceptible), trimethoprim-sulfamethoxazole, or an active cephalosporin.

The major approach to preventing *Haemophilus* disease is through active immunization with purified capsular PRP. As discussed previously, the use of conjugated vaccines has been remarkably successful in reducing the incidences of both *H. influenzae* type b disease and colonization. Currently, it is recommended that children re-

TABLE 34-2 **Differential Characteristics of Common Members of the Family Pasteurellaceae**

ORGANISM	GROWTH FACTOR REQUIREMENT		HEMOLYSIS	ENHANCED GROWTH WITH CO$_2$	CATALASE	FERMENTATION OF:			
	X	V				GLUCOSE	SUCROSE	LACTOSE	MANNOSE
Haemophilus									
H. influenzae	+	+	−	−	+	+	−	−	−
H. haemolyticus	+	+	+	−	+	+	−	−	−
H. parainfluenzae	−	+	−	−	±	+	+	−	+
H. parahaemolyticus	−	+	+	+	+	+	+	−	+
H. aphrophilus	−	−	−	+	−	+	+	+	+
H. paraphrophilus	−	+	−	+	+	+	+	+	+
H. ducreyi	+	−	−	−	−	−	−	−	−
Actinobacillus actino-mycetemcomitans	−	−	−	+	+	+	−	−	+
Pasteurella multocida	−	−	−	−	+	+	+	−	+

ceive four doses of vaccine against *H. influenzae* type b disease before the age of 2 years.

Passive immunization with hyperimmune globulins active against *H. influenzae* type b is successful in protecting high-risk children after exposure to the organism, but its use has been limited. Further trials are necessary to define the circumstances when this measure should be used.

Antibiotic chemoprophylaxis is used to eliminate the carriage of *H. influenzae* type b in children at high risk for disease (e.g., children younger than 2 years of age in a family or day-care center where systemic disease is documented). Rifampin prophylaxis has been used in these settings.

ACTINOBACILLUS

Actinobacillus species are small, facultatively anaerobic, gram-negative bacilli that grow slowly (generally requiring 2 to 3 days of incubation). Three species cause infections in humans, with *A. actinomycetemcomitans* the most important (Table 34-3). The cumbersome name derives from the fact that this organism is frequently associated with (*comitans,* from the Latin word for "accompanying") *Actinomyces.*

Members of the genus *Actinobacillus* colonize the oropharynx of humans and animals and are associated with oral disease (periodontitis), bite wounds, or endocarditis. Virtually all patients with *Actinobacillus* endocarditis have underlying cardiac disease, with the organism spreading from the oral cavity after dental procedures or from periodontitis. An interesting characteristic of *Actinobacillus* is that the bacteria are sticky, adhering to the surface of blood culture bottles in much the same way they adhere to damaged heart valves and initiate chronic endocarditis. Most serious infections are treated with

TABLE 34-3 **Actinobacillus Species Associated with Human Disease**

SPECIES	PRIMARY DISEASES
A. actinomycetemcomitans	Endocarditis, periodontitis, bite wounds
A. ureae	Opportunistic infections (bacteremia, meningitis, pneumonia)
A. hominis	Opportunistic infections (bacteremia, pneumonia)

ampicillin, either alone or in combination with an aminoglycoside. Cephalosporins can be substituted for ampicillin if resistance is encountered.

PASTEURELLA

Pasteurella are small (ranging from cocci to small bacilli), facultatively anaerobic, fermentative bacteria commonly found as commensals in the oropharynx of healthy animals. Most human infections result from animal contact (e.g., animal bites, scratches, shared food). *P. multocida* is the most common human pathogen, with the other species infrequent causes of infections (Table 34-4). Three general forms of disease are reported: (1) a localized cellulitis and lymphadenitis that occur after an animal bite or scratch; (2) an exacerbation of chronic respiratory tract disease in patients with underlying pulmonary dysfunction (presumably related to colonization of the patients' oropharynx followed by the aspiration of oral secretions); and (3) a systemic infection in immuno-

TABLE 34-4	*Pasteurella* Species Associated with Human Disease
SPECIES	**PRIMARY DISEASES**
P. multocida	Bite wounds, chronic pulmonary disease, bacteremia, meningitis
P. betti	Opportunistic infections (abscesses, bite wounds, urogenital infections, bacteremia)
P. caballi	Wound infections
P. dagmatis	Bite wounds
P. stomatis	Bite wounds

compromised patients, particularly those with underlying hepatic disease.

P. multocida can be readily isolated on blood or chocolate agar but not MacConkey agar. Large, buttery colonies can be seen after overnight incubation and have a characteristic musty odor caused by the production of indole. They can be readily identified, as indicated in Table 34-2. The organism is susceptible to a variety of antibiotics, with penicillin the antibiotic of choice and tetracycline or a cephalosporin acceptable alternatives.

CASE STUDY AND QUESTIONS

A 78-year-old man confined to a nursing home awoke with a severe headache and stiff neck. Because the man had a high fever and signs of meningitis, the nursing home staff took him to a local emergency room. CSF was cloudy. Analysis revealed 400 white blood cells/mm^3 (95% polymorphonuclear neutrophils), a protein concentration of 75 mg/dl, and a glucose concentration of 20 mg/dl. Small gram-negative bacilli were seen on Gram stained of the CSF, and cultures of CSF and blood were positive for *H. influenzae*.

1. Discuss the epidemiology of *H. influenzae* meningitis and compare it with the epidemiology of meningitis caused by *S. pneumoniae* and by *Neisseria meningitidis*.

2. What other diseases are caused by this organism? What other *Haemophilus* species cause disease and what are the diseases?

3. Why is chocolate agar needed for the isolation of *Haemophilus* organisms?

4. What diseases are caused by *Actinobacillus* organisms? What is the source of this organism?

5. What diseases are caused by *Pasteurella multocida*? What is the source of this organism?

Bibliography

Adams W et al: Decline of childhood *Haemophilus influenzae* type b (Hib) disease in the Hib vaccine era, *JAMA* 269:221-226, 1993.

Albritton WL: Infections due to *Haemophilus* species other than *H. influenzae*, *Ann Rev Microbiol* 36:199-216, 1982.

Brenner DJ et al: Biochemical, genetic, and epidemiologic characterization of *Haemophilus influenzae* biogroup *aegyptius* (*Haemophilus aegyptius*) strains associated with Brazilian purpuric fever, *J Clin Microbiol* 26:1524-1534, 1988.

Campos J: *Haemophilus*. In Murray P et al, editors: *Manual of clinical microbiology*, Washington, DC, 1995, American Society of Microbiology.

Daum R et al.: Epidemiology, pathogenesis, and prevention of *Haemophilus influenzae* disease, *J Infect Dis* 165(suppl):1-206, 1992.

Farley M et al: Incidence and clinical characteristics of invasive *Haemophilus influenzae* disease in adults, *J Infect Dis* 165 (suppl):42-43, 1992.

Holst E et al: Characterization and distribution of *Pasteurella* species recovered from infected humans, *J Clin Microbiol* 30:2984-2987, 1992.

Jordens J, Slack M: *Haemophilus influenzae*: then and now, *Eur J Clin Microbiol Infect Dis* 14:935-948, 1995.

Kaplan AH et al: Infection due to *Actinobacillus actinomycetemcomitans*: 15 cases and review, *Rev Infect Dis* 11:46-63, 1989.

Morse SA: Chancroid and *Haemophilus ducreyi*, *Clin Microbiol Rev* 2:137-157, 1989.

Totten P, Stamm W, Morris S: How to detect *Haemophilus ducreyi* in genital ulcers and why you should care, *Clin Microbiol Newsletter* 18:145-150, 1996.

Urwin G et al: Invasive disease due to *Haemophilus influenzae* serotype f: clinical and epidemiologic characteristics in the *H. influenzae* serotype b vaccine era, *Clin Infect Dis* 22:1069-1076, 1996.

Miscellaneous Gram-Negative Bacilli

Gram-negative bacilli are an extremely diverse group of organisms. Miscellaneous gram-negative organisms that cause human disease are discussed in this chapter (Table 35-1).

LEGIONELLA

In the summer of 1976, public attention was focused on an outbreak of severe pneumonia that caused many deaths in members of the American Legion convention in Philadelphia. After months of intensive investigations, a previously unknown gram-negative bacillus was isolated. In subsequent studies this organism, named *Legionella pneumophila*, was found to be the cause of multiple epidemic and sporadic infections. This organism was previously not known to exist because it stains poorly with conventional dyes and does not grow on common laboratory media. Despite the initial problems with the isolation of *Legionella* organisms, it is now recognized to be a ubiquitous aquatic saprophyte.

Taxonomic studies have shown that the family Legionellaceae consists of one genus, *Legionella*, which includes 39 species and 3 subspecies. A total of 19 species have been implicated in human disease, with the others found in environmental sources. *L. pneumophila* is the cause of almost 85% of all infections, with serotype 1 isolated most commonly (Figure 35-1).

Physiology and Structure

Members of the genus are slender, pleomorphic, gram-negative bacilli measuring 0.3 to 0.9 × 2 to 5 μm. The organisms characteristically appear as short coccobacilli in tissue but are very pleomorphic on artificial media (Figure 35-2). Legionellae in clinical specimens do not stain with common reagents but can be seen in tissues stained with Dieterle's silver stain. One species, *L. micdadei*, can also be stained with weak acid-fast stains, but the organism loses this property when it grows in culture.

Legionellae are nutritionally fastidious; their growth is enhanced with iron salts and depends on the supplementation of media with L-cysteine. The organisms are nonfermentative and derive energy from the metabolism of amino acids. Most species are motile and catalase positive, liquefy gelatin, and do not reduce nitrate or hydrolyze urea. The selective growth properties of this family have been used as the basis for the preliminary identification of clinical isolates.

Pathogenesis and Immunity

Respiratory tract disease caused by *Legionella* species develops in susceptible people who inhale infectious aerosols. Legionellae are facultative intracellular parasites that can multiply in alveolar macrophages and monocytes. The replicative cycle is initiated by binding complement to an outer membrane porin protein and depositing C3b on the bacterial surface. This permits the bacteria to bind to CR3 receptors on mononuclear phagocytes, after which they penetrate into the cell through endocytosis. The bacteria are not killed in the

TABLE 35-1	Miscellaneous Gram-Negative Bacilli and Their Diseases
ORGANISM	**DISEASE**
Legionella species	Legionnaires' disease, Pontiac fever
Bartonella species	Cat-scratch disease, Oroya fever, bacteremia, bacillary angiomatosis, bacillary peliosis
Calymmatobacterium granulomatis	Granuloma inguinale (donovanosis)
Capnocytophaga species	Periodontitis, septicemia, endocarditis, bite wound infections
Cardiobacterium hominis	Endocarditis
Eikenella corrodens	Human bite wound infection, head and neck infections, respiratory tract infections, bacteremia
Kingella species	Septic arthritis, endocarditis
Spirillum minus	Rat-bite fever
Streptobacillus moniliformis	Rat-bite fever

cells through exposure to toxic superoxide, hydrogen peroxide, and hydroxyl radicals because phagolysosome fusion is inhibited. The bacilli then proliferate and produce proteolytic enzymes, phosphatase, lipase, and nuclease, which eventually kill the host cell. Immunity to disease is primarily cell mediated, with humoral immunity playing a minor role. The bacteria are not killed until sensitized T cells activate the parasitized macrophages.

Epidemiology

Sporadic and epidemic legionellosis has a worldwide distribution (Box 35-1). The bacteria are commonly present in natural bodies of water such as lakes and streams, as well as in air conditioning cooling towers and condensers, and water systems (e.g., showers, hot tubs). The organisms can survive in moist environments for a long time, at relatively high temperatures, and in the presence of disinfectants such as chlorine. One reason for this is that the bacteria can parasitize ameba in the water and replicate in this protected environment (similar to in vivo replication in macrophages).

The incidence of infections caused by *Legionella* species is unknown because it is difficult to document disease. The number of cases has steadily increased during the past decade, with more than 1000 cases reported each year (Figure 35-3). However, serological studies have also shown that a significant proportion of the pop-

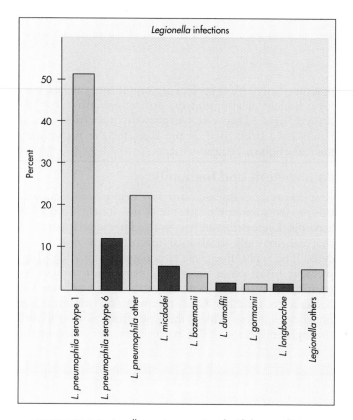

FIGURE 35-1 *Legionella* species associated with human disease.

FIGURE 35-2 *L. pneumophila* grown on buffered charcoal-yeast extract agar.

BOX 35-1 **Summary of *Legionella* Infections**

BACTERIAL FACTORS

Diseases—legionnaires' disease, Pontiac fever.
Virulence factors—facultative intracellular pathogen, inhibition of phagolysosome fusion.
Bacteria can survive in moist environments and relatively high temperatures for prolonged periods; they can replicate in amoeba.

TRANSMISSION

Common in lakes, streams, air conditioning cooling towers and condensers, and water systems.
Inhalation of infectious aerosols.
No person-to-person transmission; no animal reservoir or vector.

WHO IS AT RISK?

Elderly.
Patients with compromised cellular immunity (e.g., renal and cardiac transplant recipients) or pulmonary function (e.g., smokers).

GEOGRAPHY/SEASON

Worldwide.
Most epidemics occur in late summer and autumn.

MODES OF CONTROL

Erythromycin (drug of choice), rifampin, and fluoroquinolones.
Hyperchlorination of water supply and higher water temperatures are moderately successful in prevention.

ulation has acquired immunity to this group of organisms. Based on these studies and the knowledge that legionellae are ubiquitous aquatic saprophytes, it is reasonable to conclude that contact with the organism and acquisition of immunity after an asymptomatic infection are common, and the incidence of true disease is certainly underestimated.

Although sporadic outbreaks of the disease occur throughout the year, most epidemics of the infection occur in the late summer and autumn, presumably because the organism proliferates in water reservoirs during the warm months. The elderly are at greatest risk for disease because of their decreased cellular immunity and compromised pulmonary function. Person-to-person spread or an animal reservoir has not been demonstrated.

Clinical Syndromes

Asymptomatic *Legionella* infections are relatively common and can be detected by low levels of antibodies directed against the organism. Symptomatic infections primarily affect the lungs and present in one of two forms (Table 35-2): an influenza-like illness (referred to as **Pontiac fever**) or a severe form of pneumonia (e.g., **legionnaires' disease**).

Pontiac Fever

L. pneumophila was responsible for causing a self-limited, febrile illness in people working in the Pontiac, Michigan, Public Health Department in 1968. The disease was characterized by fever, chills, myalgia, malaise, and headache but no clinical evidence of pneumonia. The symptoms developed over a 12-hour period, persisted for 2 to 5 days, and then resolved spontaneously, with minimal morbidity and no deaths. Additional epidemics of Pontiac fever have been documented, and the incidence of disease has been high in those exposed.

Legionnaires' Disease

Legionnaires' disease (legionellosis) is characteristically more severe and causes considerable morbidity leading to death unless prompt therapy is initiated. After an incubation period of 2 to 10 days, systemic signs of an acute illness appear abruptly (e.g., fever; chills; a dry, nonproductive cough; headache). Multiorgan disease involving the gastrointestinal tract, central nervous system, liver, and kidneys is common. The primary manifestation is pneumonia with multilobe consolidation and inflammation and microabscesses in lung tissue observed on histopathological studies. Pulmonary function steadily deteriorates in susceptible patients with untreated disease. The overall mortality rate is 15% to 20% but can be much higher in patients with severely depressed cell-mediated immunity (e.g., renal or cardiac transplant recipients).

Laboratory Diagnosis

Microscopy

Legionellae in clinical specimens stain poorly with the Gram stain. Nonspecific staining methods such as those using the Dieterle silver or Gimenez stain can be used to visualize the organisms but are of little value if the speci-

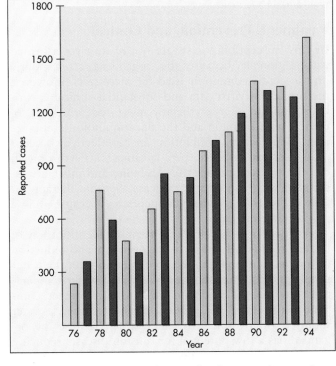

FIGURE 35-3 Reported cases of *Legionella* infections in the United States from 1976 to 1995. (From *MMWR* 44:40, 1996.)

TABLE 35-2   Comparison of Diseases Caused by *Legionella*

	LEGIONNAIRES' DISEASE	PONTIAC FEVER
EPIDEMIOLOGY		
Presentation	Epidemic, sporadic	Epidemic
Attack rate	<5%	>90%
Person-to-person spread	No	No
Underlying pulmonary disease	Yes	No
Time of onset	Epidemic disease in late summer or autumn; endemic disease throughout year	Throughout year
CLINICAL MANIFESTATIONS		
Incubation period	2-10 days	1-2 days
Pneumonia	Yes	No
Course	Requires antibiotic therapy	Self-limited
Mortality	15%-20%, higher if diagnosis is delayed	<1%

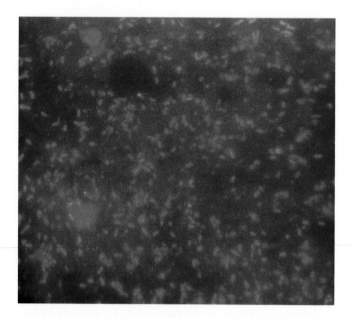

FIGURE 35-4 Direct fluorescent antibody stain of *Legionella micdadei.*

mens are contaminated with normal oral bacteria. The most sensitive way of detecting legionellae microscopically in clinical specimens is to use the direct fluorescent antibody (DFA) test, in which fluorescein-labeled monoclonal or polyclonal antibodies directed against *Legionella* species are used (Figure 35-4). The test is specific, with false-positive reactions observed only rarely. However, the sensitivity of the DFA test is low because the antibody preparations are serotype or species specific and many organisms must be present for detection. The latter problem is due to the relatively small size and predominantly intracellular location of the bacteria. Positive test results revert to negative after about 4 days of treatment. The primary advantage of microscopy over other diagnostic tests is that a positive result can be obtained rapidly.

Culture

Although legionellae were initially difficult to grow, it is now easy to do using commercially available media. As mentioned earlier, legionellae require L-cysteine, and their growth is enhanced with iron (supplied in hemoglobin or ferric pyrophosphate). The medium most commonly used for the isolation of legionellae is buffered charcoal-yeast extract (BCYE) agar, although other supplemented media have also been used. Antibiotics can be added to suppress the growth of rapidly growing contaminating bacteria. Legionellae grow in air or 3% to 5% carbon dioxide at 35° C after 3 to 5 days. Their small (1 to 3 mm) colonies have a ground-glass appearance.

Antigen Detection

Enzyme-linked immunoassays, radioimmunoassays, the agglutination of antibody-coated latex particles, and nu-

cleic acid hybridization studies have all been used to detect legionellae in respiratory specimens and urine. Although the immunological assays are relatively sensitive, the serotype-specific reagents limit the clinical usefulness of the test. In addition, antigen may be excreted in urine for as long as 1 year after the infection has resolved.

Serology

Legionellosis is commonly diagnosed using the indirect fluorescent antibody test to measure a serological response to infection. A fourfold or greater increase in the antibody titer (to a level of 128 or greater) is considered diagnostic. However, the response may be delayed, with a significant increase in the titer typically not seen until after 3 weeks of illness. High titers can occasionally persist for prolonged periods.

Identification

It is easy to identify an isolate as *Legionella* by the finding of typical morphology and specific growth requirements. Legionellae appear as weakly staining, pleomorphic, thin, gram-negative bacilli. Their growth on BCYE, but not on BCYE without L-cysteine or on enriched blood agar media, is presumptive evidence that the organism is *Legionella*. Specific staining with fluorescein-labeled antibodies can confirm the identity of the organisms. In contrast to the identification of the genus, however, species classification is problematic and generally relegated to reference laboratories. Although biochemical tests and the ability of bacilli to fluoresce under long-wave ultraviolet light are useful for differentiating species, the species can be definitively identified only by analyzing the major branched-chain fatty acids in the cell wall and DNA homology.

Treatment, Prevention, and Control

In vitro susceptibility tests are not routinely performed with legionella because the organisms grow poorly on the media commonly used for these tests. However, the limited in vitro data and substantial clinical experience indicate that erythromycin is the antibiotic of choice, with rifampin and the fluoroquinolones also active. Beta-lactam antibiotics are ineffective because most isolates produce beta-lactamases. Erythromycin can substantially reduce the morbidity and mortality associated with legionnaires' disease. Specific therapy for Pontiac fever is generally unnecessary because it is a self-limiting disease.

Prevention of legionellosis requires identification of the environmental source of the organism and reduction of the microbial burden. Hyperchlorination of the water supply and the maintenance of elevated water temperatures have proved moderately successful. However, complete elimination of *Legionella* organisms from a water supply is often difficult or impossible. Because the organism has a low potential for causing disease, reducing the number of organisms in the water supply is frequently an adequate control measure.

TABLE 35-3	*Bartonella* Species Associated with Human Infections
SPECIES	**DISEASES**
B. bacilliformis	Oroya fever (bartonellosis, Carrión's disease)
B. quintana	Trench fever (5-day fever), bacillary angiomatosis, bacillary peliosis, endocarditis
B. henselae	Cat-scratch disease, bacteremia, bacillary angiomatosis, bacillary peliosis, endocarditis
B. elizabethae	Endocarditis (rare)

BARTONELLA

As with many groups of bacteria studied in the past 10 years, analysis of the 16S ribosomal RNA has led to the reorganization of the genus *Bartonella*. The genus *Rochalimaea* was transferred into the genus *Bartonella*, which now consists of eight species, including four that cause human disease (Table 35-3). The bacteria are short (0.3 to 0.5 × 1.0 to 1.7 μm), gram-negative, aerobic bacilli with fastidious growth requirements. Although the organisms can grow on enriched blood agar, prolonged incubation (1 to 6 weeks) in a humid, 37° C atmosphere supplemented with carbon dioxide is required for their initial recovery.

Members of the genus are found in a variety of animal reservoirs and typically present without evidence of disease. Insect vectors have also been shown or implicated as vectors in human infections. Because these organisms fail to cause disease in other hosts, an animal model is not available for studying the pathogenesis of these infections.

B. bacilliformis, the original member of this genus, is responsible for causing bartonellosis, an acute febrile illness consisting of severe anemia (**Oroya fever**) followed by a chronic cutaneous form (**verruga**). Bartonellosis is restricted to Peru, Ecuador, and Colombia, the endemic regions of the sandfly vector, *Phlebotomus.* After the bite of an infected sandfly, the bacteria enter the bloodstream, multiply, and penetrate into erythrocytes. This process increases the fragility of the infected cells and facilitates their clearance by the reticuloendothelial system, leading to acute anemia. Myalgias, arthralgias, and headaches are also common. This stage of illness ends with the development of humoral immunity. In the chronic stage of bartonellosis, 1- to 2-cm cutaneous nodules appear over the course of 1 to 2 months and may persist for months to years.

B. quintana was originally described as the causative organism of **trench fever** ("5-day" fever), a disease prevalent during World War I. Infection can vary from asymptomatic to a severe, debilitating illness. Typically, patients have severe headaches, fever, weakness, and pain in the long bones (particularly the tibia). The fever can recur at 5-day intervals, hence the name of the disease. Although trench fever does not cause death, the illness can be very severe. No animal reservoir for this disease has been identified. Rather, disease is spread person to person by the human body louse.

More recently, *B. quintana* has been associated with other illnesses, namely **bacillary angiomatosis** and **bacillary peliosis hepatitis** in immunocompetent and immunocompromised patients (e.g., transplant recipients, patients with the human immunodeficiency virus), as well as in patients with endocarditis. Bacillary angiomatosis is a vascular proliferative disorder of the skin and visceral organs; patients with bacillary peliosis develop cystic, blood-filled spaces in the liver. The etiological role of *B. quintana* and other *Bartonella* species in "culture-negative" **endocarditis** is supported by serological studies.

B. henselae is also responsible for causing bacillary angiomatosis, bacillary peliosis hepatitis, and endocarditis. In addition, there is convincing evidence that this organism is responsible for most cases of **cat-scratch disease.** The disease is acquired after exposure to cats (e.g., scratches, bites, possible contact with cat fleas). Typically, this is a benign infection in children, characterized by chronic regional adenopathy of the lymph nodes draining the site of contact. Although bacilli can be seen in the lymph node tissues, culture is usually negative for organisms. A definitive diagnosis is based on the characteristic presentation and serological evidence of a recent infection. In contrast to cat-scratch disease, *B. henselae* can be isolated from blood collected from patients with **chronic bacteremia** if the cultures are incubated for 2 weeks or more. The reason this organism can be isolated in one disease but not the other is not understood.

Treatment of *Bartonella* infections is complicated because minimal information is available about the in vitro susceptibility of the organism. Cat-scratch disease does not appear to respond to antimicrobial therapy. Trench fever, bacillary angiomatosis and peliosis, and endocarditis can be treated with gentamicin, either alone or with erythromycin. Broad-spectrum cephalosporins appear to be effective, and erythromycin or doxycycline have been used with initial success, but the bacteriostatic antibiotics have a high rate of relapse.

CALYMMATOBACTERIUM

Calymmatobacterium (Donovania) granulomatis is the etiological agent of **granuloma inguinale,** a granulomatous disease affecting the genitalia and inguinal area. The organism was discovered by Donovan and subsequently renamed to reflect its encapsulated appearance in tissues (*kalymma* is Greek for "hood" or "veil"). *C. granulomatis* has been isolated once in a monocyte culture system but does not appear to grow in cell-free systems. The laboratory diagnosis is made by staining infected tis-

FIGURE 35-5 Electron micrograph of *C. granulomatis* within a mononuclear cell phagosome. Note the prominent capsule surrounding the cell, surface projections *(arrow)*, and typical gram-negative trilaminar membrane structure *(inset)*. (From Kuberski T et al: *J Infect Dis* 142:744-749, 1980.)

sues with Wright's or Giemsa stain. The organisms appear as small (0.5 to 1.0 × 1.5 μm) bacilli in the cytoplasm of histiocytes, polymorphonuclear leukocytes, and plasma cells. From 1 to 25 bacteria per phagocytic cell can be seen; a prominent capsule surrounds the organisms (Figure 35-5).

Granuloma inguinale is a rare disease in the United States but is encountered in tropical areas such as the Caribbean and New Guinea. It can be transmitted after repeated exposure through sexual intercourse or nonsexual trauma to the genitalia. After a prolonged incubation of weeks to months, subcutaneous nodules appear on the genitalia or in the inguinal area. The nodules subsequently break down, revealing one or more painless granulomatous lesions that can extend and coalesce.

Laboratory confirmation of granuloma inguinale is made by scraping the border of the lesion, by spreading the collected tissue on a slide, and by staining it with Giemsa or Wright's stain. Pathognomonic "Donovan bodies" are observed within mononuclear phagocytes.

Tetracyclines, erythromycin, and trimethoprim-sulfamethoxazole have been used successfully for treatment, although relapses have occurred. Antibiotic prophylaxis has not proved effective in preventing and controlling infection.

CAPNOCYTOPHAGA

Capnocytophaga strains are filamentous gram-negative bacilli capable of aerobic and anaerobic growth in the presence of carbon dioxide. The genus is subdivided into two groups: dysgonic fermenter 1 (DF-1), with three species, and dysgonic fermenter 2 (DF-2), with two species. DF-1 strains colonize the human oropharynx and are associated with periodontitis, bacteremia, and

rarely endocarditis. DF-2 strains colonize the dog oropharynx and are associated with bite wounds. Overwhelming sepsis can occur in patients who have undergone splenectomy or who have compromised hepatic function (e.g., cirrhosis). Most *Capnocytophaga* infections can be treated with broad-spectrum cephalosporins, fluoroquinolones, or penicillin; strains are typically resistant to the aminoglycosides.

CARDIOBACTERIUM

Cardiobacterium hominis, named for the predelection of this bacterium to cause endocarditis in humans, is the only member of the genus. *C. hominis* isolates are nonmotile, characteristically small (1 × 1 to 2 μm) but sometimes pleomorphic, gram-negative bacilli. The bacteria are fermentative, indole and oxidase positive, and catalase negative.

Endocarditis caused by *C. hominis* is uncommon, with fewer than 50 cases reported in the literature. However, many cases are unreported or undiagnosed because of the low virulence of this organism and its slow growth in vitro. *C. hominis* is present in the upper respiratory tract of almost 70% of healthy people.

Endocarditis is the only human disease caused by *C. hominis.* Most patients with *C. hominis* endocarditis have preexisting heart disease and either have a history of oral disease or have undergone dental procedures before the clinical symptoms developed. The organisms are able to enter the bloodstream from the oropharynx, adhere to the damaged heart tissue, and then slowly multiply. The course of disease is insidious and subacute, with patients typically having symptoms (fatigue, malaise, and low-grade fever) for months before seeking medical care. Complications are rare, and complete recovery after appropriate antibiotic therapy is common.

The isolation of *C. hominis* from blood cultures confirms the diagnosis of endocarditis. The organism grows slowly in culture. It takes 1 to 2 weeks before growth is detected, which is the reason that infections with these organisms are not confirmed in some patients. *C. hominis* appears in broth cultures as discrete clumps that can be easily overlooked. The organism requires enhanced carbon dioxide and humidity to grow on agar media, with pinpoint (1-mm) colonies seen on blood or chocolate agar plates after 3 days of incubation. The organism does not grow on MacConkey agar or other selective media commonly used for gram-negative bacilli. *C. hominis* can be readily identified by its growth properties, microscopic morphology, and reactivity in biochemical tests.

C. hominis is susceptible to multiple antibiotics, and most infections are successfully treated with penicillin or ampicillin for 2 to 6 weeks. *C. hominis* endocarditis in people with preexisting heart disease is prevented by the maintenance of good oral hygiene and the use of antibiotic prophylaxis at the time of dental procedures. A long-acting penicillin is effective prophylaxis, but erythromycin should not be used because resistance is common.

EIKENELLA

Eikenella corrodens is a moderate-sized (0.2 × 2 μm), nonmotile, non-spore-forming, facultatively anaerobic gram-negative bacillus. The organism is named after Eiken, who characterized the bacterium and observed the ability of the organism to pit or "corrode" agar. *E. corrodens* is a normal inhabitant of the human upper respiratory tract, but because of its fastidious growth requirements, it is difficult to detect unless specific selective culture media are used. It is an opportunistic pathogen that causes infections in immunocompromised patients and patients with diseases or trauma of the oral cavity. *E. corrodens* has been implicated as the causative agent in human bite wounds or fistfight injuries (frequently complicated by septic arthritis or osteomyelitis if initially treated improperly), sinusitis, meningitis, brain abscesses, pneumonia, lung abscesses, and endocarditis. Because most infections originate from the oropharynx, polymicrobial mixtures of aerobic and anaerobic bacteria are frequently present in cultures. Failure to cure the infection unless specific therapy is administered confirms that *Eikenella* is the causative agent in these infections.

E. corrodens is a slow-growing, fastidious organism that requires 5% to 10% carbon dioxide to grow. Small (0.5- to 1-mm) colonies are observed on common laboratory media after 48 hours of incubation. Pitting in agar is a useful differential characteristic, but fewer than half of all isolates exhibit this characteristic.

E. corrodens is susceptible to penicillin and ampicillin but resistant to oxacillin, first-generation cephalosporins, clindamycin, and the aminoglycosides. Thus *E. corrodens* is resistant to many antibiotics that are selected empirically to treat bite wound infections.

KINGELLA

Kingella species are small, gram-negative coccobacilli that morphologically resemble *Neisseria* species and reside in the human oropharynx. The bacteria are facultatively anaerobic, ferment carbohydrates, and have fastidious growth requirements. *K. kingae*, the most commonly isolated species, has been primarily responsible for causing septic arthritis in children and endocarditis in patients of all ages. Because the organism grows slowly, it may take at least 3 days of incubation before the organism can be recovered in clinical specimens. Most strains are susceptible to beta-lactam antibiotics, including penicillin and aminoglycosides.

STREPTOBACILLUS AND SPIRILLUM

Streptobacillus moniliformis and *Spirillum minus* are the causative agents of two distinct diseases referred to collectively as **rat-bite fever** (Table 35-4). *S. moniliformis* is a long, thin (0.1 to 0.5 × 1 to 5 μm), gram-negative bacillus that tends to stain poorly and be more pleomorphic in older cultures. Granules and bulbous swellings, which resemble a string of beads, may be seen. *S. minus* is a spiral, gram-negative bacillus (0.2 to 0.5 × 3 to 5 μm).

Both *Streptobacillus* and *Spirillum* organisms are found in the nasopharynx of rats and other small rodents, as well as transiently in animals that feed on rodents (e.g., dogs, cats). Turkeys exposed to rats and mice, as well as contaminated water and milk, have also been implicated in *Streptobacillus* infections.

Although the epidemiology and clinical syndrome of recurrent fevers are similar for both *Streptobacillus* and *Spirillum*, distinct differences have been observed. For example, the incubation period for *Streptobacillus* infections is shorter than that for *Spirillum* infections, and the

TABLE 35-4 Comparison of *Streptobacillus* and *Spirillum* Species		
	STREPTOBACILLUS MONILIFORMIS	**SPIRILLUM MINUS**
Distribution	Worldwide	Worldwide, primarily Asia
Reservoir	Rats and other small rodents	Rats and other small rodents
Transmission	Bite of rat or another rodent, contact with animals that feed on rodents, consumption of water or other contaminated food or fluid	Bite of rat or another rodent, contact with animals that feed on rodents
Disease	Rat-bite fever (Haverhill fever)	Rat-bite fever (sodoku)
Incubation period	<10 days	2 weeks
Clinical presentation	Abrupt onset; high fever; chills, headache, myalgias, rash, arthritis or arthralgia; recurrent fevers if untreated	Abrupt onset; fever, chills, rash, lymphangitis, lymphadenopathy; recurrent fevers if untreated
Mortality	10% if untreated	6% if untreated
Treatment	Penicillin	Penicillin
Diagnosis	Culture, serological tests	Darkfield examination, Wright's- or Giemsa-stained blood smears, animal inoculation

clinical course in patients with *Spirillum* infections does not usually include the myalgias, arthralgias, and frank arthritis. Patients with one form of *S. moniliformis* infection, **Haverhill fever** or **erythema arthriticum epidemicum**, typically have fever, rash, arthralgia, chills, vomiting, and gastrointestinal and respiratory symptoms. Ulceration at the bite site with lymphadenopathy and lymphangitis is observed in patients with *Spirillum* rat-bite infections (also known as *sodoku*). Recurrent febrile episodes are observed in patients with untreated disease caused by either organism.

S. moniliformis, but not *S. minus*, can be cultured in vitro. Blood and joint fluid should be collected for this purpose and mixed with citrate to prevent clotting during transport to the laboratory. The organism can grow on enriched media supplemented with 15% blood, 20% horse or calf serum, or 5% ascitic fluid. *S. moniliformis* is slow growing, taking at least 3 days to be isolated. When grown in broth, it has the appearance of "puffballs"; small round colonies are seen on agar, as are cell wall–defective forms with their typical fried-egg appearance. It is difficult to identify the organisms because they are relatively inactive, although acid is produced from glucose and other selected carbohydrates. The serological tests that can detect antibodies against *Streptobacillus* antigens are available in reference laboratories. A titer greater than or equal to 80 or a fourfold rise in the titer is considered diagnostic, although this test has not been standardized or extensively evaluated for cross-reactivity.

S. minus, which is more common in countries outside the United States, has not been cultured in vitro. Dark-field examination of blood, ulcer exudates, or lymph node aspirates is used to detect *S. minus*. Blood smears can be stained with Giemsa or Wright's stain. *S. minus* can also be detected in the blood of rodents 1 to 3 weeks after the intraperitoneal inoculation of the clinical specimen. Penicillin is the antibiotic of choice for treating rat-bite fever. Tetracycline can be used in penicillin-allergic patients.

CASE STUDY AND QUESTIONS

A 73-year-old man was admitted to the hospital because of breathing difficulties, chest pain, chills, and fever of several days' duration. He was well until 1 week before admission, when he noted the onset of a persistent headache and a productive cough. The patient smoked 2 packs of cigarettes a day for more than 50 years and drank a 6-pack of beer daily; he also had a history of bronchitis. Physical examination revealed an elderly man in severe respiratory distress with a temperature of 39.0° C, pulse

of 120 beats/min, respiratory rate of 36 breaths/min, and blood pressure of 145/95 mm Hg. Chest examination revealed an infiltrate in the middle and lower lobes of the right lung. The white blood cell count was 14,000 cells/mm³ (80% polymorphonuclear neutrophils). Gram stain of the sputum showed neutrophils but no bacteria, and routine bacterial cultures of sputum and blood were negative for organisms. Infection with *L. pneumophila* was suspected.

1. What laboratory tests can be used to confirm this diagnosis? Why was the routine culture and Gram stained specimen negative for *Legionella* organisms?
2. How are *Legionella* species able to survive phagocytosis by the alveolar macrophages?
3. What environmental factors are implicated in the spread of *Legionella* infections? How can this risk be eliminated or minimized?
4. What infections are caused by *Bartonella* species? *Calymmatobacterium*? *Capnocytophaga*? *Cardiobacterium*? *Eikenella*? *Kingella*? *Spirillum*? *Streptobacillus*? What is the source of each of these human pathogens?

Bibliography

Adal K, Cockerell C, Petri W: Cat scratch disease, bacillary angiomatosis, and other infections due to *Rochalimaea*, *N Engl J Med* 330:1509-1515, 1994.

Hensel D, Slater L: The genus *Bartonella*, *Clin Microbiol Newsletter* 17:9-14, 1995.

Hookey J et al: Phylogeny of Legionellaceae based on small subunit ribosomal DNA sequences and proposal of *Legionella lytica* comb. nov. for *Legionella*-like amoebal pathogens, *Int J Syst Bacteriol* 46:526-531, 1996.

Kharsany A et al: Culture of *Calymmatobacterium granulomatis*, *Clin Infect Dis* 22:391, 1996.

Kuberski T, Papadimitriou JM, Phillips P: Ultrastructure of *Calymmatobacterium granulomatis* in lesions of granuloma inguinale, *J Infect Dis* 142:744-749, 1980.

Maurin M, Raoult D: *Bartonella (Rochalimaea) quintana* infections, *Clin Microbiol Rev* 9:273-292, 1996.

Reingold AL: Role of legionellae in acute infections of the lower respiratory tract, *Rev Infect Dis* 10:1018-1028, 1988.

Spach D et al: *Bartonella (Rochalimaea)* species as a cause of apparent "culture-negative" endocarditis, *Clin Infect Dis* 20:1044-1047, 1995.

Stoloff AL, Gillies ML: Infections with *Eikenella corrodens* in a general hospital: a report of 33 cases, *Rev Infect Dis* 8:50-53, 1986.

Wormser GP, Bottone EJ: *Cardiobacterium hominis*: review of microbiologic and clinical features, *Rev Infect Dis* 5:680-691, 1983.

Anaerobic Gram-Positive Cocci and Nonspore-Forming Bacilli

The anaerobic, gram-positive cocci and nonspore-forming bacilli are a heterogeneous group of bacteria that characteristically colonize the skin and mucosal surfaces. These opportunistic pathogens are frequently recovered in mixed cultures and in patients with foreign bodies (e.g., catheter, prosthesis). They generally have fastidious nutritional requirements and grow slowly on laboratory media.

ANAEROBIC GRAM-POSITIVE COCCI

Although the taxonomic classifications of most bacteria have become more complex in recent years, that of the anaerobic cocci has been simplified. Even though species from at least five genera are found on the human skin and mucosal surfaces, the only genus of clinical significance is *Peptostreptococcus*. More than 25% of the anaerobes isolated in clinical specimens are members of this genus. These gram-positive cocci normally colonize the oral cavity, gastrointestinal tract, genitourinary tract, and skin and cause infections by spreading from these sites to adjacent sterile areas. Infections include pleuropulmonary infections, which occur after the aspiration of oral secretions; sinusitis and brain abscesses, which occur after the spread of the organisms from the oropharynx or the lungs; intraabdominal sepsis with abscess formation, which occurs after spread of the organisms from the intestines; pelvic infections (endometritis, pelvic abscess, puerperal sepsis, salpingitis, bacterial vaginosis); soft tissue infections (e.g., Meleney's gangrene, synergistic necrotizing cellulitis); endocarditis; and osteomyelitis (Figure 36-1).

Most infections are polymicrobial mixtures of aerobic and anaerobic bacteria. Only about 1% of all anaerobic bacteremias are caused by gram-positive cocci, with most caused by peptostreptococci originating from the genital tract in women. This is because anaerobic gram-positive cocci are one of the predominant organisms in the vagina, in contrast with other body sites where anaerobic gram-negative bacilli predominate. Bone and joint infections caused by anaerobes, particularly *P. magnus,* are usually a complication of surgical procedures (e.g., hip replacement). These chronic, indolent infections are caused by bacteria residing on the skin that contaminate the prosthesis.

Laboratory confirmation of infections with peptostreptococci is complicated by three factors. First, care must be taken to prevent contamination of the clinical specimen with peptostreptococci that normally colonize the mucosal surface. Second, the collected specimen must be transported in an oxygen-free container to prevent loss of the organisms. Third, specimens should be cultured on nutritionally enriched media for a prolonged period (i.e., 5 to 7 days). This is in contrast with other anaerobic bacteria that can grow in 1 to 2 days.

Members of the genus *Peptostreptococcus* are usually susceptible to penicillin, the cephalosporins, imipenem, and chloramphenicol. They have intermediate susceptibility to clindamycin, erythromycin, the tetracyclines, and metronidazole and are resistant to the aminoglycosides (as are all anaerobes). Specific therapy is generally indicated in monomicrobic infections but may not be necessary in polymicrobial infections.

ANAEROBIC, NONSPORE-FORMING, GRAM-POSITIVE BACILLI

The nonspore-forming, gram-positive bacilli are a diverse collection of facultatively anaerobic or strictly anaerobic bacteria that colonize the skin and mucosal surfaces (Table 36-1). *Actinomyces, Mobiluncus, Lactobacillus,* and *Propionibacterium* are well-recognized opportunistic pathogens, whereas *Bifidobacterium, Eubacterium,* and *Rothia* organisms rarely cause human disease.

Actinomyces

Physiology and Structure

Actinomyces organisms are facultatively anaerobic or strictly anaerobic, gram-positive bacilli. They are not acid-fast (in contrast with the morphologically similar *Nocardia* species), grow slowly in culture, and tend to produce chronic, slowly developing infections. They typically form delicate filamentous forms or hyphae, similar to fungi when detected in clinical specimens or isolated in culture (Figure 36-2). In fact, the name *Actinomyces*

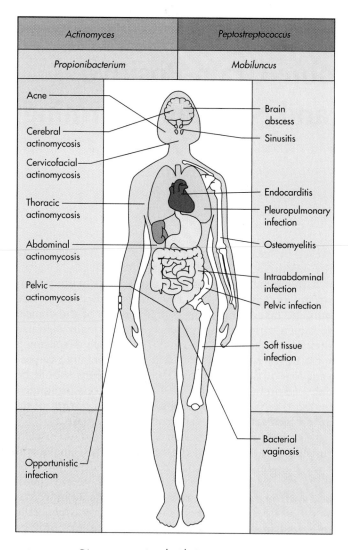

FIGURE 36-1 Diseases associated with *Peptostreptococcus, Actinomyces, Propionibacterium,* and *Mobiluncus* organisms.

TABLE 36-1	**Anaerobic, Nonspore-Forming, Gram-Positive Bacilli**

ANAEROBIC BACILLI	HUMAN DISEASE
Actinomyces species	Actinomycosis (cervicofacial, thoracic, abdominal, pelvic, central nervous system), dental caries, periodontal disease
Propionibacterium species	Acne, actinomycosis, lacrimal canaliculitis, opportunistic infections
Mobiluncus species	Bacterial vaginosis, opportunistic infections
Lactobacillus species	Endocarditis, opportunistic infections
Eubacterium species	Opportunistic infections
Bifidobacterium species	Opportunistic infections
Rothia species	Opportunistic infections

FIGURE 36-2 Gram stain of *Actinomyces* organisms in pus, demonstrating its irregularly stained, beaded, branching filaments. (From Smith EP: In Lambert H, Farrar W, editors: *Infectious diseases illustrated*, London, 1982, Gower.)

comes from Greek language and means "ray fungus." However, these organisms are true bacteria in that they lack mitochondria and a nuclear membrane, reproduce by fission, and are inhibited by penicillin but not antifungal antibiotics. Seventeen species are currently recognized, with *A. israelii, A. naeslundii, A. viscosus, A. odontolyticus, A. pyogenes,* and *A. meyeri* responsible for human disease.

Pathogenesis and Immunity

Actinomyces colonize the upper respiratory tract, gastrointestinal tract, and female genital tract. The organisms have a low virulence potential and cause disease only when the normal mucosal barriers are disrupted by trauma, surgery, or infection. Actinomycosis is the most common disease, and dental caries and periodontal disease are seen less frequently. **Actinomycosis** is characterized by the development of multiple abscesses connected by sinus tracts. Macroscopic colonies of organisms resembling grains of sand can frequently be seen in the affected tissues and the sinus tracts. These colonies, called *sulfur granules* because they appear yellow or orange, are masses of filamentous organisms bound together by calcium phosphate. The areas of suppuration are surrounded by fibrosing granulation tissue, which gives the surface overlying the involved tissues a hard or woody consistency.

Epidemiology

Actinomycosis is an endogenous infection with no evidence of person-to-person spread or disease originating from an external source such as soil or water. Disease is classified by the organ systems involved. **Cervicofacial** infections are seen in patients with poor oral hygiene or those who have had an invasive dental procedure or oral trauma. Patients with **thoracic** infections generally have a history of aspiration, with the disease becoming estab-

FIGURE 36-3 The female genital tract is normally colonized with *Actinomyces* species. The organisms can colonize the surface of foreign bodies such as this intrauterine device, leading to the development of pelvic actinomycosis. (From Smith E: In Lambert H, Farrar W, editors: *Infectious diseases illustrated*, London, 1982, Gower.)

FIGURE 36-4 Sulfur granule collected from the sinus tract in a patient with actinomycosis. Note the delicate filamentous bacilli *(arrow)* at the periphery of the crushed granule.

lished in the lungs and then spreading to adjoining tissues. **Abdominal** infections most commonly occur in patients who have undergone surgery or suffered trauma to the bowel. **Pelvic** infections can be a secondary manifestation of abdominal actinomycosis or may be a primary infection in women with intrauterine devices (Figure 36-3). **Central nervous system** infections usually represent secondary spread from another focus.

Clinical Syndromes

Most cases of actinomycosis are the cervicofacial type. The disease may occur as an acute pyogenic infection or more commonly as a slowly evolving, relatively painless process. The finding of tissue swelling with fibrosis and scarring, with open, draining sinus tracts along the angle of the jaw and neck, should alert the physician to the possibility of actinomycosis. Symptoms of thoracic actinomycosis are nonspecific. Abscesses may form in the lung tissue early in the disease and then spread into adjoining tissues as the disease progresses. Abdominal actinomycosis can spread throughout the abdomen, potentially involving virtually every organ system. Pelvic actinomycosis can occur as a relatively benign form of vaginitis, or there can be more extensive tissue destruction, including the development of tuboovarian abscesses or ureteral obstruction. The most common manifestation of central nervous system actinomycosis is a solitary brain abscess, but meningitis, subdural empyema, and epidural abscess are also seen.

Laboratory Diagnosis

Laboratory confirmation of actinomycosis is frequently difficult. Care must be used when collecting clinical specimens to not contaminate them with actinomyces that are part of the normal bacterial population on mucosal surfaces, because the significance of actinomyces isolated from contaminated specimens cannot then be deter-

FIGURE 36-5 Molar tooth appearance of *A. israelii* after incubation for 1 week. This colonial morphology serves as a reminder that the bacteria are normally found in the mouth.

mined. Because the organisms are concentrated in sulfur granules and are sparse in involved tissues, a large amount of tissue or pus should be collected. If sulfur granules are detected in a sinus tract or in tissue, the granule should be crushed between two glass slides, stained, and examined microscopically. Thin, gram-positive, branching bacilli can be seen along the periphery of the granules (Figure 36-4). Actinomyces are fastidious and grow slowly under anaerobic conditions; it can take 2 weeks or more before the organisms are isolated. Colonies appear white and have a domed surface that can become irregular after incubation for a week or more, resembling the top of a molar (Figure 36-5). Actinomyces are identified through the selective use of differential biochemical tests. Although the organisms are biochemically active, their slow growth frequently delays definitive test results.

Treatment, Prevention, and Control

Treatment for actinomycosis involves the combination of surgical debridement of the involved tissues and the prolonged administration of antibiotics. Actinomyces are uniformly susceptible to penicillin (considered the antibiotic of choice) as well as to tetracycline, erythromycin, and clindamycin. An undrained focus should be suspected in patients with infections that do not appear to respond to prolonged therapy (e.g., 4 to 12 months). The clinical response is generally good even in patients who have suffered extensive tissue destruction. It is difficult to prevent these endogenous infections. However, the maintenance of good oral hygiene and the use of appropriate antibiotic prophylaxis when the mouth or gastrointestinal tract is penetrated can do much to lower the risk of infection.

Propionibacterium

Propionibacteria are small gram-positive bacilli that are frequently arranged in short chains or clumps (Figure 36-6). They are commonly found on the skin, conjunctiva, and external ear and in the oropharynx and female genital tract. The organisms are anaerobic or aerotolerant, nonmotile, and catalase positive, and they ferment carbohydrates, producing propionic acid as their major by-product (hence the name). The two most commonly isolated species are *P. acnes* and *P. propionicus*.

Disease caused by *P. acnes* is observed in two populations: It causes acne (as the name implies) in teenagers and young adults and opportunistic infections in patients with prosthetic devices (e.g., artificial heart valves or joints) or intravascular lines (e.g., catheters, cerebrospinal fluid shunts). Propionibacteria are also commonly isolated in blood cultures, but this usually represents contamination with bacteria on the skin at the phlebotomy site.

The central role of *P. acnes* in acne is to stimulate an inflammatory response. Production of a low-molecular-weight peptide by the bacilli residing in sebaceous fol-

FIGURE 36-6 *Gram stain of* Propionibacterium *organisms.*

licles attracts leukocytes. The bacilli are then phagocytosed, followed by the release of hydrolytic enzymes that, together with bacterial lipases, proteases, neuraminidase, and hyaluronidase, precipitate the inflammatory response, leading to rupture of the follicle. *P. propionicus* causes actinomycosis, lacrimal canaliculitis (inflammation of the tear duct), and abscesses when injected into experimental animals. Because of the role this organism plays in actinomycosis, some investigators have proposed that it be included in the genus *Actinomyces.*

Propionibacteria can grow on most common media, although it may take 2 to 5 days before growth is observed. Care must be taken to avoid contamination of the specimen with the organisms normally found on the skin. The significance of the recovery of an isolate must also be interpreted in light of the clinical presentation (e.g., a catheter or other foreign body can serve as a focus for these opportunistic pathogens).

Acne is unrelated to the effectiveness of skin cleansing because the lesion develops within the sebaceous follicles. For this reason, acne is primarily managed through the topical application of benzoyl peroxide and antibiotics. Antibiotics such as erythromycin and clindamycin have proved effective.

Mobiluncus

Members of the genus *Mobiluncus* are obligate anaerobic, gram-variable or gram-negative, curved bacilli with tapered ends. Despite their appearance in Gram-stained specimens, they are classified as gram-positive bacilli because they have a gram-positive cell wall, lack endotoxin, and are susceptible to vancomycin, clindamycin, erythromycin, and ampicillin but resistant to colistin. The organisms are fastidious, growing slowly even on enriched media supplemented with rabbit or horse serum.

Two species, *M. curtisii* and *M. mulieris,* have been identified in humans. The organisms colonize the genital tract in low numbers but are abundant in women with bacterial vaginosis (vaginitis). Their microscopic appearance is a useful marker for this disease, but the precise role of these organisms in the pathogenesis of bacterial vaginosis is unclear.

Lactobacillus

Lactobacillus organisms are facultatively anaerobic or strictly anaerobic bacilli, found as part of the normal flora of the mouth, stomach, intestines, and genitourinary tract. Despite the ubiquitous nature of these organisms, they rarely are responsible for causing disease. Organisms are most commonly isolated in urine specimens and blood cultures. Because lactobacilli are the most common organism in the urethra, their recovery in urine cultures invariably stems from contamination of the specimen, even when large numbers of the organisms are present. Blood culture isolates typically originate from either a transient bacteremia with a genitourinary source (e.g., after childbirth or a gynecological procedure) or endocarditis. Treatment of endocarditis is difficult because lactobacilli are resistant to vancomycin, and other antibiotics inhibit but do not kill the organisms. A combination of penicillin with an aminoglycoside is required for bactericidal activity.

Bifidobacterium, Eubacterium, and *Rothia*

Bifidobacterium, Eubacterium, and *Rothia* species are commonly found in the oropharynx, large intestine, and vagina. These bacteria can be isolated in clinical specimens but have a very low virulence potential and usually represent clinically insignificant contaminants. To confirm their etiological role in an infection, they should be isolated repeatedly in large numbers and in the absence of other pathogenic organisms.

CASE STUDY AND QUESTIONS

A 42-year-old man entered the university hospital for the treatment of a chronically draining wound in the jaw. The patient had had many teeth extracted 3 months before admission and had poor oral hygiene and fetid breath at the time of admission. Multiple pustular nodules were seen overlying the carious teeth, and some nodules had ruptured. The drainage material consisted of serosanguineous fluid containing small, hard granules.

1. The diagnosis of actinomycosis is considered. How would you collect and transport specimens for confirmation of this diagnosis? What diagnostic tests can be performed?
2. Describe the epidemiology of actinomycosis. What is the risk factor for this patient?
3. What diseases are caused by *Propionibacterium*? What is the source of this organism?

Bibliography

Bayer A et al: Lactobacillemia: report of nine cases—important clinical and therapeutic considerations, *Am J Med* 64:808-813, 1978

Bourgault AM, Rosenblatt JE, Fitzgerald RH: *Peptococcus magnus:* significant human pathogen, *Ann Intern Med* 93:244-248, 1980.

Brook I, Frazier EH: Infections caused by *Propionibacterium* species, *Rev Infect Dis* 3:819-822, 1991.

Finegold SM, Baron EJ, Wexler HM: *A clinical guide to anaerobic infections,* Belmont, Calif, 1992, Star.

Hofstad T: Current taxonomy of medically important nonsporing anaerobes, *Rev Infect Dis* 12(suppl):122-126, 1990.

Hollick G: Isolation and identification of aerobic actinomycetes, *Clin Microbiol Newsletter* 17:25-29, 1995.

Patel R et al: Lactobacillemia in liver transplant patients, *Clin Infect Dis* 18:207-212, 1994.

Pochi PE: The pathogenesis and treatment of acne, *Ann Rev Med* 41:187-198, 1990.

Saxelin M et al: Lactobacilli and bacteremia in Southern Finland, 1989-1992, *Clin Infect Dis* 22:564-566, 1996.

Smego RA: Actinomycosis of the central nervous system, *Rev Infect Dis* 9:855-865, 1987.

Spiegel CA: Bacterial vaginosis, *Clin Microbiol Rev* 4:485-502, 1991.

Tiveljung A, Forsum U, Monstein H-J: Classification of the genus *Mobiluncus* based on comparative partial 16S rRNA gene analysis, *Int J Syst Bacteriol* 46:332-336, 1996.

CHAPTER

37

Clostridium

The genus *Clostridium* includes all anaerobic, gram-positive bacilli capable of forming endospores. Although most members of the genus are strict anaerobes, some are aerotolerant (e.g., *C. tertium, C. histolyticum*) and can grow on agar media exposed to air. Some clostridia appear to be gram-negative (e.g., *C. ramosum, C. clostridiiforme*), and spores may not be observed in some species (*C. perfringens, C. ramosum*). Thus an isolate is classified into the genus *Clostridium* on the basis of a combination of diagnostic tests, including the demonstration of spores, optimal growth anaerobically, a complex pattern of biochemical reactivity, and the findings yielded by analysis of the metabolic by-products by gas chromatography. Fortunately, most of the clinically important isolates fall within a few species (Table 37-1). At least 113 species have been described; however, recent analysis of the 16S ribosomal RNA gene sequences of these species showed that this heterogeneous collection of organisms can be subdivided into 14 groups. Although proposals to reclassify these organisms have been made, definitive action has not been taken.

The organisms are ubiquitous, present in soil, water, and sewage and as part of the normal microbial flora in the gastrointestinal tract of animals and humans. Most clostridia are harmless saprophytes, but some are well-recognized human pathogens with a clearly documented history of causing diseases such as tetanus (*C. tetani*), botulism (*C. botulinum, C. barati, C. butyricum*), and gas gangrene (*C. perfringens, C. novyi, C. septicum, C. histolyticum, C. sordellii*).

Despite the notoriety of these diseases, we now know that clostridia are more commonly associated with skin and soft tissue infections, food poisoning, and antibiotic-associated diarrhea and colitis. Their remarkable capacity for causing diseases is attributed to their ability to survive adverse environmental conditions through spore formation; their rapid growth in a nutritionally enriched, oxygen-deprived environment; and their production of numerous histolytic toxins, enterotoxins, and neurotoxins. The most important human pathogens are discussed in this chapter.

CLOSTRIDIUM PERFRINGENS
Physiology and Structure

C. perfringens, the clostridial species most frequently isolated in clinical specimens, can be associated with simple colonization or can cause severe, life-threatening disease. *C. perfringens* is a large, rectangular, gram-positive bacillus, with spores rarely observed in vivo or after in vitro cultivation (Figure 37-1). This organism is one of the few nonmotile clostridia, but rapidly spreading growth on laboratory media (resembling the growth of motile organisms) is characteristic (Figure 37-2). The organism grows rapidly in tissues and in culture, is hemolytic, and is metabolically active, which makes rapid identification possible in the laboratory. The production of four major lethal toxins of *C. perfringens* (alpha, beta, epsilon, and iota toxins) is used to subdivide isolates into five types (A through E). Type A *C. perfringens* causes most of the human infections.

Pathogenesis and Immunity

C. perfringens can cause a spectrum of diseases, from a self-limited gastroenteritis to an overwhelming destruction of tissue (e.g., clostridial myonecrosis) associated with a very high mortality, even in patients who receive early medical intervention. This pathogenic potential is attributed primarily to the 12 toxins and enzymes produced by this organism (Table 37-2). **Alpha toxin,** the most important toxin and the one produced by all types of *C. perfringens*, is a lecithinase (phospholipase C) that lyses erythrocytes, platelets, leukocytes, and endothelial cells (Figure 37-3). This toxin is associated with increased vascular permeability with massive hemolysis and bleeding, tissue destruction (as found in myonecrosis), hepatic toxicity, and myocardial dysfunction (bradycardia, hypotension). The largest quantities of alpha toxin are produced by *C. perfringens* type A. **Beta toxin** is responsible for causing the necrotic lesions in **necrotizing enteritis** (enteritis necroticans, pig-bel). **Epsilon toxin** is a protoxin that is activated by trypsin and that increases the vascular permeability of the gastrointestinal wall. **Iota toxin,** the fourth major lethal toxin produced

TABLE 37-1 Major Pathogenic Clostridia and Their Associated Human Diseases

SPECIES	ASSOCIATED DISEASE
C. barati	Botulism
C. botulinum	Botulism
C. butyricum	Botulism
C. difficile	Antibiotic-associated diarrhea, pseudomembranous colitis
C. histolyticum	Gas gangrene
C. novyi	Gas gangrene
C. perfringens	Gas gangrene, soft tissue infections (e.g., cellulitis, fasciitis), food poisoning, necrotic enteritis, septicemia
C. septicum	Gas gangrene, septicemia
C. sordelli	Gas gangrene
C. tertium	Opportunistic infections
C. tetani	Tetanus

TABLE 37-2 Virulence Factors Associated with C. perfringens

VIRULENCE FACTORS	BIOLOGICAL ACTIVITY
MAJOR LETHAL TOXINS	
Alpha toxin	Phospholipase C (lecithinase); increases vascular permeability; hemolytic; produces necrotizing activity
Beta toxin	Necrotizing activity; induces hypertension by causing release of catecholamines
Epsilon toxin	Increases permeability of gastrointestinal wall
Iota toxin	Binary toxin responsible for necrotizing activity and increased vascular permeability
Enterotoxin	Alters membrane permeability (cytotoxic, enterotoxic)
MINOR TOXINS	
Delta toxin	Hemolytic
Theta toxin	Hemolytic; cytolytic
Kappa toxin	Collagenase, gelatinase; necrotizing activity
Lambda toxin	Protease
Mu toxin	Hyaluronidase
Nu toxin	Deoxyribonuclease; hemolytic; necrotizing activity
Neuraminidase	Alters cell surface ganglioside receptors; promotes capillary thrombosis

FIGURE 37-1 Gram stain of C. perfringens.

FIGURE 37-2 Growth of C. perfringens on sheep blood agar. Note the flat, rapidly spreading colonies and the hemolytic activity of the organism. C. perfringens can be identified preliminarily by the finding of a zone of complete hemolysis (caused by the theta toxin) and a wider zone of partial hemolysis (caused by the alpha toxin), combined with the characteristic microscopic morphology.

FIGURE 37-3 Growth of C. perfringens on egg-yolk agar. The alpha toxin (lecithinase) hydrolyzes phospholipids in serum and egg yolk, producing an opaque precipitate (right). This is not observed when the organism is grown in the presence of antibodies against the toxin (left). This reaction (Nagler's reaction) is characteristic for C. perfringens.

by *C. perfringens,* has necrotic activity and increases vascular permeability.

Enterotoxin is a heat-labile protein produced in the colon and released during spore formation. Trypsin treatment enhances the toxin activity threefold. The toxin is produced primarily by type A strains but also by a few type C and D strains. It disrupts ion transport in the ileum (primarily) and jejunum by inserting into the cell membrane and altering membrane permeability. Many vegetative cells must be ingested with the contaminated food to produce the enterotoxic effects. Antibodies to enterotoxin, indicating previous exposure, are commonly found in adults, but these are not protective. The activities of the minor toxins of *C. perfringens* are summarized in Table 37-2.

Epidemiology

C. perfringens type A commonly inhabits the intestinal tract of humans and animals and is widely distributed in nature, particularly in soil and water contaminated with feces (Box 37-1). This organism forms spores under adverse environmental conditions and can survive for prolonged periods. Types B to E strains do not survive in soil but rather colonize the intestinal tract of animals and occasionally humans. *C. perfringens* type A primarily causes gas gangrene, soft tissue infections, and food poisoning, whereas type C causes enteritis necroticans.

Clinical Syndromes

Myonecrosis

Myonecrosis (gas gangrene) is a life-threatening disease that illustrates the full virulence potential of histotoxic clostridia. The onset of disease, characterized by intense pain, generally develops within 1 week after clostridia are introduced into tissue by trauma or surgery. This is followed rapidly by extensive muscle necrosis, shock, renal failure, and death, frequently within 2 days of initial onset. Macroscopic examination of muscle reveals devitalized necrotic tissue, with gas found in the tissue caused by the metabolic activity of the rapidly dividing bacteria (hence the name *gas gangrene*). Microscopically, abundant rectangular, gram-positive bacilli in the absence of inflammatory cells (resulting from lysis by clostridial toxins) are seen. The clostridial toxins characteristically cause extensive hemolysis and bleeding. Clostridial myonecrosis is most commonly caused by *C. perfringens,* although other species can also produce this disease (e.g., *C. septicum, C. histolyticum, C. sordelli,* and *C. novyi*).

Cellulitis, Fasciitis, and Other Soft Tissue Infections

Clostridial species can colonize wounds and skin with no clinical consequences. Indeed, most isolates of *C. perfringens* and other clostridial species from wound cultures are insignificant. However, these organisms can also initiate **cellulitis** (Figure 37-4), or a rapidly progressive, destructive process in which the organisms spread through fascial planes **(fasciitis),** causing suppuration and the formation of gas. Fasciitis is distinguished from myonecrosis by the absence of muscle involvement, but it too has a dismal outcome. Surgical intervention is generally unsuccessful because of the rapidity with which the organisms spread. Most infections are caused by *C. perfringens* or *C. septicum.*

Food Poisoning

Clostridial food poisoning, a relatively common but underappreciated bacterial disease, is characterized by a short incubation period (8 to 24 hours); a clinical presentation that includes abdominal cramps and watery diarrhea but not fever, nausea, or vomiting; and a clinical

---

BOX 37-1   Summary of *C. perfringens* Infections

BACTERIAL FACTORS

Diseases—gas gangrene; soft tissue infections (cellulitis, fasciitis), food poisoning, necrotizing enteritis, septicemia.
Virulence factors—see Table 37-2.
Organism is present in soil, water, sewage; normal resident of gastrointestinal tract.
Spore formation allows organism to survive in environment.
Rapid growth occurs in vivo and in vitro.

TRANSMISSION

Exogenous infections from exposure to organisms from external source (in soil and food or introduced by trauma or surgery); endogenous spread from gastrointestinal tract to normally sterile areas (tissues, blood).
Exogenous exposure more common than endogenous spread.

WHO IS AT RISK?

Surgical patients; patients after trauma with soil contamination.
People who ingest contaminated meat products (without proper refrigeration or reheating to inactivate endotoxin).

GEOGRAPHY/SEASON

Ubiquitous and worldwide.
No seasonal incidence.

MODES OF CONTROL

Rapid treatment is essential for serious infections.
Systemic infection: surgical debridement and high-dose penicillin.
For localized infection, treatment involves debridement and penicillin.
For gastroenteritis, treatment is symptomatic only.

course of less than 24 hours. Disease results from the ingestion of meat products contaminated with large numbers (10^8 to 10^9 organisms) of type A *C. perfringens*. Enterotoxin produced after the germination of the spores acts as a superantigen, stimulating the release of cytokines from lymphocytes. The refrigeration of food after preparation prevents enterotoxin production. Alternatively, reheating of the food can destroy the toxin.

Necrotizing Enteritis

Necrotizing enteritis is a rare, acute necrotizing process in the jejunum characterized by abdominal pain, bloody diarrhea, shock, and peritonitis. The mortality in patients with the infection approaches 50%. Beta toxin–producing *C. perfringens* type C is responsible for causing this disease.

Septicemia

The isolation of *C. perfringens* or other clostridial species in blood cultures can be alarming. However, more than half of the isolates are clinically insignificant, representing a transient bacteremia or, more likely, contamination of the culture with clostridia colonizing the skin. The significance of an isolate must be viewed in the light of other clinical findings.

Laboratory Diagnosis

The laboratory performs only a confirmatory role in the diagnosis of clostridial disease because therapy must be

FIGURE 37-4 Clostridial cellulitis. Clostridia can be introduced into tissue during surgery or by a traumatic injury. This patient suffered a compound fracture of the tibia. Five days after the injury, the skin became discolored, and bullae and necrosis developed. There was a serosanguineous exudate and subcutaneous gas but no evidence of muscle necrosis. The patient made an uneventful recovery. (From Lambert H, Farrar W, editors: *Infectious diseases illustrated*, London, 1982, Gower.)

initiated immediately in affected patients. The microscopic detection of gram-positive bacilli in clinical specimens, usually in the absence of leukocytes, can be a very useful finding because these organisms have a characteristic morphology. It is also relatively simple to culture these anaerobes, with *C. perfringens* detected on simple media after incubation for 1 day or less. Under appropriate conditions, *C. perfringens* can divide every 8 to 10 minutes, so growth on agar media or in blood culture broths can be detected after incubation for only a few hours. The role of *C. perfringens* in food poisoning is documented by recovery of more than 10^5 organisms per gram of food or 10^6 bacteria per gram of feces collected within 1 day of the onset of disease.

Treatment, Prevention, and Control

Systemic *C. perfringens* infections such as fasciitis and myonecrosis must be treated aggressively with surgical debridement and high-dose penicillin therapy. The use of antiserum against alpha toxin (antitoxin) and treatment in a hyperbaric oxygen chamber (presumably to inhibit growth of the anaerobe) have poorly defined benefits. Despite all therapeutic efforts, the prognosis in patients with these diseases is poor, with mortality reported from 40% to almost 100%. Less serious, localized clostridial diseases can be successfully treated with penicillin, with resistance only rarely reported for species other than *C. perfringens*. Antibiotic therapy for clostridial food poisoning is unnecessary.

Prevention and control of *C. perfringens* infections are difficult because of the ubiquitous distribution of the organisms. Disease requires introduction of the organism into devitalized tissues and maintenance of an anaerobic environment favorable for bacterial growth. Thus proper wound care and the judicious use of prophylactic antibiotics can do much to prevent most infections.

CLOSTRIDIUM TETANI
Physiology and Structure

C. tetani is a small, motile, spore-forming bacillus that frequently stains gram-negative. The organism produces round, terminal spores that give it the appearance of a drumstick (Figure 37-5). Unlike *C. perfringens*, *C. tetani* is difficult to grow and identify because it is extremely sensitive to oxygen toxicity and is relatively inactive metabolically.

Pathogenesis and Immunity

C. tetani produces two toxins: an oxygen-labile hemolysin (**tetanolysin**) and a plasmid-encoded, heat-labile neurotoxin (**tetanospasmin**) (Table 37-3). Tetanolysin is serologically related to other clostridial hemolysins and streptolysin O. The clinical significance of this enzyme is unknown, however, because it is inhibited by oxygen and serum cholesterol.

Tetanospasmin is produced during the stationary phase of growth, released when the cell is lysed, and re-

FIGURE 37-5 Gram stain of *C. tetani*. Note the terminal spores.

TABLE 37-3	**Virulence Factors Associated with *C. tetani***
VIRULENCE FACTORS	**BIOLOGICAL ACTIVITY**
Tetanospasmin	Neurotoxin blocks release of neurotransmitters for inhibitory synapses
Tetanolysin	Oxygen-labile hemolysin (unknown significance)
Spore formation	Allows organism to survive in unfavorable environments

sponsible for causing the clinical manifestations of tetanus. Tetanospasmin (an A-B toxin) is synthesized as a single 151,000-Da peptide that is cleaved into a light (A chain) and a heavy (B chain) subunit by an endogenous protease when the cell releases the neurotoxin. The two chains are held together by a disulfide bond and noncovalent forces. The carboxy-terminal portion of the heavy (100,000-Da) chain binds to a surface receptor on neuronal membranes. The light chain of the toxin, a zinc endopeptidase, is then internalized and moves from the peripheral nerve terminals to the central nervous system by retrograde axonal transport. It is released from the postsynaptic dendrites, crosses the synaptic cleft, and is localized within vesicles in the presynaptic nerve terminals. Tetanospasmin acts by blocking the release of neurotransmitters (e.g., gamma-aminobutyric acid [GABA], glycine) for inhibitory synapses, thus causing excitatory synaptic activity to be unregulated (spastic paralysis). It does not affect acetylcholine transmission (in contrast with *C. botulinum*). The toxin binding is irreversible, so recovery depends on whether new axonal terminals form.

Epidemiology

C. tetani is ubiquitous. It is found in fertile soil and colonizes the gastrointestinal tract of many animals, including humans (Box 37-2). The vegetative forms of *C. tetani* are extremely susceptible to oxygen toxicity, but the organisms sporulate readily and can survive in nature for a long time. Disease is relatively rare in the United States because of the high incidence of immunity brought about by vaccination. Fewer than 50 cases are reported annually and occur primarily in elderly patients with waning immunity (Figure 37-6). However, tetanus is still responsible for causing many deaths in people living in underdeveloped areas where vaccination is unavailable or medical practices are lax. It is estimated that more than 1 million cases occur worldwide, with a mor-

BOX 37-2	**Summary of *C. tetani* Infections**

BACTERIAL FACTORS

Diseases—see Table 37-4.

Virulence factors—see Table 37-3.

Organism is present in soil and in gastrointestinal tract of many animals, including humans (transiently).

Spore formation allows organism to survive in environment.

TRANSMISSION

Exogenous infection acquired by exposure to contaminated soil.

Most disease associated with minor trauma (e.g., skin break with contaminated splinter or another foreign body).

WHO IS AT RISK?

People with inadequate vaccine-induced immunity (particularly children and elderly people).

GEOGRAPHY/SEASON

Ubiquitous and worldwide distribution in soil.

Although exposure is common, disease is rare unless patient is inadequately immunized.

Disease is relatively common in underdeveloped areas where there is poor vaccination compliance or medical care is inadequate.

No seasonal incidence.

MODES OF CONTROL

Control involves debridement of wounds, administration of metronidazole, passive immunization with human tetanus immunoglobulin, and vaccination with tetanus toxoid.

Vaccination with three doses of tetanus toxoid is given, with boosters given every 10 years.

tality rate ranging from 20% to 50%. At least half the deaths occur in neonates.

Clinical Syndromes

The clinical symptoms of tetanus are summarized in Table 37-4. The incubation period for tetanus varies from a few days to weeks. The duration of the incubation period is directly related to the distance of the primary wound infection from the central nervous system.

Generalized tetanus is the most common form. Involvement of the masseter muscles (**trismus** or lockjaw) is the presenting sign in most patients. The characteristic sardonic smile that results from the sustained contraction of the facial muscles is known as *risus sardonicus* (Figure 37-7). Other early signs include drooling, sweating, irritability, and persistent back spasms (**opisthotonos**) (Figure 37-8). The autonomic nervous system is involved in patients with more severe disease; the signs and symptoms include cardiac arrhythmias, fluctuations in blood pressure, profound sweating, and dehydration.

Another form of *C. tetani* disease is **localized tetanus** in which the disease remains confined to the musculature at the site of primary infection. A variant is **cephalic tetanus,** in which the primary site of infection is the head. In contrast with the prognosis for patients with localized tetanus, the prognosis for patients with cephalic tetanus is very poor.

Neonatal tetanus (tetanus neonatorum) is typically associated with an initial infection of the umbilical stump, which then progresses to generalized. The mortality in infants exceeds 90%, and developmental defects are present in survivors.

Laboratory Diagnosis

The diagnosis of tetanus, as with most other clostridial diseases, is made on the basis of the clinical presentation. The microscopic detection or isolation of *C. tetani* is useful but frequently unsuccessful. Only about 30% of patients with tetanus have positive cultures because disease can be caused by relatively few organisms and the slow-growing bacteria are killed rapidly when exposed to

TABLE 37-4	Clinical Manifestations of Tetanus
DISEASE	**CLINICAL MANIFESTATIONS**
Generalized	Involvement of bulbar and paraspinal muscles (trismus or lockjaw, risus sardonicus, difficulty swallowing, irritability, opisthotonos); involvement of autonomic nervous system (sweating, hyperthermia, cardiac arrhythmias, fluctuations in blood pressure)
Cephalic	Primary infection in head, particularly ear; isolated or combined involvement of cranial nerves, particularly seventh cranial nerve; very poor prognosis
Localized	Involvement of muscles in area of primary injury; infection may precede generalized disease; favorable prognosis
Neonatal	Generalized disease in neonates; infection typically originates from umbilical stump; very poor prognosis in infants whose mothers are nonimmune

FIGURE 37-7 Risus sardonicus in tetanus caused by sustained spasms of the masseter muscles. (From Emond RT, Rowland HAK, Welsby P: *Colour atlas of infectious diseases,* ed 3, London, 1995, Wolfe.)

FIGURE 37-6 Age-specific prevalence of immunity to tetanus and incidence of disease, 1988 to 1991. The total number of *C. tetani* infections reported during this time was 221. (Data from *MMWR* annual summaries and Gergen P et al: *N Engl J Med* 332:761-766, 1995.)

FIGURE 37-8 A child with tetanus and opisthotonos resulting from persistent spasms of the back muscles. (From Emond RT, Rowland HAK, Welsby P: *Colour atlas of infectious diseases,* ed 3, London, 1995, Wolfe.)

air. The production of toxin by an isolate is confirmed by tetanus antitoxin neutralization tests in mice (a procedure performed only in public health reference laboratories).

Treatment, Prevention, and Control

The mortality associated with tetanus has steadily decreased during the past century, resulting in large part from the decreased incidence of tetanus in the United States. The highest mortality is in newborns and in patients with an incubation period of less than 1 week before the disease develops.

Treatment of tetanus requires debridement of the primary wound (which may appear innocuous), use of metronidazole, passive immunization with human tetanus immunoglobulin, and vaccination with tetanus toxoid. Wound care and metronidazole therapy eliminate the vegetative bacteria that produce toxin, and the antitoxin antibodies work by binding free tetanospasmin molecules. Metronidazole and penicillin have equivalent activity against *C. tetani*; however, penicillin acts like tetanospasmin by inhibiting GABA activity. Toxin bound to nerve endings is protected from antibodies. Thus the toxic effects must be controlled symptomatically until the normal regulation of synaptic transmission is restored. Vaccination with a series of three doses of tetanus toxoid and booster doses every 10 years is highly effective in preventing tetanus.

CLOSTRIDIUM BOTULINUM
Physiology and Structure

C. botulinum (Lat. *botulus,* "sausage"), the etiological agent of botulism, is a heterogeneous group of fastidious, spore-forming, anaerobic bacilli. The organisms are sub-

divided into four groups (I to IV) on the basis of the type of toxin produced and their proteolytic activity. Most human disease is caused by types I and II strains. Seven antigenically distinct **botulinum toxins** (A to G) have been described, with human disease associated with types A, B, E, and F. Only one toxin is produced by most individual isolates. Like tetanus toxin, *C. botulinum* toxin is a 150- to 165-kDa progenitor protein (A-B toxin) consisting of the neurotoxin subunit (light or A chain) and one or more nontoxic subunits (B or heavy chain). The nontoxic subunit(s) protect the neurotoxin from being inactivated by stomach acids.

Pathogenesis and Immunity

Botulinum toxin is similar in structure and function to tetanus toxin, differing only in the target neural cell. This toxin is very specific for cholinergic nerves. It blocks neurotransmission at peripheral cholinergic synapses by preventing release of the neurotransmitter acetylcholine. Like tetanus, recovery of function requires regeneration of the nerve endings. *C. botulinum* also produces a binary toxin consisting of two components that combine to disrupt vascular permeability.

Epidemiology

C. botulinum is commonly isolated in soil and water samples throughout the world (Box 37-3). In the United States, type A strains are found mainly in neutral or alkaline soil west of the Mississippi River; type B strains are found primarily in the eastern part of the country in rich, organic soil; and type E strains are found only in wet soil. Even though *C. botulinum* is commonly found in soil, disease is uncommon in the United States. Three forms of botulism have been identified: classical or foodborne, infant, and wound botulism. Fewer than 50

BOX 37-3   ## Summary of *C. botulinum* Infections

BACTERIAL FACTORS

Diseases—foodborne botulism, infant botulism, wound botulism.

Virulence factors—botulinum toxin (types A to G) blocks peripheral cholinergic synapses by preventing release of acetylcholine; binary toxin disrupts vascular permeability; spore formation allows organism to survive in environment.

TRANSMISSION

Present in soil.

Exogenous infection.

Ingestion of toxin in contaminated food (intoxication).

Inoculation of *C. botulinum* through skin with subsequent localized production of neurotoxin.

Infant ingestion of *C. botulinum* in food (e.g., honey), causing organism to colonize gastrointestinal tract, with subsequent production of neurotoxin.

WHO IS AT RISK?

People who eat contaminated foods (particularly home-canned produce).

Infants exposed to *C. botulinum*.

GEOGRAPHY/SEASON

Ubiquitous and worldwide.

Disease in United States is relatively rare (fewer than 50 cases annually).

No seasonal incidence.

MODES OF CONTROL

Treatment involves administration of metronidazole or penicillin, trivalent botulinum antitoxin, and ventilatory support.

Spore germination is prevented by maintaining food in an acid pH, by high sugar content (e.g., fruit preserves), or by storing it at 4° C or colder.

Toxin is destroyed by heating food for 20 minutes at 80° C.

Infant botulism is associated with consumption of contaminated foods, particularly honey. Infants younger than 1 year should not be given honey or food with honey in it.

---

cases of foodborne botulism are seen annually; most are associated with the consumption of home-canned foods (types A and B toxins) and occasionally with the consumption of preserved fish (type E toxin). The food may not appear spoiled, but even a small taste can cause full-blown clinical disease. Botulism in infants is more common (although fewer than 100 cases are reported annually) and has been associated with the consumption of foods (particularly honey) contaminated with botulinum spores. The incidence of wound botulism is unknown, but it is certainly very rare.

Clinical Syndromes

Foodborne Botulism

Patients with foodborne botulism typically become weak and dizzy 1 to 2 days after consuming the contaminated food. The initial signs include blurred vision with fixed dilated pupils, dry mouth (indicative of the anticholinergic effects of the toxin), constipation, and abdominal pain. Fever is absent. Bilateral descending weakness of the peripheral muscles develops in patients with progressive disease **(flaccid paralysis),** with death most commonly attributed to respiratory paralysis. Patients maintain a clear sensorium throughout the disease. Despite aggressive management of the patient's condition, the disease may continue to progress because of the neurotoxin's irreversible binding and long-term inhibitory effect on the release of excitatory neurotransmitters. Complete recovery in patients who survive this initial period frequently requires many months to years, until the affected nerve endings regrow. Mortality in patients with foodborne botulism, which once approached 70%, has

been reduced to 10% through the use of better supportive care, particularly in the management of respiratory complications.

Infant Botulism

Infant botulism was first recognized in 1976 and is now the most common form of botulism in the United States. In contrast with foodborne botulism, this disease is caused by neurotoxin produced in vivo by *C. botulinum* colonizing the gastrointestinal tract of young infants. Although adults certainly are exposed to the organism in their diet, *C. botulinum* cannot survive and proliferate in their intestines. However, in the absence of competitive bowel microbes, the organism can become established in the gastrointestinal tract of infants. The disease typically affects infants younger than 1 year (most between 1 to 6 months), and the symptoms are initially nonspecific (e.g., constipation, weak cry, or "failure to thrive"). Progressive disease with flaccid paralysis and respiratory arrest can develop; however, mortality in documented cases of infant botulism is very low (1% to 2%). Some infant deaths attributed to other conditions (e.g., sudden infant death syndrome) may actually be caused by botulism.

Wound Botulism

As the name implies, wound botulism develops from in vitro toxin production by *C. botulinum* in contaminated wounds. Although the symptoms of disease are identical to those of foodborne disease, the incubation period is generally longer (4 days or more), and the gastrointestinal tract symptoms are less prominent.

Laboratory Diagnosis

The clinical diagnosis of botulism is confirmed if the organism is isolated or toxin activity is shown. Toxin activity is most likely to be found early in the disease, and the organism can be grown in cultures and toxin activity detected for more than a month after the onset of the disease. An attempt should be made to culture *C. botulinum* from the feces of patients with foodborne disease and from the implicated food if it is available (Figure 37-9). Isolation of *C. botulinum* from specimens contaminated with other organisms can be improved by heating the specimen for 10 minutes at 80° C to kill all vegetative cells. Culture of the heated specimen on nutritionally enriched anaerobic media allows the heat-resistant *C. botulinum* spores to germinate. *C. botulinum* produces lipase, which appears as an iridescent film on colonies grown on egg-yolk agar.

The food, stool specimen, and patient's serum should also be tested for toxin activity. Typically, this is done at a public health reference laboratory using the mouse bioassay. The specimen is divided, and one portion is mixed with antitoxin. Both portions are then inoculated intraperitoneally into mice. If antitoxin treatment protects the mice, toxin activity is confirmed.

The diagnosis of infant botulism is supported if *C. botulinum* is isolated from feces or toxin activity is detected in feces or serum. The organism can be isolated from stool cultures in virtually all patients because carriage of the organism may persist for many months even after a baby has recovered. Wound botulism is confirmed by isolation of the organism from the wound or by detection of toxin activity in wound exudate or serum.

Treatment, Prevention, and Control

Patients with botulism require adequate ventilatory support, elimination of the organism from the gastrointestinal tract through the judicious use of gastric lavage and metronidazole or penicillin therapy, and use of trivalent botulinum antitoxin (versus toxins A, B, and E) to bind toxin circulating in the bloodstream. The role of ventilatory support in significantly reducing mortality is unquestioned. Protective levels of antibodies do not develop after disease, so patients are susceptible to secondary infections.

Disease is prevented by destroying the spores in food (virtually impossible for practical reasons), preventing spore germination (by maintaining the food in an acid pH or storage at 4° C or colder), or destroying the preformed toxin (by heating the food for 20 minutes at 80° C). Infant botulism has been associated with the consumption of honey contaminated with *C. botulinum* spores, so children younger than 1 year should not eat honey.

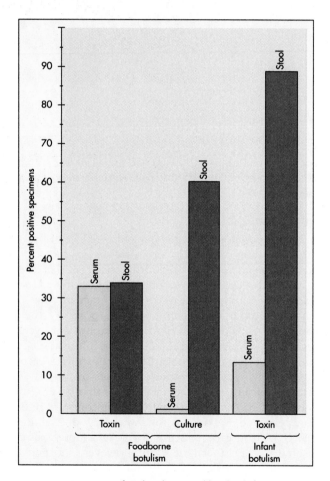

FIGURE 37-9 Detection of *C. botulinum* and botulinal toxin in serum and stool specimens collected from patients with foodborne botulism and infant botulism. Confirmation of foodborne disease requires testing the implicated food and the patient's serum and stool specimen for botulinal toxin activity, and the food and stool specimen must be cultured for the organism. No single test for foodborne botulism has a sensitivity greater than 60%. Serum and stool specimens from infants with botulism should be tested for toxin activity and the stool specimen cultured. (Data from Dowell V et al: *JAMA* 238:1829, 1977; and Hatheway C, McCroskey L: *J Clin Microbiol* 25:2334-2338, 1987.)

CLOSTRIDIUM DIFFICILE

Until the mid-1970s the clinical importance of *C. difficile* was not appreciated. This organism was infrequently isolated in fecal cultures and rarely associated with human disease. However, systematic studies now clearly show that toxin-producing *C. difficile* is responsible for causing antibiotic-associated gastrointestinal diseases ranging from a relatively benign, self-limiting diarrhea to severe, life-threatening pseudomembranous colitis (Figures 37-10 and 37-11).

C. difficile produces two toxins (Table 37-5): an **enterotoxin** (toxin A) and a **cytotoxin** (toxin B). Although these toxins are immunologically distinct, purification has proved difficult. The enterotoxin is chemotactic for neutrophils, with infiltration of polymorphonuclear neutrophil leukocytes into the ileum, resulting in the release of cytokines, hypersecretion of fluid, and development of hemorrhagic necrosis. The cytotoxin causes actin to depolymerize, with the resultant destruction of the cellular cytoskeleton both in vivo and in vitro. The precise role that each toxin plays in the pathogenesis of disease is still unclear because both toxins are produced in clostridia associated with disease (Box 37-4). Other *C. difficile* virulence factors are summarized in Table 37-5.

C. difficile is part of the normal intestinal flora in a small number of healthy people and hospitalized patients. The disease develops in people taking antibiotics because the agents alter the normal enteric flora, permitting the overgrowth of these relatively resistant organisms or making the patient more susceptible to the exogenous acquisition of *C. difficile*. The disease develops if the organisms proliferate in the colon and produce their toxins there.

The diagnosis of *C. difficile* infection is confirmed if the organisms are isolated from cultures of feces on highly selective media, the cytotoxin is detected by an in vitro cytotoxicity assay with tissue culture cells, or enterotoxin is detected by immunoassays. The most specific test for *C. difficile* disease is the **cytotoxicity assay.** A combination of diagnostic tests is performed to maximize the sensitivity used to detect colonization.

Discontinuation of the implicated antibiotic (e.g., ampicillin, clindamycin) is generally sufficient to alleviate mild disease. However, specific therapy with metronidazole or vancomycin is necessary for the management of serious disease. Relapses may occur in as many

TABLE 37-5	Virulence Factors Associated with *C. difficile*
VIRULENCE FACTORS	**BIOLOGICAL ACTIVITY**
Enterotoxin (toxin A)	Produces chemotaxis; induces cytokine production with hypersecretion of fluid; produces hemorrhagic necrosis
Cytotoxin (toxin B)	Induces depolymerization of actin with loss of cellular cytoskeleton
Adhesin factor	Mediates binding to human colonic cells
Hyaluronidase	Produces hydrolytic activity
Spore formation	Permits survival for months in hospital environment

FIGURE 37-11 Antibiotic-associated colitis. Histological section of colon showing an intense inflammatory response, with the characteristic "plaque" *(black arrow)* overlying the intact intestinal mucosa *(white arrow).* (Hematoxylin & eosin.) (From Lambert HP, Farrar WE, editors: *Infectious diseases illustrated,* London, 1982, Gower.)

FIGURE 37-10 Antibiotic-associated colitis: gross section of the lumen of the colon. Note the white plaques of fibrin, mucus, and inflammatory cells overlying the normal intestinal mucosa *(red).*

BACTERIAL FACTORS

Diseases—asymptomatic colonization, antibiotic-associated diarrhea, pseudomembranous colitis.
Virulence factors—see Table 37-5.
Present in soil, water, and sewage.
Part of normal microbial flora of gastrointestinal tract of some humans (typically present in low concentration).

TRANSMISSION

Exogenous infections spread person to person in hospital.
Endogenous infections with overgrowth of toxin-producing strains after treatment with antibiotics.
Exogenous infections, which may be more common than endogenous spread.
Spores that can remain infectious for many weeks or months.

WHO IS AT RISK?

Hospitalized patients receive antibiotics (particularly beta-lactams and clindamycin).
People in whom antibiotic exposure permits overgrowth of C. difficile.

GEOGRAPHY/SEASON

Ubiquitous and worldwide.
No seasonal incidence.

MODES OF CONTROL

Implicated antibiotic is discontinued in mild disease.
Treatment with metronidazole or vancomycin occurs in severe disease.
Relapse is common because spores are resistant to antibiotics.
Careful cleaning of hospital rooms should be done after infected patient is discharged.

FIGURE 37-12 *C. septicum.* Note spores within the bacilli.

as 20% to 30% of patients after the completion of therapy because spores of *C. difficile* are resistant to antibiotic treatment. Retreatment with the same antibiotic is frequently successful. It is difficult to prevent the disease because the organism commonly exists in hospitals, particularly in areas adjacent to infected patients. The spores of *C. difficile* are difficult to destroy; thus the organism can contaminate an environment for many months and be a major source of nosocomial outbreaks of *C. difficile* disease.

OTHER CLOSTRIDIAL SPECIES

Many other clostridia have been associated with clinically significant disease. Their virulence is due to their ability to survive exposure to oxygen by forming spores and producing many diverse toxins and enzymes. The virulence factors produced by some of the more important clostridia are summarized in Table 37-6. *C. septicum* (Figure 37-12) is a particularly important pathogen because it is a cause of nontraumatic myonecrosis and frequently exists in patients with occult colon cancer, acute leukemia, and diabetes. If the integrity of the bowel mucosa is compromised and the patient's body is less able to mount an effective response to the organism, *C. septicum* can spread into tissue and rapidly proliferate there. Most patients have a fulminant course, dying within 1 to 2 days after initial presentation.

TABLE 37-6   Virulence Factors Associated with Other Clostridial Species

VIRULENCE FACTORS	BIOLOGICAL ACTIVITY
C. SEPTICUM	
Alpha toxin	Necrotizing, hemolytic toxin
Beta toxin	Heat-stable deoxyribonuclease
Gamma toxin	Hyaluronidase
Delta toxin	Oxygen-labile hemolysin
Neuraminidase	Alters cell membrane glycoproteins
C. SORDELLII	
Lecithinase	Phospholipase C
Hemolysin	Oxygen-labile hemolytic activity
Fibrinolysin	Tissue destruction
Lethal (beta) toxin	Necrotic enterotoxin activity
Hemorrhagic toxin	Hemorrhagic cytotoxin activity
C. HISTOLYTICUM	
Alpha toxin	Necrotizing (not hemolytic) toxin
Beta toxin	Collagenase
Gamma toxin	Protease
Delta toxin	Elastase
Epsilon toxin	Oxygen-labile hemolysin
C. NOVYI	
Alpha toxin	Necrotizing toxin
Beta toxin	Lecithinase, necrotizing, hemolytic toxin
Gamma toxin	Lecithinase, necrotizing, hemolytic toxin
Delta toxin	Oxygen-labile hemolysin
Epsilon toxin	Lipase
Zeta toxin	Hemolysin
Eta toxin	Tropomyosinase
Theta toxin	Lecithinase
C. BARATI	
Botulinum toxin	Neurotoxin
C. BUTYRICUM	
Botulinum toxin	Neurotoxin

CASE STUDY AND QUESTIONS

A 61-year-old woman with left-sided face pain came to the emergency department of a local hospital. She was unable to open her mouth because of facial muscle spasms and had been unable to eat for 4 days because of severe pain in her jaw. Her attending physician noted trismus and risus sardonicus. She reported that 1 week before she incurred a puncture wound to her toe while walking in her garden. She cleaned the wound and removed small pieces of wood from it, but she did not seek medical attention. Although she received tetanus immunizations as a child, she had not received a booster vaccination since she was 15 years old. The presumptive diagnosis of tetanus was made.

1. How should this diagnosis be confirmed?
2. What is the recommended procedure for treating this patient? Should management wait until the laboratory results are available? What is the long-term prognosis for this patient?
3. Compare the mode of action of the toxins produced by *C. tetani* and *C. botulinum*.
4. What virulence factors are produced by *C. perfringens*? What diseases are caused by this organism?
5. What disease is caused by *C. difficile*? Why are infections caused by this organism difficult to manage?

Bibliography

Bongaerts G, Lyerly D: Role of toxins A and B in the pathogenesis of *Clostridium difficile* disease, *Microb Pathog* 17:1-12, 1994.
Collins M et al: The phylogeny of the genus *Clostridium:* proposal of five new genera and eleven new species combinations, *Int J Syst Bacteriol* 44:812-826, 1994.
Gergen P et al: A population-based serologic survey of immunity to tetanus in the United States, *N Engl J Med* 332:761-766, 1995.
Hatheway CL: Toxigenic clostridia, *Clin Microbiol Rev* 3:66-98, 1990.
Hatheway CL, McCroskey LM: Examination of feces and serum for diagnosis of infant botulism in 336 patients, *J Clin Microbiol* 25:2334-2338, 1987.
Knoop F, Owens M, Crocker I: *Clostridium difficile:* clinical disease and diagnosis, *Clin Microbiol Rev* 6:251-265, 1993.
Kornbluth AA, Danzid JB, Bernstein LH: *Clostridium septicum* infection and associated malignancy, *Medicine* 68:30-37, 1989.
Lyerly DM: *Clostridium difficile* testing, *Clin Microbiol Newsletter* 17:17-22, 1995.
Montecucco C, Schiavo G: Mechanism of action of tetanus and botulinum neurotoxins, *Mol Microbiol* 13:1-8, 1994.
Samore M et al: Clinical and molecular epidemiology of sporadic and clustered cases of nosocomial *Clostridium difficile* diarrhea, *Am J Med* 100:32-40, 1996.
Sanford J: Tetanus: forgotten but not gone, *N Engl J Med* 332:812-813, 1995 (editorial).
Schiavo G et al: Tetanus and botulinum neurotoxins are zinc proteases specific for components of the neuroexocytosis apparatus, *Ann N Y Acad Sci* 710:65-75, 1994.
Simpson L: Botulinum toxin: a deadly poison sheds its negative image, *Ann Intern Med* 125:616-617, 1996 (editorial).
Stevens DL et al: Spontaneous, nontraumatic gangrene due to *Clostridium septicum, Rev Infect Dis* 12:286-296, 1990.
Woodruff B et al: Clinical and laboratory comparison of botulism from toxin types A, B, and E in the United States, 1975-1988, *J Infect Dis* 166:1281-1286, 1992.

CHAPTER

38

Anaerobic Gram-Negative Bacilli

At least eight genera of anaerobic gram-negative bacilli and three genera of anaerobic gram-negative cocci colonize the human upper respiratory tract, gastrointestinal tract, and genitourinary tract (Box 38-1). Anaerobes are the predominant bacteria at each of these sites, outnumbering aerobic bacteria by 10- to 1000-fold. The anaerobic species are also numerous, with as many as 50 different species of gram-negative anaerobes present in these anatomical locations. The most common bacteria are listed in Table 38-1. Despite the abundance and diversity of these bacteria, most infections are caused by relatively few genera (Table 38-2). Among these pathogens, the most important is *Bacteroides fragilis*, the prototypical endogenous anaerobic pathogen.

PHYSIOLOGY AND STRUCTURE

At one time the genus *Bacteroides* consisted of almost 50 species, but some of these species have now been transferred to new genera. Species of pigmented, asaccharolytic bacilli were reclassified as *Porphyromonas* (from the Greek word for "purple"), and saccharolytic, bile-sensitive bacilli were transferred into the genus *Prevotella*. The genus *Bacteroides* now consists of only anaerobes previously categorized into the *B. fragilis* group and some closely related species. *B. fragilis*, the most important member of this genus, is pleomorphic in size and shape, resembling a mixed population of organisms in a casually examined Gram stain (Figure 38-1). Other gram-negative bacilli can be very small (e.g., *Prevotella* species) or elongated (e.g., *Fusobacterium*, so-named because the type species, *F. nucleatum*, is long and thin—"fusiform" shaped) (Figure 38-2). Most gram-negative anaerobes Gram stain weakly, so stained specimens must be carefully examined. Although *Bacteroides* organisms grow rapidly in culture, the other anaerobic, gram-negative bacilli are fastidious and may have to be incubated for 3 days or more before they can be detected.

TABLE 38-1	Predominant Anaerobic Gram-Negative Bacteria Colonizing Humans
SITE OF ISOLATION	**SPECIES**
Upper respiratory tract	*Bacteroides gracilis*
	Bacteroides ureolyticus
	Fusobacterium nucleatum
	Fusobacterium alocis
	Fusobacterium sulci
	Prevotella melaninogenica
	Prevotella intermedia
	Prevotella oralis
	Veillonella atypica
	Veillonella dispar
	Veillonella parvula
Gastrointestinal tract	*Bacteroides thetaiotaomicron*
	Bacteroides vulgatus
	Bacteroides capillosus
	Bacteroides coagulans
	Bacteroides putredinis
	Bacteroides ureolyticus
	Bacteroides ovatus
Genitourinary tract	*Porphyromonas asaccharolytica*
	Prevotella bivia
	Prevotella disiens
	Prevotella melaninogenica

BOX 38-1	Anaerobic Gram-Negative Bacteria

ANAEROBIC BACILLI

Bacteroides species
Bilophila species
Desulfomonas species
Fusobacterium species
Mitsuokella species
Porphyromonas species
Prevotella species
Tissierella species

ANAEROBIC COCCI

Acidaminococcus species
Megasphaera species
Veillonella species

Bacteroides organisms have a typical gram-negative cell wall structure, which can be surrounded by a polysaccharide capsule. A major component of the cell wall is a surface lipopolysaccharide (LPS). However, in contrast with the LPS molecules in *Fusobacterium* organisms and the aerobic gram-negative bacilli, the *Bacteroides* glycolipid has little or no endotoxin activity. This is because the lipid A component of LPS lacks phosphate groups on the glucosamine residues and the number of fatty acids linked to the amino sugars is reduced. Both factors are correlated with the loss of pyrogenic activity.

The anaerobic cocci are rarely isolated in clinical specimens, except when present as a contaminant. *Veillonella* species is the predominant anaerobe in the oropharynx, but it represents less than 1% of all anaerobes isolated in clinical specimens. The other cocci are rarely isolated.

PATHOGENESIS AND IMMUNITY

Despite the variety of anaerobic species that colonize the human body, relatively few are responsible for causing disease (Box 38-2). For example, *B. distasonis* and *B. thetaiotaomicron* are the predominant species of *Bacteroides* found in the gastrointestinal tract; however, more than 80% of intraabdominal infections are associated with *B. fragilis,* an organism that is a minor member of the gastrointestinal flora. The enhanced virulence of this and other pathogenic anaerobes is attributed to a variety of virulence factors that facilitate adherence of the organisms to host tissues, protection from the host immune response, and tissue destruction (Table 38-3).

Adhesins

Encapsulated *B. fragilis* and *Prevotella melaninogenica* strains can adhere to peritoneal surfaces more effectively than nonencapsulated strains. *Bacteroides* species and *Porphyromonas gingivalis* also possess fimbriae that mediate attachment to host cells.

Protection Against Oxygen Toxicity and Phagocytosis

Anaerobes capable of causing disease can generally tolerate exposure to oxygen. Catalase and superoxide dismutase, which inactivate hydrogen peroxide and the superoxide free radicals (O_2^-), respectively, are present in many pathogenic strains. In addition, the short-chain fatty acids produced during anaerobic metabolism inhibit phagocytosis and degranulation, and the capsular polysaccharide is antiphagocytic. Proteases that degrade immunoglobulins are found in *Porphyromonas* and *Prevotella* species.

TABLE 38-2 **Predominant Anaerobic Gram-Negative Bacteria Responsible for Human Disease**

INFECTION	BACTERIA
Head and neck	*Bacteroides ureolyticus*
	Fusobacterium nucleatum
	Fusobacterium necrophorum
	Porphyromonas asaccharolytica
	Porphyromonas gingivalis
	Prevotella intermedia
	Prevotella melaninogenica
Intraabdominal	*Bacteroides fragilis*
	Bacteroides thetaiotaomicron
	Prevotella melaninogenica
Gynecological	*Bacteroides fragilis*
	Prevotella bivia
	Prevotella disiens
Skin and soft tissue	*Bacteroides fragilis*
Bacteremia	*Bacteroides fragilis*
	Bacteroides thetaiotaomicron
	Fusobacterium species

FIGURE 38-1 *B. fragilis.* Organisms appear as faintly staining, pleomorphic, gram-negative bacilli.

FIGURE 38-2 *F. nucleatum.* Organisms are elongated with tapered ends (e.g., fusiform).

BOX 38-2   Summary of Anaerobic, Gram-Negative Bacterial Infections

BACTERIAL FACTORS

Diseases—chronic sinusitis, chronic otitis, periodontal diseases, brain abscess, pleuropulmonary infections after aspiration, intraabdominal infections, pelvic inflammatory disease, pelvic abscesses, endometritis, gynecological wound infections, skin and soft tissue infections, bacteremia.

Virulence factors—see Table 38-3.

TRANSMISSION

Endogenous spread to normally sterile tissues or fluids.

WHO IS AT RISK?

Surgical and trauma patients.
Patients with disruption of normal mucosa.
Patients who aspirate oral secretions.

GEOGRAPHY/SEASON

Ubiquitous and worldwide.
No seasonal incidence.

MODES OF CONTROL

Surgical drainage of abscesses and antibiotic therapy (metronidazole, clindamycin, imipenem, penicillin, if susceptible).

Prophylactic antibiotics are used if a medical procedure will disrupt the mucosa or if disruption of the mucosa has resulted from trauma.

TABLE 38-3   Virulence Factors in Anaerobic Gram-Negative Bacilli

VIRULENCE FACTOR	BACTERIA
ADHESINS	
Capsule	B. fragilis, P. melaninogenica
Fimbriae	B. fragilis, P. gingivalis
Hemagglutinin	P. gingivalis
Lectin	F. nucleatum
RESIST OXYGEN TOXICITY	
Superoxide dismutase	Many species
Catalase	Many species
ANTIPHAGOCYTIC	
Capsule	B. fragilis, P. melaninogenica
IgA, IgM, IgG proteases	Porphyromonas species, Prevotella species
Lipopolysaccharide	B. fragilis, Fusobacterium species
Volatile fatty acids	Many species
TISSUE DESTRUCTION	
Phospholipase C	F. necrophorum
Hemolysins	Many species
Proteases	Many species
Collagenase	Many species
Fibrinolysin	Many species
Neuraminidase	Many species
Heparinase	Many species
Chondroitin sulfatase	Many species
Glucuronidases	Many species
N-Acetylglucosaminidase	Many species
Volatile fatty acids	Many species

Modified from Duerden B: *Clin Infect Dis* 18(suppl 4):S253-259, 1994; and Lorber B: In *Mandell, Douglas and Bennett's principles and practice of infectious diseases,* ed 4, New York, 1995, Churchill Livingstone.

Tissue Destruction

A variety of enzymes have been associated with gram-negative anaerobes (Table 38-3). Many of these enzymes are found in both virulent and avirulent isolates. Nonetheless, the ability of these organisms to cause tissue destruction and inactivate immunoglobulins, as well as resist oxygen toxicity (superoxide dismutase), most likely plays an important role in the pathogenesis of anaerobic infections.

EPIDEMIOLOGY

As already stated, anaerobic gram-negative cocci and bacilli colonize the human body in large numbers. Their numerous important functions at these sites include stabilizing the resident bacterial flora, preventing colonization by pathogenic organisms from exogenous sources, and aiding in the digestion of food. When these organisms are responsible for disease, they originate from an endogenous source. That is, the organisms in the resident flora are able to spread by trauma or disease from the normally colonized mucosal surfaces to sterile tissues or fluids. As expected, these endogenous infections are characterized by the presence of a polymicrobial mixture of organisms. It is important to realize, however, that the mixture of organisms present on healthy mucosal surfaces differs from that in diseased tissues. This relates to the virulence potential of pathogenic organisms and their ability to increase from relatively small numbers on mucosal surfaces to be the predominant organism at the site of infection. For example, *B. fragilis* is commonly associated with pleuropulmonary, intraabdominal, and genital infections. However, the organism constitutes less than 1% of the colonic flora and is rarely isolated from the oropharynx or genital tract of healthy people unless highly selective techniques are used.

CLINICAL SYNDROMES
Respiratory Tract Infections

Up to half of the chronic infections of the sinuses and ears and virtually all periodontal infections involve mixtures of gram-negative anaerobes, with *Prevotella, Porphyromonas, Fusobacterium,* and non-*fragilis Bacteroides* organisms most commonly isolated. Anaerobes are less commonly associated with infections of the lower respiratory tract unless there is a history of aspiration of oral secretions.

Brain Abscess

Anaerobic infections of the brain are typically associated with a history of chronic sinusitis or otitis. This is confirmed by radiologic evidence of direct extension into the brain. A less common cause of such infections is bacteremic spread from a pulmonary source. In this case, multiple abscesses are present. The most common anaerobes in these polymicrobial infections are species of *Prevotella, Porphyromonas,* and *Fusobacterium* (as well as *Peptostreptococcus* and aerobic cocci).

Intraabdominal Infections

Despite the diverse population of bacteria that colonizes the gastrointestinal tract, relatively few species are associated with intraabdominal infections. Anaerobes are recovered in virtually all of these infections, with *B. fragilis* the most common organism. Other important anaerobes include *B. thetaiotaomicron* and *P. melaninogenica,* as well as the peptostreptococci and aerobic bacteria.

Gynecological Infections

Mixtures of anaerobes are frequently responsible for causing infections of the female genital tract (e.g., pelvic inflammatory disease, abscesses, endometritis, surgical wound infections). Although a variety of anaerobes can be isolated in patients with these infections, *Prevotella bivia* and *P. disiens* are the most important; *B. fragilis* is frequently responsible for abscess formation.

Skin and Soft Tissue infections

Although anaerobic gram-negative bacteria are not part of the normal flora of the skin (in contrast with *Peptostreptococcus* and *Propionibacterium* organisms), they can be introduced by a bite or as the result of contamination of a traumatized surface. In some cases the organisms may simply colonize a wound but not produce disease; at other times colonization may quickly progress to life-threatening disease such as myonecrosis. *B. fragilis* is the organism most commonly associated with significant disease.

Bacteremia

Anaerobes were at one time responsible for more than 20% of all clinically significant bacteremias; however, these organisms now cause less than 5% of these infections. The reduced incidence of disease is not completely understood but probably attributed to the widespread use of broad-spectrum antibiotics. The anaerobes most frequently isolated in blood cultures are *B. fragilis, B. thetaiotaomicron,* and *Fusobacterium* species.

LABORATORY DIAGNOSIS
Microscopy

Microscopic examination of specimens from patients with suspected anaerobic infections can be useful. Although the bacteria may stain faintly and irregularly, the finding of pleomorphic, gram-negative bacilli can be useful preliminary information.

Culture

Specimens should be collected and transported to the laboratory in an oxygen-free system, promptly inoculated onto specific media for the recovery of anaerobes, and incubated in an anaerobic environment. Because most anaerobe infections are endogenous, it is important to collect specimens so that they are not contaminated with the normal bacterial population present on the adjacent mucosal surface. Specimens should also be maintained in a moist environment because drying causes significant bacterial loss. Most *Bacteroides* organisms grow rapidly and should be detected within 2 days; however, other gram-negative anaerobes may have to be incubated longer. In addition, it is sometimes difficult to recover all clinically significant bacteria because of the different organisms present in polymicrobial infections. The use of selective media has facilitated the recovery of most important anaerobes (Figure 38-3).

FIGURE 38-3 Growth of *B. fragilis* on *Bacteroides* bile-esculin agar. Most aerobic and anaerobic bacteria are inhibited by bile and gentamicin in this medium, whereas the *B. fragilis* group of organisms is stimulated by bile, resistant to gentamicin, and able to hydrolyze esculin, producing a black precipitate.

Biochemical Identification

The preliminary identification of the *B. fragilis* group can be made by Gram stain and colonial morphology; resistance to kanamycin, vancomycin, and colistin; and stimulated growth in 20% bile. The definitive identification of this group and other gram-negative anaerobes is accurately made using commercially prepared biochemical systems that measure the activity of preformed enzymes. Gas chromatography has occasionally proved to be a useful, simple technique for detecting metabolic byproducts (short-chain fatty acids) and can be used to supplement biochemical testing.

TREATMENT, PREVENTION, AND CONTROL

Antibiotic therapy combined with surgical intervention is the main approach for managing serious anaerobic infections. Beta-lactamase is produced by virtually all members of the *B. fragilis* group, many *Prevotella* and *Porphyromonas* species, and some *Fusobacterium* isolates, which renders the bacteria resistant to penicillin and many cephalosporins. However, high concentrations of some penicillins (e.g., carbenicillin, piperacillin), as well as beta-lactamase inhibitors and other selected beta-lactam antibiotics (e.g., cefoxitin, imipenem), can be used to treat these infections. Clindamycin resistance in *Bacteroides* organisms, which is plasmid mediated, has become more prevalent in recent years, with an average of 7% to 10% of the isolates in the United States resistant. Metronidazole is active against *Bacteroides* species and other gram-negative bacilli and is the antibiotic of choice for treating infections caused by these organisms. The anaerobic cocci are usually susceptible to penicillin, cephalosporins, clindamycin, chloramphenicol, and metronidazole. However, it is often unnecessary to use specific therapy against them.

Because *Bacteroides* species constitute an important part of the normal microbial flora and infections result from the endogenous spread of the organisms, disease is virtually impossible to control. However, it is important to recognize that diagnostic or surgical procedures disrupting the natural barriers around the mucosal surfaces can introduce these organisms into normally sterile sites. If these barriers are invaded, prophylactic treatment with antibiotics may be indicated.

CASE STUDY AND QUESTIONS

A 65-year-old man entered the emergency department of a local hospital. He appeared to be acutely ill, with abdominal tenderness and a temperature of 40.0° C. Because appendicitis was suspected, the patient was taken to surgery. A ruptured appendix surrounded by approximately 20 ml of gross, foul-smelling pus was found at laparotomy. The pus was drained and submitted for aerobic and anaerobic bacterial cultures, as well as Gram staining. After surgery the patient was started on antibiotic therapy. Gram stain revealed a polymicrobial mixture of organisms, and culture was positive for *B. fragilis*, *Escherichia coli*, and *Enterococcus faecalis*.

1. Which organism or organisms are responsible for causing the abscess formation? What virulence factors are responsible for causing abscess formation?
2. *B. fragilis* causes infections at what other body sites?
3. What antibiotics should be selected to manage this polymicrobial infection?
4. What other anaerobic gram-negative bacilli can cause human disease?

Bibliography

Bjornson AB: Role of humoral factors in host resistance to the *Bacteroides fragilis* group, *Rev Infect Dis* 12:S161-168, 1990.

Cuchural GJ et al: Susceptibility of the *Bacteroides fragilis* group in the United States: analysis by site of isolation, *Antimicrob Agents Chemother* 32:717-722, 1988.

Duerden B: Virulence factors in anaerobes, *Clin Infect Dis* 18(suppl 4):S253-S259, 1994.

Finegold SM, Baron EJ, Wexler HM: *A clinical guide to anaerobic infections*, Belmont, Calif, 1992, Star.

Jousimies-Somer H, Summanen P, Finegold S: *Bacteroides, Porphyromonas, Prevotella, Fusobacterium,* and other anaerobic gram-negative bacteria. In Murray P et al, editors: *Manual of clinical microbiology*, ed 6, Washington, DC, 1995, ASM.

Lindberg AA et al: Structure-activity relationships in lipopolysaccharides of *Bacteroides fragilis, Rev Infect Dis* 12:S133-S140, 1990.

Tessier F et al: Antigenic relationships among *Bacteroides* species studied by rocket-line immunoelectrophoresis, *Int J Syst Bacteriol* 43:191-195, 1993.

39

Nocardia, Rhodococcus, and Related Actinomycetes

The aerobic actinomycetes are gram-positive, catalase-positive bacilli that are found in soil, decaying vegetation, and ventilation systems and that colonize animals and humans. Some actinomycetes have delicate filamentous forms (also called *hyphae*), similar to fungal hyphal forms, in clinical specimens and in culture. However, the cell wall structure and antimicrobial susceptibility patterns are typical of bacteria. The **mycolic acid**–containing members of this group consist of three families: Corynebacteriaceae (see Chapter 26), Nocardiaceae, and Mycobacteriaceae (see Chapter 40). Four genera are currently placed in the family Nocardiaceae: *Nocardia, Rhodococcus, Tsukamurella,* and *Gordona*. Organisms from all four genera stain irregularly with Gram stain and are **partially acid-fast** (resistant to decolorization with weak acid solutions). Numerous other genera of actinomycetes have been described, but the genera most commonly isolated in clinical specimens or associated with human disease are listed in Box 39-1. The spectrum of the diseases associated with these organisms is extensive and includes insignificant colonization (many genera), pulmonary disease *(Nocardia, Rhodococcus),* systemic infections *(Nocardia, Rhodococcus),* mycetoma *(Actinomadura, Nocardiopsis, Streptomyces,* and *Nocardia),* other opportunistic cutaneous infections (most genera), Whipple's disease *(Tropheryma),* and allergic pneumonitis (thermophilic actinomycetes).

NOCARDIA
Physiology and Structure

The genus *Nocardia* was named after Nocard, who was the first to describe bovine disease characterized by pyogenic pulmonary and cutaneous lesions. The organisms are strict aerobic bacilli that form branched hyphae in tissues and culture. The organisms are gram-positive, although many stain poorly and appear to be gram-negative with intracellular gram-positive beads (Figure 39-1). *Nocardia* organisms have a cell wall structure that is similar to mycobacteria with mycolic acids present and, like mycobacteria, are acid-fast (Figure 39-2). This acid-fastness is a helpful characteristic for distinguishing *Nocardia* organisms from morphologically similar organisms such as *Actinomyces*. *Nocardia* species are catalase positive, use carbohydrates oxidatively, and can grow on most nonselective laboratory media; however, isolation can require at least a week of incubation. The morphology of colonies varies from dry to waxy and from white to orange. Phylogenetic analysis of 16s rDNA has identified 10 species of *Nocardia*. Unfortunately, it is difficult to distinguish many of these species on the basis of their phenotypic properties (e.g., reactivity in biochemical tests). The species most commonly associated with human disease are *N. asteroides, N. brasiliensis, N. otitidiscaviarum,* and *N. farcinica*. However, the role that *N. farcinica* plays in the pathogenesis of human disease is certainly underestimated because most laboratories classify it within the *N. asteroides* complex.

Pathogenesis and Immunity

Organisms in the *N. asteroides* complex cause approximately 90% of human *Nocardia* infections. They cause bronchopulmonary disease in immunocompromised patients, with a high predilection for hematogenous spread to the central nervous system or skin. Patients at greatest risk for disease are those with T-cell deficiencies produced by disease (e.g., leukemia, acquired immunodeficiency syndrome) or immunosuppressive therapy (e.g., patients receiving corticosteroids, such as renal and cardiac transplant recipients). Disease can also occur in patients with chronic pulmonary diseases such as bronchitis, emphysema, asthma, bronchiectasis, and alveolar proteinosis. *N. brasiliensis* and *N. otitidiscaviarum* most commonly cause primary cutaneous infections (e.g., mycetoma, lymphocutaneous infections, superficial abscesses, cellulitis) in immunocompetent patients, with infrequent hematogenous dissemination.

Bronchopulmonary infections develop after the initial colonization of the oropharynx by inhalation and then aspiration of oral secretions into the lower airways. Primary cutaneous nocardiosis develops after traumatic introduction of organisms into subcutaneous tissues. Disease is characterized by necrosis and abscess formation, similar to that caused by other pyogenic bacteria. Chronic infections with sinus tract formation can occur, particularly with primary cutaneous infections. Although

FIGURE 39-1 Gram stain of *N. asteroides* in expectorated sputum. Note that the delicate beaded filaments cannot be distinguished from *Actinomyces* organisms (see Chapter 36).

FIGURE 39-2 Acid-fast stain of *N. asteroides* in expectorated sputum. This genus does not uniformly retain the stain ("partially acid-fast").

BOX 39-1	**Pathogenic Aerobic Actinomycetes**

ACTINOMYCETES WITH MYCOLIC ACIDS

Corynebacteriaceae
Nocardiaceae
   Nocardia species
   Rhodococcus species
   Gordona species
   Tsukamurella species
Mycobacteriaceae

ACTINOMYCETES WITH NO MYCOLIC ACIDS

Actinomadura species
Nocardiopsis species
Streptomyces species
Dermatophilus species
Oerskovia species
Rothia species
Tropheryma species
Thermophilic actinomycetes
   Saccharopolyspora species
   Saccharomonospora species
   Thermoactinomyces species

sulfur granules are observed with *Actinomyces* species, they are uncommon with *Nocardia* and seen only with cutaneous involvement. Colonization of the oropharynx or wounds can occur, so the significance of isolating *Nocardia* organisms in clinical specimens must be judged in light of the clinical presentation.

Epidemiology

Nocardia infections are exogenous (i.e., caused by organisms not part of the normal human flora). Despite the ubiquitous presence of the organism in soil rich with organic matter and the abundance of immunocompromised patients in hospitals, fewer than 1000 infections are documented annually in the United States. However, most investigators believe that the actual number is much larger. Most reported cases are sporadic and acquired outside the hospital and primarily occur in adult patients (Box 39-2).

Clinical Syndromes

Bronchopulmonary infections caused by *Nocardia* species cannot be distinguished from infections caused by other pyogenic organisms, although *Nocardia* infections tend to develop more slowly. Signs such as cough, dyspnea, and fever are usually present but are not diagnostic. Cavitation and spread into the pleura are common. Even though the clinical picture is not specific for *Nocardia*, these organisms should be considered when immunocompromised patients develop pneumonia with cavitation, particularly if there is evidence of dissemination to the central nervous system or subcutaneous tissues. **Cutaneous infections** may be primary infections (e.g., mycetoma, lymphocutaneous infections, cellulitis, subcutaneous abscesses) or may result from the spread of organisms from a primary pulmonary infection. **Actinomycotic mycetoma** is a painless, chronic infection characterized by localized subcutaneous swelling, suppuration, and the formation of multiple sinus tracts (Figure 39-3). The underlying connective tissues, muscle, and bone can be involved, and draining sinus tracts usually open on the skin surface. A variety of organisms can cause mycetoma, although *N. brasiliensis* is the most common cause in North America, Central America, and South America. **Lymphocutaneous infections** involve the regional lymph nodes, with cutaneous involvement along the lymphatics. These infections resemble cutaneous infections caused by species of mycobacteria and by the fungus *Sporothrix schenckii*. *Nocardia* can also cause **chronic ulcerative lesions**, **subcutaneous abscesses**, and **cellulitis**.

BOX 39-2   *Summary of Nocardia Infections*

BACTERIAL FACTORS

Gram-positive, partially acid-fast, filamentous bacilli; cell wall with mycolic acid.

Virulence factors—not well characterized; opportunistic pathogen.

Diseases—bronchopulmonary, cutaneous (mycetoma, lymphocutaneous and subcutaneous abscesses, cellulitis, secondary spread from primary pulmonary infection), central nervous system (chronic meningitis, brain abscesses), ocular.

TRANSMISSION

Exogenous infections acquired by inhalation (pulmonary), traumatic introduction (cutaneous), or opportunistic exposure (ocular).

WHO IS AT RISK?

Immunocompetent patients with chronic pulmonary disease (bronchitis, emphysema, bronchiectasis, alveolar proteinosis).

WHO IS AT RISK?—cont'd

People who have suffered skin wounds through which the organisms could be introduced into subcutaneous tissues.

Immunocompromised patients with T-cell deficiencies (transplant recipients, patients with malignancies, patients infected with the human immunodeficiency virus, patients receiving corticosteroids).

GEOGRAPHY/SEASON

Ubiquitous and worldwide.

No seasonal incidence.

MODES OF CONTROL

Antibiotic therapy with sulfonamides or antibiotics with proven in vivo activity.

Proper wound care.

As many as one third of all patients with *N. asteroides* infections have central nervous system involvement, most commonly involving the formation of single or multiple brain abscesses. The disease can present initially as chronic meningitis.

Nocardia organisms also cause **ocular infections** in immunocompetent and immunocompromised patients. These opportunistic infections result from the inadequate care of contact lenses or ophthalmological manipulations.

Laboratory Diagnosis

The specimens collected for the isolation of *Nocardia* organisms are dictated by the patient's clinical presentation. Multiple sputum specimens should be collected from patients with pulmonary disease because the slow growth of the organism and the presence of contaminating organisms make recovery unreliable. Because *Nocardia* organisms are usually distributed throughout the tissue and abscess material, it is relatively easy to detect them in microscopic studies and isolate them in vitro in patients with cutaneous or central nervous system disease. The delicate hyphae of *Nocardia* organisms in tissues cause them to resemble *Actinomyces* organisms; however, *Nocardia* organisms stain poorly with Gram stain, and most isolates are partially acid-fast (Figures 39-1 and 39-2). The organisms grow on most laboratory media incubated in an atmosphere of 5% to 10% carbon dioxide, but the presence of these slow-growing organisms may be obscured by more rapidly growing commensal bacteria. If a specimen is received potentially contaminated with rapidly growing bacteria (e.g., sputum), selective media should be inoculated. Success has been

FIGURE 39-3 Mycetoma caused by *N. brasiliensis.* The foot is grossly enlarged and covered with multiple draining sinus tracts. (From Binford CH, Connor DH, editors: *Pathology of tropical and extraordinary diseases,* vol 2, Washington, DC, 1976, Armed Forces Institute of Pathology.)

achieved with the medium used for the isolation of *Legionella* species (buffered charcoal-yeast extract [BCYE] agar) and other selective media. *Nocardia* organisms occasionally grow on media used for the isolation of mycobacteria and fungi. It is important to notify the laboratory that nocardiosis is suspected because most laboratories do not routinely incubate clinical specimens for more than 1 to 3 days. It takes more time (i.e., as long as 1 week) for *Nocardia* species to be isolated.

The preliminary identification of *Nocardia* organisms is uncomplicated. The species can be initially classified on the basis of detecting filamentous acid-fast bacilli. However, definitive identification is frequently delayed because *N. asteroides* complex, the species group most commonly isolated, is nonreactive with most differential tests used for biochemical classification (Table 39-1).

Treatment, Prevention, and Control

Nocardia infections are treated with the combination of antibiotics and appropriate surgical intervention. Sulfonamides are the antibiotics of choice for treating nocardiosis. Tobramycin, amikacin, and some of the newer beta-lactams also have good in vitro activity, but their in vivo effectiveness is unproved. Of the clinically important *Nocardia* species, *N. farcinica* is the most resistant to antibiotics, including sulfa drugs. Antibiotic therapy should be extended for 6 weeks or more. Whereas the clinical response is favorable in patients with localized infections, the prognosis is poor for immunocompromised patients with disseminated disease.

Because *Nocardia* organisms are ubiquitous, it is impossible to avoid exposure to them. However, bronchopulmonary disease is uncommon in immunocompetent persons, and primary cutaneous infections can be prevented through proper wound care. The complications associated with disseminated disease can be minimized if nocardiosis is considered in the differential diagnosis for immunocompromised patients with cavitary pulmonary disease.

RHODOCOCCUS

The genus *Rhodococcus* ("red-pigmented coccus") consists of 15 species of gram-positive, obligate aerobic actinomycetes. The cell wall of these catalase-positive coccobacilli is similar to that of *Nocardia* and *Mycobacterium*: It contains mycolic acid and tuberculostearic acid, rendering the organisms acid-fast. *R. equi* (formerly *Corynebacterium equi*) is a well-recognized veterinary pathogen, particularly in herbivores, and has been associated in recent years with human disease. People at greatest risk for infection include those who have contact with farm animals, particularly immunocompromised patients (e.g., patients with malignancies or transplants, those receiving corticosteroids, those infected with the human immunodeficiency virus). However, despite the recovery of this organism from colonized and infected herbivores as well as from soil contaminated with herbivore manure, most infected patients do not have a history of contact with grazing animals. The recent increase in the incidence of human infection is most likely related to the increase in the number of patients with immunosuppressive diseases and to the enhanced awareness of the organism.

R. equi is a facultative, intracellular organism that survives in macrophages and causes granulomatous inflammation, which leads to abscess formation. Although numerous putative virulence factors have been identified, the precise pathophysiology of the infections is incompletely understood. Immunocompromised patients most typically present with invasive pulmonary disease (e.g., pneumonia, lung abscesses), with evidence of dissemination to distal sites (lymph nodes, meninges, pericardium, and skin) commonly observed. Rhodococci usually cause opportunistic infections in immunocompetent patients (e.g., posttraumatic cutaneous infections, peritonitis and chronic dialysis patients, traumatic endophthalmitis).

Rhodococcus organisms grow readily on nonselective media incubated aerobically, although the characteristic

TABLE 39-1   Identification Tests for Common *Nocardia* Species

TESTS	N. ASTEROIDES COMPLEX*	N. BRASILIENSIS	N. OTITIDIS-CAVIARUM
Decomposition of:			
Casein	−	+	−
Tyrosine	−	+	−
Xanthine	−	−	+
Gelatin	−	+	−
Starch	−	−	−
Urea	+	+	+
Acid from:			
Glucose	+	+	+
Rhamnose	+/−	−	−

Nocardia asteroides complex includes *N. asteroides*, *N. farcinica*, and *N. nova*.

pigment may not be obvious for 4 days or more. They appear as pleomorphic, gram-positive coccobacilli that can stain weakly acid-fast. The organism can be identified by biochemical tests, although it is relatively inert.

Rhodococcus infections have proved difficult to treat. Although in vitro tests and tests in animal models have identified specific combinations of drugs as effective, only limited success has been realized in the treatment of human infections using these agents, particularly in immunocompromised patients. Currently, treatment with erythromycin and rifampin is recommended, but relapses are frequently observed.

GORDONA AND TSUKAMURELLA

Gordona and *Tsukamurella* organisms were previously classified with *Rhodococcus* because they are morphologically similar, contain mycolic acids, and are partially acid-fast. The organisms are present in soil and are rare opportunistic pathogens in humans. *G. bronchialis* has been associated with pulmonary and cutaneous infections, as well as nosocomial infections such as those resulting from contaminated intravascular catheters. *T. paurometabolum* is often recovered as an environmental contaminant or associated with a catheter infection.

ACTINOMADURA, NOCARDIOPSIS, AND STREPTOMYCES

Mycetoma can be caused by fungi, as well as by bacteria in the genera *Actinomadura, Nocardiopsis, Streptomyces,* and *Nocardia.* The precise etiology of this disease can be determined only by cultivation because many of these organisms resemble fungi when seen in tissue and the diseases are clinically indistinguishable. Infection usually results from the traumatic introduction of the bacteria or fungi into tissue, most commonly in an extremity. Chronic cutaneous and subcutaneous infections with abscess and sinus tract formation then develop. These pathogens can be isolated on Sabouraud's dextrose agar (typically considered a fungal medium) or on nonselective bacterial media. It may take as long as 3 weeks of incubation before growth is apparent. The isolates are identified on the basis of morphological criteria and the results of selected biochemical tests. Effective therapy includes both surgical debridement and appropriate antibiotics, such as trimethoprim-sulfamethoxazole, streptomycin, rifampin, dapsone, or a combination of these agents. Because the clinical diagnosis is noncontributory and culture results may be delayed for 3 weeks or more, empirical therapy for bacterial and fungal infection must be initiated. Broad-spectrum antibiotics that are effective against all potential pathogens should be chosen.

OTHER ACTINOMYCETES

Dermatophilus, an actinomycete found in the soil, causes infections in humans (e.g., slaughterhouse workers, butchers, hunters, dairy farmers, veterinarians) exposed to infected animals or contaminated animal products. The disease is an exudative dermatitis with encrustations that typically involve the hands or feet. This organism is susceptible to many antibiotics, and most infections are treated with the combination of penicillin and an aminoglycoside.

Oerskovia is an opportunistic human pathogen associated with peritonitis in patients receiving chronic peritoneal dialysis, traumatic endophthalmitis, central nervous system shunt infections, catheter-associated bacteremia, and endocarditis occurring after the placement of a homograft. Most infections do not respond to antibiotics unless the foreign body is removed.

Rothia is part of the normal bacterial flora of the oropharynx and is associated with dental plaque. Invasive disease has been rarely reported.

Tropheryma whippelii is a newly classified bacterium believed to cause **Whipple's disease,** a disease characterized by arthralgia, diarrhea, abdominal pain, weight loss, lymphadenopathy, fever, and increased skin pigmentation. Historically the disease was diagnosed on the basis of the clinical presentation and the finding of periodic acid–Schiff—positive inclusions in foamy macrophages that infiltrated the lamina propria of the small intestine. Recently, analysis of the rDNA of these bacteria revealed that they are members of the actinomycetes. Although techniques to culture these organisms have not been developed, polymerase chain reaction–based diagnostic tests are now available.

Allergic pneumonitis ("farmer's lung") is a hypersensitivity reaction to repeated exposure to **thermophilic actinomycetes** commonly found in decaying vegetation. The clinically significant genera are *Thermoactinomyces* (three species), *Saccharopolyspora* (one species), and *Saccharomonospora* (one species). Patients with the disease have granulomatous changes in the lung, with pulmonary edema, eosinophilia, and elevated IgE levels. Clinical diagnosis is confirmed by detecting specific precipitin antibodies to these agents in serum.

CASE STUDY AND QUESTIONS

A 47-year-old renal transplant recipient who had been receiving prednisone and azathioprine for 2 years was admitted to the university medical center. Two weeks before, the patient noticed the development of a dry, persistent cough. Five days before admission, the cough became productive, and pleuritic chest pain developed. One day before admission, the patient was in mild respiratory arrest, and chest radiographs revealed a patchy right upper lobe infiltrate. Sputum specimens were initially sent for bacterial culture, which were reported as negative for organisms after 2 days of incubation. Antibiotic therapy with cephalothin was ineffective, so additional specimens were collected for the culture of bacteria, mycobacteria, *Legionella* species, and fungi. After 4 days of incubation, *Nocardia* organims were isolated on the media inoculated for mycobacteria, *Legionella* species, and fungi.

1. Why did the organism fail to grow on media for bacteria? What can be done to correct this problem?
2. What is the most likely species of *Nocardia* involved in this infection? If this organism disseminates, what two target tissues are most likely to be involved?
3. What diseases are caused by *N. asteroides* complex? *N. brasiliensis*? *N. otitidiscaviarum*?
4. What disease is caused by *Rhodococcus* organisms in immunocompromised patients? What diagnostic property does this organism share with *Nocardia* organisms? Which two other genera discussed in this chapter share the same property?
5. Which bacteria cause mycetoma?

Bibliography

Chun J, Goodfellow M: A phylogenetic analysis of the genus *Nocardia* with 16S rRNA gene sequences, *Int J Syst Bacteriol* 45:240-245, 1995.

Dobbins W: The diagnosis of Whipple's diseases, *N Engl J Med* 332:390-392, 1995 (editorial).

Harvey RL, Sunstrum JC: *Rhodococcus equi* infection in patients with and without human immunodeficiency virus infection, *Rev Infect Dis* 13:139-145, 1991.

Lerner P: Nocardiosis, *Clin Infect Dis* 22:891-905, 1996.

Maiwald M et al: Reassessment of the phylogenetic position of the bacterium associated with Whipple's disease and determination of the 16S-23S ribosomal intergenic spacer sequence, *Int J Syst Bacteriol* 46:1078-1082, 1996.

McNeil M, Brown J: The medically important aerobic actinomycetes: epidemiology and microbiology, *Clin Microbiol Rev* 7:357-417, 1994.

Prescott JF: *Rhodococcus equi:* an animal and human pathogen, *Clin Microbiol Rev* 4:20-34, 1991.

Relman D et al: Identification of the uncultured bacillus of Whipple's disease, *N Engl J Med* 327:293-301, 1992.

Smego RA, Gallis HA: The clinical spectrum of *Nocardia brasiliensis* infection in the United States, *Rev Infect Dis* 6:164-180, 1984.

CHAPTER ·········· 40

Mycobacterium

The genus *Mycobacterium* consists of nonmotile, non-spore-forming, aerobic bacilli that are 0.2 to 0.6 × 1 to 10 μm in size. The bacilli occasionally form branched filaments, but these can be readily disrupted. The cell wall is rich in lipids, making the surface hydrophobic and the mycobacteria resistant to many disinfectants as well as to common laboratory stains. Once stained, the bacilli also cannot be decolorized with acid solutions, hence the name **acid-fast bacilli.** Because the mycobacterial cell wall is complex and this group of organisms is fastidious, most mycobacteria grow slowly, dividing every 12 to 24 hours. Isolation of the slow-growing organisms (*M. tuberculosis, M. arium-intracellulare*) can require 3 to 8 weeks of incubation whereas the more "rapidly growing" mycobacteria (e.g., *M. fortuitum, M. chelonae, M. abscessus*) require incubation for 3 days or more. *M. leprae,* the etiological agent of leprosy, cannot be grown in cell-free cultures.

Mycobacteria are still a significant cause of morbidity and mortality, particularly in countries with limited medical resources. Currently, 74 species of mycobacteria have been identified, with 23 species of slow-growing and 5 species of rapid-growing mycobacteria associated with human disease (Table 40-1). Despite the abundance of mycobacterial species, more than 95% of all human infections are caused by only seven species or groups: *M. tuberculosis, M. leprae, M. avium-intracellulare* complex, *M. kansasii, M. fortuitum, M. chelonae,* and *M. abscessus.*

PHYSIOLOGY AND STRUCTURE

Bacteria are classified in the genus *Mycobacterium* on the basis of their acid-fastness, the presence of mycolic acids containing 60 to 90 carbons that are cleaved by pyrolysis to C22 to C26 fatty acid methyl esters, and a high (61% to 71%) G+C content in their DNA. Although other species of bacteria can be acid-fast (i.e., *Nocardia, Rhodococcus, Tsukamurella, Gordona*), they stain less intensely (are partially acid-fast), their mycolic acids chains are shorter, and their G+C content is lower.

Mycobacteria possess a complex, lipid-rich cell wall. This cell wall is responsible for many of the characteristic properties of the bacteria (e.g., acid-fastness, slow growth, resistance to detergents, resistance to common antibacterial antibiotics, antigenicity). The basic structure of the cell wall is typical of gram-positive bacteria: an inner cytoplasmic membrane overlayed with a thick peptidoglycan layer and no outer membrane. However, the peptidoglycan skeleton is covalently linked with arabinogalactan-mycolic acid molecules and is overlayed with free lipids and polypeptides (Figure 40-1). The surface glycolipids, including species-specific mycosides (peptidoglycolipids, oligoliposaccharides) and phenolic glycolipids, are highly antigenic. They constitute 25% of the dry weight of the cell wall and contribute to the hydrophobic properties of mycobacteria. Another cell wall lipid, **cord factor** (6´6´-dimycolate of trehalose), is responsible for producing the parallel alignment of rows of bacilli ("cord" formation), a characteristic of virulent strains of *M. tuberculosis.*

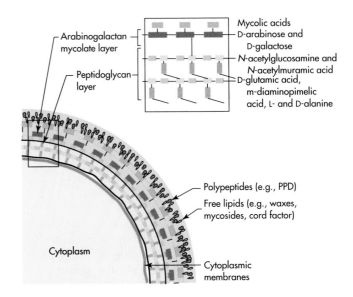

FIGURE 40-1 Mycobacterial cell wall structure. Mycolic acids are attached to the arabinose-galactose layer at the arabinose side chain. Phosphodiester linkage binds the arabinogalactan layer to the underlying peptidoglycan layer at the muramic acid subunit. *PPD,* Purified protein derivative. (Redrawn from Kubica GP, Wayne LG, editors: *The mycobacteria: a sourcebook,* New York, 1984, Marcel Dekker.)

FIGURE 40-2 *M. tuberculosis* colonies on Löwenstein-Jensen agar after 8 weeks of incubation. (From Baron EJ, Peterson LR, Finegold SM: *Bailey and Scott's diagnostic microbiology,* ed 9, St Louis, 1994, Mosby.)

FIGURE 40-3 *M. kansasii* colonies on Middlebrook agar 1 day after exposure to light. (From Baron EJ, Peterson LR, Finegold SM: *Bailey and Scott's diagnostic microbiology,* ed 9, St Louis, 1994, Mosby.)

TABLE 40-1   Classification of Mycobacteria Pathogenic for Humans

ORGANISM	PATHOGENICITY	FREQUENCY IN UNITED STATES	ORGANISM	PATHOGENICITY	FREQUENCY IN UNITED STATES
M. TUBERCULOSIS COMPLEX			**RUNYON GROUP III**		
M. tuberculosis	Strictly pathogenic	Common	M. avium	Strictly pathogenic	Common
M. leprae	Strictly pathogenic	Uncommon	M. intracellulare	Strictly pathogenic	Common
M. africanum	Strictly pathogenic	Rare	M. genavense	Strictly pathogenic	Uncommon
M. bovis	Strictly pathogenic	Rare	M. haemophilum	Usually pathogenic	Uncommon
M. ulcerans	Strictly pathogenic	Rare	M. malmoense	Usually pathogenic	Rare
			M. shimoidei	Sometimes pathogenic	Rare
RUNYON GROUP I			M. celatum	Sometimes pathogenic	Rare
M. kansasii	Usually pathogenic	Common	M. branderi	Sometimes pathogenic	Rare
M. marinum	Usually pathogenic	Uncommon			
M. simiae	Usually pathogenic	Uncommon	**RUNYON GROUP IV**		
M. asiaticum	Usually pathogenic	Rare	M. fortuitum	Sometimes pathogenic	Common
M. intermedium	Sometimes pathogenic	Rare	M. chelonae	Sometimes pathogenic	Common
			M. abscessus	Sometimes pathogenic	Uncommon
RUNYON GROUP II			M. mucogenicum	Sometimes pathogenic	Uncommon
M. szulgai	Usually pathogenic	Uncommon	M. peregrinum	Sometimes pathogenic	Rare
M. scrofulaceum	Sometimes pathogenic	Uncommon			
M. xenopi	Sometimes pathogenic	Uncommon			
M. lentiflavum	Sometimes pathogenic	Rare			
M. interjectum	Unknown	Rare			

The peptide chains in the outer layer constitute 15% of the cell wall weight and are biologically important antigens, stimulating the patient's cellular immune response to infection. Extracted and partially purified preparations of these protein derivatives are used as a skin test reagent to measure exposure to *M. tuberculosis.* Similar preparations from other mycobacteria have been used as species-specific skin test reagents.

Growth properties and colonial morphology are used for the preliminary identification of mycobacteria. As noted earlier, *M. tuberculosis* and closely related species are slow-growing bacteria. The colonies are nonpigmented or buff colored (Figure 40-2). Runyon classified the other mycobacteria into four groups on the basis of their rate of growth and their ability to produce pigments in the presence or absence of light. The pigmented mycobacteria produce intensely yellow carotenoids. Photochromogens (Runyon group I) produce these pigments only after exposure to light (Figure 40-3), whereas scotochromogenic organisms (Runyon group II) pro-

BOX 40-1   **Summary of *M. tuberculosis* Infections**

BACTERIAL FACTORS

Diseases—localized pulmonary infections or dissemination to other body sites such as bone marrow, spleen, kidneys, central nervous system. Bacteria may multiply to produce symptomatic disease or become dormant after initial replication. Dormant bacilli can be reactivated, followed by progression to disease with declining immunity or late in life.

Virulence factors—organism able to replicate in nonactivated macrophages; can survive for years in dormant state. Pathology depends on host's response to infection rather than produced by bacterial toxins or enzymes.

Lipid-rich cell wall makes mycobacteria resistant to disinfectants, detergents, common antibacterial antibiotics, and traditional stains.

TRANSMISSION

Humans, the only natural reservoir.

Person-to-person exposure by means of infectious aerosols.

WHO IS AT RISK?

Anyone exposed to person with active tuberculosis, particularly immunocompromised patients, the homeless, drug and alcohol abusers, and institutionalized people.

Risk of disease related to infectious dose and patient's immunological competence.

GEOGRAPHY/SEASON

Worldwide, with highest incidence in underdeveloped countries.

No seasonal incidence.

MODES OF CONTROL

Therapy prolonged with combination of effective antibiotics. (Resistance develops rapidly if single antibiotic is used.)

Prophylaxis with isoniazid or another effective antibiotic for exposed people with a positive skin test result.

Vaccination with bacille Calmette-Guérin used as immunoprophylaxis in areas with high incidence of endemic disease.

Implementation of appropriate public health measures to ensure prompt detection and treatment of newly infected patients.

---

duce the pigments in the dark and the light. The slow-growing, nonpigmented mycobacteria are classified as Runyon group III, whereas the relatively rapidly growing mycobacteria are classified as Runyon group IV. The Runyon classification can be used to differentiate the most common mycobacterial isolates (Table 40-1).

MYCOBACTERIUM TUBERCULOSIS
Pathogenesis and Immunity

Tuberculosis is the classic human mycobacterial disease (Box 40-1). The infection is acquired through the inhalation of aerosolized infectious particles, which then travel to the terminal airways. At this site the bacteria penetrate into unactivated alveolar macrophages and replicate freely. The infected phagocytic cells are eventually destroyed, after which there are further cycles of phagocytosis by macrophages, mycobacterial replication, and cell lysis. Although phagocytosis is initiated by alveolar macrophages, circulating macrophages and lymphocytes are attracted to the infectious focus by the bacilli, cellular debris, and host chemotactic factors (e.g., complement component C5a). The histological characteristic of this focus is formation of multinucleated giant cells of fused macrophages, also called **Langhans' cells.** Infected macrophages can also spread during the initial phase of disease to the local lymph nodes, as well as into the bloodstream and other tissues (e.g., bone marrow, spleen, kidneys, central nervous system).

The intracellular replication of mycobacteria stimulates both helper (CD4+) T cells and cytotoxic (CD8+) T cells. Activation of CD4+ cells leads to antibody production, but this is ineffective in controlling mycobacterial disease because the bacteria are protected in their intracellular location. T cells also release gamma-interferon and other cytokines that activate macrophages. Activated macrophages can engulf and kill mycobacteria. The cytotoxic T cells can also lyse phagocytic cells with replicating mycobacteria, thus permitting phagocytosis and bacterial killing by activated phagocytic cells. If a small antigenic burden is present at the time that the macrophages are stimulated, the bacilli are destroyed with minimal tissue damage. However, if many bacilli are present, the cellular immune response results in tissue necrosis. Multiple host factors are involved in this process, including cytokine toxicity, local activation of the complement cascade, ischemia, and exposure to macrophage-derived hydrolytic enzymes and reactive oxygen intermediates. No known mycobacterial toxin or enzyme has been associated with tissue destruction.

The effectiveness of bacillary elimination is in part related to the size of the focus of infection. Localized collections of activated macrophages (**granulomas**) prevent further spread of the bacilli. These macrophages can penetrate into small granulomas (less than 3 mm) and kill all the bacilli contained in them. However, larger necrotic or caseous granulomas become encapsulated with fibrin that effectively protects the bacilli from macrophage killing. The bacilli can remain dormant in this stage or be reactivated years later when the patient's immunological responsiveness wanes as the result of old age or immunosuppressive disease or therapy. This is the reason that disease may not develop until late in life in patients with a history of exposure to tuberculosis.

Epidemiology

Although tuberculosis can be established in primates and laboratory animals such as guinea pigs, humans are the only natural reservoir. The disease is spread by close person-to-person contact through the inhalation of infectious aerosols. Large particles are trapped on mucosal surfaces and removed by the ciliary action of the respiratory tree. However, small particles containing one to three tubercle bacilli can reach the alveolar spaces and establish infection.

It is estimated that one third of the world's population, including 10 million in the United States, are infected with *M. tuberculosis*. Each year 8 million new cases and 3 million deaths are reported worldwide. Although the incidence of tuberculosis in the United States had steadily decreased since the early 1900s, this trend changed in 1984 (Figure 40-4). This problem is attributed to the immigration of people from countries with endemic tuberculosis and to increased infections in the homeless, drug and alcohol abusers, prisoners, and people infected with the human immunodeficiency virus (HIV). Because it is difficult to eradicate disease in these patients, spread of the infection to other populations, including health care workers, poses a significant public health problem. This is particularly true for drug-resistant *M. tuberculosis* because patients treated inadequately may remain infectious for a long time. However, the incidence of tuberculosis is again decreasing as the result of dedicated public health efforts.

Clinical Syndromes

Although tuberculosis can involve any organ, most infections are restricted to the lungs. The initial pulmonary focus is the middle or lower lung fields, where the tubercle bacilli can multiply freely. The patient's cellular immunity is activated and mycobacterial replication ceases in most patients within 3 to 6 weeks of exposure to the organism. However, approximately 5% of patients exposed to *M. tuberculosis* will progress to active disease within 2 years, and another 5% to 10% will develop disease sometime later in life. The likelihood of infection progressing to active disease is a function of the infectious dose and the patient's immune competence. For example, active disease will develop in approximately 10% of HIV-infected patients within 1 year of exposure, compared with a 10% risk of disease during the lifetime of a non–HIV-infected patient. In HIV-infected patients, disease usually appears before the onset of other opportunistic infections, is twice as likely to spread to extrapulmonary sites, and can progress rapidly to death.

The clinical signs and symptoms of tuberculosis reflect the site of infection, with primary disease usually re-

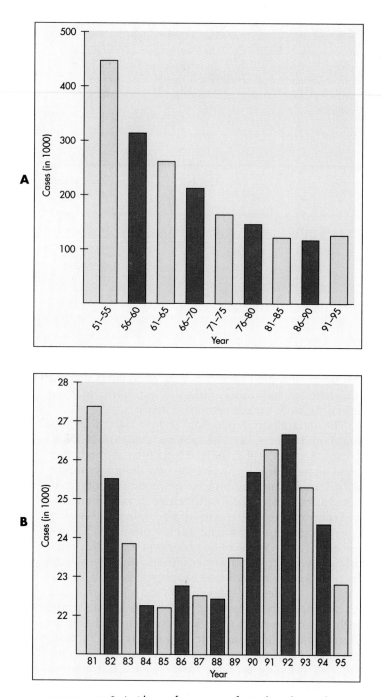

FIGURE 40-4 A, Incidence of new cases of *M. tuberculosis* in the United States since 1951. **B,** Annual incidence of disease since 1981. (Redrawn from *MMWR* 44:1-87, 1995.)

stricted to the lower respiratory tract. The disease is insidious in onset, with patients typically having nonspecific complaints of malaise, weight loss, cough, and night sweats. Sputum production may be scant or bloody and purulent. Sputum production with hemoptysis is associated with tissue destruction (e.g., cavitary disease). The clinical diagnosis is supported by radiographic evidence of pulmonary disease, positive skin test reactivity, and the laboratory detection of mycobacteria either by microscopy or in cultures. One or both upper lobes of the lungs are usually involved in patients with active disease that includes pneumonitis or abscess formation and cavitation.

As noted earlier, extrapulmonary tuberculosis can occur as the result of the hematogenous spread of the bacilli during the initial phase of multiplication. There may be no evidence of pulmonary disease in patients with disseminated or **miliary** tuberculosis.

MYCOBACTERIUM LEPRAE
Pathogenesis and Immunity

Leprosy (also called **Hansen's disease**) is caused by *M. leprae* (Box 40-2). Leprosy presents clinically as tuberculoid leprosy or lepromatous leprosy, with intermediate forms also recognized. Like infection with *M. tuberculosis,* the clinical manifestations of leprosy depend on the patient's immune reaction to the bacilli. Patients with **tuberculoid leprosy** have a strong cellular immune reaction but a weak humoral antibody response. Infected tissues typically have many lymphocytes and granulomas but relatively few bacilli (Table 40-2). Like *M. tuberculosis* infections in immunocompetent patients, the bacteria produce cytokines (e.g., interferon-gamma, IL-2) that mediate macrophage activation, phagocytosis, and bacillary clearance. Patients with **lepromatous leprosy,** on the other hand, have a strong antibody response but a specific defect in their cellular response to *M. leprae* antigens. Thus an abundance of bacilli are typically observed in dermal macrophages and the Schwann cells of the peripheral nerves. This is the most infectious form of leprosy.

Epidemiology

Leprosy is a relatively rare mycobacterial disease in the United States; approximately 250 cases are reported annually. However, more than 12 million cases are recognized worldwide, with most in Asia and Africa. Less than 10% of the infections in the United States are in native-born Americans; most are in immigrants from Mexico, Asia, the Pacific Islands, and Africa. The largest number of cases in the United States are reported in California, Hawaii, and Texas: leprosy is endemic in these states as well as in Louisiana. Endemic disease is found in armadillos, which represent a potential domestic reservoir of infection.

Disease is spread by person-to-person contact. Although the most important route of infection is unknown, it is believed that *M. leprae* is spread either through the inhalation of infectious aerosols or through skin contact with respiratory secretions and wound exudates. Numerous *M. leprae* are found in the nasal secretions from patients with lepromatous leprosy.

M. leprae cannot grow in cell-free cultures. Thus laboratory confirmation of leprosy requires histopathological findings consistent with the clinical disease and skin test reactivity to lepromin or requires acid-fast bacilli found in the lesions.

Clinical Syndromes

As noted earlier, leprosy presents clinically as tuberculoid or lepromatous disease; each manifests typical clinical and immunological characteristics (Table 40-2 and Fig-

---

BOX 40-2   Summary of *M. leprae* Infections

BACTERIAL FACTORS

Disease—leprosy (also called *Hansen's disease*): tuberculoid form and lepromatous form, with intermediate presentations common.

Virulence factors—disease manifestations depend on patient's immune response to infection; bacterial factors not prominent.

Bacteria do not grow in culture. Diagnosis is made by specific skin test (tuberculoid form) or positive acid-fast stain with typical clinical presentation (lepromatous form).

TRANSMISSION

Lepromatous leprosy: highly infectious; infectivity of tuberculoid leprosy: low.

Person-to-person spread by inhalation or direct contact with lesions.

Armadillos: naturally infected.

WHO IS AT RISK?

People in close contact with patients with the lepromatous form of disease.

GEOGRAPHY/SEASON

Worldwide (e.g., Mexico, Asia, Pacific Islands, Africa); rare in United States (primarily in California, Hawaii, Texas). No seasonal incidence.

MODES OF CONTROL

Treatment with effective antimicrobials, such as dapsone, rifampin, and clofazimine or ethionamide, for a minimum of 2 years.

Control effected by prompt recognition and treatment of infected people.

TABLE 40-2	Clinical and Immunological Manifestations of Leprosy	
FEATURES	**TUBERCULOID LEPROSY**	**LEPROMATOUS LEPROSY**
Skin lesions	Few erythematous or hypopigmented plaques with flat centers and raised, demarcated borders; peripheral nerve damage with complete sensory loss; visible enlargement of nerves	Many erythematous macules, papules, or nodules; extensive tissue destruction (e.g., nasal cartilage, bones, ears); diffuse nerve involvement with patchy sensory loss; lack of nerve enlargement
Histopathology	Infiltration of lymphocytes around center of epithelial cells; presence of Langhans' cells; few or no acid-fast bacilli observed	Predominantly "foamy" macrophages with few lymphocytes; lack of Langhans' cells; numerous acid-fast bacilli in skin lesions and internal organs
Infectivity	Low	High
Immune response		
Delayed hypersensitivity	Reactivity to lepromin	Nonreactivity to lepromin
Immunoglobulin levels	Normal	Hypergammaglobulinemia
Erythema nodosum leprosum	Absent	Usually present

A   **B**

FIGURE 40-5 A, Tuberculoid leprosy. Early tuberculoid lesions are characterized by anesthetic macules with hypopigmentation. **B,** Lepromatous leprosy with extensive infiltration, edema, and corrugation of the face. (From Peters W, Gilles HM: *Color atlas of tropical medicine and parasitology,* ed 4, London, 1995, Wolfe.)

ure 40-5). Lepromatous leprosy is the form characteristically associated with disfiguring skin lesions.

MYCOBACTERIUM AVIUM-INTRACELLULARE

M. avium-intracellulare is a common environmental isolate present in soil, water, and food. Before the acquired immunodeficiency syndrome (AIDS) epidemic, recovery of the organism in clinical specimens typically represented a transient colonization in asymptomatic patients. When disease was observed, it was generally restricted to patients with compromised pulmonary function (e.g., patients with chronic bronchitis or obstructive pulmonary disease, previous pulmonary damage as the result of infection or other disease) and was clinically identical to pulmonary tuberculosis. However, a new spectrum of disease has arisen, making infection with *M. avium-intracellulare* the most common mycobacterial disease in AIDS patients in the United States. (*M. tuberculosis* infections are more common in countries where tuberculosis is highly endemic.) In contrast with disease in other groups of patients, *M. avium-intracellulare* infection in these patients is typically disseminated, and virtually no organ is spared. The magnitude of these infections is remarkable, with the tissues of some patients literally filled with the mycobacteria (Figure 40-6) and hundreds to thousands of bacilli per milliliter of blood. Overwhelming disseminated infections with *M. avium-intracellulare* are particularly common in AIDS patients in the terminal stages of their immune disorder.

M. avium-intracellulare disease in AIDS patients is believed to develop after the ingestion of contaminated food or water. The mycobacteria then multiply in localized lymph nodes and spread systemically. The clinical manifestations of disease are not observed until the mass of replicating bacilli impair normal organ function. Person-to-person transmission is not seen. *M. avium-intracellulare* infections are summarized in Box 40-3.

OTHER SLOW-GROWING MYCOBACTERIA

Many other slow-growing mycobacteria can cause human disease, and new species continue to be reported as better diagnostic test methods are developed. The spectrum

Summary of *M. avium-intracellulare* Infections

BACTERIAL FACTORS

Diseases—asymptomatic colonization; chronic, localized pulmonary disease; disseminated disease, particularly in patients with AIDS in whom many bacteria are present in the blood and tissues.

Virulence factors—pathology caused by organ dysfunction resulting from abundance of bacteria in tissues and host response to infection.

TRANSMISSION

Acquired primarily through ingestion of contaminated food or water; inhalation of infectious aerosols believed to play a minor role, except in patients with localized pulmonary disease.

WHO IS AT RISK?

Immunocompromised patients or people with long-standing pulmonary disease.

GEOGRAPHY/SEASON

Worldwide.
No seasonal incidence.

MODES OF CONTROL

Ubiquitous presence of organism in nature makes control of exposure difficult.

High prevalence of drug resistance necessitates empirical trial of therapy.

Successful management of individual patients requires aggressive diagnostic and therapeutic efforts (e.g., surgery, antibiotic).

of diseases produced by these mycobacteria also continues to expand, in large part because diseases such as AIDS and malignancies have left a population of patients highly susceptible to organisms with relatively low virulence potentials. In some cases, these mycobacteria produce disease identical to pulmonary tuberculosis (e.g., *M. bovis*, *M. kansasii*), other species commonly cause infections localized to lymphatic tissue *(M. scrofulaceum)*, and others that grow optimally at cool temperatures primarily produce cutaneous infections *(M. ulcerans, M. marinum, M. haemophilum)*. However, disseminated disease can be observed in AIDS patients infected with these same species as well as relatively uncommon mycobacteria (e.g., *M. genavense, M. simiae*). Most of these mycobacteria have been isolated in soil and water and occasionally from infected animals (e.g., *M. bovis* causes bovine tuberculosis). Frequently, the isolation of these mycobacteria in clinical specimens simply represents a transient colonization with organisms that the patient ingested. With the exception of *M. bovis* and other mycobacteria closely related to *M. tuberculosis*, person-to-person spread of these mycobacteria does not occur.

RAPID-GROWING MYCOBACTERIA

The many mycobacteria have been subdivided into slow-growing species and rapid-growing species (growth in less than 7 days). The latter group currently contains 39 species, with 5 responsible for human infections (Table 40-1). The most common isolates are *M. fortuitum, M. chelonae,* and *M. abscessus*. It is important to distinguish between the rapid-growing and slow-growing mycobacteria because the rapid-growing species have a relatively low virulence potential, stain irregularly with traditional

FIGURE 40-6 *M. avium-intracellulare*–infected tissue from an AIDS patient photographed under low *(top)* and high *(bottom)* magnification.

BOX 40-4   Summary of Infections with Rapid-Growing Mycobacteria

BACTERIAL FACTORS

Diseases—asymptomatic colonization; iatrogenic infections (e.g., infections related to bronchoscopy, surgical wounds, peritoneal dialysis, intravenous lines); traumatic wound infections (e.g., after farming accident).

Virulence factors—pathology depends on host's response to infection.

TRANSMISSION

Environmental source of organism.

Contamination of open lesion or medical device.

WHO IS AT RISK?

People exposed to organism.

Infectious dose significantly reduced if a foreign body is present (e.g., intravascular catheter, soil).

GEOGRAPHY/SEASON

Worldwide.

No seasonal incidence for iatrogenic infections; infections caused by environmental accident are more common in warm months.

MODES OF CONTROL

Effective antibiotics and surgical debridement (removal of foreign body) and drainage necessary for management of infections.

Use of appropriate infection-control practices can control exposure to mycobacteria in hospital. Organisms are ubiquitous in environmental sources, so contamination of traumatic wounds is not uncommon.

BOX 40-5   Laboratory Diagnosis of Mycobacterial Disease

DETECTION

Skin test

Microscopy
  Carbol fuchsin acid-fast stain
  Fluorochrome acid-fast stain
Direct nucleic acid probes
Culture
  Solid agar- or egg-based media
  Broth-based media

IDENTIFICATION

Morphological properties
Biochemical reactions
Analysis of cell wall lipids
Nucleic acid probes
Nucleic acid sequencing

mycobacterial stains, and are more susceptible to "conventional" antibacterial antibiotics than to drugs used to treat mycobacterial infections.

The rapid-growing mycobacteria rarely cause disseminated infections. Rather, they are most commonly associated with disease occurring after bacteria are introduced into the deep subcutaneous tissues by trauma or iatrogenic infections (e.g., infections associated with an intravenous catheter, contaminated wound dressing, prosthetic device such as a heart valve, peritoneal dialysis, and bronchoscopy). Unfortunately, the incidence of infections with these organisms is increasing as more invasive procedures are performed in hospitalized patients

and advanced medical care lengthens the life spans of immunocompromised patients. The rapid-growing mycobacteria infections are summarized in Box 40-4.

Laboratory Diagnosis

The various laboratory tests used in the diagnosis of infections caused by rapid-growing mycobacteria are listed in Box 40-5.

Skin Test

Reactivity to an intradermal injection of mycobacterial antigens can differentiate between infected and noninfected people (Box 40-5). The only evidence of infection with mycobacteria in most patients is a lifelong positive skin test reaction and radiographic evidence of calcification of the initial active foci in the lungs or other organs. Tests with protein antigens extracted from *M. tuberculosis* have been used most commonly and are the best-standardized ones, although skin tests with other species-specific mycobacterial antigens have also been developed.

The methods of antigen preparation and skin inoculation have been changed many times since the tests were first developed. The currently recommended tuberculin antigen is the purified protein derivative (**PPD**) of the cell wall. In this test, tuberculin is inoculated into the intradermal layer of the patient's skin either by injecting a specific amount of antigen (0.1 μg [5 tuberculin units] of PPD) or by placing a drop of the antigen on the skin and then injecting the antigen using a multiprong inoculator (**tine test**). The latter test is not recommended, however, because the amount of antigen injected into the intradermal layer cannot be accurately controlled. Skin test reactivity is measured 48 hours later. Positive reactivity is defined differently depending on the population (Table 40-3). A positive PPD reaction usually develops 3 to 4 weeks after infection. Exposure to other

| TABLE 40-3 | Criteria Defining Positive PPD Reactivity in Patients Exposed to *M. tuberculosis* |

REACTIVITY TO PPD	POPULATIONS
≥5 mm of induration	Very high-risk people, including HIV-infected patients and people with abnormal chest x-ray study and recent close contact with patient with tuberculosis
≥10 mm of induration	Other high-risk people, including foreign-born people: HIV-negative IV drug users; medically underserved, low-income people; residents of long-term-care facilities; and immunocompromised patients
≥15 mm of induration	All other people

FIGURE 40-7 Acid-fast stains of *M. tuberculosis*. **A,** Stained with carbolfuchsin using the Kinyoun method. **B,** Stained with the fluorescent dyes auramine and rhodamine using the Truant fluorochrome method.

mycobacteria may cause a patient to show a reactivity with tuberculin, but this is generally less than a 10-mm induration. Patients infected with *M. tuberculosis* may not show a response to the tuberculin skin test if they are anergic (particularly true in HIV-infected patients); thus control antigens should always be used with tuberculin tests.

Reactivity to lepromin, which is prepared from inactivated *M. leprae*, is valuable for confirming the clinical diagnosis of tuberculoid leprosy. Papular induration develops 3 to 4 weeks after the intradermal injection of the antigen. This test is not useful for identifying patients with lepromatous leprosy because these patients are anergic to the antigen.

Microscopy

The microscopic detection of acid-fast bacilli in clinical specimens is the most rapid way to confirm mycobacterial disease. The clinical specimen is stained with carbolfuchsin (Ziehl-Nielsen or Kinyoun methods) or fluorescent auramine-rhodamine dyes (Truant fluorochrome method), decolorized with an acid-alcohol solution, and then counterstained. The specimens are examined with a light microscope or, if fluorescent dyes are used, a fluorescent microscope (Figure 40-7). The Truant fluorochrome method is more sensitive because the specimen can be scanned rapidly under low magnification for fluorescent areas and then the acid-fact bacilli confirmed using higher magnification.

Approximately one third to one half of all culture-positive specimens have bacilli detected by acid-fast microscopy. The sensitivity of this test is high with respiratory specimens (particularly from patients with radiographic evidence of cavitation) and specimens with many mycobacteria isolated in culture. The specificity of the test is greater than 95%.

Nucleic Acid Probes

Although microscopy provides useful information regarding the presence of mycobacterial disease, it cannot identify the particular mycobacterial species involved. For this reason, techniques have been developed to detect specific mycobacterial nucleic acid sequences present in clinical specimens. Because only a few bacteria may be present, a variety of amplification techniques are used (e.g., polymerase chain reaction, ligase chain reaction, transcription-mediated amplification). The procedures currently used are specific for *M. tuberculosis* but relatively insensitive. However, with further refinements, these procedures will most likely prove to be useful diagnostic tools.

Culture

Mycobacteria that cause pulmonary disease, particularly in patients with evidence of cavitation, are abundant in the respiratory secretions (e.g., 10^8 bacilli or more). Recovery of the organisms is virtually assured in patients from whom early morning respiratory specimens are collected for 3 consecutive days. It is more difficult, however, to isolate *M. tuberculosis* and other mycobacteria from other sites in patients with disseminated disease (e.g., genitourinary tract, tissues, cerebrospinal fluid). In such cases, additional specimens must be collected for cultures, and a large volume of fluid must be processed.

The in vitro growth of mycobacteria is complicated by the fact that most isolates grow slowly and can be obscured by the rapid-growing bacteria that normally colonize people. Thus specimens such as sputum are initially treated with a decontaminating reagent (e.g., 2% sodium hydroxide) to remove organisms that could confound results. Mycobacteria can tolerate brief alkali treatment, which kills the rapid-growing bacteria and permits the selective isolation of mycobacteria. Extended decontamination of the specimen kills mycobacteria, so the procedure is not performed when normally sterile specimens are being tested or when few mycobacteria are expected.

When specimens were inoculated onto egg-based (e.g., Löwenstein-Jensen) and agar-based (e.g., Middlebrook) media, it generally took a long time before *M. tuberculosis*, *M. avium-intracellulare*, and other important slow-growing mycobacteria could be detected. However, this time has been shortened through the use of specially formulated broth cultures that support the rapid growth of most mycobacteria. Thus the average time to grow mycobacteria has been decreased from 3 to 4 weeks to 10 to 14 days.

Preliminary Identification

Growth properties and colonial morphology can be used for the preliminary identification of the most common species of mycobacteria. This is important because only mycobacteria in the *M. tuberculosis* complex are transmitted from person to person. Thus only patients infected with these organisms must be isolated and their close contacts given prophylactic antibiotics. The preliminary identification of an isolate can also be used to guide empirical antimicrobial therapy.

Definitive Identification

The mycobacteria can be identified definitively using a variety of techniques. Biochemical tests are a standard way to identify mycobacteria (Table 40-4), but results

are not available for at least 3 weeks. Mycobacterial species can also be identified through chromatographic analysis of their characteristic cell wall lipids. However, species-specific molecular probes are the most useful means for identifying commonly isolated mycobacteria (e.g., *M. tuberculosis*, *M. avium-intracellulare* complex, *M. kansasii*). Because many organisms are present after in vitro cultivation, it is not necessary to amplify the target genomic sequence. The commercially prepared probe identification systems currently used are rapid (test time, 2 hours), sensitive, and specific. An additional way to identify mycobacterial species for which probes are not available involves the amplification of the species-specific, hypervariable regions of the 16S ribosomal RNA genes followed by sequence analysis to identify the species. This method is rapid (2 days) and is not limited by the availability of specific probes. It is likely that this method will eventually replace biochemical methods of identifying many mycobacterial species.

Treatment, Prevention, and Control

Treatment

Slow-growing mycobacteria are resistant to most antibiotics used to treat other bacterial infections. In general, patients must take multiple antibiotics for an extended period (e.g., a minimum of 6 to 9 months), or antibiotic-resistant strains will develop. In 1990 the first outbreaks of multidrug-resistant *M. tuberculosis* were observed in AIDS patients and the homeless in New York and Miami. This multidrug resistance has seriously complicated the treatment of tuberculosis in these populations. At present, the recommended treatment regimen consists of isoniazid (INH), rifampin, and pyrazinamide for 2 months, followed by an additional 4 months of therapy with INH and rifampin alone. If the patient is from a community with drug-resistant tuberculosis, ethambutol or streptomycin is added to the initial therapy. Treatment is more prolonged in HIV-infected patients.

M. avium-intracellulare is resistant to most common antimycobacterial agents. For therapy to be effective, patients must receive a combination of clarithromycin,

---

TABLE 40-4	Selected Biochemical Reactions for Five Commonly Isolated Mycobacteria						
ORGANISM	NIACIN	NITRATE REDUCTASE	HEAT-STABLE CATALASE	TWEEN-80 HYDROLYSIS	IRON UPTAKE	ARYLSULFATASE	UREASE
M. tuberculosis	+	+	−	−		−	+
M. kansasii	−	+	+	+		−	+
M. avium-intracellulare	−	−	±	−		−	−
M. fortuitum	−	+	+	V	+	+	+
M. chelonae	V	−	V	V	−	+	+

Based on data from Murray PR et al, editors: *Manual of clinical microbiology*, ed 6, Washington DC, 1995, ASM.
V, Variable.

ethambutol, and rifabutin for a lengthy period. Unfortunately, the toxic effects of this combination of agents are significant. For this reason other combinations are being evaluated.

Unlike the slow-growing mycobacteria, the rapid-growing species are resistant to most commonly used antimycobacterial agents but are susceptible to antibiotics such as amikacin, imipenem, clarithromycin, and the sulfonamides. The specific activity of these agents must be determined by in vitro tests. Because infections with these mycobacteria are generally confined to the skin or associated with prosthetic devices, surgical debridement or removal of the prosthesis is also necessary.

Treatment in patients with *M. leprae* infections is based on clinical experience because in vitro testing is not possible and in vivo testing with animal models (e.g., mouse footpad inoculations) is not practical. The organism rapidly becomes resistant to single agents, and for this reason it is recommended that primary therapy consist of dapsone, rifampin, and clofazimine or ethionamide. If this disease is diagnosed early and treatment is initiated promptly, the clinical response can be satisfactory. However, delays in treatment can have devastating consequences. Therapy is administered for a minimum of 2 years, and it can be lifelong in some patients.

Chemoprophylaxis

Prophylaxis with INH for 6 to 12 months is advocated for people who have been significantly exposed to drug-susceptible *M. tuberculosis* or shown a recent conversion in their skin test reactivity. Prophylactic regimens for people exposed to drug-resistant tuberculosis are being evaluated. In reality, however, this treatment is aimed at treating subclinical infection rather than prophylaxis. Hepatotoxicity, particularly in older persons, is associated with INH prophylaxis. Because *M. avium-intracellulare* infections are common in AIDS patients, chemoprophylaxis is recommended in patients whose CD4+ counts fall below 75 cells. A combination of clarithromycin or azithromycin with rifabutin is recommended. Chemoprophylaxis is unnecessary for patients with other mycobacterial infections.

Immunoprophylaxis

Vaccination with attenuated *M. bovis* (bacille Calmette-Guérin [**BCG**]) is commonly used in countries where tuberculosis is endemic and responsible for causing significant morbidity and mortality. This practice can lead to a significant reduction in the incidence of tuberculosis if administered to people when they are young (it is less effective in adults). Unfortunately, BCG immunization cannot be used in immunocompromised patients (e.g., HIV-infected patients). Thus it is unlikely to be useful in controlling the spread of drug-resistant tuberculosis. An additional problem with BCG immunization is that positive skin test reactivity develops in all patients; thus skin testing cannot be used to detect previous exposure to *M. tuberculosis*. For these reasons BCG immunization is not widely done in the United States or in other countries where the incidence of tuberculosis is low.

Control

It was estimated that tuberculosis would be eliminated in the United States by the end of the twentieth century. This seemed reasonable until the mid-1980s, when a dramatic change in the incidence of disease occurred (Figure 40-4). With the increased prevalence of disease in immunocompromised patients, homeless, and abusers of drugs or alcohol, the control of tuberculosis has become a medical and a social problem. A high index of clinical suspicion and rapid diagnostic tests are required for the prompt identification of appropriate therapy.

CASE STUDY AND QUESTIONS

A 35-year-old man with a history of intravenous drug use entered the local health clinic with complaints of a dry, persistent cough; fever; malaise; and anorexia. Over the preceding 4 weeks he had lost 15 pounds and experienced chills and sweats. The chest radiograph revealed patchy infiltrates throughout the lung fields. Because the patient had a nonproductive cough, sputum was induced and submitted for bacterial, fungal, and mycobacterial cultures, as well as examination for *Pneumocystis* organisms. Blood cultures, as well as serological tests for HIV infection, were performed. The patient was found to be HIV positive. The results of the tests for *Pneumocystis* species were negative, as are all cultures after 2 days of incubation; however, cultures were positive for *M. tuberculosis* after an additional 1 week of incubation.

1. Why is *M. tuberculosis* more virulent in HIV-infected patients compared with non–HIV-infected patients?
2. What is unique about the cell wall of mycobacteria and what biological effects can be attributed to the cell wall structure?
3. What are the two clinical presentations of *M. leprae* infections? How do the diagnostic tests differ for these two presentations?
4. What is the definition of a positive skin test (PPD) result for *M. tuberculosis*?
5. Why do mycobacterial infections have to be treated for 6 months or more? What is the recommended therapy for *M. tuberculosis*? *M. avium-intracellulare*? *M. fortuitum*?

Bibliography

Bloch AB et al: Nationwide survey of drug-resistant tuberculosis in the United States, *JAMA* 271:665-671, 1994.

Cantwell MF et al: Epidemiology of tuberculosis in the United States, 1985-1992, *JAMA* 272:535-539, 1994.

Centers for Disease Control and Prevention: Guidelines for preventing the transmission of *Mycobacterium tuberculosis* in health-care facilities, *MMWR* 43(RR-13):1-132, 1994.

Cohn ZA, Kaplan G: Hansen's disease, cell-mediated immunity, and recombinant lymphokines, *J Infect Dis* 163:1195-1200, 1991.

Ellner JJ: Multidrug-resistant tuberculosis, *Adv Intern Med* 40:155-198, 1995.

Hastings RC et al: Leprosy, *Clin Microbiol Rev* 1:330-348, 1988.

Huebner RE, Castro KG: The changing face of tuberculosis, *Ann Rev Med* 46:47-55, 1995.

Inderlied CB, Kemper CA, Bermudez LEM: The *Mycobacterium avium* complex, *Clin Microbiol Rev* 6:266-310, 1993.

Ingram CW et al: Disseminated infection with rapidly growing mycobacteria, *Clin Infect Dis* 16:463-471, 1993.

Kiehn TE, Armstrong D: Current topic: mycobacteriology, *Eur J Clin Microbiol Infect Dis* 13:881-1006, 1994.

Kim JH, Langston AA, Gallis HA: Miliary tuberculosis: epidemiology, clinical manifestations, diagnosis, and outcome, *Rev Infect Dis* 12:583-590, 1990.

Kubica GP, Wayne LG: *The mycobacteria: a sourcebook*, New York, 1984, Marcel Dekker.

Lipsky BA et al: Factors affecting the clinical value of microscopy for acid-fast bacilli, *Rev Infect Dis* 6:214-222, 1984.

Nolte FS, Metchock B. *Mycobacterium*. In Murray PR et al, editors: *Manual of clinical microbiology*, Washington, DC, 1995, ASM.

Raviglione MC, Snider DE, Kochi A: Global epidemiology of tuberculosis: morbidity and mortality of a worldwide epidemic, *JAMA* 273:220-226, 1995.

Salyers AA, Whitt DD: *Bacterial pathogenesis: a molecular approach*, Washington, DC, 1994, ASM.

Saubolle MA et al: *Mycobacterium haemophilum*: microbiology and expanding clinical and geographic spectra of disease in humans, *Clin Microbiol Rev* 9:435-447, 1996.

Sepkowitz KA et al: Tuberculosis in the AIDS era, *Clin Microbiol Rev* 8:180-199, 1995.

Summary of notifiable diseases, United States, 1995, *MMWR* 44:1-87, 1995.

Verdon R et al: Tuberculous meningitis in adults: review of 48 cases, *Clin Infect Dis* 22:982-988, 1996.

Woods GL, Washington JA II: Mycobacteria other than *Mycobacterium tuberculosis*: review of microbiologic and clinical aspects, *Rev Infect Dis* 9:275-294, 1987.

41

Treponema, Borrelia, and Leptospira

The bacteria in the order Spirochaetales have been grouped together on the basis of their common morphological properties. These spirochetes are thin, helical (0.1 to 0.5 × 5 to 20 μm), gram-negative bacteria (Figures 41-1 and 41-2). The order Spirochaetales is subdivided into two families and seven genera, of which three *(Treponema, Borrelia,* and *Leptospira)* are responsible for human disease (Table 41-1).

TREPONEMA

The two treponemal species that cause human disease are *T. pallidum* (with three subspecies) and *T. carateum.* All are morphologically identical, produce the same serological response in humans (e.g., positive reactivity in the Venereal Disease Research Laboratory [VDRL], fluorescent treponemal antibody absorption [FTA-ABS], and microhemagglutination test for *T. pallidum* [MHA-TP] tests), and are susceptible to penicillin. The organisms are distinguished by their epidemiological characteristics and clinical manifestations of disease. *T. pallidum* subspecies *pallidum* (referred to as *T. pallidum* in this chapter) is the etiological agent of the venereal disease **syphilis,** *T. pallidum* subspecies *endemicum* causes endemic syphilis, or **bejel,** T. pallidum subspecies *pertenue* causes **yaws,** and *T. carateum* causes **pinta.** Bejel, yaws, and pinta are nonvenereal diseases. Syphilis is discussed initially; the other treponemal diseases are discussed at the end of the section.

Physiology and Structure

Syphilis is a sexually transmitted disease that has plagued humans for centuries. The spirochete that causes this disease is a strict human pathogen. Natural syphilis is not found in any other species, and experimental syphilis has been established only in rabbits. *T. pallidum* is a thin, coiled spirochete (0.1 × 5 to 15 μm) that cannot be grown in cell-free cultures. Limited growth of the organisms has been achieved in cultured rabbit epithelial cells, but replication is slow (doubling time is 30 hours) and can be maintained only for a few generations. The spirochetes were once considered strict anaerobes; however, it is now known that they can use glucose oxidatively.

The spirochetes are too thin to be seen with light microscopy in specimens stained with Gram or Giemsa stain. Motile forms can be visualized by darkfield illumination or by staining with specific antitreponemal antibodies labeled with fluorescent dyes.

Pathogenesis and Immunity

The inability to grow *T. pallidum* to high concentrations in vitro has limited detection of specific virulence factors in this organism. However, several investigators have now cloned *T. pallidum* genes in *Escherichia coli* and isolated the protein products. Several gene products have been associated specifically with virulent strains, although their role in pathogenesis remains to be delineated. The outer membrane proteins are associated with adherence to the surface of host cells, and virulent spirochetes produce hyaluronidase, which may facilitate perivascular infiltration. Virulent spirochetes are also coated with host cell fibronectin, which can protect against phagocytosis.

The tissue destruction and lesions observed in syphilis are primarily the consequence of the patient's immune response to infection. The clinical course of syphilis evolves through three phases. The initial, or primary, phase is characterized by one or more skin lesions **(chancres)** at the site where the spirochete penetrated. Although spirochetes are disseminated in the bloodstream soon after infection, the chancre represents the primary site of initial replication. Histological examination of the lesion reveals endarteritis and periarteritis (characteristic of syphilitic lesions at all stages) and infiltration of the ulcer with polymorphonuclear leukocytes and macrophages. Spirochetes are ingested by the phagocytic cells, but the organisms frequently survive. In the secondary phase the clinical signs of disseminated disease appear, with prominent skin lesions dispersed over the entire body surface (Figure 41-3). Spontaneous remission may occur after the primary or secondary stages, or the patient may develop late manifestations of disease in which virtually all tissues may be involved. Each phase repre-

TABLE 41-1 **Order Spirochaetales**

SPIROCHAETALES	HUMAN DISEASE	ETIOLOGICAL AGENT
FAMILY SPIROCHAETACEAE		
Genus *Cristispira*	None	—
Genus *Serpulina*	None	—
Genus *Spirochaeta*	None	—
Genus *Treponema*	Syphilis	*T. pallidum* subspecies *pallidum*
	Bejel	*T. pallidum* subspecies *endemicum*
	Yaws	*T. pallidum* subspecies *pertenue*
	Pinta	*T. carateum*
Genus *Borrelia*	Epidemic relapsing fever	*B. recurrentis*
	Endemic relapsing fever	Many *Borrelia* species
	Lyme borreliosis	*B. burgdorferi, B. garinii, B. afzelii*
FAMILY LEPTOSPIRACEAE		
Genus *Leptonema*	None	—
Genus *Leptospira*	Leptospirosis	*L. interrogans*

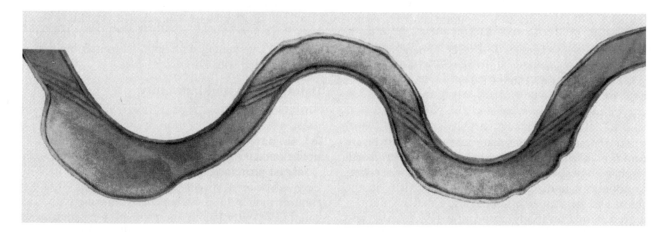

FIGURE 41-1 Helical arrangement of *Treponema pallidum*. The name *spirochete* is derived from the Greek words for "coiled hair." This is an appropriate term for bacteria that are longer than most others associated with human disease and that are frequently too thin to be seen by light microscopy. Note the periplasmic flagella that run along the length of the spirochete. (From Binford CH, Connor DH: *Pathology of tropical and extraordinary diseases*, vol 1, 1976, Washington, DC, 1976, Armed Forces Institute of Pathology.)

FIGURE 41-2 Electron micrograph and drawing of cross section through *Borrelia burgdorferi,* the agent that causes Lyme borreliosis. The protoplasmic core of the bacterium is enclosed in a cytoplasmic membrane and conventional cell wall. This in turn is surrounded by an outer envelope, or sheath. Between the protoplasmic core and outer sheath are periplasmic flagella (also called *axial fibrils*), which are anchored at either end of the bacterium and wrap around the protoplasmic core. From 2 to more than 100 flagella are present, with the number characteristic of individual species. These flagella are essential for motility. (From Steere AC et al: *N Engl J Med* 308:733-740, 1983.)

FIGURE 41-3 Disseminated rash in secondary syphilis. (From Habif TP: *Clinical dermatology: a color guide to diagnosis and therapy,* St Louis, 1996, Mosby.)

BOX 41-1 **Summary of *Treponema* Infections**

BACTERIAL FACTORS

Diseases—venereal syphilis *(T. pallidum* subspecies *pallidum)*, endemic syphilis or bejel *(T. pallidum* subspecies *endemicum)*, yaws *(T. pallidum* subspecies pertenue), pinta *(T. carateum)*.

Virulence factors—outer membrane proteins promote adherence to host cells; hyaluronidase may facilitate perivascular infiltration; coating of fibronectin protects against phagocytosis.

Tissue destruction primarily results from host's immune response to infection.

TRANSMISSION

Humans are the only host.

Venereal syphilis transmitted by sexual contact or congenitally.

Other *Treponema* infections transmitted by contact of mucous membranes with infectious lesions; congenital infections rare.

WHO IS AT RISK?

Venereal syphilis: sexually active adolescents and adults; children born of mothers with active disease.

Other *Treponema* infections: children or adults in contact with infectious lesions.

GEOGRAPHY/SEASON

Venereal syphilis is worldwide.

Endemic syphilis (bejel) occurs in desert and temperate regions of North Africa, Middle East, and Northern Australia.

Yaws occurs in tropical or desert regions of Africa, South America, and Indonesia.

Pinta occurs in tropical areas of Central and South America.

No seasonal incidence.

MODES OF CONTROL

Penicillin is drug of choice; tetracycline, erythromycin, chloramphenicol are administered if patient is allergic to penicillin.

Safe sex practices should be emphasized, and treatment of sexual partners of infected patients.

Endemic syphilis, yaws, and pinta can be eliminated through organized public health measures (treatment, education); however, these efforts have been inconsistently applied.

sents localized multiplication of the spirochete and tissue destruction. Although replication is slow, numerous organisms are present in the initial chancre as well as in the secondary lesions after the spirochetes are disseminated in the bloodstream.

Epidemiology

Syphilis is found worldwide and is the third most common sexually transmitted bacterial disease in the United States (after *Neisseria gonorrhoeae* and *Chlamydia* infections) (Box 41-1). Although the incidence of disease has steadily decreased with the advent of penicillin therapy in the early 1940s, a significant number of infections are still documented each year (Figure 41-4). In 1995, almost 70,000 cases of syphilis were reported in the United States. However, numerous infections go unreported, which contributes to a gross underestimation of the true incidence of this disease.

Because natural syphilis is exclusive to humans and has no other known natural hosts, the most common route of spread is by direct sexual contact. *T. pallidum* is extremely labile, unable to survive exposure to drying or disinfectants. Thus syphilis cannot be spread through contact with inanimate objects such as toilet seats. The disease can also be acquired congenitally or by transfusion with contaminated blood. Syphilis is not highly contagious; the risk of a person contracting the disease after a single sexual contact is estimated to be 30%. However,

contagiousness is influenced by the stage of disease in the infectious person. As mentioned previously, the spirochetes cannot survive on dry skin surfaces. Thus *T. pallidum* is transferred primarily during the early stages of disease when there are many organisms present in moist cutaneous or mucosal lesions. Congenital transmission to the fetus can take place soon after the mother is infected because bacteremia characteristically occurs early in the disease. A woman with untreated disease can have spontaneous bacteremia for as long as 8 years; the spirochetes are transmitted to fetal tissues if the woman becomes pregnant during this period. After 8 years, the disease can remain active, but bacteremia is not believed to occur.

With the advent of effective antimicrobial therapy, the incidence of late (tertiary) syphilis has markedly decreased. Although antibiotic therapy has led to a decrease in the length of infectivity in infected people, the incidence of primary and secondary syphilis has remained high because of sexual practices, particularly prostitution to support drug habits. The incidence of congenital syphilis corresponds to the pattern of syphilis in women of childbearing age.

Clinical Syndromes

The natural history of untreated acquired syphilis is illustrated in Figure 41-5.

Primary Syphilis

As noted earlier, the initial syphilitic chancre develops at the site where the spirochete is inoculated. Multiple chancres can be observed in immunocompromised patients such as those infected with the human immunodeficiency virus. The lesion starts as a papule but then erodes to become a painless ulcer with raised borders. In most patients a painless regional lymphadenopathy develops 1 to 2 weeks after the appearance of the chancre, which represents a local focus for the proliferation of spirochetes. Abundant spirochetes are present in the chancre and can be disseminated throughout the patient by way of the lymphatic system and bloodstream. The fact that this ulcer heals spontaneously within 2 months gives the patient a false sense of relief.

Secondary Syphilis

The clinical evidence of disseminated disease marks the second stage of syphilis. In this stage, patients typically experience a flulike syndrome with sore throat, headache, fever, myalgias, anorexia, lymphadenopathy, and a generalized mucocutaneous rash. The flulike syndrome and lymphadenopathy generally appear first and then are followed a few days later by the disseminated skin lesions. The rash can be variable (macular, papular, pustular), can cover the entire skin surface (including the palms and soles), and may resolve slowly over a period of weeks to months. As with the primary chancre, the rash in secondary syphilis is highly infectious. Gradually the rash and symptoms resolve spontaneously, and the patient enters the latent or clinically inactive stage of disease.

Late Syphilis

A small proportion of patients can progress to the tertiary stage of syphilis. The diffuse, chronic inflammation characteristic of late syphilis can cause a devastating destruction of virtually any organ or tissue (e.g., arteritis, dementia, blindness). Granulomatous lesions (**gummas**) may be found in bone, skin, and other tissues. The nomenclature of late syphilis reflects the organs of primary involvement (e.g., neurosyphilis, cardiovascular

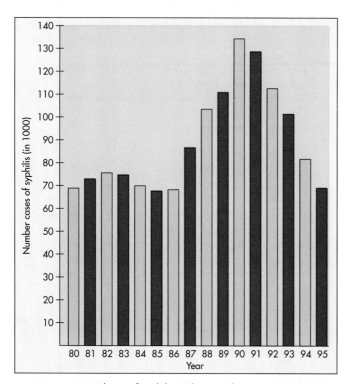

FIGURE 41-4 Incidence of syphilis in the United States, 1980-1995. (From *MMWR* 44:74-79, 1996.)

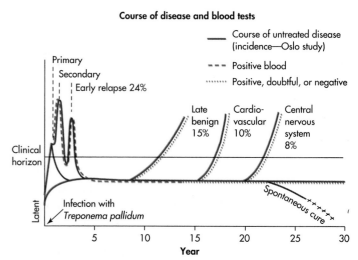

FIGURE 41-5. The natural history of untreated acquired syphilis was carefully chronicled at the University of Oslo. (Modified from Morgan H:*South Med J* 26:18-22, 1933; incidence data from Clark E, Danbolt N: *J Chron Dis* 2:311-344, 1955.)

syphilis). An increased incidence of neurosyphilis despite adequate therapy for early syphilis has been documented in patients with acquired immunodeficiency syndrome (AIDS).

Congenital Syphilis

In utero infections can lead to serious fetal disease, resulting in the death of the fetus, multiorgan malformations, or latent infections. Most infected infants are born without clinical evidence of the disease, but then rhinitis develops and is followed by a widespread desquamating maculopapular rash. Late bony destruction and cardiovascular syphilis are common in untreated infants who survive the initial course of disease.

Laboratory Diagnosis

Microscopy

The diagnosis of primary, secondary, or congenital syphilis can be made rapidly by darkfield examination of the exudate from skin lesions (Table 41-2 and Figure 41-6). However, the test is reliable only when clinical material with actively motile spirochetes is examined immediately by an experienced microscopist. The spirochetes do not survive transport to the laboratory,

and tissue debris can be mistaken for spirochetes. Material collected from oral lesions should not be examined because nonpathogenic oral spirochetes can contaminate the specimen. *T. pallidum* can be identified specifically using fluorescein-labeled antitreponemal antibodies. Histological staining of tissue lesions may be beneficial in showing the organisms; silver stains are used most commonly.

Culture

Efforts to culture *T. pallidum* in vitro should not be attempted because the organism does not grow in artificial cultures.

Serology

Syphilis is diagnosed in most patients on the basis of serological tests. The two general types of tests used are biologically nonspecific (nontreponemal) tests and the specific treponemal tests (Table 41-3).

FIGURE 41-6 *T. pallidum* in a darkfield microscopy study. (From Peters W, Gilles HM: *A color atlas of tropical medicine and parasitology,* ed 4, London, 1995, Wolfe.)

TABLE 41-2	**Diagnostic Tests for Syphilis**
DIAGNOSTIC TEST	**METHOD OR EXAMINATION**
Microscopy	Darkfield
	Direct fluorescent-antibody staining
Culture	Not available
Serology	Nontreponemal tests
	VDRL
	RPR
	Treponemal tests
	FTA-ABS
	MHA-TP

TABLE 41-3	**Sensitivity and Specificity of Serological Tests for Syphilis**				
	SENSITIVITY (%)				
TEST	**PRIMARY**	**SECONDARY**	**LATENT**	**LATE**	**SPECIFICITY (%)**
NONTREPONEMAL					
VDRL	78 (74-87)	100	95 (88-100)	71 (37-94)	98 (96-99)
RPR	86 (77-100)	100	98 (95-100)	73	98 (93-99)
TREPONEMAL					
FTA-ABS	84 (70-100)	100	100	96	97 (94-100)
MHA-TP	76 (69-90)	100	97 (97-100)	94	99 (98-100)

Based on data from Larsen S, Steiner B, Rudolph A: *Clin Microbiol Rev* 8:1-21, 1995.
RPR, Rapid plasma reagin.

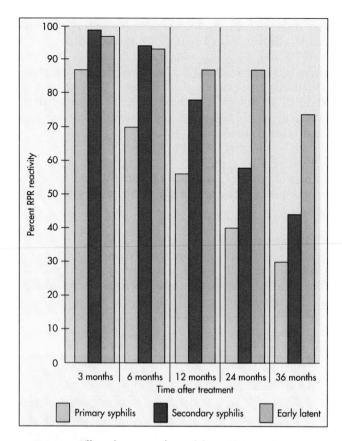

FIGURE 41-7 Effect of treatment for syphilis on RPR reactivity. (Data from Romanowski B et al: *Ann Intern Med* 114:1005-1009, 1991.)

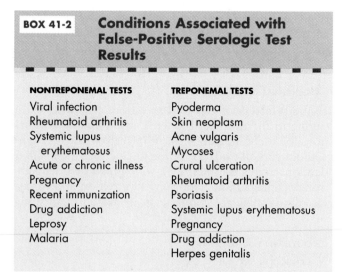

BOX 41-2 Conditions Associated with False-Positive Serologic Test Results

NONTREPONEMAL TESTS	TREPONEMAL TESTS
Viral infection	Pyoderma
Rheumatoid arthritis	Skin neoplasm
Systemic lupus erythematosus	Acne vulgaris
	Mycoses
Acute or chronic illness	Crural ulceration
Pregnancy	Rheumatoid arthritis
Recent immunization	Psoriasis
Drug addiction	Systemic lupus erythematosus
Leprosy	Pregnancy
Malaria	Drug addiction
	Herpes genitalis

Nontreponemal tests measure IgG and IgM antibodies (also called *reagin antibodies*) developed against lipids released from damaged cells during the early stage of disease and also present on the cell surface of treponemes. The antigen used for the nontreponemal tests is cardiolipin, which is derived from beef heart. The two tests used most commonly are the **VDRL** test and the rapid plasma reagin (**RPR**) test. Both tests measure the flocculation of cardiolipin antigen by the patient's serum. Both tests can be done rapidly, although complement in serum must be inactivated for 30 minutes before the VDRL test can be performed. Only the VDRL test should be used to test cerebrospinal fluid from patients with suspected neurosyphilis.

Treponemal tests are specific antibody tests used to confirm positive reactions with the VDRL or RPR tests. The treponemal tests can also be positive before the nontreponemal tests become positive in early syphilis, or they can remain positive when the nonspecific tests revert to negative in some patients who have late syphilis. The tests most commonly used are the **FTA-ABS** test and **MHA-TP**. The MHA-TP test is technically easier to perform and the results easier to interpret than the FTA-ABS test. The Western blot assay with whole-cell *T. pallidum* as the antigen recently has been used successfully as a confirmatory treponeme-specific test.

Because positive reactions with the nontreponemal tests develop late during the first phase of disease, the serological findings are negative in many patients who initially have chancres. However, serological results are positive within 3 months in all patients and remain positive in untreated patients with secondary syphilis. The antibody titers slowly decrease in patients with untreated syphilis, and serological results are negative in approximately 25% to 30% of patients with late syphilis. Although the results of treponemal tests generally remain positive for the life of the person who has syphilis, a negative test is unreliable in AIDS patients.

Successful treatment of primary or secondary syphilis, and to a lesser extent, late syphilis, leads to reduced titers measured in the VDRL and RPR tests (Figure 41-7). Thus these tests can be used to monitor the effectiveness of therapy, although seroreversion is slowed in patients in an advanced stage of disease, those with high initial titers, and those who have had syphilis previously. The treponemal tests are influenced less by therapy than the VDRL and RPR tests are, with seroconversion observed in less than 25% of patients successfully treated during the primary stage of the disease.

The specificity of the nontreponemal tests is at least 98%. However, transient false-positive reactions are seen in patients with acute febrile diseases, after immunizations, and in pregnant women. Long-term false-positive reactions occur most often in patients with chronic autoimmune diseases or infections that involve the liver or that cause extensive tissue destruction. The specificity of the treponemal tests is 97% to 99%, with most false-positive reactions observed in patients with elevated gamma-globulin levels and autoimmune diseases (Box 41-2). Many of the false-positive reactions can be resolved using the Western blot assay, which may become the preferred confirmatory test.

Positive serological tests in infants of infected mothers can represent a passive transfer of antibodies or a specific immunological response to infection. These two possibilities are distinguished by measuring the antibody titers in the sera of the infant over a 6-month period. The antibody titers in noninfected infants decrease to undetectable levels within 3 months of birth but remain elevated in infants who have congenital syphilis.

Treatment, Prevention, and Control

Penicillin is the drug of choice for treating infections with *T. pallidum.* Long-acting benzathine penicillin is used for the early stages of syphilis, and penicillin G is recommended for congenital and late syphilis. Tetracycline or doxycycline can be used as alternative antibiotics for patients allergic to penicillin. Only penicillin can be used for the treatment of patients with neurosyphilis, so penicillin-allergic patients must undergo desensitization. This is also true for pregnant women, who should not be treated with the tetracyclines.

Because protective vaccines are not available, syphilis can only be controlled through the practice of safe sex techniques and the adequate contact and treatment of the sex partners of patients who have documented infections. In recent years the control of syphilis and other venereal diseases has been complicated by an increase in prostitution in drug abusers.

OTHER TREPONEMES

Three other nonvenereal treponemal diseases are important: bejel, yaws, and pinta. These diseases are primarily observed in impoverished children. *T. pallidum* subspecies *endemicum* is responsible for bejel, also called *endemic syphilis.* Disease is spread person to person by the use of contaminated eating utensils. The initial oral lesions are rarely observed, but secondary lesions include oral papules and mucosal patches. Gummas of the skin, bones, and nasopharynx are late manifestations. The disease is present in Africa, Asia, and Australia.

T. pertenue is the etiological agent of **yaws,** a granulomatous disease in which patients have skin lesions early in the disease (Figure 41-8) and then late destructive lesions of the skin, lymph nodes, and bones. The disease is present in primitive, tropical areas of South America, Central Africa, and Southeast Asia and is spread by direct contact with infected skin lesions.

T. carateum is responsible for causing **pinta,** a disease that primarily affects the skin. Small pruritic papules develop on the skin surface after a 1- to 3-week incubation period. These lesions enlarge and persist for months to years before resolving. Disseminated, recurrent, hypopigmented lesions can develop over years, resulting in scarring and disfigurement. Pinta is present in Central and South America and is also spread by direct contact with infected lesions.

Bejel, yaws, and pinta are diagnosed by their typical clinical presentation in an endemic area. The diagnoses of yaws and pinta are confirmed by the detection of spirochetes in skin lesions by darkfield microscopy, but this test cannot be used to detect spirochetes in patients with the oral lesions of bejel. The results of serological

FIGURE 41-8 Yaws. The elevated papillomatous nodules characteristic of early yaws are widely distributed and painless. They contain numerous spirochetes, which are easily seen on darkfield microscopy studies. (From Peters W, Gilles HM: *A color atlas of tropical medicine and parasitology,* ed 4, London, 1995, Wolfe.)

tests for syphilis are also positive but may develop only late in the disease.

Penicillin, tetracycline, and chloramphenicol have been used to treat these diseases. The disease is controlled through the treatment of infected people and the elimination of person-to-person spread.

BORRELIA

Members of the genus *Borrelia* cause two important human diseases: relapsing fever and Lyme disease. **Relapsing fever** is a febrile illness characterized by recurrent episodes of fever and septicemia separated by afebrile periods. Two forms of the disease are recognized. *B. recurrentis* is the etiological agent of **epidemic** or **louse-borne relapsing fever** and is spread person to person by the human body louse *(Pediculus humanus).* **Endemic relapsing fever** is caused by as many as 15 species of borreliae and is spread by infected soft ticks of the genus *Ornithodoros.*

The history of Lyme disease begins in 1977, when an unusual cluster of children with arthritis was noted in Lyme, Connecticut. Five years later the spirochete responsible for this disease was discovered by Burgdorfer. **Lyme disease** is a tick-borne disease with protean manifestations, including dermatological, rheumatological, neurological, and cardiac abnormalities. The best clinical marker for the disease is the initial skin lesion, **erythema migrans,** which occurs in 60% to 70% of infected adults and less frequently in children. Until recently, all cases of Lyme disease (or Lyme borreliosis) were believed to be caused by one organism, *B. burgdorferi.* However, more recent studies of the DNA relatedness among isolates have identified at least three species: *B. burgdorferi,* found in the United States and Europe; *B. garinii,* found in Europe and Japan; and *B. afzelii,* also found in Europe

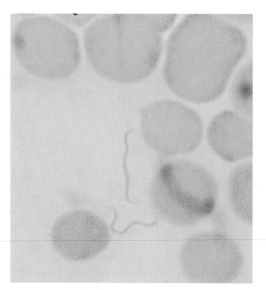

FIGURE 41-9 *Borrelia* organisms present in the blood of a patient with endemic relapsing fever. (Giemsa stain.)

Infection	Reservoir	Vector
Relapsing fever Epidemic (louse-borne)	Humans	Body louse
Relapsing fever Endemic (tick-borne)	Rodents, soft-shelled ticks	Soft-shelled tick
Lyme disease	Rodents, deer, domestic pets, hard-shelled ticks	Hard-shelled tick

FIGURE 41-10 Epidemiology of *Borrelia* infections.

BOX 41-3   Summary of *Borrelia* Infections

BACTERIAL FACTORS

Epidemic relapsing fever—etiological agent is *B. recurrentis;* vector is human body louse *(Pediculus humanus)* human reservoir.

Endemic relapsing fever—etiological agent is at least 15 species of *Borrelia;* vector is soft-shell tick *(Ornithodoros);* reservoirs are rodents, small mammals, and ticks.

For Lyme disease, *B. burgdorferi* causes disease in the United States; *B. burgdorferi, B. garinii, B. afzelii,* and other species cause disease in Europe and Asia. Vectors are hard-shell ticks: *Ixodes scapularis (I. dammini)* in Eastern and Midwestern United States, *I. pacificus* in the western United States, *I. ricinus* in Europe, and *I. persulcatus* in Eastern Europe and Asia. White-footed mouse is most important reservoir in United States.

Periodic febrile and afebrile periods result from antigenic variation in *Borrelia* that cause relapsing fever.

TRANSMISSION

Epidemic relapsing fever: transmitted person to person by the human body louse.

Endemic relapsing fever: transmitted by soft ticks from rodents to humans.

Lyme disease: transmitted by hard ticks from mice to humans.

WHO IS AT RISK?

Relapsing fever: people exposed to lice (epidemic disease) in crowded or unsanitary conditions; people exposed to ticks (endemic disease) in rural areas.

Lyme disease: people exposed to ticks.

GEOGRAPHY/SEASON

Epidemic relapsing fever is endemic in Central and East Africa and South America (Bolivia, Peru).

Endemic relapsing fever has worldwide distribution and is in western states of United States.

Lyme disease has worldwide distribution.

Seasonal incidence corresponds to feeding patterns of vectors; most cases of Lyme disease in United States occur in late spring and early summer (feeding pattern of nymphs).

MODES OF CONTROL

For relapsing fever, treatment is with tetracycline or erythromycin.

For Lyme disease, treatment is with amoxicillin, tetracycline, or ceftriaxone.

Exposure to insect vector can be decreased through use of insecticides and insect repellents applied to clothing and wearing of protective clothing that reduces exposure of skin to insects; recombinant ospC vaccine is being developed for Lyme disease.

and Japan. It is likely that more species will be identified as additional isolates are characterized. For the purposes of this chapter, until the taxonomy is defined better, all strains are referred to as *B. burgdorferi.*

Physiology and Structure

Members of the genus *Borrelia* are weakly staining, gram-negative bacilli that resemble other spirochetes. They tend to be larger than other spirochetes (0.2 to 0.5 × 3 to 30 μm), stain well with aniline dyes (e.g., Giemsa or Wright stain), and can be easily seen in smears of peripheral blood from patients with relapsing fever (Figure 41-9) but not those with Lyme disease. From 7 to 20 periplasmic flagella (depending on the species) are present between the periplasmic cylinder and the outer envelope and are responsible for the organism's twisting motility. Borreliae are microaerophilic and have complex nutritional requirements, making it difficult to recover them in culture. The species that have been successfully cultured have generation times of 18 hours or longer. Because culture is generally unsuccessful, diagnosis of diseases caused by borreliae is by microscopy (relapsing fever) or serology (Lyme disease).

Pathogenesis and Immunity

After a person is exposed to infected arthropods, borreliae spread in the bloodstream to multiple organs. Members of the genus do not produce recognized toxins and are rapidly removed when a specific antibody response is mounted. The periodic febrile and afebrile cycles of relapsing fever stem from the ability of the borreliae to undergo antigenic variation. When specific IgM antibodies are formed, agglutination with complement-mediated lysis occurs, and the borreliae are rapidly cleared from the bloodstream. However, organisms residing in internal tissues can alter their serotype-specific outer envelope proteins through gene rearrangement and emerge as antigenically novel organisms. The clinical manifestations of relapsing fever are in part a response to the release of endotoxin by the organism.

B. burgdorferi are present in low numbers in the skin when erythema migrans develops. This has been shown by culture of the organism from skin lesions or detection of bacterial nucleic acids by polymerase chain reaction (PCR) amplification. Spirochetes are infrequently isolated from clinical material late in the disease. It is not known whether the viable organisms cause these late manifestations of disease or whether they represent immunological cross-reactivity to *Borrelia* antigens. Although the immune response to the organism is depressed at the time that skin lesions initially develop, antibodies develop over months to years and are responsible for producing the complement-mediated clearance of the borreliae.

Epidemiology

The etiological agent of louse-borne epidemic relapsing fever is *B. recurrentis,* the vector is the human **body louse,** and humans are the only reservoir (Box 41-3 and Figure 41-10). Lice become infected after feeding on an infected person. The organisms are ingested, pass through the wall of the gut, and multiply in hemolymph. Disseminated disease is not believed to occur in lice, so human infection occurs when the lice are crushed during feeding. Infected lice do not survive for more than a few months, so maintenance of the disease requires crowded, unsanitary conditions (e.g., wars, natural disasters) that permit frequent human contact with infected lice. Louse-borne relapsing fever is endemic in tropical and temperate regions of the world, particularly Central and Eastern Africa and South America.

Several features distinguish endemic relapsing fever from epidemic disease. Tick-borne endemic relapsing fever is a zoonotic disease, with rodents, small mammals, and **soft ticks** (*Ornithodoros* species) the main reservoirs, and many species of *Borrelia* responsible for the disease. Unlike the louse-borne infections, the borreliae that cause endemic disease produce a disseminated infection in ticks. However, the arthropods can survive and maintain an endemic reservoir of infection by transovarian transmission. Furthermore, ticks can survive for months to years between feedings. A history of a tick bite may also not be elicited because the soft ticks are primarily nocturnal feeders and remain attached for only a few minutes. The ticks contaminate the bite wound with borreliae present in saliva or feces. Tick-borne disease is found worldwide, corresponding to the distribution of the *Ornithodoros* tick. In the United States, disease is primarily found in the Western states.

Despite the relatively recent recognition of Lyme disease in the United States, retrospective studies have shown that the disease was present for many years in this and other countries. Lyme disease has now been described on 6 continents, in at least 20 countries, and in 46 states of the United States. The incidence of disease has risen dramatically since 1982, when 497 cases were reported, to 1995, when more than 11,600 cases were reported (Figure 41-11). Lyme disease is the leading vector-borne disease in the United States. The three principal foci of infection in the United States are the Northeast (Massachusetts to Maryland), the upper Midwest (Minnesota and Wisconsin), and the Pacific West (California and Oregon). Hard ticks are the major vectors of Lyme disease: *Ixodes scapularis* (*Ixodes dammini*) in the Northeast and Midwest and *I. pacificus* on the West Coast. *I. ricinus* is the major tick vector in Europe and *I. persulcatus* in Eastern Europe and Asia. The major reservoir hosts in the United States are the white-footed mouse and white-tailed deer. The white-footed mouse is the primary host of larval and nymph forms of *Ixodes* species, and the adult *Ixodes* species infest the white-tailed deer. Because the nymph stage causes more than 90% of the cases of documented disease, the mouse host is more relevant for human disease.

Ixodes larvae become infected when they feed on the mouse reservoir. The larva molts to a nymph in late spring and takes a second blood meal; in this case the hu-

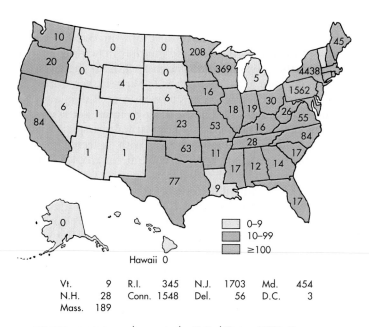

Vt. 9   R.I. 345   N.J. 1703   Md. 454
N.H. 28   Conn. 1548   Del. 56   D.C. 3
Mass. 189

FIGURE 41-11 Lyme disease in the United States, 1995. (From *MMWR* 45:481, 1996.)

man can be the accidental host. Although the borreliae are transmitted in the tick's saliva during a prolonged period of feeding (48 hours or more), most patients do not remember having had a specific tick bite. The nymphs mature into adults in the late summer and take a third feeding. Although the white-tailed deer is the natural host, humans can also be infected at this stage.

Clinical Syndromes

Relapsing Fever

The clinical presentations of epidemic louse-borne and endemic tick-borne relapsing fever are essentially the same, although a small pruritic eschar may develop at the site of the tick bite (Figure 41-12). After a 1-week incubation period, the disease is heralded by the abrupt onset of shaking chills, fever, muscle aches, and headache. Splenomegaly and hepatomegaly are common. These symptoms correspond to the bacteremic phase of the disease and resolve after 3 to 7 days, when the borreliae are cleared from the blood. Bacteremia and fever return after a 1-week afebrile period. The clinical symptoms are generally milder and last a shorter time during this and subsequent febrile episodes. A single relapse is characteristic of epidemic louse-borne disease, and multiple relapses are common in endemic tick-borne disease. The clinical course and outcome of epidemic relapsing fever tend to be more severe than they are in those with endemic disease, but this may be related to the patients' underlying poor state of health. Mortality with endemic disease is less than 5% but can be 4% to 40% in epidemic disease.

Lyme Disease

Clinical diagnosis of Lyme disease is complicated by the varied presentations and the lack of reliable diagnostic tests. The clinical and laboratory definitions of Lyme dis-

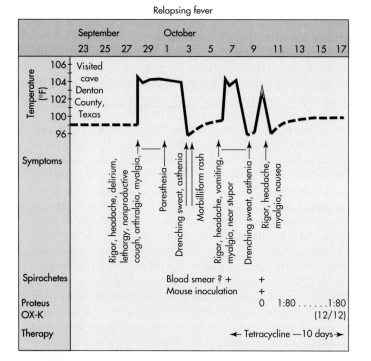

FIGURE 41-12 The clinical evolution of tick-borne relapsing fever in a 14-year-old boy. The initial febrile episode is typically the most severe. Subsequent episodes tend to be shorter and less intense. Although nonspecific reactivity with *Proteus* OX-K antigens is frequently observed, the specific diagnosis is made on the basis of the observation of borreliae in peripheral blood smears. These are positive for organisms only during the febrile periods. (Modified from Southern P, Sanford J: *Medicine* 48:129-149, 1969.)

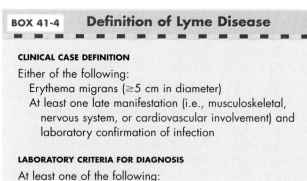

BOX 41-4   **Definition of Lyme Disease**

CLINICAL CASE DEFINITION

Either of the following:
Erythema migrans (≥5 cm in diameter)
At least one late manifestation (i.e., musculoskeletal, nervous system, or cardiovascular involvement) and laboratory confirmation of infection

LABORATORY CRITERIA FOR DIAGNOSIS

At least one of the following:
Isolation of *B. burgdorferi*
Demonstration of diagnostic levels of IgM or IgG antibodies to the spirochetes
Significant increase in antibody titer between acute and convalescent serum samples

ease by the Centers for Disease Control and Prevention are summarized in Box 41-4.

After an incubation period of 3 to 30 days, one or more skin lesions typically develop at the site of the tick bite. The lesion (erythema migrans) begins as a small macule or papule and then enlarges over the next few weeks, ultimately covering an area ranging from 5 cm to more than 50 cm in diameter (Figure 41-13). The lesion typically has a red, flat border and central clearing as it develops; however, erythema, vesicle formation, and central necrosis can also be seen. The lesion fades and disappears within weeks, although new, transient lesions may subsequently appear. Other early signs and symptoms of Lyme disease include malaise, severe fatigue, headache, fever, chills, musculoskeletal pains, myalgias, and lymphadenopathy. These last for an average of 4 weeks.

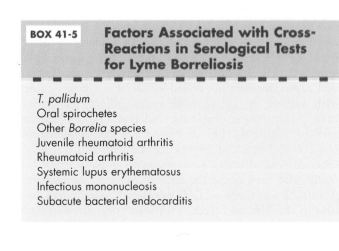

| BOX 41-5 | **Factors Associated with Cross-Reactions in Serological Tests for Lyme Borreliosis** |

T. pallidum
Oral spirochetes
Other *Borrelia* species
Juvenile rheumatoid arthritis
Rheumatoid arthritis
Systemic lupus erythematosus
Infectious mononucleosis
Subacute bacterial endocarditis

FIGURE 41-13 Erythema migrans rash on the arm of a patient with Lyme borreliosis.

Late manifestations develop in almost 80% of patients with untreated Lyme disease. These can develop from within a week of the onset of disease to more than 2 years later. There are two phases of the late stage. The first involves neurological symptoms (meningitis, encephalitis, peripheral nerve neuropathy) and cardiac dysfunction (heart block, myopericarditis, congestive heart failure). These symptoms are seen in 10% to 15% of patients and can last for days to months. The second phase is characterized by arthralgias and arthritis. These complications can persist for months to years, during which spirochetes are only rarely visualized in the involved tissue or isolated in culture.

Laboratory Diagnosis

Microscopy

Because of their relatively large size, borreliae that cause relapsing fever can be seen during the febrile period on Giemsa- or Wright-stained preparation of blood. This is the most sensitive method for diagnosing relapsing fever, with smears positive for organisms in more than 70% of patients. The sensitivity of the test can be improved by inoculating a mouse with blood from infected patients and then after 1 to 10 days examining the mouse's blood for the presence of borreliae. The microscopic examination of blood or tissues from patients with Lyme disease is not recommended because *B. burgdorferi* is rarely seen in clinical specimens.

Culture

Some borreliae, including *B. recurrentis* and *B. hermsii* (a common cause of endemic relapsing fever in the United States), can be cultured in vitro on specialized media. However, the cultures are rarely performed in most clinical laboratories because the media are not readily available and the organisms grow slowly on them. There has been limited success with the culture of *B. burgdorferi,* although isolation of the organism has been improved through the use of specialized media. However, the sensitivity of culture is low for all specimens except the initial skin lesion, which is pathognomonic, thus making culture rarely necessary.

Serology

Serological tests are not useful in the diagnosis of relapsing fever because the borreliae that cause this condition undergo antigenic phase variation. In contrast, serological testing is an important confirmatory test for patients with suspected Lyme disease. The tests most commonly used are the immunofluorescence assay and the enzyme-linked immunosorbent assay (ELISA). ELISA is preferred because it is more sensitive and specific for all stages of Lyme disease. Unfortunately, all serological tests are relatively insensitive during the early acute stage of disease. IgM antibodies appear 2 to 4 weeks after the onset of erythema migrans in untreated patients; the levels peak after 6 to 8 weeks of illness and then decline to a normal range after 4 to 6 months. The IgM level may remain elevated in some patients with a persistent infection. The IgG antibodies appear later. Their levels peak after 4 to 6 months of illness and persist during the late manifestations of the disease. Thus most patients with late complications of Lyme disease have detectable antibodies to *B. burgdorferi,* although the antibody level may be ablated in patients treated with antibiotics. Detection of antibodies in cerebrospinal fluid is strong evidence for neuroborreliosis.

Although cross-reactions are uncommon, positive serological results must be interpreted carefully, particularly if the titers are low (Box 41-5). Most false-positive reactions occur in patients with *T. pallidum* infections. These can be excluded by performing a nontreponemal test for syphilis; the result is negative in patients with Lyme disease.

Western blot analysis has been used to confirm the specificity of a positive ELISA reaction. The 41-kD flagellar antigen (common to many spirochetes) is the major target of IgM antibodies. IgG antibodies against other antigens (e.g., 31-kD outer surface protein A [ospA], 34-kD ospB, 21-kD ospC, 60-kD common heat shock protein) develop late in disease. However, specific reactions with antigens unique to *B. burgdorferi* need to be detected for this test to be considered useful.

If multiple *Borrelia* species are found to cause Lyme disease in the United States, as is the case in Europe and Asia, then interpretation of the ELISA and Western blot tests would need to be reassessed. At present, serological tests should be considered confirmatory and should not be performed in the absence of an appropriate history and clinical symptoms of Lyme disease. Preliminary studies have shown that the detection of *Borrelia*-specific DNA amplified by the PCR may be an effective diagnostic test for Lyme disease. However, this test is not yet commercially available.

Treatment, Prevention, and Control

Relapsing fever has been treated most effectively with tetracycline or erythromycin. Tetracycline is the drug of choice but is contraindicated for pregnant women and young children. A **Jarisch-Herxheimer reaction** (shocklike picture with rigors, leukopenia, an increase in temperature, and a decrease in blood pressure) can occur in patients within a few hours after therapy is started and must be carefully managed. This reaction corresponds to the rapid killing of borreliae and the possible release of toxic products such as endotoxin.

The early manifestations of Lyme disease are effectively managed with orally administered doxycycline or amoxicillin. Therapy also lessens the likelihood and the severity of late complications. Despite this intervention, Lyme arthritis and other complications occur in a small number of patients. Ceftriaxone, doxycycline, or amoxicillin has been used for the treatment of these manifestations. Patients with neurological and musculoskeletal disease typically require prolonged treatment, and relapses may necessitate retreatment.

Prevention of tick-borne *Borrelia* diseases includes the avoidance of ticks and their natural habitats, the wearing of protective clothing such as long pants tucked into socks, and the use of insect repellents. Rodent control is also important in the prevention of endemic relapsing fever. Epidemic louse-borne disease is controlled through the use of delousing sprays and improvements in hygienic conditions. Vaccines are not available for relapsing fever. A whole-cell, inactivated *B. burgdorferi* vaccine and a recombinant vaccine directed against the ospA antigen elicit protective antibodies in experimental animals. The recombinant vaccine is being evaluated in human subjects.

LEPTOSPIRA
Physiology and Structure

The taxonomy of the genus *Leptospira* is undergoing some changes. It has been proposed that the genus should be subdivided into 11 species; however, because this nomenclature has not been universally adopted, the more traditional subdivision into two species is used here: *L. biflexa* (63 serovars) and *L. interrogans* (210 serovars). The species names are derived from the fact that *Leptospira* are thin, coiled bacilli (0.1 × 6 to 12 μm) with a hook at one or both ends (*biflexa,* for "twice bent"; *interrogans,* meaning "shaped like a question mark") (Figure 41-14). *L. biflexa* is a free-living saprophyte found in moist environmental sites and is not associated with disease. *L. interrogans* is pathogenic for many wild and domestic animals, as well as humans. About 22 serotypes of *L. interrogans* cause human disease in the United States, with serotypes *icterohaemor-*

FIGURE 41-14 *L. interrogans* serotype *icterohaemorrhagiae.* Silver staining of organisms grown in culture. Notice the tightly coiled body with hooked ends. (From Emond R, Rowland H: *Color atlas of infectious diseases,* ed 3, London, 1995, Wolfe.)

rhagiae, canicola, pomona, and *autumnalis* the most common. Some serotypes have been historically associated with specific clinical presentations (*icterohaemorrhagiae,* Weil's disease; *pomona,* swineherd's disease; *autumnalis,* Fort Bragg fever or pretibial eruptions), but it is now recognized that the illnesses are not serotype specific.

The pathogenic leptospires are obligatively aerobic and motile by means of two periplasmic flagella, each anchored at opposite ends of the bacterium. They utilize fatty acids and alcohols as sources of carbon and energy. The leptospires can be grown on specially formulated media enriched with rabbit serum or bovine serum albumin.

Pathogenesis and Immunity

L. interrogans can cause subclinical infection, a mild influenza-like febrile illness, or severe systemic disease **(Weil's disease),** with renal and hepatic failure, extensive vasculitis, myocarditis, and death. The severity of the disease is influenced by the number of infecting organisms, the host's immunological defenses, and the virulence of the infecting strain.

Because leptospires are thin and highly motile, they can penetrate intact mucous membranes or skin through small cuts or abrasions. They can then spread in the bloodstream into all tissues, including the central nervous system. *L. interrogans* multiplies rapidly and damages the endothelium of small blood vessels, which is responsible for the major clinical manifestations of disease (e.g., meningitis, hepatic and renal dysfunction, hemorrhage). Organisms can be found in blood and cerebrospinal fluid early in the disease and in urine during the later stages. Clearance of leptospires occurs when hu-

moral immunity develops. However, some clinical manifestations may stem from immunological reactions with the organisms. For example, meningitis develops after the organisms have been removed from the cerebrospinal fluid and immune complexes have been detected in renal lesions.

Epidemiology

Leptospirosis has a worldwide distribution (Box 41-6). Fewer than 100 human infections are normally documented in the United States each year (Figure 41-15), with most cases reported from Hawaii. However, the incidence of disease is significantly underestimated because most infections are mild and misdiagnosed as a "viral syndrome" or viral aseptic meningitis. Because many states failed to report this disease to the public health service, mandatory reporting was discontinued in 1995. Thus it will be impossible to determine the true prevalence of this disease in the future.

Many wild and domestic animals are colonized with leptospires. Rodents (particularly rats), dogs, and farm animals are the most common sources of human disease in the United States. Serological studies have shown a high incidence of exposure to leptospires in urban youths. This is attributed to their contact with the urine of infected rats. Chronic carriage in humans has not been demonstrated.

Leptospires usually cause asymptomatic infections in their reservoir host, in which the spirochetes colonize the renal tubules and are shed in urine in large numbers. Streams, rivers, standing water, and moist soil can be contaminated with urine from infected animals and serve as a source for human infection, with organisms surviv-

---

BOX 41-6 Summary of *Leptospira* Infections

BACTERIAL FACTORS

Diseases—mild viral-like syndrome, leptospirosis, Weil's disease.

Virulence factors—direct invasion and replication in tissues; immune complex glomerulonephritis.

TRANSMISSION

U.S. reservoirs: rodents (particularly rats), dogs, farm animals, and wild animals.

Humans: accidental, end-stage host.

Organism that can penetrate skin through minor breaks in epidermis.

People infected with leptospires through exposure to water contaminated with urine from an infected animal and handling of tissues from infected animal.

WHO IS AT RISK?

People exposed during recreational activities in urine-contaminated streams, rivers, and standing water.

WHO IS AT RISK—CONT'D

Occupational exposure to infected animals: farmers, meat handlers, veterinarians.

GEOGRAPHY/SEASON

Worldwide.

Infection is rare in United States.

Disease is more common during warm months (recreational exposure).

MODES OF CONTROL

Treatment of severe infections involves intravenous penicillin or ampicillin; mild infections involves oral ampicillin, amoxicillin, or doxycycline.

Doxycycline but not the penicillins are used for prophylaxis.

Vaccination of herds and domestic pets should be done.

Rats should be controlled.

ing for as long as 6 weeks in such sites. Leptospires require a moist, alkaline environment to survive. Most human infections result from recreational exposure to contaminated water or occupational exposure to infected animals (farmers, slaughterhouse workers, and veterinarians). Most human infections occur during the warm months, when recreational exposure is greatest. Person-to-person spread has not been documented.

Clinical Syndromes

Most infections with *L. interrogans* are clinically inapparent and detected only through the demonstration of specific antibodies. Symptomatic infections develop after a 1- to 2-week incubation period (Figure 41-16). The initial presentation is similar to an influenza-like illness, with fever and myalgias. During this phase, the patient is bacteremic with the leptospires, and the organisms can frequently be isolated in cerebrospinal fluid, even though no meningeal symptoms are present. The fever and myalgias may remit after 1 week, or the patient may develop a more advanced disease—including aseptic meningitis—or a generalized illness with headache, rash, vascular collapse, thrombocytopenia, hemorrhage, and hepatic and renal dysfunction (Weil's disease).

Leptospirosis confined to the central nervous system can be mistaken for viral meningitis because the course of the disease is generally uncomplicated with a very low mortality rate. Culture of cerebrospinal fluid is usually negative at this stage. In contrast, the icteric form of

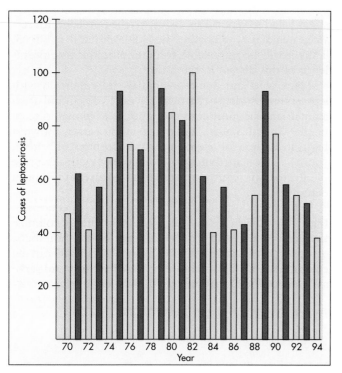

FIGURE 41-15 Leptospirosis in the United States from 1970 to 1994. (From *MMWR* 44:74-79, 1996.)

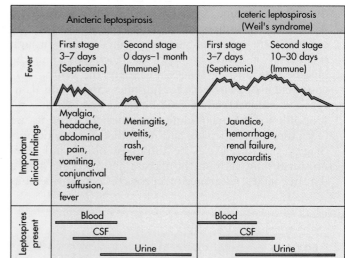

FIGURE 41-16 Stages of icteric and anicteric leptospirosis. *CSF,* Cerebrospinal fluid. (Redrawn from Feigin R, Anderson D: *CRC Crit Rev Clin Lab Sci* 5:413, 1975.)

TABLE 41-4	**Diagnostic Tests for *Leptospirosis***	
DIAGNOSTIC TEST	**METHOD**	**TEST ACCURACY**
Microscopy	Gram stain	Organisms too thin to be detected
	Darkfield examination	Insensitive, nonspecific
	Silver stain	Insensitive, nonspecific
	Direct fluorescent antibody	Insensitive, specific
Culture	Blood	Positive during first 10 days
	Cerebrospinal fluid	Positive during first 10 days
	Urine	Positive after first week
Nucleic acid probes	Direct hybridization	Insensitive, specific
	Amplification (e.g., PCR)	Sensitive, specific
Serology	Microscopic agglutination test	Sensitive, specific, reference laboratory test, serovar specific
	Indirect hemagglutination, slide agglutination, ELISA	Insensitive, nonspecific

generalized disease (approximately 10% of all symptomatic infections) is more severe and is associated with a mortality approaching 10%. Although hepatic involvement with jaundice is striking in patients with severe leptospirosis, hepatic necrosis is not seen, and surviving patients do not suffer permanent hepatic damage. Similarly, most patients recover full renal function.

Congenital leptospirosis can also occur. This disease is characterized by the sudden onset of headache, fever, myalgias, and a diffuse rash.

Laboratory Diagnosis

The tests used to diagnose leptospirosis are summarized in Table 41-4.

Microscopy

Because leptospires are thin, they are at the limit of the resolving power of a light microscope, so they cannot be seen easily by conventional light microscopy. Neither Gram stain nor silver stain is reliable in the detection of leptospires. Darkfield microscopy is also relatively insensitive and can yield nonspecific findings. Although leptospires can be seen in blood specimens early in the disease, protein filaments from erythrocytes can be easily mistaken for organisms. Fluorescein-labeled antibody preparations have been used to stain leptospires but are not available in most clinical laboratories.

Culture

Leptospires can be cultured on specially formulated media (Fletcher, EMJH, or Tween 80–albumin). They grow slowly (generation time, 6 to 16 hours), requiring incubation at 28° to 30° C for as long as 4 months; however, most cultures are positive within 2 weeks. *L. interrogans* can be recovered in blood or cerebrospinal fluid during the first 10 days of infection and in urine after the first week and for as long as 3 months. The concentration of organisms in blood, cerebrospinal fluid, and urine may be low, so multiple specimens should be collected if leptospirosis is suspected. In addition, inhibitors present in blood and urine may delay or prevent recovery of leptospires.

Nucleic Acid Probes

Preliminary work with the detection of leptospires using nucleic acid probes has had measured success. Techniques using nucleic acid amplification (e.g., PCR) are more sensitive than direct hybridization methods. Unfortunately, commercial molecular diagnostic systems are not currently available.

Serology

Because of the need for specialized media and prolonged incubation, most laboratories do not attempt to culture leptospires and thus rely on serological techniques. The reference method for all serological tests is the microscopic agglutination test (MAT). This test measures the ability of the patient's serum to agglutinate live leptospires. Because the test is directed against specific serotypes, it is necessary to use pools of leptospiral antigens. In this test, serial dilutions of the patient's serum are mixed with the test antigens and then examined microscopically for agglutination. Agglutinins appear in the blood of untreated patients during the second week of illness, although this response may be delayed for as long as several months. Infected patients have a titer of at least 100, and it may be 25,000 or higher. Patients treated with antibiotics may have a diminished antibody response and nondiagnostic titers. Agglutinating antibodies are detectable for many years after the acute illness, so their presence may represent either a blunted antibody response in a treated patient with acute disease or residual antibodies is a person with a distant, unrecognized infection with leptospires. Because the MAT uses live organisms, it is only performed in reference laboratories. Alternative tests such as indirect hemagglutination, slide agglutination, and ELISA are less sensitive and specific and are not recommended.

Treatment, Prevention, and Control

Leptospirosis is usually not fatal, particularly in the absence of icteric disease. Patients with severe disease should be treated with intravenously administered penicillin or ampicillin, and patients with less severe disease can be treated with orally administered doxycycline, ampicillin, or amoxicillin. Doxycycline but not the penicillins can be used to prevent disease in people exposed to infected animals or water contaminated with urine. It is difficult to eradicate leptospirosis because the disease is widespread in wild and domestic animals. However, the vaccination of livestock and pets has proved successful in reducing the incidence of disease in these populations and therefore subsequent human exposure. Rodent control is also effective in eliminating leptospirosis in communities.

CASE STUDY AND QUESTIONS

A 18-year-old woman seen by her physician complained of knee pain that started 2 weeks before. Three months earlier, soon after vacationing in Connecticut, she noticed a circular area of redness on her lower leg that was approximately 10 cm in diameter. Over the next 2 weeks the area enlarged, and the border became more clearly demarcated. However, the rash gradually disappeared. A few days after the rash disappeared, she experienced the onset of headaches, an inability to concentrate, and nausea. These symptoms also gradually abated. The pain in her knee developed approximately 1 month after these symptoms disappeared. On examination of the knee, mild tenderness and pain were noted. A small amount of serous fluid was aspirated from the joint, and it had a white blood cell count of 45.0×10^7/ml. Antibodies to *B. burgdorferi* were present in the patient's serum (titers of 32 and 1024 for IgM and IgG, respectively), confirming the clinical diagnosis of Lyme arthritis.

1. What are the initial and late manifestations of Lyme disease?

2. What are the limitations of the following diagnostic tests for Lyme disease: microscopy, culture, and serology? How does this compare with the diagnostic tests for other relapsing fevers?

3. Name two examples each of nontreponemal and treponemal tests for syphilis. What reactions would you expect for those tests in patients with primary, secondary, and late syphilis?

4. What are the reservoir and vectors for syphilis, epidemic and endemic relapsing fever, Lyme disease, and leptospirosis?

5. What diagnostic tests can be used for the diagnosis of leptospirosis?

BIBLIOGRAPHY

Balmelli T, Piffaretti J: Analysis of the genetic polymorphism of *Borrelia burgdorferi sensu lato* by multilocus enzyme electrophoresis, *Int J Syst Bacteriol* 46:167-172, 1996.

Baranton G et al: Delineation of *Borrelia burgdorferi sensu stricto, Borrelia garinii* sp. nov., and Group VS461 associated with Lyme borreliosis, *Int J Syst Bacteriol* 42:378-383, 1992.

Barbour AG, Hayes SF: Biology of *Borrelia species, Microbiol Rev* 50:381-400, 1986.

Butler T et al: Infection with *Borrelia recurrentis:* pathogenesis of fever and petechiae, *J Infect Dis* 140:665-672, 1979.

Centers for Disease Control and Prevention: CDC 1993 Sexually transmitted diseases treatment guidelines, *MMWR* 42:27-46, 1993.

Duffey P, Salugsugan J: Serodiagnosis of Lyme borreliosis, *Clin Microbiol Newslett* 15:81-86, 1993.

Heath CW, Alexander AD, Galton MM: Leptospirosis in the United States: analysis of 483 cases in man, 1949-1961, *N Engl J Med* 273:857-864, 915-922, 1965.

Johnson B et al: Serodiagnosis of Lyme disease: accuracy of a two-step approach using a flagella-based ELISA and immunoblotting, *J Infect Dis* 174:346-353, 1996.

Larsen S, Steiner B, Rudolph A: Laboratory diagnosis and interpretation of tests for syphilis, *Clin Microbiol Rev* 8:1-21, 1995.

Mouritsen C et al: Polymerase chain reaction detection of Lyme disease: correlation with clinical manifestations and serologic responses, *Am J Clin Pathol* 105:647-654, 1996.

Nocton J, Steere A: Lyme disease, *Adv Intern Med* 40:69-115, 1995.

Ras N et al: Phylogenesis of relapsing fever *Borrelia* spp., *Int J Syst Bacteriol* 46:859-865, 1996.

Rolfs R: Treatment of syphilis, 1993, *Clin Infect Dis* 20(suppl 1):S23-S38, 1995.

Rolfs RT, Nakashima AK: Epidemiology of primary and secondary syphilis in the United States, 1981 through 1989, *JAMA* 264:1432-1437, 1990.

Romanowski B et al: Serologic response to treatment of infectious syphilis, *Ann Intern Med* 114:1005-1009, 1991.

Sigal L, editor: National clinical conference on Lyme disease, *Am J Med* 98 (4A):S1-S84, 1995.

Southern PM, Sanford JP: Relapsing fever: a clinical and microbiological review, *Medicine* 48:129-149, 1969.

Spach D et al: Tick-borne diseases in the United States, *N Engl J Med* 329:936-947, 1993.

Van Dam A et al: Different genospecies of *Borrelia burgdorferi* are associated with distinct clinical manifestations of Lyme borreliosis, *Clin Infect Dis* 17:708-717, 1993.

Vinetz J et al: Sporadic urban leptospirosis, *Ann Intern Med* 125:794-798, 1996.

White DJ et al: The geographic spread and temporal increase of the Lyme disease epidemic, *JAMA* 266:1230-1236, 1991.

Wormser G: A vaccine against Lyme disease? *Ann Intern Med* 123:627-629, 1995.

CHAPTER 42

Mycoplasma and *Ureaplasma*

The class of organisms Mollicutes is subdivided into three families, with the human pathogens placed in the family Mycoplasmataceae. This family contains two genera, *Mycoplasma* and *Ureaplasma*, with 11 of the species colonizing or causing disease in humans (Table 42-1). *M. pneumoniae* (also called **Eaton's agent** after the investigator who originally isolated it) causes respiratory tract disease, and *M. hominis*, *M. genitalium*, and *U. urealyticum* cause genitourinary tract diseases. These and other mycoplasmas that colonize humans have been associated with a variety of other maladies (e.g., infertility, spontaneous abortion, vaginitis, cervicitis, epididymitis, prostatitis). However, their etiological role in these diseases remains unknown.

PHYSIOLOGY AND STRUCTURE

Mycoplasma and *Ureaplasma* organisms are the smallest free-living bacteria (Table 42-2). They are unique among bacteria because they do not have a cell wall and the cell membrane contains sterols. In contrast, other cell wall–deficient bacteria (also called **L forms**) do not have sterols in their cell membrane and can form cell walls under the appropriate growth conditions. The absence of the cell wall renders the mycoplasmas resistant to penicillins, cephalosporins, vancomycin, and other antibiotics that interfere with synthesis of the cell wall. The mycoplasmas form pleomorphic filaments with an average diameter of 0.1 to 0.3 μm, and many can pass through the 0.45-μm filters used to remove bacteria from solutions. For these reasons the mycoplasmas were originally thought to be viruses. However, the organisms divide by binary fission (typical of all bacteria), grow on artificial cell-free media, contain both RNA and DNA, and are gram negative. Mycoplasmas are facultatively anaerobic (except *M. pneumoniae*, which is a strict aerobe) and require exogenous sterols supplied by animal serum added to the growth medium. The mycoplasmas grow slowly, with a generation time of 1 to 6 hours, and most form small colonies that have a fried-egg appearance (Figure 42-1). Colonies of *Ureaplasma* organisms (also called **T strains,** for tiny strains) are extremely small, 10 to 50 μm in diameter.

Because these organisms do not have a cell wall, the major antigenic determinants are membrane glycolipids and proteins. These antigens cross-react with human tissues and other bacteria.

Pathogenesis and Immunity

M. pneumoniae is an extracellular pathogen that adheres to the respiratory epithelium by means of a specialized terminal protein attachment factor. This 168-kD terminal adhesin protein, called **P1,** interacts specifically with glycoprotein receptors at the base of cilia on the epithelial cell surface. Ciliostasis then occurs, after which the superficial layer of epithelial cells is destroyed. The loss of these cells interferes with the normal clearance of the upper airways and permits the lower respiratory tract to become contaminated with microbes and mechanically irritated. This process is responsible for causing the persistent cough present in patients with symptomatic disease. *M. pneumoniae* functions as a superantigen, stimu-

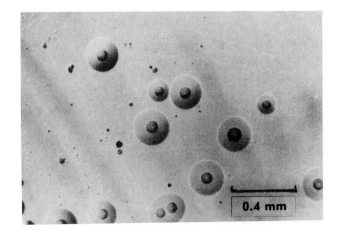

FIGURE 42-1 Fried-egg appearance of colonies of mycoplasmas. All mycoplasmas except *M. pneumoniae* typically show this morphology. *M. pneumoniae* has a strict aerobic atmosphere requirement. It is one of the slowest-growing mycoplasmas, and it appears as homogeneous granular colonies after incubation for 1 week or more. The other mycoplasmas generally grow within 1 to 4 days. (From Razin S, Oliver O: *J Gen Microbiol* 24:225-237, 1961.)

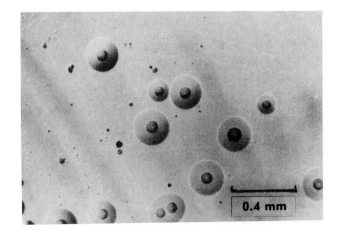
0.4 mm

TABLE 42-1   Mycoplasmataceae Isolated in Humans

ORGANISM	SITE	DISEASE
M. pneumoniae	Respiratory tract	Upper respiratory tract disease, tracheobronchitis, atypical pneumonia
M. hominis	Genitourinary tract	Pyelonephritis, pelvic inflammatory disease, postpartum fever
M. genitalium	Genitourinary tract	Nongonococcal urethritis
M. orale	Respiratory tract	Unknown
M. salivarium	Respiratory tract	Unknown
M. buccale	Respiratory tract	Unknown
M. faucium	Respiratory tract	Unknown
M. lipophilum	Respiratory tract	Unknown
M. pimatum	Respiratory tract, genitourinary tract	Unknown
M. fermentans	Genitourinary tract	Unknown
U. urealyticum	Genitourinary tract	Nongonococcal urethritis

Modified from Baum S. In Mandell G, Bennett J, Dolin R: *Principles and practice of infectious diseases,* New York, 1995, Churchill Livingstone.

TABLE 42-2   Properties of *Mycoplasma* and *Ureaplasma* Organisms

PROPERTIES	CHARACTERISTICS
Size	0.1 to 0.3 μm
Cell wall	Absent
Growth	
Atmosphere	Facultatively anaerobic*
Nutritional requirement	Sterols
Nutritional supplements	Vitamins, amino acids, nucleic acid precursors
Other	Cell-free growth
Replication	Binary fission
Generation time	1 to 6 hours
Antibiotic susceptibility	
Penicillins	Resistant
Cephalosporins	Resistant
Tetracycline	Susceptible
Erythromycin	Susceptible†

*M. pneumoniae is an obligate aerobe.
†M. hominis is resistant.

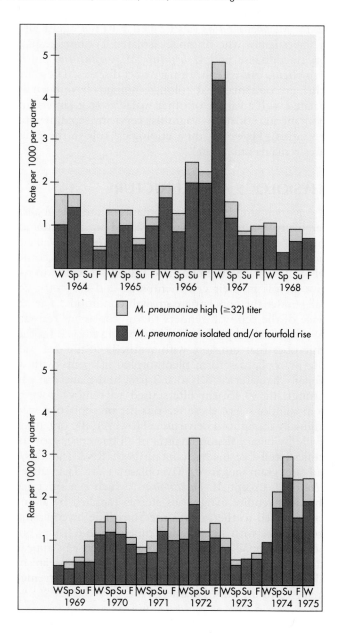

FIGURE 42-2 *M. pneumoniae* infections in children younger than 15 years were seen throughout the 12 years of this study in Seattle. No seasonal incidence was observed, but year-to-year fluctuations were common. *W,* Winter; *Sp,* spring; *Su,* summer; *F,* fall. (Redrawn from Foy HM et al: *J Infect Dis* 139:681-687, 1979.)

BOX 42-1   Summary of *M. pneumoniae* Infections

BACTERIAL FACTORS

Diseases—upper respiratory tract disease, tracheobronchitis, atypical pneumonia.

Virulence factors—terminal adhesin protein (P1), stimulation of cytokine release.

M. pneumoniae is smallest free-living bacterium.

Absence of cell wall and requirement for sterols are unique among bacteria.

Replication by binary fission and presence of DNA and RNA distinguish mycoplasmas from viruses.

TRANSMISSION

Inhalation of aerosolized droplets by means of close contact.
Human pathogen.

WHO IS AT RISK?

Primarily children and young adults.

GEOGRAPHY/SEASON

Worldwide.

No seasonal incidence although year-to-year fluctuations in incidence of disease.

MODES OF CONTROL

Erythromycin, doxycycline, and fluoroquinolones.

Immunity to reinfection is not lifelong, and vaccines are ineffective.

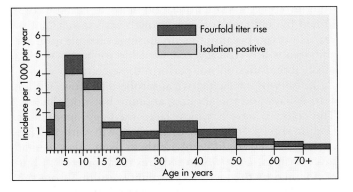

FIGURE 42-3 Incidence of pneumonia with *M. pneumoniae* in different age groups. The greatest number of infections is in 5- to 15-year-old patients. (From Foy H et al: *J Infect Dis* 139:681-687, 1979.)

lating inflammatory cells to migrate to the site of infection and release cytokines, initially TNF-alpha and IL-1 and later IL-6. This contributes to both the clearance of the bacteria as well as the observed pathology.

Epidemiology

Pneumonia caused by *M. pneumoniae* occurs worldwide throughout the year, with no consistent increase in seasonal activity (Figure 42-2). However, because pneumonia caused by other infectious agents (e.g., *Streptococcus pneumoniae*, viruses) is frequently more common during the cold months, *M. pneumoniae* disease is proportionally more common during the summer and fall (Box 42-1). Epidemic disease occurs every 4 to 8 years. Disease is most common in school-age children and young adults (Figure 42-3), with disease uncommon in children younger than 5 years or adults older than 20 years. *M. pneumoniae* is the most common cause of pneumonia in children from 5 to 15 years of age.

In 1987, it was estimated that 11 to 15 million cases of *M. pneumoniae* infection occur annually in the United States. This is not a reportable disease, and specific diagnostic tests are not readily available, so the true incidence is not known. It has been reported that *M. pneumoniae* causes an average of 15% to 20% of all community-acquired pneumonias. Although infections in adults are more severe than those in children, normally adults with infection do not need to be hospitalized. Infection is spread by nasal secretions. Close contact is necessary for spread to occur, and the infection usually occurs among classmates or family members. The attack rate is higher in children than in adults (overall average, approximately 60%). The incubation period and time of infectivity are prolonged. Thus disease can persist for months among classmates or family members.

Infants, particularly girls, are colonized with *M. hominis*, *M. genitalium*, and *Ureaplasma* species at birth, with *Ureaplasma* organisms isolated more frequently. Although carriage of these mycoplasmas usually does not persist, a small proportion of prepubertal children remain colonized. The incidence of genital mycoplasmas increases after puberty, corresponding to sexual activity. Approximately 15% of sexually active men and women are colonized with *M. hominis*, and 45% to 75% are colonized with *Ureaplasma* organisms. The incidence of carriage in adults who are sexually inactive is no greater than that in prepubertal children.

Clinical Syndromes

Infection with *M. pneumoniae* typically produces mild **upper respiratory tract disease.** Low-grade fever, malaise, headache, and a dry, nonproductive cough develop in the patient 2 to 3 weeks after exposure. Symptoms gradually worsen over the next few days and can persist for 2 weeks or more. More severe disease with lower respiratory tract symptoms develops in less than 10% of patients. **Tracheobronchitis** can occur, and in this infection the bronchial passages primarily become infiltrated with lymphocytes and plasma cells. Pneumonia (**primary atypical pneumonia** or **walking pneumo-**

nia) can also develop, with a patchy bronchopneumonia seen on chest radiographs that is typically more impressive than the physical findings. Myalgias and gastrointestinal tract symptoms are uncommon. Secondary complications include otitis media, erythema multiforme (Stevens-Johnson syndrome), hemolytic anemia, myocarditis, pericarditis, and neurological abnormalities. The disease resolves slowly. Secondary infections can occur because immunity is incomplete.

The role of other mycoplasmas in human disease is less clearly defined. *M. genitalium* and *U. urealyticum* can cause nongonococcal urethritis, and *M. hominis* has been implicated as a cause of pyelonephritis, pelvic inflammatory disease, and postpartum fever. The evidence implicating the organisms in these diseases is based on recovery of the bacteria from specimens from infected patients, a serological response to the organism, clinical improvement after treatment with specific antibiotics, pathology demonstrated in animal models, or a combination of these findings. However, it is common for the genitourinary tract to be colonized with these organisms, and their presence can mask a more important pathogen.

Laboratory Diagnosis

The diagnostic tests for *M. pneumoniae* infections are summarized in Table 42-3 and Figure 42-4.

Microscopy

Although mycoplasmas are taxonomically classified as gram-negative bacteria, they stain poorly because they have no cell wall.

Culture

Unlike other mycoplasmas, *M. pneumoniae* is a strict aerobe. This mycoplasma can be isolated from throat washings or expectorated sputum, although most infected patients produce scant amounts of sputum. The specimen should be inoculated into special media supplemented with serum (provides cholesterol), yeast extract (for nucleic acid precursors), glucose, a pH indicator, and penicillin (to inhibit other bacteria). The organisms grow slowly in culture, with a generation time of 6 hours, and a positive culture is a relatively insensitive finding. In one well-designed study, 36% of the isolates were detected within 2 weeks, whereas the remaining isolates had to be incubated for as long as 6 weeks. In another study, only 64% of the patients with serological evidence of an acute *Mycoplasma* infection were culture positive. Growth of the organisms in culture is indicated by the metabolism of glucose with a corresponding pH change. Colonies of *M. pneumoniae* are small and have a homogeneous granular appearance, unlike the fried-egg morphology of other mycoplasmas. Identification of isolates can be confirmed by inhibition of their growth with specific antisera. However, because this organism is difficult to grow and results are typically not available for many weeks, most laboratories do not perform these cultures.

M. hominis is a facultative anaerobe that grows within 1 to 4 days and metabolizes arginine but not glucose. The colonies have a typical large fried-egg appearance (Figure 42-1). Inhibition of their growth with specific antisera is used to differentiate them from other genital mycoplasmas. *Ureaplasma* requires urea for growth but is inhibited by the increased alkalinity resulting from the metabolism of urea. Thus the growth medium must be supplemented with urea and highly buffered. Even if this is done, these mycoplasmas die rapidly after initial isolation.

TABLE 42-3	Diagnostic Tests for *M. pneumoniae* Infections
TEST	**ASSESSMENT**
Microscopy	Test is not useful because organisms do not have a cell wall and are too small to be seen by light microscopy.
Culture	Test is slow (2-6 weeks before positive) and insensitive; it is not available in most laboratories.
Serology	
Complement fixation	Titers peak within 4 weeks and persist for 6-12 months; diagnostic titer is ≥32, or a fourfold increase; it has good sensitivity but can be nonspecific.
ELISA or immunofluorescence	Test is sensitive and easier to perform than complement fixation; nonspecific reactions can occur.
Cold agglutinins	Diagnostic titer is ≥128, or a fourfold increase; seroconversion occurs in 34% to 68% (insensitive); test is nonspecific.

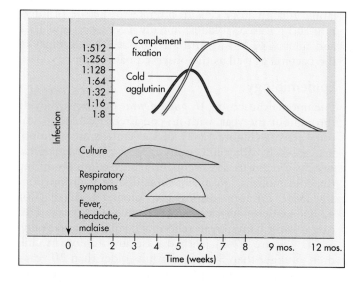

FIGURE 42-4 Correlation between clinical course of *M. pneumoniae* infection and results of diagnostic tests.

Serology

Serological tests are available only for *M. pneumoniae*. It is generally not useful to detect the local production of IgA because the antibody rapidly disappears after the onset of infection. Detection of IgA by complement fixation is more useful. The antibody is initially detected soon after the onset of infection. The titer peaks within 4 weeks and persists for 6 to 12 months. This is the standard diagnostic test for *M. pneumoniae* infections. One study reported a significant increase in antibody titers or an initial titer of at least 32 in 90% of patients with a positive culture. Because the antibodies are directed against outer membrane glycolipids common to other organisms and tissues, false-positive reactions are observed. These occur in patients with other mycoplasmas, in the presence of some plant antigens, and in patients with bacterial meningitis, syphilis, or pancreatitis. Complement fixation tests are cumbersome, and most laboratories now use tests such as enzyme-linked immunosorbent assays and immunofluorescence.

It is also possible to measure nonspecific reactions to the outer membrane glycolipids. The most useful of these is the production of cold agglutinins (e.g., IgM antibodies that bind the I antigen on the surface of human erythrocytes at 4° C). The cold agglutinin assay is positive in approximately 65% of patients with *M. pneumoniae* infections, particularly those who are symptomatic. Because this test is not specific for *M. pneumoniae*, cross-reactions are observed in patients with respiratory tract diseases caused by other organisms (e.g., infectious mononucleosis, adenovirus). Strongly reactive cold agglutinin titers of at least 128 or a significant increase in the titer constitutes presumptive evidence of *Mycoplasma* disease.

Treatment, Prevention, and Control

Erythromycin and tetracycline (or doxycycline) are equally effective in treating *M. pneumoniae* infections, although the tetracyclines are reserved for the treatment of adults with infection. Tetracyclines, which have the advantage of also being active against *Chlamydia* organisms, a common cause of nongonococcal urethritis, are also active against most other mycoplasmas. Erythromycin or spectinomycin are active antibiotics that can be used to treat infections caused by some strains of *Ureaplasma* resistant to tetracyclines. Unlike the other mycoplasmas, *M. hominis* is resistant to erythromycin and occasionally to the tetracyclines. Clindamycin has been used to treat infections caused by these resistant strains.

The prevention of *Mycoplasma* disease is problematic. *M. pneumoniae* infections are spread by close contact; thus the isolation of infected people could theoretically reduce the risk of infection. However, this is impractical because of the prolonged infectivity of the patient, even while receiving appropriate antibiotics. Inactivated vaccines, as well as attenuated live vaccines, have also proved disappointing. The protective immunity conferred has been low. Infections with *M. hominis*, *M. genitalium*, and *Ureaplasma* species are transmitted by sexual contact. Thus the disease can be prevented by avoiding sexual activity or using proper barrier precautions.

CASE STUDY AND QUESTIONS

Increased lethargy, headache, cough, a low-grade fever, and chills and sweats at night developed in a 21-year-old student. When she was seen at the student health center, she had a nonproductive cough and dyspnea on exertion. Her pulse rate was 95 beats/min, and her respiratory rate was 28 breaths/min. Her pharynx was erythematous; scattered rhonchi and rales but no consolidation were noted on auscultation. A chest radiograph showed patchy infiltrates. A Gram stain of sputum contained many white blood cells but no organisms. A *Mycoplasma* complement fixation titer on admission was 8 and was found to have increased to 32 a week later. She was treated with erythromycin and responded slowly during the next 2 weeks.

1. Should cultures of induced sputum have been performed to confirm the serological diagnosis? When would the results be available?
2. How do *Mycoplasma* species differ from other bacteria?
3. Describe the epidemiology of *M. pneumoniae* infections. What is characteristic about this patient?
4. What other mycoplasmas cause human disease? What diseases?

Bibliography

Barile MF et al: Current topics in mycoplasmology, *Rev Infect Dis* 4:1-277, 1982.

Cassell GH, Cole BC: *Mycoplasmas* as agents of human disease, *N Engl J Med* 304:80-89, 1981.

Cole B, Sawitzke A: Mycoplasmas, superantigens and autoimmune arthritis. In Henderson B et al, editors: *Mechanisms and models in rheumatoid arthritis*, San Diego, 1996, Academic.

Foy HM et al: Long-term epidemiology of infections with *Mycoplasma pneumoniae*, *J Infect Dis* 139:681-687, 1979.

Kenny GE et al: Diagnosis of *Mycoplasma pneumoniae* pneumonia: sensitivities and specificities of serology with lipid antigen and isolation of the organism on soy peptone medium for identification of infections, *J Clin Microbiol* 28:2087-2093, 1990.

Lo S: New understandings of mycoplasmal infections and diseases, *Clin Microbiol Newslett* 17:169-173, 1995.

Luby JP: Pneumonia caused by *Mycoplasma pneumoniae* infection, *Clin Chest Med* 12:237-244, 1991.

Maniloff J et al, editors: *Mycoplasmas: molecular biology and pathogenesis*, Washington, DC, 1992, American Society of Microbiologists.

McMahon DK, Dummer JS, Pasculle AW: Extragenital *Mycoplasma hominis* infections in adults, *Am J Med* 89:275-281, 1990.

Waites K et al: Laboratory diagnosis of mycoplasmal and ureaplasmal infections, *Clin Microbiol Newslett* 18:105-112, 1996.

Rickettsia, Ehrlichia, and Coxiella

Rickettsia, Ehrlichia, and *Coxiella* are aerobic, gramnegative bacilli that are obligate intracellular parasites. Although they are commonly classified in a single family, analysis of their DNA sequences has revealed that this is invalid. They are therefore discussed as distinct, unrelated genera in this chapter.

These bacteria were originally thought to be viruses because they were small (0.3×1 to 2 μm), stained poorly with the Gram stain, and grew only in the cytoplasm of eukaryotic cells. However, they are now known to be structurally similar to gram-negative bacilli; to contain DNA, RNA, and enzymes for the Krebs cycle and ribosomes for protein synthesis; to multiply by binary fission; and to be inhibited by antibiotics (e.g., tetracycline, chloramphenicol).

The pathogenic species of these three genera are maintained in animal and arthropod reservoirs and transmitted by arthropod vectors (e.g., ticks, mites, lice, fleas). Humans are accidental hosts. The species that cause human disease are summarized in Table 43-1 and Figure 43-1.

PHYSIOLOGY AND STRUCTURE

The structure of the cell wall in these bacteria is typical of gram-negative bacilli, with a peptidoglycan layer and lipopolysaccharide (LPS). However, the peptidoglycan layer is minimal in some bacteria, and the LPS has only weak endotoxin activity (or is absent as in *Ehrlichia* species). The bacteria do not have flagella and are surrounded by a loosely adherent slime layer. All organisms are seen best with Giemsa or Gimenez stain and react weakly with Gram stain. All bacteria are strict intracellular parasites, but their intracellular location varies: *Rickettsia* species are found free in the cytoplasm, whereas *Coxiella* and *Ehrlichia* species multiply in cytoplasmic vacuoles.

The bacteria enter eukaryotic cells by stimulating phagocytosis. After engulfment, the *Rickettsia* species must degrade the phagosome membrane by producing phospholipase A and be released into the cytoplasm, or the organisms will not survive. Multiplication by binary fission is slow (generation time, 9 to 12 hours). *R. prow-*

azekii accumulates in the cell until it lyses; in contrast, *R. rickettsii* and *R. tsutsugamushi* are continually released from cells through long cytoplasmic projections.

After *Coxiella* species enters the cell, it remains in the phagolysosome, where the organism has become adapted to growing in the acidic environment. In contrast, *Ehrlichia* species are killed if lysosomes fuse with their cytoplasmic vacuoles. Figure 43-2 illustrates the growth cycle of *Ehrlichia* species, which includes three stages of growth: elementary body, initial body, and morula. Figure 43-3 is an electron micrograph of a canine monocyte infected with *E. canis.*

The reason that these bacteria must grow inside eukaryotic cells is not understood. The bacteria are capable

Disease	Organism	Vector	Reservoir
Rocky Mountain spotted fever	R. rickettsii	Tick-borne	Ticks, wild rodents
Ehrlichiosis	E. chaffeensis		Ticks
Rickettsialpox	R. akari	Mite-borne	Mites, wild rodents
Scrub typhus	R. tsutsugamushi		Mites (chiggers), wild rodents
Epidemic typhus	R. prowazekii	Louse-borne	Humans, squirrel fleas, flying squirrels
Trench fever	R. quintana		Humans
Murine typhus	R. typhi	Flea-borne	Wild rodents
Q fever	C. burnetii	None*	Cattle, sheep, goats, cats

FIGURE 43-1 Epidemiology of common *Rickettsia, Ehrlichia,* and *Coxiella* infections.

of protein synthesis and can produce adenosine triphosphate (ATP) by means of the tricarboxylic acid cycle. It appears that the bacteria are energy parasites that use the host cell ATP as long as it is available. They also use the host cell coenzyme A, nicotinamide adenine dinucleotide, and available amino acids.

Once these bacteria are released from the host cell, they are unstable and die quickly. The exception is *Coxiella* species, which is highly resistant to desiccation and remains viable in the environment for months to years. This characteristic is extremely important in the epidemiology of *Coxiella* infections.

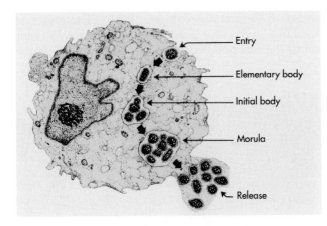

FIGURE 43-2 The growth of *Ehrlichia* organisms in an infected cell. (From McDade JE: *J Infect Dis* 161:609-612, 1990.)

FIGURE 43-3 Electron micrograph of *E. canis* in the cytoplasm of a canine monocyte (bar = 1 μm). (From McDade JE: *J Infect Dis* 161:609-612, 1990.)

TABLE 43-1   **Distribution of *Rickettsia, Ehrlichia,* and *Coxiella* Species Associated with Human Disease**

ORGANISM	HUMAN DISEASE	DISTRIBUTION
Rickettsia organisms		
Spotted fever group		
R. rickettsii	Rocky Mountain spotted fever	Western hemisphere
R. conorii	Boutonneuse fever	Mediterranean countries, Africa, India, Southwest Asia
R. sibirica	Siberian tick typhus	Siberia, Mongolia, northern China
R. australis	Australian tick typhus	Australia
R. akari	Rickettsialpox	United States, former Soviet Union
R. japonica	Oriental spotted fever	Japan
Typhus group		
R. prowazekii	Epidemic typhus	South America and Africa
	Recrudescent typhus	Worldwide
	Sporadic typhus	United States
R. typhi	Murine typhus	Worldwide
Scrub typhus group		
R. tsutsugamushi	Scrub typhus	Asia, northern Australia, Pacific Islands
Ehrlichia organisms		
E. canis group		
E. chaffeensis	Human monocytic ehrlichiosis	Southeast and South Central United States
E. phagocytophila group		
E. equi	Human granulocytic ehrlichiosis	Northeastern and Upper Midwestern United States, Northern California
E. sennetsu group		
E. sennetsu	Sennetsu fever	Japan
Coxiella burnetii	Q fever	Worldwide

RICKETTSIA RICKETTSII
Pathogenesis and Immunity

There is no evidence that *R. rickettsii* produces toxins or that the host's immune response is responsible for producing the pathology of Rocky Mountain spotted fever. The primary clinical manifestations appear to result from the replication of bacteria in endothelial cells, with subsequent damage to the cells and leakage of the blood vessels. Hypovolemia and hypoproteinemia caused by the loss of plasma into the tissue can lead to reduced perfusion of various organs and organ failure.

Epidemiology

R. rickettsii is responsible for Rocky Mountain spotted fever, which is the most common rickettsial disease in the United States, with 400 to 700 documented cases reported annually (Box 43-1 and Figure 43-4). Although the disease was first described in Idaho and later in Montana, most cases are now seen in the Southeast Atlantic and South Central states (Figure 43-5). The reason for this shift is unknown, but it could result from a reduction in the tick population or a decrease in the propor-

FIGURE 43-4. Annual incidence of Rocky Mountain spotted fever in the United States, 1961 to 1995. (Redrawn from *MMWR* 44:74-79, 1996.)

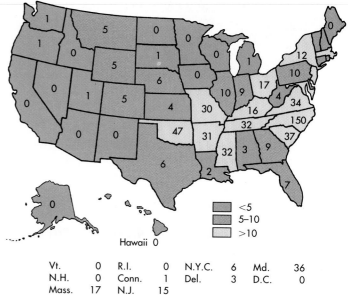

Vt.	0	R.I.	0
N.H.	0	Conn.	1
Mass.	17	N.J.	15

N.Y.C.	6	Md.	36
Del.	3	D.C.	0

FIGURE 43-5. Distribution of Rocky Mountain spotted fever in the United States, 1995. (Redrawn from *MMWR* 44:8, 1996.)

BOX 43-1   Summary of *R. rickettsii* Infections

BACTERIAL FACTORS

Disease—Rocky Mountain spotted fever.
Virulence factors—intracellular parasite; replicates in endothelial cells, with resulting vasculitis.
R. rickettsii is most common rickettsial disease in United States.

TRANSMISSION

Hard ticks (*D. andersoni* and *D. variabilis* in the United States) are primary reservoirs and vectors.
Transmission requires prolonged contact (24 to 48 hours).

WHO IS AT RISK?

People in contact with infected ticks.

GEOGRAPHY/SEASON

Distribution in Western hemisphere; in United States, infection is most common in Southeast Atlantic and South Central states.
Disease is most frequent from April through September.

MODES OF CONTROL

Antibiotics administered include the tetracyclines and chloramphenicol.
People should avoid tick-infected areas, wear protective clothing, and use effective insecticides.
People should remove attached ticks immediately.
No vaccine is currently available.

tion of infected ticks. The principal reservoir for *R. rickettsii* is infected hard ticks: the wood tick *(Dermacentor andersoni)* in Rocky Mountain states and the dog tick *(Dermacentor variabilis)* in the southeastern states and the West Coast. Other tick reservoirs are *Rhipicephalus sanguineus* in Mexico, and *Amblyomma cajennense* in Central and South America. It is not clear whether the Lone Star tick *(Amblyomma americanum)* in the South Central states is a reservoir. The rickettsiae are maintained in the tick population by transovarian transmission. Mammals such as wild rodents can also serve as reservoirs, but this is considered an uncommon source for tick-to-human infections.

Rickettsial infections are spread to humans by the adult ticks when they feed. More than 90% of all infections occur from April through September, corresponding to the period of greatest tick activity. To become infected a person must be exposed to the tick for a lengthy period (e.g., 24 to 48 hours). The dormant avirulent rickettsiae are activated by the warm blood meal, then must be released from the tick salivary glands and penetrate the bloodstream of the human host.

Clinical Syndromes

Clinically symptomatic disease develops 2 to 14 days (average, 7 days) after the tick bite (Table 43-2). The patient may not recall the painless tick bite. The disease is heralded by fever, chills, headache, and myalgias. A rash develops after 3 or more days and can evolve from a macular to petechial form (Figure 43-6). The rash can develop late in the disease and is not observed in about 10% of infected patients. Complications of Rocky Mountain spotted fever can include gastrointestinal symptoms, respiratory failure, encephalitis, and renal failure. Complications increase and the prognosis is worse when the characteristic rash does not develop or develops late in the disease because the diagnosis is delayed.

Laboratory Diagnosis

Although the rickettsiae stain poorly with Gram stain, they can be stained with Giemsa or Gimenez stain. Specific fluorescein-labeled antibodies can also be used to stain biopsy tissue specimens; however, this procedure is less sensitive in patients who have received effective antibiotics.

The rickettsiae can be isolated in tissue culture or embryonated eggs. However, bacterial isolation is primarily performed in reference laboratories because the bacteria grow slowly and their recovery is traditionally considered a hazardous procedure.

The primary diagnostic procedure for Rocky Mountain spotted fever is serology. Although the Weil-Felix test (which involves the differential agglutination of *Proteus* antigens) has been used historically for the diagnosis of rickettsial infections, it is not now recommended because it is insensitive and nonspecific. Tests for detecting *Rickettsia*-specific antibodies have been developed and include the complement fixation (CF) test, the indirect flu-

TABLE 43-2 **Clinical Course of Human Diseases Caused by *Rickettsia, Ehrlichia,* and *Coxiella* Species**

DISEASE	AVERAGE INCUBATION PERIOD (DAYS)	CLINICAL PRESENTATION	RASH	ESCHAR	MORTALITY
Rocky Mountain spotted fever	7	Abrupt onset; fever, chills, headache, myalgia	>90%; macular; centripetal spread	No	20%*
Rickettsialpox	9 to 14	Abrupt onset; fever, headache, chills, myalgia, photophobia	100%; papulovesicular; generalized	Yes	<1%
Epidemic typhus	8	Abrupt onset; fever, headache, chills, myalgia, arthralgia	40% to 80%; macular; centrifugal spread	No	Variable
Endemic typhus	7 to 14	Gradual onset; fever, headache, myalgia, cough	>55%; maculopapular rash on trunk	No	1% to 2%
Scrub typhus	10 to 12	Abrupt onset; fever, headache, myalgia	<50%; maculopapular rash; centrifugal	No	7%*
Ehrlichiosis	12	Abrupt onset; fever, headache, myalgia, malaise, leukopenia, thrombocytopenia	20%; nonspecific	No	5%
Q fever (acute)	20	Abrupt onset; fever, headache, chills, myalgia; granulomatous hepatitis	No	No	1%
Q fever (chronic)	Months to years	Chronic disease with subacute onset; endocarditis, hepatic dysfunction	No	No	High

*Mortality in untreated patients.

FIGURE 43-6. The rash of Rocky Mountain spotted fever consists of a generally distributed, sharply defined maculopapular rash that becomes purpuric macules. The rash initially involves the extremities and then spreads to the trunk; the palms and soles can be involved. (From Binford CH, Connor DH, editors: *Pathology of tropical and extraordinary diseases: an atlas*, vol 1, Washington, DC, 1976, Armed Forces Institute of Pathology.)

orescent antibody (IFA) test, and latex agglutination. However, the CF test is insensitive and antibodies are detected relatively late in the disease, so it is rarely used. The IFA test is both sensitive (94% to 100%) and specific (100%), with the finding of a fourfold rise in the antibody titers or an initial titer of 64 or more considered a positive result. The initial antibody response is detected 2 to 3 weeks after the onset of disease, and antibodies remain detectable for a long time. The latex agglutination test is positive earlier than the IFA test (e.g., 1 to 2 weeks after onset), but the result rapidly reverts to negative. The test may also be slightly less sensitive than the IFA test.

The direct detection of rickettsial antigens in skin biopsy specimens is a rapid, specific method for confirming the clinical diagnosis of Rocky Mountain spotted fever. This can be done using specific antibodies labeled with fluorescent dyes that can stain the intracellular bacteria. Alternatively, nucleic acid probes are also an accurate method for detecting rickettsiae. Unfortunately, both antigen tests are offered only in reference laboratories, so there is some delay before test results are available.

Treatment, Prevention, and Control

Rickettsiae are susceptible to the tetracyclines and chloramphenicol. The prompt diagnosis and instituition of appropriate therapy usually result in a satisfactory prognosis. Unfortunately, this may not happen if key clinical signs (such as the rash) develop late or not at all. In addition, the serological findings frequently are not available until 2 to 4 weeks after the onset of disease, which can also delay the start of treatment. The morbidity and mortality are high if the diagnosis or specific therapy is considerably delayed. There is no vaccine for Rocky Mountain spotted fever. Thus avoidance of tick-infested areas, the use of protective clothing and insect repellents, and the prompt removal of attached ticks are the best preventive measures. It is virtually impossible to elimi-

nate the tick reservoir because the tick can survive for as long as 4 years without feeding.

OTHER SPOTTED FEVER RICKETTSIAE

At least five other rickettsial species in the spotted fever group cause human disease (Table 43-1). *R. akari*, the agent responsible for causing **rickettsialpox,** is occasionally isolated in the United States. Infections with *R. akari* are maintained in the rodent population through the bite of mouse ectoparasites (e.g., mites) and in mites by transovarian transmission. Humans become accidental hosts when bitten by infected mites.

Clinical infection with *R. akari* is biphasic. First, a papule develops at the site where the mite has bitten the host. This occurs approximately 1 week after the bite and quickly progresses to ulceration and then eschar formation. During this period, the rickettsiae spread systemically. After an incubation period of 7 to 24 days (average, 9 to 14 days), the second phase of the disease develops abruptly with high fever, severe headache, chills, sweats, myalgias, and photophobia. A generalized papulovesicular rash forms within 2 to 3 days. A poxlike progression of the rash is then seen, in which vesicles form and then crust over. Despite the appearance of the disseminated rash, rickettsialpox is usually mild and uncomplicated, with untreated patients completely healed within 2 to 3 weeks. Specific therapy with tetracycline or chloramphenicol speeds the process.

RICKETTSIA PROWAZEKII
Epidemiology

R. prowazekii is the etiological agent of **epidemic typhus,** also called **louse-borne typhus,** and the principal vector is the human body louse, *Pediculus humanus* (Box 43-2). In contrast to most other rickettsial diseases, hu-

BOX 43-2   Summary of *R. prowazekii* Infections

BACTERIAL FACTORS

Diseases—epidemic (louse-borne) typhus, recrudescent typhus (Brill-Zinsser disease), sporadic typhus.

Virulence factors—intracellular parasite; replicates in endothelial cells, with resulting vasculitis.

TRANSMISSION

Epidemic typhus spread person to person by louse vector.

Sporadic disease believed to be spread from squirrels to humans by squirrel fleas.

WHO IS AT RISK?

People in crowded, unsanitary conditions (epidemic typhus).

Recrudescent disease in previously infected patients (particularly immigrants from Eastern Europe) that can develop years after initial infection.

WHO IS AT RISK—CONT'D

People who come in contact with flying squirrels (sporadic typhus).

GEOGRAPHY/SEASON

Infection occurs most commonly in Central and South America and Africa and less commonly in United States; sporadic disease is present in eastern states of United States. No seasonal incidence.

MODES OF CONTROL

Antibiotic therapy includes administration of tetracyclines or chloramphenicol.

Reduction of lice population is achieved by use of insecticides.

Inactivated vaccine is available for high-risk populations.

mans are the primary reservoir of typhus. Epidemic typhus occurs among people living in crowded, unsanitary conditions that favor the spread of body lice, conditions such as those that arise during wars, famines, and natural disasters. Lice die from their infection within 2 to 3 weeks, and this prevents the transovarian transmission of *R. prowazekii.* The disease is present in Central and South America, Africa, and less commonly in the United States. The incidence of the disease in the United States is unknown because it is not classified as a disease reportable to public health departments. Sporadic disease in the United States is primarily restricted to rural areas of the eastern states. It occurs in this area because flying squirrels, as well as squirrel fleas and lice, are infected with *R. prowazekii.* Squirrel lice do not feed on humans, but the fleas are less discriminating and may be responsible for transmitting the *Rickettsia* organism from squirrels to humans. Epidemiological and serological evidence supports this hypothesis, but such transmission has not been documented.

Recrudescent disease with *R. prowazekii* (**Brill-Zinsser disease**) can occur in people years after their initial infection. Such people in the United States are primarily Eastern European immigrants who were exposed to epidemic typhus during World War II.

Clinical Syndromes

In a recent study of epidemic typhus in Africa, clinical disease was found to develop after a 2- to 30-day incubation period (average, 8 days). Most of the patients initially had nonspecific symptoms; then within 1 to 3 days, high fever, severe headache, and other symptoms such as chills, myalgias, arthralgia, and anorexia developed. Less than 40% of the patients had a petechial or macular rash, but darkly pigmented skin can obscure the rash. Complications of epidemic typhus can include myocarditis and central nervous system dysfunction; a mortality rate

as high as 66% has been reported in some epidemics. This high mortality rate undoubtedly stems from the poor general health, nutrition, and hygiene of the population, together with the lack of antibiotic therapy and proper supportive medical care. In patients with uncomplicated disease, the temperature returns to normal within 2 weeks, but complete convalescence may take 3 months or more.

As noted earlier, reactivation or recrudescent epidemic typhus (Brill-Zinsser disease) can occur years after the initial disease. However, the course is generally milder than epidemic typhus, and the convalescence is shorter.

Laboratory Diagnosis

CF testing with species-specific *R. prowazekii* antigens has been used but is insensitive. This test has been replaced now with IFA and agglutination tests.

Treatment, Prevention, and Control

The tetracyclines and chloramphenicol are highly effective in the treatment of epidemic typhus. However, antibiotic treatment must be combined with effective louse-control measures for the management of an epidemic. A formaldehyde-inactivated typhus vaccine is available, and its use is recommended in high-risk populations.

RICKETTSIA TYPHI
Epidemiology

Endemic or **murine typhus** is caused by *R. typhi.* Approximately 40 to 60 cases are reported annually in the United States from the Gulf states (especially Texas) and Southern California (Box 43-3). Endemic disease continues to be reported in people living in the temperate and subtropical coastal areas of Africa, Asia, Australia,

---

Europe, and South America. Rodents are the primary reservoir worldwide, and the rat flea (*Xenopsylla cheopis*) is the principal vector. However, the cat flea (*Ctenocephalides felis*), which inhabits cats, opossums, raccoons, and skunks, is considered an important vector for disease in the United States. Most cases occur during the warm months.

Clinical Syndromes

The incubation period for *R. typhi* disease is 7 to 14 days. The symptoms appear abruptly, with fever, severe headache, chills, myalgia, and nausea most common. A rash develops in approximately half of infected patients, most commonly late in the illness. It is typically restricted to the chest and abdomen but may extend to the palms and soles. The course of disease is generally uncomplicated, lasting less than 3 weeks even in untreated patients.

Laboratory Diagnosis

An *R. typhi*–specific IFA test is used to confirm the diagnosis of murine typhus. A fourfold increase in the titer or a single titer of at least 128 is diagnostic. Significant titers are usually detectable within 1 to 2 weeks of the onset of disease.

Treatment, Prevention, and Control

Tetracycline, doxycycline, or chloramphenicol is effective in the treatment of murine typhus, and patients respond promptly to these agents. It is difficult to control and prevent endemic typhus because the reservoir and vector are widely distributed. Any such efforts should be directed at controlling the rodent reservoir. An effective vaccine is not available.

RICKETTSIA TSUTSUGAMUSHI

R. tsutsugamushi is the etiological agent for **scrub typhus,** a disease transmitted to humans by mites (chiggers, red mites). The reservoir for this *Rickettsia* species is the mite population, in which the rickettsiae are transmitted by transovarian means. Infection is also present in the rodent population, which can serve as a reservoir for mite infections. Because mites feed only once during their life span, rodents are not believed to be an important reservoir for human disease. Scrub typhus is present in people living in eastern Asia, Australia, and Japan and other Western Pacific islands. It can also be imported into the United States.

R. tsutsugamushi disease develops suddenly after a 6- to 18-day incubation period (average, 10 to 12 days), with severe headache, fever, and myalgias. A macular to papular rash develops on the trunk in less than half of patients and spreads centrifugally to the extremities. Generalized lymphadenopathy, splenomegaly, central nervous system complications, and heart failure can occur. Fever in untreated patients disappears after 2 to 3 weeks, whereas patients who receive appropriate treatment with tetracycline, doxycycline, or chloramphenicol respond promptly. No vaccine is available, so the disease is prevented by avoiding exposure to chiggers (i.e., the wearing of protective clothing, the use of insect repellents).

EHRLICHIA
Pathogenesis and Immunity

Bacteria in the genus *Ehrlichia* (organisms named after Paul Ehrlich, one of the fathers of microbiology) are leukocytic organisms that parasitize lymphocytes, neutrophils, and monocytes. They spare erythrocytes. The intracellular location of the organisms protects them from the host's antibody response.

Epidemiology

The genus *Ehrlichia* is subdivided into three genogroups, with species that cause human disease found in each group (Table 43-3). *E. sennetsu*, primarily restricted to Japan, causes **Sennetsu fever** and was the first species found to cause human disease (Box 43-4). Tick-borne ehrlichiosis was first recognized in the United States in

Summary of Human *Ehrlichia* Infections

BACTERIAL FACTORS

Diseases—human monocytic ehrlichiosis *(E. chaffeensis);* human granulocytic ehrlichiosis *(E. equi* or related organism); Sennetsu fever *(E. sennetsu).*

Virulence factors—intracellular replication; ability to sequester or destroy infected circulating cells.

TRANSMISSION

Ticks: important reservoir and vector of monocytic and granulocytic ehrlichiosis; white-tailed deer: possible reservoir for granulocytic disease.

WHO IS AT RISK?

People in contact with ticks in endemic area.

GEOGRAPHY/SEASON

Sennetsu fever is restricted to Japan.

Human monocytic ehrlichiosis is found primarily in Southeastern, mid-Atlantic, and South Central states.

Human granulocytic ehrlichiosis is found primarily in Wisconsin, Minnesota, and Connecticut.

Disease is most common during warm months when ticks feed.

MODES OF CONTROL

Antibiotic therapy includes administration of doxycycline.

People should decrease contact with ticks, wear protective clothing and insect repellents, and remove embedded ticks immediately.

Vaccines are not available.

1986. The disease, **human monocytic ehrlichiosis,** was initially believed to be caused by *E. canis;* however, a serologically distinct species, *E. chaffeensis,* is now recognized to be the etiological agent. This organism was first isolated from an Army reservist at Fort Chaffee, Arkansas (hence the species name). More than 360 infections with this pathogen were reported from 1987 to 1995, predominantly in the southeastern, mid-Atlantic, and South Central areas of the United States (e.g., Oklahoma, Texas, Arkansas, Missouri, Georgia, South Carolina). This corresponds to the geographic distribution of the Lone Star tick *(A. americanum),* which is the primary reservoir-vector responsible for transmitting the organism. Clearly the prevalence of this disease has been underestimated. Serological studies have shown that antibodies to *E. chaffeensis* are at least as common as antibodies to *R. rickettsii,* which has a similar geographic distribution. Likewise, the prevalence of **human granulocytic ehrlichiosis** is unknown. The agent that causes this disease is either *E. equi* or a closely related species. Disease has been documented in Wisconsin, Minnesota, and Connecticut, and there is evidence of a broader distribution. The ticks associated with the transmission of this disease are the deer tick *(Ixodes scapularis)* and the dog tick *(D. variabilis),* and it is likely that deer are an important reservoir for this *Ehrlichia* species. The incidence of human disease in the United States is highest between May and July.

Clinical Syndromes

Patients with Sennetsu fever typically have an acute febrile illness that includes lethargy, cervical lymphadenopathy, and an increased number of peripheral mononuclear cells and atypical lymphocytes.

Human monocytic ehrlichiosis and granulocytic ehrlichiosis have similar manifestations and resemble Rocky Mountain spotted fever. Approximately 12 days after the tick bite (range, 1 to 3 weeks), a high fever, headache, malaise, and myalgia develop. Leukopenia, caused by the

TABLE 43-3	**Classification of *Ehrlichia* Species**
SPECIES	**DISEASE**
E. canis genogroup	
E. canis	Canine monocytic ehrlichiosis
E. chaffeensis	Human monocytic ehrlichiosis
E muris	Murine monocytic ehrlichiosis
E. ewingii	Canine granulocytic ehrlichiosis
E. phagocytophila genogroup	
E. phagocytophila	Ruminant granulocytic ehrlichiosis
E. equi	Equine granulocytic ehrlichiosis
	Canine granulocytic ehrlichiosis
	Human granulocytic ehrlichiosis
E. platys	Canine thrombocytic ehrlichiosis
E. sennetsu genogroup	
E. sennetsu	Sennetsu fever
E. risticii	Equine monocytic ehrlichiosis

destruction of leukocytes, and thrombocytopenia are also observed. A rash develops in only 20% of patients. Indeed, the absence of a rash has been partly responsible for the difficulty in diagnosing these diseases. Mortality is less than 5% in patients with monocytic ehrlichiosis and approaches 10% in those with granulocytic ehrlichiosis. Complications and death are most common in elderly patients. However, the prognosis is generally good in treated patients, with complete recovery the norm.

Laboratory Diagnosis

Microscopy and culture have not proved useful for the diagnosis of human ehrlichiosis. Intracellular organisms (morula) are rarely observed when peripheral blood smears are examined. Likewise, although the etiological agents of both forms of ehrlichiosis have been cultured in vitro, this is difficult to do and would not be performed in a clinical laboratory. The most common methods used for confirming the clinical diagnosis of ehrlichiosis are serology and DNA probe tests. An increase in the antibody titer is typically observed 2 or more weeks after the initial presentation. Species-specific reagents are now available, so the reactivity is specific. Species-specific DNA can also be characterized. Although this is primarily a research tool at present, it is believed that this will be the preferred test in the future.

Treatment, Prevention, and Control

Patients with suspected ehrlichiosis should be treated with doxycycline. Therapy should not be delayed pending laboratory confirmation of the disease because the incidence of complications and death is increased in patients whose treatment is delayed. Although chloramphenicol has been used, it is not believed to be effective. Infection is prevented by avoiding tick-infested areas, wearing protective clothing, and using insect repellents. Embedded ticks should be removed promptly. Vaccines are not available.

COXIELLA BURNETII
Pathogenesis and Immunity

Our understanding of the pathogenesis of **Q fever** is limited because acute disease is typically self-limiting and there is no animal model for the chronic disease. Human infection most commonly occurs after the inhalation of airborne particles from a contaminated environmental source rather than from the bite of an arthropod vector, as occurs in *Rickettsia* and *Ehrlichia* infections. *Coxiella* organisms proliferate locally in the respiratory tract and then disseminate to other organs. Pneumonia and granulomatous hepatitis develop in patients with severe, acute infections. Disease is associated with an antigenic

shift in the cell wall LPS (phase variation). Antibodies develop initially against the phase II antigen, and this response is a useful marker for acute disease. High antibody titers to phase I and II antigens are detected in patients with chronic infections. Despite the presence of antibodies, clinical improvement is associated with cellular immunity. The high antibody titers observed in patients with chronic disease lead to the formation of immune complexes and are in part responsible for producing some of the signs and symptoms of this disease.

Epidemiology

C. burnetii is extremely stable in harsh environmental conditions and can survive in soil for months to years. The range of hosts for *C. burnetii* is wide, with infections found in mammals, birds, and numerous different genera of ticks (Box 43-5). Sheep, cattle, and goats, as well as recently infected cats, dogs, and rabbits, are the primary reservoirs for human disease. The bacteria can reach high concentrations in the placenta of infected livestock. Thus dried placentas left on the ground after parturition, feces, urine, and tick feces can contaminate soil, which in turn can serve as a focus for infection if these bacteria become airborne and are inhaled. *C. burnetii* is also excreted in milk, so people who consume contaminated unpasteurized milk can become infected.

Q fever has a worldwide distribution. Although only 20 to 30 cases are reported annually in the United States, this is certainly an underestimation of the actual prevalence of this disease. Infection is common in the livestock in the United States; however, actual disease is very rare. Human exposure, particularly for ranchers, veterinarians, and food handlers, is frequent, and experimental studies have shown that the infectious dose of *C. burnetii* is small. Thus most human infections are mild or asympto-

---

BOX 43-5 **Summary of Human *C. burnetii* Infections**

BACTERIAL FACTORS

Disease—acute Q fever (influenza-like syndrome, atypical pneumonia, hepatitis, pericarditis, myocarditis, meningoencephalitis); chronic Q fever (endocarditis, hepatitis, pulmonary disease, infection of pregnant women).

Virulence factors—intracellular replication; formation of immune complexes in chronic disease; extremely stable in environment.

TRANSMISSION

Many reservoirs and hosts, including mammals, birds, and ticks.

Most human infections associated with contact with infected cattle, sheep, goats, dogs, and cats.

Most disease acquired through inhalation; possible disease from consumption of contaminated milk.

WHO IS AT RISK?

People exposed to infected livestock: farmers, ranchers, veterinarians, meat handlers.

Patients with previous cardiac damage: possible endocarditis.

GEOGRAPHY/SEASON

Worldwide; disease is relatively uncommon in United States.

No seasonal incidence.

MODES OF CONTROL

Doxycycline is used in acute disease; combination of doxycycline or trimethoprim-sulfamethoxazole with rifampin is used in chronic disease.

People should minimize contact with infected animals, although avoidance is not always possible because many animals are asymptomatic.

Use of vaccines is under evaluation.

matic. This is confirmed by serological studies, which have shown that more than half of all recent seroconverters do not have a history of disease. Infections also go undiagnosed because *C. burnetii* is frequently not considered in patients who have symptomatic disease.

Clinical Syndromes

C. burnetii infections can present in an acute or a chronic fashion. Acute disease is characterized by a long incubation period (average, 20 days), followed by the sudden onset of severe headache, high fever, chills, and myalgias. Respiratory symptoms are generally mild, mimicking the "atypical pneumonia" caused by *Mycoplasma* species (see Chapter 42) and *Chlamydia* organisms (see Chapter 44) but can be severe. Hepatosplenomegaly is present in approximately half of patients. Histologically diffuse granulomas are seen in the liver of most patients who have acute Q fever. The most common presentation of chronic Q fever is subacute endocarditis, generally on a prosthetic or previously damaged heart valve. The incubation period for chronic Q fever can be months to years, and the presentation is insidious. Unfortunately, chronic disease frequently progresses in an unrelenting fashion, and the prognosis is poor.

Laboratory Diagnosis

At present, Q fever can be diagnosed by culture (not commonly performed) or by specific serological tests. *C. burnetii* undergoes phase variation, characterized by the development of phase I and II antigens. The phase I antigens are only weakly antigenic. In acute Q fever, IgM and IgG antibodies are developed primarily against phase II antigens. Acute Q fever is diagnosed on the basis of a fourfold increase in antibody titers, an IgM titer of at least 50, or an IgG titer of at least 200. The IgM complement fixation titer in untreated patients is first positive after 2 weeks and then reverts to negative after 12 weeks. The IgG titer is positive after 12 weeks and persists for more than 1 year in 90% of patients. A diagnosis of chronic Q fever is confirmed by the demonstration of antibodies against both phase I and II antigens, with the titers to the phase I antigen typically higher.

Treatment, Prevention, and Control

Acute Q fever can be managed with oral tetracyclines (e.g., doxycycline). Chronic disease, such as Q fever endocarditis, should be treated for a prolonged period with a bactericidal combination of drugs such as rifampin and either doxycycline or trimethoprim-sulfamethoxazole. The difficulty in the treatment of patients with these infections is that antibiotic activity is suboptimal against the bacteria replicating in intracellular, acidic vacuoles.

An inactivated vaccine for Q fever has been developed but is not commercially available in the United States. Although it is protective for humans, the duration of immunity is unknown. The vaccine is poorly accepted for the immunization of livestock herds because infected animals are asymptomatic and it is unknown if animal immunization will alter the incidence of human disease.

CASE STUDY AND QUESTIONS

A 37-year-old man came to the local emergency room because of fever, arthralgias, myalgias, and malaise. He was well until 4 days before admission, when he developed a temperature to 40° C, a diffuse headache, photophobia, nausea, and vomiting. His family physician examined him and prescribed a cephalosporin antibiotic, but the patient did not experience any relief in symptoms. Physical examination in the emergency room revealed a critically ill man with a temperature of 39.7° C, pulse of 110 beats/min, respiratory rate of 28 breaths/min, and blood pressure of 100/60 mm Hg. A dermatological evaluation revealed no ulcerations, rashes, or petechiae. The patient recalled having had numerous tick bites 2 weeks before the onset of symptoms. Serological tests for *Rickettsia* species yielded negative findings; however, tests for *E. chaffeensis* were positive with a titer of 64.

1. What rickettsial and ehrlichial infections are observed in the United States? What are the organisms responsible, the reservoirs, and the vectors for each disease?
2. How are *Rickettsia*, *Coxiella*, and *Ehrlichia* organisms able to survive phagocytosis?
3. What are the major differences in clinical diseases caused by *R. rickettsii* and *E. chaffeensis*?
4. Describe the epidemiology of Q fever. How does the etiological agent for it differ from that for rickettsial infection?

Bibliography

Archibald L, Sexton D: Long-term sequelae of Rocky Mountain spotted fever, *Clin Infect Dis* 20:1122-1125, 1995.

Bakken J et al: Human granulocytic ehrlichiosis in the upper Midwest United States: a new species emerging? *JAMA* 272:212-218, 1994.

Dumler JS: Laboratory diagnosis of human rickettsial and ehrlichial infections, *Clin Microbiol Newslett* 18:57-61, 1996.

Dumler JS, Bakken JS: Ehrlichial diseases of humans: emerging tick-borne infections, *Clin Infect Dis* 20:1102-1110, 1995.

Dumler JS, Taylor JP, Walker DH: Clinical and laboratory features of murine typhus in South Texas, 1980 through 1987, *JAMA* 266:1365-1370, 1991.

Fishbein D, Dawson J, Robinson L: Human ehrlichiosis in the United States, 1985 to 1990, *Ann Intern Med* 120:736-743, 1994.

Magnarelli L, Dumler J: Ehrlichioses: emerging infectious diseases in tick-infected areas, *Clin Microbiol Newslett* 18:81-83, 1996.

Perine PL et al: A clinico-epidemiological study of epidemic typhus in Africa, *Clin Infect Dis* 14:1149-1158, 1992.

Raoult D, Marrie T: Q fever, *Clin Infect Dis* 20:489-496, 1995.

Reimer L: Q fever, *Clin Microbiol Rev* 6:193-198, 1993.

Rikihisa Y: The tribe Ehrlichieae and ehrlichial diseases, *Clin Microbiol Rev* 4:286-308, 1991.

Spach D et al: Tick-borne diseases in the United States, *N Engl J Med* 329:936-947, 1993.

Walker DH: *Biology of rickettsial diseases*, Boca Raton, Fla, 1988, CRC.

Winkler HH: *Rickettsia* species, *Ann Rev Microbiol* 44:131-153, 1990.

Chlamydia

The family Chlamydiaceae consists of one genus, *Chlamydia*, with four species: *C. trachomatis, C. psittaci, C. pneumoniae,* and *C. pecorum*. The first three are well-recognized human pathogens, but *C. pecorum* is rarely isolated and is not discussed further here. The chlamydiae were once considered to be viruses because they are small enough to pass through 0.45-μm filters and are obligate intracellular parasites. However, chlamydiae possess inner and outer membranes similar to those of gram-negative bacteria; contain both DNA and RNA; possess prokaryotic ribosomes; synthesize their own proteins, nucleic acids, and lipids; and are susceptible to numerous antibiotics. Unlike other bacteria, however, chlamydiae lack a peptidoglycan layer. Properties that differentiate the three common species are summarized in Table 44-1.

PHYSIOLOGY AND STRUCTURE

Chlamydiae exist in two morphologically distinct forms: the small (300- to 400-nm) infectious **elementary body** (EB) and the larger (800- to 1000-nm) noninfectious **reticulate body** (RB). Much like a spore, the EB is resistant to many harsh environmental factors. Despite the fact that these bacteria lack the rigid peptidoglycan layer found in most other bacteria, the outer membrane proteins are extensively cross-linked by disulfide bonds between cysteine residues. Although chlamydiae do not replicate in the EB form, they are infectious in this form; that is, they can bind to receptors on host cells and stimulate uptake by the infected cell. The RB is the metabolically active, replicating chlamydial form. Because the extensive cross-linked proteins are absent in the RBs, this form is osmotically fragile; however, the RBs are protected by their intracellular location. Other important structural components of chlamydiae include a genus-specific lipopolysaccharide (LPS) that can be detected in a complement fixation (CF) test and species- and strain-specific antigens in the outer membrane. Chlamydiae are nonmotile and nonpiliated.

Chlamydiae replicate by a unique growth cycle that occurs within susceptible host cells (Figure 44-1). The cycle is initiated when the infectious EBs become attached to the microvilli of susceptible cells, followed by active penetration into the host cell. After they are internalized, the chlamydiae remain within cytoplasmic phagosomes, where the replicative cycle proceeds. The fusion of cellular lysosomes with the EB-containing phagosome and subsequent intracellular killing are specifically inhibited. Phagolysosomal fusion is prevented if the outer membrane is intact. If the outer membrane is damaged or the chlamydiae are inactivated with heat or coated with antibodies, the bacteria are rapidly killed after phagolysosomal fusion. In addition, if other bacteria are phagocytosed with the chlamydiae, they are eliminated, so the protection is not a generalized phenomenon.

Within 6 to 8 hours after entering the cell, the EBs reorganize into the metabolically active RBs. RBs are able to synthesize their own DNA, RNA, and protein but lack the necessary metabolic pathways to produce their own high-energy phosphate compounds. Chlamydiae have been termed *energy parasites* because of this defect. Some strains may also depend on the host to provide specific amino acids. The RBs replicate by binary fission, which continues for the next 18 to 24 hours. The phagosome with accumulated RBs is called an **inclusion** and can be readily detected by histological stains. Approximately 18 to 24 hours after infection, the RBs begin reorganizing into the smaller EBs, and between 48 and 72 hours, the cell ruptures and then releases the infective EBs.

CHLAMYDIA TRACHOMATIS

C. trachomatis has a very limited host range, with infections restricted to humans and one strain that causes mouse pneumonitis. The species has been subdivided into three **biovars:** trachoma, LGV (lymphogranuloma venereum), and a third biovar that contains the mouse pneumonitis agent. It is thought that the mouse strain belongs in a separate species, although this reclassification has not yet occurred. The human biovars (Table 44-2) have been further divided into 15 serotypes (commonly called *serological variants,* or **serovars**) on the basis of antigenic differences in the major outer membrane protein (MOMP). The LGV biovar consists of three

TABLE 44-1	**Differentiation of Chlamydia Species that Cause Human Disease**			

PROPERTY	C. TRACHOMATIS	C PNEUMONIAE	C. PSITTACI
Host range	Primarily human pathogen	Primarily human pathogen	Primarily animal pathogen; occasionally infects humans
Biovars	LGV; trachoma; mouse pneumonitis	TWAR	Many
Diseases	LGV: lymphogranuloma venereum; trachoma: ocular trachoma, oculogenital disease, infant pneumonia	Bronchitis, pneumonia, sinusitis, pharyngitis, coronary artery disease(?)	Pneumonia (psittacosis)
EB morphology	Round, narrow periplasmic space	Pear-shaped, large periplasmic space	Round, narrow periplasmic space
Inclusion body morphology	Single, round inclusion per cell	Multiple, uniform inclusions per cell	Multiple, variably sized inclusions per cell
Plasmid DNA	Yes	No	Yes
Iodine-staining glycogen in inclusions	Yes	No	No
Susceptibility to sulfonamides	Yes	No	No

TABLE 44-2	**Clinical Spectrum of *C. trachomatis* Infections**

SEROVARS	DISEASES
A, B, Ba, C	Trachoma
B, Ba, D to K	Oculogenital disease (conjunctivitis, urethritis, proctitis, cervicitis); infant pneumonia
L_1, L_2, L_3	LGV

serovars (L_1, L_2, L_3), with the remaining 12 serovars (A, B, Ba, C to K) in the trachoma biovar.

Pathogenesis and Immunity

There is a limited range of cells that *C. trachomatis* can infect. Receptors for EBs are primarily restricted to non-ciliated columnar, cuboidal, or transitional epithelial cells, which are found on the mucous membranes of the urethra, endocervix, endometrium, fallopian tubes, anorectum, respiratory tract, and conjunctivae. The LGV biovar replicates in mononuclear phagocytes present in the lymphatic system. The clinical manifestations of chlamydial infections are due to the direct destruction of cells during replication and the host inflammatory response.

Chlamydiae gain access through minute abrasions or lacerations. In LGV the lesions form in the lymph nodes draining the site of primary infection (Figure 44-2). Granuloma formation is characteristic. The lesions may become necrotic, attract polymorphonuclear leukocytes, and cause the inflammatory process to spread to surrounding tissues. Subsequent rupture of the lymph node causes abscesses or sinus tracts to form. Infection with

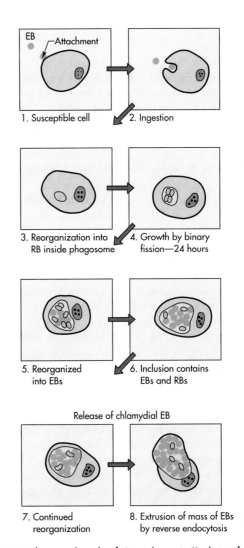

FIGURE 44-1 The growth cycle of *C. trachomatis*. (Redrawn from Batteiger B, Jones R: *Infect Dis Clin North Am* 1:55-81, 1987.)

FIGURE 44-2 Patient with lymphogranuloma venereum, showing bilateral inguinal buboes *(arrows)* with adenopathy above and below the inguinal ligament on one side (the groove sign) and thinning of the skin over the adenopathy on the opposite side, where the node is about to rupture. (From Holmes KK et al, editors: *Sexually transmitted diseases,* New York, 1984, McGraw-Hill.)

non-LGV serotypes of *C. trachomatis* stimulates a severe inflammatory response consisting of neutrophils, lymphocytes, and plasma cells. True lymphoid follicles with germinal centers eventually are induced.

Infection does not confer long-lasting immunity. Rather, reinfection characteristically induces a vigorous inflammatory response with subsequent tissue damage. This response produces the vision loss in patients with ocular infections and scarring with sterility and sexual dysfunction in patients with genital infections.

Epidemiology

C. trachomatis is found worldwide and causes trachoma (chronic keratoconjunctivitis), oculogenital disease, pneumonia, and LGV (Table 44-2). An estimated 500 million people worldwide are infected with the serovar trachoma, with 7 to 9 million blinded as a result. Trachoma is endemic in the Middle East, North Africa, and India. Infections occur predominantly in children, who are the chief reservoir of *C. trachomatis* in endemic areas. The incidence of infection is decreased in older children and adolescents; however, the incidence of blindness continues to increase through adulthood as the disease progresses. Trachoma is transmitted eye to eye by droplet, hands, contaminated clothing, and eye-seeking flies, which transmit ocular discharges from the eyes of infected children to the eyes of uninfected children. Because a high percentage of children in endemic areas harbor *C. trachomatis* in their respiratory and gastrointestinal tracts, the pathogen may also be transmitted by respiratory droplet or through fecal contamination. Trachoma generally is endemic in communities where the living conditions are crowded, sanitation is poor, and the personal hygiene of the people is poor—risk factors that promote the transmission of infections.

Most cases of *C. trachomatis* adult inclusion conjunctivitis occur in people who are 18 to 30 years of age, with genital infection probably preceding eye involvement. Autoinoculation and oral-genital contact are believed to be the routes of transmission. A third form of *C. trachomatis* eye infections is inclusion conjunctivitis in the newborn, an infection acquired during passage of the infant through an infected birth canal. *C. trachomatis* conjunctivitis develops in approximately 25% of infants whose mothers have active genital infections.

Pulmonary infection with *C. trachomatis* also occurs in newborns. A diffuse interstitial pneumonia develops in 10% to 20% of infants exposed to the pathogen at birth.

C. trachomatis is thought to be the most common sexually transmitted bacterial disease in the United States, with an estimated 4 million new cases per year. It is estimated that 50 million new infections occur each year worldwide. Most genital tract infections are caused by serotypes D through K. *Neisseria gonorrhoeae* and chlamydiae are the most common causes of epididymitis in sexually active men, and gram-negative bacilli (e.g., *Escherichia coli, Pseudomonas* species) are more common in men older than 35 years. As much as 15% of the cases of proctitis in homosexual men are caused by *C. trachomatis.*

LGV is a chronic sexually transmitted disease caused by *C. trachomatis* serotypes L_1, L_2, and L_3. It occurs sporadically in North America, Australia, and Europe but is highly prevalent in Africa, Asia, and South America. In the United States, 200 to 500 cases have been reported annually during the past decade, with male homosexuals the major reservoir of disease. Acute LGV is seen more frequently in men, primarily because symptomatic infection is less common in women.

Clinical Syndromes

C. trachomatis causes a wide range of clinical diseases (Box 44-1).

Trachoma

Trachoma is a chronic disease caused by serovars A, B, Ba, and C. Initially, patients have a follicular conjunctivitis with diffuse inflammation that involves the entire conjunctiva. The conjunctivae become scarred as the disease progresses, causing the patient's eyelids to turn inward. The inturned eyelashes in turn abrade the cornea, which eventually results in corneal ulceration, scarring, pannus formation (invasion of vessels into the cornea), and loss of vision. It is common for trachoma to recur after apparent healing, most likely the result of subclinical infections that have been documented in children in endemic areas and in U.S. immigrants who acquired trachoma during their childhoods in their native countries.

Adult Inclusion Conjunctivitis

An acute follicular conjunctivitis caused by the *C. trachomatis* strains associated with genital infections (B, Ba, D to K) has been documented in sexually active adults. The infection is characterized by mucopurulent discharge, keratitis, corneal infiltrates, and occasionally

BOX 44-1   Summary of *C. trachomatis* Infections

BACTERIAL FACTORS

Diseases—trachoma biovar: ocular trachoma, adult inclusion conjunctivitis, neonatal conjunctivitis, infant pneumonia, urogenital infections; LGV biovar: LGV, ocular LGV.

Virulence factors—intracellular replication, prevention of phagolysosomal fusion, survival of infectious EBs as a result of cross-linkage of membrane proteins.

Pathology in trachoma and the complications in genital disease result from reinfection.

TRANSMISSION

Sexually transmitted; most frequent bacterial pathogen in United States.

Infected patients, who may be asymptomatic.

Inoculation through break in skin or membranes.

Passage to newborn at birth.

Trachoma spread to eye by means of contaminated hand, droplets, clothing, and flies.

WHO IS AT RISK?

People with multiple sexual partners.

Homosexuals, who are more at risk for LGV.

WHO IS AT RISK—cont'd

Newborns born of infected mothers.

Reiter's syndrome: young white men.

Trachoma: children, particularly those in crowded living conditions where sanitation and hygiene are poor.

GEOGRAPHY/SEASON

Urogenital infections are worldwide.

LGV is highly prevalent in Africa, Asia, and South America.

Trachoma is endemic in Middle East, North Africa, and India.

No seasonal incidence.

MODES OF CONTROL

In LGV, doxycycline or erythromycin is given, and fluctuant lymph nodes are drained.

In ocular and genital diseases, azithromycin, doxycycline, or ofloxacin is administered.

In neonatal conjunctivitis and pneumonia, erythromycin is given.

Safe sex practices and prompt treatment of patient and sexual partners help control infection.

---

some corneal vascularization. Corneal scarring has been observed in patients with chronic infection.

Neonatal Conjunctivitis

Eye infections can also develop in infants exposed to *C. trachomatis* at birth. After an incubation of 5 to 12 days, the infant's eyelids swell, hyperemia occurs, and copious purulent discharge appears. Untreated infections may run a course as long as 12 months, during which time conjunctival scarring and corneal vascularization occur. Infants who are untreated or treated with topical therapy only are at risk for *C. trachomatis* pneumonia.

Infant Pneumonia

The incubation period for infant pneumonia is variable, but the onset generally occurs 2 to 3 weeks after birth. Rhinitis is initially observed in such infants, after which a distinctive staccato cough develops. The child remains afebrile throughout the clinical illness, which can last for several weeks. Radiographic signs of infection can persist for months.

Ocular Lymphogranuloma Venereum

The LGV serotypes of *C. trachomatis* have been implicated as a cause of Parinaud's oculoglandular conjunctivitis, which is a conjunctival inflammation associated with preauricular, submandibular, and cervical lymphadenopathy.

Urogenital Infections

Most genital tract infections in women are asymptomatic (as many as 80%) but can nevertheless become sympto-

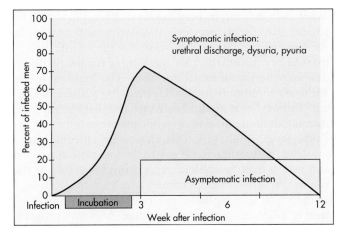

FIGURE 44-3 Time course of untreated chlamydial urethritis in men.

matic; the clinical manifestations include cervicitis, endometritis, urethritis, salpingitis, bartholinitis, and perihepatitis. Chlamydial infection may be overlooked in asymptomatic patients. A mucopurulent discharge and hypertrophic ectopy are seen in patients with symptomatic infection, and generally yield more organisms on cultures than in those with asymptomatic infections. Urethritis caused by *C. trachomatis* may occur with or without a concurrent cervical infection. As noted earlier, most genital infections in men caused by *C. trachomatis* are symptomatic; however, as many as 25% of chlamydial infections in men may be asymptomatic (Figure 44-3). Approximately 35% to 50% of cases of **nongonococcal**

urethritis are caused by *C. trachomatis*. **Postgonococcal urethritis** results from coinfection with both *Neisseria gonorrhoeae* and *C. trachomatis*. The symptoms of the chlamydial infection develop after successful treatment of the gonorrhea because the incubation period is longer. Although there is less purulent exudate in patients with chlamydial urethral infections, infections cannot be reliably differentiated from gonorrhea.

Reiter's syndrome (urethritis, conjunctivitis, polyarthritis, and mucocutaneous lesions) is believed to be initiated by genital infection with *C. trachomatis*. Although chlamydiae have not been isolated from the synovial fluid of such patients, EBs have been observed in the fluid or tissue from men with sexually acquired reactive arthritis. The disease usually occurs in young white men. Approximately 50% to 65% of patients with Reiter's syndrome have a chlamydial genital infection at the onset of arthritis, and serological studies indicate that more than 80% of men with Reiter's syndrome have evidence of a preceding or concurrent infection with *C. trachomatis*.

Lymphogranuloma Venereum

After an incubation of 1 to 4 weeks, a primary lesion appears at the site of infection (e.g., penis, urethra, glans, scrotum, vaginal wall, cervix, vulva) in patients with LGV. The lesion is often overlooked, however, because it is small, painless, and inconspicuous and heals rapidly. The patient may experience fever, headache, and myalgia at the time of the lesion. The second stage of infection is marked by inflammation and swelling of the lymph nodes draining the site of initial infection. The inguinal nodes are most commonly involved, becoming painful, fluctuant "buboes" that gradually enlarge and that can rupture, forming draining fistulas. Systemic manifestations may include fever, chills, anorexia, headache, meningismus, myalgias, and arthralgias. Proctitis is common in women and results from lymphatic spread from the cervix or the vagina. Proctitis develops in men after anal intercourse or as the result of lymphatic spread from the urethra. Untreated LGV may resolve at this stage, or it may progress to a chronic ulcerative phase in which genital ulcers, fistulas, strictures, or genital elephantiasis develops.

Laboratory Diagnosis

C. trachomatis infection can be diagnosed on the basis of cytological, serological, or culture findings; through the direct detection of antigen in clinical specimens; and through the use of molecular probes. The sensitivity of each method depends on the patient population examined, the site where the specimen is obtained, and the nature of the disease. For example, symptomatic infections are generally easier to diagnose than asymptomatic infections because more chlamydiae are present in the specimen. The quality of the specimen is also important. Because chlamydiae are obligate intracellular bacteria, specimens must be obtained from the involved site (e.g., urethra, cervix, rectum, oropharynx, conjunctiva). A specimen of pus or an urethral exudate is inadequate. It has been estimated that 30% of the specimens submitted for study in patients with suspected *Chlamydia* infection are inappropriate.

Cytology

Examination of Giemsa-stained cell scrapings for the presence of inclusions was the first method used for the diagnosis of *C. trachomatis* infection. However, this method is insensitive compared with culture or direct immunofluorescence. Likewise, Papanicolaou's staining of cervical material has been found to be an insensitive and nonspecific method.

Culture

The isolation of *C. trachomatis* in cell culture remains the most specific method of diagnosing *C. trachomatis* infections. The bacteria infect a restricted range of cell lines in vitro (e.g., HeLa-229, McCoy, BHK-21, Buffalo green monkey kidney cells), similar to the narrow range of cells they infect in vivo. The test sensitivity has been improved as the result of modifications in the culture procedures. These modifications include pretreatment of the specimen with chemical inhibitors of host cell metabolism (e.g., cycloheximide), centrifugation of the specimen onto the cell monolayers (modifies the host cell), use of the shell vial technique (growth of the host cell monolayer on glass coverslips rather than in small microtiter wells), multiple passages or subcultures of infected cells, and the use of iodine stains or fluorescein-conjugated antibodies to detect intracellular inclusions (iodine stains glycogen-containing *C. trachomatis* inclusions; Figure 44-4). Despite these improvements, the sensitivity of culture is compromised if inadequate specimens are used and if chlamydial viability has been lost during transport of the specimen. It has been estimated that the sensitivity of the findings yielded by a single endocervical specimen may be only 70% to 85%.

FIGURE 44-4 Iodine-stained *C. trachomatis* inclusion bodies *(arrows)*.

Antigen Detection

Two general approaches have been used to detect chlamydial antigens in clinical specimens: direct immunofluorescence staining (DFA) with fluorescein-conjugated monoclonal antibodies (Figure 44-5) and enzyme-linked immunoassays. In both assays, antibodies are used that have been prepared against either the chlamydial MOMP or the cell wall LPS. Because antigenic determinants on LPS may be shared with other bacteria, particularly those in fecal specimens, antibody tests that target the LPS antigen are considered less specific. The sensitivity of each assay method has been reported to vary enormously, but neither is considered as sensitive as culture, particularly if male urethral specimens or specimens from asymptomatic patients are used. The latter pose a problem because relatively few chlamydiae may be present.

Nucleic Acid Probes

Three different nucleic acid probe tests are currently available. One measures for the presence of a species-specific sequence of 16S rRNA. The advantage of this test is that the nucleic acid does not have to be amplified. The other two tests are based on the amplification of target nucleic acids, one by the polymerase chain reaction (**PCR**) and the other by the ligase chain reaction (**LCR**). Both amplification techniques are highly sensitive (generally reported to be 90% to 98% sensitive) and may rapidly replace culture or the antigen detection methods in the laboratory diagnosis of *C. trachomatis* infection.

Serology

The skin test for LGV (**Frei test**) is of historical interest only because it was found to be both insensitive and nonspecific. LGV is currently diagnosed on the basis of the CF test, which measures complement-fixing antibodies directed against the LPS genus-specific antigen. Unfortunately, because the test is positive in patients exposed to other strains of *C. trachomatis,* it is not specific for LGV. Serological testing is of limited value in the diagnosis of other chlamydial urogenital infections in adults because the test cannot differentiate between current and past infection. Most adults with infection have been previously exposed to *C. trachomatis* and thus are seropositive. Although IgM may not always be produced, the presence of a high titer of IgM (e.g., at least 128) indicates a recent infection. A negative serological test may be used as the basis for excluding infection; however, antibodies are not detected early in the disease, and the response may be diminished in patients who have received antibiotic therapy. Detection of IgM to *C. trachomatis* is useful in the diagnosis of neonatal infection.

Treatment, Prevention, and Control

It is recommended that patients with LGV be treated with doxycycline for 21 days, with erythromycin or sulfisoxazole recommended for pregnant women or patients unable to tolerate doxycycline. Ocular and genital infections in adults should be treated with one dose of azithromycin, doxycycline for 7 days, or ofloxacin for 7 days. Doxycycline and azithromycin cannot be used in pregnant women. Antibiotic therapy without improved sanitation is of limited value in areas where trachoma is endemic. The surgical correction of lid deformities reduces the likelihood of trachoma-induced blindness. Newborn conjunctivitis and pneumonia should be treated with erythromycin for 10 to 14 days.

It is difficult to prevent *C. trachomatis* infections because the population with endemic disease frequently has limited access to medical care. The blindness associated with advanced stages of this disease can be prevented only by prompt treatment of early disease and the prevention of reexposure. Although treatment can be successful in individuals living in areas where the disease is endemic, it is difficult to eradicate the disease within a population and to prevent reinfections. *Chlamydia* conjunctivitis and genital infections are prevented through the use of safe sexual practices and the prompt treatment of symptomatic patients and their sexual partners.

CHLAMYDIA PNEUMONIAE

C. pneumoniae was first isolated from the conjunctiva of a child in Taiwan. It was initially considered a psittacosis strain because of the morphology of the inclusions produced in cell culture. However, it was shown subsequently that the Taiwan isolate (TW-183) is serologically related to a pharyngeal isolate designated AR-39, and the strain was designated TWAR. DNA homology studies have shown that the TWAR strain is a species distinct from both *C. trachomatis* and *C. psittaci,* and it is now called *C. pneumoniae.* Only a single serotype has been identified. Infection is transmitted by respiratory secretions; no animal reservoir has been identified.

C. pneumoniae is an important cause of bronchitis, pneumonia, sinusitis, and possibly atherosclerosis (Box

FIGURE 44-5 Fluorescent-stained elementary bodies *(arrows)* in a clinical sample.

BOX 44-2 Summary of *C. pneumoniae* Infections

BACTERIAL FACTORS

Diseases—bronchitis, pneumonia, sinusitis, pharyngitis, atherosclerosis(?).

Virulence factors—intracellular replication; prevention of phagolysosome fusion; ability to infect and destroy ciliated epithelial cells of respiratory tract, smooth muscle cells, endothelial cells, and macrophages; extracellular survival of infectious EBs.

TRANSMISSION

Person-to-person spread by inhalation of infectious aerosols. No animal reservoir.

WHO IS AT RISK?

High prevalence of infections throughout life; most infections asymptomatic.
Disease most common in adults.

GEOGRAPHY/SEASON

Worldwide.
No seasonal incidence.

MODES OF CONTROL

Treatment is with tetracycline or erythromycin; failures are common, so retreatment may be required.

44-2). Infection is believed to be common; an estimated 200,000 to 300,000 cases of *C. pneumoniae* pneumonia are reported annually, with disease most common in adults. More than 50% of people have serological evidence of past infections. Most *C. pneumoniae* infections are asymptomatic or mild and include a persistent cough and malaise; patients do not need to be hospitalized. More severe respiratory tract infections typically involve a single lobe of the lungs. These infections cannot be differentiated from other atypical pneumonias, such as those caused by *Mycoplasma pneumoniae*, *Legionella pneumoniae*, and respiratory viruses.

The role of *C. pneumoniae* in the pathogenesis of atherosclerosis remains to be defined. The disease is believed to result from an inflammatory response to chronic infection. It is known that *C. pneumoniae* can infect and grow in smooth muscle cells, endothelial cells of the coronary artery, and macrophages. The organism has also been demonstrated in biopsy specimens of atherosclerotic lesions by culture, PCR amplification, immunohistological staining, electron microscopy, and in situ hybridization. It is possible that the organism is responsible for the endovascular pathology.

Diagnosis of *C. pneumoniae* infections is difficult. The organisms cannot grow in the cell lines used for the isolation of *C. trachomatis*. However, it has recently been shown that *C. pneumoniae* can infect and grow in the HL cell line, as well as in HEp-2 cells. Culture is positive in 50% to 75% of patients with serological evidence of a recent infection. PCR amplification of chlamydial nucleic acids is approximately 25% more sensitive than culture. However, this test is primarily a research tool and is not currently available in a commercially prepared kit. CF testing or microimmunofluorescence can be used to make a serological diagnosis. Because the CF test uses a genus-specific antigen, it is not specific for *C. pneumoniae* infection; the microimmunofluorescence test uses *C. pneumoniae* EBs as antigen, so it is specific. A four-fold increase in the titer of IgM or IgG is diagnostic, whereas an IgM titer of 16 or more or an IgG titer of

512 or more is suggestive of recent infection. However, the microimmunofluorescence test is available only in a few specialized laboratories.

Tetracycline or erythromycin administered for 10 to 14 days has been used to treat infections. Unfortunately, it is relatively common for treatment to fail, necessitating retreatment. Control of exposure to *C. pneumoniae* is likely to be difficult because the bacterium is ubiquitous.

CHLAMYDIA PSITTACI

C. psittaci is the cause of **psittacosis (parrot fever),** which can be transmitted to humans. The disease was first observed in parrots, thus the name *psittacosis* (*psittakos* is the Greek word for "parrot"). In reality, however, the natural reservoir of *C. psittaci* is virtually any species of birds, and the disease has been referred to more appropriately as *ornithosis* (derived from the Greek word *ornithos* for "bird"). Other animals such as sheep, cows, and goats, as well as humans, can become infected. The organism is present in the blood, tissues, feces, and feathers of infected birds that may appear either ill or healthy.

Infection occurs by means of the respiratory tract, after which the bacteria spread to the reticuloendothelial cells of the liver and spleen (Box 44-3). The organisms multiply in these sites, producing focal necrosis. The lung and other organs are then seeded as the result of hematogenous spread, which causes a predominantly lymphocytic inflammatory response in the alveolar and interstitial spaces. Edema, thickening of the alveolar wall, infiltration of macrophages, necrosis, and occasionally hemorrhage occur at these sites. Mucous plugs develop in the bronchioles, causing cyanosis and anoxia.

Approximately 50 to 100 cases of the disease are reported annually in the United States, with most infections in adults (Figure 44-6). However, this number certainly is an underestimation of the true prevalence of disease because human infections may be asymptomatic or mild, exposure to an infected bird may not be sus-

---

> **BOX 44-3   Summary of *C. psittaci* Infections**
>
> **BACTERIAL FACTORS**
>
> Diseases—psittacosis (ornithosis).
> Virulence factors—intracellular parasite, prevention of phagolysosomal fusion, survival of infectious EBs as result of cross-linkage of membrane proteins.
>
> **TRANSMISSION**
>
> Infection acquired by contact with infected bird or animal (may appear healthy).
> Person-to-person infection very uncommon.
>
> **WHO IS AT RISK?**
>
> Disease most common in adults.
> Occupations at increased risk include veterinarians, zookeepers, pet shop workers, and employees in poultry-processing plants.
>
> **GEOGRAPHY/SEASON**
>
> Worldwide.
> No seasonal incidence, although periodic outbreaks are observed.
>
> **MODES OF CONTROL**
>
> Tetracycline or erythromycin is used for treatment.
> Infections should be controlled in domestic and imported pet birds using chlortetracycline.

---

pected, convalescent serum may not be collected so that the clinical diagnosis can be confirmed, and antibiotic therapy may blunt the antibody response. Further, because of the serological cross-reactions with *C. pneumoniae,* specific estimates of the prevalence of disease will remain unreliable until a definitive diagnostic test is developed.

The bacterium is usually transmitted to humans through the inhalation of dried bird excrement. Person-to-person transmission is rare. Veterinarians, zookeepers, pet shop workers, and employees of poultry-processing plants are at increased risk for this infection.

The illness develops after an incubation of 7 to 15 days and is usually manifested by headache, high fever, and chills (Figure 44-7). Other early manifestations include malaise, anorexia, myalgia, arthralgia, and occasionally a pale macular rash. Pulmonary signs include a nonproductive cough, rales, and consolidation. Central nervous system involvement is common, usually consisting of headache, but encephalitis, convulsions, coma, and death may occur in severe cases. Patients may suffer gastrointestinal tract symptoms such as nausea, vomiting, and diarrhea. Other systemic symptoms include carditis, hepatomegaly, splenomegaly, and follicular keratoconjunctivitis.

Psittacosis is usually diagnosed on the basis of serological findings. A fourfold increase in titer, shown by the CF testing of paired acute and convalescent phase sera, is diagnostic. Titer increases are usually observed by the end of the second week of illness. A single CF titer of at least 32 is evidence of recent infection. *C. psittaci* can be isolated in cell culture (e.g., L cells) after 5 to 10 days of incubation, although this is rarely done in clinical laboratories. Genus-specific antigen tests and molecular probes can also be used to confirm the clinical diagnosis.

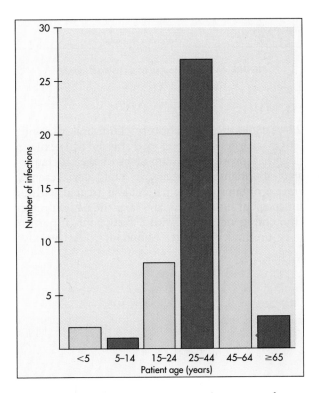

FIGURE 44-6 Age of patients with documented *C. psittaci* infections, 1995. (Data from *MMWR* 44:10, 1996.)

Infections can be treated successfully with tetracycline or erythromycin. Psittacosis can be prevented only through the control of infections in domestic and imported pet birds. This can be done by treating birds with chlortetracycline hydrochloride for 45 days. No vaccine currently exists for this disease.

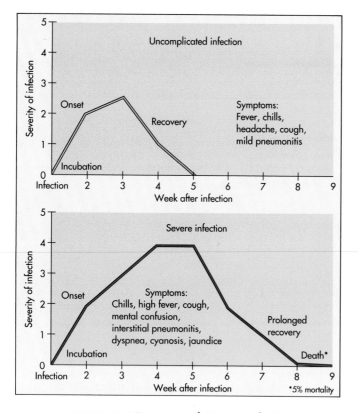

FIGURE 44-7 Time course of *C. psittaci* infection.

but no organisms were observed on Gram stain. Culture of the discharge was negative for *N. gonorrhoeae* but positive for *C. trachomatis.*

1. Why was penicillin ineffective against *Chlamydia*? What antibiotic can be used to treat the chlamydial infection in this patient?
2. Describe the growth cycle of *Chlamydia* organisms. What structural features make the EBs and RBs well suited for their environment?
3. Describe the differences among the three chlamydial species that cause human disease.
4. Compare the epidemiology of psittacosis with respiratory infections caused by the other chlamydial species.

CASE STUDIES AND QUESTIONS

A 22-year-old man had a history of urethral pain and purulent discharge. This developed after he had sexual contact with a prostitute. Gram stain of the discharge revealed abundant gram-negative diplococci resembling *Neisseria* organisms. The patient was treated with penicillin and sent home. Two days later the patient returned to the emergency room with a complaint of persistent, watery urethral discharge. Abundant white blood cells

BIBLIOGRAPHY

Batteiger BE, Jones RB: Chlamydial infections, *Infect Dis Clin North Am* 1:55-81, 1987.

Black C: Current methods of laboratory diagnosis of *Chlamydia trachomatis* infections, *Clin Microbiol Rev* 10:160-184, 1997.

Gasdos C et al: Phylogenetic relationship of *Chlamydia pneumoniae* to *Chlamydia psittaci* and *Chlamydia trachomatis* as determined by analysis of 16S ribosomal DNA sequences, *Int J Syst Bacteriol* 43:610-612, 1993.

Grayston J et al: Evidence that *Chlamydia pneumoniae* causes pneumonia and bronchitis, *J Infect Dis* 168:1231-1235, 1993.

Oldach D et al: Rapid diagnosis of *Chlamydia psittaci* pneumonia, *Clin Infect Dis* 17:338-343, 1993.

Ramirez J and the *Chlamydia pneumoniae* Atherosclerosis Study Group: Isolation of *Chlamydia pneumoniae* from the coronary artery of a patient with coronary atherosclerosis, *Ann Intern Med* 125:979-982, 1996.

Schacter J: *Biology of* Chlamydia trachomatis. In Holmes KK et al, editors: *Sexually transmitted diseases*, New York, 1984, McGraw-Hill.

Scieux C et al: Lymphogranuloma venereus: 27 cases in Paris, *J Infect Dis* 160:662-668, 1989.

CHAPTER 45

Role of Bacteria in Disease

A summary of the bacteria most commonly associated with human disease is presented in this chapter. The biology of individual groups of bacteria was examined in Chapters 22 through 44. However, human diseases occur not as discrete groups of organisms but rather as pathogenic processes in one or more organ systems. The clinical management of infections is therefore predicated on the ability to develop a differential diagnosis. That is, it is critically important to know the organisms most commonly associated with a particular infectious process (e.g., bacteremia, pneumonia, gastroenteritis) or epidemiological situation (e.g., foodborne or waterborne diseases, arthropod-associated infections).

The development of an infection depends on the complex interactions of the host's susceptibility to infection, the organism's virulence potential, and the opportunity for interaction between host and organism. It is impossible to summarize in a single chapter the complex interactions that lead to the development of disease in each organ system. That is the domain of texts in infectious disease. Rather, this chapter is intended to serve as a very broad overview of the bacteria commonly associated with infections at specific body sites and with specific diseases (Tables 45-1 to 45-4). Because many factors influence the relative frequency with which specific organisms cause disease (e.g., age, underlying disease, epidemiological factors, host immunity), no attempt is made to define all the factors associated with disease caused by specific organisms. That material is provided in the preceding chapters. Furthermore, the roles of fungi, viruses, and parasites are not considered here but rather in the respective sections of this book. For additional information about organ-oriented infections, see the texts listed in the bibliography.

Bibliography

Balows A, Truper HG, editors: *The prokaryotes,* ed 2, New York, 1992, Springer-Verlag.

Finegold SM, George WL: *Anaerobic infections in humans,* San Diego, 1989, Academic.

Kelley WN et al: *Textbook of internal medicine,* Philadelphia, 1989, JB Lippincott.

Mandell GL, Bennett JE, Dolin R, editors: *Principles and practice of infectious diseases,* ed 4, New York, 1995, Churchill Livingstone.

Murray PR et al, editors: *Manual of clinical microbiology,* ed 6, Washington, DC, 1995, ASM.

TABLE 45-1   Summary of Bacteria Associated with Human Disease

SYSTEM AFFECTED	COMMON PATHOGENS	UNCOMMON PATHOGENS
BLOOD		
Bacteremia	Coagulase-negative *Staphylococcus* species, *Staphylococcus aureus*, *Enterococcus* species, *Streptococcus pneumoniae*, *Escherichia coli*, *Klebsiella pneumoniae*, *Enterobacter* species, *Proteus mirabilis*, *Pseudomonas aeruginosa*	Many aerobic and anaerobic bacteria, *Mycobacterium avium*, other mycobacteria
Catheter-related sepsis	Coagulase-negative *Staphylococcus*, *Staphylococcus aureus*, *Corynebacterium* species, *Propionibacterium* species	—
Endocarditis	Viridans group *Streptococcus*, coagulase-negative *Staphylococcus*, *Staphylococcus aureus*	*Enterococcus* species, *Streptococcus pneumoniae*, HACEK group (*Haemophilus aphrophilus*, *Actinobacillus* species, *Cardiobacterium hominis*, *Eikenella corrodens*, *Kingella* species), *Coxiella burnetii*, *Chlamydia psittaci*, *Pseudomonas* species, *Serratia* species, other enteric gram-negative bacilli, *Bartonella* species
Septic thrombophlebitis	*Staphylococcus aureus*, *Klebsiella* species, *Enterobacter* species, *Pseudomonas* species, *Bacteroides* species, *Fusobacterium* species	—
CENTRAL NERVOUS SYSTEM		
Acute meningitis	*Streptococcus pneumoniae*, *Neisseria meningitidis*, group B *Streptococcus*, *Escherichia coli*	*Haemophilus influenzae*, *Listeria monocytogenes*, *Leptospira* species, *Staphylococcus aureus*, enteric gram-negative bacilli, *Nocardia* species, *Rickettsia* species, *Ehrlichia* species
Chronic meningitis	*Mycobacterium tuberculosis*, *Nocardia* species	*Borrelia burgdorferi*, *Brucella* species, other mycobacteria, *Treponema pallidum*
Encephalitis	—	*Rickettsia* species, *Ehrlichia* species, *Coxiella* species, *Mycoplasma pneumoniae*, *Listeria* species, *Nocardia* species, *Actinomyces* species
Brain abscess	Oral aerobic and anaerobic bacteria, *Staphylococcus aureus*, Enterobacteriaceae	*Clostridium* species, *Nocardia* species, *Mycobacterium tuberculosis*, *Streptococcus pneumoniae*
Subdural empyema	*Staphylococcus aureus*	*Streptococcus pneumoniae*, mixed anaerobes, *Haemophilus* species, group B *Streptococcus*, *Neisseria meningitidis*
UPPER RESPIRATORY TRACT		
Sinusitis	*Streptococcus pneumoniae*, *Moraxella catarrhalis*, *Haemophilus influenzae*, anaerobes, *Staphylococcus aureus*	Group A *Streptococcus*
Pharyngitis	Group A *Streptococcus*	Group C *Streptococcus*, *Arcanobacterium haemolyticum*, *Mycoplasma pneumoniae*, *Chlamydia pneumoniae*, *Neisseria gonorrhoeae*, *Corynebacterium diphtheriae*, *Corynebacterium ulcerans*, mixed anaerobes (Vincent's angina)
Tracheobronchitis	*Mycoplasma pneumoniae*	—
Epiglottitis	—	*Haemophilus influenzae*, nonencapsulated *Haemophilus* species, *Streptococcus pneumoniae*, *Staphylococcus aureus*
Otitis externa	*Pseudomonas aeruginosa*	*Staphylococcus aureus*, group A *Streptococcus*, *Proteus mirabilis*

TABLE 45-1 **Summary of Bacteria Associated with Human Disease—cont'd**

SYSTEM AFFECTED	COMMON PATHOGENS	UNCOMMON PATHOGENS
UPPER RESPIRATORY TRACT—cont'd		
Otitis media	Streptococcus pneumoniae, Haemophilus influenzae, Moraxella catarrhalis, anaerobes	Staphylococcus aureus, group A Streptococcus
LOWER RESPIRATORY TRACT		
Bronchitis	Haemophilus influenzae, Streptococcus pneumoniae, Moraxella catarrhalis, Mycoplasma pneumoniae, Chlamydia pneumoniae	Enteric gram-negative bacilli, Bordetella pertussis
Acute pneumonia	Streptococcus pneumoniae, Staphylococcus aureus, Mycoplasma pneumoniae, Chlamydia species, Klebsiella pneumoniae, Legionella species, Pseudomonas aeruginosa, mixed anaerobes	Many aerobic bacteria
Chronic pneumonia	Mycobacterium tuberculosis, Nocardia species, mixed anaerobes	Actinomyces species, Burkholderia pseudomallei, Mycobacterium species
Pleural effusion/empyema	Staphylococcus aureus, Streptococcus pneumoniae, group A Streptococcus, mixed anaerobes	—
Lung abscess	Staphylococcus aureus, Klebsiella pneumoniae, mixed anaerobes, Pseudomonas aeruginosa, group A Streptococcus, Nocardia species, Mycobacterium tuberculosis	Enteric gram-negative bacilli, Rhodococcus species
EYE		
Conjunctivitis	Streptococcus pneumoniae, Staphylococcus aureus, Haemophilus influenzae (H. aegyptius), Neisseria gonorrhoeae, Chlamydia trachomatis	—
Keratitis	Staphylococcus aureus, Streptococcus pneumoniae, group A Streptococcus, Pseudomonas aeruginosa, Moraxella species	—
Endophthalmitis	Staphylococcus aureus, Pseudomonas aeruginosa, Bacillus species, Streptococcus pneumoniae	Coagulase-negative Staphylococcus
INTRAABDOMINAL		
Spontaneous peritonitis	Escherichia coli, Klebsiella pneumoniae, Streptococcus pneumoniae, Enterococcus species	Staphylococcus aureus, anaerobes, Neisseria gonorrhoeae, Chlamydia trachomatis, Mycobacterium tuberculosis
Secondary peritonitis	Escherichia coli, Enterococcus species, Bacteroides fragilis, other enteric anaerobes, Pseudomonas aeruginosa	Staphylococcus aureus, Neisseria gonorrhoeae, Mycobacterium tuberculosis
Dialysis-associated peritonitis	Coagulase-negative Staphylococcus, Staphylococcus aureus, Corynebacterium species, Escherichia coli, Klebsiella species, Enterobacter species, Proteus species	Enteric gram-negative bacilli
Intraabdominal abscess	Escherichia coli, Bacteroides fragilis group, Enterococcus species	Enteric gram-negative bacilli, Actinomyces species
GASTROINTESTINAL		
Gastritis	Helicobacter pylori	—
Gastroenteritis	Campylobacter species, Salmonella species, Shigella species, Yersinia species, Aeromonas species, Plesiomonas shigelloides, Escherichia coli (enterotoxic, enteroinvasive, enteropathogenic, enterohemorrhagic), Vibrio cholerae, Vibrio parahaemolyticus, Bacillus cereus, Pseudomonas aeruginosa, Clostridium perfringens, Clostridium difficile	—

Continued

TABLE 45-1	**Summary of Bacteria Associated with Human Disease—cont'd**	
SYSTEM AFFECTED	**COMMON PATHOGENS**	**UNCOMMON PATHOGENS**
GASTROINTESTINAL—cont'd		
Proctitis	Neisseria gonorrhoeae, Chlamydia trachomatis, Treponema pallidum	—
Intoxication (toxin in food)	Staphylococcus aureus, Bacillus cereus, Clostridium botulinum, Pseudomonas aeruginosa	—
GENITAL		
Urethritis	Neisseria gonorrhoeae, Chlamydia trachomatis, Ureaplasma urealyticum	Neisseria meningitidis
Bacterial vaginosis	Synergistic infection with anaerobes (e.g., Mobiluncus species, Bacteroides species, Peptostreptococcus species)	—
Cervicitis	Neisseria gonorrhoeae, Chlamydia trachomatis	Actinomyces species, Mycobacterium tuberculosis
Genital ulcers	Treponema pallidum, Haemophilus ducreyi, Chlamydia trachomatis (lymphogranuloma venereum), Calymmatobacterium granulomatosis	Francisella tularensis
URINARY TRACT		
Cystitis	Escherichia coli, Proteus mirabilis, Klebsiella species, Enterococcus species, Staphylococcus saprophyticus	Staphylococcus aureus, Corynebacterium ureolyticus
Pyelonephritis	Escherichia coli, Proteus mirabilis, Klebsiella species, Staphylococcus aureus	Enterococcus species, Corynebacterium ureolyticus
Prostatitis	Escherichia coli, Proteus mirabilis, Klebsiella species, Enterobacter species, Enterococcus species	Neisseria gonorrhoeae, Chlamydia trachomatis, Mycobacterium tuberculosis
Urinary calculi	Proteus mirabilis, Klebsiella pneumoniae, Corynebacterium urealyticum, Staphylococcus saprophyticus	—
Renal abscess	Staphylococcus aureus, mixed anaerobes	—
BONES AND JOINTS		
Arthritis	Staphylococcus aureus, Neisseria gonorrhoeae, Streptococcus pneumoniae	Brucella species, Haemophilus influenzae, enteric gram-negative bacilli, Nocardia species, Mycobacterium species
Osteomyelitis	Staphylococcus aureus, groups A and B Streptococcus, Pseudomonas aeruginosa, Escherichia coli, Salmonella species, other enteric gram-negative bacilli	Mycobacterium tuberculosis, anaerobes
Prosthesis-associated infections	Staphylococcus aureus, coagulase-negative Staphylococcus, group A Streptococcus, viridans group Streptococcus	Corynebacterium species, Propionibacterium species, Peptostreptococcus species
SKIN AND SOFT TISSUE		
Impetigo	Group A Streptococcus, Staphylococcus aureus	—
Folliculitis	Staphylococcus aureus, Pseudomona aeruginosa	—
Furuncles and carbuncles	Staphylococcus aureus	—
Paronychia	Staphylococcus aureus, group A Streptococcus, Pseudomonas aeruginosa	—
Erysipelas	Group A Streptococcus	—
Cellulitis	Group A Streptococcus, Staphylococcus aureus, Haemophilus influenzae	—

TABLE 45-1   Summary of Bacteria Associated with Human Disease—cont'd

SYSTEM AFFECTED	COMMON PATHOGENS	UNCOMMON PATHOGENS
SKIN AND SOFT TISSUE—cont'd		
Necrotizing cellulitis and fasciitis	Group A *Streptococcus, Clostridium perfringens,* other clostridial species, *Bacteroides fragilis,* other anaerobes, Enterobacteriaceae, *Pseudomonas aeruginosa*	—
Bacillary angiomatosis	*Bartonella henselae, Bartonella quintana*	—
Infections of burns	*Pseudomonas aeruginosa, Enterobacter* species, *Enterococcus* species, *Staphylococcus aureus,* group A *Streptococcus*	Many aerobic and anaerobic bacteria
Bite wounds	Mixed anaerobes, *Eikenella corrodens, Pasteurella multocida* (animal bites), *Staphylococcus aureus,* group A *Streptococcus*	Many gram-negative bacilli
Surgical wounds	*Staphylococcus aureus,* groups A and B *Streptococcus, Clostridium perfringens, Corynebacterium* species, coagulase-negative *Staphylococcus*	Many gram-negative bacilli
Traumatic wounds	Many gram-negative bacilli, *Bacillus* species, *Staphylococcus aureus*	—

TABLE 45-2   Selected Bacteria Associated with Foodborne Disease

ORGANISM	IMPLICATED FOODS
Aeromonas species	Meats, produce, dairy products
Bacillus cereus	Fried rice, meats, vegetables
Brucella species	Unpasteurized dairy products, meat
Campylobacter species	Poultry, unpasteurized dairy products
Clostridium botulinum	Vegetables, fruits, fish, honey
Clostridium perfringens	Beef, poultry, pork, gravy
Escherichia coli	
Enterohemorrhagic	Beef, unpasteurized milk, fruit juices
Enterotoxigenic	Lettuce, fruits, vegetables
Enteroinvasive	Lettuce, fruits, vegetables
Francisella tularensis	Rabbit meat
Listeria monocytogenes	Unpasteurized dairy products, coleslaw, poultry
Plesiomonas shigelloides	Seafood
Salmonella species	Poultry, unpasteurized dairy products
Shigella species	Eggs, lettuce
Staphylococcus aureus	Ham, poultry, egg dishes, pastries
Streptococcus, group A	Egg dishes
Vibrio cholerae	Shellfish
Vibrio parahaemolyticus	Shellfish
Yersinia enterocolitica	Unpasteurized dairy products, pork

TABLE 45-3   Selected Bacteria Associated with Waterborne Diseases

ORGANISM	DISEASE
Aeromonas species	Gastroenteritis, wound infections, septicemia
Campylobacter species	Gastroenteritis
Francisella tularensis	Tularemia
Legionella species	Respiratory disease
Leptospira species	Systemic disease
Mycobacterium marinum	Cutaneous infection
Plesiomonas shigelloides	Gastroenteritis
Pseudomonas species	Dermatitis
Salmonella species	Gastroenteritis
Shigella species	Gastroenteritis
Vibrio species	Gastroenteritis, wound infection, septicemia
Yersinia enterocolitica	Gastroenteritis

TABLE 45-4   Arthropod-Associated Diseases

ARTHROPOD	ORGANISM	DISEASE
Tick	*Borrelia burgdorferi*	Lyme disease
	Borrelia garinii	Lyme disease
	Borrelia afzelii	Lyme disease
	Borrelia, other species	Endemic relapsing fever
	Coxiella burnetii	Q fever
	Ehrlichia chaffeensis	Human monocytic ehrlichiosis
	Ehrlichia equi	Human granulocytic ehrlichiosis
	Francisella tularensis	Tularemia
	Rickettsia rickettsii	Rocky Mountain spotted fever
	Rickettsia conorii	Mediterranean spotted fever
	Rickettsia sibirica	Siberian tick typhus
	Rickettsia australis	Australian tick typhus
	Rickettsia japonica	Oriental spotted fever
Flea	*Rickettsia conorii*	Mediterranean spotted fever
	Rickettsia prowazekii	Sporadic typhus
	Rickettsia typhi	Murine typhus
	Yersinia pestis	Plague
Lice	*Bartonella quintana*	Trench fever
	Borrelia recurrentis	Epidemic relapsing fever
	Rickettsia prowazekii	Epidemic typhus
Mite	*Rickettsia akari*	Rickettsialpox
	Rickettsia tsutsugamushi	Scrub typhus
Sandfly	*Bartonella bacilliformis*	Bartonellosis (Carrión's disease)

SECTION

Virology

Mechanisms of Viral Pathogenesis

Viruses cause disease after they break through the natural protective barriers of the body, evade immune control, and either kill cells of an important tissue (e.g., brain) or trigger a destructive immune and inflammatory response. The outcome of a viral infection is determined by the nature of the virus-host interaction and the host's response to the infection (Box 46-1). The immune response is the best treatment, but it is also a major factor in the pathogenesis of a viral infection. The tissue targeted by the virus determines the nature of the disease and its symptoms, whereas many viral and host factors determine the severity of the disease. These factors include the strain of virus, the inoculum size, and the general health of the infected person. The effectiveness of the infected person's immune response determines the severity and duration of the disease.

A particular disease may be caused by several viruses that have a common tissue **tropism** (preference) (e.g., hepatitis, liver; common cold, upper respiratory tract; encephalitis, central nervous system). On the other hand, a particular virus may cause several different diseases or no observable symptoms. For example, herpes simplex virus type 1 can cause gingivostomatitis, pharyngitis, herpes labialis (cold sores), genital herpes, encephalitis, or keratoconjunctivitis, depending on the affected cell type, or it can cause no disease at all. Although normally benign, this virus can be life-threatening in a newborn or an immunocompromised person.

Many viruses encode activities (**virulence factors**) that promote the efficiency of viral replication, viral transmission, the access and binding of the virus to target tissue, or the escape of the virus from host defenses and immune resolution (see Chapter 14). These activities may not be essential for viral growth in tissue culture but are necessary for the pathogenicity or the survival of the virus in the host. Loss of these virulence factors results in **attenuation** of the virus. Many live-virus vaccines are attenuated virus strains.

The discussion in this chapter focuses on viral disease at the cellular level (cytopathogenesis), the host level (mechanisms of disease), and the population level (epidemiology and control). The antiviral immune response is discussed here and in Chapter 14.

INFECTION OF THE TARGET TISSUE

The virus gains entry into the body through breaks in the skin or through the mucoepithelial membranes that line the orifices of the body (eyes, respiratory tract, mouth, genitalia, and gastrointestinal tract). The skin is an otherwise excellent barrier to infection, and the orifices are protected by tears, mucus, ciliated epithelium, stomach acid, bile, and immunoglobulin A (see Chapters 14 and 19). *Inhalation is probably the most common route of viral infection.*

On entry into the body, the virus replicates in cells that express viral receptors and that have the appropriate biosynthetic machinery. *Many viruses can initiate infection in the oral mucosa or upper respiratory tract.* Symptoms may accompany viral replication at the primary site. The virus may replicate and remain at the primary site, may disseminate to other tissues via the bloodstream or the mononuclear phagocyte and lymphatic system, or may disseminate through neurons (Figure 46-1).

The bloodstream and the lymphatic system are the predominant means of viral transfer in the body. The virus may gain access to these after tissue damage, by means of phagocytosis, or as the result of active transport mechanisms. Many viruses can infect and be transported across the mucoepithelial cells of the oropharynx, gastrointestinal tract, vagina, and anus. Several enteric viruses (picornaviruses and reoviruses) bind to receptors on M cells, which translocate the virus to the underlying Peyer's patches of the lymphatic system.

The transport of virus in the blood is termed **viremia.** The virus may be either free in the plasma or cell associated in lymphocytes or macrophages. Viruses taken up by phagocytic macrophages may be inactivated, may replicate, or may be delivered to other tissues by way of the mononuclear phagocyte system (e.g., lymph nodes, spleen, liver, other tissues). Replication of a virus in macrophages, the endothelial lining of blood vessels, or the liver can cause the infection to be amplified and initiate the development of a secondary viremia. In many cases a secondary viremia precedes delivery of the virus to the target tissue (e.g., liver, skin) and the manifestation of symptoms.

Viruses can gain access to the **central nervous system** or brain from the bloodstream, from infected meninges or cerebrospinal fluid, by the migration of infected macrophages, or by the infection of peripheral and sensory (olfactory) neurons. Viruses in the blood may infect and disrupt the endothelial cell lining and exit the blood vessels or traverse the blood-brain barrier to infect the central nervous system. The meninges are accessible to many of the viruses spread by viremia, which may provide access to neurons. Herpes simplex, varicella-zoster, and rabies viruses initially infect mucoepithelium, skin, or muscle and then the peripheral innervating neuron, which transports the virus to the central nervous system or brain.

VIRAL PATHOGENESIS
Cytopathogenesis

There are three potential outcomes from a viral infection of a cell: failed infection (**abortive infection**), cell death (**lytic infection**), and infection without cell death (**persistent infection**) (Box 46-2 and Table 46-1). Viral mutants, which cause abortive infections, do not multiply and therefore disappear. *Persistent infections include chronic (nonlytic, productive), latent (limited viral macromolecular but no virus synthesis), recurrent, and transforming (immortalizing) infections.* The nature of the infection is determined by both viral and cellular characteristics. A **nonpermissive** cell does not allow replication of a particular type or strain of virus. A **per-**

missive cell provides the biosynthetic machinery (e.g., transcription factors, posttranslational processing enzymes) to support the complete replicative cycle of the virus. A **semipermissive** cell may be very inefficient or support some but not all steps in viral replication.

Replication of the virus can initiate changes in cells that lead to cytolysis or to alterations in the cell's appearance, functional properties, or antigenicity. The effects on the cell may result from viral takeover of macro-

FIGURE 46-1 A, The stages of viral infection. The virus is released from one person, is acquired by another, replicates, and initiates a primary infection at the site of acquisition. Depending on the virus, it may then spread to other body sites and finally to a target tissue characteristic of the disease. The cycle is continued by the release of new virus. The thickness of the arrow denotes the degree to which the original virus inoculum is amplified on replication. The boxes indicate a site or cause of symptoms. **B,** Time course of viral infection. The time course of symptoms and the immune response correlate with the stage of viral infection and depend on whether the virus causes symptoms at the primary site or whether it causes symptoms only after dissemination to another (secondary) site. *HIV,* Human immunodeficiency virus; *HBV,* hepatitis B virus; *CMV,* cytomegalovirus.

BOX 46-2 Determinants of Viral Pathogenesis

INTERACTION OF VIRUS WITH TARGET TISSUE

Access of virus to target tissue
  Stability of virus in the body
    Temperature
    Acid and bile of the gastrointestinal tract
  Ability to cross skin or mucous epithelial cells (e.g., cross the gastrointestinal tract into the bloodstream)
  Ability to establish viremia
  Ability to spread through the reticuloendothelial system
Target tissue
  Specificity of viral attachment proteins
  Tissue-specific expression of receptors

CYPTOPATHOLOGICAL ACTIVITY OF THE VIRUS

Efficiency of viral replication in the cell
  Optimum temperature for replication
  Permissiveness of temperature for replication
Cytotoxic viral proteins
Inhibition of cell's macromolecular synthesis
Accumulation of viral proteins and structures (inclusion bodies
Altered cell metabolism (e.g., cell immortalization)

IMMUNE RESPONSE

Nonspecific antiviral immune responses
  Interferon
  Natural killer cells and macrophages
Antigen-specific immune responses
  T-cell responses
  Antibody responses
Viral mechanisms of escape of immune responses

IMMUNOPATHOLOGY

Interferon: influenza-like symptoms
T-cell responses: delayed-type hypersensitivity
Antibody: complement, antibody-dependent cellular cytotoxicity, immune complexes
Other inflammatory responses

TABLE 46-1 Types of Viral Infections at the Cellular Level

TYPE	VIRUS PRODUCTION	FATE OF CELL
Abortive	−	No effect
Cytolytic	+	Death
Persistent		
Productive	+	Senescence
Latent	−	No effect
Transforming		
DNA viruses	−	Immortalization
RNA viruses	+	Immortalization

molecular synthesis, the accumulation of viral proteins or particles, or a modification or disruption of cellular structures (Table 46-2).

Lytic Infections

Viral replication is often incompatible with the maintenance of essential cell functions and viability. Some viruses prevent the synthesis of cellular macromolecules or produce degradative enzymes and toxic proteins. This prevents cellular growth and repair and leads to death of the cell. For example, herpes simplex and other viruses produce proteins that inhibit the synthesis of cellular DNA and messenger RNA (mRNA) and synthesize other proteins that degrade host DNA to provide sub-

strates for viral genome replication. Cellular protein synthesis may be actively blocked (e.g., poliovirus inhibits translation of 5′ capped cellular mRNA) or passively blocked (e.g., through the production of much viral mRNA that successfully competes for ribosomes) (see Chapter 6).

Replication of the virus and the accumulation of viral components and progeny within the cell can disrupt the structure and function of the cell or disrupt lysosomes, causing autolysis. The expression of viral antigens on the cell surface and disruption of the cytoskeleton can cause the cell-to-cell interactions and cellular appearance to change and can make the cell a target for immunocytolysis.

Cell surface expression of the glycoproteins of some paramyxoviruses, herpesviruses, and retroviruses triggers the fusion of neighboring cells into multinucleated giant cells called **syncytia**. Cell-to-cell fusion may occur in the absence of new protein synthesis (fusion from without), as occurs in infections with Sendai and other paramyxoviruses, or may require new protein synthesis (fusion from within), as occurs in infection with the herpes simplex virus. Syncytia formation allows the virus to spread from cell to cell and escape antibody detection. The syncytia formation that occurs in infection with the human immunodeficiency virus (HIV) also causes death of the cells.

Some viral infections cause characteristic changes in the appearance and properties of the target cells. For example, chromosomal aberrations and degradation can

TABLE 46-2	**Mechanisms of Viral Cytopathogenesis**
MECHANISM	**EXAMPLES**
Inhibition of cellular protein synthesis	Polioviruses, herpes simplex virus, togaviruses, poxviruses
Inhibition and degradation of cellular DNA	Herpesviruses
Alteration of cell membrane structure	
Glycoprotein insertion	All enveloped viruses
Syncytia formation	Herpes simplex virus, varicella–zoster virus, paramyxoviruses, human immunodeficiency virus
Disruption of cytoskeleton	Nonenveloped viruses (accumulation), herpes simplex virus
Permeability	Togaviruses, herpesviruses
Inclusion bodies	
Negri bodies (intracytoplasmic)	Rabies
Owl's eye (intranuclear)	Cytomegalovirus
Cowdry type A (intranuclear)	Herpes simplex virus, subacute sclerosing panencephalitis (measles) virus
Intranuclear basophilic	Adenoviruses
Intracytoplasmic acidophilic	Poxviruses
Perinuclear cytoplasmic acidophilic	Reoviruses
Toxicity of virion components	Adenovirus fibers

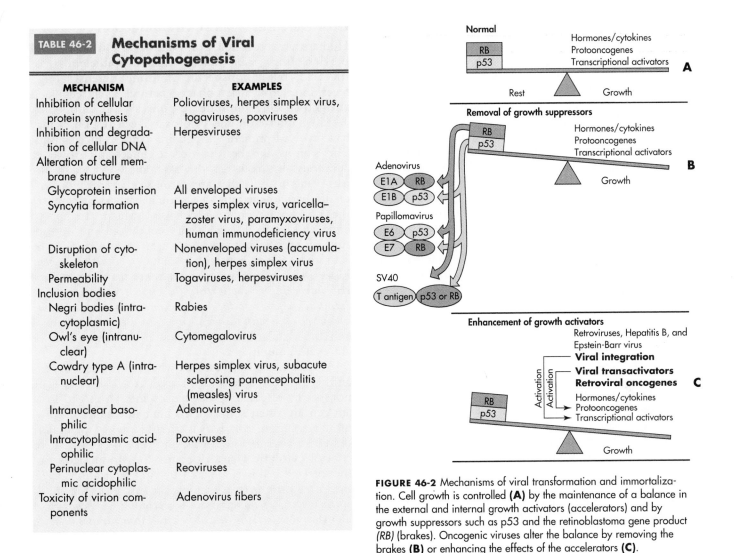

FIGURE 46-2 Mechanisms of viral transformation and immortalization. Cell growth is controlled (**A**) by the maintenance of a balance in the external and internal growth activators (accelerators) and by growth suppressors such as p53 and the retinoblastoma gene product (*RB*) (brakes). Oncogenic viruses alter the balance by removing the brakes (**B**) or enhancing the effects of the accelerators (**C**).

occur, and these can be detected by histological staining (e.g., marginated chromatin ringing the nuclear membrane in herpes simplex virus–infected and adenovirus-infected cells). In addition, new, stainable structures called **inclusion bodies** may appear within the nucleus or cytoplasm. These may result from virus-induced changes in the membrane or chromosomal structure or may represent the sites of viral replication or accumulations of viral capsids. The nature and location of these inclusion bodies are characteristic of particular viral infections and facilitate laboratory diagnosis (Table 46-2). Viral infection may also cause vacuolization, or rounding of the cells, and other nonspecific histological changes indicative of sick cells.

Nonlytic Infections

A **persistent** infection occurs in an infected cell that is not killed by the virus. Some viruses cause such a persistent productive infection because the virus is released gently from the cell by exocytosis or by budding from the plasma membrane. *DNA virus infections in which the cell restricts or lacks the machinery for transcribing all the viral genes cause a **latent** or **immortalizing** infection.* The specific transcription factors required by such a virus may be expressed only in specific tissues, in growing but not resting cells, or after hormone or cytokine induction. For example, the herpes simplex virus establishes a latent infection in neurons that lack the nuclear factors required to transcribe the immediate early viral genes, but stress and other stimuli can activate viral replication.

Oncogenic Viruses

Some DNA viruses and retroviruses establish persistent infections that can also stimulate uncontrolled cell growth, causing the **transformation** or **immortalization** of the cell (Figure 46-2). Characteristics of transformed cells include continued growth without senescence, alterations in cell morphology and metabolism, increased cell growth rate and sugar transport, loss of cell-contact-inhibition of growth, and ability to grow in a suspension or a semisolid agar.

Different oncogenic viruses have different mechanisms for immortalizing cells. Viruses immortalize cells either by promoting or providing growth-stimulating genes or by removing the inherent braking mechanisms, which limit DNA synthesis and cell growth. Immortalization by DNA viruses occurs in semipermissive cells, which express only select viral genes but do not produce virus. The synthesis of viral DNA, late mRNA, late proteins, or virus, or a combination of these, causes cell death, which precludes immortalization. Papillomavirus, SV40 virus, and adenovirus encode proteins that bind and inactivate cell growth–regulatory proteins, such as p53 or the retinoblastoma gene product. Loss of p53 also makes the cell more susceptible to mutation. This releases the brakes on cell growth. Epstein-Barr virus immortalizes B cells by stimulating cell growth (as a B-cell mitogen) and by inducing expression of the cell's *bcl-2* oncogene, which prevents programmed cell death **(apoptosis).**

Retroviruses (RNA viruses) use two approaches to oncogenesis. Some oncoviruses encode **oncogene** proteins (e.g., *sis, ras, src, mos, myc, jun, fos*), which are almost identical to the cellular proteins involved in **cellular growth control** (e.g., components of a growth factor signal cascade- or growth-regulating transcription factors). The overproduction or altered function of these oncogene products stimulates cell growth. *These oncogenic viruses rapidly cause tumors to form.* However, no human retrovirus of this type has been identified. **Human T-cell lymphotropic virus** (HTLV-1) (the only human oncogenic retrovirus identified) uses more subtle mechanisms of leukemogenesis. It encodes a protein *(tax)* that **transactivates** gene expression, including genes for growth-stimulating lymphokines (e.g., interleukin-2). This constitutes the second approach to oncogenesis. The integration of HTLV-1 near a cellular growth-stimulating gene can also cause the gene to be activated by the strong viral enhancer and promoter sequences encoded at each end of the viral genome (LTR sequences). *HTLV-1–associated leukemias take longer to develop, occurring 20 to 30 years after infection.* Retroviruses continue to produce virus in immortalized or transformed cells.

Viral transformation is the first step but is generally not sufficient to cause oncogenesis and tumor formation. Instead, over time, these occur because immortalized cells are more likely than normal cells to accumulate other mutations or chromosomal rearrangements that promote tumor cell development. Immortalized cells may also be more susceptible to cofactors and tumor promoters (e.g., phorbol esters, butyrate), which enhance tumor formation. Approximately 15% of human cancers can be related to oncogenic viruses such as HTLV-1, hepatitis B virus, papillomaviruses 16 and 18, and Epstein-Barr virus. Herpes simplex virus type 2 may be a cofactor for human cervical cancer.

Host Defenses Against Viral Infection

Humans are protected from viral infection by **natural barriers** (e.g., skin, mucus, ciliated epithelium, gastric acid, bile), **nonspecific immune defenses** (e.g., fever, interferon, macrophages, natural killer cells), and **antigen-specific immune responses** (e.g., antibodies, T cells). Interferon and cytotoxic T-cell responses may have evolved primarily as antiviral defense mechanisms. The skin is the best barrier to infection. However, abrasions or breaks in the skin allow access of the pathogens to cells that are permissive to infection. After the virus penetrates the natural barriers, it activates the nonspecific immune defenses, which attempt to limit and control local viral replication and spread. Antigen-specific immune responses are the last to be activated and are generally systemic. *The ultimate goal of the immune response is to eliminate the virus and the cells harboring or replicating the virus (resolution). The immune response is the best and in most cases the only means of controlling a viral infection.* Both the humoral and the cellular immune responses are important for antiviral immunity.

A viral infection resolves when all infectious virus and virus-infected cells are cleared from the body. The nonspecific responses produced by interferon and local antigen are often sufficient to limit infection and promote resolution. *Antibody is effective against extracellular virus, especially viremias,* and may be sufficient to control **cytolytic viruses** because the virion factory of the infected cell is eliminated by viral replication. *Cell-mediated immunity is required for lysis of the target cell in the setting of noncytolytic infections (e.g., hepatitis A virus) and infections caused by enveloped viruses.* Failure of the infection to resolve may lead to persistent or chronic infections or death of the patient. A detailed description of the antiviral immune response is presented in Chapter 14.

Immunopathology

The hypersensitivity and inflammatory reactions initiated by antiviral immunity can be the major cause of disease-related pathological conditions (Table 46-3). First, cell damage, interferon and lymphokines, and activation of the C3 component of complement by the alternative pathway can initiate inflammatory responses early in the infection. For example, interferon and lymphokines stimulate multiple body systems to produce the systemic symptoms that are usually associated with mild viral infections (e.g., fever, runny nose, malaise, headache). These symptoms often precede **(prodrome)** the characteristic symptoms of the viral infection, especially during viremia. Later, immune complexes and complement activation (classic pathway), CD4 T-cell–induced delayed-type hypersensitivity, and immune cytolysis may induce inflammatory responses. Cell damage, complement activation, and delayed-type hypersensitivity usually initiate the local responses, which are characterized by neutrophil infiltration and more cell damage.

TABLE 46-3	**Viral Immunopathogenesis**	
IMMUNOPATHOGENESIS	**IMMUNE MEDIATORS**	**EXAMPLES**
Influenza-like symptoms	Interferon, lymphokines	Respiratory viruses, arboviruses (viremia-inducing viruses)
DTH and inflammation	T cells, PMNs	Enveloped viruses
Immune-complex disease	Antibody, complement,	Hepatitis B virus, rubella
Hemorrhagic disease	T cell, antibody, complement	Dengue virus
Postinfection cytolysis	T cells	Enveloped viruses (e.g., postmeasles encephalitis)
Immunosuppression	—	HIV, cytomegalovirus, measles virus, influenza virus

DTH, Delayed-type hypersensitivity; *PMNs,* polymorphonuclear leukocytes.

The inflammatory response initiated by cell-mediated immunity is difficult to control and damages tissue. *Enveloped virus infections in particular induce cell-mediated immune responses that usually produce more extensive immunopathological conditions.* For example, the classic symptoms of measles and mumps result from the T-cell–induced inflammatory and hypersensitivity responses rather than from viral cytopathology. The presence of large amounts of antigen in blood during viremias or chronic infections (e.g., hepatitis B virus infection) can initiate the classic immune complex hypersensitivity reactions. Immune complexes containing virus or viral antigen can activate the complement system, triggering inflammatory responses and tissue destruction. These immune complexes often accumulate in the kidney and cause renal problems.

In the case of dengue and measles viruses, partial immunity to a related strain can initiate a more severe host response and disease on challenge with a new strain. This is because antigen-specific T-cell and antibody responses are enhanced and induce significant inflammatory and hypersensitivity damage to infected endothelial cells (dengue hemorrhagic fever) or skin and the lung (atypical measles). In addition, a nonneutralizing antibody can facilitate the uptake of dengue and yellow fever viruses into macrophages through Fc receptors, where they can replicate.

Children generally have a less active cell-mediated immune response than adults and therefore generally have milder symptoms during infections caused by some viruses (e.g., measles, mumps, Epstein-Barr, and varicella-zoster viruses). However, in the case of hepatitis B virus, mild or no symptoms correlate with an inability to resolve the infection, and this results in chronic disease.

Viral Disease

The relative susceptibility of a person and the severity of the disease depend on factors such as the nature of the exposure; the immune status, age, and general health of the person; the viral dose; and the genetics of the virus and the host. Once the host is infected, however, the host's immune status is probably the major factor that determines whether a viral infection causes a life-threatening disease, a benign lesion, or no symptoms at all.

TABLE 46-4	**Incubation Periods of Common Viral Infections**
DISEASE	**INCUBATION PERIOD***
Influenza	1-2 days
Common cold	1-3 days
Bronchiolitis, croup	3-5 days
Acute respiratory disease (adenoviruses)	5-7 days
Dengue	5-8 days
Herpes simplex	5-8 days
Enteroviruses	6-12 days
Poliomyelitis	5-20 days
Measles	9-12 days
Smallpox	12-14 days
Chickenpox	13-17 days
Mumps	16-20 days
Rubella	17-20 days
Mononucleosis	30-50 days
Hepatitis A	15-40 days
Hepatitis B	50-150 days
Rabies	30-100 days
Papilloma (warts)	50-150 days
HIV (acquired immunodeficiency syndrome)	1-10 years

Modified from White DO, Fenner F: *Medical virology,* ed 3, New York, 1986, Academic.
*Until first appearance of prodromal symptoms. Diagnostic signs (e.g., rash, paralysis) may not appear until 2 to 4 days later.

The stages of viral infection are shown in Figure 46-2. The initial period before the characteristic symptoms of a disease are detected is termed the **incubation period.** During this period, the virus is replicating but has not reached the target tissue or induced sufficient damage to cause the disease. *The incubation period is relatively short if infection of the primary site produces the characteristic symptoms of the disease.* During the **prodrome,** nonspecific or influenza-like symptoms may precede the characteristic symptoms of the disease. The incubation periods for many common viral infections are listed in Table 46-4. Specific viral diseases are discussed in subsequent chapters and reviewed in Chapter 65.

Viral infections may be apparent or inapparent and may cause acute or chronic disease. The nature and severity of the symptoms of a viral disease are related to the function of the infected target tissue (e.g., liver, hepatitis; brain, encephalitis) and the extent of the immunopathology triggered by the infection. The ability and speed with which a person's immune system controls and resolves a viral infection usually determine whether acute or chronic disease ensues and the severity of the symptoms (Figure 46-3).

Inapparent infections result if the infected tissue is undamaged, if the infection is controlled before the virus reaches its target tissue, if the target tissue is expendable, if the damaged tissue is rapidly repaired, or if the degree of damage is below a functional threshold for that particular tissue. For example, many infections of the brain are inapparent or are below the threshold of severe loss of function, but encephalitis results if the loss of function becomes significant. However, *asymptomatic infections are major sources of contagion*. Such inapparent infections are frequently detected in people by the finding of virus-specific antibody. For example, although 97% of

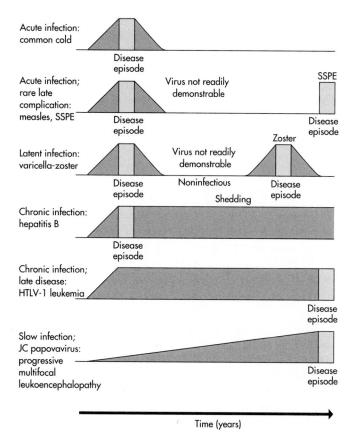

FIGURE 46-3 Acute infection and various types of persistent infection, as illustrated by the diseases indicated in the column at the left. Vertical box *(green)* illustrates disease episode. *SSPE*, Subacute sclerosing panencephalitis. (Redrawn from White DO, Fenner F: *Medical virology*, ed 3, New York, 1986, Academic.)

adults have antibody (seropositive) to varicella-zoster virus, less than half remember having had chickenpox.

EPIDEMIOLOGY

Infection of a population is similar to infection of a person in that the virus must spread through the population and is controlled by immunization of the population (Box 46-3). To endure, viruses must continue to infect new, immunologically naive, susceptible hosts.

Exposure

People are exposed to viruses throughout their lives. However, some situations, vocations, life-styles, and living arrangements increase the likelihood of a person coming in contact with certain viruses. In addition, many viruses are ubiquitous, as borne out by the fact that evidence of exposure (antibodies to the virus) can be detected in most young children (herpes simplex virus type 1, human herpesvirus 6, varicella-zoster virus, parvovirus B19) or by early adulthood (Epstein-Barr virus and many respiratory and enteric viruses). Poor hygiene and crowded living, school, and job conditions promote exposure to respiratory and enteric viruses. Day-care centers are consistent sources of viral infections, especially viruses spread by the respiratory and fecal-oral routes. Travel, summer camp, and vocations that bring people in contact with a virus vector, such as mosquitos, put them at particular risk for infection by arboviruses and other zoonoses. Sexual promiscuity also promotes the spread and acquisition of several viruses. Health care workers such as physicians, dentists, nurses, and technicians are frequently exposed to respiratory and other viruses but are especially at risk for acquiring viruses from contaminated blood (hepatitis B virus, HIV) or vesicle fluid (herpes simplex virus).

Transmission of Viruses

Viruses are transmitted by direct contact (including sexual contact), injection with contaminated fluids or blood or the transplantation of organs, and the respiratory and fecal-oral routes (Table 46-5). *The route of transmission depends on the source of the virus (the tissue site of viral replication and secretion) and the ability of the virus to endure the hazards and barriers of the environment and the body en route to the target tissue*. For example, viruses that replicate in the respiratory tract (e.g., influenza A virus) are released in aerosol droplets, whereas enteric viruses (e.g., picornaviruses and reoviruses) are passed by the fecal-oral route. Cytomegalovirus is transmitted in most bodily secretions because it infects mucoepithelial, secretory, and other cells found in the skin, secretory glands, lungs, liver, and other organs. Togaviruses and rhabdoviruses can be introduced into human hosts by means of arthropod or animal bites.

The presence or absence of an envelope is the major structural determinant of the mode of viral transmission.

Nonenveloped viruses can withstand drying, the effects of detergents, and extremes of pH and temperature, whereas enveloped viruses generally cannot. Specifically, most nonenveloped viruses can withstand the acidic environment of the stomach and the detergent-like bile of the intestines, as well as mild disinfection and insufficient sewage treatment. These viruses are generally transmitted by the respiratory and fecal-oral routes and can often be acquired from contaminated objects, termed **fomites.** For example, hepatitis A virus, a picornavirus, is a nonenveloped virus that is transmitted by the fecal-oral route and acquired from contaminated water, shellfish, and food. Rhinoviruses and many other nonenveloped viruses can be spread by contact with fomites such as handkerchiefs or toys.

Unlike the sturdy nonenveloped viruses (naked capsid viruses), enveloped viruses are comparatively fragile. They require an intact envelope for infectivity. These viruses must remain wet and are spread in respiratory droplets, blood, mucus, saliva, or semen; by injection; or in organ transplants. Most enveloped viruses are also labile in response to acid and detergents, which precludes their being transmitted by the fecal-oral route. Exceptions are hepatitis B virus and coronaviruses.

Animals can also act as **vectors** that spread viral disease to other animals and humans and even to other lo-

TABLE 46-5	**Viral Transmission**
MODE	**EXAMPLES**
Respiratory transmission	Paramyxoviruses, influenza viruses, picornaviruses, rhinoviruses, enteroviruses, varicella-zoster virus, B19 virus
Fecal-oral transmission	Picornaviruses, rotavirus, reovirus, caliciviruses, Norwalk virus, adenovirus
Contact (lesions, saliva, fomites)	Herpes simplex virus, rhinoviruses, poxviruses, adenovirus
Zoonoses (animals, insects)	Togaviruses (alpha), flaviviruses, bunyaviruses, orbiviruses, arenaviruses, rabies virus
Transmission via blood	HIV, HTLV-1, hepatitis B virus, hepatitis C virus, hepatitis delta virus, cytomegalovirus
Sexual contact	Blood-borne viruses, herpes simplex virus, human papillomavirus
Maternal-neonatal transmission	Rubella virus, cytomegalovirus, B19 virus, echovirus, herpes simplex virus, varicella-zoster virus
Genetic	Prions, retroviruses

BOX 46-3   Viral Epidemiology*

MECHANISMS OF VIRAL TRANSMISSION†

Aerosols
Fomites (e.g., tissues, clothes)
Direct contact with secretions (e.g., saliva, semen)
Sexual contact
Blood transfusion or organ transplant
Zoonoses (animals, insects [arboviruses])

DISEASE AND VIRAL FACTORS THAT PROMOTE TRANSMISSION

Stability of virion in response to the environment (e.g., drying, drinking water, detergents, temperature)
Replication and secretion of virus into transmissible aerosols and secretions (e.g., saliva, semen)
Asymptomatic transmission
Transience or ineffectiveness of immune response to control reinfection or recurrence

RISK FACTORS

Age
Health
Immune status
Occupation: contact with agent or vector

RISK FACTORS—cont'd

Travel history
Life-style
Children in day-care centers

CRITICAL COMMUNITY SIZE

Seronegative, susceptible people

GEOGRAPHY AND SEASON

Presence of cofactors or vectors in the environment
Habitat and season for arthropod vectors (mosquitos)
School session: close proximity and crowding
Home-heating season

MODES OF CONTROL

Quarantine
Elimination of the vector
Immunization
    Natural infection
    Vaccination
Treatment

*Infection of a population instead of a person.
†See also Table 46-5.

cales. They can also be reservoirs for the virus that maintain and amplify the virus in the environment. Viral diseases that are shared by animals or insects and humans are called **zoonoses**. Arthropods, including mosquitos, ticks, and sandflies, can act as vectors for togaviruses, flaviviruses, bunyaviruses, and reoviruses. These viruses are often referred to as **arboviruses** because they are *ar*thropod *bo*rne. Most arboviruses have a very broad host range, which may include specific insects, birds, reptiles, and mammals, in addition to humans. Raccoons, foxes, dogs, and cats are vectors for the rabies virus.

Other factors that can promote the transmission of viruses include the potential for asymptomatic infection, crowded living conditions, certain occupations, certain life-styles, day-care centers, and travel. With regard to the first of these conditions, many viruses (e.g., HIV, varicella-zoster virus) are released before symptoms appear, making it difficult to restrict transmission. Viruses that cause persistent productive infections (e.g., cytomegalovirus, HIV) are a particular problem because the infected person is a continual source of virus that may result in spread to immunologically naive people. Viruses with many different serotypes (rhinoviruses) or viruses capable of changing their antigenicity (influenza and HIV) also readily find immunologically naive populations.

Maintenance of a Virus in the Population

The persistence of a virus in a community depends on the availability of a critical number of immunologically naive (seronegative), susceptible people. The efficiency of the route of transmission determines the size of the susceptible population necessary for continuation. *Immunization, produced by natural means or by vaccination, is the best way of reducing the number of such susceptible people.*

Age

The age of the person is an important factor in determining his or her susceptibility to viral infections. Infants, children, adults, and the elderly are susceptible to different viruses and have different symptomatic responses to the infection. This may result from differences in body size, tissue characteristics, recuperative abilities, and most important, immune status in people in these various age groups. Differences in life-styles, habits, school environments, and job settings at different ages also determine when people are exposed to viruses.

Infants and children acquire a series of respiratory and exanthematous viral diseases because they have not yet been exposed to them and are therefore immunologically naive. Infants are especially prone to more serious presentations of paramyxovirus respiratory infections and gastroenteritis because of their small size and physiological requirements (e.g., nutrients, water, electrolytes). However, children generally do not mount as severe an immunopathological response as adults, and some diseases (herpesviruses) are more benign in children.

The elderly are especially susceptible to new viral infections and the reactivation of latent viruses. Because they are less able to initiate a new immune response, repair damaged tissue, and recover, they are therefore more susceptible to outbreaks of the new strains of the influenza A and B viruses. The elderly are also more prone to zoster (shingles), a recurrence of varicella-zoster virus.

Immune Status

The competence of a person's immune response and his or her immune history determine how quickly and efficiently the infection is resolved, but these factors can also determine the severity of the symptoms. The rechallenge of a person with prior immunity usually results in asymptomatic or mild disease without transmission. However, people who are in an immunosuppressed state as a result of acquired immunodeficiency syndrome, cancer, or immunosuppressive therapy are at greater risk of suffering more serious disease on primary infection (measles, vaccinia) and more prone to suffer recurrences of infections with latent viruses (e.g., herpesviruses, papovaviruses).

Other Host Factors

As noted earlier, the general health of a person plays an important role in determining the competence and nature of his or her immune response. For example, poor nutrition compromises a person's immune system and decreases his or her tissue regenerative capacity. Immunosuppressive diseases and therapies allow viral replication or recurrence to proceed unchecked. A person's genetic makeup also plays an important role in determining the response of his or her immune system to viral infection. Specifically, genetic differences in immune-response genes, genes for viral receptors, and other genetic loci affect the person's susceptibility to a viral infection and the severity of the infection.

Geographical and Seasonal Considerations

The geographical distribution of a virus is usually determined by whether the requisite cofactors or vectors are present or whether there is an immunologically naive, susceptible population. For example, many of the arboviruses are limited to the ecological niche of their arthropod vectors. However, extensive global transportation is eliminating many of the geographically determined restrictions to virus distribution.

Seasonal differences in the occurrence of viral disease correspond with behaviors that promote the spread of the virus. For example, respiratory viruses are more prevalent in the winter because of crowding and temperature and humidity conditions that facilitate the spread of or stabilize the extracorporeal virus. Enteric viruses, on the other hand, are more prevalent during the summer, possibly because hygiene is less effective during this season. The seasonal differences in arboviral diseases reflect the life cycle of the arthropod vector or its reservoir (e.g., birds).

Outbreaks, Epidemics, and Pandemics

Outbreaks of a viral infection often result from the introduction of a virus (such as hepatitis A) into a new location. The outbreak originates from a common source (e.g., food preparation), and often the epidemic can be stopped once the source is identified. Epidemics occur over a larger geographical area and generally result from the introduction of a new strain of virus into an immunologically naive population. **Pandemics** are worldwide epidemics, usually resulting from the introduction of a new virus (e.g., HIV). Pandemics of influenza A have occurred approximately every 10 years as the result of the introduction of new strains of the virus.

CONTROL OF VIRAL SPREAD

The spread of a virus can be controlled by **quarantine**, good hygiene, changes in life-style, elimination of the vector, or **immunization** of the population. Quarantine was once the only means of limiting epidemics of viral infections and is most effective for limiting the spread of viruses that always cause symptomatic disease (e.g., smallpox). It is now used especially in hospitals to limit the nosocomial spread of viruses, especially to high-risk patients (e.g., immunosuppressed people). The proper sanitation of contaminated items and disinfection of the water supply are means of limiting the spread of enteric viruses. Changes in life-style have made a difference in the spread of sexually transmitted viruses such as HIV, hepatitis B virus, and herpes simplex virus. Elimination of the arthropod or its ecological niche (e.g., drainage of the swamps it inhabits) has proved effective for controlling arboviruses.

The best way to limit viral spread, however, is to immunize the population. Such immunization produced by natural infection or vaccination protects the person and reduces the size of the immunologically naive, susceptible population necessary to promote the spread of the virus.

QUESTIONS

1. List the routes by which viruses gain entry into the body, the barriers to infection at each route, and a virus that infects by each route.
2. Describe or draw the path of a virus that is transmitted by an aerosol and causes lesions on the skin (similar to varicella).
3. Identify the structures that elicit a protective antibody response to adenovirus, influenza A virus, poliovirus, and rabies virus.
4. Describe the major roles of each of the following in promoting resolution of a viral infection: interferon, macrophage, natural killer cells, CD4 T cells, CD8 T cells, and antibody.
5. Why are alpha- and beta-interferons produced before gamma-interferon?
6. How does the nucleoprotein of influenza virus become an antigen for cytolytic CD8 T cells?
7. What events occur during the prodromal periods of a respiratory virus disease (e.g., parainfluenza virus) and encephalitis (e.g., St. Louis encephalitis virus)?
8. List the viral characteristics (structure, replication, target tissue) that would promote transmission by the fecal-oral route, by arthropods, by fomites, by mother's milk, and by sexual activity.
9. Describe the different mechanisms by which oncogenic viruses immortalize cells.

Bibliography

Belshe RB: *Textbook of human virology,* ed 2, St Louis, 1991, Mosby.

Ellner PD, Neu HC: *Understanding infectious disease,* St Louis, 1992, Mosby.

Emond RT, Rowland HAK, Welsby P: *Color atlas of infectious diseases,* ed 3, St Louis, 1995, Mosby.

Fields BN , Knipe DM, Howley PM, editors: *Virology,* ed 3, New York, 1996, Lippincott-Raven.

Gorbach SL, Bartlett JG, Blacklow NR: *Infectious diseases,* Philadelphia, 1992, WB Saunders.

Hart CA, Broadhead RL: *Color atlas of pediatric infectious diseases,* St Louis, 1992, Mosby.

Haukenes G, Haaheim LR, Pattison JR: *A practical guide to clinical virology,* New York, 1989, John Wiley & Sons.

Krugman S et al: *Infectious diseases of children,* ed 9, St Louis, 1992, Mosby.

Mandell GL, Douglas RG Jr, Bennett JE: *Principles and practice of infectious disease,* ed 3, New York, 1990, Churchill Livingstone.

Mims CA, White DO: *Viral pathogenesis and immunology,* Oxford, 1984, Blackwell.

Richman DD, Whitley RJ, Hayden FG: *Clinical virology,* New York, 1997, Churchill Livingston.

Shulman ST, Phair JP, Sommers HM: *The biologic and clinical basis of infectious diseases,* ed 4, Philadelphia, 1992, WB Saunders.

White DO, Fenner FJ: *Medical virology,* ed 4, Orlando, Fla, 1994, Academic.

Antiviral Agents

The development of antiviral chemotherapy has lagged significantly behind the development of antibacterial drugs. Antibacterial drugs, such as the beta-lactam and aminoglycoside antibiotics, are targeted at enzymes and structures unique to almost all prokaryotes and essential to their viability. However, viruses, unlike most bacteria, are obligate intracellular parasites that use the host cell's biosynthetic machinery and enzymes for replication (see Chapter 6). Hence it is more difficult to inhibit viral replication without it also being toxic to the host.

Early antiviral drugs were selective poisons that targeted cells with extensive DNA and RNA synthesis, similar to the activity of cancer chemotherapies. Newer antiviral drugs are targeted toward viral encoded enzymes or structures of the virus that are important for replication. Many of these compounds are classic biochemical inhibitors of viral encoded enzymes. Unlike the activity of antibacterial drugs, the activity of antiviral drugs is generally limited to specific families of viruses. Newer antiviral therapies are directed at blocking the expression of the viral genome and promoting immune resolution of the viral infection (e.g., with interferon). Antiviral drugs have been developed against viruses that cause significant morbidity and mortality and also provide reasonable targets for drug action (Box 47-1). As has occurred with antibacterial drugs, however, resistance to antiviral drugs is becoming more of a problem because of the increased long-term treatment of immunocompromised people (e.g., patients with acquired immunodeficiency syndrome [AIDS]).

TARGETS FOR ANTIVIRAL DRUGS

Analysis of the steps of the viral replication cycle has identified potential targets for antiviral drugs (e.g., structures, enzymes, or processes important or essential for virus production). These targets are described in this chapter, and examples of antiviral drugs developed to target these sites are also given. These targets and their respective antiviral agents are listed in Table 47-1 and shown in Figure 6-10.

Attachment is the first step in viral replication. It is mediated by the interaction of a viral attachment protein with its cell surface receptor. This interaction can be blocked by **neutralizing antibodies,** which bind and coat the virion, or by **receptor antagonists.** The administration of specific antibodies **(passive immunization)** is the oldest form of antiviral therapy. Receptor antagonists include peptide or sugar analogues of the cell receptor or the viral attachment protein that competitively block the interaction of the virus with the cell. Specific peptides of the human immunodeficiency virus (HIV) glycoprotein gp120 or its receptor, the CD4 molecule of T cells, block infection and are being investigated for their clinical potential. Acidic polysaccharides, such as heparan and dextran sulfate, interfere with viral binding and have been suggested for the treatment of infection with herpes simplex virus (HSV), HIV, or other viruses.

Penetration and uncoating of the virus are required to deliver the viral genome into the cytoplasm of the host cell. After uptake of many viruses, the acidic environment of the endocytic vesicle is used to initiate uncoating. Specifically, the acidic pH promotes conformational changes in attachment proteins that promote fusion or membrane disruption. **Amantadine, rimantadine,** and other hydrophobic amines (weak organic bases) are antiviral agents that can neutralize the pH of these compartments and inhibit virion uncoating. Tromantadine, a derivative of amantadine, inhibits penetration of HSV. Arildone, disoxaril, and other methylisoxazole compounds block uncoating by fitting into a cleft in the receptor-binding canyon of the picornavirus capsid.

Amantadine and rimantadine have a more specific activity against influenza A. These compounds bind to and block the H^+ channel formed by the M_2 protein. Without the influx of H^+ the M_1 matrix proteins do not dissociate from the nucleocapsid (uncoating), preventing movement of the nucleocapsid to the nucleus, transcription, and replication. Blockage of this proton pore also disrupts the proper processing of the hemagglutinin protein late in the replication cycle. In the absence of a functional M_2 proton pore, the hemagglutinin inopportunely changes its conformation into its "fusion form" and is inactivated as it traverses the normally acidic Golgi environment.

Although messenger RNA (mRNA) synthesis is essential for the production of virus, it is difficult to inhibit viral mRNA synthesis without affecting cellular mRNA synthesis. In particular, DNA viruses use the host cell's transcriptases for mRNA synthesis, making this a poor target for antiviral drugs. In addition, the RNA polymerases encoded by RNA viruses may not be sufficiently different enough from host cell transcriptases to allow the development of antiviral drugs that selectively inhibit this activity. Alternatively, the high rate at which RNA viruses mutate may result in the generation of many drug-resistant strains. Guanidine and 2-hydroxybenzyl-benzimidine are two compounds that can block picornavirus RNA synthesis by binding to the 2C picornavirus protein, which is essential for RNA synthesis.

The proper processing (splicing) and translation of viral mRNA can be inhibited by **interferon, antisense oligonucleotides,** and other agents. Viral infection of an interferon-treated cell triggers a cascade of biochemical events that block viral replication. Specifically, the degradation of viral and cellular mRNA is enhanced, and mRNA binding to the ribosome is blocked, preventing protein synthesis and viral replication. Interferon is described further in Chapter 14. Interferon and artificial interferon inducers (Ampligen: poly rI:rC) have been approved for clinical use (papilloma, hepatitis B and C) or are in clinical trials. Antisense oligonucleotides are short, oligomeric sequences (20 nucleotides) that are complementary to specific sequences of the viral genome. These oligomers are chemically synthesized from nucleotide

---

BOX 47-1   Viruses Treatable with Antiviral Drugs

Herpes simplex virus
Varicella-zoster virus
Cytomegalovirus
Human immunodeficiency virus
Influenza A virus
Respiratory syncytial virus
Hepatitis A, B, and C viruses*
Papillomavirus*

*Experimental protocols are available.

TABLE 47-1   Examples of Targets for Antiviral Drugs

REPLICATION STEP OR TARGET	AGENT	TARGETED VIRUS*
Attachment	Peptide analogues of attachment protein	Human immunodeficiency virus (gp 120/CD4 receptor)
	Neutralizing antibodies	Most viruses
	Dextran sulfate, heparin	Human immunodeficiency virus; herpes simplex virus
Penetration and uncoating	Amantadine, rimantadine	Influenza A virus
	Tromantadine	Herpes simplex virus
	Arildone, disoxaril	Picornaviruses
Transcription	Interferon	Hepatitis A, B, and C viruses; papillomavirus
	Antisense oligonucleotides	Papillomavirus
Protein synthesis	Interferon	Hepatitis A, B, and C viruses; papillomavirus
DNA replication (polymerase)	Nucleotide analogues	Herpesviruses; human immunodeficiency virus; hepatitis B virus
	Phosphonoformate, phosphonoacetic acid	Herpesviruses
Nucleoside biosynthesis	Ribavirin	Respiratory syncytial virus
Nucleotide scavenging (thymidine kinase)	Nucleoside analogues	Herpes simplex virus; varicella-zoster virus
Glycoprotein processing	—	Human immunodeficiency virus
Assembly (protease)	Hydrophobic substrate analogues	Human immunodeficiency virus
Virion integrity	Nonoxynol-9	Human immunodeficiency virus; herpes simplex virus

*Therapies may not have received approval for human use.

analogues and are resistant to nuclease digestion. The binding of antisense oligonucleotides to newly transcribed viral RNA prevents its being processed (spliced) into mRNA in the nucleus, its delivery to the cytoplasm, and its binding to the ribosome. RO 24-7429 is an antisense oligonucleotide that inhibits the tat transactivation function and prevents activation of the transcription of HIV mRNA and HIV replication. Isatin-beta-thiosemicarbazone induces mRNA degradation in poxvirus-infected cells and was used as a treatment for smallpox.

Viral DNA polymerases (including reverse transcriptases) are the **prime target** for antiviral drugs because they are *essential* for virus replication. Most antiviral drugs are **nucleoside analogues,** which are nucleosides with modifications of the base, sugar, or both (Figure 47-1). Before being used by the polymerase, the nucleoside analogues must be phosphorylated to the triphosphate form by viral enzymes (e.g., HSV thymidine kinase), cellular enzymes, or both. For example, the thymidine kinase of HSV and varicella-zoster virus (VZV) applies the first phosphate to **acyclovir (ACV)** and the cellular enzymes apply the rest. HSV mutants lacking thymidine kinase activity are resistant to ACV. **Azidothymidine (AZT)** and many other nucleoside analogues are phosphorylated by cellular enzymes.

Nucleotide analogues selectively inhibit viral polymerases because these enzymes are less accurate than host cell enzymes and bind a nucleotide analogue with modifications of the base, sugar, or both, several hundred-fold better than the host cell enzyme. These drugs **prevent chain elongation or proper recognition** and **base pairing** (Figure 47-1). Antiviral drugs that cause termination of the DNA chain because of modified nucleoside sugar residues include **ACV, ganciclovir (GCV), valacyclovir, famciclovir, adenosine arabinoside (Vidarabine; Ara A), zidovudine (AZT), dideoxycytidine,** and **dideoxyinosine.** Antiviral drugs that become incorporated into the viral genome and cause errors in replication (mutation) and transcription (inactive mRNA and proteins) because of modified nucleoside bases include **5(-iododeoxyuridine (Idoxuridine)** and **trifluorothymidine (trifluridine).** The rapid rate and large extent of nucleotide incorporation during viral replication make DNA viral replication especially susceptible to these drugs. A variety of other nucleoside analogues are also being developed as antiviral drugs.

Pyrophosphate analogues resembling the by-product of the polymerase reaction, such as **phosphonoformic acid (Foscarnet [PFA])** and **phosphonoacetate,** are classic inhibitors of the herpesvirus polymerases. Nevirapine, delaviradine, and other **nonnucleoside reverse transcriptase inhibitors** do not bind to the substrate site and are noncompetitive inhibitors of the enzyme.

Deoxyribonucleotide scavenging enzymes (e.g., the thymidine kinase and ribonucleotide reductase of the herpesviruses) are also enzyme targets of antiviral drugs. These enzymes provide nucleotide substrates to facilitate the replication of the DNA virus genome.

Cellular enzymes or pathways important to viral replication but not to cell viability are also targets for antiviral drugs. **Ribavirin** is such an agent. It resembles guanosine monophosphate and inhibits nucleoside biosynthesis,

FIGURE 47-1 *Structure of nucleoside analogues that are antiviral drugs. The chemical distinctions between the natural deoxynucleoside and the antiviral drug analogues are highlighted. Arrows indicate related drugs. Valacyclovir (not shown) is the L-valylester of acyclovir. Famciclovir (not shown) is the diacetyl 6-deoxyanalogue of penciclovir. Both of these drugs are metabolized to the active drug in the liver or intestinal wall.*

mRNA capping, and other processes important to the replication of many viruses.

Although bacterial protein synthesis is the target for several antibacterial compounds, viral protein synthesis is a poor target for antiviral drugs because the virus uses host cell ribosomes and synthetic mechanisms. However, viral replication can be inhibited through inhibition of the posttranslational modification of proteins, such as the proteolysis of a viral polyprotein, glycoprotein processing (castanospermine, deoxynojirimycin), or phosphorylation (D609:xanthate). Agents that inhibit the glycoprotein processing of HIV or HSV block viral release and inhibit glycoprotein functions such as attachment and fusion, thereby preventing both the production and spread of the virus.

The **HIV protease** is unique and *essential* to the assembly of virions and the production of infectious virions. Computer-assisted molecular modeling has been used to design inhibitors of the HIV protease such as **saquinavir, ritonavir,** and **indinavir** by modeling inhibitors that would fit into the active site of the enzyme. The enzyme structures were defined by x-ray crystallographic and molecular biological studies. Proteases of other viruses are also targets for antiviral drugs.

Preventing the acquisition of the virus, preventing the spread of the virus, and promoting the antiviral immune response of the host also have therapeutic potential. For example, enveloped viruses are susceptible to certain lipid and detergent-like molecules that disperse or disrupt the envelope membrane, thereby preventing acquisition of the virus. Nonoxynol-9, a detergent-like component in birth control jellies, can inactivate HSV and HIV and prevent sexual acquisition of the virus. Antibodies, acquired naturally or by passive immunization (see Chapter 15), prevent both the acquisition and spread of the virus. Interferon, interferon inducers, and other immunomodulatory biological response modifiers are agents that stimulate resolution of the infection by the host. Biological response modifiers under investigation include adjuvants consisting of bacterial components, mismatched polynucleotides (e.g., Ampligen:poly rI:rC), and immunomodulatory chemicals. These agents stimulate the production and release of interferon and other lymphokines, which have antiviral activity and activate natural killer and killer cell immune responses.

ANTIVIRAL DRUGS AVAILABLE FOR CLINICAL USE

Most of the antiviral drugs approved by the U.S. Food and Drug Administration (Table 47-2) are nucleoside analogues that inhibit viral polymerases. These drugs are generally activated by phosphorylation by cellular or viral kinases. Selective inhibition of viral replication results from enhanced nucleoside phosphorylation, preferential binding of the drug to viral rather than cellular DNA polymerases, or the more rapid synthesis of DNA in infected cells.

Acyclovir, Valacyclovir, and Famciclovir

ACV (acycloguanosine) differs from the nucleoside guanosine by having an acyclic (hydroxyethoxymethyl) side chain instead of a ribose or deoxyribose sugar. ACV has selective action against HSV and VZV, the herpesviruses that encode a thymidine kinase (Figure 47-2). The viral thymidine kinase activates the drug by phosphorylation, and host cell enzymes complete the progression to the diphosphate and finally to the triphosphate form. Because there is no initial phosphorylation in uninfected cells, there is no active drug to inhibit cellular DNA synthesis or to cause toxicity. The ACV triphosphate competes with the guanosine triphosphate inhibiting the enzyme, causes termination of the growing viral DNA chain because there is no 3'-hydroxyl group on the ACV molecule to allow chain elongation, and inactivates the DNA polymerase. The selectivity and minimal toxicity of ACV are also a result of its 100-fold or greater use by the viral DNA polymerase than by cellular DNA polymerases. However, mutations in either the **thymidine kinase** or the **polymerase** can generate ACV-resistant strains, which are less virulent than the parent strain but can still cause disease in immunocompromised patients, especially those with AIDS.

ACV is effective against HSV infections such as encephalitis, disseminated herpes, and other serious herpes presentations. The fact that it is not toxic to uninfected cells allows its use as a prophylactic treatment to prevent recurrent outbreaks, especially in immunosuppressed people. A recurrent episode may be prevented if it is treated within 48 hours of the stimulus of recurrence, before the onset of inflammatory responses. ACV inhibits the replication of HSV but cannot resolve the latent HSV infection.

ACV can also be used for the treatment of VZV infection, but higher doses are required because VZV is less sensitive to ACV. ACV is phosphorylated less efficiently by the VZV thymidine kinase. **Valacyclovir,** the valyl ester derivative of ACV, is more efficiently absorbed after oral administration and rapidly converted into ACV, increasing the bioavailability of ACV for the treatment of serious varicella or zoster disease. Similarly, **famciclovir** is a derivative of **penciclovir,** which is well absorbed orally and then converted to the active drug in the liver or intestinal lining. Penciclovir inhibits VZV and HSV in the same way that ACV does but is concentrated and persists in the infected cells to a greater extent than ACV. Penciclovir also has some activity toward the Epstein-Barr virus and cytomegalovirus (CMV).

Ganciclovir

GCV (dihydroxypropoxymethyl guanine) differs from ACV by the addition of a single hydroxymethyl group in the acyclic side chain (Figure 47-1). The remarkable result of this is that it confers considerable activity against CMV. CMV does not encode a thymidine kinase, but a viral encoded protein kinase phosphorylates GCV. Once activated by phosphorylation, GCV inhibits all her-

Acyclovir

FIGURE 47-2 Activation of ACV (acycloguanosine) in herpes simplex virus–infected cells. ACV is converted to acycloguanosine monophosphate (acyclo GMP) by herpes-specific viral thymidine kinase and then to acycloguanosine triphosphate by cellular kinases.

ATP | Viral thymidine kinase

**Acycloguanosine monophosphate
(acyclo GMP)**

2 ATP →

Cellular kinases

**Acycloguanosine triphosphate
(acyclo GTP)**

TABLE 47-2   **Antiviral Drug Therapies Approved by the U.S. Food and Drug Administration**

VIRUS	ANTIVIRAL DRUG	TRADE NAME
HSV	Acyclovir*	Zovirax
	Adenosine arabinoside (Ara A)	Vidarabine, Vira A
	Iododeoxyuridine†	Stoxil (idoxuridine)
	Trifluorothymidine†	Viroptic (trifluridine)
VZV	Valacyclovir‡	Valtrex
	Famciclovir‡	Famvir
Cytomegalovirus	Ganciclovir	Cytovene
	Phosphonoformate	Foscarnet, Foscavir
HIV		
Nucleoside analogue reverse transcriptase inhibitors	Azidothymidine	Zidovudine, Retrovir
	Dideoxyinosine	Didanosine
	Dideoxycytidine	Zalcitabine
	d4T	Stavudine
	3TC	Lamivudine
Nonnucleoside reverse transcriptase inhibitors	Nevirapine	—
	Delavirdine	—
Protease inhibitors	Saquinavir	Invirase
	Ritonavir	Norvir
	Indinavir	Crixivan
	Nelfinavir	—
Influenza A virus	Amantadine	Symmetrel
	Rimantadine	
Hepatitis C virus	Interferon-alpha	Interferon-alpha-2a:Roferon A
		Interferon-alpha-2b:Intron A
Papillomavirus	Interferon-alpha	—
Respiratory syncytial virus, Lassa virus	Ribavirin	Virazole

*Also active against VZV.
†Topical use only.
‡Also active against HSV.

pesvirus DNA polymerases. The viral DNA polymerases have nearly 30 times greater affinity for the drug than the cellular DNA polymerase.

GCV is effective in the treatment of CMV retinitis in patients with AIDS. Studies are also in progress to determine its efficacy in the treatment of CMV esophagitis, colitis, and pneumonia. It is currently available only for intravenous administration. Because the drug can cause bone marrow toxicity, its use is primarily limited to the treatment of CMV infections in AIDS patients. Interestingly, this potential toxicity has been used as the basis for the development of an antitumor therapy. In one application, an HSV thymidine kinase gene was incorporated into the cells of a brain tumor using a retrovirus vector. These cells became susceptible to the GCV and die because the retrovirus replicated only in the growing cells and the thymidine kinase was expressed only in the tumor cells.

Adenine Arabinoside

Ara A (Vidarabine) is a purine nucleoside analogue identical in structure to adenosine except that arabinose is substituted for ribose as the sugar moiety (Figure 47-1). It is phosphorylated by cellular enzymes (especially adenosine kinase), even in uninfected cells, and thus has a greater potential for causing toxicity than ACV. Although both cellular and viral DNA polymerases are inhibited by Ara A triphosphate, the viral enzyme is 6 to 12 times more sensitive. This is the basis for a somewhat favorable therapeutic/toxic ratio. Ara A is incorporated into viral as well as cellular DNA.

Ara A was the principal antiviral drug used in the treatment of herpesvirus infections until ACV was introduced. Ara A is also active against VZV but not the Epstein-Barr virus or CMV. The drug is rapidly deactivated by host cell enzymes to produce an inactive metabolite and is relatively insoluble in physiological solutions. These properties make it difficult to deliver an effective inhibitory dose. Resistance can develop as a result of the mutation of the viral DNA polymerase.

Azidothymidine

First developed as an anticancer drug, AZT was the first useful therapy for HIV infection. AZT (Retrovir, Zidovudine), a nucleoside analogue of thymidine, inhibits the reverse transcriptase of HIV (Figure 47-1). Like other nucleosides, AZT must be phosphorylated, in this case by host cell enzymes. However, it lacks the 3′ hydroxyl necessary for DNA chain elongation. The selective therapeutic effect of AZT stems from the 100-fold-lower sensitivity of the host cell DNA polymerase as compared with the sensitivity of the HIV reverse transcriptase.

Continuous oral AZT treatment is administered to HIV-infected people with depleted CD4 T-cell counts (less than 500 cells per milliliter) to prevent progression of disease. AZT treatment of pregnant HIV-infected women can prevent the transmission of or reduce the likelihood of transmitting the virus to the baby. Toxicity to AZT ranges from nausea to life-threatening bone marrow toxicity.

The same characteristic that makes HIV sensitive to AZT also promotes the development of resistance. Specifically, the high error rate of the HIV polymerase creates extensive mutations and promotes the development of resistant strains. This problem is being addressed by the administration of multiple-drug therapy as initial therapy. It is more difficult for the HIV to develop resistance to multiple drugs, and any multiple drug-resistant HIV strains are likely to be much weaker than the parent strains.

Dideoxyinosine Dideoxycytidine, Stavudine, and Lamivudine

Several other nucleoside analogues have been approved as anti-HIV agents. **Dideoxyinosine (Didanosine)** is a nucleoside analogue that is converted to dideoxyadenosine triphosphate to inhibit the HIV reverse transcriptase (Figure 47-1). Like AZT, dideoxyinosine, **dideoxycytidine,** and **stavudine** lack a 3′ hydroxyl group and inhibit the HIV reverse transcriptase by preventing DNA chain elongation and inhibit HIV replication in a similar manner. **Lamivudine** (2′-deoxy-3′-thiacytidine) also has a modified sugar attached to the nucleotide base and prevents DNA chain elongation. These drugs are available for the treatment of AIDS patients unresponsive to AZT therapy or can be given in combination with AZT.

Ribavirin

Ribavirin is an analogue of the nucleoside guanosine (Figure 47-1) but differs from guanosine in that its base ring is incomplete and open. Like other nucleoside analogues, ribavirin must be phosphorylated. The drug is active in vitro against a broad range of viruses.

Ribavirin monophosphate resembles guanosine monophosphate and inhibits nucleoside biosynthesis, mRNA capping, and other processes important to the replication of many viruses. Ribavirin depletes the cellular stores of guanine by inhibiting inosine monophosphate dehydrogenase, an enzyme important in the synthetic pathway of guanosine. It also prevents the synthesis of the mRNA 5′ cap by interfering with the guanylation and methylation of the nucleic acid base. In addition, ribavirin triphosphate inhibits RNA polymerases. Its multiple sites of action may explain the lack of ribavirin-resistant mutants of respiratory syncytial virus or influenza A virus.

Ribavirin is administered in an aerosol for the treatment of children with severe respiratory syncytial virus bronchopneumonia and potentially adults with severe influenza or measles. The drug may be effective for the treatment of Lassa fever and Korean and Argentine hemorrhagic fevers, in which cases it is administered orally or intravenously.

Other Nucleoside Analogues

Iododeoxyuridine (idoxuridine), trifluorothymidine (trifluridine) (Figure 47-1), and **fluorouracil** are analogues of thymidine. These drugs inhibit the biosynthesis of thymidine, a nucleotide essential for DNA synthesis, or replace thymidine and become incorporated into the viral DNA. This action inhibits further synthesis of the virus or causes extensive misreading of the genome, leading to mutation and inactivation of the virus. These drugs target cells in which extensive DNA replication is taking place, as occurs in cells infected with HSV.

Iododeoxyurine was the first anti-HSV drug approved for human use. It was at one time used for the topical treatment of herpes keratitis but has been replaced by trifluridine and other more effective, less toxic agents. Fluorouracil is an antineoplastic drug that kills rapidly growing cells but has also been used for the topical treatment of warts caused by human papillomaviruses.

Many other nucleoside analogues that have antiviral activity are being investigated for clinical use against the herpesviruses, hepatitis B virus, and HIV. These compounds include modified pyrimidines such as bromovinyldeoxyuridine with a modified base, fluoroiodoaracytosine with a modified base and a 2-fluoro arabinose sugar instead of ribose, and 2-fluoromethylarauridine with the same modified sugar as fluoroiodoaracytosine. Researchers have also developed purine analogues that lack or have alternate sugar residues attached to the nucleoside base, similar in concept to ACV.

Nonnucleoside Polymerase Inhibitors

Foscarnet (PFA) and the related **phosphonoacetic acid** (PAA) are simple compounds that resemble py-rophosphate (Figure 47-3). These drugs inhibit viral replication by binding to the pyrophosphate-binding site of the DNA polymerase to block nucleotide binding. PFA and PAA do not inhibit cellular polymerases at pharmacological concentrations, but they can cause renal and other problems because of their ability to chelate divalent metal ions (e.g., calcium) and become incorporated into bone. PFA inhibits the DNA polymerase of all herpesviruses and the HIV reverse transcriptase without having to be phosphorylated by nucleotide kinases (e.g., thymidine kinase). PFA has been approved for the treatment of CMV retinitis in AIDS patients.

Nevirapine, delavirdine, and other **nonnucleoside reverse transcriptase inhibitors** bind to sites on the enzyme different from the substrate. Because these drugs' mechanisms of action differ from those of the nucleoside analogues, the mechanism of HIV resistance to the agents is also different. As a result, these drugs may become very useful in combination with nucleoside analogues for the treatment of HIV infection.

Protease Inhibitors

The unique structure of the HIV protease and its essential role in the production of a functional virion has made this enzyme a good target for antiviral drugs. **Saquinavir, indinavir,** and **ritonavir** are such agents and work by slipping into the hydrophobic active site of the enzyme to inhibit its action. As occurs with the other anti-HIV drugs, drug-resistant strains may arise as the result of mutation. The combination of a protease inhibitor with AZT and a second nucleotide analogue can reduce blood levels of HIV to undectable levels. Development of resistance to a "cocktail" of anti-HIV drugs is also less likely than that to a single drug.

Amantadine and Rimantadine

Amantadine and rimantadine are amphipathic amine compounds with clinical efficacy against the influenza A virus but not the influenza B or other viruses (Figure 47-3). Amantadine has several effects on influenza A replication. Both compounds are acidotrophic and concentrate in and buffer the contents of the endosomal vesicles involved in the uptake of the influenza virus. This can inhibit the acid-mediated change in conformation in the hemagglutinin protein required for fusion of the viral envelope with cell membranes. However, the specificity of the amantadine stems from its ability to bind to and block the proton channel formed by the M_2 matrix protein of the influenza A virus. Influenza A strains with an altered M_2 matrix or hemagglutinin protein may be resistant to these drugs.

Amantadine is effective in preventing influenza A and may be useful in ameliorating the infection if taken within 48 hours of exposure. It is also useful as a prophylactic treatment in lieu of vaccination. In addition, it is an alternative therapy for Parkinson's disease. Its principal toxic effect is on the central nervous system, with

FIGURE 47-3 Structures of nonnucleoside antiviral drugs.

patients experiencing nervousness, irritability, and insomnia.

Interferon

Genetically engineered forms of interferon-alpha have been approved for human use. Interferon-alpha is normally produced by leukocytes in response to viral challenge. Interferons work by binding to cell surface receptors and initiating a cellular antiviral response. In addition, interferons stimulate the immune response and promote the immune clearance of viral infection. Interferon-alpha is active toward many viral infections, including hepatitis A and B, HSV, papillomavirus, and rhinovirus. It has been approved for the treatment of condyloma acuminatum (genital warts, a presentation of papillomavirus) and hepatitis C. Interferon causes the influenza-like symptoms observed during many viremic and respiratory tract infections and causes similar side effects during treatment. Interferon is discussed further in Chapter 14.

QUESTIONS

1. List the steps in viral replication that are poor targets for antiviral drugs. Why?
2. List the viruses that can be treated with an antiviral drug. Distinguish the viruses treatable with an antiviral nucleoside analogue.
3. A mutation in the gene for which enzymes or proteins would confer resistance to the following antiviral drugs: ACV, Ara A, phosphonoformate, amantadine, AZT?
4. A patient has been exposed to influenza A virus and is in his third day of symptoms. He has heard that an antiinfluenza drug is available and requests therapy. You tell him that therapy is not appropriate. To what therapeutic agent is the patient referring, and why did you decline to use the treatment?
5. After treatment of an AIDS patient prophylactically with ACV for 6 months, viral disease becomes evident. The ACV treatment is stopped for 2 weeks and then resumed. No virus is observed on resumption of therapy. Which virus is being treated by the ACV? Why did the treatment become ineffective? Why did the disease disappear after the break in therapy?

Bibliography

Baron S et al: The interferons: mechanisms of action and clinical applications, *JAMA* 266:1375-1383, 1991.

Fischl MA et al: The efficacy of azidothymidine (AZT) in the treatment of patients with AIDS and AIDS-related complex: a double-blind, placebo-controlled trial, *N Engl J Med* 317:185-191, 1987.

Havlichek DH, Neu HC: Antiviral drugs. In Wingard LB Jr et al, editors: *Human pharmacology: molecular to clinical,* St Louis, 1991, Mosby.

Mills J, Volberding PA, Corey L: Antiviral chemotherapy, *Adv Exp Med Biol* vol 394, 1996 (entire issue).

Minor JR, Hay AJ, Belshe RB: *Antiviral drug therapy.* In Belshe RB, editor: *Textbook of human virology,* ed 2, St Louis, 1991, Mosby.

Pharmaceutical Manufacturer's Association. *1991 survey report on AIDS medicines in development: AIDS patient care,* Washington, DC, 1992, The Association.

Richman DD: Antiviral therapy of HIV infection, *Annu Rev Med* 42:69-90, 1991.

CHAPTER 48

Laboratory Diagnosis of Viral Diseases

The patient's history and symptoms provide the first clues to the diagnosis of a viral infection, but the diagnostic process also includes the exclusion of other types of infection (e.g., bacterial, fungal). Results from viral laboratory studies can confirm the diagnosis by identifying the viral agent of infection. Appropriate therapy can be chosen once this is known. Identification of a viral agent is also useful for defining the disease process, for monitoring the disease epidemiologically, and for educating physicians and patients.

A clinical diagnosis of a viral infection can be confirmed in the laboratory through the observation of virus-induced **cytopathological effects (CPEs)** on cells, electron microscopic detection of viral particles, isolation and growth of the virus, detection of viral components (e.g., proteins, enzymes, nucleic acids), and evaluation of the patient's immune response to the virus (serology). The molecular and immunological techniques used for many of these procedures are described in Chapters 17 and 18. Virus, viral antigens, and CPEs can be detected by means of cytological examinations of clinical specimens or of tissue culture cells grown and infected in the laboratory (Box 48-1).

CYTOLOGY

The cytological examination of specimens can furnish information that can be used to make a rapid initial diagnosis of infections caused by viruses that produce a characteristic CPE. Characteristic CPEs include changes in cell morphology, cell lysis, vacuolation, syncytia (Figure 48-1), and inclusion bodies. **Inclusion bodies** constitute either histological changes in the cells caused by viral components or virus-induced changes in cell structures. For example, Cowdry type A inclusions in single cells or in large syncytia (multiple cells fused together) are a characteristic finding in cells infected with herpes simplex virus (HSV) or varicella-zoster virus (VZV) (Figure 48-2). Nuclear, owl-eye inclusion bodies are found in the cells of tissues with cytomegalovirus (CMV) or in the sediment of urine from patients with the infection. Rabies may be detected by the finding of Negri bodies (rabies virus inclusions) in brain tissue (Figure 48-3).

ELECTRON MICROSCOPY

Electron microscopy is not a standard clinical laboratory technique, but it can be used to detect and identify some viruses if sufficient viral particles are present. The addition of virus-specific antibody to a sample can cause viral particles to clump and thereby facilitate the detection and simultaneous identification of the virus (immuno-electron microscopy). This method is useful for the detection of enteric viruses, such as rotavirus, which are produced in abundance and have a characteristic morphology. Appropriately processed tissue from a biopsy or clinical specimen can also be examined for the presence of viral structures.

VIRAL ISOLATION AND GROWTH

The "gold standard" for proving a viral etiology of a syndrome is the recovery and growth of the infecting agent. The patient's symptoms and travel history, the season of the year, and a presumptive diagnosis help determine the appropriate procedures to be used to isolate a viral agent (Table 48-1). For example, cerebrospinal fluid and urine are appropriate specimens to be obtained in a patient who has symptoms of central nervous system disease after parotitis because the mumps virus that can cause such disease can be isolated in these specimens. A focal encephalitis with a temporal lobe localization preceded by headaches and disorientation suggests HSV infection, in which case biopsy of the brain should be performed to obtain tissue for cytological studies and viral isolation. The development of meningitis symptoms during the summer indicates an enterovirus etiology, in which case cerebrospinal fluid, a throat swab, and stool should be collected.

The selection of the appropriate specimen for viral culture is often complicated because several viruses may cause the same clinical disease. For example, aseptic meningitis can be caused by many agents, so it may be necessary to obtain several types of specimens to identify the causal virus.

Specimens should be collected early in the acute phase of infection before the virus ceases to be shed. For example, respiratory viruses may be shed for only 3 to 7 days and lapse before the symptoms cease. HSV and VZV may not be recoverable from lesions more than 5 days after the onset of symptoms. It may be possible to isolate an enterovirus from the cerebrospinal fluid for only 2 to 3 days after the onset of the central nervous system manifestations. In addition, antibody produced in response to the infection may block the detection of virus.

The shorter the interval between the collection of a specimen and its delivery to the laboratory, the greater the potential for isolating a virus. This is because many viruses are labile and the samples are also susceptible to bacterial and fungal overgrowth. Viruses are best transported and stored on ice and in special media that contain antibiotics and proteins such as serum albumin or gelatin. Significant losses in infectious titers occur when enveloped viruses (e.g., HSV, VZV, influenza virus) are

FIGURE 48-1 Syncytium formation by measles virus. Multinucleated giant cell *(arrow)* visible in a histological section of lung biopsy tissue from a measles virus–induced giant cell pneumonia in an immunocompromised child. (From Hart C, Broadhead RL: *A color atlas of pediatric infectious diseases,* London, 1992, Wolfe.)

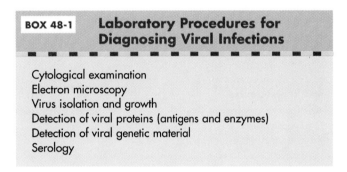

BOX 48-1   **Laboratory Procedures for Diagnosing Viral Infections**

Cytological examination
Electron microscopy
Virus isolation and growth
Detection of viral proteins (antigens and enzymes)
Detection of viral genetic material
Serology

A

B

FIGURE 48-2 HSV-induced CPE. A biopsy specimen of an HSV-infected liver shows an eosinophilic Cowdry type A intranuclear inclusion body *(A)* surrounded by a halo and a ring of marginated chromatin at the nuclear membrane. An infected cell *(B)* exhibits a smaller condensed nucleus (pyknotic). (Courtesy Dr. J.I. Pugh, St. Albans; from Emond RT, Rowland HAK: *A color atlas of infectious diseases,* ed 3, London, 1995, Mosby.)

FIGURE 48-3 Negri bodies caused by rabies. **A,** A section of brain from a patient with rabies shows Negri bodies *(arrow)*. **B,** Higher magnification from another biopsy specimen. (**A** from Hart C, Broadhead RL: *A color atlas of pediatric infectious diseases,* London, 1992, Wolfe.)

TABLE 48-1	Specimens for Viral Diagnosis	
COMMON PATHOGENIC VIRUSES	**SPECIMENS FOR CULTURE**	**COMMENTS**
RESPIRATORY TRACT		
Adenovirus; influenza virus; enterovirus (picornavirus); rhinovirus; paramyxovirus; rubella virus; HSV	Nasal washing, throat swab, nasal swab, sputum	Enterovirus is also shed in stool.
GASTROINTESTINAL TRACT		
Reovirus; rotavirus; adenovirus; Norwalk virus, calicivirus	Stool, rectal swab	Samples are analyzed by electron microscopy and antigen detection (ELISA); viruses are not cultured.
MACULOPAPULAR RASH		
Adenovirus; enterovirus (picornavirus)	Throat swab, rectal swab	—
Rubella virus; measles virus	—	Rubella and measles viruses may be detected in urine.
VESICULAR RASH		
Coxsackievirus; echovirus; HSV; VZV	Vesicle fluid, scraping or swab, enterovirus in stool	Initial diagnosis of HSV and VZV can be obtained from vesicle scraping (Tzanck smear).
CENTRAL NERVOUS SYSTEM (ASEPTIC MENINGITIS, ENCEPHALITIS)		
Enterovirus (picornavirus)	Stool	—
Arboviruses (e.g., togaviruses, bunyavirus)	Rarely cultured	Diagnosis is by serological tests.
Rabies virus	Tissue, saliva, brain biopsy	Diagnosis is by immunofluorescence analysis for antigen.
HSV; CMV; mumps virus; measles virus	Cerebrospinal fluid, brain immunofluorescence analysis	Virus isolation and antigen are assayed.
URINARY TRACT		
Adenovirus; CMV	Urine	Cytomegalovirus may be shed without apparent disease.
BLOOD		
HIV; human T-cell leukemia virus; hepatitis B, C, and D viruses	Blood	Serological antigen or antibody detection (ELISA), polymerase chain reaction (PCR), and reverse transcriptase PCR are done.

Data from Cherneskey MA, Ray CG, Smith TF: *Cumitech 15: laboratory diagnosis of viral infections,* Washington, DC, 1982, American Society for Microbiology; and Hsiung GD: *Diagnostic virology,* New Haven, Conn, 1982, Yale.

BOX 48-2   Systems for the Propagation of Viruses

People
Animals: cows (e.g., Jenner's cowpox vaccine), chickens, mice, rats, suckling mice
Embryonated eggs
Organ and tissue culture
  Organ culture
  Primary tissue culture
  Cell lines: diploid
  Tumor or immortalized cell line

BOX 48-3   Viral Cytopathological Effects

Cell death
  Cell rounding
  Degeneration
  Aggregation
  Loss of attachments to substrate
Characteristic histological changes: inclusion bodies in the nucleus or cytoplasm, margination of chromatin
Syncytia: multinucleated giant cells caused by virus-induced cell-cell fusion
Cell surface changes
  Viral antigen expression
  Hemadsorption (hemagglutinin expression)

---

kept at room temperature or frozen at $-20°$ C. This is not the case for nonenveloped viruses (e.g., adenoviruses, enteroviruses).

Viral Growth

Virus can be grown in tissue culture, embryonated eggs, or experimental animals (Box 48-2). However, although embryonated eggs are still used for the growth of virus for some vaccines (e.g., influenza), they have been replaced by cell cultures for routine virus isolation in clinical laboratories. Experimental animals are rarely used in clinical laboratories for the purpose of isolating viruses.

Cell Culture

Different types of tissue culture cells are used to grow viruses. **Primary cell cultures** are obtained by dissociating specific animal organs with trypsin or collagenase. The cells yielded by this method are then grown as monolayers (fibroblast or epithelial) or in suspension (lymphocyte) in artificial media supplemented with bovine serum or another source of growth factors. Primary cells can be dissociated with trypsin and passed or transferred to become secondary cell cultures. **Diploid cell strains** are cultures of a single cell type that are capable of being passed a large but finite number of times before they senesce, or undergo a significant change in their characteristics. **Tumor cells** and cells immortalized by viruses or chemicals can be grown as cell lines and consist of a single cell type that can be passed continuously without senescing.

Primary monkey kidney cells are excellent for the recovery of myxoviruses, paramyxoviruses, many enteroviruses, and some adenoviruses. Human fetal diploid cells, which are generally fibroblastic cells, support the growth of a broad spectrum of viruses (e.g., HSV, VZV, adenoviruses, picornaviruses) and are the only cells in which CMV can be recovered. HEp-2 cells, a continuous line of epithelial cells derived from a human cancer, are excellent for the recovery of respiratory syncytial virus, adenoviruses, and HSV. Many clinically significant viruses can be recovered in at least one of these cell cultures.

Viral Detection

A virus can be detected and initially identified by observation of the virus-induced CPE in the cell monolayer (Box 48-3 and Figure 48-4). For example, a single virus may cause a focus of cytopathology (**plaque**). The type of cell culture, the characteristics of the CPE, and the rapidity of viral growth can be used to initially identify many clinically important viruses. This approach to identifying viruses is similar to that used in the identification of bacteria, which is based on the growth and morphology of colonies on selective differential media.

Some viruses grow slowly or not at all or do not readily cause a CPE in cell lines typically used in clinical virology laboratories. Some cause conditions that are hazardous or not routinely available. These viruses are most frequently diagnosed on the basis of serological findings or through the detection of viral genomes or antigens.

Characteristic viral properties can also be used to identify viruses that do not cause a classic CPE. For example, the rubella virus may not cause a CPE, but it does prevent (interfere with) the replication of picornaviruses in a process known as *heterologous interference*, which can be used to identify the virus. Cells infected with the influenza virus, parainfluenza virus, mumps virus, and togavirus express a viral glycoprotein (hemagglutinin) that binds erythrocytes of defined animal species to the infected cell surface (**hemadsorption**) (Figure 48-5). When released into the cell culture medium, such viruses can be detected by the agglutination of erythrocytes, a process termed **hemagglutination.** The strain of virus can be identified by blocking the hemagglutination with a specific antibody, a process called **hemagglutination inhibition (HI).**

The amount of virus can be quantitated by determining the titer of virus that causes cytopathology in tissue culture (**tissue culture dose [TCD50]**); that kills 50%

FIGURE 48-5 Hemadsorption of erythrocytes to cells infected with influenza viruses, mumps virus, parainfluenza viruses, or togaviruses express a hemagglutinin on their surfaces that binds erythrocytes of selected animal species.

FIGURE 48-4 CPE of HSV infection. **A,** Uninfected Vero cells, an African green monkey kidney cell line. **B,** HSV-1–infected Vero cells showing rounded cells, multinucleated cells, and loss of the monolayer.

of a set of test animals (**lethal dose [LD50]**); or that initiates a detectable symptom, antibody, or other response in 50% of a set of test animals (**infectious dose [ID50]**). The number of infectious viruses can also be evaluated by a count of the plaques produced by tenfold dilutions of sample (**plaque-forming units**). The ratio of viral particles to plaque-forming units is always greater than 1 because numerous defective viral particles are produced during viral replication.

Interpretation of Culture Results

In general the detection of any virus in host tissues, cerebrospinal fluid, blood, or vesicular fluid can be considered a highly significant finding. However, viral shedding may also be induced by an underlying condition (e.g., another infection, an immunosuppressed state, stress) and unrelated to the disease symptoms. Certain viruses can be intermittently shed without the affected person manifesting symptoms for periods ranging from weeks (enteroviruses in feces) to many months or years (HSV or CMV in the oropharynx and vagina; adenoviruses in the oropharynx and intestinal tract). Virus will not be isolated if the sample is improperly handled, there is neu-

tralizing antibody in the sample, or the sample is acquired before or after viral shedding.

DETECTION OF VIRAL PROTEINS

Enzymes and other proteins are produced during viral replication and can be detected by biochemical, immunological, and molecular biological means (Box 48-4). The viral proteins can be separated by electrophoresis and their patterns used to identify and distinguish different viruses. For example, the electrophoretically separated HSV-infected cell proteins and virion proteins exhibit different patterns for different types and strains of HSV-1 and HSV-2.

The detection and assay of characteristic enzymes or activities can identify and quantitate specific viruses. For example, the presence of reverse transcriptase in serum or cell culture indicates the presence of a retrovirus. Similarly, hemagglutination or hemadsorption can be used to easily assay the hemagglutinin produced by the influenza virus.

Antibodies can be used as sensitive and specific tools to detect, identify, and quantitate the virus and viral antigen in clinical specimens or cell cultures (immunohistochemistry). Specifically, monoclonal or monospecific antibodies are useful for distinguishing among viral strains and mutants. Viral antigens on the cell surface or within the cell can be detected by **immunofluorescence** and **enzyme immunoassay (EIA)** (see Figures 18-2 and 18-3). Virus or antigen released from infected cells can be detected by **enzyme-linked immunosorbent assay (ELISA)**, **radioimmunoassay (RIA)**, and **latex agglutination (LA)**.

The detection of CMV can be enhanced using a combination of cell culture and immunological methods. In this method, the clinical sample is centrifuged onto cells grown on a coverslip or the bottom of a shell vial. This

BOX 48-4 **Assays for Viral Proteins and Nucleic Acids**

PROTEINS

Protein patterns (electrophoresis)
Enzyme activities (e.g., reverse transcriptase)
Hemagglutination and hemadsorption
Antigen detection (e.g., indirect fluorescence, enzyme-linked immunosorbent assay, Western blot)

NUCLEIC ACIDS

Restriction endonuclease cleavage patterns
Electrophoretic mobilities of RNA for segmented RNA viruses (electrophoresis)
DNA genome hybridization in situ (cytochemistry)
Southern, Northern, and dot blots
Polymerase chain reaction (DNA)
Reverse transcriptase polymerase chain reaction (RNA)

increases the efficiency of the method and accelerates virus entry into the cells on the coverslip. The cells can then be analyzed by immunofluorescence or EIA for early viral antigens, which are detectable within 24 hours instead of the 7 to 14 days it takes for a CPE to become evident.

DETECTION OF VIRAL GENETIC MATERIAL

The genome structure and genetic sequence are major distinguishing characteristics of the family, type, and strain of virus (Box 48-4). The electrophoretic patterns of RNA (influenza, reovirus) or restriction endonuclease fragment lengths from DNA viral genomes are like genetic fingerprints for these viruses. Different strains of HSV-1 and HSV-2 can be distinguished in this way by restriction fragment length polymorphism.

DNA probes with sequences complementary to specific regions of a viral genome can be used, like antibodies, as sensitive and specific tools for detecting a virus. These probes can detect the virus even in the absence of viral replication. DNA probe analysis is especially useful for detecting slowly replicating or nonproductive viruses such as CMV and human papillomavirus. Specifically, DNA probes are used to detect specific viral genetic sequences in fixed, permeabilized tissue biopsy specimens by **in situ hybridization,** or they are used to detect viral genomes in clinical samples using **dot** or **Southern blot analysis** of electrophoretically separated restriction endonuclease cleavage fragments of the genome blotted onto nitrocellulose filters. Electrophoretically separated viral RNA (**Northern blot**–RNA:DNA probe hybridization) blotted onto a nitrocellulose filter can be detected in a similar manner. The viral nucleic acids are detected by autoradiography or by fluorescent or EIA-like meth-

ods. Many viral probes and kits for detecting viruses are now commercially available.

DNA probes are especially useful for detecting and locating viral genomes in patient samples in which there is no CPE or in which either the viral antigen level is below the level of detection or the antigen cannot be detected using the specific immunological tests available. DNA probes are also useful for studying the expression of specific viral genes in different cell types (see Figure 17-3).

The **polymerase chain reaction (PCR)** and **reverse transcriptase PCR (RT-PCR)** are becoming very important for viral detection. Use of the appropriate primers can promote a million-fold amplification of a target sequence in a few hours. This technique is especially useful for detecting latent and integrated virus sequences, such as the sequences of retroviruses, herpesviruses, papillomaviruses, and other papovaviruses, as well as those of viruses present in low concentrations. RT-PCR uses the retroviral reverse transcriptase to convert viral RNA to DNA to allow PCR amplification of the viral nucleic acid sequences. This approach was very useful for identifying and distinguishing the hantaviruses which caused the outbreak in New Mexico in 1993.

VIRAL SEROLOGY

The humoral immune response provides a history of a patient's infections. Serology can be used to identify the virus and its strain or serotype, evaluate the course of an infection, and determine whether it is a primary infection or a reinfection and whether it is acute or chronic. Serological data on a viral infection are provided by the antibody type and titer and the nature of the antigenic targets. Serological studies are used for the identification of viruses that are difficult to isolate and grow in cell culture and of viruses that cause diseases with slow courses (see Box 18-2).

The detection of virus-specific IgM antibody, which is present during the first 2 to 3 weeks of a primary infection, generally indicates a recent primary infection. Seroconversion is indicated by at least a fourfold increase in the antibody titer between the titer determined in the serum obtained during the acute phase of disease and that determined in the serum obtained at least 2 to 3 weeks later, during the convalescent phase. Reinfection or recurrence later in life causes an anamnestic (secondary or booster) response. Antibody titers may remain high in patients who suffer frequent recurrence of a disease (e.g., herpesviruses).

Because of the inherent imprecision of serological assays based on twofold serial dilutions, a fourfold increase in the antibody titer between acute and convalescent sera is required to indicate seroconversion. For example, samples with 512 units and 1023 units of antibody would both give a signal on a 512-fold dilution but not a 1024-fold dilution and would be reported as 512. On the other hand, samples with 1020 and 1030 units are not significantly different but would be reported as titers of 512 and 1024, respectively.

The course of a chronic infection can also be determined by a serological profile. Specifically, the presence of antibodies to several key viral antigens and their titers can be used to identify the stage of disease caused by certain viruses. This is especially useful for the diagnosis of viral diseases with slow courses (e.g., hepatitis B, infectious mononucleosis caused by Epstein-Barr virus). In general the first antibodies to be detected are directed against the antigens most available to the immune system (e.g., on the virion or infected-cell surfaces). Later in the infection, when cells have been lysed by the infecting virus or the cellular immune response, antibodies directed against the intracellular viral proteins and enzymes are detected. For example, antibodies to the envelope and capsid antigens of Epstein-Barr virus are detected first. Then, during convalescence, antibodies to nuclear antigens, such as the Epstein-Barr virus nuclear antigen, are detected.

A serological battery or panel consisting of assays for several viruses may be used for the diagnosis of certain diseases. Local epidemiological factors, the time of year, patient factors such as immunocompetency, the patient's travel history, and the patient's age influence the choice of virus assays to be included on a panel. For example, HSV and mumps, western and eastern equine encephalitis, St. Louis encephalitis, and California encephalitis viruses may be included in a panel of tests for central nervous system diseases (see Box 18-2).

Serological Test Methods

The serological tests used in virology are listed in Box 18-1 and described further in Chapter 18. **Neutralization** and **HI** tests assay antibody on the basis of its recognition of and binding to virus. The antibody coating of the virus

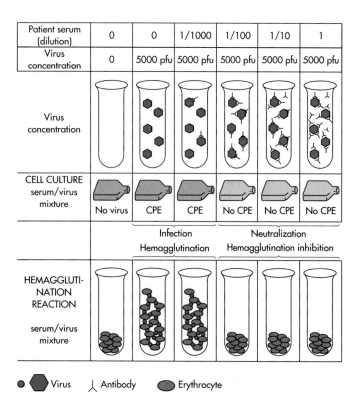

FIGURE 48-6 Neutralization, hemagglutination, and hemagglutination inhibition assays. In the assay shown, tenfold dilutions of serum were incubated with virus. Aliquots of the mixture were then added to cell cultures or erythrocytes. In the absence of antibody, the virus infected the monolayer (indicated by CPE) and caused hemagglutination (i.e., formed a gel-like suspension of erythrocytes). In the presence of the antibody, infection was blocked (neutralization), and hemagglutination was inhibited, allowing the erythrocytes to pellet. The titer of antibody in the serum was 100. *pfu,* Plaque-forming units.

Strip	Interpretation	Bands present
2	Indeterminate	p24, p55, gp160
5	Indeterminate	p24, p55
6	Indeterminate	p24, gp41, p55, p66, gp120, gp160
7	Positive	p17, p24, p31, gp41, p51, p55, p66, gp120, gp160

FIGURE 48-7 Western blot analysis of HIV antigens and antibody. HIV protein antigens are separated by electrophoresis and blotted onto nitrocellulose paper strips. The strip is incubated with patient antibody, washed to remove the unbound antibody, and then reacted with enzyme conjugated antihuman antibody and chromophoric substrate. Serum from an HIV-infected person binds and identifies the major antigenic proteins of HIV. Of the four sera shown, only serum 7 recognizes all the antigens and is definitively positive. (From Belshe RB, editor: *Textbook of human virology,* ed 2, St Louis, 1991, Mosby.)

blocks its binding to indicator cells (Figure 48-6). For neutralization, antibody inhibits infection and cytopathology in tissue culture cells. A neutralization antibody response is virus and strain specific. The response often develops with the onset of symptoms and persists for long periods. HI is used for the identification of viruses that can selectively agglutinate erythrocytes of various animal species (e.g., chicken, guinea pig, human). Antibody in serum prevents a standardized amount of virus from binding to and agglutinating erythrocytes.

The indirect fluorescent antibody test and solid-phase immunoassays such as LA , ELISA, and RIA are commonly used to detect and quantitate specific antibody-virus antigen immune complexes. These tests can detect both viral antigen and antiviral antibody. Western blot analysis has become very important to confirm seroconversion and hence infection with the human immunodeficiency virus (HIV). Patient antibody recognition of specific viral proteins separated by electrophoresis, transferred (blotted) onto a filter paper (e.g., nitrocellulose, nylon), and visualized with an enzyme-conjugated antihuman antibody confirms the ELISA-indicated diagnosis of HIV infection (Figure 48-7).

Limitations to the Use of Serology

The presence of an antiviral antibody indicates previous infection but is not sufficient to indicate when the infection occurred. The finding of virus-specific IgM, a fourfold increase in the antibody titer between the acute and convalescent sera, or specific antibody profiles is indicative of recent infection. False-positive or false-negative test results may also confuse the diagnosis. In addition, patient antibody may be bound with viral antigen (as occurs in patients with hepatitis B) in immune complexes, thereby preventing its detection. Serological cross-reactions between different viruses may also confuse the identity of the infecting agent (e.g., parainfluenza and mumps express related antigens). Conversely, the antibody used in the assay may be too specific (many monoclonal antibodies) and may not recognize other viruses from the same family, giving a false-negative result (e.g., rhinovirus). A good understanding of the clinical symptoms and a knowledge of the limitations and potential problems with serological assays will aid in making the diagnosis.

QUESTIONS

1. Brain tissue is obtained at autopsy from a person who died of rabies. What procedures could be used to confirm the presence of rabies virus–infected cells in the brain tissue?
2. A cervical Papanicolaou smear is taken from a woman with a vaginal papilloma (wart). Certain types of papilloma have been associated with cervical carcinoma. What method, or methods, would be used to detect and identify the type of papilloma in the cervical smear?
3. A legal case would be settled by identification of the source of an HSV infection. Serum and viral isolates are obtained from the infected person and two contacts. What methods could be used to determine whether the person is infected with HSV-1 or HSV-2? What methods could be used to compare the type and strain of HSV obtained from all three people?
4. Serum is taken when the disease presents and 3 weeks later from a 50-year-old man experiencing influenza-like symptoms. The HI data for the current strain of influenza A (H3N2) are presented at the top, right-hand side. Hemagglutination is indicated by the filled circle. Is the patient infected with the current strain of influenza A?

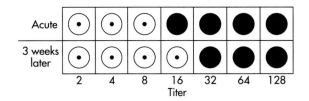

5. A policeman accidentally sticks his finger with a drug addict's syringe needle. He is concerned that he may be infected with HIV. Samples are taken from the policeman a month later for analysis. What assays would be appropriate to determine whether the man is infected with the virus? In this case, it may be too early to detect an antibody response to the virus. What procedures would be appropriate to assay for virus or viral components?

Bibliography

Baron EJ, Peterson LR, Finegold SM: *Bailey and Scott's diagnostic microbiology,* ed 9, St Louis, 1994, Mosby.

Chernesky MA, Ray CG, Smith TF: *Laboratory diagnosis of viral infections,* Washington, DC, 1982, American Society for Microbiology.

Hsiung GD: *Diagnostic virology,* ed 3, New Haven, 1982, Yale.

Lennette EH, editor: *Laboratory diagnosis of viral infections,* New York, 1985, Marcel Dekker.

Lennette DA, Spector S, Thompson KD, editors: *Infections: the role of the clinical laboratory,* Baltimore, 1979, University Park.

Menegus MA: *Diagnostic virology.* In Belshe RB, editor: *Textbook of human virology,* ed 2, St Louis, 1991, Mosby.

Specter S, Lancz G, editors: *Clinical virology manual,* ed 2, New York, 1992, Elsevier.

49

Papovaviruses

The papovavirus family (Papovaviridae) includes the papillomaviruses and polyomaviruses (Table 49-1). Papovaviruses are capable of causing lytic, chronic, latent, and transforming infections, depending on the host cell. Human papillomaviruses (HPVs) cause **warts,** and several genotypes are associated with human cancer (e.g., **cervical carcinoma**). BK and JC viruses, members of the *Polyomavirus* genus, usually cause asymptomatic infection but are associated with renal disease and progressive multifocal leukoencephalopathy, respectively, in immunosuppressed people. Simian virus-40 (SV-40) is the prototype polyomavirus. Although these two genera are in the same family, the viruses differ in size, antigenic determinants, and biological properties.

The papovaviruses are small, nonenveloped icosahedral capsid viruses with double-stranded circular DNA genomes (Box 49-1). They encode proteins that promote cell growth. This facilitates lytic viral replication in a permissive cell type. However, these proteins may also oncogenically transform a cell that is nonpermissive. The polyomaviruses, especially SV-40, have been studied extensively as model oncogenic viruses.

HUMAN PAPILLOMAVIRUSES
Structure and Replication

Classification of the HPVs is based on their DNA relatedness because these viruses cannot be grown readily in tissue culture. On the basis of the DNA sequence homology exhibited by different HPVs, at least 58 types have been identified and classified into 1 of 16 (A through P) groups. HPV can be distinguished further as **cutaneous HPV** or **mucosal HPV** on the basis of the tissue susceptible to the virus. This determines the site of the infection and the lesion. Viruses in similar groups frequently cause similar types of warts.

The icosahedral capsid of HPVs is 50 to 55 nm in diameter and consists of two structural proteins forming 72 capsomeres (Figure 49-1). The HPV genome is circular and has approximately 8000 base pairs. The HPV DNA encodes seven or eight early genes (E1 to E8), depending on the virus, and two late or structural (L1 and L2) genes as well as an origin of transcription and repli-

cation, all located on one strand (the plus strand) (Figure 49-2).

HPV replication is very dependent on the host cell's transcriptional machinery. The virus remains latent in a plasmid form in the basal layer of cells but replicates in the differentiating epithelial cells of the skin or mucosa. The specific nuclear factors expressed in the different layers and types of skin and mucosa control transcription of viral genes and the replication of the genome. As a result, the replication of virus correlates with the expression of specific keratins.

Pathogenesis

Papillomaviruses infect and replicate in the squamous epithelium of skin **(warts)** and mucous membranes **(genital, oral, and conjunctival papillomas)** to induce epithelial proliferation. Infected cells undergo nuclear changes and have large perinuclear vacuoles surrounded by dense cytoplasm, an appearance termed **koilocytosis.** It usually takes 3 to 4 months for the wart to develop. The viral infection remains local and generally regresses spontaneously but can recur (Figure 49-3; see also Figure 40-6, *A*). The HPV pathogenic mechanisms are summarized in Box 49-2.

The oncogenic potential of HPV has been extensively studied. Viral DNA has been found in benign and malignant tumors, especially mucosal papillomas. HPV-16 and HPV-18 cause cervical papillomas and dysplasia, and at least 85% of cervical carcinomas contain **integrated HPV-DNA** rather than plasmidlike DNA. Integration often causes the E1 and E2 genes to be inactivated, thereby limiting viral replication and allowing expression of the E6 and E7 genes. The E6 and E7 proteins of HPV-16 and HPV-18 have been identified as **oncogenes,** which bind and inactivate the cellular growth-suppressor (transformation-suppressor) proteins, p53 and p105 retinoblastoma gene product (p105RB). **E6 binds the p53 protein, and E7 binds to RB.** Without these brakes on cell growth, the cell is more susceptible to mutation, chromosomal aberrations, or the action of a cofactor and develops into cancer.

The mechanism by which papillomas resolve is not known. However, it is known that cell-mediated immu-

FIGURE 49-1 Computer reconstruction of cryoelectron micrographs of HPV. *Left,* View of the surface of HPV shows 72 capsomeres arranged in an icosahedron. All the capsomeres (pentons and hexons) appear to form a head with a regular five-point–star shape. *Right,* Computer cross-section of the capsid shows the interaction of the capsomeres and channels in the capsid. (From Baker TS et al: *Biophysical J* 60:1445-1456, 1991.)

BOX 49-1   **Unique Properties of Papovaviruses**

There is a small **icosahedral** capsid virion.
Double-stranded circular DNA genome is replicated and assembled in the nucleus.
There are two major genera:
   Papilloma: **HPV** types 1 to 58+ (as determined by genotype; types defined by DNA homology, tissue tropism, and association with oncogenesis)
   Polyoma: SV-40, **JC virus,** and **BK virus**
Viruses have defined tissue tropisms determined by receptor interactions and the transcriptional machinery of the cell.
Viruses encode proteins that promote cell growth by binding to the cellular growth-suppressor proteins p53 and p105RB. Polyoma T antigen binds to p105RB and p53. **E6 binds to p53, and E7 binds to p105RB.**
Viruses can cause lytic infections in permissive cells but cause abortive, persistent, or latent infections or **immortalize (transform)** nonpermissive cells.

Genome is a double-standed circular molecule.

E1 protein binds DNA at ori and promotes viral DNA replication (like T antigen of SV-40). E2 protein binds DNA, helps E1, and activates viral mRNA synthesis.

E6 and E7 of HPV-16 and HPV-18 can become immortalizing genes; HPV-16 is associated with human cervical cancer.

L1 and L2 gene products are late structural (capsid) proteins.

| Enhancer promotor | Immortalize, growth promoting | Viral DNA replication | Transcriptional and replication regulator | Minor capsid | Major capsid |

FIGURE 49-2 Genome of HPV-16. DNA is normally a double-stranded circular molecule but is shown here in its linear, integrated form. *E6,* Oncogene protein that binds p53; *E7,* oncogene protein that binds p105RB; *rep ori,* origin of replication; *L1,* major capsid protein; *L2,* minor capsid protein. (Courtesy Tom Broker, MD, Baltimore.)

TABLE 49-1   **Human Papovaviridae and Their Diseases**

VIRUS	DISEASE
Papillomavirus	Warts
Polyomavirus	
BK virus	Renal disease*
JC virus	Progressive multifocal leukoencephalopathy*

*Disease occurs in immunosuppressed patients.

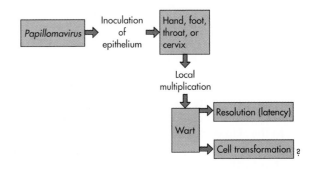

FIGURE 49-3 Progression of HPV infection.

BOX 49-2   Disease Mechanisms of Papovaviruses

PAPILLOMAVIRUSES

Virus is acquired by **close contact** and infects the epithelial cells of the skin or mucous membranes.

Tissue tropism and disease presentation depend on the papillomavirus type.

Viral replication depends on the epithelial cell differentiation stage: It is persistent in the basal layer and active in differentiated keratinocytes.

Viruses cause benign outgrowth of cells into **warts.**

Warts resolve spontaneously, possibly resulting from immune response.

Certain types are associated with **dysplasia** that may become **cancerous** with the action of cofactors.

DNA of specific HPV types is present (integrated) in the tumor cell chromosomes.

POLYOMAVIRUSES (JC AND BK VIRUSES)

Virus is probably acquired through the respiratory route and spread by viremia to the kidneys early in life.

Infections are **asymptomatic.**

Virus establishes **persistent** and **latent** infection in organs such as the kidneys and lungs.

In **immunocompromised** people, JC virus is activated, spreads to the brain, and causes progressive multifocal leukoencephalopathy **(PML),** a conventional slow virus disease.

In PML, JC virus partially transforms astrocytes and kills oligodendrocytes, causing characteristic lesions and sites of demyelination.

BK virus is ubiquitous but is not associated with serious disease.

BOX 49-3   Epidemiology of Papovaviruses

DISEASE/VIRAL FACTORS

Capsid virus is resistant to inactivation.

Virus persists in host.

Asymptomatic shedding is likely.

TRANSMISSION

Papillomavirus: **direct contact, sexual contact** (sexually transmitted disease) for certain virus types, or passage through infected birth canal for laryngeal papillomas (types 6 and 11).

Polyoma: inhalation of infectious aerosols.

WHO IS AT RISK?

Papilloma: warts are common; sexually active people are at risk for infection with HPV types correlated with oral and genital cancers.

WHO IS AT RISK?—cont'd

Polyoma: ubiquitous; immunocompromised people at risk for progressive multifocal leukoencephalopathy.

GEOGRAPHY/SEASON

Viruses are found worldwide.

There is no seasonal incidence.

MODES OF CONTROL

There are no modes of control.

---

nity is an important factor, as shown by the fact that immunosuppressed people have recurrences and more severe presentations of papillomavirus and other papovavirus infections.

Epidemiology

HPV resists inactivation and can be transmitted on fomites, such as the surfaces of counters or furniture, bathroom floors, and towels (Box 49-3). Asymptomatic shedding may promote transmission. HPV infections are transmitted by direct contact and acquired through small breaks in the skin or mucosa. Inoculation can occur during sexual intercourse, while an infant is passing through an infected birth canal, or as the result of chewing warts (a childhood habit).

Common, plantar, and flat warts are most common in children and young adults. The lower incidence in adults may result from acquired immunity. Laryngeal papillomas occur in young children and middle-aged adults.

HPV is a **sexually transmitted disease** common among sexually active people. Findings from recent studies indicate that genital HPV infections may occur in 10% to 20% of women. HPV-16, HPV-18, and several other types of HPV are closely linked to cervical carcinoma, the second leading cause of cancer death in women (approximately 500,000 deaths per year).

Clinical Syndromes

The clinical syndromes and the HPV types that cause them are summarized in Table 49-2.

TABLE 49-2   **Clinical Syndromes Associated with Papillomaviruses**

	HPV TYPES	
SYNDROME	**COMMON**	**UNCOMMON**
SKIN WARTS		
Plantar wart	1	2, 4
Common wart	2, 4	1, 7, 26, 29
Flat wart	3, 10	27, 28, 41
Epidermodysplasia verruciformis	5, 8, 17, 20, 36	9, 12, 14, 15, 19, 21-25, 38, 46
BENIGN HEAD AND NECK TUMORS		
Laryngeal papilloma	6, 11	—
Oral papilloma	6, 11	2, 16
Conjunctival papilloma	11	—
ANOGENITAL WART		
Condyloma acuminatum	6, 11	1, 2, 10, 16, 30, 44, 45
Cervical intraepithelial neoplasia, cancer	16, 18	11, 31, 33, 35, 42-44

Modified from Balows A et al: *Laboratory diagnosis of infectious diseases: principles and practice,* vol 2, New York, 1988, Springer-Verlag.

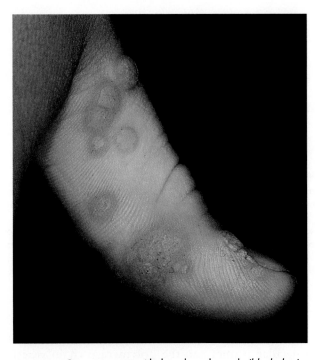

FIGURE 49-4 Common warts with thrombosed vessels *(black dots).* (From Habif TP: *Clinical dermatology: a color guide to diagnosis and therapy,* St Louis, 1985, Mosby.)

Skin Warts

Most people with HPV infection have the common types of the virus (HPV-1 through HPV-4), which infect keratinized surfaces, usually on the hands and feet (Figure 49-4). Initial infection occurs in childhood or early adolescence. The incubation period before a wart develops may be as long as 3 to 4 months. The appearance of the wart (dome shaped, flat, or plantar) depends on the HPV type and the infected site.

Benign Head and Neck Tumors

Single oral papillomas are the most benign epithelial tumors of the oral cavity. They are pedunculated with a fibrovascular stalk, and their surface usually has a rough papillary appearance. They can occur in people of any age group, are usually solitary, and rarely recur after surgical excision. **Laryngeal papillomas** are commonly associated with HPV-6 and HPV-11 and are the most common benign epithelial tumors of the larynx. However, laryngeal papillomatosis is usually considered a life-threatening condition in children because of the danger of the papillomas obstructing the airway. Occasionally, papillomas may extend down the trachea and into the bronchi.

Anogenital Warts

Genital warts **(condyloma acuminatum)** occur almost exclusively on the squamous epithelium of the external genitalia and perianal areas. Approximately 90% are caused by HPV-6 and HPV-11. Anogenital lesions infected with these types of HPV rarely become malignant in otherwise healthy people.

Cervical Dysplasia and Neoplasia

HPV infection of the genital tract is now recognized as a common sexually transmitted disease. Cytological changes characteristic of this viral infection **(koilocytotic cells)** are detected in approximately 5% of all **Papanicolaou-stained cervical smears** (Figure 49-5). Infection of the female genital tract by HPV-16 and HPV-18 and,

FIGURE 49-5 Papanicolaou stain of the exfoliated cervicovaginal squamous epithelial cells showing the perinuclear cytoplasmic vacuolization termed *koilocytosis* (vacuolated cytoplasm) characteristic of HPV infection. (×400.)

TABLE 49-3	Laboratory Diagnosis of *Papillomavirus* Infections

TEST	DETECTS
Cytology	Koilocytotic cells
In situ DNA probe analysis*	Viral nucleic acid
Polymerase chain reaction*	Viral nucleic acid
Southern blot hybridization	Viral nucleic acid
Immunofluorescent and immunoperoxidase staining	Viral structural antigens
Electron microscopy	Virus
Culture	Not useful

*Method of choice.

FIGURE 49-6 A, Comparison of normal skin and a papilloma (wart). HPV infection promotes the outgrowth of prickle cells (acanthosis), which causes the skin to thicken and promotes the production of keratin (hyperkeratosis), thereby causing epithelial spikes to form (papillomatosis). The virus replicates in the granular cells close to the final keratin layer. **B,** DNA probe analysis of an HPV-6–induced anogenital condyloma. A biotin-labeled DNA probe was localized by horseradish peroxidase–conjugated avidin conversion of the substrate to a chromogen precipitate. Dark staining is seen over the nuclei of koilocytotic cells. (**A** modified from Jenson AB et al: *Papillomavirus etiology of oral cavity papillomas.* In Hooks J, Jordan, W, editors: *Viral infections in oral medicine,* New York, 1982, North Holland-Elsevier. **B** from Belshe RB, editor: *Textbook of human virology,* ed 2, St Louis, 1991, Mosby.)

rarely, by other types of HPV is associated with intraepithelial cervical neoplasia and cancer. The first neoplastic changes noted by light microscopy are termed **dysplasia.** Approximately 40% to 70% of the mild dysplasias spontaneously regress.

Cervical cancer is thought to develop through a continuum of progressive cellular changes, from mild (cervical intraepithelial neoplasia [CIN I]) to moderate neoplasia (CIN II) to severe dysplasia or carcinoma in situ. This sequence of events can occur over a 1- to 4-year period.

Laboratory Diagnosis

A wart can be confirmed microscopically on the basis of its characteristic histological appearance, which consists of hyperplasia of the **prickle cells** and an excess production of keratin (**hyperkeratosis**) (Figure 49-6). Papillomavirus infection can be detected in **Papanicolaou smears** by the presence of koilocytotic (vacuolated cytoplasm) squamous epithelial cells, which are rounded and

occur in clumps (Figure 49-5 and Table 49-3). **DNA molecular probes** and the **polymerase chain reaction** (PCR) are the methods of choice for establishing the diagnosis of HPV infection using cervical swabs and tissue specimens. Papillomaviruses do not grow in cell cultures, and tests for HPV antibodies are rarely used except in research surveys.

Treatment, Prevention, and Control

Warts spontaneously regress, but this may take many months to years. Warts are removed because of pain and discomfort, cosmetic reasons, and potential spread to other parts of the body or to other people. They are removed using surgical cryotherapy, electrocautery, or chemical means, although recurrences are common. Injection of interferon is also beneficial. Surgery may be necessary for the removal of laryngeal papillomas.

At present the best way to prevent transmission is to avoid coming in direct contact with infected tissue. Proper precautions (e.g., the use of condoms) can prevent the sexual transmission of HPV.

POLYOMAVIRUSES

The human polyomaviruses (**BK** and **JC viruses**) are ubiquitous but usually do not cause disease. They are difficult to grow in cell cultures. SV-40 and murine polyomaviruses in particular have been studied extensively as models of tumor-causing viruses.

Structure and Replication

The polyomaviruses are smaller (45 nm in diameter), contain less nucleic acid (5000 base pairs), and are less complex than the papillomaviruses (Box 49-1). The genomes of BK virus, JC virus, and SV-40 are closely related and are divided into early, late, and noncoding regions (Figure 49-7). The early region on one strand codes for nonstructural **T (transformation) proteins** (including large T antigen), and the late region, which is on the other strand, codes for three viral capsid proteins (**VP1, VP2,** and **VP3**) (Box 49-4). The noncoding region contains the origin of DNA replication and the site of the transcriptional control sequences for both early and late genes.

After viral entry into the cell, the DNA is uncoated and delivered to the nucleus. The early genes encode the large T and small t antigens, proteins that promote cell growth. Viral replication requires the transcriptional and DNA replication machinery provided by a growing cell. The large T antigens of the SV-40, JC virus, and BK virus have several functions. For example, the T antigen of SV-40 binds to DNA and controls early and late gene transcription, as well as viral DNA replication. In addition, the T antigen binds to the two major cellular growth-suppressor proteins, p53 and p105RB, which promotes cell growth.

As is the case with the HPVs, polyomavirus replication is very dependent on host cell factors. Permissive cells allow the transcription of late viral mRNA and viral replication, which results in cell death. However, some nonpermissive cells allow only the early genes, including T antigen, to be expressed, potentially leading to oncogenic transformation of the cell.

The polyomavirus genome is used very efficiently. The noncoding region of the genome contains the initiation sites for the early and late mRNAs as well as the origin for DNA replication. The three late proteins are produced from mRNAs, which have the same initiation site, and then are processed into three unique mRNAs.

The viral DNA is maintained and replicated bidirectionally, similar to the way in which a bacterial plasmid is

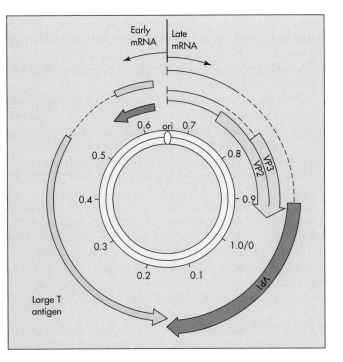

FIGURE 49-7 Genome of the SV-40 virus. The genome is a prototype of that of other polyomaviruses and contains an early, late, and noncoding region. The noncoding region contains the star sequence for the early and late genes and for DNA replication (*ori*). The individual early and late mRNAs are processed from the larger nested transcripts. (Redrawn from Butel JS, Jarvis DL: *Biochem Biophys Acta* 865:171-195, 1986.)

BOX 49-4   **Polyomavirus Proteins**

EARLY

Large T: Regulation of early and late mRNA transcription; DNA replication; cell growth promotion and transformation

Small t: Viral DNA replication

LATE

VP1: Major capsid protein and viral attachment protein
VP2: Minor capsid protein
VP3: Minor capsid protein

maintained and replicated. DNA replication precedes late mRNA transcription and protein synthesis. The virus is assembled in the nucleus, and virus is released by cell lysis.

Pathogenesis

Each polyomavirus is limited to specific hosts and cell types within that host. For example, JC and BK viruses are human viruses that probably enter the respiratory tract, after which they infect lymphocytes and then the kidney with a minimal cytopathological effect. The BK virus establishes latent infection in the kidney, and the JC virus establishes infection in the kidneys, in B cells, and in monocytes-lineage cells. Replication is blocked in immunocompetent people.

In immunocompromised patients such as those with acquired immunodeficiency syndrome (AIDS), reactivation of the virus in the kidney leads to viral shedding in the urine and potentially severe urinary tract infections (BK virus) or viremia and central nervous system infection (JC virus) (Figure 49-8). JC virus crosses the blood-brain barrier by replicating in the endothelial cells of capillaries. An abortive infection of astrocytes results in partial transformation, yielding enlarged cells with abnormal nuclei resembling glioblastomas. Productive lytic infections of oligodendrocytes cause demyelination (Box 49-3). Like the SV-40 virus, the BK and JC viruses cause tumors to form in hamsters; however, these viruses are not associated with any human tumors.

Epidemiology

Polyomavirus infections are ubiquitous, and most people are infected with both the JC and BK viruses by the age of 15 years (Box 49-3). Respiratory transmission is the probable mode of spread. Latent infections can be reactivated in people whose **immune systems are suppressed** as a result of AIDS, organ transplantation, or pregnancy.

Early batches of poliomyelitis vaccine were contaminated with SV-40, a simian polyomavirus that was undetected in the primary monkey cell cultures used to prepare the vaccine. Although many people were vaccinated with the contaminated vaccines, no SV-40–related tumors have ever been reported.

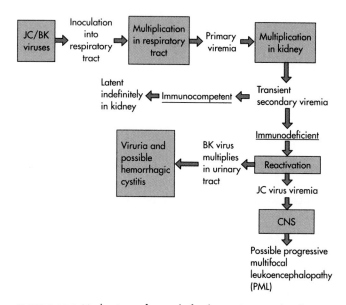

FIGURE 49-8 Mechanisms of spread of polyomaviruses within the body.

Clinical Syndromes

Primary infection is virtually always asymptomatic. The BK and JC viruses are commonly found to be excreted in the urine of as many as 40% of immunocompromised patients. The viruses are also reactivated during pregnancy, but no effects on the fetus have been established.

The ureteral stenosis observed in renal transplant recipients appears to be associated with BK virus, as is the hemorrhagic cystitis observed in bone marrow transplant recipients.

Progressive multifocal leukoencephalopathy is a rare syndrome. This subacute demyelinating disease occurs in immunocompromised patients, including those with AIDS, and is caused by the **JC virus.** As the name implies, patients may have multiple neurological symptoms unattributable to a single anatomical lesion. Speech, vision, coordination, mentation, or a combination of these functions is impaired, followed by paralysis of the arms and legs and finally death. The cerebrospinal fluid is normal, however, and does not contain antibody to the JC virus.

Laboratory Diagnosis

Progressive multifocal leukoencephalopathy is definitively diagnosed on the basis of the findings yielded by the histological examination of brain tissue obtained by biopsy or at autopsy. Foci of demyelination surrounded by oligodendrocytes with inclusions adjacent to areas of demyelination are observed in such tissue. Electron microscopy, **PCR,** or **DNA probe analysis** can be used to detect virus in brain tissue. The term *leukoencephalopathy* refers to the presence of lesions in only the white matter. There is little if any inflammatory cell response. Magnetic resonance imaging or computed tomographic scans may show evidence of lesions.

Urine cytological tests can reveal the presence of JC or BK virus infection by revealing the existence of enlarged cells with dense basophilic intranuclear inclusions resembling those induced by cytomegalovirus. Cytomegalovirus inclusions, however, are smaller and have a larger halo effect (i.e., a clear zone around the inclusion but within the nuclear membrane).

It is difficult to isolate BK and JC viruses in tissue cultures, and therefore this is not routinely attempted.

Quicker methods of analysis now include in situ immunofluorescence, immunoperoxidase, DNA probe analysis, and PCR analysis of cerebrospinal fluid, urine, or biopsy material for the particular genetic sequences.

Treatment, Prevention, and Control

No specific treatment for polyomavirus infection is available, other than to decrease the immunosuppression responsible for allowing the polyomavirus to be reactivated and symptoms to occur. The ubiquitous nature of polyomaviruses and the lack of understanding of their modes of transmission make it unlikely that the primary infection can be prevented.

CASE STUDY AND QUESTIONS

A 25-year-old carpenter notices the appearance of several hyperkeratotic papules (warts) on the palm side of his index finger. They do not change in size and cause him only minimal discomfort. After a year, they spontaneously disappear.

1. Will this virus infection spread to other body sites?
2. After its disappearance, is the infection likely to be completely resolved or persist in the host?
3. What viral, cellular, and host conditions regulate the replication of this virus and other HPVs?
4. How would the papillomavirus type causing this infection be identified?
5. Is it likely that this type of HPV is associated with human cancer? If not, which types are associated with cancer and which cancers are they?

Bibliography

Arthur RR et al: Association of BK viruria with hemorrhagic cystitis in recipients of bone marrow transplants, *New Engl J Med* 315:230-234, 1986.

Crum CP, Barber S, Roche JK: Pathobiology of papillomavirus-related cervical diseases, *Clin Microbiol Rev* 4:270-285, 1991.

Fields BN, Knipe DM, Howley PM, editors: *Virology,* ed 3, New York, 1996, Lippincott-Raven.

Gorbach SL, Bartlett JG, Blacklow NR, editors: *Infectious diseases,* Philadelphia, 1992, WB Saunders.

Howley PM: Role of the human papillomaviruses in human cancer, *Cancer Res* 51(suppl 18):5019S-5022S, 1991.

Hseuh C, Reyes CV: Progressive multifocal leukoencephalopathy, *Am Fam Physician* 37:129-132, 1988.

Major EO et al: Pathogenesis and molecular biology of progressive multifocal leukoencephalopathy, *Clin Microb Rev* 5:49-73, 1992.

Mandell GL, Bennett JE, Dolin R: *Principles and practice of infectious diseases,* ed 4, New York, 1995, Churchill Livingstone.

Miller DM, Brodell RT: Human papillomavirus infection: treatment options for warts, *Am Fam Physician* 53:135-143, 1996.

Morrison EA: Natural history of cervical infection with human papillomavirus, *Clin Infect Dis* 18:172-180, 1994.

White DO, Fenner FJ: *Medical virology,* ed 4, New York, 1994, Academic.

zur-Hausen H: Viruses in human cancers, *Science* 254:1167-1173, 1991.

zur-Hausen H: *Human pathogenic papillomaviruses,* vol 186, *Current Topics in Microbiology and Immunology,* New York, 1994, Springer-Verlag.

CHAPTER 50

Adenoviruses

denoviruses were first isolated in 1953 in a human adenoid cell culture. Since then, approximately 100 serotypes, at least 42 of which infect humans, have been recognized. All human serotypes are included in a single genus within the family Adenoviridae. On the basis of the findings from DNA homology studies and the hemagglutination patterns, the 42 serotypes have been found to belong to one of six subgroups (A to F) (Table 50-1). The viruses in each subgroup share many properties.

The first human adenoviruses to be identified, numbered 1 to 7, are the most common. Common disorders caused by the adenoviruses include **respiratory tract infection, conjunctivitis, hemorrhagic cystitis,** and **gastroenteritis.** Several adenoviruses have an oncogenic potential in animals and for this reason have been extensively studied by molecular biologists. These studies have elucidated many viral and eukaryotic intracellular processes. For example, analysis of the gene for the adenovirus hexon led to the discovery of introns and the splicing of eukaryotic messenger RNAs (mRNAs). Adenovirus is also being used for gene replacement therapy (e.g., cystic fibrosis).

STRUCTURE AND REPLICATION

Adenoviruses are double-stranded DNA viruses with a genome molecular weight of 20 to 25×10^6 daltons. The adenovirus genome is a linear, double-stranded DNA with a terminal protein (molecular weight, 55,000 daltons) covalently attached at each 5' end. The virions are nonenveloped icosadeltahedrons with a diameter of 70 to 90 nm (Figure 50-1 and Box 50-1). The capsid comprises 240 capsomeres, which consist of **hexons** and **pentons.** The 12 pentons, which are located at each of the vertices, contain a penton base and a fiber. The fiber contains the **viral attachment proteins** and can act as a hemagglutinin. The penton base and fiber are toxic to cells. The pentons and fibers also contain type-specific antigens.

The core complex within the capsid includes viral DNA and at least two major proteins. At least 11 polypeptides are contained in the adenovirus virion, 9 of which have an identified structural function (Table 50-2).

A map of the adenovirus genome shows the locations of the viral genes (Figure 50-2). The genes are transcribed from both DNA strands and in both directions at different times during the replication cycle. Most of the RNA transcribed from the adenovirus genome is processed into several individual mRNAs in the nucleus. Early proteins promote cell growth and include a **DNA polymerase** that is involved in the replication of the genome. Adenovirus also encodes proteins that suppress host immune and inflammatory responses. Late proteins, which are synthesized after the onset of viral DNA replication, are primarily structural in function.

The replication of adenoviruses has been studied extensively in HeLa cell cultures. One virus cycle takes approximately 32 to 36 hours and produces 10,000 virions. In this process the viral fiber proteins interact with cell surface receptors (approximately 100,000 fiber receptors are present on each cell), and virons enter the cell by means of endocytosis. The virus lyses the endosomal vesicle, and the capsid delivers the DNA genome to the nucleus. The penton and fiber proteins of the capsid are toxic to the cell and can inhibit cellular macromolecular synthesis.

Early transcriptional events lead to the formation of gene products that can stimulate cell growth and promote viral DNA replication. As is the case for the papovaviruses, several adenovirus mRNAs will share the same promoter but are produced through the splicing out of different introns. Transcription of the E1A gene, processing of the primary transcript (splicing out of introns to yield three mRNAs), and translation produce the transactivator proteins required for transcription of the other early proteins. Other early proteins include more DNA-binding proteins, the DNA polymerase, and proteins to help the virus escape the immune response. The **E1A** and **E1B proteins** stimulate cell growth by binding to the cellular growth-suppressor proteins **p53** (E1B) and **RB** (retinoblastoma gene product) (E1A). In permissive cells, growth of the cells facilitates transcription and replication of the genome, which ultimately causes cell death. In nonpermissive cells, the virus establishes latency, or for rodent cells, the E1A and E1B may promote cell growth without cell death and promote oncogenicity.

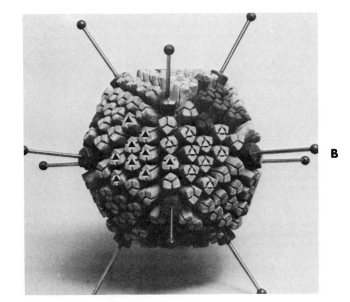

FIGURE 50-1 A, Electron micrograph of adenovirus virion with fibers. **B,** Model of adenovirus virion with fibers. (**A** from Valentine RC, Periera HG: *J Molecular Biol* 13:13-20, 1965; **B** from Ginsberg HS: *The adenoviruses,* New York, 1984, Plenum.)

BOX 50-1   Unique Features of Adenovirus

Naked icosadeltahedral capsid has **fibers** (viral attachment proteins) at vertices.

Linear double-stranded genome has 5′ terminal proteins.

Virus encodes proteins to promote mRNA and DNA synthesis, including its own **DNA polymerase.**

Human adenoviruses are grouped A through F by DNA homologies and by serotype (more than 42 types).

Serotype is mainly due to differences in the penton base and fiber protein, which determine the nature of tissue tropism and disease.

Virus causes **lytic, persistent,** and **latent** infections in humans, and some strains can **immortalize certain animal cells.**

TABLE 50-1   Illnesses Associated with Adenoviruses

ILLNESS CATEGORY	MOST COMMON SEROTYPES
Endemic respiratory disease	1, 2, 5
Acute respiratory disease of military recruits	3, 4, 7, 14, 21
Adenoviral pneumonias	3, 4, 7b, 14, 21
Epidemic keratoconjunctivitis	8, 19
Pharyngoconjunctival fever	3, 7
Less common syndromes	
Pertussis syndrome	1-3, 5
Acute hemorrhagic cystitis	1, 4, 7, 11, 21
Hepatic disorders	3, 7
Gastroenteritis	9, 12, 13, 18, 25-28, 40-42
Intussusception	1, 2, 5
Musculoskeletal disorders	7
Genital infections	19
Skin infections	2, 4, 7, 21
Infections in immunocompromised hosts	32, 34-36

From Liu C: *Adenoviruses.* In Belshe RB, editor, *Textbook of human virology,* ed 2, St Louis, 1991, Mosby.

Viral DNA replication occurs in the nucleus and by a viral DNA polymerase from both strands of the DNA. The polymerase uses a primer consisting of a 55,000-dalton viral protein (terminal protein) and a cytosine monophosphate.

Late gene transcription starts after DNA replication. Most of the individual late mRNAs are generated from a large (83% of the genome) primary transcript encoded by the right strand of the genome that is processed into individual mRNAs.

Capsid proteins are produced in the cytoplasm and then transported to the nucleus for viral assembly. Empty capsids first assemble, and then the viral DNA and core

TABLE 50-2   **Major Adenovirus Proteins**

PROTEIN	NUMBER	MOLECULAR WEIGHT (KD)	FUNCTION
Early gene products*			
E1A			Activates viral gene transcription
			Binds cellular growth suppressor: RB105 promotes transformation
			Deregulates cell growth
			Inhibits activation of interferon response elements
E1B			Binds cellular growth suppressor: p53 promotes transformation
			Blocks apotosis
E2			Activates some promoters
			Is terminal protein on DNA
			DNA polymerase
E3			Prevents tumor necrosis factor–alpha cytotoxicity
E4			Limits viral cytopathological effect
VA RNAs			Inhibit interferon response
Capsid			
	II	120	Hexon protein
			Contains family antigen and some serotyping antigens
	III	85	Penton base protein
			Toxic to tissue culture cells
	IV	62	Fiber
			Responsible for attachment and hemagglutination; contains some serotyping antigens
	VI	24	Hexon-associated proteins
	VIII	13	Penton-associated proteins
	IX	12	
	IIIa	66	
Core			
	V	48	Core protein 1: DNA-binding protein
	VII	18	Core protein 2: DNA-binding protein

*Early genes encode several mRNA and proteins by alternative splicing patterns.

FIGURE 50-2 Simplified genome map of adenovirus type 2. Genes are transcribed from both strands (l and r) in opposite directions. The early genomes are transcribed from four promoter sequences. All of the late genes are transcribed from one promoter sequence. Alternative splicing patterns of primary RNA transcripts produce the full repertoire of viral proteins. The splicing pattern for the E2 transcript is shown as an example. *E,* Early protein; *L,* late protein. (Based on data from Jawetz E, Melnick JL, Adelberg EA, editors: *Review of medical microbiology,* ed 17, Norwalk, Conn, 1987, Appleton & Lange.)

proteins enter the capsid through an opening at one of the vertices. Cleavage of several of the capsid proteins and of the terminal protein attached to the DNA causes the particle to mature into a stable and infectious virion. Because the replication and assembly process is inefficient and error prone (11 to 2300 particles produced per plaque-forming unit), DNA, protein, and numerous defective particles accumulate in nuclear inclusion bodies. The virus remains in the cell until the cell degenerates and lyses.

PATHOGENESIS AND IMMUNITY

Adenoviruses are capable of causing lytic (e.g., mucoepithelial cells), latent (e.g., lymphoid and adenoid cells), and transforming (hamster, not human) infections. These viruses infect **epithelial cells** lining respiratory and enteric organs (Box 50-2). Viremia may occur after local replication of the virus, with subsequent spread of the virus to visceral organs (Figure 50-3). This dissemination is more likely to occur in immunocompromised patients than in immunocompetent people. The viral fiber proteins determine the target cell specificity among adenovirus serotypes. The toxic activity of the penton base protein can result in inhibition of cellular mRNA transport and protein synthesis, cell rounding, and tissue damage.

The virus has a propensity to become **latent** in lymphoid tissue, such as adenoids, tonsils, or Peter's patches, and can be reactivated in patients in an immunosuppressed state or infected with other agents. Although certain adenoviruses (groups A and B) can transform and are **oncogenic in rodent cells,** adenovirus transformation of human cells has not been observed. The time course of adenovirus infection is shown in Figure 50-4.

The histological hallmark of adenovirus infection is a dense, central intranuclear inclusion within an infected epithelial cell that consists of viral DNA and protein (Figure 50-5). These inclusions may resemble those seen in cells infected with cytomegalovirus, but adenovirus does not cause cellular enlargement (cytomegaly). Mononuclear cell infiltrates and epithelial cell necrosis are seen with the characteristic inclusions.

Antibody is important for causing lytic adenovirus infections to resolve and protects the person from reinfection with the same serotype. Cell-mediated immunity is important in limiting virus outgrowth, as borne out by the fact that immunosuppressed people suffer recurrent disease.

Adenovirus encodes several early proteins that help the virus **avoid immune defenses.** For example, during viral replication, a short RNA segment is produced; this

> **BOX 50-2**   **Disease Mechanisms of Adenoviruses**
>
> Virus is spread by **aerosol, close contact, or fecal-oral** means to establish pharyngeal infection. Fingers spread virus to eyes.
> Virus infects **mucoepithelial cells** in the respiratory tract, gastrointestinal tract, and conjunctiva or cornea, causing cell damage directly.
> Virus **persists** in lymphoid tissue (e.g., tonsils, adenoids, Peyer's patches).
> **Antibody** is important for prophylaxis and resolution.
> Disease is determined by the tissue tropism of the specific group or serotype of the virus strain.

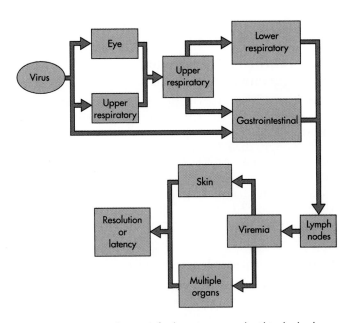

FIGURE 50-3 Mechanism of adenovirus spread within the body.

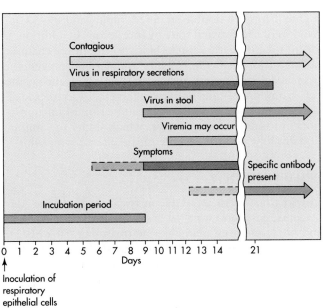

FIGURE 50-4 Time course of adenovirus respiratory infection.

BOX 50-3 **Epidemiology of Adenoviruses**

DISEASE/VIRAL FACTORS

Capsid virus is resistant to inactivation by gastrointestinal tract and drying.

Disease symptoms may resemble those of other respiratory virus infections.

Virus may cause asymptomatic shedding.

TRANSMISSION

Direct contact via respiratory droplets and fecal matter, on hands, on fomites (e.g., towels, contaminated medical instruments), close contact, and inadequately chlorinated swimming pools.

WHO IS AT RISK?

People in day-care centers, military training camps, and swimming clubs.

GEOGRAPHY/SEASON

Virus is found worldwide.

There is no seasonal incidence.

MODES OF CONTROL

Live vaccine for serotypes 4 and 7 is available for military use.

FIGURE 50-5 Histological appearance of adenovirus-infected cells. Inefficient assembly of virions yields dark basophilic nuclear inclusion bodies containing DNA, proteins, and capsids.

segment forms a double-stranded duplex and blocks activation of the antiviral state by interferon. In addition, a 19,000-dalton early protein binds to the heavy chain of class I major histocompatibility antigen and prevents it from reaching the cell membrane, thus preventing the cell from presenting antigenic targets to cytotoxic T cells. Several proteins inhibit the induction of inflammation by tumor necrosis factor, which limits the immunopathology and the severity of the disease symptoms.

EPIDEMIOLOGY

Adenovirus virions are stable in response to drying, detergents, gastrointestinal tract secretions (acid, protease, and bile), and even mild chlorine treatment (Box 50-3). This allows their spread by the fecal-oral route, by fingers, by **fomites** (including towels and medical instruments), and in poorly chlorinated swimming pools.

Adenoviruses are spread exclusively by human-to-human transmission, mainly by **respiratory or fecal-oral contact,** with no apparent animal reservoirs for the virus.

Close interaction among people, as occurs in classrooms and military barracks, promotes spread of the virus. Adenoviruses may be shed intermittently and over long periods from the pharynx and especially in feces. Most infections are asymptomatic, which greatly facilitates their spread in the community.

Adenoviruses 1 through 7 are the most prevalent serotypes. From 5% to 10% of cases of pediatric respiratory tract disease are caused by adenovirus types 1, 2, and 5. Serotypes 4 and 7 seem especially able to spread among military recruits because the prevalence of antibody to these serotypes is low in young adults.

CLINICAL SYNDROMES

Adenoviruses primarily infect children and less commonly infect adults. Infection with reactivated virus occurs in immunocompromised children and adults. Several distinct clinical syndromes are associated with adenovirus infection (Table 50-1).

Acute Febrile Pharyngitis and Pharyngoconjunctival Fever

Adenovirus causes pharyngitis, which is often accompanied by conjunctivitis **(pharyngoconjunctival fever).** Pharyngitis alone occurs in young children, particularly those younger than 3 years of age, and may mimic streptococcal infection. Affected patients have mild influenza-like symptoms, including nasal congestion, cough, coryza, malaise, fever, chills, myalgia, and headache, which may last 3 to 5 days. Pharyngoconjunctival fever occurs more often in outbreaks that involve older children.

Acute Respiratory Tract Disease

Acute respiratory tract disease is a syndrome of fever, cough, pharyngitis, and cervical adenitis. It occurs primarily among military recruits because of serotypes 4 and 7.

FIGURE 50-6 Conjunctivitis caused by adenovirus.

Other Respiratory Tract Diseases

Adenoviruses cause coldlike symptoms, laryngitis, croup, and bronchiolitis. They can also cause a pertussis-like illness in children and adults that consists of a prolonged clinical course and true viral pneumonia.

Conjunctivitis and Epidemic Keratoconjunctivitis

Adenoviruses cause a follicular conjunctivitis in which the mucosa of the palpebral conjunctiva becomes pebbled or nodular and both conjunctivae (palpebral and bulbar) become inflamed (Figure 50-6). Such conjunctivitis may occur sporadically or in outbreaks that can be traced to a common source (e.g., swimming pools). Epidemic keratoconjunctivitis may be an occupational hazard for industrial workers, with the most striking epidemic occurring in people working in the naval shipyards of Pearl Harbor, where it caused more than 10,000 cases during 1941 and 1942. Irritation of the eye by a foreign body, dust, debris, and the like is a risk factor for the acquisition of this infection.

Gastroenteritis and Diarrhea

Adenovirus is a major cause of acute viral gastroenteritis; 15% of the cases of gastroenteritis in hospitalized patients are caused by this virus. Adenovirus serotypes 40, 41, and 42 have been grouped as enteric adenoviruses (group F) and appear to be responsible for causing episodes of diarrhea in infants. These enteric adenoviruses do not replicate in the same tissue culture cells as other adenoviruses and rarely cause fever or respiratory tract symptoms.

Other Presentations

Adenovirus has also been associated with a pertussis-like illness, intussusception in young children, acute hemorrhagic cystitis with dysuria and hematuria in young boys, musculoskeletal disorders, and genital and skin infections.

Systemic Infection in Immunocompromised Patients

Immunocompromised patients are at risk for serious adenovirus infections, although not as much as they are for infections caused by herpesviruses. Diseases caused by these viruses in immunocompromised patients include pneumonia and hepatitis. Infection can originate from exogenous or endogenous (reactivation) sources.

LABORATORY DIAGNOSIS

The isolation of most adenovirus types is best accomplished in cell cultures derived from epithelial cells (e.g., primary human embryonic kidney cells, continuous [transformed] lines such as HeLa or human epidermal carcinoma cells). The virus causes a lytic infection with characteristic inclusion bodies within 2 to 20 days. Recovery of virus from cell culture requires an average of 6 days.

For the results of virus isolation to be significant, the isolate should be obtained from a site or secretion relevant to the disease symptoms. Isolation of adenovirus from the throat of a patient with pharyngitis is usually diagnostic if laboratory findings eliminate other common causes of pharyngitis, such as *Streptococcus pyogenes*.

Immunoassays, including fluorescent antibody and enzyme-linked immunosorbent assays, the polymerase chain reaction (PCR), and DNA probe analysis, can be used to detect and type and group the virus in clinical samples and tissue cultures. Enzyme immunoassay, PCR, DNA probe analysis, and immunoelectron microscopy are used to identify enteric adenovirus serotypes 40, 41, and 42, which do not grow readily in available cell cultures. These serotypes may be responsible for diarrhea in infants. The characteristic intranuclear inclusions can be seen in infected tissue during histological examination. However, such inclusions are rare and must be distinguished from those produced by cytomegalovirus.

Serological assays such as complement fixation, hemagglutination inhibition, enzyme immunoassay, and neutralization techniques have been used to detect type-specific antibodies after adenovirus infection. However, a fourfold rise in the antibody level between acute and convalescent serum specimens, or seroconversion, must occur for active infection to be diagnosed. Serological testing is rarely used except to confirm the significance of a fecal or upper respiratory tract isolate by identifying its serotype.

TREATMENT, PREVENTION, AND CONTROL

There is no known treatment for adenovirus infection. Live oral vaccines have been used to prevent infections with adenovirus 4 and 7 in military recruits, but they are not used in civilian populations. The widespread use of live adenovirus vaccines is unlikely because members of some species of the adenovirus family are oncogenic. However, genetically engineered subunit vaccines could be prepared and used in the future.

CASE STUDY AND QUESTIONS

A 7-year-old boy attending summer camp complains of sore throat, headache, cough, red eyes, and tiredness and is sent to the infirmary. His temperature is 40° C. Within hours other campers and counselors visit the infirmary with similar symptoms. Symptoms last for 5 to 7 days. All the patients have gone swimming in the camp pond. More than 50% of the people in the camp complain of symptoms similar to the initial case. The public health department identifies the agent as adenovirus serotype 3.*

1. Toward which adenovirus syndrome do the symptoms point?
2. An outbreak as large as this indicates a common source of infection. What was the most likely source or sources? What were the most likely routes by which the virus was spread?
3. What physical properties of the virus facilitate its transmission?

*Modified from *MMWR* 41:342-344, 1991.

4. What precautions or actions should the camp owners take to prevent other outbreaks?
5. What sample or samples would have been used by the public health department to identify the infectious agent and what tests would be required to diagnose the infection?

Bibliography

Balows, Hausler WJ Jr, Lennette EH, editors: *Laboratory diagnosis of infectious diseases: principles and practice*, vol 2, New York, 1988, Springer-Verlag.

Belshe RB, editor: *Textbook on human virology*, ed 2, St Louis, 1991, Mosby.

Doerfleur W, Böhm P, editors: *The molecular repertoire of adenoviruses I, II, III, Current topics in microbiology and immunology* 199, New York, 1995, Springer-Verlag (monographs).

Fields BN, Knipe DM, Howley PM, editors: *Virology*, ed 3, New York, 1996, Lippincott-Raven.

Ginsberg HS: *The adenoviruses*, New York, 1984, Plenum.

Gorbach SL, Bartlett JG, Blacklow NR, editors: *Infectious diseases*, Philadelphia, 1992, WB Saunders.

Mandell GL, Bennett JE, Dolin R: *Principles and practice of infectious diseases*, ed 4, New York, 1995, Churchill Livingstone.

White DO, Fenner FJ: *Medical virology*, ed 4, New York, 1994, Academic.

CHAPTER 51

Human Herpesviruses

The human herpesviruses are grouped into three subfamilies on the basis of differences in viral characteristics (genome structure, tissue tropism, cytopathology, and site of latent infection) as well as the pathogenesis of the disease and disease presentation (Table 51-1). The human herpesviruses include herpes simplex viruses (HSV) types 1 and 2, varicella-zoster virus (VZV), Epstein-Barr virus (EBV), cytomegalovirus (CMV), human herpesvirus 6 (HHV6), human herpesvirus 7 (HHV7), and the recently discovered human herpesvirus 8 (HHV8) associated with Kaposi's sarcoma.

The herpesviruses are a diverse group of large DNA viruses that share a common virion morphology, a basic mode of replication, and the capacity to establish latent and recurrent infections. Cell-mediated immunity is also important for controlling infection with these viruses and causing symptoms. Herpesviruses encode proteins and enzymes that facilitate the replication and interaction of the virus with the host. The herpesviruses can cause lytic, persistent, latent/recurrent, and in the case of EBV, immortalizing infections (Box 51-1).

Herpesvirus infections are common, and the viruses are **ubiquitous.** Although these viruses usually cause benign disease, they can also be associated with significant morbidity and mortality, especially in immunosuppressed people. Fortunately some herpesviruses encode enzymes, including deoxyribonucleotide-scavenging enzymes (e.g., HSV thymidine kinase). These enzymes are targets for antiviral agents. The U.S. Food and Drug Administration (FDA) has approved a live-virus vaccine for VZV.

STRUCTURE OF HERPESVIRUSES

The herpesviruses are **large, enveloped** viruses that contain **double-stranded DNA.** The virion is approximately 150 nm in diameter and has the characteristic morphology shown in Figure 51-1. The DNA core is surrounded by an **icosadeltahedral capsid** containing 162 capsomeres. This is enclosed by a glycoprotein-containing envelope. Herpesviruses encode several glycoproteins for viral attachment, fusion, and immune escape. The space between the envelope and the capsid is called the *tegument* and contains viral proteins and enzymes that help initiate replication. As enveloped viruses the herpesviruses are sensitive to acid, solvents, detergents, and drying.

Herpesvirus genomes are linear, double-stranded DNA but differ in size and gene orientation (Figure 51-2). Direct or inverted repeat sequences bracket unique regions of the genome (unique long [U_L], unique short [U_S]), allowing circularization and recombination within the genome. Recombination among inverted repeats of HSV, CMV, and VZV allows large portions of the genome to switch the orientation of their U_L and U_S gene segments with respect to each other.

REPLICATION OF THE HERPESVIRUSES

Herpesvirus replication is initiated by the interaction of viral glycoproteins with cell surface receptors. The tropism of some herpesviruses (e.g., EBV) is restricted by the tissue-specific expression of receptors. The nucleocapsid is then released into the cytoplasm through fusion of the envelope with the plasma membrane. Enzymes and transcription factors are carried into the cell in the tegument of the virion. The nucleocapsid docks with the nuclear membrane and delivers the genome into the nucleus, where the genome is transcribed and replicated.

Transcription of the viral genome and viral protein synthesis proceed in a coordinated and regulated manner in three phases: first, **immediate early proteins** (alpha), consisting of DNA-binding proteins important for the regulation of gene transcription; then **early proteins** (beta), consisting of more transcription factors and enzymes, including the DNA polymerase; and finally **late proteins** (gamma), consisting mainly of structural proteins. These proteins are generated after viral genome replication has begun.

The viral genome is transcribed by cellular DNA-dependent RNA polymerases and *is regulated by viral-encoded and cellular nuclear factors. The interplay of these factors determines whether the infection is lytic, persistent, or latent.* Cells that promote latent infection restrict transcription to specific genes without genome replication. Progression to early and late gene expression results in cell death and lytic infection.

TABLE 51-1   Properties Distinguishing the Herpesviruses

SUBFAMILY	VIRUS	PRIMARY TARGET CELL	SITE OF LATENCY	MEANS OF SPREAD
ALPHAHERPESVIRINAE				
Human herpesvirus 1	Herpes simplex type 1	Mucoepithelial cells	Neuron	Close contact
Human herpesvirus 2	Herpes simplex type 2	Mucoepithelial cells	Neuron	Close contact (sexually transmitted disease)
Human herpesvirus 3	Varicella-zoster virus	Mucoepithelial cells	Neuron	Respiratory and close contact
GAMMAHERPESVIRINAE				
Human herpesvirus 4	Epstein-Barr virus	B cells and epithelial cells	B cell	Saliva (kissing disease)
Human herpesvirus 8	Kaposi's sarcoma–related virus	—	—	Saliva
BETAHERPESVIRINAE				
Human herpesvirus 5	Cytomegalovirus	Monocyte, lymphocyte, and epithelial cells	Monocyte, lymphocyte, and ?	Close contact, transfusions, tissue transplant, and congenital
Human herpesvirus 6	Herpes lymphotropic virus	T cells and ?	T cells and ?	Respiratory and close contact?
Human herpesvirus 7	Human herpesvirus 7	T cells and ?	T cells and ?	?

? indicates that other cells may also be the primary target or site of latency.

A

B

FIGURE 51-1 Electron micrograph **(A)** and general structure **(B)** of the herpesviruses. The DNA genome of the herpesvirus in the core is surrounded by an icosadeltahedral capsid and an envelope. Glycoproteins are inserted into the envelope.

Herpesviruses have large, enveloped icosadelta-hedral capsids containing **double-stranded DNA genomes.**

Herpesviruses encode many proteins that regulate messenger RNA and DNA synthesis and the shutoff of the host cell DNA, RNA, and protein synthesis.

Herpesviruses encode enzymes (**DNA polymerase**) that promote viral DNA replication and that are good targets for **antiviral drugs.**

DNA replication and assembly occur in the nucleus; virus buds from nuclear membrane and is released by exocytosis and cell lysis.

Herpesviruses can cause **lytic, persistent, latent,** and for EBV, **immortalizing infections.**

Herpesviruses are ubiquitous. Cell-mediated immunity is required for control.

FIGURE 51-2 Herpesvirus genomes. The genomes of the herpesvirus are doubled-stranded DNA. The length and complexity of the genome differ for each virus. Inverted repeats in HSV, VZV, and CMV allow the genome to recombine with itself to form isomers. Large genetic repeat sequences are boxed. The genomes of HSV and CMV have two sections, the unique long (U_L) and the unique short (U_S), each of which is bracketed by two sets of inverted repeats of DNA. The inverted repeats facilitate the replication of the genome but also allow the U_L and U_S regions to invert independently of each other to yield four different genomic configurations, or isomers. VZV has only one set of inverted repeats and can form two isomers. EBV exists in only one configuration, with several unique regions surrounded by direct repeats. *Purple,* Direct repeat DNA sequences; *green,* inverted repeat DNA sequences.

Replication of the viral genome is performed by the viral-encoded DNA polymerase. Viral-encoded scavenging enzymes provide deoxyribonucleotide substrates for the polymerase and are targets of antiviral drugs. These enzymes facilitate replication of the virus in nongrowing cells that lack sufficient substrates for viral DNA synthesis (e.g., neurons).

Empty procapsids assemble in the nucleus, are filled with DNA, acquire an envelope at the nuclear membrane, and exit the cell by exocytosis or by lysis of the cell. Transcription, protein synthesis, glycoprotein processing, and exocytotic release from the cell are performed by cellular machinery. The replication of HSV is discussed in more detail later.

HERPES SIMPLEX VIRUS

HSV was the first human herpesvirus to be recognized. The name *herpes* is derived from a Greek word meaning "to creep." "Cold sores" were described in antiquity, and their viral etiology was established in 1919.

The two types of HSV, 1 and 2, share many characteristics, including DNA homology, antigenic determinants, tissue tropism, and disease symptoms. However, they can still be distinguished by differences in these properties.

Structure

The HSV genome is large enough to encode approximately 80 proteins. Only half are required for viral replication; the others facilitate the virus' interaction with different host cells and the immune response. The HSV genome encodes enzymes, including a DNA-dependent DNA polymerase and scavenging enzymes such as deoxyribonuclease, thymidine kinase, ribonucleotide reductase, protease, and other enzymes. Ribonucleotide reductase converts ribonucleotides to deoxyribonucleotides, and thymidine kinase phosphorylates the deoxyribonucleotides to provide substrates for replication of the viral genome. The substrate specificities of these enzymes and the DNA polymerase differ significantly from their cellular analogue and thus represent potentially good targets for antiviral chemotherapy.

HSV encodes at least 11 glycoproteins that serve as viral attachment proteins (gB, gC, gD, gH), fusion proteins (gB), structural proteins, immune escape proteins (gC, gE, gI), and other functions. For example, the C3 component of the complement system binds to gC and is depleted from serum. The Fc portion of IgG binds to a gE/gI complex, thereby camouflaging the virus and virus-infected cells. These actions reduce the antiviral effectiveness of antibody.

Replication

HSV can infect most types of human cells and even cells of other species. The virus generally causes lytic infections of fibroblasts and epithelial cells and latent infections of neurons (see Figure 6-6 for diagram).

HSV-1 binds initially to heparan sulfate, a proteoglycan found on the outside of many cell types, and then interacts with a receptor protein closer to the cell surface. The major route by which HSV penetrates the host cell is through fusion at the cell surface membrane. On fusion the virion releases a protein that promotes the initiation of viral gene transcription, a viral-encoded protein kinase, and cytotoxic proteins into the cytoplasm.

The immediate early gene products include DNA-binding proteins, which stimulate DNA synthesis and promote the transcription of the early viral genes. During a latent infection a specific region of the genome is transcribed to produce **latency-associated transcripts (LATs)**. These are the only detectable viral products synthesized in these cells, and viral replication does not proceed further.

The early proteins consist mostly of enzymes, including the DNA-dependent polymerase. As catalytic proteins, relatively few copies of these enzymes are required to promote replication. Other early proteins inhibit the production and initiate the degradation of cellular messenger RNA and DNA. Expression of the early and late genes generally leads to cell death.

The genome starts to replicate as soon as the polymerase is synthesized. Circular, end-to-end concatameric forms of the genome are made initially. Later in the infection the DNA is replicated by a rolling circle mechanism to produce a linear string of genomes resembling a roll of toilet paper in concept. The concatamers cleave into individual genomes as the DNA is sucked into a procapsid.

Genome replication triggers transcription of the late genes by which the structural proteins are encoded. Many copies of these proteins are required. The capsid proteins are then transported to the nucleus, where they are assembled into empty procapsids and filled with DNA. The glycoproteins are synthesized and then receive the high-mannose, *n*-linked glycan precursor at the endoplasmic reticulum. After this, the glycoproteins diffuse to the contiguous nuclear membrane. DNA-containing capsids associate and bud from viral glyco-

protein-modified portions of the nuclear membrane. The virus then buds into the endoplasmic reticulum and is transferred in a vesicle to the Golgi apparatus, where the glycoproteins are processed. The virus is released by exocytosis or cell lysis. The virus is also spread by cell-cell fusion and through intracellular bridges.

Pathogenesis and Immunity

The mechanisms involved in the pathogenesis of HSV-1 and HSV-2 are very similar (Box 51-2). Both viruses initially infect and replicate in mucoepithelial cells and then establish latent infection of the innervating neurons. The site of infection and the nature of the subsequent disease are predominantly dependent on the means by which the virus is acquired. HSV-1 is usually associated with infections above the waist and HSV-2 with infections below the waist (Figure 51-3). Other differences between the two types include differences in their receptor specificity, growth characteristics, and antigenicity. HSV-2 has a greater potential to cause viremia and associated systemic influenza-like symptoms.

HSV can cause **lytic** infections of most cells, persistent infections of lymphocytes and macrophages, and **latent** infection of neurons. Cytolysis generally results from the virus-induced inhibition of cellular macromolecular syn-

BOX 51-2   Disease Mechanisms for HSV

Disease is initiated by direct contact and depends on infected tissue (e.g., oral, genital, brain).
Virus causes direct cytopathology.
Virus avoids antibody by cell-to-cell spread (syncytia).
Virus establishes latency in neurons (hides from immune response).
Virus reactivates from latency by stress or immune suppression.
Cell-mediated immunity is *required* for resolution with limited role for antibody.
Cell-mediated immunopathology contributes to symptoms.

FIGURE 51-3 Disease syndromes of HSV. HSV-1 and HSV-2 can infect the same tissues and cause similar diseases but have a predilection for the sites and diseases indicated.

thesis, the degradation of host cell DNA, membrane permeation, cytoskeletal disruption, and senescence of the cell. In addition, changes in the nuclear structure and margination of the chromatin occur, and **Cowdry type A acidophilic intranuclear inclusion bodies** are produced. Many strains of HSV also initiate **syncytia** formation. In tissue culture, HSV rapidly infects and kills cells.

HSV initiates infection of the mucosal membranes or enters through breaks in the skin. The virus replicates in the cells at the base of the lesion and infects the innervating neuron, traveling by retrograde transport to the ganglion (the trigeminal ganglia for oral HSV and the sacral ganglia for genital HSV). The virus then returns to the initial site of infection and may be inapparent or produce **vesicular lesions.** The vesicle fluid contains infectious virions. Tissue damage is caused by a combination of viral pathology and immunopathology. The lesion generally heals without producing a scar.

Humoral and cellular immunity are necessary for the HSV infection to be controlled and resolve. During the primary infection, interferon and natural killer cells limit the progression of the infection. Delayed-type hypersensitivity and cytotoxic killer T-cell responses as well as activated macrophages kill infected cells and resolve the current disease. However, the immunopathology caused by the cell-mediated and inflammatory responses is also a major cause of the symptoms. Antibody directed against the glycoproteins of the virus neutralizes extracellular virus, limiting its spread. However, the virus can escape such antibody neutralization and clearance by direct cell-to-cell spread and latent infection of the neuron. In addition, the virion and virus-infected cells express antibody (Fc) and complement receptors that weaken these humoral defenses. As a result, the **cell-mediated immune response is essential for controlling and resolving HSV infections.** In the absence of functional cell-mediated immunity, HSV infection may disseminate to the vital organs and the brain.

Latent infection occurs in neurons and results in no detectable damage. A **recurrence** can be activated by various stimuli (e.g., stress, trauma, fever, sunlight). In this event the virus travels back down the nerve, causing lesions to develop at the dermatome and at the same spot each time. The stress triggers reactivation by promoting replication of the virus in the nerve, by transiently depressing cell-mediated immunity, or by inducing both processes. The virus can be reactivated despite the presence of antibody. However, recurrent infections are generally less severe, more localized, and of shorter duration than the primary episodes because of the existence of memory immune responses.

Epidemiology

Because HSV can establish latency with the potential for asymptomatic recurrence, the infected person is a lifelong source of contagion (Box 51-3). As an enveloped virus, HSV is very labile and is readily inactivated by drying, detergents, and the conditions of the gastrointestinal tract. Although HSV can infect animal cells, HSV infection is exclusively a human disease.

HSV is transmitted in vesicle fluid, saliva, and vaginal secretions (the **"mixing and matching of mucous membranes"** MMMM). Both types of HSV can cause oral and genital lesions. HSV-1 is usually spread by oral contact (kissing) or through the sharing of glasses, toothbrushes, or other saliva-contaminated items. HSV-1

BOX 51-3   Epidemiology of HSV Infection

DISEASE/VIRAL FACTORS

Virus causes lifelong infection.
Recurrent disease is source of contagion.
Virus may cause asymptomatic shedding.

TRANSMISSION

Virus is transmitted in saliva, in vaginal secretions, and by contact with lesion fluid.
Virus is transmitted orally and sexually and by placement into eyes and breaks in skin.
HSV-1 is generally transmitted orally; HSV-2 is generally transmitted sexually.

WHO IS AT RISK?

Children and sexually active people: at risk for classic presentations of HSV-1 and HSV-2, respectively.
Physicians, nurses, dentists, and others in contact with oral and genital secretions: at risk for infections of fingers (herpetic whitlow). *wrestlers too*

WHO IS AT RISK?—cont'd

Immunocompromised people and neonates: at risk for disseminated, life-threatening disease.

GEOGRAPHY/SEASON

Virus is found worldwide.
There is no seasonal incidence.

MODES OF CONTROL

Antiviral drugs are available.
No vaccine is available.
Health care workers should wear gloves to prevent herpetic whitlow.
Patients with active genital lesions should refrain from intercourse until lesions are completely reepithelialized.

FIGURE 51-4 Clinical course of genital herpes infection. The time course and symptoms of primary and recurrent genital infection with HSV-2 are compared. *Top,* Primary infection. *Bottom,* Recurrent disease. (Data from Corey L et al: *Ann Intern Med* 98:958-973, 1983.)

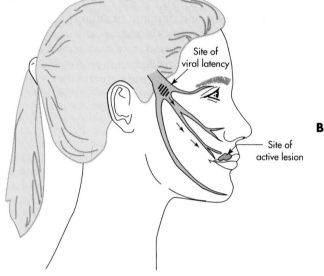

FIGURE 51-5 A, Primary herpes gingivostomatitis. **B,** HSV establishes latent infection and can recur from the trigeminal ganglia. (**A** from Hart CA, Broadhead RL: *A color atlas of pediatric infectious diseases,* London, 1992, Wolfe; B modified from Straus SE: *Herpes simplex virus and its relatives.* In Schaechter M, Eisenstein BI, Medoff G: *Mechanisms of microbial disease,* ed 2, Baltimore, 1993, Williams & Wilkins.)

infection of the fingers or body can result from mouth-to-skin contact, with the virus in this case entering through a break in the skin. Autoinoculation may also cause infection of the eyes.

HSV-1 infection is common. More than 90% of people living in underdeveloped areas have the antibody to HSV-1 by 2 years of age. This may result from crowded living conditions or poor hygiene.

HSV-2 is spread mainly by sexual contact or autoinoculation or from an infected mother to her infant at birth. Depending on a person's sexual practices and hygiene, HSV-2 may infect the genitalia, anorectal tissues, or oropharynx. The virus may then cause symptomatic or asymptomatic primary infection or recurrences. A neonate may become infected during a primary HSV-2 infection in the mother during pregnancy. This results from an ascending in utero infection. More likely, the infant of an infected mother becomes infected as a result of the excretion of HSV-2 from the cervix during vaginal delivery. Perinatal and neonatal infections are associated with similar morbid outcomes.

Initial infection with HSV-2 occurs later in life than infection with HSV-1 and correlates with increased sexual activity. Seropositivity to HSV-2 ranges from less than 1% in college freshmen to 15% to 20% in people in the middle and higher socioeconomic brackets to 40% to 60% in the members of lower socioeconomic groups to 80% in prostitutes.

HSV-2 is seroepidemiologically associated with human cervical cancer, possibly as a cofactor with human papillomavirus or another infectious agent. Partial inac-

tivation of the HSV-2 genome with ultraviolet light causes the virus to immortalize cells in tissue culture.

Clinical Syndromes

HSV-1 and HSV-2 are common human pathogens that can cause painful but benign presentations and recurrent disease. In the classic presentation the lesion is a clear vesicle on an erythematous base (dewdrop on a rose petal) and then progresses to pustular lesions, ulcers, and crusted lesions (Figure 51-4). However, both viruses can cause **significant morbidity and mortality on infection of the eye or brain and on disseminated infection in an immunosuppressed person or a neonate.**

Oral herpes can be caused by HSV-1 or HSV-2. Primary herpetic gingivostomatitis in toddlers and children

FIGURE 51-6 Cold sore of recurrent herpes labialis. It is less severe than that of primary disease. (From Hart CA, Broadhead RL: *A color atlas of pediatric infectious diseases,* London, 1992, Wolfe.)

FIGURE 51-7 Herpetic whitlow. (From Emond RTD, Rowland HAK: *A color atlas of infectious diseases,* ed 3, London, 1995, Mosby.)

is almost always caused by HSV-1, whereas young adults may be infected with HSV-1 or HSV-2. The lesions begin as clear vesicles that rapidly ulcerate. These whitish areas may be widely distributed throughout the mouth, involving the palate, pharynx, gingivae, buccal mucosa, and tongue (Figure 51-5).

People may experience recurrent mucocutaneous HSV infection (**cold sores**) (Figure 51-6) even though they never had clinically apparent primary infection. The virus is generally activated from the trigeminal ganglia. As noted earlier, the symptoms of a recurrent episode are less severe, more localized, and of shorter duration than those of a primary episode. **Herpes pharyngitis** is becoming a prevalent diagnosis in young adults with sore throats caused by viral infections. Severe HSV **stomatitis,** resembling a primary gingivostomatitis, may occur in patients who are immunosuppressed as the result of disease or therapy.

Herpetic keratitis is almost always limited to one eye. It can cause recurrent disease, leading to permanent scarring, corneal damage, and blindness.

Herpetic whitlow is an infection of the finger, and herpes gladiatorum is an infection of the body. The virus establishes infection through cuts or abrasions in the skin. Herpetic whitlow often occurs in nurses or physicians who attend patients with HSV infections, in thumb-sucking children (Figure 51-7), and in people who have genital HSV infections. Herpes gladiatorum is often acquired during wrestling.

Eczema herpeticum is acquired by children with active eczema. The underlying disease promotes the spread of the infection along the skin and potentially to the adrenal glands, liver, and other organs.

Genital herpes is usually caused by HSV-2 but can also be caused by HSV-1 (responsible for 10% of genital infections). Most primary genital infections are asymptomatic. When present, the lesions vary in number and are usually painful. In male patients the lesions typically develop on the glans or shaft of the penis and occasionally

in the urethra. In female patients the lesions may be seen on the vulva, vagina, cervix, perianal area, or inner thigh and are frequently accompanied by itching and a mucoid vaginal discharge. In patients of both sexes a primary infection may be accompanied by fever, malaise, myalgia, and inguinal adenitis, which are symptoms related to a transient viremia. **HSV proctitis** is a painful disease in which the lesions are found in the lower rectum and anus. The presence of antibody to HSV-1 lessens the symptoms. The symptoms and time course of primary and recurrent genital herpes are compared in Figure 51-4.

Recurrent genital HSV disease is shorter in duration and less severe than the primary episode. Recurrences result from reactivation of the latent virus in a sacral ganglion. Almost all recurrent genital infections are caused by HSV-2. Recurrences in approximately half of patients are preceded by a characteristic prodrome of burning or tingling in the area in which the lesions eventually erupt. Episodes of recurrence may be as frequent as every 2 to 3 weeks or may be infrequent. Unfortunately, any infected patient may shed virus asymptomatically. These people may be important vectors for spread of this virus.

Herpes encephalitis is an acute febrile disease that is usually caused by HSV-1. The lesions are generally limited to one of the temporal lobes. The viral pathology and immunopathology cause the destruction of the temporal lobe and give rise to erythrocytes in the cerebrospinal fluid, seizures, focal neurological abnormalities, and other characteristics of viral encephalitis. Herpes encephalitis is the most common viral cause of sporadic encephalitis and causes significant morbidity and mortality even in patients who receive appropriate treatment. The disease occurs at all ages and at any time of the year. Fortunately there are only 300 to 1000 cases per year. **HSV meningitis** is most often a complication of genital HSV-2 infection, and symptoms resolve on their own.

HSV infection in the neonate and newborn is a devastating and usually fatal disease caused most often by **HSV-2.** It may be acquired in utero but more frequently is contracted during passage of the infant through the genital canal when the mother is shedding herpesvirus at the time of delivery. In the absence of a developed cell-mediated immune response, HSV **disseminates** to the liver, lung, and other organs, as well as to the central nervous system.

Laboratory Diagnosis

Cytology and Histology

Characteristic cytopathological effects (CPEs) can be identified in a **Tzanck smear** (a scraping of the base of a lesion), Papanicolaou smear, or biopsy specimen (Table 51-2). These include syncytia, "ballooning" cytoplasm, and Cowdry type A intranuclear inclusions (see Figure 48-2). The cytological findings are indicative but not definitive, however. A rapid, definitive determination of HSV can be made by demonstrating viral antigen (using immunofluorescence or the immunoperoxidase method) or DNA (using in situ hybridization) in the tissue.

Virus Isolation

Virus isolation is the most definitive assay for the diagnosis of HSV infection. Virus can be obtained from vesicles but not crusted lesions. Specimens are collected by aspirating the lesion fluid or by applying a cotton swab to the vesicles and then inoculating the material collected directly into cell cultures.

HSV produces a CPE within 1 to 3 days in HeLa cells, HEp-2 cells, human embryonic fibroblasts, or rabbit kidney cells. Infected cells become enlarged and appear ballooned (see Figure 48-4). Some isolates induce fusion of neighboring cells, giving rise to multinucleated giant cells (syncytia).

HSV isolates can be typed by biochemical, biological, or immunological methods. The restriction endonuclease cleavage patterns of the DNA of HSV-1 and HSV-2 are unique and allow unequivocal typing of the isolates. HSV type-specific DNA probes and antibodies are also available for detecting and differentiating HSV-1 and HSV-2.

Serology

Serological procedures are useful only for diagnosing a primary HSV infection and for epidemiological studies. They are not useful for diagnosing recurrent disease because a significant rise in antibody titers does not usually accompany recurrent disease.

Treatment, Prevention, and Control

HSV encodes several target enzymes for antiviral drugs (Box 51-4) (see Chapter 47). Most antiherpes drugs are nucleotide analogues or inhibitors of the viral DNA polymerase, an enzyme essential for viral replication and the best antiviral drug target. FDA-approved anti-HSV drugs include **acyclovir** (ACV), vidarabine (adenosine arabinoside [Ara A]), idoxuridine (iododeoxyuridine),

---

TABLE 51-2   Laboratory Diagnosis of HSV Infections

APPROACH	TEST/COMMENT
Direct microscopic examination of cells from base of lesion	**Tzanck smear** shows **multinucleated giant cells** and **Cowdry type A inclusion bodies.**
Cell culture	HSV replicates and causes identifiable CPE in most cell cultures.
Assay of tissue biopsy, smear, or vesicular fluid for HSV antigen	Enzyme immunoassay, immunofluorescent stain, and in situ DNA probe analysis are used.
HSV type distinction (HSV-1 vs. HSV-2)	Type-specific antibody, DNA maps of restriction enzyme, SDS–gel protein patterns, and DNA probe analysis are used.
Serology	Serology is not useful except for epidemiology.

SDS, Sodium dodecyl sulfate.

BOX 51-4   FDA-Approved Antiviral Treatments for Herpesvirus Infections

HSV-1 AND HSV-2
Acyclovir
Famciclovir
Valacyclovir
Adenosine arabinoside
Iododeoxyuridine
Trifluridine

VZV
Acyclovir
Famciclovir
Valacyclovir
Varicella-zoster immune globulin (VZIG)
Zoster immune plasma (ZIP)
Live vaccine

EBV
None

CMV
Ganciclovir*
Foscarnet*

*Also inhibits HSV and VZV.

and trifluridine. **Famciclovir** (a derivative of **penciclovir**) and **valacyclovir** (the valyl ester of ACV) are FDA approved and are related to ACV in their mechanism of action but have different pharmacological properties.

ACV is the most prescribed anti-HSV drug. ACV, and penciclovir are activated by the viral thymidine kinase and then used as a substrate by the viral DNA polymerase. These drugs are then incorporated into and prevent the elongation of the viral DNA. These drugs are effective in treating serious presentations of HSV disease and first episodes of genital herpes; they are also used for prophylactic treatment. ACV is relatively nontoxic and has been administered for long-term prophylaxis. The most prevalent form of **resistance** to these drugs results from mutations that inactivate the **thymidine kinase,** thereby reducing conversion of the drug to its active form. Mutation of the **viral DNA polymerase** can also produce resistance. Fortunately, resistant strains appear to be less virulent.

Ara A is also approved for the treatment of HSV infection. However, it is less soluble, less potent, and more toxic than ACV. Trifluridine and ACV have replaced iododeoxyuridine as topical agents for the treatment of herpetic keratitis. Tromantadine, an amantadine derivative, is approved for topical use in countries other than the United States and works by inhibiting penetration and syncytia formation. None of the treatments, however, can eliminate a latent infection.

HSV-1 is transmitted most often from an active mucocutaneous lesion, so avoidance of direct contact with this reduces the risk of infection. Unfortunately, the symptoms may be inapparent, and thus the virus can be transmitted unknowingly.

Physicians, nurses, dentists, and technicians must be especially careful when handling potentially infected tissue or fluids. The wearing of gloves can prevent the acquisition of infections of the fingers (herpetic whitlow). People with recurrent herpetic whitlow disease are very contagious and can spread the infection to patients. The virus is readily disinfected by washing with soap.

Patients who have a history of genital HSV infection must be instructed to refrain from sexual intercourse while they have prodromal symptoms or lesions and to resume sexual intercourse only after lesions are completely reepithelialized because virus can be isolated even from lesions that have crusted over. Condoms may be useful and are undoubtedly better than nothing but may not be fully protective.

A pregnant woman who has active genital HSV infection or who is asymptomatically shedding the virus in the vagina at term may transmit HSV to the neonate if the infant is delivered vaginally. Such transmission can be prevented by delivering the infant by cesarean section.

No vaccine is currently available for HSV. However, killed, subunit, vaccinia hybrid, and DNA vaccines are being developed to prevent acquisition of the virus or to treat infected people.

VARICELLA-ZOSTER VIRUS

VZV causes **chickenpox** (varicella) and with recurrence causes herpes zoster, or **shingles.** VZV shares many characteristics with HSV, including (1) the ability to establish latent infection of neurons and recurrent disease at the innervated dermatome, (2) the importance of cell-mediated immunity in controlling and preventing serious disease, and (3) the characteristic blisterlike lesions that form. Like HSV, VZV encodes a **thymidine kinase** and is susceptible to **antiviral drugs.** Unlike HSV, the predominant means by which VZV is spread is by the **respiratory route.** Viremia occurs after local replication of the virus in the respiratory tract, leading to the formation of skin lesions over the entire body.

Structure and Replication

VZV has the smallest genome of the human herpesviruses, but each gene in VZV is represented by a counterpart in HSV. VZV replicates slower and in fewer types of cells than HSV. Human diploid fibroblasts in vitro and epithelial cells in vivo can support VZV replication. VZV establishes a latent infection of neurons, as does HSV.

Pathogenesis and Immunity

Primary VZV infection begins in the mucosa of the respiratory tract and then progresses via the bloodstream and lymphatic system to the cells of the reticuloendothelial system (Box 51-5 and Figures 51-8 and 51-9). A secondary viremia occurs after 11 to 13 days and spreads the virus throughout the body and to the skin. The virus causes a dermal vesiculopustular rash that develops in successive crops. Fever and systemic symptoms occur with the rash.

The virus becomes latent in the dorsal root or cranial nerve ganglia after the primary infection. The virus can

---

BOX 51-5   Disease Mechanisms of VZV

Initial replication is in the respiratory tract.

VZV infects epithelial cells and fibroblasts.

VZV can form syncytia and spread directly from cell to cell.

Virus is spread by viremia to skin and causes lesions in successive crops.

VZV can escape antibody clearance, and cell-mediated immune response is essential to control infection. Disseminated, life-threatening disease can occur in immunocompromised people.

Virus establishes latent infection of neurons, usually dorsal root and cranial nerve ganglia.

Herpes zoster may result from depression of cell-mediated immunity and other mechanisms of viral activation.

FIGURE 51-8 Mechanism of spread of VZV within the body. VZV initially infects the respiratory tract and is spread by the reticuloendothelial system and by viremia to other parts of the body.

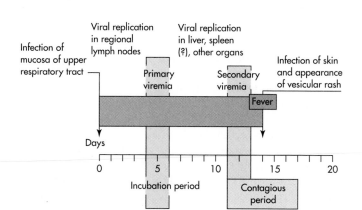

FIGURE 51-9 Time course of varicella (chickenpox). The course in young children, as presented in this figure, is generally shorter and less severe than that of adults.

BOX 51-6 **Epidemiology of VZV Infection**

DISEASE/VIRAL FACTORS

Virus causes lifelong infection.
Recurrent disease is source of contagion.

TRANSMISSION

Virus is transmitted mainly by respiratory droplets but also by direct contact.

WHO IS AT RISK?

Children (age, 5-9): mild classic disease.
Teens and adults: at risk for more severe disease with potential pneumonia. *can be fatal*
Immunocompromised people and newborns: at risk for life-threatening pneumonia, encephalitis, and progressive-disseminated varicella.
Elderly and immunocompromised people: at risk for recurrent disease (zoster [shingles]).

GEOGRAPHY/SEASON

Virus is found worldwide.
There is no seasonal incidence.

MODES OF CONTROL

Antiviral drugs are available.
Immunity is lifelong.
Varicella-zoster immunoglobulin is available for immunocompromised people and staff exposed to virus as well as newborns of mothers showing symptoms within 5 days of birth.
Live vaccine (Oka strain) is available.

---

be reactivated in older adults or in patients with impaired cellular immunity. On reactivation the virus migrates along neural pathways to the skin, where a vesicular rash known as *herpes zoster,* or *shingles,* develops.

Antibody is important in limiting the viremic spread of VZV, but cell-mediated immunity is essential for limiting the progression of and resolving the disease. The overzealous cell-mediated immune response that occurs in adults is responsible for causing more extensive cell damage and a more severe presentation (especially in the lung) on primary infection than that seen in children. The virus causes more disseminated and serious disease in the absence of cell-mediated immunity.

Epidemiology

VZV is extremely communicable, with rates of infection exceeding 90% among susceptible household contacts (Box 51-6). The disease is spread principally by the respiratory route but may also be spread through contact with skin vesicles. Patients are contagious before and during symptoms. Primary VZV infection occurs throughout childhood, and more than 90% of adults in developed countries have the VZV antibody. Herpes zoster results from the reactivation of a patient's latent endogenous virus, not as an epidemic outbreak. Zoster develops in approximately 10% to 20% of the population infected with VZV, with the incidence increasing with age. Zoster lesions contain viable virus and therefore may be a source of varicella infection in a nonimmune person (child).

Clinical Syndromes

Varicella is one of the five **classic childhood exanthems;** rubella, roseola, fifth disease, and measles constitute the remaining four.

Varicella (chickenpox) results from a primary infection with VZV; it is usually a mild disease of childhood and is usually symptomatic, although asymptomatic infection may occur (Figure 51-9). Varicella is characterized by fever and a maculopapular rash that appear after an incubation period of about 14 days (Figure 51-10). Within hours, each maculopapular lesion forms a thin-walled vesicle on a maculopapular base (dewdrop on a rose petal) that measures approximately 2 to 4 mm in diameter. This vesicle is the hallmark of varicella. Within 12 hours the vesicle becomes pustular and begins to crust, after which scabbed lesions appear. Successive crops of lesions appear for 3 to 5 days, and at any given time all stages of skin lesions can be observed.

The rash is generalized, more severe on the trunk than on the extremities, and notably present on the scalp, which distinguishes it from many other diseases. The lesions itch and cause scratching, which may lead to bacterial superinfection and scarring. Lesions on the mucous membrane typically occur in the mouth, conjunctivae, and vagina. Thrombocytopenia may also develop occasionally, but in this case the rash may be hemorrhagic.

Primary infection in adults is usually more severe than that in children. **Interstitial pneumonia** may occur in 20% to 30% of adult patients and may be fatal.

As noted earlier, **herpes zoster** (*zoster* means "belt" or "girdle") is a recurrence of a latent varicella infection acquired earlier in the patient's life. Severe pain in the area innervated by the nerve usually precedes the appearance of the chickenpox-like lesions. The rash is usually limited to a dermatome. The lesions are typically small, closely spaced, and maculopapular and have an erythematous base, in contrast with the more diffuse pattern of vesicles characteristic of varicella (Figure 51-11). A chronic pain syndrome called **postherpetic neuralgia,** which can persist for months to years, occurs in as many as 30% of patients older than 65 years in whom zoster develops.

VZV infection in immunocompromised patients or neonates can result in serious, progressive, and potentially fatal disease. Defects in cell-mediated immunity in such patients increase the risk for dissemination of the virus to the lungs, brain, and liver, which may be fatal.

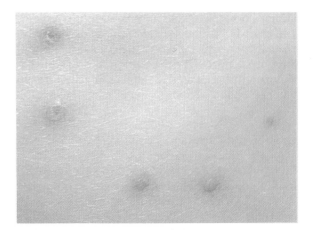

FIGURE 51-10 Characteristic skin rash of varicella in all stages of its evolution. (From Hart CA, Broadhead RL: *A color atlas of pediatric infectious diseases,* London, 1992, Wolfe.)

FIGURE 51-11 Herpes zoster in a thoracic dermatome.

This may occur in response to a primary exposure to varicella or as disseminated herpes zoster.

Laboratory Diagnosis
Cytology

The CPE in VZV-infected cells is similar to that seen in HSV-infected cells and include Cowdry type A intranuclear inclusions and syncytia. These cells may be seen in skin lesions, respiratory specimens, or organ biopsy specimens. Syncytia may also be seen in Tzanck smears of scrapings of a vesicle's base. Direct fluorescent antibody methods can also be used to examine skin lesion scrapings or biopsy specimens for membrane antigens (FAMA). Antigen detection is more sensitive than virus isolation as a means of diagnosing VZV infection.

Virus Isolation

It is difficult to isolate VZV in cell cultures because the virus is labile during transport to the laboratory and replicates poorly in vitro. Cultures of material from skin lesions that are crusted over (5 or more days after onset) are usually negative for the virus. Human diploid fibroblasts can support VZV replication and exhibit a CPE similar to that seen in HSV-infected cells but after a longer incubation period.

Serology

Serological tests that detect antibodies to VZV are used to screen people for immunity to VZV. However, antibody levels are normally low, so sensitive tests such as immunofluorescence or enzyme-linked immunosorbent assay (ELISA) must be performed to detect the antibody. IgM and a significant increase in the antibody level can be detected in people experiencing herpes zoster.

Treatment, Prevention, and Control

Treatment may be appropriate for adults and immunocompromised patients with VZV infections and for people with shingles, but no treatment is usually necessary for children with varicella. **ACV, famciclovir,** and **valacyclovir** have been approved for the treatment of VZV infections. The VZV DNA polymerase is much less sensitive to treatment requiring large doses of ACV or the improved pharmacodynamics of famciclovir and valacyclovir (Box 51-4).

Like other respiratory viruses, it is difficult to limit the transmission of VZV. Because VZV infection in children is generally mild and induces lifelong immunity, exposure of children to VZV early in life is often encouraged. However, high-risk people (e.g., immunosuppressed children) should be protected from exposure to VZV.

VZV disease may be prevented or ameliorated in immunosuppressed patients susceptible to severe disease through the administration of varicella-zoster immunoglobulin (VZIG). VZIG is prepared by pooling plasma from seropositive people. It is ineffective, however, as a therapy for patients suffering from active varicella or herpes zoster disease.

A live attenuated vaccine for VZV (Oka strain) has been licensed for use in the United States and is administered on the same schedule as the measles, mumps, and rubella (MMR) vaccine. The vaccine induces the production of protective or ameliorating antibody and cell-mediated immunity. It is effective as a prophylactic treatment in people even after exposure to VZV. Most significantly, it promotes protection in immunodeficient children.

EPSTEIN-BARR VIRUS

EBV was discovered by electron microscopic observation of characteristic herpes virions in biopsy specimens of an African Burkitt's lymphoma (AfBL). However, its association with infectious mononucleosis was discovered accidentally when serum collected from a laboratory technician convalescing from infectious mononucleosis was found to contain the antibody that recognized AfBL cells. This finding was later confirmed in a large serological study performed on college students.

EBV causes **heterophile antibody-positive infectious mononucleosis** and has been causally **associated with AfBL (endemic Burkitt's lymphoma) and nasopharyngeal carcinoma.** EBV has also been associated with B-cell lymphomas in patients with acquired or congenital immunodeficiencies. EBV is a mitogen for B cells and **immortalizes B cells** in tissue culture.

Structure and Replication

EBV is a gammaherpesvirus with a very limited host range and a tissue tropism defined by the limited cellular expression of its receptor. This receptor is also the receptor for the C3d component of the complement system (also called *CR2* or *CD21*). It is expressed on B cells of humans and New World monkeys and on epithelial cells of the oropharynx and nasopharynx.

EBV infection has three potential outcomes: The virus can replicate in epithelial cells permissive for EBV replication; it can cause latent infection of B cells in the presence of competent T cells, or it can stimulate and immortalize B cells, which are semipermissive for EBV replication.

Different viral transcription programs are initiated for the latent and lytic infections. During a latent infection, infected cells contain a small number of circular, plasmidlike EBV genomes that replicate only during cell division. Select immediate early genes are expressed; these include Epstein-Barr nuclear antigens (EBNAs) 1, 2, 3A, 3B, and 3C; latent proteins (LPs); latent membrane proteins (LMPs) 1 and 2; and two small Epstein-Barr–encoded RNA (EBER) molecules, EBER1 and EBER2. The EBNAs and latent proteins are DNA-binding proteins that are essential for establishing an infection (EBNA-1), immortalization (EBNA-2), and other purposes. The LMPs are membrane proteins with oncogene-like activities.

Permissive cells allow the transcription and translation of the ZEBRA peptide, which activates the early genes of the virus and the lytic cycle. After synthesis of the DNA polymerase and DNA replication, the viral capsid and glycoproteins are synthesized. These include gp350/220 (related glycoproteins of 350,000 and 220,000 daltons), which is the viral attachment protein, and gp85 (85,000 daltons).

Pathogenesis and Immunity

The virus establishes a productive infection in the epithelial cells of the oropharynx (Box 51-7 and Figure 51-12). The virus is then shed into the saliva and accesses B cells in lymphatic tissue and blood. Lytic infection leads to the production of EBV proteins, including the early antigens, viral capsid antigen, and the glycoproteins of the membrane antigen (Table 51-3).

EBV is a B-cell mitogen that stimulates growth, prevents apoptosis (programmed cell death), and immortalizes the cells. EBV infection of the B cell also alters the way in which it interacts with the rest of the immune system. EBV enhances the expression of cell surface proteins such as histocompatibility leukocyte antigen, adhesion proteins, and the CD23 blast antigen and encodes an analogue of interleukin-10 (BCRF-1). BCRF-1 promotes immune escape by inhibiting TH1 helper T cells, including interferon-gamma secretion and early T-cell responses to the virus while promoting B-cell growth and

FIGURE 51-12 Progression of EBV infection. Infection may result in lytic or immortalizing infection, which can be distinguished by the production of virus and the expression of different viral proteins and antigens. T cells limit the outgrowth of the EBV-infected cells. *EA,* Early antigen; *VCA,* viral capsid antigen; *MA,* membrane antigen; *LYDMA,* lymphocyte-defined membrane antigen.

BOX 51-7   Disease Mechanisms of EBV

Virus in saliva initiates infection of oral epithelia and spreads to B cells in lymphatic tissue.

There is productive infection in epithelial cells.

Virus promotes growth of B cells (immortalizes).

T cells kill and limit B-cell outgrowth and promote latency in B cells. They are *required for controlling infection.* Antibody role is limited.

T-cell response (lymphocytosis) contributes to symptoms of **infectious mononucleosis.**

There is causative association with lymphoma and leukemia in T-cell–deficient people and African children living in malarial regions (African Burkitt's lymphoma) and with nasopharyngeal carcinoma in China.

TABLE 51-3   Markers of EBV Infection

NAME	ABBREVIATION	CHARACTERISTICS	BIOLOGICAL ASSOCIATION	CLINICAL ASSOCIATION
EBV nuclear antigen	EBNA	Nuclear	EBNA is a nonstructural antigen and is first antigen to appear; EBNA is seen in all infected and transformed cells, and it binds to cell DNA.	Anti-EBNA develops late in infection.
Early antigen	EA-R	Only cytoplasmic	EA-R appears before EA-D; its appearance is first sign that infected cell has entered lytic cycle.	Anti–EA-R is seen in Burkitt's lymphoma.
	EA-D	Diffuse in cytoplasm and nucleus	—	Anti–EA-D is seen in infectious mononucleosis.
Viral capsid antigen	VCA	Cytoplasmic	VCA is a late antigen; it is found in virus producer cells.	Anti-VCA IgM is transient; anti-VCA IgG is persistent.
Lymphocyte-defined membrane antigen	LYDMA	—	LYDMA is not found on Burkitt's lymphoma cells; it is found on cells infected in vitro, and is found on nonproducer cells	LYDMA is not detectable by antibody.
Membrane antigen	MA	Cell surface	MAs are the envelope glycoproteins.	Same as VCA.
Heterophile antibody		Recognition of Paul-Bunnell antigen on sheep, horse, or bovine erythrocytes	EBV-induced B-cell proliferation promotes production of heterophile antibody.	Early symptoms occur in more than 50% of patients.

IgG synthesis. Continued B-cell proliferation in conjunction with the effects of other cofactors may result in the development of lymphoma.

Infectious mononucleosis results from a *civil war* between the EBV-infected B cells and the protective T cells. The classic **lymphocytosis** (increase in mononuclear cells) associated with infectious mononucleosis results mainly from the activation and proliferation of T cells. These appear as atypical lymphocytes (also called **Downey cells**) (Figure 51-13). They increase in number in the peripheral blood during the second week of infection, accounting for 10% to 80% of the total white cell count at this time. The large T-cell response causes the swollen lymph glands, spleen, and liver, which occur later in the disease.

T cells limit the proliferation of EBV-infected B cells in tissue culture and are essential in controlling the disease (Figure 51-14). It is difficult for EBV infections to resolve in people with impaired cell-mediated immunity, and B-cell lymphoproliferative diseases may result.

Epidemiology

EBV is transmitted in saliva (Box 51-8). More than 90% of EBV-infected people intermittently shed the virus for life, even when totally asymptomatic. Children can acquire the virus at an early age by sharing contaminated drinking glasses. They generally have subclinical disease. Saliva sharing between adolescents and young adults often occurs during kissing, thus the nickname the *kissing disease*. Disease in these people may go unnoticed or present in varying degrees of severity. Approximately 70% of the population of the United States is infected by age 30.

The geographical distribution of EBV-associated neoplasms indicate a possible association with potential cofactors. The immunosuppressive potential of malaria has been suggested as a cofactor in the progression of chronic or latent EBV infection to AfBL. The restriction

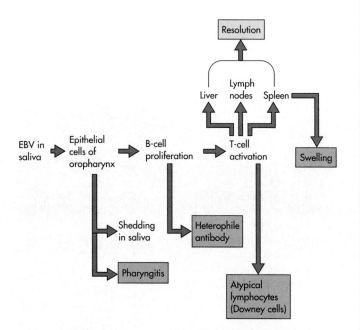

FIGURE 51-13 Atypical T-cell (Downey cell) characteristic of infectious mononucleosis. The cells have a more basophilic and vacuolated cytoplasm than normal lymphocytes, and the nucleus may be oval, kidney shaped, or lobulated. The cell margin may seem to be indented by neighboring red blood cells.

FIGURE 51-14 Pathogenesis of EBV. EBV is acquired by close contact between persons through saliva and infects the B cells. The resolution of the EBV infection and many of the symptoms of infectious mononucleosis result from the activation of T cells in response to the infection.

BOX 51-8   Epidemiology of EBV Infection

DISEASE/VIRAL FACTORS

Virus causes lifelong infection.
Recurrent disease is cause of contagion.
Virus may cause asymptomatic shedding.

TRANSMISSION

Tranmission occurs via saliva, close oral contact (kissing disease), or sharing of items such as toothbrushes and cups.

WHO IS AT RISK?

Children, who may be asymptomatic or have mild symptoms.
Teenagers and adults: at risk for infectious mononucleosis.
Immunocompromised people: at highest risk for life-threatening neoplastic disease.

GEOGRAPHY/SEASON

There is worldwide distribution of infectious mononucleosis.
There is causative association with AfBL in malarial belt of Africa.
There is no seasonal incidence.

MODES OF CONTROL

There are no modes of control.

of nasopharyngeal carcinoma to people living in certain regions of China has indicated a possible genetic predisposition to the cancer or possibly the presence of cofactors in the food or environment.

Transplant recipients, patients with acquired immunodeficiency syndrome (AIDS), and genetically immunodeficient people are at high risk for lymphoproliferative disorders initiated by EBV. These may appear as polyclonal and monoclonal B-cell lymphomas. These people are also at high risk for a productive infection in the form of hairy oral leukoplakia.

Clinical Syndromes

Heterophile Antibody-Positive Infectious Mononucleosis

Like infections caused by other herpesviruses, EBV infection in a child is much milder than infection in an adolescent or adult. In fact, infection in children is usually subclinical. Infectious mononucleosis is characterized by high fever, malaise, pharyngitis, lymphadenopathy (swollen glands), and often hepatosplenomegaly. A rash may occur, especially after ampicillin treatment. The major complaint of people with infectious mononucleosis is fatigue (Figure 51-15). The disease is rarely fatal in healthy people but can cause serious complications resulting from neurological disorders, laryngeal obstruction, or rupture of the spleen. Neurological complications can include meningoencephalitis and the Guillain-Barré syndrome. Heterophile-negative "mononucleosis" is likely to be caused by CMV if the patient is 25 years of age or older.

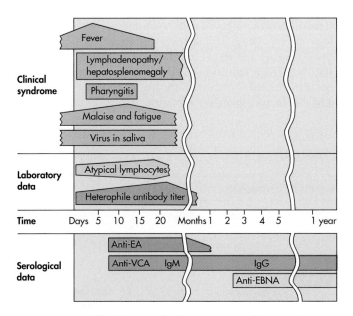

FIGURE 51-15 Clinical course of infectious mononucleosis and laboratory findings of those with the infection. EBV infection may be asymptomatic or produce the symptoms of mononucleosis. The incubation period can last as long as 2 months. *EA,* Early antigen; *VCA,* viral capsid antigen.

Chronic Disease

EBV can cause cyclical recurrent disease in some people. These patients experience chronic tiredness and may also have low-grade fever, headaches, and sore throat. This is different from chronic fatigue syndrome, which has another etiology.

Epstein-Barr Virus–Induced Lymphoproliferative Diseases

People lacking T-cell immunity are likely to suffer life-threatening polyclonal leukemia-like B-cell proliferative disease and lymphoma instead of infectious mononucleosis on infection with EBV. People with congenital deficiencies of T-cell function are likely to suffer the life-threatening **X-linked lymphoproliferative disease.** Transplant recipients undergoing immunosuppressive treatment are at high risk for **posttransplant lymphoproliferative disease** instead of infectious mononucleosis after exposure to the virus or on reactivation of latent virus. Similar diseases are seen in patients with AIDS.

AfBL (endemic lymphoma) is a poorly differentiated monoclonal B-cell lymphoma of the jaw and face that is endemic in children living in the malarial regions of Africa. The tumors contain EBV DNA sequences but express only the EBNA-1 viral antigen. Virions can occasionally be seen in electron micrographs of infected material. In addition to EBV DNA, the tumor cells contain chromosomal translocations that juxtapose the C-*myc* oncogene to a very active promoter such as immunoglobulin gene promoter [t(8;14), t(8;22), t(8;2)]. The tumor cells are also relatively invisible to immune control. It is not known how malaria acts to promote EBV involvement with AfBL. EBV is also associated with Burkitt's lymphomas in people living in other parts of the world but to a much lesser extent. A large percentage of **Hodgkin's lymphomas** also contain EBV DNA sequences.

As noted earlier, **nasopharyngeal carcinoma** is endemic in the Orient, occurs in adults, and contains EBV DNA within the tumor cells. Unlike Burkitt's lymphoma, in which the tumor cells are derived from lymphocytes, the tumor cells of nasopharyngeal carcinoma are of epithelial origin.

Hairy Oral Leukoplakia

Hairy oral leukoplakia is an unusual presentation of a productive EBV infection of epithelial cells characterized by lesions of the mouth. It is an opportunistic presentation that afflicts AIDS patients.

Laboratory Diagnosis

EBV-induced infectious mononucleosis is usually documented by the finding of atypical lymphocytes, **lymphocytosis** (mononuclear cells constituting 60% to 70% of the white blood cell count with 30% atypical lymphocytes), heterophile antibody, and antibody to viral antigens. Virus isolation is not practical. DNA probe analysis and immunofluorescent identification of viral antigens are used to detect evidence of infection.

Atypical lymphocytes are probably the earliest detectable indication of an EBV infection. These cells appear with the onset of symptoms and disappear with resolution of the disease.

Heterophile antibody results from the nonspecific, mitogen-like activation of B cells by EBV and the production of a wide repertoire of antibodies. These antibodies include an IgM heterophile antibody that recognizes the Paul-Bunnell antigen on sheep, horse, and bovine erythrocytes but not that on guinea pig kidney cells. The heterophile antibody response can usually be detected by the end of the first week of the illness and lasts for as long as several months. It is an excellent indication of EBV infection in adults but is not as reliable in indicating infection in children or infants. The monospot test and ELISA are rapid and widely used for the detection of the heterophile antibody.

Serological tests for antibody to viral antigens are useful in patients whose EBV infections cannot be diagnosed on the basis of the usual clinical criteria and the results of heterophile antibody tests (Figure 51-15 and Table 51-4). Recent EBV infection is indicated by the finding of any of the following: (1) IgM antibody to the viral capsid antigen (VCA), (2) the presence of VCA antibody and the absence of EBNA antibody, (3) a rising EBNA titer, or (4) an elevated VCA and early antigen antibodies. The finding of *both* VCA and EBNA antibodies in serum indicates that the person has had a past infection.

Treatment, Prevention, and Control

No effective treatment or vaccine is available for EBV disease (Box 51-4). The ubiquitous nature of the virus and the potential for asymptomatic shedding make control of infection difficult. However, infection elicits lifelong immunity. Therefore the best means of preventing infectious mononucleosis is to be exposed to the virus early in life because the disease is more benign in children.

CYTOMEGALOVIRUS

CMV is a common human pathogen, infecting 0.5% to 2.5% of all newborns and approximately 50% of the adult population in developed countries. It is the most common viral cause of **congenital defects.** CMV becomes particularly important as a pathogen in **immunocompromised patients.**

Structure and Replication

CMV is a member of the betaherpesviruses and is considered lymphotropic. It has the largest genome of the human herpesviruses. Human CMV replicates only in human cells. Fibroblasts, epithelial cells, and macrophages are permissive for CMV replication. CMV establishes latent infection in mononuclear lymphocytes, the stromal cells of the bone marrow, and other cells.

Pathogenesis and Immunity

In general the pathogenesis of CMV disease is similar to that of disease caused by other herpesviruses (Box 51-9). As just noted, the virus establishes latent infection in mononuclear leukocytes and in organs such as the kidneys and heart. Such infection appears to be reactivated by immunosuppression (e.g., corticosteroids, infection with human immunodeficiency virus) and possibly by allogeneic stimulation (i.e., the host response to transfused or transplanted cells). Cell-mediated immunity is essential for resolving and controlling the outgrowth of CMV infection.

In most cases the virus replicates and is shed without causing symptoms (Table 51-5). Replication of CMV in ductal epithelial cells promotes excretion of the virus in most body fluids. CMV is highly cell associated and is transmitted by infected cells, including lymphocytes and leukocytes, which also spread the virus throughout the body (Figure 51-16). This close cell association protects the virus from antibody-mediated inactivation. Virus can be transmitted in cells by means of blood transfusions and organ transplants. Activation and replication of the

---

TABLE 51-4   **Serological Profile for EBV Infections**

PATIENT'S CLINICAL STATUS	HETEROPHILE ANTIBODIES	EBV-SPECIFIC ANTIBODIES				COMMENT
		VCA-IgM	VCA-IgG	EA	EBNA	
Susceptible	−	−	−	−	−	—
Acute primary	+	+	+	±	−	—
Chronic primary	−	−	+	+	−	—
Past infection	−	−	+	−	+	—
Reactivation infection	−	−	+	+	+	EA restricted or diffuse
Burkitt's lymphoma	−	−	+	+	+	EA restricted only
Nasopharyngeal carcinoma	−	−	+	+	+	EA diffuse only

VCA, Viral capsid antigen; *EA,* early antigen.

Modified from Balows A, Hausler WJ Jr, Lennette EH, editors: *Laboratory diagnosis of infectious diseases: principles and practices,* New York, 1988, Springer-Verlag.

virus in the kidney and secretory glands promote its secretion in urine and bodily secretions, including semen and milk.

Epidemiology and Clinical Syndromes

CMV can be isolated from urine, blood, throat washings, saliva, tears, breast milk, semen, stool, amniotic fluid, vaginal and cervical secretions, and tissues obtained for transplantation (Table 51-6 and Box 51-10). The congenital, oral, and sexual routes; blood transfusion; and tissue transplantation are the major means by which CMV is transmitted.

Congenital Infection

CMV is the most prevalent viral cause of congenital disease. A significant percentage (0.2% to 2.0%) of all newborns in the United States are infected with CMV at birth, and a large percentage are infected within the first months of life. Approximately 10% of these newborns (4000 per year) show clinical evidence of disease, such as microcephaly, intracerebral calcification, hepatosplenomegaly, and rash (cytomegalic inclusion disease). Unilat-

eral or bilateral hearing loss and mental retardation are common consequences of congenital CMV infection. The mothers of almost all infants who have these birth defects have had primary infections during their pregnancies.

Fetuses are infected by virus in the mother's blood (primary infection) or by virus ascending from the cervix (after a recurrence). The symptoms of congenital infection are less severe or can be prevented in the fetus of a seropositive mother. Congenital CMV infection is best

FIGURE 51-16 CMV-infected cell with basophilic nuclear inclusion body.

TABLE 51-5   Sources of CMV Infection

AGE GROUP	SOURCE
Neonate	Transplacental transmission, intrauterine infections, cervical secretions
Baby or child	Body secretions: breast milk, saliva, tears, urine
Adult	Sexual transmission (semen), blood transfusion, organ graft

BOX 51-9   Disease Mechanisms of CMV

CMV is acquired from blood, tissue, and most body secretions.

CMV causes productive infection of epithelial and other cells.

CMV establishes latency in T cells, macrophages, and other cells.

Cell-mediated immunity is required for resolution and contributes to symptoms. Antibody role is limited.

Suppression of cell-mediated immunity allows recurrence and severe presentation.

CMV generally causes subclinical infection.

TABLE 51-6   CMV Syndromes

TISSUE	CHILDREN/ADULTS	IMMUNOSUPPRESSED PATIENTS
Predominant nature of disease	**Inapparent infection (prominent presentation of disease)**	**Disseminated disease, severe disease**
Eyes	—	Chorioretinitis
Lungs	—	Pneumonia
Gastrointestinal tract	—	Esophagitis, colitis
Nervous system	Polyneuritis, myelitis	Meningitis and encephalitis, myelitis
Lymphoid system	Mononucleosis syndrome, posttransfusion syndrome	Leukopenia, lymphocytosis
Major organs	Carditis,* hepatitis*	Hepatitis
Neonates	**Deafness, mental retardation**	—

*Complication of mononucleosis or postperfusion syndrome.

BOX 51-10   Epidemiology of CMV Infection

DISEASE/VIRAL FACTORS

Virus causes lifelong infection.
Recurrent disease is source of contagion.
Virus may cause asymptomatic shedding.

TRANSMISSION

Transmission occurs via blood, organ transplants, and all secretions, including urine, saliva, semen, cervical secretions, breast milk, and tears.
Virus is transmitted orally and sexually, in blood transfusions,
in tissue transplants, in utero, at birth, and by nursing.

WHO IS AT RISK?

Babies.
Babies of mothers who seroconvert during term: at high risk
for congenital defects.

WHO IS AT RISK?—cont'd

Sexually active people.
Blood and organ recipients.
Burn patients.
Immunocompromised people, who may have symptomatic
and recurrent disease.

GEOGRAPHY/SEASON

Virus is found worldwide.
There is no seasonal incidence.

MODES OF CONTROL

Antiviral drugs are available for patients with AIDS.
Screening potential blood and organ donors for CMV reduces transmission of virus.

---

documented by isolating the virus from the infant's urine during the first week of life.

Perinatal Infection

In the United States as many as 20% of pregnant women harbor CMV in their cervix at term and are likely to experience reactivation of the virus during pregnancy. Approximately half the neonates born through an infected cervix acquire CMV infection and become excreters of the virus at 3 to 4 weeks of age. Neonates may also acquire CMV from maternal milk or colostrum. Perinatal infection causes no clinically evident disease in healthy full-term infants.

Another means by which neonates can acquire CMV is through blood transfusions. Of the seronegative babies who are exposed to blood from seropositive donors, 13.5% acquire CMV infection in the immediate postnatal period. Significant clinical infection may occur in the premature infants who acquire CMV from transfused blood, with pneumonia and hepatitis the major manifestations.

Infection in Children and Adults

Only 10% to 15% of adolescents are infected with CMV, but this number increases to 50% by 35 years of age. CMV is a **sexually transmitted disease.** It has been isolated from the cervix of 13% to 23% of women at venereal disease clinics, and the titer of the CMV in semen is the highest of that in any body secretion. CMV is more prevalent among people in low socioeconomic brackets living in crowded conditions and in people living in underdeveloped countries.

Although most CMV infections acquired in young adulthood are asymptomatic, patients may show a **heterophile-negative mononucleosis syndrome,** with symptoms similar to those of EBV infection but with less severe pharyngitis and lymphadenopathy (Figure 51-17). Although CMV infection promotes a T-cell outgrowth (atypical lymphocytosis) similar to that seen in EBV infection, heterophile antibody is not present. This reflects differences between CMV and EBV in terms of the target cell and the action of the virus on the target cell. CMV disease should be suspected in a patient with heterophile-negative mononucleosis or signs of hepatitis but with negative results to tests for hepatitis A, B, and C.

Transfusion and Transplantation Transmission

Transmission of CMV by blood most often results in an asymptomatic infection; if symptoms are present, they typically resemble those of mononucleosis. Fever, splenomegaly, and atypical lymphocytosis usually begin 3 to 5 weeks after transfusion. Pneumonia and mild hepatitis may also occur. CMV may also be transmitted by organ transplantation (e.g., kidneys, bone marrow), and CMV infection is often reactivated in transplant recipients during periods of intense immunosuppression.

Infection in the Immunocompromised Host

CMV is a prominent opportunistic infectious agent in immunocompromised people, in whom it causes recurrent disease. Primary infection with CMV may also occur in these patients.

CMV disease of the **lung** is a common outcome in immunosuppressed patients and can be fatal if not treated. In addition, CMV often causes **retinitis** in patients who are severely immunodeficient (e.g., in as many as 10% to 15% of patients with AIDS). Interstitial pneumonia and encephalitis may also be caused by CMV but may be difficult to distinguish from such infections caused by other opportunistic infectious agents. CMV **colitis** or **esophagitis** may develop in as many as 10% of AIDS patients. CMV esophagitis may mimic candidal esophagitis. A smaller percentage of immunocompromised patients may experience CMV infection of the gastrointestinal tract. Patients with CMV colitis usually have diarrhea, weight loss, anorexia, and fever. CMV is also responsible for causing the failure of many kidney transplants.

Laboratory Diagnosis

Histology

The histological hallmark of CMV infection is the cytomegalic cell, which is an enlarged cell (25 to 35 mm) that contains a dense, central, **"owl's eye,"** basophilic intranuclear inclusion body (Table 51-7 and Figure 51-16). These infected cells may be found in any tissue of the body and in urine and are thought to be epithelial in origin. These inclusions are readily seen with Papanicolaou or hematoxylin-eosin stains.

Immune and DNA Probe Techniques

A rapid, sensitive diagnosis can be obtained by histological means using antibodies (especially monoclonal) and **DNA probes** to directly detect the CMV antigens and the genome in tissues (see Figure 17-3). Enzyme immunoassay and fluorescence methods detect the probes.

Culture

Culture has generally been regarded as the definitive method for detecting CMV infection. It is especially reliable in immunocompromised patients because they often have high titers of virus in their secretions. For example, in the semen of AIDS patients, titers of viable virus may be greater than 10^6.

CMV grows only in diploid-fibroblast cell cultures and must be maintained for at least 4 to 6 weeks because the characteristic CPE develops very slowly in specimens with very low titers of the virus. More rapid results may be achieved by **culture amplification** of a specimen. In this procedure, specimens are inoculated by centrifuging them in a shell vial seeded with diploid fibroblast cells. Specimens are examined after 1 to 2 days of incubation by indirect immunofluorescence for the presence of either immediate early antigen or a combination of immediate early antigen and early antigen.

Serology

Seroconversion is usually an excellent marker for primary CMV infection. Titers of CMV-specific IgM antibody may be very high in AIDS patients. However, CMV-specific IgM antibody may also develop during the reactivation of CMV and is therefore not a dependable indicator of primary infection.

Treatment, Prevention, and Control

Ganciclovir (dihydroxypropoxymethyl guanine; Cytovene) and **foscarnet** (phosphonoformic acid) have been approved by the FDA for the treatment of CMV infections and are especially useful for immunosuppressed pa-

TABLE 51-7	**Laboratory Tests for Diagnosing CMV Infection**
TEST	**FINDING**
Cytology and histology*	"Owl's eye" inclusion body
	Antigen detection
	In situ DNA probe hybridization
Cell culture	Cytological effect in human diploid fibroblasts
	Immunofluorescence detection of early antigens
Serology	Primary infection

*Samples taken for analysis include urine, saliva, blood, bronchoalveolar lavage specimens, and tissue biopsy specimens.

tients (Box 51-4). Ganciclovir is structurally similar to ACV, but unlike ACV, it can be activated by phosphorylation by a CMV enzyme to inhibit the viral DNA polymerase. However, it is more toxic than ACV. Ganciclovir can be used to treat severe CMV infections in immunocompromised patients. Foscarnet is a simple molecule that inhibits the viral DNA polymerase by mimicking the pyrophosphate portion of nucleotide triphosphates. It has been approved as an alternative to ganciclovir.

CMV is spread mainly by the sexual route and the tissue transplant and transfusion routes, and spread by these means is preventable. Semen is a major vector for the sexual spread of CMV to both heterosexual and homosexual contacts. The use of condoms or abstinence from anal intercourse would limit spread. Transmission of the virus can also be reduced through the screening of potential blood and organ donors for CMV seronegativity. This is especially important for donors of blood transfusions to be given to infants. Although congenital and perinatal transmission of CMV cannot effectively be prevented, a seropositive mother is least likely to produce a baby with symptomatic CMV disease. No vaccine for CMV is available.

HUMAN HERPESVIRUSES 6 AND 7

HHV6 was first isolated from the blood of AIDS patients and grown in T-cell cultures. It was identified as a herpesvirus because of the characteristic morphology of these viruses within infected cells. Like EBV and CMV, it is lymphotropic and ubiquitous. At least 45% of children are seropositive for HHV6 by age 2. In 1988, HHV6 was serologically associated with a common disease of children, **exanthema subitum,** commonly known as **roseola**.

HHV7 was isolated in a similar manner from the T cells of an AIDS patient also infected with HHV6. However, it remains an orphan virus with no disease association.

FIGURE 51-17 Time course of symptoms of exanthema subitum (roseola) caused by HHV6. Compare these symptoms and this time course with those of fifth disease, which is caused by parvovirus B19 (see Chapter 53).

Pathogenesis and Immunity

HHV6 infection occurs very early in life, indicating that it must be shed and spread readily. It is present in the saliva of most adults and is spread by oral secretions.

The only target cell of the virus that has been identified is the T cell. HHV6 establishes a latent infection in T cells but may be activated and replicate on mitogen stimulation of the cells. Cells in which the virus is replicating appear large and refractile and have occasional intranuclear and intracytoplasmic inclusion bodies. T-cell leukemia cell lines also support replication of the virus. Resting lymphocytes and lymphocytes of normal immune people are resistant to infection, however.

Like the replication of EBV and CMV, the replication of HHV6 is controlled by cell-mediated immunity. The virus is likely to become activated in AIDS patients and others with lymphoproliferative and immunosuppressive disorders.

Clinical Syndromes

Exanthema subitum, or roseola, is a common benign exanthematous disease of children, one of the five **classic childhood exanthems** (Figure 51-17). It is characterized by the rapid onset of high fever of a few days' duration, which is followed by a generalized rash that lasts only 24 to 48 hours. The presence of infected T cells or the activation of delayed-type hypersensitivity T cells in the skin may cause the rash. The disease is effectively controlled and resolved by cell-mediated immunity, but the virus establishes a lifelong latent infection of T cells.

HHV6 may also cause a mononucleosis syndrome and lymphadenopathy and may be a cofactor in the pathogenesis of AIDS.

OTHER HUMAN HERPESVIRUSES

HHV8 DNA sequences were discovered in biopsy specimens of Kaposi's sarcomas and a rare type of B-cell lymphoma from AIDS patients using polymerase chain reaction analysis. HHV8 was also present in the saliva of a large percentage of AIDS patients. Genome sequence analysis showed that the virus was unique but related to the Gammaherpesvirinae (like EBV). HHV8 DNA is present and associated with peripheral blood lymphocytes, most likely B cells, in approximately 10% of immunocompetent people. HHV8 may only be associated with significant disease in people who are immunocompromised.

Herpesvirus simiae-B virus is the simian counterpart of HSV and is indigenous to Asian monkeys. The virus is transmitted by monkey bites or saliva or even by tissues and cells widely used in virology laboratories. Once infected, a human may have pain, localized redness, and vesicles at the site of the virus' entrance. An encephalopathy develops in patients and is frequently fatal; most who survive have serious brain damage. Virus isolation or serological tests can be used to establish the diagnosis of B virus infections.

CASE STUDIES AND QUESTIONS

A 2-year-old child with fever for 2 days was not eating and was crying often. On examination the physician noted that the mucous membranes of the mouth were covered with numerous shallow, pale ulcerations. A few red papules and blisters were also observed around the border of the lips. The symptoms worsened over the next 5 days and then slowly resolved, with complete healing after 2 weeks.

1. The physician suspects that this is an HSV infection. How would the diagnosis be confirmed?
2. How could you determine whether this infection was caused by HSV-1 or HSV-2?
3. What immune responses were most helpful in resolving this infection and when were they activated?
4. HSV escapes complete immune resolution by causing latent and recurrent infections. What was the site of latency in this child and what might promote future recurrences?
5. What were the most probable means by which the baby was infected with HSV?
6. Which antiviral drugs are available for the treatment of HSV infections? What are their targets? Were they indicated for this child? If not, why not?

A 17-year-old high school student has had low-grade fever and malaise for several days, followed by sore throat, swollen cervical lymph nodes, and increasing fatigue. The patient also noted some discomfort in the left upper quadrant of the abdomen. The sore throat, lymphadenopathy, and fever gradually resolved over the next 2 weeks, but his full energy level did not return for another 6 weeks.

1. What laboratory tests would confirm the diagnosis of EBV-induced infectious mononucleosis and distinguish it from CMV infection?
2. To what characteristic diagnostic feature of the disease does *mononucleosis* refer?
3. What causes the swollen glands and fatigue?
4. Who is at greatest risk for a serious outcome from an EBV infection? What is it? Why?

Bibliography

Belshe RB: *Textbook of human virology,* ed 2, St Louis, 1991, Mosby.

Fields BN, Knipe DM, Howley PM, editors: *Virology,* ed 3, New York, 1996, Lippincott-Raven.

Garcia-Blanco MA, Cullen BR: Molecular basis of latency in pathogenic human viruses, *Science* 254:815-820, 1991.

Gorbach SL, Bartlett JG, Blacklow NR, editors: *Infectious diseases,* Philadelphia, 1992, WB Saunders.

Mandell GL, Bennett JE, Dolin R: *Principles and practice of infectious diseases,* ed 4, New York, 1995, Churchill Livingstone.

McGeoch DJ: The genomes of the human herpesviruses: contents, relationships and evolution, *Annu Rev Microbiol* 43:235-265, 1989.

White DO, Fenner FJ: *Medical virology,* ed 4, New York, 1994, Academic.

Herpes Simplex Virus

Arbesfeld DM, Thomas I: Cutaneous herpes simplex infections, *Am Fam Physician* 43:1655-1664, 1991.

Dawkins BJ: Genital herpes simplex infections, *Prim Care* 17:95-113, 1990.

Landy HJ, Grossman JH III: Herpes simplex virus, *Obstet Gynecol Clin North Am* 16:495-515, 1989.

Rouse BT: Herpes simplex virus: pathogenesis, immunobiology and control, *Curr Top Microbiol Immunol* 179:1-179, 1992.

Varicella-Zoster Virus

Arvin AM, Moffat JF, Redman R: Varicella-zoster virus: aspects of pathogenesis and the host response to natural infection and varicella vaccine, *Adv Virus Res* 46:263-309, 1996.

Croen KD, Strauss SE: Varicella zoster latency, *Annu Rev Microbiol* 45:265-282, 1991.

Ostrove JM: Molecular biology of varicella zoster virus, *Adv Virus Res* 38:45-98, 1990.

Epstein-Barr Virus

Basgoz N, Preiksaitis JK: Post-transplant lymphoproliferative disorder, *Infect Dis Clin North Am* 9:901-923, 1995.

Englund JA: The many faces of Epstein-Barr virus, *Postgrad Med* 83:167-179, 1988.

Khanna R, Burrows SR, Moss DJ: Immune regulation in EBV-associated diseases, *Microbiol Rev* 59:387-405, 1995.

Sugden B: EBV's open sesame, *Trends Biochemical Sci* 17:239-240, 1992.

Thorley-Lawson DA: Epstein-Barr virus and the B cell: that's all it takes, *Trends Microbiol* 4:204-208, 1996.

Cytomegalovirus and Human Herpesviruses 6, 7, and 8

Ablashi DV et al: Human herpesvirus-6 (HHV6) (short review), *In Vivo* 5:193-200, 1991.

Bigoni B et al: Human herpesvirus 8 is present in the lymphoid system of healthy persons and can reactivate in the course of AIDS, *J Infect Dis* 173:542-549, 1996.

McDougall JK: Cytomegalovirus, *Curr Top Microbiol Immunol* 154:1-279, 1990.

Pellet PE, Black JB, Yamamoto Y: Human herpesvirus 6: the virus and the search for its role as a human pathogen, *Adv Virol* 41:1-52, 1992.

Plachter B, Sinzger C, Jahn G: Cell types involved in replication and distribution of human cytomegalovirus, *Adv Virus Res* 46:197-264, 1996.

Proceedings of a conference on pathogenesis of cytomegalovirus diseases, *Transplant Proc* 23(suppl 3):1-182, 1991.

Wyatt LS, Frenkel N: Human herpesvirus 7 is a constitutive inhabitant of adult human saliva, *J Virol* 66:3206-3209, 1992.

Yamanishi K et al: Identification of human herpesvirus-6 as a causal agent for exanthema subitum, *Lancet* 1:1065-1067, 1988.

CHAPTER 52

Poxviruses

The poxviruses include the human viruses **variola (smallpox)** *(Orthopoxvirus)*, **molluscum contagiosum** *(Molluscipoxvirus)*, and poxviruses in other genera that naturally infect animals but can cause incidental infection in humans (zoonosis). Many of these viruses share antigenic determinants with smallpox, allowing the use of an animal poxvirus for a human vaccine.

In eighteenth century England, smallpox accounted for 7% to 12% of all deaths and the deaths of one third of children. However, the development of the first live vaccine in 1796 and the later worldwide distribution of this vaccine led to the **eradication** of smallpox by 1980. As a result, reference stocks of smallpox virus in two World Health Organization (WHO) laboratories were destroyed in 1996 after an international agreement to do so had been reached.

It is still important, however, to study the poxvirus family for the following reasons: (1) The mechanisms of spread of variola virus within the body represent a model for the spread of other viral infections, (2) poxviruses other than variola virus cause human disease, and (3) vaccinia virus has become an excellent vector that can be used for the development of hybrid vaccines containing the genes of other infectious agents.

STRUCTURE AND REPLICATION

The structure of the vaccinia virus and the way in which the virus replicates are representative of the structure and replication of other poxviruses. Poxviruses are the largest viruses, almost visible on light microscopy (Box 52-1). They measure 230×300 nm and are ovoid to brick shaped (Figure 52-1). An outer membrane and envelope enclose the core and core membrane, which are flanked by two lateral bodies and contain many enzymes and other proteins. The viral genome consists of a large double-stranded, linear DNA, which is fused at both ends. The genome of vaccinia virus consists of 86,000 base pairs (molecular weight, approximately 120×10^6 daltons).

The replication of poxviruses is unique among the DNA-containing viruses in that the entire multiplication cycle takes place within the host cell cytoplasm (Figure 52-2). As a result, *poxviruses must encode the enzymes re-*

quired for messenger RNA (mRNA) and DNA synthesis as well as the activities the other DNA viruses normally obtain from the host cell.

Viral penetration occurs within phagocytic vacuoles. After this, the outer membrane is removed in the vacuole, and early gene transcription is initiated. The virion core contains a specific transcriptional activator and all the enzymes necessary for transcription, including a multisubunit RNA polymerase, and enzymes for polyadenylate addition and capping. Among the early proteins produced is an uncoating protein that removes the core membrane, thereby liberating viral DNA into the cell cytoplasm. After this, viral DNA replicates in electron-dense cytoplasmic inclusions (Guarnieri's inclusion bodies) referred to as *factories*. Late viral mRNA is translated into structural and virion proteins. Unlike other viruses, the poxvirus membranes assemble around the core factories. About 10,000 viral particles are produced per infected cell and are released on cell lysis.

As noted earlier, the vaccinia virus is being used as an expression vector to produce live recombinant/hybrid vaccines for more virulent infectious agents (Figure 52-3). In this process the foreign gene, which encodes

---

BOX 52-1   Unique Properties of Poxviruses

Poxviruses are the largest, most complex viruses.

Poxviruses have complex, oval to brick-shaped morphology with internal structure.

Poxviruses have a linear, double-stranded DNA genome with fused ends.

Poxviruses are **DNA viruses that replicate in the cytoplasm.**

Virus encodes and carries all proteins necessary for mRNA synthesis.

Virus also encodes proteins for functions such as DNA synthesis, nucleotide scavenging, and immune escape mechanisms.

Virus is assembled in inclusion bodies (Guarnieri's bodies), where it acquires its outer membranes.

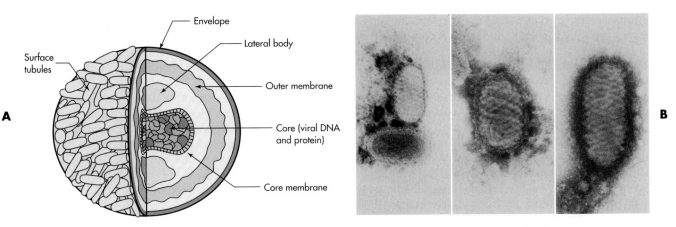

FIGURE 52-1 **A,** Structure of the vaccina virus. Within the virion, the core assumes the shape of a dumbbell because of the large lateral bodies. Virions have a double membrane; the "outer membrane" assembles around the core in the cytoplasm, and the envelope is acquired on exit from the cell. **B,** Electron micrographs of orf virus. Notice its complex structure.

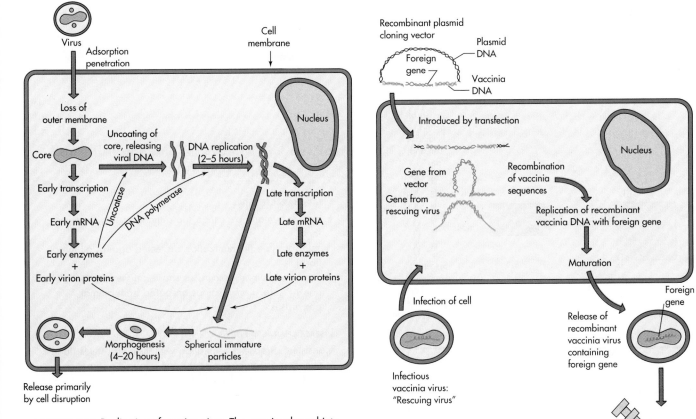

FIGURE 52-2 Replication of vaccina virus. The core is released into the cytoplasm, where virion enzymes initiate transcription. A viral encoded "uncoatase" enzyme then causes the release of DNA. Viral polymerase replicates the genome, and late transcription occurs. DNA and protein are assembled into cores with the core membrane. An outer membrane shrouds the core containing the lateral bodies and the enzymes required for infectivity. The virion buds through the plasma membrane or is released by cell lysis. *mRNA,* Messenger RNA.

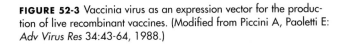

FIGURE 52-3 Vaccinia virus as an expression vector for the production of live recombinant vaccines. (Modified from Piccini A, Paoletti E: *Adv Virus Res* 34:43-64, 1988.)

the immunizing molecule, and specific vaccinia gene sequences are added to a plasmid. This recombinant plasmid is next inserted into a host cell that is then infected with vaccinia virus. The foreign gene is directed into the "rescuing" vaccinia virus genome because of the homologous vaccinia sequences included on the plasmid. Immunization with the recombinant vaccinia virus results from expression of the foreign gene and its presentation to the immune response almost as if by infection with the other agent. Experimental vaccines for human immunodeficiency virus, hepatitis B, influenza, and other agents have been prepared using these techniques. The potential for producing other vaccines in this manner is unlimited.

PATHOGENESIS AND IMMUNITY

Smallpox virus was inhaled and replicated in the upper respiratory tract (Figure 52-4). Dissemination occurred via lymphatic and cell-associated viremic spread. Internal and dermal tissues were inoculated after a second, more intense viremia. Molluscum contagiosum and the other poxviruses, on the other hand, are acquired by direct contact with lesions and do not spread extensively.

The poxviruses encode many proteins that facilitate their replication and pathogenesis in the host. These include proteins that initially stimulate host cell growth and then lead to cell lysis and viral spread. Molluscum contagiosum causes a wartlike lesion rather than a lytic infection.

Cell-mediated immunity is essential for resolving a poxvirus infection. However, poxviruses encode proteins that help the virus evade immune control. These include the cell-to-cell spread of the virus to avoid antibody and proteins that impede the interferon, complement, and inflammatory responses. The disease mechanisms of poxviruses are summarized in Box 52-2.

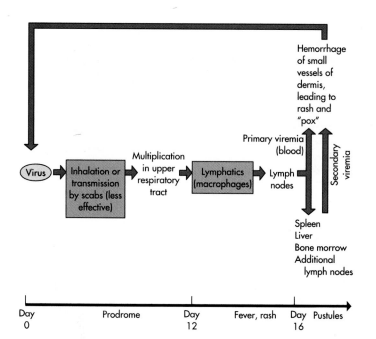

FIGURE 52-4 Spread of smallpox within the body. The virus enters and replicates in the respiratory tract without causing symptoms or contagion. The virus infects macrophages, which enter the lymphatic system and carry the virus to regional lymph nodes. The virus then replicates and initiates a viremia, causing the infection to spread to the spleen, bone marrow, lymph nodes, liver, and all organs, followed by the skin (rash). A secondary viremia causes the development of additional lesions throughout the host, followed by death or recovery with or without sequelae. Recovery was associated with prolonged immunity and lifelong protection.

BOX 52-2   Disease Mechanisms of Poxvirus

Smallpox was initiated by respiratory tract infection and was spread mainly by the lymphatic system and cell-associated viremia.

Molluscum contagiosum and zoonoses are transmitted by contact.

Virus may cause initial stimulation of cell growth and then cell lysis.

Virus encodes immune escape mechanisms.

Cell-mediated and humoral immunity are important for resolution.

BOX 52-3   Properties of Smallpox that Led to Its Eradication

VIRAL CHARACTERISTICS

Exclusive human host range (no animal reservoirs or vectors)

Single serotype (immunization protected against all infections)

Animal and human poxviruses share antigenic determinants ("safe" live vaccines prepared from animal poxviruses)

DISEASE CHARACTERISTICS

Consistent disease presentation with visible pustules (Identification of sources of contagion allowed quarantine and vaccination of contacts.)

VACCINE

Stable, inexpensive, easy-to-administer vaccine
Presence of scar indicating successful vaccination

PUBLIC HEALTH SERVICE

Successful WHO worldwide program combining vaccination and quarantine.

EPIDEMIOLOGY

Most of the poxviruses of importance to humans are primary pathogens in vertebrates rather than humans (e.g., cow, sheep, goats) and infect humans only through accidental occupational exposure (zoonosis). The exception is molluscum contagiosum and *was* smallpox.

Smallpox (variola) was very contagious and, as just noted, was spread primarily by the respiratory route. It was also spread less efficiently through close contact with dried virus on clothes or other materials. Despite the severity of the disease and its tendency to spread, several factors contributed to its elimination (Box 52-3).

CLINICAL SYNDROMES

The diseases associated with poxviruses are listed in Table 52-1.

Smallpox

Two variants of smallpox existed: variola major, which was associated with a mortality of 15% to 40%, and variola minor, which was associated with a mortality of 1%. Smallpox was usually initiated by infection of the respiratory tract with subsequent involvement of local lymph glands, which in turn led to viremia. The incubation period ranged from 5 to 17 days and averaged 12 days. The symptoms and course of the disease are presented in Figure 52-4, and the characteristic rash is shown in Figure 52-5.

Smallpox was usually diagnosed clinically but was confirmed by growth of the virus in embryonated eggs or cell cultures. Characteristic lesions (pocks) appeared on the chorioallantoic membrane of embryonated eggs.

Smallpox was the first disease to be controlled by immunization, and its eradication is one of the greatest triumphs of medical epidemiology. It resulted from a massive WHO campaign to vaccinate all susceptible people, especially those exposed to anyone with the disease, and thereby interrupt the chain of human-to-human transmission. This campaign, which began in 1967, succeeded, with the last case of naturally acquired infection reported in 1977 and eradication acknowledged in 1980.

Variolation constituted an initial attempt at immunization and involved the inoculation of susceptible people with the virulent smallpox pus. It was first performed in the Far East and later in England. Cotton Mather subsequently introduced the practice to the United States. Variolation was associated with a fatality rate of approximately 1%, a better risk than that associated with smallpox itself. In 1796, Jenner developed and then popularized a vaccine using the less virulent cowpox virus, which shares antigenic determinants with smallpox.

As smallpox began to be totally eradicated, it became apparent that the rate of serious reactions to vaccination (see the discussion of vaccinia) exceeded the risk of infection in the developed world. Therefore smallpox vaccination began to be discontinued in the 1970s, with its use totally discontinued after 1980.

FIGURE 52-5 Child with smallpox. Note the characteristic rash.

TABLE 52-1	**Diseases Associated with Poxviruses**		
VIRUS	**DISEASE**	**SOURCE**	**LOCATION**
Variola	Smallpox (now extinct)	Humans	Extinct
Vaccinia	Used for smallpox vaccination	Laboratory product	—
Orf	Localized lesion	Zoonosis—sheep, goats	Worldwide
Cowpox	Localized lesion	Zoonosis—rodents, cats, cows	Europe
Pseudocowpox	Milker's nodule	Zoonosis—dairy cows	Worldwide
Monkeypox	Generalized disease	Zoonosis—monkeys, squirrels	Africa
Bovine papular stomatitis virus	Localized lesion	Zoonosis—calves, beef cattle	Worldwide
Tanapox	Localized lesion	Rare zoonosis—monkeys	Africa
Yabapos	Localized lesion	Rare zoonosis—monkeys, baboons	Africa
Molluscum contagiosum	Many skin lesions	Humans	Worldwide

Modified from Balows A, Hausler WJ Jr, Lennette EH, editors: *Laboratory diagnosis of infectious diseases: principles and practice,* vol 2, New York, 1988, Springer-Verlag.

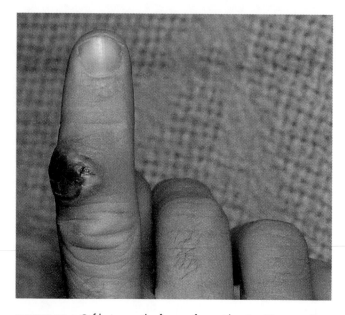

FIGURE 52-6 Orf lesion on the finger of a taxidermist. (Courtesy Joe Meyers, MD, Akron, Ohio.)

Vaccinia

The virus used for the smallpox vaccine was the vaccinia virus, and the vaccination procedure consisted of scratching live virus into the patient's skin and then observing for the development of vesicles and pustules to confirm a "take." However, as the incidence of smallpox waned, it became apparent that there were more complications related to vaccination than cases of smallpox. Several of these complications were severe and even fatal and included encephalitis and progressive infection (**vaccinia necrosum**); the latter occurred occasionally in immunocompromised patients who were inadvertently vaccinated. The relative ease with which vaccinia virus infections were spread person to person among unvaccinated people therefore posed a threat to the immunocompromised contacts of vaccinees.

Orf, Cowpox, and Monkeypox

The poxvirus of animals such as sheep or goats (orf) and cows (cowpox) can infect humans, usually as a result of accidental direct contact with the lesions. In these instances, nodular lesions usually form on the fingers or face and are hemorrhagic (cowpox) or granulomatous (orf or pseudocowpox) (Figure 52-6). Vesicular lesions frequently develop and then regress in 25 to 35 days, generally without scar formation. The lesions may be mistaken for anthrax. The etiological viruses can be grown in culture or seen directly with electron microscopy.

More than 100 cases of illnesses resembling smallpox have been attributed to the monkeypox virus. All have occurred in western and central Africa, especially Zaire.

Molluscum Contagiosum

The lesions of molluscum contagiosum differ significantly from pox lesions in that they are nodular to wart-

FIGURE 52-7 Molluscum contagiosum. **A,** Skin lesion. **B,** Microscopic view; epidermis is filled with molluscum bodies. ($\times$100.)

like (Figure 52-7, *A*). They begin as papules and then become pearly, umbilicated nodules that are 2 to 10 mm in diameter and have a central caseous plug that can be readily expressed (squeezed out). They are most common on the trunk, genitalia, and proximal extremities and usually occur in a cluster of 5 to 20 nodules. The incubation period for molluscum contagiosum is 2 to 8 weeks, and the disease is spread by direct contact (e.g., sexual contact, wrestling) or fomites (e.g., towels). Molluscum contagiosum cannot be grown in tissue culture or animal models.

The diagnosis of molluscum contagiosum is confirmed histologically by the finding of very characteristic large, eosinophilic cytoplasmic inclusions (**molluscum bodies**) in epithelial cells (Figure 52-7, *B*). These can be seen in biopsy specimens or in the expressed caseous core.

Lesions of molluscum contagiosum disappear in 2 to 12 months, presumably as a result of acquired immune responses. Treatment, if required, consists of curettage and the application of liquid nitrogen or iodine solutions.

QUESTIONS

1. The structure of poxviruses is more complex than that of most other viruses. What problems does this create for viral replication?
2. Poxviruses replicate in the cytoplasm. What problems does this create for viral replication?
3. How does the immune response to smallpox infection in an immunologically naive person differ from that in a vaccinated person? When is antibody present in each case? What stage, or stages, of viral dissemination are blocked in each case?
4. What characteristics of smallpox facilitated its elimination?
5. Vaccinia virus is being used as a vector for the development of hybrid vaccines. Why is vaccinia virus well suited to this task? Which infectious agents would be appropriate for a vaccinia hybrid vaccine and why?

Bibliography

Belshe RB, editor: *Textbook of human virology,* ed 2, St Louis, 1991, Mosby.

Fenner F: A successful eradication campaign: global eradication of smallpox, *Rev Infect Dis* 4(5):916-930, 1982.

Fields BN, Knipe DM, Howley PM, editors: *Virology,* ed 3, New York, 1996, Lippincott-Raven.

Gorbach SL, Bartlett JG, Blacklow NR, editors: *Infectious diseases,* Philadelphia, 1992, WB Saunders.

Mandell GL, Bennett JE, Dolin R: *Principles and practice of infectious diseases,* ed 4, New York, 1995, Churchill Livingstone.

Moyer RW, Turner PC: Poxviruses, *Curr Top Microbiol Immunol* 163:1-211, 1990.

Piccini A, Paoletti E: Vaccinia: virus, vector, vaccine, *Adv Virus Res* 34:43-64, 1988.

White DO, Fenner FJ. *Medical virology,* ed 4, New York, 1994, Academic.

Parvoviruses

The Parvoviridae are the smallest of the DNA viruses. Their small size and limited genetic repertoire make them dependent on the host cell or a helper virus to replicate, more so than any other DNA virus.

Only one member of the Parvoviridae, **B19,** a member of the *Parvovirus* genus, is known to cause human disease. B19 normally causes **erythema infectiosum,** or **fifth disease,** a mild febrile exanthematous disease that occurs in children. It goes by the latter name because it was the fifth of the childhood exanthems, with the first four comprising varicella, rubella, roseola, and measles. B19 is also responsible for causing episodes of aplastic crisis in patients with chronic hemolytic anemia and is associated with acute polyarthritis in adults. Intrauterine infection of a fetus may cause abortion. Other parvoviruses such as RA-1 (isolated from a person with rheumatoid arthritis) and fecal parvoviruses have not been shown to cause human disease. Feline and canine parvoviruses do not cause human disease and are preventable by vaccination of the pet.

Adeno-associated viruses, members of the ***Dependovirus* genus,** commonly infect humans but only in association with a second "helper" virus, usually an adenovirus. Dependoviruses neither appear to cause illness nor modify infection by their helper viruses. A third genus of the family, *Densovirus,* infects only insects.

STRUCTURE AND REPLICATION

The parvoviruses are extremely small (18 to 26 nm in diameter) and have a nonenveloped, icosahedral virion (Box 53-1 and Figure 53-1). The B19 virus genome contains one linear, single-stranded DNA molecule with a molecular weight of 1.5 to 1.8×10^6 d (5.5 kilobases in length) (Box 53-2). Plus or minus DNA strands are packaged separately into virions. Two structural, one nonstructural, and several smaller proteins are encoded by the overlapping of reading frames on the plus-stranded genome. **Only one serotype of B19 is known to exist.**

B19 virus replicates in **mitotically active** cells and prefers cells of the **erythroid lineage,** such as fresh human bone marrow cells, erythroid cells from fetal liver, and erythroid leukemia cells (Figure 53-2). After binding to the erythrocyte blood group P antigen (globoside) and its internalization, the virion is uncoated, and the single-stranded DNA genome is delivered to the nucleus. Factors available only during the S phase of the cell's growth cycle and cellular DNA polymerases are required to generate a complementary DNA strand. A double-stranded DNA version of the virion genome is required for transcription and replication. Inverted repeat sequences of DNA at both ends of the genome facilitate viral DNA synthesis. These ends fold back and hybridize with the genome to create a primer for the cell's DNA polymerase.

BOX 53-1 **Unique Properties of Parvoviruses**

Smallest DNA virus
Naked icosahedral capsid
Single-stranded DNA genome
Requirement of growing cells (B19) or helper virus (dependovirus) for replication

---

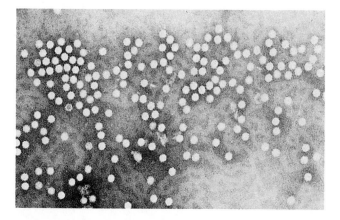

FIGURE 53-1 Electron micrograph of parvovirus. Parvoviruses are small (18 to 26 nm), nonenveloped viruses with single-stranded DNA. (Courtesy Centers for Disease Control and Prevention, Atlanta.)

Messenger RNA (mRNA) for the nonstructural regulatory and structural capsid proteins is generated from the same promoter by differential splicing of the primary transcript. Viral proteins synthesized in the cytoplasm then return to the nucleus, where the virion is assembled. The nuclear and cytoplasmic membrane degenerates, and the virus is released on cell lysis.

PATHOGENESIS AND IMMUNITY

B19 targets and is cytolytic for erythroid precursor cells (Box 53-3). B19 disease is determined by the direct killing of these cells and the subsequent immune response to the infection (rash and arthralgia).

Studies performed in volunteers suggest that B19 virus first replicates in the upper respiratory tract, then spreads by viremia to the bone marrow and elsewhere, where it replicates and kills erythroid precursor cells (Figure 53-3). The disease has a biphasic course. The **initial febrile stage** is the infectious stage. During this time, erythrocyte production is stopped for approximately 1 week as the result of the viral killing of erythroid precursor cells. Viremia occurs within 8 days of infection and is accompanied by nonspecific influenza-like symptoms. High titers of virus are also released into oral and respiratory secretions. Antibody stops the viremia, leading to resolution of the disease. The **second symptomatic stage** appears to be immune mediated. The rash and arthralgia seen in this stage coincide with the appearance of virus-specific IgM, the disappearance of detectable B19 virus, and the formation of immune complexes.

Hosts with chronic hemolytic anemia (e.g., sickle cell anemia) infected with B19 are at risk for a life-threaten-

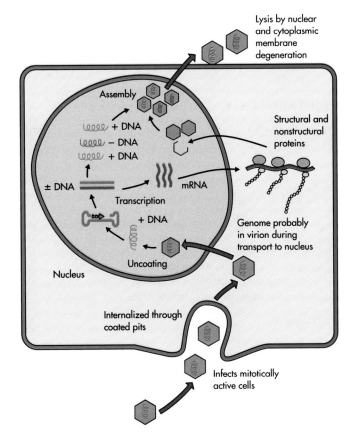

FIGURE 53-2 Postulated replication of parvovirus (B19) based on information from related viruses (minute virus of mice). The internalized parvovirus delivers its genome to the nucleus, where the single-stranded (plus or minus) DNA is converted to double-stranded DNA by host factors and DNA polymerases present only in growing cells. Transcription, replication, and assembly occur in the nucleus. Virus is released by cell lysis.

BOX 53-2   Parvovirus Genome

Single-stranded linear DNA genome
  Approximately 5.5 kilobases in length
    Plus and minus strands packaged into separate B19 virions with approximately equal frequency
  Ends of the genome having inverted repeats that hybridize to form hairpin loops and a primer for DNA synthesis

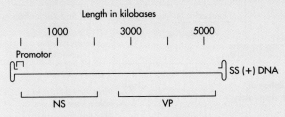

Coding region for B19 on plus strand
Separate coding regions for nonstructural and structural proteins transcribed from one promoter

---

BOX 53-3   Disease Mechanisms of B19 Parvovirus

Virus is spread by **respiratory** and **oral** secretions.
Virus **infects mitotically active erythroid precursor** cells in bone marrow and establishes lytic infection.
Virus establishes large **viremia** and can **cross the placenta.**
Antibody is important for resolution and prophylaxis.
Virus causes **biphasic disease:**
  Initial phase is related to viremia:
    Influenza-like symptoms and viral shedding
  Later phase is related to immune response:
    Circulating immune complexes of antibody and virions that do not fix complement
    Result: erythematous maculopapular rash, arthralgia, and arthritis
Depletion of erythroid precursor cells and destabilization of erythrocytes initiate **aplastic crisis in people with chronic anemia.**

ing reticulocytopenia, which is referred to as an **aplastic crisis.** This results from the combination of B19 depletion of the red blood cell precursors and the shortened life span of the erythrocytes caused by underlying anemia.

EPIDEMIOLOGY

As much as 65% of the adult population is infected with B19 by 40 years of age (Box 53-4). Erythema infectio-

sum is most common in children and adolescents aged 4 to 15 years, and it tends to occur in late winter and spring. The virus is most likely transmitted by respiratory droplets and oral secretions. Parenteral transmission of the virus by blood-clotting factor concentrate has also been described.

CLINICAL SYNDROMES

As already noted, B19 virus is the cause of **erythema infectiosum** (fifth disease) (Box 53-5). Infection starts with an unremarkable prodromal period, during which the person is contagious. Infection of a normal host may cause no noticeable symptoms or may cause fever and nonspecific symptoms such as sore throat, malaise, and myalgia and a slight decrease in hemoglobin levels (Figure 53-4). This is followed by a distinctive rash on the cheeks that looks as though the person has been slapped.

BOX 53-4   **Epidemiology of B19 Parvovirus Infection**

DISEASE/VIRAL FACTORS

Capsid virus is resistant to inactivation.
Contagious period precedes symptoms.
Virus crosses placenta and infects fetus.

TRANSMISSION

Respiratory droplets.

WHO IS AT RISK?

Children, especially elementary school age: erythema infectiosum (fifth disease).
Parents of children with B19 infection.
Pregnant women: fetal infection and disease.
People with chronic anemia: aplastic crisis.

GEOGRAPHY/SEASON

Virus is worldwide.
Fifth disease is more common in late winter and spring.

MODES OF CONTROL

There are no modes of control.

BOX 53-5   **Clinical Consequences of Parvovirus (B19) Infection**

Mild influenza-like illness (fever, headache, chills, myalgia, malaise)
Erythema infectiosum (fifth disease)
Aplastic crisis in people with chronic anemia
Arthropathy (polyarthritis: symptoms in many joints)
Risk of fetal loss as a result of B19 virus crossing the placenta, causing anemia-related pathology but not congenital anomalies

---

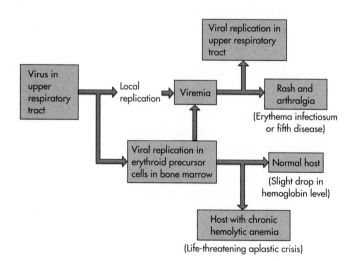

FIGURE 53-3 Mechanism of spread of parvovirus within the body.

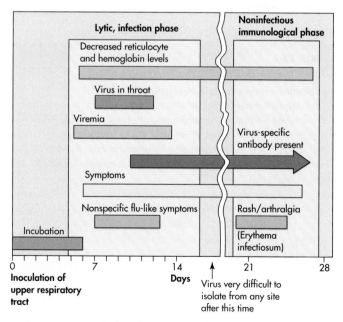

FIGURE 53-4 Time course of parvovirus (B19) infection. B19 causes biphasic disease: first, an initial, lytic infection phase characterized by febrile, influenza-like symptoms and then a noninfectious immunological phase characterized by a rash and arthralgia.

The rash then usually spreads, especially to exposed skin such as the arms and legs (Figure 53-5), and then subsides over 1 to 2 weeks. Relapse of the rash may occur often.

B19 infection in adults causes **polyarthritis.** Arthritis of the hands, wrists, knees, and ankles predominates, and the rash may precede the arthritis but often does not occur. B19 infection of immunocompromised people may result in chronic disease.

The most serious complication of parvovirus infection is the **aplastic crisis** that occurs in patients with chronic hemolytic anemia (sickle cell anemia). Infection in these people causes a transient reduction in erythropoiesis in the bone marrow. This results in a transient reticulocytopenia that lasts 7 to 10 days and a decrease in hemoglobin level. An aplastic crisis is accompanied by fever and nonspecific symptoms of malaise, myalgia, chills, and itching. A maculopapular rash with arthralgia and some joint swelling may also be present.

B19 infection of a seronegative mother increases the risk for fetal death. The virus can infect the fetus and kill erythrocyte precursors, causing anemia and congestive heart failure **(hydrops fetalis).** Infection of seropositive pregnant women often has no adverse effect on the fetus. There is no evidence that B19 causes congenital abnormalities (Box 53-4).

LABORATORY DIAGNOSIS

The diagnosis of erythema infectiosum is usually based on the clinical presentation. For B19 disease to be definitively diagnosed, however, specific IgM or viral DNA must be detected (e.g., to distinguish the rash of B19 from that of rubella in a pregnant woman). Enzyme-linked immunosorbent assays for B19 IgM and IgG have recently become available. The polymerase chain reaction is a very sensitive method for detecting the B19 genome in clinical samples but requires adequate controls. Virus isolation is not performed.

TREATMENT, PREVENTION, AND CONTROL

No specific antiviral treatment or means of control are available. Vaccines are available for dog and cat parvoviruses.

CASE STUDY AND QUESTIONS

Mrs. Doe called the pediatrician, complaining that her daughter had a rash. The daughter's face appeared as if it had been slapped. She had no fever or other notable symptom. On questioning, Mrs. Doe reported that her daughter had a mild cold within the previous 2 weeks and that she (the mother) was currently having more joint pain than usual and is very tired.

1. What features of this history indicate a parvovirus B19 etiology?
2. Was the child infectious at presentation? If not, when was she contagious?
3. What caused the symptoms?
4. Were the symptoms of the mother and daughter related?
5. What underlying condition would put the daughter at increased risk for serious disease after B19 infection? The mother?
6. Why is quarantine a poor means of limiting the spread of B19 parvovirus?

Bibliography

Anderson LJ: Human parvoviruses, *J Infect Dis* 161:603-608, 1990.

Anderson MJ: Parvoviruses. In Belshe RB, editor: *Textbook of human virology,* ed 2, St Louis, 1991, Mosby.

Balows A, Hausler WJ Jr, Lennette EH, editors: *Laboratory diagnosis of infectious diseases: principles and practice,* vol 2, New York, 1988, Springer-Verlag.

Berns KI: *The parvoviruses,* New York, 1984, Plenum.

Berns KI: Parvovirus replication, *Microbiol Rev* 54:316-329, 1990.

Chorba T et al: The role of parvovirus B19 in aplastic crisis and erythema infectiosum (fifth disease), *J Infect Dis* 154:383-393, 1986.

Fields BN, Knipe DM, Howley PM, editors: *Virology,* ed 3, New York, 1996, Lippincott-Raven.

Gorbach SL, Bartlett JG, Blacklow NR, editors: *Infectious diseases,* Philadelphia, 1992, WB Saunders.

Mandell GL, Bennett JE, Dolin R: *Principles and practice of infectious diseases,* ed 4, New York, 1995, Churchill Livingstone.

Naides SJ et al: Rheumatologic manifestations of human parvovirus B19 infection in adults, *Arthritis Rheum* 33:1297-1309, 1990.

Török TJ: Parvovirus B19 and human disease, *Adv Intern Med* 37:431-455, 1992.

Ware RE: *Parvovirus infections.* In Krugman SK et al: *Infectious diseases of children,* ed 9, St Louis, 1992, Mosby.

White DO, Fenner FJ: *Medical virology,* ed 4, New York, 1994, Academic.

FIGURE 53-5 A "slapped cheek" appearance is typical of the rash for erythema infectiosum. (From Hart CA, Broadhead RL: *A color atlas of pediatric infectious diseases,* London, 1992, Wolfe.)

Picornaviruses

$\mathbf{P}$icornaviridae is one of the largest families of viruses and includes some of the most important human and animal viruses (Box 54-1). As the name indicates, these viruses are **small** *(pico)* **RNA** viruses that have a **naked capsid** structure. The family includes more than 230 members and are divided into four genera: *Enterovirus, Rhinovirus, Cardiovirus,* and *Aphthovirus.* Of these, only **enteroviruses** and **rhinoviruses** cause human disease. The enteroviruses can be distinguished from the rhinoviruses by the stability of the capsid at a pH 3, the optimum temperature for growth, their mode of transmission, and the diseases they cause (Box 54-2).

At least 72 serotypes of human enteroviruses exist, including the polioviruses, coxsackieviruses, and echoviruses. Hepatitis A virus is also classified in this group (enterovirus 72) but is discussed separately in Chapter 62. The capsids of these viruses are very *resistant* to harsh environmental conditions (sewage systems) and the conditions in the gastrointestinal tract, a fact that facilitates their transmission by the fecal-oral route. However, although they may initiate infection in the gastrointestinal tract, the enteroviruses rarely cause enteric disease. Infections are usually asymptomatic. Several different disease syndromes may be caused by a specific serotype of enterovirus. Likewise, several different serotypes may cause the same disease, depending on the target tissue affected. The most well-known and well-studied picornavirus is poliovirus, of which there are three serotypes.

Coxsackieviruses are named after the town of Coxsackie, New York, where they were first isolated. They are divided into two groups, A and B, on the basis of certain biological and antigenic differences and further subdivided into numerical serotypes on the basis of additional antigenic differences.

The name *echovirus* is derived from *e*nteric *c*ytopathic *h*uman *o*rphan because these agents were not initially thought to be associated with clinical disease. Now 32 serotypes are recognized. Since 1967, newly isolated enteroviruses have been distinguished numerically.

The human rhinoviruses include at least 100 serotypes and are the major cause of the common cold. They are **sensitive to acidic pH** and **replicate poorly at temperatures above 33° C.** This sensitivity usually limits rhinoviruses to causing upper respiratory tract infections.

STRUCTURE

The plus-strand RNA of the picornaviruses is surrounded by an icosahedral capsid approximately 30 nm in diameter. The icosahedral capsid has 12 pentameric vertices, each of which is composed of five protomeric units of proteins. The protomers are made of four virion polypeptides (VP1 to VP4). VP2 and VP4 are generated by the cleavage of a precursor, VP0. VP4 in the virion solidifies the structure, but it is not generated until the genome is incorporated into the capsid. It is released on binding of the virus to the cellular receptor. The capsids are stable in the presence of heat and detergent and, except for the rhinoviruses, are also stable in acid. The capsid structure is so regular that paracrystals of virions often form in infected cells (Figures 54-1 and 54-2).

The genome of the picornaviruses resembles a messenger RNA (mRNA) (Figure 54-3). It is a **single strand of plus-sense RNA** of approximately 7400 bases that has a poly A at the 3′ end and a small protein, VPg (22 to 24 amino acids), attached to the 5′ end. The poly

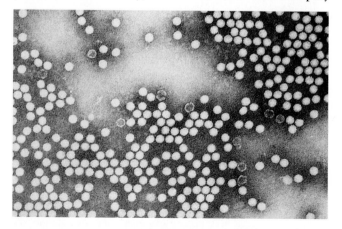

FIGURE 54-1 Electron micrograph of poliovirus. (Courtesy Centers for Disease Control and Prevention, Atlanta.)

Enterovirus
   Poliovirus types 1, 2, and 3
   Coxsackie A virus types 1 to 22 and 24
   Coxsackie B virus types 1 to 6
   Echovirus (ECHO virus) types 1 to 9, 11 to 27, and 29
      to 34
   Enterovirus 68 to 72 (72 is hepatitis A virus)
Rhinovirus types 1 to 100+
Cardiovirus
Aphthovirus

Virus is **naked, small** (25 to 30 nm) **icosahedral** capsid enclosing a single-stranded positive RNA genome:
   Enteroviruses are resistant to pH 3 to 9, detergents, mild sewage treatment, and heat.
   Rhinoviruses are labile at acidic pH; optimum growth temperature is 33° C.
Genome is an mRNA.
Naked genome is sufficient for infection.
Virus replicates in cytoplasm.
Viral RNA is translated into polyprotein, which is then cleaved into enzymatic and structural proteins.
Most viruses are **cytolytic.**

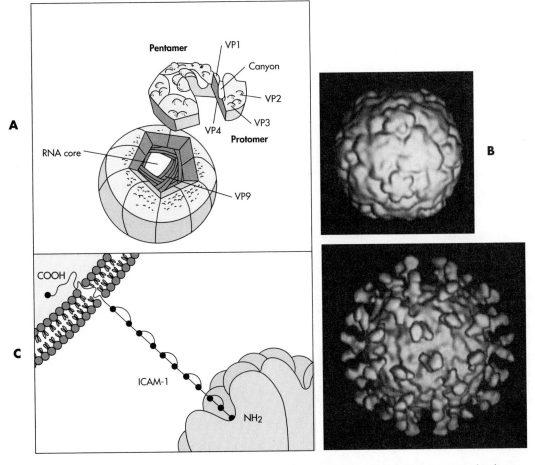

FIGURE 54-2 A, Structure of the human rhinovirus and its interaction with the ICAM-1 receptor-binding canyon surrounding the starlike structure at the vertices. **B,** Cryoelectron microscopy computer-generated reconstruction of the human rhinovirus 16. **C,** Interaction of ICAM-1 molecule with the virion. **D,** Cryoelectron microscopy reconstruction of the interaction of a soluble form of ICAM-1 with human rhinovirus 16. NOTE: There is one ICAM-1 per capsomere. *ICAM-1,* Intercellular adhesion molecule 1. (**B** and **D** courtesy Tim Baker, Purdue University.)

FIGURE 54-3 Structure of the picornavirus genome. The genome is translated as a polyprotein, which is cleaved by viral-encoded and cellular proteases into individual proteins. *g'*, Guanidine resistance marker (a genic locus involved in the initiation of RNA synthesis); *Poly A*, polyadenylate.

A sequence enhances the infectivity of the RNA, and the VPg may be important in packaging the genome into the capsid and initiating viral RNA synthesis. *The naked picornavirus genome is sufficient to infect a cell.*

The genome encodes a polyprotein that is proteolytically cleaved to produce the enzymatic and structural proteins of the virus. In addition to the capsid proteins and VPg, the picornaviruses encode at least one protease and an RNA-dependent RNA polymerase. Poliovirus also produces a protease that degrades the 200,000-dalton cap-binding protein of eukaryotic ribosomes, thereby blocking the translation of cellular mRNA.

REPLICATION

The specificity of the picornavirus interaction for cellular receptors is the major determinant of their target tissue tropism and disease (see Figure 6-12). The VP1 proteins at the vertices of the virion contain a canyon structure to which the receptor binds. The site of binding is protected from antibody neutralization. Arildone and related antiviral compounds contain a 3-methylisoxazole group that binds to the floor of this canyon and alters its conformation to prevent the uncoating of the virus.

The picornaviruses have been categorized into several receptor families. The receptors for polioviruses and rhinoviruses have recently been identified as tissue-specific cellular adhesion molecules. These molecules are members of the immunoglobulin superfamily. Their primary function is to promote normal and immunological cell-to-cell interactions. At least 80% of the rhinoviruses and several serotypes of coxsackievirus recognize intercellular adhesion molecule 1 (ICAM-1), which is expressed on epithelial cells, fibroblasts, and endothelial cells. Poliovirus binds to a molecule of similar structure and presumably of similar function. The cells in which the poliovirus receptor is expressed correlate directly with the limited range of poliovirus infection.

On binding to the receptor, the VP4 is released and the virion weakened. Either the genome is then injected directly across the membrane through a channel created at one of the vertices of the virion, or the virus is internalized by receptor-mediated endocytosis, followed by release of the genome as the virion dissociates in the acidic environment of the endosome. The genome binds directly to ribosomes despite the lack of a 5′ cap structure. The ribosomes recognize a unique internal RNA loop in the genome. A polyprotein containing all the viral protein sequences is synthesized within 10 to 15 minutes of infection. This polyprotein is cleaved by viral proteases encoded in the polyprotein. The viral RNA-dependent RNA polymerase generates a negative-strand RNA template from which the new mRNA/genome and templates can be synthesized. The amount of viral mRNA increases rapidly in the cell, with the number of viral RNA molecules reaching 400,000 per cell.

Several picornaviruses inhibit cellular RNA and protein synthesis during infection. For example, cleavage of the 200,000-dalton cap-binding protein of the ribosome by a poliovirus protease prevents most cellular mRNA from binding to the ribosome. Permeability changes induced by picornaviruses also reduce the ability of cellular mRNA to bind to the ribosome. In addition, viral mRNA can outcompete cellular mRNA for the factors required in protein synthesis. These activities contribute to the cytopathological effect of the virus on the target cell.

As the viral genome is being replicated and translated, the structural proteins VP0, VP1, and VP3 are cleaved from the polyprotein by a viral-encoded protease and assembled into subunits. A total of 5 subunits associate into pentamers, and 12 pentamers associate to form the procapsid. After insertion of the genome, VP0 is cleaved into VP2 and VP4 to complete the capsid. The virion is usually released on cell lysis.

ENTEROVIRUSES
Pathogenesis and Immunity

Enterovirus infections are usually asymptomatic but can cause symptoms ranging from coldlike symptoms to paralytic disease (Box 54-3). Contrary to their name, enteroviruses do not usually cause enteric disease but are transmitted by the fecal-oral route. Differences in the nature of the diseases produced by the enteroviruses result mainly from differences in tissue tropism and the cytolytic capacity of the virus (Figure 54-4). Poliovirus has been studied extensively and is the prototype for the pathogenesis of the enteroviruses.

The upper respiratory tract, the oropharynx, and the intestinal tract are the portals of entry for enteroviruses. The virions are impervious to stomach acid, proteases, and bile. Viral replication is initiated in the mucosa and lymphoid tissue of the tonsils and pharynx, and the virus later infects lymphoid cells of Peyer's patches underlying the intestinal mucosa. Primary viremia spreads the virus to receptor-bearing target tissues, where a second phase of viral replication may occur, resulting in symptoms and a secondary viremia. In the case of poliovirus, the virus must cross the blood-brain barrier or may gain access to the brain by infecting skeletal muscle and traveling up the innervating nerves to the brain, somewhat like rabies

Disease Mechanisms of Picornaviruses

Enteroviruses enter via the oropharynx, intestinal mucosa, or upper respiratory tract and infect the underlying lymphatic tissue; rhinoviruses are restricted to the upper respiratory tract.

In the absence of serum antibody, enterovirus spreads by viremia to cells of a receptor-bearing target tissue.

Different picornaviruses bind to different receptors, many of which are members of the immunoglobulin superfamily (i.e., ICAM-1).

The infected target tissue determines the subsequent disease.

Viral, rather than immune, pathology is usually responsible for causing disease symptoms.

The secretory antibody response is transitory but can prevent the initiation of infection.

Serum antibody blocks viremic spread to target tissue, preventing symptoms.

Enterovirus is shed in feces for long periods.

Infection is usually asymptomatic or causes mild influenza-like or upper respiratory tract disease.

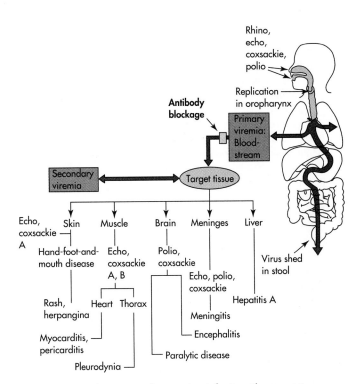

FIGURE 54-4 Pathogenesis of enterovirus infection. The target tissue infected by the enterovirus determines the predominant disease caused by the virus. *Rhino,* Rhinovirus; *echo,* echovirus; *coxsackie,* coxsackievirus; *polio,* polio virus.

does (see Chapter 58). Viral shedding from the oropharynx can be detected for a short time before symptoms begin, whereas viral production and shedding from the intestine may last for 30 days or longer, even in the presence of a humoral immune response.

Poliovirus has one of the narrowest tissue tropisms, recognizing a receptor expressed on anterior horn cells of the spinal cord, dorsal root ganglia, motor neurons, skeletal muscle cells, lymphoid cells, and few other cells. Coxsackieviruses and echoviruses recognize receptors expressed on more cell types and tissues and cause a broader repertoire of diseases (Table 54-1). Receptors for these enteroviruses are present on cells of the central nervous system, heart, lung, pancreas, mucosa, and other tissues.

Most enteroviruses are **cytolytic,** replicating rapidly and causing direct damage to the target cell. The hepatitis A virus is the exception. It is not very cytolytic, and the kinetics of the immune response to hepatitis A correlate with the appearance of symptoms.

Antibody is the major protective immune response to the enteroviruses. Secretory antibody can prevent the initial establishment of infection in the oropharynx and gastrointestinal tract, and serum antibody prevents viremic spread to the target tissue and therefore disease. The time course for antibody development after a mock infection with a live vaccine is presented in Figure 54-10.

Cell-mediated immunity is not usually involved in protection but may play a role in pathogenesis. Hepatitis A virus is the exception in that T cells are also important for the resolution of the disease. T cells appear to contribute to the pathogenesis of coxsackie B virus–induced myocarditis in mice.

Epidemiology

The enteroviruses are exclusively human pathogens (Box 54-4). As the name implies, these viruses are primarily spread by the **fecal-oral** route. **Asymptomatic shedding** can occur for up to a month. Poor sanitation and crowded living conditions foster transmission of the viruses (Figure 54-5). Sewage contamination of water supplies can result in enterovirus epidemics. Outbreaks of enterovirus disease are seen in schools and day-care settings. Summer is the major season for such disease. The coxsackieviruses and echoviruses may also be spread in aerosol droplets and cause respiratory tract infections.

With the success of the polio vaccines, the wild-type poliovirus has been eliminated from the Western Hemisphere (Figure 54-6). Five to ten cases of vaccine-related polio disease occur per year, and these result from the reversion of the vaccine virus and its reestablishing neurovirulence. In areas where the vaccine is not available or in communities where vaccination is contrary to religious beliefs or other teachings, paralytic polio still may occur. Polioviruses are spread most often during the summer and autumn.

Paralytic polio was once considered a middle-class disease because good hygiene would delay exposure of a person to the virus until late childhood, the adolescent

TABLE 54-1 Summary of Clinical Syndromes Associated with Major Enterovirus Groups

SYNDROME	OCCURRENCE	POLIOVIRUSES	COXSACKIE A VIRUSES	COXSACKIE B VIRUSES	ECHOVIRUSES
Paralytic disease	Sporadic	+	+	+	+
Encephalitis, meningitis	Outbreaks	+	+	+	+
Carditis	Sporadic		+	+	+
Neonatal disease	Outbreaks			+	+
Pleurodynia	Outbreaks			+	
Herpangina	Common		+		
Hand-foot-and-mouth disease	Common		+		
Rash disease	Common		+	+	+
Acute hemorrhagic conjunctivitis	Epidemics		+		
Respiratory tract infections	Common	+	+	+	+
Undifferentiated fever	Common	+	+	+	+
Diarrhea, gastrointestinal disease	Uncommon				+
Diabetes, pancreatitis	Uncommon			+	
Orchitis	Uncommon			+	
Disease in immunodeficient patients	—	+	+		+
Congenital anomalies	Uncommon		+	+	

BOX 54-4 Epidemiology of Enterovirus Infections

DISEASE/VIRAL FACTORS

Infection is often asymptomatic, with viral shedding.
Virion is resistant to environmental conditions (detergents, acid, drying, mild sewage treatment, and heat).

TRANSMISSION

Fecal-oral route: poor hygiene, dirty diapers (especially in day-care settings).
Ingestion via contaminated food and water.
Contact with infected hands and fomites.
Inhalation of infectious aerosols.

WHO IS AT RISK?

Young children: at risk for polio (asymptomatic or mild disease).
Older children and adults: at risk for polio (asymptomatic to paralytic disease).

WHO IS AT RISK?—cont'd

Newborns and neonates: at highest risk for serious coxsackievirus and enterovirus disease. (Nature of disease correlates with specific enterovirus types and age of person.)

GEOGRAPHY/SEASON

Viruses have worldwide distribution; wild-type polio is virtually eradicated in developed countries because of vaccination program.
Disease is more common in summer.

MODES OF CONTROL

For polio, live oral polio vaccine (trivalent OPV) or inactivated trivalent vaccine (IPV) is administered.
For other enteroviruses, there is no vaccine; good hygiene limits spread.

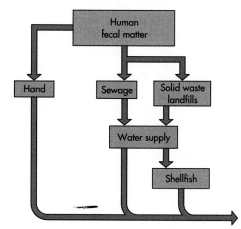

FIGURE 54-5 Transmission of enteroviruses. The capsid structure is resistant to mild sewage treatment, saltwater, detergents, and temperature changes, allowing these viruses to be transmitted by fecal-oral routes and on hands.

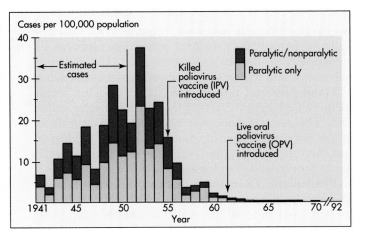

FIGURE 54-6 Incidence of polio in the United States. Killed (inactivated) poliovirus vaccine *(IPV)* was introduced in 1955 and live (oral) poliovirus vaccine *(OPV)* in 1961 and 1962. (Courtesy Centers for Disease Control: *Immunization against disease: 1972,* Washington, DC, 1973, US Government Printing Office.)

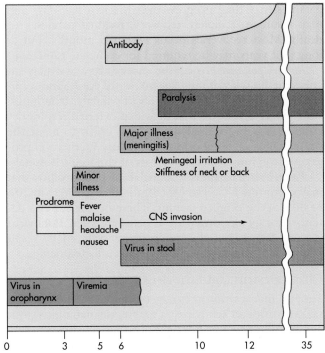

FIGURE 54-7 Progression of poliovirus infection. Infection may be asymptomatic or progress to minor or major disease. *CNS,* Central nervous system.

years, or adulthood, when infection would produce the most severe symptoms. Infection during early childhood generally results in asymptomatic or very mild disease.

Like poliovirus infection, coxsackie A virus disease in adults is generally more severe than that in children. However, coxsackie B virus and some of the echoviruses (especially echo 11) can be particularly harmful to infants. Differences in the susceptibility to and severity of poliovirus and coxsackievirus infection with age may result from differences in the distribution and amount of receptor expression or other factors.

Clinical Syndromes

The clinical syndromes produced by the enteroviruses are determined by several factors, including the viral serotype; the infecting dose; tissue tropism; the portal of entry; the patient's age, gender, and state of health; and pregnancy. The incubation period for enterovirus disease varies from 1 to 35 days, depending on the virus, the target tissue, and the person's age. Viruses that affect oral and respiratory sites have the shortest incubation periods.

Poliovirus Infections

Wild-type polio infections are becoming rarer because of the success of the polio vaccines (Figure 54-6). However, as noted earlier, vaccine-associated cases of polio do occur, and some populations remain unvaccinated, putting them at risk for infection. Poliovirus may cause one of four outcomes in unvaccinated people, depending on the progression of the infection (Figure 54-7):

Asymptomatic illness results if the viral infection is limited to the oropharynx and the gut. At least 90% of poliovirus infections are asymptomatic.

Abortive poliomyelitis, the **minor illness,** is a nonspecific febrile illness occurring in approximately 5% of infected people. Fever, headache, malaise, sore throat, and vomiting occur in such people within 3 to 4 days of exposure.

Nonparalytic poliomyelitis or **aseptic meningitis** occurs in 1% to 2% of patients with poliovirus infections. In this case the virus progresses into the central nervous system and the meninges, causing back pain and muscle spasms in addition to the symptoms of the minor illness.

Paralytic polio, the **major illness,** occurs in 0.1% to 2.0% of persons with poliovirus infections and is the most severe outcome. It appears 3 to 4 days after the minor illness has subsided, thereby producing a biphasic illness. In this disease the virus spreads from the blood to the **anterior horn cells** of the spinal cord and the motor cortex of the brain. The severity of the paralysis is determined by the extent of the neuronal infection and the neurons affected. Spinal paralysis may involve one or more limbs, whereas bulbar (cranial) paralysis may involve a combination of cranial nerves and even the medullary respiratory center.

Paralytic poliomyelitis is characterized by an asymmetrical flaccid paralysis with no sensory loss. Poliovirus type 1 is responsible for 85% of the cases of paralytic polio disease. Types 2 and 3 may cause vaccine-associated disease because of reversion of the virus from an attenuated form to virulence.

The degree of paralysis varies in that it may involve only a few muscle groups (e.g., one leg) or there may be complete flaccid paralysis of all four extremities. The paralysis may then progress over the first few days and may result in complete recovery, residual paralysis, or death. Most recoveries occur within 6 months, but as long as 2 years may be required for complete remission.

Bulbar poliomyelitis can be more severe and may involve the muscles of the pharynx, vocal cords, and respiration and result in death in 75% of patients. Iron lungs, which were chambers that provided external respiratory compression, were used during the 1950s to assist the breathing of such polio patients. Before vaccination programs, iron lungs filled the wards of children's hospitals.

Postpolio syndrome is a sequelae of poliomyelitis that may occur much later in life (30 to 40 years later) in 20% to 80% of the original victims. These people suffer a deterioration of the originally affected muscles. Poliovirus is not present, but the syndrome is believed to result from a loss of neurons in the initially affected nerves.

Coxsackievirus and Echovirus Infections

Several clinical syndromes may be caused by either a coxsackievirus or an echovirus (e.g., aseptic meningitis), but certain illnesses are especially associated with coxsackieviruses. Coxsackie A viruses are associated with diseases with vesicular lesions (e.g. herpangina), whereas coxsackie B serotypes (*B for body*) are most frequently associated with myocarditis and pleurodynia. These viruses can also cause a polio-like paralytic disease. The most common results of infection are lack of symptoms or a mild upper respiratory tract or influenza-like disease.

Herpangina is inappropriately named because it has no relation to herpesvirus. Rather, it is caused by several types of coxsackie A virus. Fever, sore throat, pain on swallowing, anorexia, and vomiting characterize this disorder. The classic finding is vesicular ulcerated lesions around the soft palate and uvula (Figure 54-8). Less typically the lesions affect the hard palate. The virus can be recovered from the lesions or from feces. The disease is self-limited and requires only symptomatic management.

Hand-foot-and-mouth disease is a vesicular exanthem caused by an enterovirus, usually coxsackievirus A16. The name is descriptive because the main features of this infection consist of vesicular lesions of the hands, feet, mouth, and tongue (Figure 54-9). The patient is mildly febrile, and the illness subsides in a few days.

Pleurodynia (Bornholm disease), also known as the *devil's grip,* is an acute illness in which patients have a sudden onset of fever and unilateral low thoracic, pleuritic chest pain, which may be excruciating. Abdominal pain and even vomiting may also occur, and muscles on the involved side may be extremely tender. Pleurodynia lasts an average of 4 days but may relapse after the condition has been asymptomatic for several days. Coxsackie B virus is the causative agent.

Myocardial and pericardial infections caused by coxsackie B virus occur sporadically in older children and adults but are most threatening in newborns. Neonates with these infections have febrile illnesses and the sudden and unexplained onset of heart failure. Cyanosis, tachycardia, cardiomegaly, and hepatomegaly occur. Electrocardiographic changes are found in patients with myocarditis. The mortality associated with the infection is high, and autopsy typically reveals the involvement of other organ systems, including the brain, liver, and pancreas. **Acute benign pericarditis** affects young adults but may be seen in older people. The symptoms resemble those of myocardial infarction but fever is more severe.

FIGURE 54-8 Herpangina. Characteristic discrete vesicles are seen on the anterior tonsillar pillars. (Courtesy Dr. GDW McKendrick. From Lambert HP et al: *Infectious diseases illustrated*, London, 1982, Gower.)

FIGURE 54-9 Hand-foot-and-mouth disease caused by coxsackie A virus. Lesions initially appear in the oral cavity and then develop within 1 day on the palms and, as seen here, on the soles. (From Habif TP: *Clinical dermatology: a color guide to diagnosis and therapy*, ed 3, St Louis, 1996, Mosby.)

Viral (aseptic) meningitis is an acute febrile illness accompanied by headache and signs of meningeal irritation, including nuchal rigidity. Petechiae or a skin rash may occur in patients with enteroviral meningitis. Recovery is usually uneventful unless the illness is associated with encephalitis (meningoencephalitis) or occurs in infants younger than 1 year old. Outbreaks of picornavirus meningitis occur each year during the summer and autumn.

Fever and rash may occur in patients infected with echoviruses or coxsackieviruses. The eruptions are usually maculopapular but may occasionally be petechial or even vesicular. The petechial type of eruption must be differentiated from that of meningococcemia. The child with enteroviral infection is not as ill or as toxic as and has a less intense leukocytosis than the child with meningococcemia.

Some strains of coxsackie B virus and echovirus can be transmitted transplacentally to the neonate. Infection of an infant by this or another route may produce severe disseminated disease.

Other Enterovirus Diseases

Enterovirus 70 and a variant of coxsackievirus A24 have recently been associated with an extremely contagious ocular disease, **acute hemorrhagic conjunctivitis.** The infection causes subconjunctival hemorrhages and conjunctivitis. The disease has a 24-hour incubation period and resolves within 1 or 2 weeks.

Respiratory tract disease, hepatitis, and diabetes are some of the syndromes attributed to enteroviruses. Coxsackieviruses A21 and A24 and echoviruses 11 and 20 can cause rhinovirus-like coldlike symptoms if the upper respiratory tract becomes infected. Enterovirus 72 causes hepatitis A disease (see Chapter 62). Coxsackie B infections of the pancreas have been suspected of causing insulin-dependent diabetes because they cause destruction of the islets of Langerhans.

Laboratory Diagnosis
Clinical Chemistry

Cerebrospinal fluid (CSF) from poliovirus or enterovirus aseptic meningitis reveals a predominantly lymphocytic pleocytosis (presence of 25 to 500 cells). In contrast with bacterial meningitis, in viral meningitis the CSF glucose level is usually normal or slightly low. The CSF protein level is normal to slightly elevated. The CSF is rarely positive for the virus.

Culture

Polioviruses may be isolated from the patient's pharynx during the first few days of illness and from the feces for as long as 30 days but rarely from the CSF. The virus grows well in monkey kidney tissue culture. Coxsackieviruses and echoviruses can usually be isolated from the throat and stool during infection and often from the CSF in patients with meningitis. Virus is rarely isolated in patients with myocarditis, however, because the symp-toms occur several weeks after the initial infection. The coxsackie B viruses can be grown on primary monkey or human embryo kidney cells. Many coxsackie A virus strains do not grow in tissue culture, however, and must still be grown in suckling mice. The specific type of enterovirus can be determined only by using specific antibody and assays (e.g., neutralization, immunofluorescence, ELISA).

Serology

Serological confirmation of an enterovirus infection can be made by the detection of specific immunoglobulin M (IgM) or the finding of a fourfold increase in the antibody titer between the time of the acute illness and the period of convalescence. The many serotypes of echovirus and coxsackievirus make this approach difficult, but it may be useful in documenting poliovirus infection.

Treatment, Prevention, and Control

No specific antiviral therapy is available for enterovirus infections. Supportive therapy is extremely important for patients with paralytic disease to assist in their potential recovery.

The prevention of paralytic poliomyelitis is one of the triumphs of modern medicine. By 1979, infections with the wild-type poliovirus disappeared from the United States, with the number of cases of polio decreasing from 21,000 per year in the prevaccine era to 18 in unvaccinated patients in 1977. Unfortunately, health care delivery systems in underdeveloped countries are unable to provide adequate vaccine administration for their people; for this reason, wild-type viral disease still exists in Africa, the Middle East, and Asia.

Two types of poliovirus vaccine exist: the **inactivated polio vaccine (IPV),** developed by Jonas Salk, and a **live attenuated oral polio vaccine (OPV),** developed by Albert Sabin. Both vaccines incorporate the three strains of polio, are stable, are relatively inexpensive, and induce a protective antibody response (Figure 54-10). The IPV was proved effective in 1955, but until recently, the oral vaccine has been used instead because of its ease of delivery and its capacity to elicit lifelong immunity (Box 54-5). New recommendations now encourage use of the IPV for the initial immunizations of babies.

The OPV was attenuated (i.e., rendered less virulent) by passage in human or monkey cell cultures. Attenuation yielded a virus that can replicate in the oropharynx and intestinal tract but cannot infect neuronal cells. A further advantage of the live vaccine strain is that it is shed in feces for weeks and may be spread to close contacts. This will immunize or reimmunize them, which promotes mass immunization. The major drawback of the live vaccine is that there is a remote potential for the virus to revert to its virulent form and cause paralytic disease. The incidence of this is estimated to be 1 per 4 million doses administered (versus 1 in 100 people infected with the wild-type poliovirus). The risk of vaccine-asso-

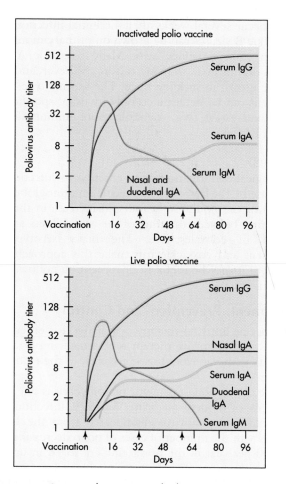

FIGURE 54-10 Serum and secretory antibody response to intramuscular inoculation of IPV and to live attenuated OPV. Note the presence of secretory IgA induced by the live polio vaccine. (Redrawn from Ogra P et al: *Rev Infect Dis* 2:352-369, 1980.)

ciated paralytic poliomyelitis is increased in immunocompromised people, but the disease is more likely to occur in susceptible adults than in susceptible children. Such vaccine-associated poliomyelitis may occur in the contacts as well as the recipients of the vaccine.

Children should receive the OPV at 2, 4, and 15 months and at 4 to 6 years of age. New guidelines suggest administration of the IPV for the first two doses to eliminate the risk of vaccine-related paralytic polio disease. The IPV instead of the OPV is administered in several European countries, with good results.

No vaccines exist for coxsackieviruses or echoviruses. Transmission of these viruses can presumably be reduced by improvements in hygiene and living conditions.

RHINOVIRUSES

Rhinoviruses are the most important cause of the **common cold** and upper respiratory tract infections. Such infections are self-limited, however, and do not cause serious disease. At least 100 serotypes of rhinovirus have been identified. At least 80% of the rhinoviruses share a common receptor, which is also used by some of the coxsackieviruses. This receptor has been identified as ICAM-1, which was discussed earlier. ICAM-1 is a member of the immunoglobulin superfamily and is expressed on epithelial, fibroblast, and B-lymphoblastoid cells.

Pathogenesis and Immunity

Unlike the enteroviruses, rhinoviruses are unable to replicate in the gastrointestinal tract (Box 54-3). The rhinoviruses are **labile to acidic pH** and **grow best at 33° C,** which may partly account for their predilection for the cooler environment of the nasal mucosa. Infec-

---

BOX 54-5   **Advantages and Disadvantages of Polio Vaccines**

LIVE (OPV)

Advantages

Effectiveness

Lifelong immunity

Induction of secretory antibody response similar to that of
   natural infection

Possibility of attenuated virus circulating in community by
   spread to contacts (indirect immunization) (herd immunity)

Ease of administration

Lack of need for repeated boosters

Disadvantages

Risk of vaccine-associated poliomyelitis in vaccine recipients
   or contacts

Spread of vaccine to contacts without their consent

Unsafe administration for immunodeficient patients

INACTIVATED (IPV)

Advantages

Effectiveness

Good stability during transport and in storage

Safe administration in immunodeficient patients

No risk of vaccine-related disease

Disadvantages

Lack of induction of local (gut) immunity

Need for booster vaccine for lifelong immunity

Fact that injection is more painful than oral administration

Fact that higher community immunization levels are needed
   than with live vaccine

tion can be initiated by as little as one infectious viral particle. During the peak of illness, concentrations of 500 to 1000 infectious virions per milliliter are in nasal secretions. The virus enters through the nose, mouth, or eyes and initiates infection of the upper respiratory tract, including the throat. Most viral replication occurs in the nose, and the onset and the severity of the symptoms correlates with the time of viral shedding and the quantity (titer) of virus shed. Infected cells release bradykinin and histamine, which cause a "runny nose."

Immunity to rhinoviruses is transient and is unlikely to prevent subsequent infection because of the numerous serotypes. Both nasal secretory IgA and serum IgG antibody are induced by a primary rhinovirus infection and can be detected within a week of infection. The secretory IgA response dissipates quickly, and immunity begins to wane approximately 18 months after infection.

Interferon, which is generated in response to the infection, may limit the progression of the infection and contribute to the symptoms. Interestingly, the release of cytokines during inflammation can promote the spread of the virus by enhancing the expression of ICAM-1 viral receptors. Cell-mediated immunity is not likely to play an important role in controlling rhinovirus infections.

Epidemiology

Rhinoviruses cause at least half of all upper respiratory tract infections (Box 54-6). Other agents that cause the symptoms of the common cold include enteroviruses, coronaviruses, and parainfluenza viruses. Rhinoviruses can be transmitted by two mechanisms: as aerosols and on fomites (e.g., by hands or on contaminated inanimate objects). Hands appear to be the major vector, and direct person-to-person contact is the predominant mode of spread. This is shown by the fact that rhinoviruses can be recovered from the hands of 40% to 90% of persons with colds but from only 6% to 15% of the inanimate objects around them. However, these nonenveloped viruses are extremely stable and can survive on such objects for many hours.

Rhinoviruses produce clinical illness in only half of those infected. Asymptomatic people are also capable of spreading the virus, even though they may produce less virus.

Rhinovirus "colds" most frequently occur in the early autumn and the late spring in people living in temperate climates. These peaks may reflect social patterns (e.g., return to school and day care) rather than any change in the virus itself.

Rates of infection are highest in infants and children. Children under 2 years of age "share" their colds with their families. Secondary infections occur in approximately 50% of family members, especially other children.

Many different rhinovirus serotypes may be found in a given community during a specific cold season, but the predominant strains are usually the newly categorized serotypes. This indicates the existence of a gradual antigenic drift (mutation), similar to that seen for the influenza virus.

Clinical Syndromes

Common cold symptoms caused by rhinoviruses cannot readily be distinguished from those caused by other viral respiratory pathogens (e.g., enteroviruses, paramyxoviruses, coronaviruses). An upper respiratory tract infection usually begins with sneezing, followed soon by rhinorrhea (runny nose). The rhinorrhea increases and is then accompanied by symptoms of nasal obstruction. Mild sore throat also occurs, along with headache and malaise. The illness peaks in 3 to 4 days, but the cough and nasal symptoms may persist for 7 to 10 days or longer. Fever and rigors sometimes accompany rhinovirus infections.

Laboratory Diagnosis

The clinical syndrome of the common cold is usually so characteristic that laboratory diagnosis is unnecessary unless the physician needs to establish which of the many respiratory viruses is causing a patient's illness. The diagnostic methods used to identify rhinoviruses include culture and serology.

Culture

Nasal washings are the best clinical specimen for recovering the virus. Rhinoviruses are grown in human diploid-fibroblast cells (e.g., WI-38). As already stated, these viruses grow best at 33° C. Virus is isolated in tis-

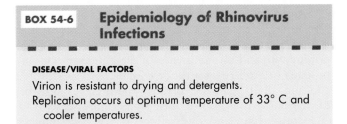

BOX 54-6   **Epidemiology of Rhinovirus Infections**

DISEASE/VIRAL FACTORS
Virion is resistant to drying and detergents.
Replication occurs at optimum temperature of 33° C and cooler temperatures.

TRANSMISSION
Direct contact via infected hands and fomites.
Inhalation of infectious droplets.

WHO IS AT RISK?
People of all ages.

GEOGRAPHY/SEASON
Virus is found worldwide.
Disease is more common in early autumn and late spring.

MODES OF CONTROL
Washing hands and disinfecting contaminating object help prevent spread.

sue culture in 1 to 7 days, with an average of 4 to 5 days. Virus is identified by typical cytopathological effect and the demonstration of acid lability. Serotyping is rarely necessary but can be done using pools of specific neutralizing sera.

Serology

The performance of serological testing to document rhinovirus infection is not practical. No antigen is common to all rhinoviruses, thus making it difficult to maintain virus stocks for testing. Furthermore, multiple serotypes of rhinovirus may circulate in the community simultaneously, increasing the difficulty of such testing.

Treatment, Prevention, and Control

There are many over-the-counter remedies for the common cold, but no specific therapy has been found effective. Nasal vasoconstrictors may provide relief, but their use may be followed by rebound congestion and a worsening of symptoms. Rigorous studies of vitamin C therapy have not shown it to be efficacious.

No antiviral drug has proved therapeutically useful in controlling rhinovirus infections. The intranasal administration of interferon can block infection for a short time after a known exposure, but its long-term use (e.g., throughout the "cold season") could cause symptoms at least as bad as those of the rhinovirus infection. Experimental antiviral drugs, such as arildone, rhodanine, disoxaril, and their analogues, contain a 3-methylisoxazole group that inserts into the base of the receptor-binding canyon and blocks uncoating of the virus. Enviroxime inhibits the viral RNA-dependent RNA polymerase. A polypeptide receptor analogue based on the ICAM-1 protein structure may have potential as an antiviral drug.

Rhinovirus is not a very good candidate for a vaccine. The multiple serotypes, the apparent antigenic drift in rhinoviral antigens, the requirement for secretory IgA production, and the transience of the antibody response pose major problems for the development of vaccines. In addition, the benefit-to-risk ratio would be very low because rhinoviruses do not cause significant disease.

Handwashing and the disinfection of contaminated objects are the best means of preventing the spread of the virus. The impregnation of nasal tissue with antiviral chemicals has been attempted, but the product was not a commercial success.

CASE STUDY AND QUESTIONS

A 6-year-old girl was brought to the office at 4:30 PM because she had a sore throat and had been unusually tired and was napping excessively. Her temperature was 39° C. She had an erythematous throat with enlarged tonsils and a faint rash on her back. At 10:30 PM the patient's mother reported that the child had vomited 3 times, continued to nap excessively, and complained of a headache when awake. You examined the child at 11:30 PM and noted that she was lethargic and aroused only when her head was turned, complaining that her back hurt. Her CSF contained no red blood cells but there were 28 white blood cells/mm³, half polymorphonuclear neutrophils and half lymphocytes. The glucose and protein levels in the CSF were normal, and Gram stain of a specimen of CSF showed no bacteria.

1. What were the key signs and symptoms in this case?
2. What was the differential diagnosis?
3. What signs and symptoms suggested an enterovirus infection?
4. How would the diagnosis be confirmed?
5. What were the most likely sources and means of infection?
6. What were the target tissue and mechanism of pathogenesis?

Bibliography

Ansardi D et al: Poliovirus assembly and encapsidation of genomic RNA, *Adv Virus Res* 46:2-70, 1996.

Fields BN, Knipe DM, Howley PM, editors: *Virology,* ed 3, New York, 1996, Lippincott-Raven.

Levandowski RA: *Rhinoviruses.* In Belshe RB, editor: *Textbook of human virology,* ed 2, St Louis, 1991, Mosby.

McKinlay MA, Pevear DC, Rossmann MG: Treatment of the picornavirus common cold by inhibitors of viral uncoating and attachment, *Ann Rev Microbiol* 46:635-654, 1992.

Melnick JL: *Live attenuated poliovaccines.* In Plotkin SA, Martin EA, editors: *Vaccines,* Philadelphia, 1988, WB Saunders.

Moore M, Morens DM: *Enteroviruses including polioviruses.* In Belshe RB, editor: *Textbook of human virology,* ed 2, St Louis, 1991, Mosby.

Racaniello VR: Picornaviruses, *Curr Top Microbiol Immunol* 161:1-192, 1990.

Ren R, Racaniello VR: Human poliovirus receptor gene expression and poliovirus tissue tropism in transgenic mice, *J Virology* 66:296-304, 1992.

Robbins FC: *Polio: historical.* In Plotkin SA, Martin EA, editors: *Vaccines,* Philadelphia, 1988, WB Saunders.

Salk J, Drucker J: *Noninfectious poliovirus vaccine.* In Plotkin SA, Martin EA, editors: *Vaccines,* Philadelphia, 1988, WB Saunders.

Wilfert CM, Lehrman SN, Katz SL: Enteroviruses and meningitis, *Pediatr Infect Dis* 2:333-341, 1983.

CHAPTER 55

Paramyxoviruses

The Paramyxoviridae include the following genera: *Morbillivirus, Paramyxovirus,* and *Pneumovirus* (Table 55-1). Human pathogens within the morbilliviruses include the **measles** virus; within the paramyxoviruses, the **parainfluenza** and **mumps** viruses; and within the pneumoviruses, the **respiratory syncytial virus** (RSV). Their virions have similar morphologies and protein components, and they share the capacity to induce **cell-cell fusion** (syncytia formation and multinucleated giant cells).

The major diseases these agents cause are well known. Measles causes a potentially serious generalized infection characterized by a maculopapular rash **(rubeola).** Parainfluenza viruses cause upper and lower respiratory tract infections, primarily in children, including pharyngitis, croup, bronchitis, bronchiolitis, and pneumonia. Mumps virus causes a systemic infection, whose most prominent clinical manifestation is parotitis. RSV causes mild upper respiratory tract infections in children and adults but can cause life-threatening pneumonia in infants.

Measles and mumps viruses have *only* one serotype, which has allowed the development of effective **live vaccines.** In the United States and other developed countries, successful vaccination programs that use live attenuated measles and mumps vaccines have made measles and mumps rare. In particular, these programs have led to the virtual elimination of the serious sequelae of measles, which remains a serious disease in the absence of vaccine-induced protection.

STRUCTURE AND REPLICATION

Paramyxoviruses consist of **negative-sense, single-stranded RNA** (5 to 8 $\times$ 10^6 daltons) in a helical nucleocapsid surrounded by a pleomorphic **envelope** of approximately 156 to 300 nm (Figure 55-1). They are similar in many respects to orthomyxoviruses but are larger and do not have the unique segmented genome of the influenzaviruses (Box 55-1). Although significant homology exists between paramyxovirus genomes, the order of the protein-coding regions differs for each genus. The gene products of the measles virus are given in Table 55-2.

The nucleocapsid consists of the negative-sense, single-stranded RNA associated with the nucleoprotein (NP), polymerase phosphoprotein (P), and large (L) protein. The L protein is the RNA polymerase, the P protein facilitates RNA synthesis, and the NP protein helps maintain genomic structure. The nucleocapsid associates with the matrix (M) protein at the base of the lipid envelope. The virion envelope contains two glycoproteins, a fusion (**F**) protein, which promotes fusion of the viral and host cell membranes, and a viral attachment protein (hemagglutinin-neuraminidase [**HN**], hemagglutinin [**H**], or **G** protein) (Box 55-1). The F protein must be activated by proteolytic cleavage, which produces F$_1$ and F$_2$ glycopeptides held together by a disulfide bond, to express membrane-fusing activity.

Replication of the paramyxoviruses is initiated by the binding of the HN, H, or G protein on the virion envelope to sialic acid on the cell surface glycolipids. The F protein promotes fusion of the envelope with the plasma membrane. Paramyxoviruses are also able to induce cell-cell fusion, thereby creating multinucleated giant cells (syncytia).

The replication of the genome occurs in a manner similar to that of other negative-strand RNA viruses (i.e., rhabdoviruses). The RNA polymerase is carried into the cell in the nucleocapsid. Transcription, protein synthesis, and replication of the genome all occur in the host cell's cytoplasm. The genome is transcribed into individual messenger RNAs (mRNAs) and a full-length positive-sense RNA template. New genomes associate with the L, N, and NP proteins to form nucleocapsids, which associate with the M proteins on viral glycoprotein–modified

TABLE 55-1	**Paramyxoviridae**
GENUS	**HUMAN PATHOGEN**
Morbillivirus	Measles virus
Paramyxovirus	Parainfluenza viruses 1 to 4
	Mumps virus
Pneumovirus	Respiratory syncytial virus

FIGURE 55-1 A, Model of paramyxovirus. The helical nucleocapsid—consisting of negative-sense, single-stranded RNA and the P protein, nucleoprotein (NP), and large (L) protein—associate with the matrix *(M)* protein at the envelope membrane surface. The nucleocapsid contains RNA transcriptase activity. The envelope contains the viral attachment glycoprotein (hemagglutinin-neuraminidase *[HN]*, hemagglutinin *[H]*, or G protein *[G]*) and the fusion *(F)* protein. **B,** Electron micrograph of a disrupted paramyxovirus showing the helical nucleocapsid. (**A** redrawn from Jawetz E, Melnick JL, Adelberg EA: *Review of medical microbiology,* ed 17, Norwalk, Conn, 1987, Appleton & Lange; **B** courtesy Centers for Disease Control and Prevention, Atlanta.)

BOX 55-1   Unique Features of the Paramyxoviridae

Large virion consists of a negative RNA genome in a helical nucleocapsid surrounded by an envelope containing a viral attachment protein (HN, paramyxovirus and mumps virus; H, measles virus; and G, respiratory syncytial virus [RSV]) and a fusion glycoprotein (F).

The three genera can be distinguished by the activities of the viral attachment protein: HN of paramyxovirus and mumps virus has hemagglutinin and neuraminidase, and H of measles virus has hemagglutinin activity, but G of RSV lacks these activities.

Virus replicates in the cytoplasm.

Virions penetrate the cell by fusion with the plasma membrane.

Viruses induce cell-cell fusion, causing multinucleated giant cells.

Paramyxoviridae are transmitted in respiratory droplets and initiate infection in the respiratory tract.

Cell-mediated immunity causes many of the symptoms but is essential for control of the infection.

TABLE 55-2   Viral-Encoded Proteins of Measles Virus

GENE PRODUCTS*	VIRION LOCATION	FUNCTION
Nucleoprotein (NP)	Major internal protein	Protection of viral RNA
Polymerase phosphoprotein (P)	Association with nucleoprotein	Possible part of transcription complex
Matrix (M)	Inside of virion envelope	Assembly of virions
Fusion factor (F)	Transmembranous envelope glycoprotein	Factor active in fusion of cells, hemolysis, and viral entry
Hemagglutinin-neuraminidase (HN): hemagglutinin (H); glycoprotein (G)	Transmembranous envelope glycoprotein	Viral attachment proteins
Large protein (L)	Association with nucleoprotein	Polymerase

Modified from Fields BN, editor: *Virology,* New York, 1985, Raven.
*In order of transcription.

FIGURE 55-2 Replication of paramyxoviruses. The virus binds to glycolipids and fuses with the cell surface. Individual mRNAs for each protein and a full-length template are transcribed from the genome. Replication occurs in the cytoplasm. The nucleocapsid associates with matrix and glycoprotein-modified plasma membranes and leaves the cell by budding. (−), Negative sense; (+), positive sense; *ER,* endoplasmic reticulum. (Redrawn from Balows A, Hausler WJ Jr, Lennette EH: *Laboratory diagnosis of infectious diseases: principles and practice,* New York, 1988, Springer-Verlag.)

plasma membranes. The glycoproteins are synthesized and processed like cellular glycoproteins. Mature virions then bud from the host cell plasma membrane and exit the cell. Replication of the paramyxoviruses is represented by the RSV infectious cycle shown in Figure 55-2.

MEASLES VIRUS

Measles is the only virus of human importance in the *Morbillivirus* genus. The infection is one of the five **classic childhood exanthems,** along with rubella, roseola, fifth disease, and chickenpox. Historically, measles was one of the most common and unpleasant viral infections. The rash, high fever, cough, conjunctivitis, and coryza

BOX 55-2   Disease Mechanisms of Measles Virus

Virus infects epithelial cells of respiratory tract.
Virus spreads systematically in lymphocytes and by **viremia.**
Virus replicates in cells of conjunctivae, respiratory tract, urinary tract, lymphatic system, blood vessels, and central nervous system.
Rash is caused by T-cell response to virus-infected epithelial cells lining capillaries.
Cell-mediated immunity is essential to control infection; antibody is not sufficient because of measles' ability to spread cell to cell.
Sequelae in central nervous system may result from immunopathogenesis (postinfectious measles encephalitis) or development of defective mutants (subacute sclerosing panencephalitis).

affected most children in the United States before 1960. Measles is still one of the most prominent causes of disease and death worldwide despite the existence of the live vaccine.

Pathogenesis and Immunity

Measles is known for its propensity to cause cell fusion, resulting in the formation of giant cells (Box 55-2). As a result, the virus can pass directly from cell to cell and escape antibody control. Inclusions occur most commonly in the cytoplasm and are composed of incomplete viral particles. Infection usually leads to cell lysis, but persistent infections without lysis can occur in certain cell types (e.g., human brain cells).

Measles is **highly contagious** and is transmitted from person to person by **respiratory droplets** (Figure 55-3). Local replication of virus in the respiratory tract precedes its spread to the lymphatic system and viremia. The wide dissemination of the virus causes infection of the conjunctiva, respiratory tract, urinary tract, small blood vessels, lymphatic system, and the central nervous system. The characteristic measles rash is caused by immune T cells targeted to measles-infected endothelial cells lining small blood vessels. Recovery follows the rash in most patients, who then have **lifelong immunity** to the virus. In some patients, a **postinfectious encephalitis,** which is believed to be immune mediated, occurs after the rash. The time course of measles infection is shown in Figure 55-4.

Cell-mediated immunity is responsible for causing most of the symptoms and is essential for the control of measles infection. T cell–deficient children infected with measles have an atypical presentation consisting of a giant cell pneumonia without a rash. Immunocompromised patients with measles may have continuing infection, resulting in death.

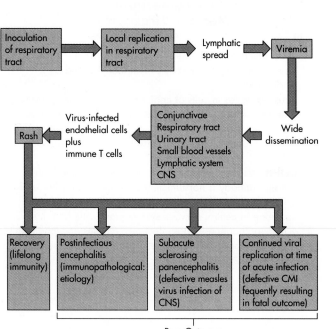

FIGURE 55-3 Mechanisms of spread of the measles virus within the body and the pathogenesis of measles. *CNS*, Central nervous system; *CMI*, cell-mediated immunity.

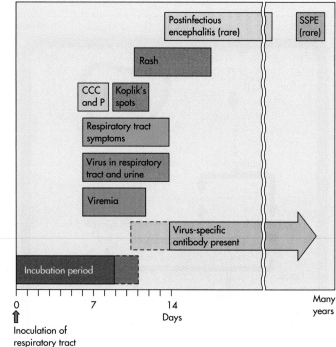

FIGURE 55-4 Time course of measles virus infection. Characteristic prodrome symptoms are cough, conjunctivitis, coryza, and photophobia *(CCC and P)*, followed by the appearance of Koplik's spots and rash. *SSPE*, Subacute sclerosing panencephalitis.

BOX 55-3   Epidemiology of Measles

DISEASE/VIRAL FACTORS

Virus has large, relatively stable virion that is easily inactivated.
Contagion period precedes symptoms.
Host range is limited to humans.
Only one serotype exists.
Immunity is lifelong.

TRANSMISSION

Inhalation of large-droplet aerosols.

WHO IS AT RISK?

Unvaccinated people.
Immunocompromised people, who have more serious outcomes.

GEOGRAPHY/SEASON

Virus is found worldwide.
Virus is endemic from autumn to spring, possibly because of crowding indoors.

MODES OF CONTROL

Live attenuated vaccine (Schwartz or Moraten variants of Edmonston B strain) can be administered.
Immune serum globulin can be administered after exposure.

Epidemiology

Measles can be spread in respiratory secretions before and after the onset of characteristic symptoms and is one of the most contagious infections known (Box 55-3). In a household, approximately 85% of exposed susceptible people become infected, and 95% of these people develop clinical disease. Epidemics tend to occur in 1- to 3-year cycles when a sufficient number of susceptible people has accumulated. Many of these cases occur in preschool-age children who have not been vaccinated and who live in large urban areas. The incidence of infection peaks in the winter and spring.

The measles virus has only one serotype and infects only humans, and infection usually presents with symptoms. These properties facilitated the development of an effective vaccine program. Since vaccination was intro-

TABLE 55-3	Clinical Consequences of Measles Virus Infection
DISORDER	**SYMPTOMS**
Measles	Characteristic maculopapular rash, cough, conjunctivitis, coryza, photophobia, Koplik's spots; *complications:* otitis media, croup, bronchopneumonia, and encephalitis
Atypical measles	Rash (most prominent in distal areas); possible vesicles, petechiae, purpura, or urticaria
Subacute sclerosing panencephalitis	Central nervous system manifestations (e.g., personality, behavior, and memory changes; myoclonic jerks; spasticity; and blindness)

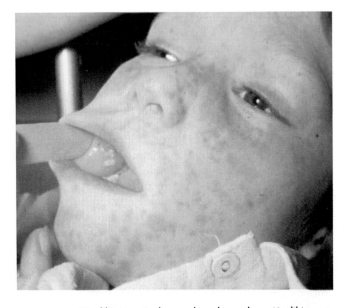

FIGURE 55-5 Koplik's spots in the mouth and exanthem. Koplik's spots usually precede the measles rash and may be seen for the first day or two after the rash appears. (Courtesy Dr. J.I. Pugh, St. Albans; from Emond RTD, Rowland HAK: *A color atlas of infectious diseases,* ed 3, London, 1995, Mosby.)

duced, the yearly incidence of measles has dropped dramatically, from 300 to 1.3 per 100,000 (U.S. statistics for 1981 to 1988). This represents a 99.5% reduction in the incidence of the infection from that in the prevaccination period of 1955 to 1962. However, a fifteenfold increase in the incidence of measles was noted between 1989 and 1991 in the United States, resulting mainly from poor compliance with vaccination programs. Measles is still common in people living in developing countries and is the most a significant cause of death in children 1 to 5 years of age in several countries.

Clinical Syndromes

Measles is a serious febrile illness (Table 55-3). The incubation period lasts 7 to 13 days, and the prodrome starts with high fever and the **three *C*'s—cough, coryza, and conjunctivitis,** in addition to **photophobia.** The patient is most infectious at this time.

After 2 days of illness, the typical mucous membrane lesions, known as **Koplik's spots** (Figure 55-5), appear. They are seen most commonly on the buccal mucosa across from the molars, but they may appear on other mucous membranes as well, including the conjunctivae and the vagina. The lesions, which last 24 to 48 hours, are usually small (1 to 2 mm) and are best described as grains of salt surrounded by a red halo. Their appearance in the mouth establishes with certainty the diagnosis of measles.

Within 12 to 24 hours after the appearance of Koplik's spots, the **exanthem** of measles starts below the ears and spreads over the body. The rash is **maculopapular** and usually very extensive, and often the lesions become confluent. The rash, which takes 1 or 2 days to cover the body, fades in the same order it appeared. The fever is highest and the patient the sickest on the day the rash appears (Figure 55-6).

One of the most feared complications of measles is **encephalitis,** which may be fatal in 15% of such patients.

FIGURE 55-6 Measles rash. (From Habif TP: *Clinical dermatology: color guide to diagnosis and therapy,* St Louis, 1985, Mosby.)

It may occur in as many as 0.5% of those infected and usually begins 7 to 10 days after the onset of illness.

Pneumonia, which can also be a serious complication, accounts for 60% of the deaths caused by measles. The mortality associated with pneumonia, like the incidence of the other complications associated with measles, is increased in the setting of malnutrition and is inversely proportional to age. **Giant cell pneumonia** without rash occurs in children lacking T-cell immunity. Bacterial superinfection is common in patients with pneumonia caused by the measles virus.

Atypical measles occurs in people who received the older inactivated measles vaccine and were subsequently exposed to the wild measles virus. It may also rarely occur in those vaccinated with the attenuated virus vaccine. Prior sensitization with insufficient protection enhances the immunopathological response to challenge by the wild measles virus. The illness begins abruptly and is a more intense presentation of measles.

Subacute sclerosing panencephalitis (SSPE) is an extremely serious, very late neurological sequela of measles that afflicts about 7 in 1 million patients. It occurs when a defective measles virus persists in the brain and acts as a **slow virus.** The virus can replicate and spread directly from cell to cell but is not released. Many months or years after clinical measles, the patient develops changes in personality, behavior, and memory. Myoclonic jerks, blindness, and spasticity follow. Unusually high levels of measles antibodies are found in the blood and cerebrospinal fluid of these patients. The incidence of SSPE has decreased markedly as the result of the measles vaccination programs.

Laboratory Diagnosis

The clinical manifestations of measles are usually so characteristic that it is rarely necessary to perform laboratory tests to establish the diagnosis. The measles virus is difficult to isolate and grow, although it can be grown in primary human or monkey cell cultures. Respiratory tract secretions, urine, blood, and brain tissue are the recommended specimens. It is best to collect respiratory and blood specimens during the prodromal stage and up until 1 to 2 days after the appearance of the rash.

Measles antigen can be detected by immunofluorescence in pharyngeal cells or urinary sediment, but this test is not generally available. Characteristic cytopathological effects, including multinucleated giant cells with cytoplasmic and nuclear inclusion bodies, can be seen in Giemsa-stained cells taken from the upper respiratory tract and urinary sediment.

Antibody, especially immunoglobulin M (IgM), can be detected when the rash is present. Measles infection can be confirmed by the finding of seroconversion or a fourfold increase in the titer of measles-specific antibodies between sera obtained during the acute stage and the convalescent stage.

Treatment, Prevention, and Control

A live attenuated measles vaccine, in use since 1963, has been responsible for a significant reduction in the incidence of measles in the United States. The current Schwartz or Moraten attenuated strains of the original Edmonston B vaccine are being used in the United States. Live attenuated vaccine is given to all children younger than 15 months of age, in combination with mumps and rubella vaccines (**MMR vaccine**) (Box 55-4). Although immunization is successful in more than 95% of vaccinees, revaccination is required in most states for children before grade school or junior high school. As noted earlier, a killed measles vaccine, which was introduced in 1963, was not protective, and its use was subsequently discontinued because recipients were at risk for the more serious atypical measles presentation on infection.

Hospitals in areas experiencing endemic measles may wish to vaccinate or check the immune status of their employees to decrease the risk of nosocomial transmission.

Exposed susceptible people who are immunocompromised should be given immune serum globulin to lessen the risk and severity of clinical illness. This product is most effective if given within 6 days of exposure. No specific antiviral treatment is available for measles.

PARAINFLUENZA VIRUSES

Parainfluenza viruses, which were discovered in the late 1950s, are respiratory viruses that usually cause **mild coldlike symptoms** but can also cause serious respiratory tract disease. Four serological types within the parainfluenza genus are human pathogens. Types 1 to 3 are second only to RSV as important causes of **severe lower respiratory tract infection in infants and young children.** They are especially associated with laryngotracheobronchitis (**croup**). Type 4 causes only mild upper respiratory tract infection in children and adults.

Pathogenesis and Immunity

Parainfluenza viruses infect epithelial cells of the upper respiratory tract (Box 55-5). The virus replicates more rapidly than measles and mumps viruses and can cause giant cell formation and cell lysis. Unlike measles and

---

BOX 55-4	**MMR Vaccine**

Composition: live attenuated virus
 Measles: Schwartz or Moraten substrains of Edmonston B strain
 Mumps: Jeryl Lynn strain
 Rubella: RA/27-3 strain
Vaccination schedule: at 15-24 months and at 4 to 6 years or before junior high school
Efficiency: 95% lifelong immunization with a single dose

Data from *MMWR* 40(RR-12), 1991.

mumps viruses, the parainfluenza viruses rarely cause viremia. The viruses generally stay in the upper respiratory tract, causing only coldlike symptoms. In approximately 25% of cases the virus spreads to the lower respiratory tract, and in 2% to 3%, disease may take the severe form of laryngotracheobronchitis.

The cell-mediated immune response is responsible for causing cell damage, as well as conferring protection. Immunoglobulin A responses are protective but short lived. Multiple serotypes and the short duration of immunity after natural infection make reinfection common, but the reinfection is milder, suggesting at least partial immunity.

Epidemiology

Paramyxoviruses are ubiquitous, and infection is common (Box 55-6). The virus is transmitted by person-to-person contact and respiratory droplets. Primary infections usually occur in infants and small children younger than 5 years. Reinfections occur throughout life, indicating that immunity is short lived. Infections with parainfluenza viruses 1 and 2, the major causes of croup, tend to occur in the autumn, whereas parainfluenza virus 3 infections occur throughout the year. All of these viruses spread readily within hospitals and can cause outbreaks in nurseries and pediatric wards.

BOX 55-5	**Disease Mechanisms of Parainfluenza Viruses**

There are four serotypes of viruses.

Infection is **limited to respiratory tract;** upper respiratory tract disease is most common, but significant disease can occur with lower respiratory tract infection.

Parainfluenza viruses are not systemic and do *not* cause viremia.

Diseases include **coldlike** symptoms, **bronchitis** (inflammation of bronchial tubes), and **croup** (laryngotracheobronchitis).

Infection induces protective immunity of short duration.

Clinical Syndromes

Parainfluenza viruses 1, 2, and 3 may cause respiratory tract syndromes ranging from a mild coldlike upper respiratory tract infection (coryza, pharyngitis, mild bronchitis, and fever) to bronchiolitis and pneumonia. Older children and adults generally experience milder infections than those seen in young children, although pneumonia may occur in the elderly. A parainfluenza virus infection in infants may be more severe than infections in adults, causing bronchiolitis, pneumonia, and most notably, croup (laryngotracheobronchitis). **Croup** results in subglottal swelling, which may close the airway. Clinically, hoarseness, a "seal bark" cough, tachypnea, tachycardia, and suprasternal retraction develop in infected patients after a 2- to 6-day incubation period. Most children recover within 48 hours. The principal differential diagnosis is epiglottitis caused by *Haemophilus influenzae.*

Laboratory Diagnosis

Parainfluenza virus that is isolated from nasal washings and respiratory secretions grows well in primary monkey kidney cells. However, like the other paramyxoviruses, the virions are labile during transit to the laboratory. The presence of virus-infected cells in aspirates or in cell culture is indicated by the finding of syncytia and is identified by immunofluorescence. Like the hemagglutinin of the influenzaviruses, the hemagglutinin of the parainfluenza viruses promotes hemadsorption and hemagglutination. The serotype of the virus can be determined using specific antibody to block hemadsorption or hemagglutination (hemagglutination inhibition).

Treatment, Prevention, and Control

Treatment includes the administration of nebulized cold or hot steam and careful monitoring of the upper airway. On rare occasions, intubation may become necessary. No specific antiviral agents are available.

Vaccination with killed vaccines is ineffective, possibly because they fail to induce local secretory antibody and appropriate cellular immunity. No live attenuated vaccine is available.

BOX 55-6	*Epidemiology of Parainfluenza Virus Infections*

DISEASE/VIRAL FACTORS

Virus has large, relatively stable virion that is easily inactivated.

Contagion period precedes symptoms and may occur in absence of symptoms.

Host range is limited to humans.

Reinfection can occur later in life.

TRANSMISSION

Inhalation of large-droplet aerosols.

WHO IS AT RISK?

Children: at risk for mild disease and croup.

Adults: at risk for reinfection with milder symptoms.

GEOGRAPHY/SEASON

Virus is ubiquitous and worldwide.

Incidence is seasonal.

MODES OF CONTROL

There are no modes of control.

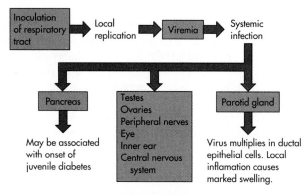

FIGURE 55-7 Mechanism of spread of mumps virus within the body.

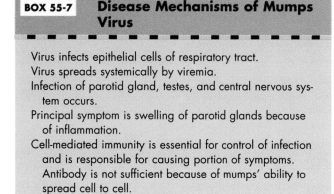

| BOX 55-7 | **Disease Mechanisms of Mumps Virus** |

Virus infects epithelial cells of respiratory tract.

Virus spreads systemically by viremia.

Infection of parotid gland, testes, and central nervous system occurs.

Principal symptom is swelling of parotid glands because of inflammation.

Cell-mediated immunity is essential for control of infection and is responsible for causing portion of symptoms. Antibody is not sufficient because of mumps' ability to spread cell to cell.

MUMPS VIRUS

Mumps virus is the cause of acute, benign viral **parotitis** (painful swelling of the salivary glands). Mumps is rarely seen in countries that promote use of the live vaccine, which is administered with the measles and rubella live vaccines.

Mumps virus was isolated in embryonated eggs in 1945 and in cell culture in 1955. The virus is a member of the Paramyxoviridae and is most closely related to parainfluenza virus 2, but there is no cross-immunity with the parainfluenza viruses.

Pathogenesis and Immunity

The mumps virus, of which only **one serotype** is known, causes a lytic infection of cells (Box 55-7). The virus initiates infection in the epithelial cells of the upper respiratory tract and infects the parotid gland either by way of Stensen's duct or by means of a viremia. The virus is spread by the viremia throughout the body to the testes, ovary, pancreas, thyroid, and other organs. Infection of the central nervous system with symptoms occurs in as many as 50% of those infected (Figure 55-7). Inflammatory responses are mainly responsible for causing the symptoms. The time course of human infection is shown in Figure 55-8. **Immunity is lifelong.**

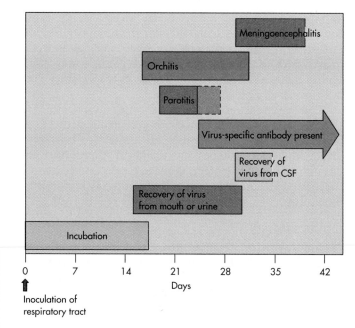

FIGURE 55-8 Time course of mumps virus infection.

Epidemiology

Mumps, like measles, is a very communicable disease with only one serotype, and it infects only humans (Box 55-8). In the absence of vaccination programs, infection occurs in 90% of people by age 15. The virus is spread by direct person-to-person contact and by respiratory droplets. The virus is present in respiratory secretions for as long as 7 days before clinical illness occurs and often does not produce symptoms, so it is virtually impossible to control the spread of the virus. Living or working in close quarters promotes the spread of the virus, and the incidence of the infection is greatest in the winter and spring.

Clinical Syndromes

Mumps infections are often asymptomatic. Clinical illness is manifested as a parotitis that is almost always bilateral and accompanied by fever. Onset is sudden. Oral examination reveals redness and swelling of the ostium of Stensen's duct. The swelling of other glands and meningoencephalitis may occur a few days after the onset of the viral infection but can occur in the absence of parotitis. The swelling resulting from mumps orchitis may cause sterility. Mumps virus involves the central nervous system in approximately 50% of patients, and 10% of them may exhibit clinical evidence of such an infection.

Laboratory Diagnosis

Virus can be recovered from saliva, urine, the pharynx, secretions from Stensen's duct, and cerebrospinal fluid. Virus is present in saliva for approximately 5 days after the onset of symptoms and in urine for as long as 2 weeks. Mumps virus grows well in monkey kidney cells,

---

BOX 55-8   **Epidemiology of Mumps Virus**

DISEASE/VIRAL FACTORS

Virus has large, relatively stable virion that is easily inactivated.

Contagion period precedes symptoms.

Virus may cause asymptomatic shedding.

Host range is limited to humans.

Only one serotype exists.

Immunity is lifelong.

TRANSMISSION

Inhalation of large-droplet aerosols.

WHO IS AT RISK?

Unvaccinated people.

Immunocompromised people, who have more serious outcomes.

GEOGRAPHY/SEASON

Virus is found worldwide.

Virus is endemic in late winter and early spring.

MODES OF CONTROL

Live attenuated vaccine (Jeryl Lynn strain) is part of MMR.

---

causing the formation of multinucleated giant cells. The hemadsorption of guinea pig erythrocytes also occurs on virus-infected cells.

A clinical diagnosis can be confirmed by serological testing. A fourfold increase in the virus-specific antibody level or the detection of mumps-specific IgM antibody indicates active infection. Hemagglutination inhibition, enzyme-linked immunosorbent assay, and immunofluorescence tests can be used to detect the mumps virus, antigen, or antibody.

Treatment, Prevention, and Control

Vaccines provide the only effective means for preventing the spread of mumps infection. Since the introduction of the live attenuated vaccine (Jeryl Lynn vaccine) in the United States in 1967 and its administration as part of the MMR vaccine, the yearly incidence of the infection has declined from 76 to 2 per 100,000. Unfortunately, use of this vaccine in the world is limited. Antiviral agents are not available.

RESPIRATORY SYNCYTIAL VIRUS

RSV, first isolated from a chimpanzee in 1956, is a member of the *Pneumovirus* genus. It is the most frequent cause of fatal acute respiratory tract infection in infants and young children. It infects virtually everyone by 4 years of age, and reinfections occur throughout life, even among the elderly.

The major structural difference between RSV and the other paramyxoviruses is that the RSV has a smaller nucleocapsid. It also lacks hemagglutinin and neuraminidase activities.

Pathogenesis and Immunity

RSV produces an infection that is localized to the respiratory tract (Box 55-9). As the name suggests, RSV induces syncytia. The pathological effect of RSV is mainly due to direct viral invasion of the respiratory epithelium, which is followed by immunologically mediated cell injury. Necrosis of the bronchi and bronchioles leads to

BOX 55-9   **Disease Mechanisms of RSV**

Virus causes localized infection of respiratory tract.

Virus does not cause viremia or systemic spread.

Pneumonia results from cytopathological spread of virus (including syncytia).

Bronchiolitis is most likely mediated by host's immune response.

Narrow airways of young infants are readily obstructed by virus-induced pathology.

Maternal antibody does not protect infant from infection.

Natural infection does not prevent reinfection.

Improper vaccination increases severity of disease.

---

the formation of "plugs" of mucus, fibrin, and necrotic material within smaller airways. The narrow airways of young infants are readily obstructed. Natural immunity does not prevent reinfection, and vaccination with killed vaccine appears to enhance the severity of subsequent disease.

Epidemiology

RSV is very prevalent in young children, with infection of 65% to 98% of children in day-care centers occurring by age 3 (Box 55-10). As many as 25% to 33% of these cases involve the lower respiratory tract, and 1% are severe enough to necessitate hospitalization (occurring in as many as 95,000 children in the United States each year).

RSV infections almost always occur in the winter. Unlike influenza, which may occasionally skip a year, RSV epidemics occur every year.

The virus is very contagious, with an incubation period of 4 to 5 days. The introduction of the virus into a nursery, especially into an intensive care nursery, can be devastating. Virtually every infant becomes infected, and the infection is associated with considerable morbidity and occasionally death. The virus is transmitted on

DISEASE/VIRAL FACTORS

Virus has large, relatively stable virion that is easily inactivated.

Contagion period precedes symptoms and may occur in absence of symptoms.

Host range is limited to humans.

TRANSMISSION

Inhalation of large-droplet aerosols.

WHO IS AT RISK?

Infants: lower respiratory tract infection (bronchiolitis and pneumonia).

WHO IS AT RISK?—cont'd

Children: spectrum of disease—mild to pneumonia.
Adults: reinfection with milder symptoms.

GEOGRAPHY/SEASON

Virus is ubiquitous and is found worldwide.
Incidence is seasonal.

MODES OF CONTROL

Immune globulin is available for high-risk infants.
Aerosol ribavirin is available for infants with serious disease.

TABLE 55-4   Clinical Consequences of RSV Infection

DISORDER	AGE
Bronchiolitis, pneumonia, or both	Fever, cough, dyspnea, and cyanosis in children younger than 1 year
Febrile rhinitis and pharyngitis	Children
Common cold	Older children and adults

hands, by fomites, and to some degree by respiratory routes.

As already noted, virtually all children are infected by RSV by the age of 4, especially in urban centers. Outbreaks may also occur among the elderly (e.g., in nursing homes). Virus is shed in respiratory secretions for many days, especially by infants.

Clinical Syndromes

RSV can cause any respiratory tract illness, from a common cold to pneumonia (Table 55-4). Upper respiratory tract infection with prominent **rhinorrhea** ("runny nose") is most common in older children and adults. A more severe lower respiratory tract illness, **bronchiolitis,** may occur in infants. Because of inflammation at the level of the bronchiole, there is air trapping and decreased ventilation. Clinically, the patient usually has low-grade fever, tachypnea, tachycardia, and expiratory wheezes over the lungs. Bronchiolitis is usually self-limited, but it can be a frightening disease to observe in an infant. It may be fatal in premature infants, those with underlying lung disease, and the immunocompromised.

Laboratory Diagnosis

RSV is difficult to isolate in cell culture. Commercially available immunofluorescence and enzyme immunoassay tests are available for direct detection of the viral antigen in infected cells and nasal washings. The finding of seroconversion or a fourfold or greater increase in the antibody titer can substantiate the diagnosis.

Treatment, Prevention, and Control

In otherwise healthy infants, treatment is supportive and includes the administration of oxygen, intravenous fluids, and nebulized cold steam. **Ribavirin,** a guanosine analogue, is approved for the treatment of patients predisposed to a more severe course (e.g., premature or immunocompromised infants). It is administered by inhalation (nebulization). Passive immunization with anti-RSV immunoglobulin is available for premature infants. Infected children must be isolated. Because hospital staff caring for infected children can transmit the virus to uninfected patients, control measures, including handwashing and the wearing of gowns, goggles, and masks, are essential.

No vaccine is currently available for RSV prophylaxis. A previously available vaccine containing inactivated RSV caused recipients to have more severe RSV infection when subsequently exposed to the live virus. This is thought to have resulted from the mounting of a heightened immunological response at the time of exposure to the wild virus.

CASE STUDIES AND QUESTIONS

An 18-year-old college freshman complained of a cough, runny nose, and conjunctivitis. The physician in the campus health center noticed small white lesions inside his mouth. The next day, a confluent red rash covered his face and neck.

1. What clinical characteristics of this case were diagnostic for measles?
2. Were any laboratory tests readily available to confirm the diagnosis? If so, what were they?
3. Is there a possible treatment for this patient?
4. When was this patient contagious?
5. Why is this disease not common in the United States?
6. Provide several possible reasons for this person's susceptibility to measles at 18 years of age.

A 13-month-old child had a runny nose, mild cough, and low-grade fever for several days. The cough got worse and sounded like "barking." The child made a wheezing sound when agitated. The child appeared well except for the cough. A lateral x-ray examination of the neck showed a subglottic narrowing.

1. What is the specific and common name for these symptoms?
2. What other agents would cause a similar clinical presentation (differential diagnosis)?
3. Were there readily available laboratory tests to confirm this diagnosis? If so, what were they?
4. Was there a possible treatment for this child?

5. When was this child contagious, and how was the virus transmitted?

Bibliography

Balows A, Hausler WJ Jr, Lennette EH: *Laboratory diagnosis of infectious diseases: principles and practice,* New York, 1988, Springer-Verlag.

Belshe RB, editor: *Textbook of human viruses,* ed 2, St Louis, 1991, Mosby.

Centers for Disease Control: Public-sector vaccination efforts in response to the resurgence of measles among preschool-aged children: United States, 1989-1991, *MMWR* 41:522-525, 1992.

Fields BN, Knipe DM, Howley PM, editors: *Virology,* ed 3, New York, 1996, Lippincott-Raven.

Galinski MS: Paramyxoviridae: transcription and replication, *Adv Virus Res* 40:129-163, 1991.

Hart CA, Broadhead RL: *Color atlas of pediatric infectious diseases,* St Louis, 1992, Mosby.

Hinman AR: Potential candidates for eradication, *Rev Infect Dis* 4:933-939, 1982.

Krugman S et al: *Infectious diseases of children,* ed 9, St Louis, 1992, Mosby.

ter Meulen V, Billeter MA: Measles virus, *Curr Top Microbiol Immunol* 191:1-196, 1995.

White DO, Fenner F: *Medical virology,* Orlando, Fla, 1986, Academic.

CHAPTER 56

Orthomyxoviruses

nfluenza A, B, and C viruses are the only members of the Orthomyxoviridae family, of which only influenza A and B viruses cause significant human disease. The orthomyxoviruses are **enveloped and have a segmented negative-sense RNA genome.** The segmented genome of these viruses facilitates the development of new strains through the mutation and reassortment of the gene segments between different human and animal strains of virus. This genetic instability is responsible for the annual **epidemics (mutation:drift)** and periodic **pandemics (reassortment:shift)** of influenza infection worldwide.

Influenza is one of the most prevalent and significant viral infections worldwide. There are even descriptions of influenza epidemics (local) that occurred in ancient times. Probably the most famous influenza pandemic is the one that swept the world in 1918 to 1919, killing 20 million people. In fact, more people died of influenza during this time than in the battles of World War I. Pandemics in recent years occurred in 1947, 1957, 1968, and 1977. Fortunately, vaccine and antiviral drug prophylaxis is now available for people at risk for serious outcomes.

Influenza viruses are respiratory viruses that cause respiratory symptoms and the classic influenza-like symptoms of fever, malaise, headache, and myalgia (body aches). The term *flu,* however, has been mistakenly used to refer to many other respiratory and viral infections (e.g., "intestinal flu").

STRUCTURE AND REPLICATION

Influenza virions are pleomorphic, appearing spherical or tubular (Box 56-1 and Figure 56-1) and ranging in diameter from 80 to 120 nm. The envelope contains two glycoproteins, **hemagglutinin (HA) and neuraminidase (NA),** and is internally lined by the **matrix (M_1)** and **membrane (M_2)** proteins. The genome of the influenza A and B viruses consists of eight different helical nucleocapsid segments, each of which contains a negative-sense RNA associated with the **nucleoprotein (NP)** and the **transcriptase (RNA polymerase components: PB1, PB2, PA)** (Table 56-1). Influenza C has only seven genomic segments.

The genomic segments in the influenza A virus range from 890 to 2340 bases. All the proteins are encoded on separate segments, with the exception of the nonstructural proteins (NS_1 and NS_2) and the M_1 and M_2 proteins, which are transcribed from one segment each.

The HA forms a spike-shaped trimer, which is activated by protease and is cleaved into two subunits held together by a disulfide bond (see Figure 6-6). The HA has several functions: It is the viral attachment protein, binding to sialic acid on epithelial cell surface receptors; it promotes fusion of the envelope to the cell membrane; it hemagglutinates (binds and aggregates) human, chicken, and guinea pig red blood cells; and it elicits the protective neutralizing antibody response. Mutation-derived changes in HA are responsible for the minor ("drift") and major ("shift") changes in antigenicity. Shifts occur only with influenza A virus, and the different HAs are designated H1, H2, and so on.

The NA glycoprotein forms a tetramer and has enzyme activity. The NA cleaves the sialic acid on glycoproteins, including the cell receptor. Cleavage of the sialic acid on virion proteins prevents clumping and appears to facilitate the release of virus from infected cells. The NA of influenza A virus also undergoes antigenic changes, and major differences acquire the designations N1, N2, and so on.

The M_1, M_2, and NP proteins are type specific and are therefore used to differentiate among influenza A, B, and C viruses. The M_1 proteins line the inside of the virion and promote assembly. The M_2 protein forms a proton channel in membranes and promotes viral release. The M_2 of influenza A is a target for the antiviral drugs amantadine and rimantadine.

Viral replication begins with the binding of HA to specific sialic acid structures on cell surface glycoproteins (Figure 56-2). The virus is then internalized into a coated vesicle and transferred to an endosome. Acidification of the endosome causes the HA to bend over and expose hydrophobic fusion–promoting regions of the protein. The viral envelope then fuses with the endosome membrane. The M_2 protein promotes acidification of the envelope contents to break the interaction between the M_1 protein and the NP to allow uncoating and

472

A

B

Hemagglutinin
Neuraminidase
Lipid bilayer
Matrix protein
Polymerase
Nucleoprotein
RNA

FIGURE 56-1 A, Model of influenza A virus. **B,** Electron micrographs of influenza A virus. (**A** from Tagawa SB. In Kaplan MM, Webster RG: The epidemiology of influenza, *Sci Am* 237:88-106, 1977; **B** from Balows A et al, editors: *Laboratory diagnosis of infectious diseases: principles and practice,* vol 2, Heidelberg, 1988, Springer-Verlag.)

BOX 56-1   Unique Features of the Influenza A and B Viruses

Enveloped virion has a genome of **eight negative-sense RNA nucleocapsid segments.**

Hemagglutinin glycoprotein is the viral attachment protein and fusion protein, and it elicits neutralizing, protective antibody responses.

Influenza transcribes and replicates its genome in the target cell nucleus but assembles and buds from the plasma membrane.

The antiviral drugs **amantadine** and **rimantadine** inhibit an uncoating step and target the M_2 membrane protein.

The segmented genome promotes **genetic diversity** caused by **mutation** and **reassortment** of segments on infection with two different strains.

TABLE 56-1   Products of Influenza Gene Segments

SEGMENT*	PROTEIN	FUNCTION
1	PB2	Polymerase component
2	PB1	Polymerase component
3	PA	Polymerase component
4	HA	Hemagglutinin, viral attachment protein, fusion protein, target of neutralizing antibody
5	NP	Nucleocapsid
6	NA	NA (cleaves sialic acid and promotes virus release)
7†	M_1	Matrix protein: viral structural protein (interacts with nucleocapsid and envelope, promotes assembly)
	M_2	Membrane protein (forms membrane channel and target for amantadine, facilitates uncoating and HA production)
8†	NS_1	Nonstructural protein (inhibits cellular mRNA translation)
	NS_2	Nonstructural protein (important but unknown function)

*Listed in decreasing order of size.
†Encodes two mRNAs.

---

delivery of the nucleocapsid into the cytoplasm. The nucleocapsid travels to the nucleus, where it is transcribed into messenger RNA (mRNA). The influenza transcriptase (PA, PB1, PB2) uses host cell mRNA as a primer for viral mRNA synthesis. In so doing, it steals the methylated cap region of the RNA, the sequence required for efficient binding to ribosomes. All the genomic segments are transcribed into 5' capped, 3' polyadenylate (poly A)

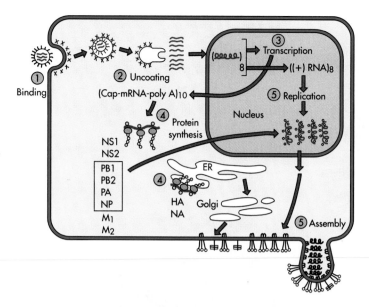

FIGURE 56-2 Replication of influenza A virus. After binding *(1)* to sialic acid–containing receptors, influenza is endocytosed and fuses *(2)* with the vesicle membrane. Unlike most other RNA viruses, transcription *(3)* and replication *(5)* of the genome occur in the nucleus. Viral proteins are synthesized *(4)*, helical nucleocapsids form and associate *(5)* with M_1 protein–lined membranes containing HA and NA glycoproteins. The virus buds from the plasma membrane. *(+)*, Positive sense; *ER*, endoplasmic reticulum.

BOX 56-2   Disease Mechanisms of Influenza A and B Viruses

Virus can establish infection of upper and lower respiratory tract.

System symptoms are due to the interferon and lymphokine response to the virus. Local symptoms are due to epithelial cell damage, including ciliated and mucus-secreting cells.

Interferon and cell-mediated immune responses (NK and T cell) are important for immune resolution and immunopathogenesis.

Infected people are predisposed to bacterial superinfection because of the loss of these natural barriers and induction of bacterial adhesion to epithelial cells.

Antibody is important for future protection against infection and is specific for defined epitopes on HA and NA.

The HA and NA of influenza A virus can undergo **major (reassortment, shift)** and **minor (mutation, drift)** antigenic changes to ensure the presence of immunologically naive, susceptible people.

Influenza B virus undergoes only minor antigenic changes.

---

containing mRNA for individual proteins, except the segments for the M and NS proteins, which are each differentially spliced (using cellular enzymes) to produce two different mRNAs. The mRNAs are translated into protein in the cytoplasm. The HA and NA glycoproteins are processed by the endoplasmic reticulum and Golgi apparatus. The M_2 protein inserts into cellular membranes, and its proton channel prevents acidification of Golgi and other vesicles. This prevents acid-induced folding and inactivation of the HA within the cell. The HA and NA are then transported to the cell surface.

Later, positive-sense RNA templates for each segment are produced, and the negative-sense RNA genome is replicated in the nucleus. The genomic segments are then transported to the cytoplasm and associate with polymerase and NP proteins to form the nucleocapsid, which interacts with the M_1 protein lining plasma membrane sections containing M_2, HA, and NA. The genomic segments are enveloped in a random manner, with about 11 segments per virion. This produces a small number of virions with a complete genome (and numerous defective particles). These particles are antigenic and can cause interference, which may limit the progression of the infection. The virus buds from the cell and is released about 8 hours after infection.

PATHOGENESIS AND IMMUNITY

Influenza initially establishes a local upper respiratory tract infection (Box 56-2). To do this, the virus first targets and kills mucus-secreting, ciliated, and other epithelial cells, causing the loss of this primary defense system. NA facilitates the development of the infection by cleaving sialic acid residues of the mucus, thereby providing access to tissue. If the virus spreads to the lower respiratory tract, the infection can cause severe desquamation (shedding) of bronchial or alveolar epithelium down to a single-cell–thick basal layer or to the basement membrane. In addition to compromising the natural defenses of the respiratory tract, influenza infection promotes bacterial adhesion to the epithelial cells. Pneumonia may result from a viral pathogenesis or from a secondary bacterial infection. Influenza may also cause a transient or low-level viremia and rarely involves tissues other than the lung.

Histologically, influenza infection leads to an inflammatory cell response of the mucosal membrane, which consists primarily of monocytes and lymphocytes and few neutrophils. Submucosal edema is present. Lung tissue may reveal hyaline membrane disease, alveolar emphysema, and necrosis of the alveolar walls (Figure 56-3).

Recovery is associated with the production of interferon and the mounting of cell-mediated immune responses. T-cell responses are important for effecting recovery and immunopathogenesis. However, influenza infection depresses macrophage and T-cell function, hindering immune resolution. Interestingly, recovery often precedes detection of antibody in serum or secretions.

Protection against reinfection is primarily associated with the development of **antibodies to HA,** but antibodies to NA are also protective. The antibody response is specific for each strain of influenza, but the **cell-medi-**

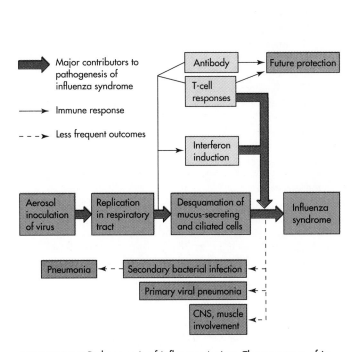

FIGURE 56-3 Pathogenesis of influenza A virus. The symptoms of influenza are caused by viral pathology and immunopathology, but the infection may promote secondary bacterial infection. *CNS,* Central nervous system.

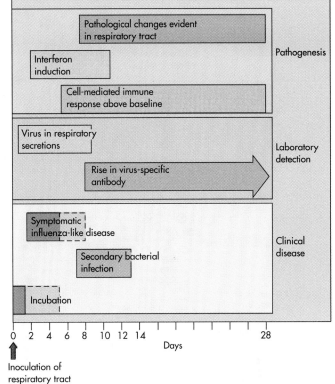

FIGURE 56-4 Time course of influenza A virus infection. The classic "flu syndrome" occurs early. Later, pneumonia may result from bacterial pathogenesis, viral pathogenesis, or immunopathogenesis.

ated immune response is more general and capable of responding to influenza strains of the same type (influenza A or B virus). Antigenic targets for T-cell responses include the nucleocapsid proteins (NP, PB2), M_1 protein, and HA.

The symptoms and time course of the disease are determined by the interferon and T-cell responses and the extent of the epithelial tissue loss. Influenza is normally a self-limited disease that rarely involves organs other than the lung. Many of the classic flu symptoms (e.g., fever, malaise, headache, and myalgia) are associated with interferon induction. Repair of the compromised tissue is initiated within 3 to 5 days of the start of symptoms but may take as long as a month. The time course of influenza virus infection is illustrated in Figure 56-4.

EPIDEMIOLOGY

Strains of influenza A virus are classified by type (A, B, and C), place of original isolation, date of original isolation, and antigen (HA and NA). For example, a current strain of influenza virus might be designated A/Bangkok/1/79 (H3N2), meaning that this is an influenza A virus first isolated in Bangkok in January 1979, containing HA (H3) and NA (N2) antigens. Strains of influenza B are designated by type, geography, date of isolation (e.g., B/Singapore/3/64) without specific mention of HA or NA antigens.

New influenza strains are generated through mutation and reassortment. The genetic diversity of influenza A is fostered by its segmented genomic structure and ability to infect and replicate in humans and many animal species, including birds and pigs. Hybrid viruses are created by coinfection of a cell with different strains of influenza A virus, allowing the genomic segments to randomly associate into new virions. A major change in the HA glycoprotein without loss of cell binding may allow a mutant virus to change its antigenicity and infect the immunologically naive population. For example, a highly pathogenic reassortant virus for seals was generated by simultaneous infection of a seal with two avian influenza viruses (Figure 56-5). This type of reassortment is postulated to be the source of pathogenic human strains. Because of the high population density and proximity of humans, pigs, and ducks in China, it is thought to be a breeding ground for new reassortant viruses and the source of many of the pandemic strains of influenza.

Minor antigenic changes resulting from mutation of the HA and NA genes are called **antigenic drift.** This occurs every 2 to 3 years, causing local outbreaks of influenza A and B infection. Major antigenic changes **(antigenic shift)** result from the reassortment of genomes between different strains, including animal strains, but this **occurs only with the influenza A virus.** Such changes are often associated with the occurrence of pandemics. Antigenic shifts occur infrequently, taking

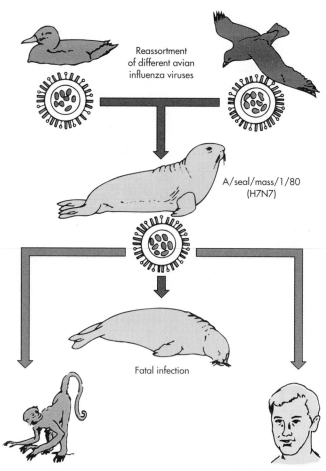

Reassortment
of different avian
influenza viruses

A/seal/mass/1/80
(H7N7)

Fatal infection

Experimental infections
(squirrel monkeys, pigs, ducks)

Accidental infection
(humans in laboratory)

FIGURE 56-5 Reassortment of genomic fragments of influenza A virus. Diagram of the origin of the seal influenza virus: A/seal/Mass/1/80 (H7N7). Since all of the eight genes of the seal influenza virus are most closely rated with those in different avian viruses, it is proposed that seals were mixedly infected with influenza viruses by fecal contamination from birds. The resulting reassortment virus had the required gene constellation to replicate in seal tissues and cause high mortality. This virus has been accidentally transmitted to humans in the laboratory, causing conjunctivitis. Experimentally, the virus has been shown to replicate preferentially in mammalian species, causing systemic infection in some squirrel monkeys and asymptomatic infection of pigs. (Modified from Fields BN, editor: *Virology*, New York, 1985, Raven.)

| BOX 56-3 | **Epidemiology of Influenza A and B Viruses** |

DISEASE/VIRAL FACTORS

Influenza is enveloped and inactivated by detergents.
Segmented genome facilitates major genetic changes, especially to targets of humoral immune response, HA and NA.
Influenza infects many vertebrate species, including other mammals and birds.
Coinfection with animal and human strains of virus can generate very different virus strains by genetic reassortment.
Transmission of virus often precedes symptoms.

TRANSMISSION

Virus is spread by inhalation of small aerosol droplets expelled during talking, breathing, and coughing.
Virus likes cool, less humid atmosphere (e.g., winter heating season).
Virus is extensively spread by school children.

WHO IS AT RISK?

Seronegative people.
Adults: classic "flu syndrome."
Children: asymptomatic to severe respiratory tract infections.
High-risk groups: elderly, immunocompromised people, and people with underlying cardiac or respiratory problems (including people with asthma and smokers).

GEOGRAPHY/SEASON

There is worldwide occurrence: Epidemics are local; pandemics are worldwide.
Disease is more common in winter.

MODES OF CONTROL

Amantadine and rimantadine have been approved for prophylaxis or early treatment.
Killed vaccine contains predicted yearly strains of influenza A and B viruses.

| TABLE 56-2 | **Influenza Pandemics Resulting from Antigenic Shift** |

YEAR OF PANDEMIC	INFLUENZA A SUBTYPE
1918	$H_{sw}N1$ Probable swine flu strain
1947	H1N1
1957	H2N2 Asian flu strain
1968	H3N2 Hong Kong flu strain
1977	H1N1

place on average every 10 years (Table 56-2). For example, the prevalent influenza A virus in 1947 was the H1N1 subtype. In 1957, there was a shift in both antigens, resulting in an H2N2 subtype. H3N2 appeared in 1968, and H1N1 reappeared in 1977. The reappearance of H1N1 is probably due to the infection of seronegative members of the population younger than 30 years of age, who were susceptible to the virus. Prior exposure and an anamnestic antibody response protected the members of the population older than 30 years. In contrast to influenza A, influenza B is predominantly a human virus and does not undergo antigenic shift.

The changing antigenic nature of influenza ensures a large proportion of immunologically naive, susceptible people (especially children) in the population (Box 56-3). An influenza outbreak can be readily detected by the increased absenteeism in schools and work and the number of emergency room visits. During the winter, influenza outbreaks occur annually in temperate climates. Fortunately, influenza virus is present in a community for only a short time (4 to 6 weeks).

Influenza infection is spread readily via small airborne droplets expelled during talking, breathing, and coughing. The virus can also survive on countertops for as long as a day.

The most susceptible population is children, and school-age children are most likely to spread the infection. Contagion precedes symptoms and lasts for a long time, especially in children. Children, immunosuppressed people (including pregnant women), the elderly, and people with heart and lung ailments (including smokers) are at highest risk for more serious disease, pneumonia, or other complications of infection.

The surveillance of influenza A and B outbreaks is extensive to identify the new strains that should be incorporated into new vaccines. The prevalence of a particular strain of influenza A or B virus changes each year and reflects the particular immunological naiveté of the population at that time. Surveillance also extends into the animal populations because of the possible presence of recombinant animal influenza A strains that can cause pandemics.

CLINICAL SYNDROMES

Depending on the degree of immunity to the infecting strain of virus and other factors, infection may range from asymptomatic to severe. Patients with underlying cardiorespiratory disease, people with immune deficiency (even that associated with pregnancy), and smokers are more prone to have a severe case.

After an incubation period of 1 to 4 days, the "flu syndrome" begins with a brief prodrome of malaise and headache lasting a few hours. This is followed by the additional abrupt onset of fever, severe myalgia, and usually a nonproductive cough. The illness persists for approximately 3 days, and unless a complication occurs, recovery is complete within 7 to 10 days. Influenza in young children resembles other severe respiratory tract infections causing bronchiolitis, croup, otitis media, and, rarely, febrile convulsions (Table 56-3). Complications of influenza include bacterial pneumonia, myositis, and Reye's syndrome. The central nervous system can also be involved. Influenza B disease is similar to influenza A.

Influenza may directly cause pneumonia, but it more commonly promotes a secondary bacterial superinfection that leads to bronchitis or pneumonia. The tissue damage caused by progressive influenza virus infection of alveoli can be extensive, leading to hypoxia and bilat-

TABLE 56-3	Diseases Associated with Influenza Virus Infection
DISORDER	**SYMPTOMS**
Acute influenza infection in adults	Rapid onset of fever, malaise, myalgia, sore throat, and nonproductive cough
Acute influenza infection in children	Acute disease similar to that in adults but with higher fever, gastrointestinal tract symptoms (abdominal pain, vomiting), otitis media, myositis, and more frequent croup

Complications of influenza virus infection	Primary viral pneumonia
	Secondary bacterial pneumonia
	Myositis and cardiac involvement
	Neurological syndromes
	  Guillain-Barré syndrome
	  Encephalopathy
	  Encephalitis
	  Reye's syndrome

eral pneumonia. Secondary bacterial infection usually involves *Streptococcus pneumoniae*, *Haemophilus influenzae*, or *Staphylococcus aureus*. In these instances, sputum usually becomes productive and purulent.

Although generally the infection is limited to the lung, certain strains of influenza can spread to other sites in certain people. For example, myositis (inflammation of muscle) may occur in children. Encephalopathy, although rare, may accompany an acute influenza illness and may be fatal. Postinfluenza encephalitis occurs 2 to 3 weeks after recovery from influenza. It is associated with evidence of inflammation and is rarely fatal.

Reye's syndrome is an acute encephalitis that affects children and occurs after a variety of acute febrile viral infections, including varicella as well as influenza B and A. Children given salicylates (aspirin) are at increased risk for this syndrome. In addition to encephalopathy, hepatic dysfunction is present. The mortality rate may be as high as 40%.

LABORATORY DIAGNOSIS

The occurrence of the characteristic symptoms of influenza in a person during a community outbreak of the infection is often sufficient to clinch the diagnosis. The laboratory can distinguish influenza from other respiratory viruses and identify its type and strain (Table 56-4).

Influenza viruses are obtained from respiratory secretions. The virus is generally isolated in primary monkey kidney cell cultures or the Madin-Darby canine kidney cell line. Nonspecific cytopathological effects may be noted within as few as 2 days (average, 4 days). Before the cytopathological effects develop, the addition of guinea pig erythrocytes may reveal **hemadsorption** (the

TABLE 56-4	Laboratory Diagnosis of Influenza Virus Infection

TEST	DETECTS
Cell culture in primary monkey kidney or Madin-Darby canine kidney cells	Presence of virus, limited cytopathological effects
Hemadsorption to infected cells	Presence of HA on cell surface
Hemagglutination	Presence of virus in secretions
Hemagglutination inhibition	Type and strain of influenza virus or specificity antibody
Antibody inhibition of hemadsorption	Identification of influenza type and strain
Immunofluorescence, ELISA	Influenza virus antigens in respiratory secretions or tissue culture
Serology: hemagglutination inhibition, hemadsorption inhibition, ELISA, immunofluorescence, complement fixation	Seroepidemiology

ELISA, Enzyme-linked immunosorbent assay.

adherence of these erythrocytes to HA-expressing infected cells). The addition of influenza virus–containing media to erythrocytes promotes the formation of a gel-like aggregate termed **hemagglutination.** Hemagglutination and hemadsorption are not specific to influenza viruses, however; parainfluenza and other viruses also exhibit these properties.

Specific identification of the influenza virus requires immunological tests such as immunofluorescence or inhibition of hemadsorption or hemagglutination with specific antibody (see Chapter 48). Enzyme immunoassay or immunofluorescence can be used to detect viral antigen in exfoliated cells, respiratory secretions, or cell culture. Serological studies are too slow to aid in the diagnosis of an influenza infection and are generally used for epidemiological purposes.

TREATMENT, PREVENTION, AND CONTROL

Hundreds of millions of dollars are spent on acetaminophen, antihistamines, and similar drugs to relieve the symptoms of influenza. The antiviral drug amantadine and its analogue rimantadine are effective for prophylaxis and for treatment during the first 24 to 48 hours after the onset of influenza A illness. These drugs inhibit an uncoating step of the influenza A virus but not the influenza B or C virus. The target for their action is the M_2 protein. Treatment cannot prevent the later host-induced immunopathogenic stages of the disease.

The airborne spread of influenza is almost impossible to limit. However, the best way to control the virus is through immunization. Natural immunization which results from prior exposure, is protective for long periods. A killed-virus vaccine representing the "strains of the year" and amantadine prophylaxis can also produce immunity.

Killed (formalin-inactivated) influenza vaccine is available every year. Killed whole-virus vaccines are prepared from virus grown in embryonated eggs and then chemically inactivated. Detergent-treated virion preparations and HA- and NA-containing detergent extracts of virus are also available. Ideally the vaccine incorporates antigens of the A and B influenza strains that will be prevalent in the community during the upcoming winter. For instance, the trivalent influenza vaccine used in 1992 and 1993 consisted of inactivated A/Texas/91-like (H1N1), A/Beijing/89-like (H3N2), and B/Panama/90-like virus strains. Vaccination is routinely recommended for the elderly and those with chronic pulmonary or heart disease.

CASE STUDY AND QUESTIONS

In late December a 22-year-old man suddenly experienced headache, myalgia, malaise, dry cough, and a fever. He basically felt lousy. After a couple of days, he had a sore throat, his cough worsened, and he started to feel nauseated and vomited. Several of his family members experienced similar symptoms during the previous 2 weeks.

1. In addition to influenza, what other agents could cause similar symptoms (differential diagnosis)?
2. How would the diagnosis of influenza be confirmed?
3. Amantadine is effective against influenza. What is its mechanism of action? Will it be effective for this patient? For uninfected family members or contacts?
4. When was the patient contagious, and how was the virus transmitted?
5. What family members were at greatest risk for serious disease and why?
6. Why is influenza so difficult to control even when there is a national vaccination program?

Bibliography

Fields BN, Knipe DM, Howley PM, editors: *Virology,* ed 3, New York, 1996, Lippincott-Raven.

Hay AJ et al: *Influenza viruses.* In Belshe RB, editor: *Textbook of human virology,* ed 2, St Louis, 1991, Mosby.

Helenius A: Unpacking the incoming influenza virus, *Cell* 69:577-578, 1992.

Stuart-Harris C: The epidemiology and prevention of influenza, *Am Sci* 69:166-172, 1981.

Webster RG et al: Evolution and ecology of influenza viruses, *Microbiol Rev* 56:152-179, 1992.

CHAPTER 57

Reoviruses

The **Reoviridae** include the orthoreoviruses, rotaviruses, orbiviruses, and coltiviruses (Table 57-1). The name *reovirus* was proposed in 1959 by Albert Sabin for a group of respiratory and enteric viruses that were not associated with any known disease process, thus the name *reovirus (respiratory, enteric, orphan)*. The Reoviridae are nonenveloped viruses with **double-layered protein capsids** containing **10 to 12 segments of the double-stranded RNA genomes**. These viruses are stable over wide pH and temperature ranges and in airborne aerosols. The **orbiviruses** and **coltiviruses** are spread by arthropods and are arboviruses.

The orthoreoviruses, also referred to as *mammalian reoviruses* or simply *reoviruses*, were first isolated in the 1950s from the stools of children. They are the prototype of this virus family, and the molecular basis of their pathogenesis has been studied extensively. In general, these viruses cause asymptomatic infections in humans.

Rotaviruses cause human infantile gastroenteritis, a very common disease. In fact, rotaviruses account for approximately 50% of all cases of diarrhea in children requiring hospitalization because of dehydration (70,000 cases per year in the United States). In underdeveloped countries, rotaviruses may be responsible for causing as many as 1 million deaths each year from uncontrolled viral diarrhea.

STRUCTURE

Rotaviruses and reoviruses share many structural, replicative, and pathogenic features. Reoviruses and rotaviruses have an icosahedral morphology with a double-layered capsid (60 to 80 nm in diameter) (Box 57-1 and Figure 57-1) and a double-stranded segmented genome (*"double:double"*). The name *rotavirus* is derived from the Latin word *rota*, meaning "wheel," which refers to the virion appearance in negative-stained electron micrographs (Figure 57-2).

The outer capsid is composed of structural proteins (Figure 57-3), which surround a nucleocapsid core that includes enzymes for RNA synthesis and 10 (reo) or 11 (rota) different double-stranded RNA genomic segments. Proteolytic cleavage of the outer capsid (as occurs in the gastrointestinal tract) activates the virus for infection and produces an **intermediate/infectious subviral particle (ISVP)**.

TABLE 57-1   **Reoviridae Responsible for Human Disease**

VIRUS	DISEASE
Orthoreovirus*	Mild upper respiratory tract illness, gastrointestinal tract illness, biliary atresia
Orbivirus/coltivirus	Febrile illness with headache and myalgia
Rotavirus	Gastrointestinal tract illness, respiratory tract illness (?)

*Reovirus is the common name for the family Reoviridae and for the specific genus Orthoreovirus.

BOX 57-1   **Unique Features of Reoviridae**

Double-layered capsid virion (60 to 80 nm) has icosahedral symmetry containing 10 to 12 **double-stranded genomic segments** (depending on the virus).

Virion is **resistant** to environmental and gastrointestinal conditions (e.g., detergents, acidic pH, drying).

Rotavirus and orthoreovirus virions are activated by mild proteolysis to intermediate/infectious subviral particles (ISVP), increasing their infectivity.

Inner capsid contains a complete transcription system, including enzymes for 5' capping and polyadenylate addition.

Viral replication occurs in the cytoplasm. Double-stranded RNA remains in the inner core.

Rotavirus inner capsid aggregates in the cytoplasm and then buds into the endoplasmic reticulum, acquiring its outer capsid and a membrane, which is then lost.

Virus is released by cell lysis.

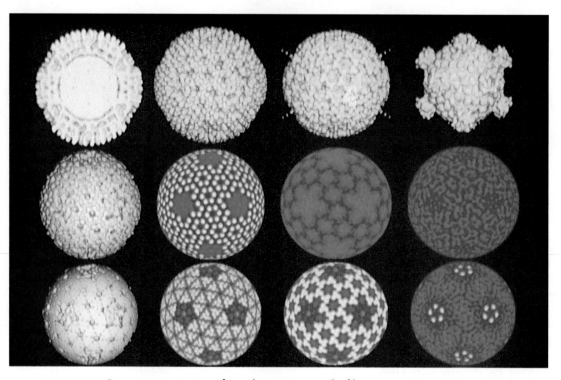

FIGURE 57-1 Computer reconstruction of cryoelectron micrograph of human reovirus type 1 (Lang). *Top left to right,* Cross section of virion, intermediate/infectious subviral particle, and core particle. The intermediate/infectious subviral particle and core particles are generated by proteolysis of the virion and play important roles in the replication cycle. *Center and bottom:* Computer-generated images of the virions at different radii after shaving off the outer layers of features. The colors help one visualize the symmetry and molecular interactions within the capsid. (Courtesy Tim Baker, Purdue University.)

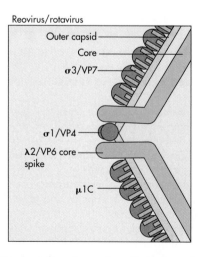

FIGURE 57-2 Structure of reovirus and rotavirus core and outer proteins. σ1/VP4, Viral attachment protein; σ3/VP7, major capsid component; λ2/VP6, major inner capsid protein; μ1C, minor outer capsid protein. (Redrawn from Sharpe AH, Fields BN: *N Engl J Med* 312:486-497, 1985.)

FIGURE 57-3 Electron micrograph of rotavirus. Bar = 100 nm. (From Fields BN, Knipe DM, Howley PM, editors: *Virology,* New York, 1985, Raven.)

TABLE 57-2 Functions of Reovirus Gene Products

GENOMIC SEGMENTS (MOLECULAR WEIGHT)	PROTEIN	FUNCTION (IF KNOWN)
Large segments (2.8×10^6)		
1	Lambda-3 (inner capsid)	Polymerase
2	Lambda-2 (outer capsid)	Capping enzyme*
3	Lambda-1 (inner capsid)	Transcriptase component
Medium segments (1.4×10^6)		
1	Mu-2 (inner capsid)	—
2	Mu-1C (outer capsid)	Cleaved from mu-1, complexes with sigma-3, promotes entry
3	Mu-NS	Promotes viral assembly†
Small segments (0.7×10^6)		
1	Sigma-1 outer capsid)	Viral attachment protein, hemagglutinin, determines tissue tropism
2	Sigma-2 (inner capsid)	Facilitates viral RNA synthesis
3	Sigma-NS	Facilitates viral RNA synthesis
4	Sigma-3 (outer capsid)	Major component of outer capsid with mu-1C

*Elicits neutralizing antibodies
†NS proteins are not found in the virion.

TABLE 57-3 Functions of Rotavirus Gene Product

GENE SEGMENT	PROTEIN (LOCATION)	FUNCTION	GENE SEGMENT	PROTEIN (LOCATION)	FUNCTION
1	VP1 (inner capsid)	Polymerase	8	NS35	—
2	VP2 (inner capsid)	Transcriptase component	9	VP7 (outer capsid)	Type-specific antigen, major outer capsid component that is glycosylated in ER and facilitates attachment and entry
3	VP3 (inner capsid)	mRNA capping			
4	VP4 (outer capsid spike protein at vertices of virion)	Activation by protease to VP5 and VP8 in ISVP, hemagglutinin, viral attachment protein			
5	NS53	RNA binding	10	NS28	Glycosylated resident in ER that promotes inner capsid binding to ER, transient envelopment, and addition of outer capsid
6	VP6 (inner capsid)	Major structural protein of inner capsid, binding to NS28 at ER to promote assembly of outer capsid			
7	NS34	—	11	NS26	—

ER, Endoplasmic reticulum.

Interestingly, rotaviruses resemble enveloped viruses in that they have glycoproteins that act as the viral attachment proteins, acquire but then lose an envelope during assembly, and appear to have a fusion protein activity that promotes direct penetration of the target cell membrane.

The genomic segments of rotaviruses and reoviruses encode structural and nonstructural proteins. The genomic segments of reovirus, the proteins they encode, and their functions are summarized in Table 57-2; those of rotavirus are summarized in Table 57-3. As with influenza A, with reoviruses, reassortment of gene segments can occur and thus create hybrid viruses.

Core proteins include enzymatic activities required for the transcription of messenger RNA (mRNA). These include a 5′-methyl guanosine mRNA capping enzyme and an RNA polymerase. The sigma-1 protein (reo) and VP4 (rota) are located at the vertices of the capsid and extend from the surface like spike proteins. They have several functions, including hemagglutination and viral attachment, and elicit neutralizing antibodies. VP4 is activated by protease cleavage, exposing a structure similar to the fusion proteins of paramyxoviruses. Its cleavage is necessary for productive entry of the virus into cells. Sigma-3 of reoviruses and VP7 of rotaviruses elicit neutralizing antibody and bind to cell surface receptors.

REPLICATION

The replication of reoviruses and rotaviruses starts with ingestion of the virus (Figure 57-4). The virion outer capsid protects the inner nucleocapsid and core from the environment, especially the acidic environment of the gastrointestinal tract. The complete virion is then partially digested in the gastrointestinal tract and presumably activated by protease cleavage and loss of the external capsid proteins (sigma-3/VP7) and cleavage of the VP4 to produce the ISVP. The sigma-1/VP4 at the vertices of the ISVP binds to sialic acid–containing glycoproteins on epithelial and other cells, which include the beta-adrenergic receptor for reovirus. The ISVP of rotavirus penetrates the target cell membrane through an unknown mechanism. Whole virions of reovirus and rotavirus can be taken up by receptor-mediated endocytosis; however, this is a dead-end pathway for rotavirus.

The ISVP releases the core into the cytoplasm, and the enzymes in the core initiate mRNA production. The **double-stranded RNA always remains in the core.** Transcription of the genome occurs in two phases, **early and late,** but before replication of the genome. The negative-sense (−) RNA strand is used as the template by virion core enzymes, which synthesize individual mRNAs complete with a 5′-methyl guanosine cap and a 3′-polyadenylate tail. The mRNA then leaves the core and is translated. Virion proteins and positive-sense (+) RNA segments associate together into corelike structures that aggregate into large cytoplasmic inclusions. The (+) RNA segments are copied to produce (−) RNAs in the new cores, which replicates the genome. The new cores can generate more (+) RNA or be assembled into virions.

FIGURE 57-4 Replication of rotavirus. Rotavirus virions are activated by protease (e.g., in the gastrointestinal tract) to an ISVP. The ISVP binds, penetrates the cell, and loses its outer capsid. The inner capsid contains the enzymes for mRNA transcription using the (−) strand as a template. Some mRNA segments are transcribed early; others are transcribed later. Enzymes in the virion cores attach 5′ cap (*G) and poly A (AAA) to mRNA. VP7 and NS28 are synthesized as glycoproteins and expressed in the endoplasmic reticulum. (+) RNA is mRNA and enclosed into inner capsids as a template to replicate the +/− segmented genome. The capsids aggregate and "dock" onto the NS28 protein in the endoplasmic reticulum, acquiring VP7 and its outer capsid and an envelope. The virus loses the envelope and leaves the cell on cell lysis.

The assembly processes for reovirus and rotavirus differ. In the assembly of reovirus, the outer capsid proteins associate with the core, and the virion leaves the cell on cell lysis. Rotavirus assembly resembles that of an enveloped virus in that the rotavirus cores associate with the NS28 viral protein on the outside of the endoplasmic reticulum (ER) and acquire its VP7 outer capsid protein and a membrane on budding into the ER. The VP7 is a glycoprotein that is in the membrane. The membrane is lost in the ER, and the virus leaves the cell on cell lysis. Reovirus inhibits cellular macromolecular synthesis within 8 hours of infection.

ORTHOREOVIRUSES (MAMMALIAN REOVIRUSES)

The orthoreoviruses are ubiquitous, having been isolated in nearly all mammals worldwide. The virions are very stable and have been detected in sewage and river water. The mammalian reoviruses occur in three serotypes, referred to as *reovirus types 1 to 3;* these serotypes are based on neutralization and hemagglutination-inhibition tests. All three serotypes share a common complement-fixing antigen.

Pathogenesis and Immunity

Orthoreoviruses do not cause significant disease in humans. However, studies of reovirus disease in mice have advanced our understanding of the pathogenesis of viral infections in humans. Depending on the reovirus strain, the virus can be neurotropic or viscerotropic in mice. The functions and virulence properties of the reovirus proteins were identified by comparing the activities of interstrain hybrid viruses that differ in only one genomic segment (encoding one protein). The new activity is attributable to the genomic segment from the other virus strain.

After ingestion and proteolytic production of the ISVP, the orthoreoviruses bind to M cells in the small intestine, which then transfer the virus to the lymphoid tissue of Peyer's patches lining the intestines. After this, the viruses replicate and initiate a viremia. Although the virus is cytolytic in vitro, it causes few if any symptoms before entering the circulation and producing infection at a distant site. In the mouse model, the outer capsid protein responsible for causing hemagglutinin activity (sigma-1) also facilitates viral spread to the mesenteric lymph nodes and determines whether the virus is neurotropic.

Mice, and presumably humans, mount protective humoral and cellular immune responses to outer capsid proteins. Although orthoreoviruses are normally lytic, they can also establish persistent infection in cell culture.

Epidemiology

As already mentioned, the orthoreoviruses have been found worldwide. Seroprevalence studies suggest that most people are probably infected during childhood, since by adulthood approximately 75% have the antibody. Antibody is also detected in most animals, including chimpanzees and monkeys. It is not known whether animals are a reservoir for human infections.

Clinical Syndromes

Orthoreoviruses infect people of all ages, but linking specific diseases to these agents has been difficult. Most infections are thought to be asymptomatic or are so mild that they go undetected. Thus far these viruses have been linked to mild upper respiratory tract illness (low-grade fever, rhinorrhea, pharyngitis), gastrointestinal tract disease, and biliary atresia.

Laboratory Diagnosis

Human orthoreovirus infection can be detected by assay of the viral antigen or RNA in clinical material, virus isolation, or serological assays for virus-specific antibody. Throat, nasopharyngeal, and stool specimens from patients with suspected upper respiratory tract or diarrheal disease are used as samples. Human orthoreoviruses can be isolated using mouse L-cell fibroblasts, primary monkey kidney cells, and HeLa cells.

Serological diagnosis of infection requires the documentation of a fourfold or greater increase in virus-specific antibody between an acute and a convalescent specimen, since antibodies to orthoreoviruses typically are present in healthy children and adults. The techniques used to detect orthoreovirus antibody include hemagglutination inhibition, neutralization, complement fixation, and indirect immunofluorescence, but these tests are not routinely performed.

Treatment, Prevention, and Control

Orthoreovirus disease is mild and self-limited. For this reason, treatment has not been necessary, and prevention and control measures have not been investigated.

ROTAVIRUSES

Rotaviruses have been implicated worldwide as common agents of infantile diarrhea. The rotaviruses are a large group of gastroenteritis-causing viruses found in many different mammals and birds.

Rotavirus virions are relatively stable at room temperature and to treatment with detergents, pH extremes of 3.5 to 10, or even repeated freezing and thawing. Infectivity is enhanced by proteolytic enzymes such as trypsin.

Human and animal rotaviruses are divided into serotypes, groups, and subgroups. Serotypes are distinguished primarily by the VP7 outer capsid protein and, to a lesser extent, on the VP4 minor outer capsid protein. Groups are determined primarily on the basis of the antigenicity of VP6 and on the electrophoretic mobility of the genomic segments. Subgroups are determined on the basis of the VP6 inner capsid protein. Seven serotypes (1 to 7), two subgroups (I and II), and at least five groups (A to E) in the human and animal rotaviruses have been so identified.

Pathogenesis and Immunity

Rotaviruses can survive the acidic environment in a buffered stomach or in a stomach after a meal (Box 57-2). Viral replication occurs after adsorption to columnar epithelial cells covering the villi of the small intestine. Approximately 8 hours after infection, cytoplasmic inclusions are seen that contain newly synthesized proteins and RNA. The virus causes cell lysis.

Studies of biopsy specimens of the small intestine from infants and of experimentally infected animals show shortening and blunting of the microvilli and mononuclear cell infiltration into the lamina propria. Infection prevents the absorption of water, causing a net secretion of water and loss of ions, which together result in a watery diarrhea. The attendant loss of fluids and electrolytes can lead to severe dehydration and even death if therapy does not include electrolyte replacement. As many as 10^{10} viral particles per gram of stool may be released during disease.

Immunity to infection requires the presence of antibody, primarily immunoglobulin A, in the lumen of the gut. Actively or passively acquired antibody (including antibody in colostrum and mother's milk) apparently lessens the severity of disease but does not consistently prevent reinfection. In the absence of antibody, the inoculation of even small amounts of virus causes infection and diarrhea. Infection in infants and small children is generally symptomatic, whereas infection in adults is usually asymptomatic, possibly a result of preexisting immunity.

Epidemiology

Rotaviruses are found worldwide. Children are infected at an early age, as shown by the early acquisition of antibody (Box 57-3). Rotaviruses are assumed to be passed from person to person by the **fecal-oral** route. Maximal shedding of the virus occurs 2 to 5 days after the start of diarrhea but can occur without symptoms. The virus survives well on fomites such as furniture and toys, as well as on hands, because it can withstand drying. Although domestic animals are known to harbor serologically related rotaviruses, they are not believed to be a common source of human infection. Outbreaks occur in preschools and day-care centers and among hospitalized infants.

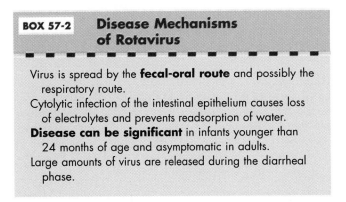

BOX 57-2   **Disease Mechanisms of Rotavirus**

Virus is spread by the **fecal-oral route** and possibly the respiratory route.

Cytolytic infection of the intestinal epithelium causes loss of electrolytes and prevents readsorption of water.

Disease can be significant in infants younger than 24 months of age and asymptomatic in adults.

Large amounts of virus are released during the diarrheal phase.

DISEASE/VIRAL FACTORS

Capsid virus is resistant to environmental and gastrointestinal conditions.

Large amounts of virus are released in fecal matter.

Asymptomatic infection can result in release of virus.

TRANSMISSION

Virus is transmitted in fecal matter, especially in day-care settings.

Respiratory transmission may be possible.

WHO IS AT RISK?
Rotavirus Type A

Infants younger than 24 months of age: at risk for infantile gastroenteritis with potential dehydration.

Older children and adults: at risk for mild diarrhea.

Undernourished people in underdeveloped countries: at risk for diarrhea, dehydration, and death.

Rotavirus Type B

Infants, older children, and adults in China: at risk for severe gastroenteritis.

GEOGRAPHY/SEASON

Virus is found worldwide.

Disease is more common in autumn, winter, and spring.

MODES OF CONTROL

Handwashing and isolation of known cases are modes of control.

Experimental live vaccines use bovine or monkey rotavirus.

Rotaviruses are **one of the most common causes of serious diarrhea in young children** worldwide. Most children have been infected by the virus by 4 years of age. In North America, outbreaks occur annually during the autumn, winter, and spring. Serotype A is the most common. Serotype B is associated with disease in older children and adults in China. More severe disease occurs in severely malnourished children. Rotavirus diarrhea is a severe life-threatening disease for infants in developing countries and occurs year round.

Clinical Syndromes

The incubation period for rotavirus diarrheal illness is estimated to be approximately 48 hours. The major clinical findings in hospitalized patients include diarrhea, vomiting, fever, and dehydration. Fecal leukocytes and blood in stool do not occur in this form of diarrhea. Rotavirus gastroenteritis is a self-limited disease, and recovery is generally complete and without sequelae. However, the infection may prove fatal in infants who live in developing countries and who are malnourished and dehydrated before the infection.

The role of rotaviruses in respiratory tract infection is controversial. Human studies have detected virus in the respiratory secretions of children with respiratory symptoms, and animal studies have documented that aerosol transmission can occur.

Laboratory Diagnosis

The clinical findings in patients with rotavirus infection resemble those of other viral diarrheas (e.g., Norwalk virus). Most patients have **large quantities of virus in stool,** making the direct detection of viral antigen the method of choice for diagnosis. **Enzyme immunoassay** and latex agglutination are quick, easy, and relatively inexpensive ways to detect rotavirus in stool. Viral particles in specimens can also be readily detected by **electron microscopy.**

The cell culture of rotavirus is difficult and not reliable for diagnostic purposes. Serological studies are primarily used for research and epidemiological purposes. Because so many people have rotavirus-specific antibody, a fourfold rise in antibody titer is necessary for the diagnosis of recent infection or active disease.

Treatment, Prevention, and Control

No specific antiviral therapy is available for a rotavirus infection. The morbidity and mortality associated with rotavirus diarrhea result from dehydration and electrolyte imbalance. The purpose of supportive therapy is to replace fluids so that the blood volume and electrolyte and acid-base imbalances are corrected.

Rotavirus vaccines are being developed to protect children, especially those in underdeveloped countries, from potentially fatal disease. Vaccines have been prepared from animal rotaviruses, such as the rhesus monkey rotavirus and the Nebraska calf diarrhea virus. These vaccines share antigenic determinants with human rotaviruses, do not cause disease in humans, and afford some protection against infection. Unfortunately, they may not protect against all serotypes of rotavirus.

Rotaviruses are acquired very early in life. The ubiquitous nature of these viruses make it unlikely that the spread of the virus and infection can be prevented. Hospitalized patients with disease must be isolated, however, to limit spread of the infection to other susceptible patients.

COLTIVIRUSES AND ORBIVIRUSES

The coltiviruses and orbiviruses infect vertebrates and invertebrates. The coltiviruses cause Colorado tick fever and related human disease. The orbiviruses mainly cause disease in animals, including blue tongue disease of sheep, African horse sickness, and epizootic hemorrhagic disease of deer.

Colorado tick fever, an acute disease characterized by fever, headache, and severe myalgia, was originally described in the nineteenth century and is now believed to be one of the most common tick-borne viral diseases in the United States. Although hundreds of infections occur annually, the exact number is not known because it is not a reportable disease.

The structure and physiology of the coltiviruses and orbiviruses are similar to those of other Reoviridae with three major exceptions: (1) The outer capsid of the orbiviruses has no discernible capsomeric structure, even though the inner capsid is icosahedral; (2) the virus causes viremia, infects erythrocyte precursors, and remains in the mature red blood cells protected from the immune response; and (3) the orbivirus life cycle includes both vertebrates and invertebrates (insects). Colorado tick fever viruses have 12 double-stranded RNA genomic segments, and orbiviruses have 10.

Pathogenesis

Colorado tick fever virus infects erythroid precursor cells without severely damaging them. The virus remains within the cells, even after they mature into red blood cells. This protects the virus from clearance. The resulting viremia can persist for weeks or months, even after symptomatic recovery. Both of these factors promote transmission of the virus to the tick vector.

Serious hemorrhagic disease can result from the infection of vascular endothelial and vascular smooth muscle cells and pericytes, thereby weakening capillary structure. This leads to leakage and hemorrhage and potentially hypotension and shock. Neuronal infection can lead to meningitis and encephalitis.

Epidemiology

Colorado tick fever occurs in western and northwestern areas of the United States and western Canada, where the wood tick *Dermacentor andersoni* is distributed (elevations of 4000 to 10,000 feet) (Figure 57-5). Ticks acquire the virus by feeding on viremic hosts and subsequently transmit the virus in saliva when they feed on a new host. Natural hosts can be one of many mammals, including squirrels, chipmunks, rabbits, and deer. Human disease is observed during the spring, summer, and autumn.

Clinical Syndromes

Colorado tick fever virus generally causes mild or subclinical infection. The symptoms of the acute disease resemble those of dengue. After a 3- to 6-day incubation period, symptomatic infections start with the sudden onset of fever, chills, headache, photophobia, myalgia, arthralgia, and lethargy (Figure 57-6). Characteristics of the infection include a biphasic fever and conjunctivitis, and possibly lymphadenopathy, hepatosplenomegaly, and a maculopapular or petechial rash. A leukopenia involving both neutrophils and lymphocytes is an important hallmark of the disease. Children occasionally have a more severe hemorrhagic disease. Colorado tick fever must be differentiated from Rocky Mountain spotted fever, a tick-borne bacterial infection characterized by a rash.

Laboratory Diagnosis

A diagnosis of Colorado tick fever can be established through the direct detection of viral antigens or by virus isolation or serological tests. The best, most rapid method is detection of viral antigen on the surface of erythrocytes in a blood smear using immunofluorescence. Laboratory tests may be available through state health departments or the Centers for Disease Control and Prevention.

The titers of antibody in acute and convalescent specimens must be compared for a serologically based diagnosis to be rendered because subclinical infections can occur and antibody may persist for a lifetime. Specific IgM is present for about 45 days after the onset of illness and is also presumptive evidence of an acute or a very recent infection. Immunofluorescence is the best technique, but complement fixation, neutralization, and enzyme immunoassay are also used to detect Colorado tick fever antibody.

Treatment, Prevention, and Control

No specific treatment is available for Colorado tick fever. The disease is generally self-limited, indicating that sup-

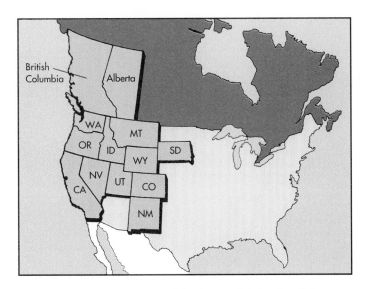

FIGURE 57-5 Geographical distribution of Colorado tick fever.

FIGURE 57-6 Time course of Colorado tick fever.

portive care is sufficient. As already mentioned, the viremia is long lasting, implying that infected patients should not donate blood soon after recovery. Prevention includes avoiding tick-infested areas, using protective clothing and tick repellents, and removing ticks before they bite. Unlike tick-borne rickettsial disease, in which prolonged feeding is required for the bacteria to be transmitted, the virus from the tick's saliva can enter the bloodstream rapidly. A formalinized Colorado tick fever vaccine has been developed and evaluated, but because of the mildness of the disease, its distribution to the general public is not warranted.

CASE STUDY AND QUESTIONS

A 6-month-old child was seen in the emergency room in January after 2 days of persistent watery diarrhea and vomiting accompanied by a low-grade fever and mild cough. The infant appeared dehydrated and required hospitalization. The patient attended a day-care center.

1. In addition to rotavirus, what other viral agents must be considered in the differential diagnosis of this infant? If the patient had been a teenager or an adult?
2. How would the diagnosis of rotavirus have been confirmed?
3. How was the virus transmitted? How long was the patient contagious?
4. Who was at risk for serious disease?

Bibliography

Balows A, Hausler WJ, Lennette EH, editors: *Laboratory diagnosis of infectious diseases: principles and practice,* New York, 1988, Springer-Verlag.

Bellamy AR, Both GW: Molecular biology of rotaviruses, *Adv Virol* 38:1-44, 1990.

Belshe RB, editor: *Textbook of human virology,* ed 2, St Louis, 1991, Mosby.

Blacklow NR, Greenberg HB: Viral gastroenteritis, *N Engl J Med* 325:252-264, 1991.

Christensen ML: Human viral gastroenteritis, *Clin Microbiol Rev* 2:51-89, 1989.

Feigin RD, Cherry JD, editors: *Textbook of pediatric infectious disease,* ed 2, Philadelphia, 1987, WB Saunders.

Fields BN, Knipe DM, Howley PM, editors: *Virology,* ed 3, New York, 1996, Lippincott-Raven.

Joklik WK, editor: *The Reoviridae,* New York, 1983, Plenum.

Nibert ML, Furlong DB, Fields BN: Mechanisms of viral pathogenesis: distinct forms of reovirus and their roles during replication in cells and host, *J Clin Invest* 88:727-734, 1991.

Ramig RF: Rotaviruses, *Curr Top Microbiol Immunol* 185:1-380, 1994.

Sharpe AH, Fields BN: Pathogenesis of viral infections: basic concepts derived from the reovirus model, *N Engl J Med* 312:486-497, 1985.

58

Rhabdoviruses

The members of the family Rhabdoviridae (from the Greek word *rhabdos*, meaning "rod") include pathogens for a variety of mammals, fish, birds, and plants. The rhabdoviruses include *Vesiculovirus* (vesicular stomatitis viruses [VSVs]); *Lyssavirus* (rabies and rabies-like viruses), an unnamed genus constituting the plant rhabdovirus group; and other ungrouped rhabdoviruses of mammals, birds, fish, and arthropods.

Rabies virus is the most significant pathogen of the rhabdoviruses. Until Louis Pasteur's development of one of the earliest killed-virus vaccines, a bite from a "mad dog" inevitably led to the characteristic symptoms of **hydrophobia** and almost certain death.

PHYSIOLOGY, STRUCTURE, AND REPLICATION

Rhabdoviruses are **bullet-shaped, enveloped virions** with a diameter of 50 to 95 nm and length of 130 to 380 nm (Box 58-1 and Figure 58-1). Spikes composed of a trimer of the glycoprotein (G) cover the surface of the virus. The G protein is the viral attachment protein and generates neutralizing antibodies. The G protein of the vesicular stomatitis virus is a simple glycoprotein with *N*-linked glycan. This G protein has been used as the prototype for studying glycoprotein processing and cell surface expression.

Within the envelope, the **helical nucleocapsid** is coiled symmetrically into a cylindrical structure, giving it the appearance of striations (Figure 58-1). The nucleocapsid is composed of one molecule of **single-stranded, negative-sense RNA** and the nucleoprotein (N), plus large (L) and nonstructural (NS) proteins. The matrix (M) protein lies between the envelope and the nucleocapsid. The N protein is the major structural protein of the virus. It protects the RNA from ribonuclease digestion and maintains the RNA in a configuration acceptable for transcription. The L and NS proteins constitute the RNA-dependent RNA polymerase.

The replicative cycle of VSV is the prototype for the rhabdoviruses and other negative-strand RNA viruses (see Figure 6-13). The viral G protein attaches to the host cell and is internalized by endocytosis. The viral envelope then fuses with the membrane of the endosome on acidification of the vesicle. This causes the nucleocapsid to be released into the cytoplasm, where replication takes place.

The RNA-dependent RNA polymerase associated with the nucleocapsid transcribes the viral genomic RNA, producing five individual mRNAs. These mRNAs are then translated into the five viral proteins. The viral genomic RNA is also transcribed into a full-length positive-sense RNA template that is used to generate new genomes. The G protein is synthesized by membrane-bound ribosomes, processed by the Golgi apparatus, and delivered to the cell surface in membrane vesicles. The M protein associates with the G protein–modified membranes.

Assembly of the virion occurs in two phases: assembly of the nucleocapsid in the cytoplasm and envelopment and release at the cell plasma membrane. The genome associates with the N protein and then with the polymerase proteins L and NS to form the nucleocapsid. Association with the M protein at the plasma membrane induces coiling of the nucleocapsid into its condensed form. The virus then buds through the plasma membrane and is released when the entire nucleocapsid is enveloped. Cell death and lysis occur after infection with most rhabdoviruses, with the important exception of rabies virus, which produces little discernible cell damage.

FIGURE 58-1 Rhabdoviridae seen by electron microscopy: rabies virus *(left)* and vesicular stomatitis virus *(right)*. (From Fields BN: *Virology,* New York, 1985, Raven.)

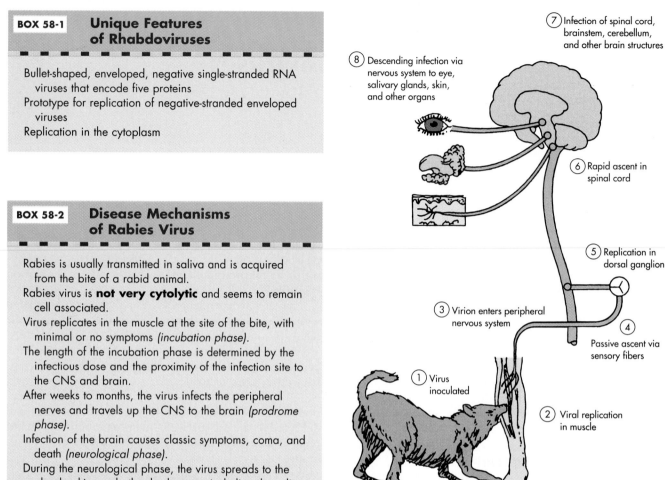

FIGURE 58-2 Pathogenesis of rabies virus infection. Numbered steps describe the sequence of events. (Redrawn from Belshe RB, editor: *Textbook of human virology,* ed 2, St Louis, 1991, Mosby.)

PATHOGENESIS AND IMMUNITY

Only the pathogenesis of rabies virus infection is discussed here (Box 58-2). Rabies infection usually results from the bite of a rabid animal. Rabies infection of the animal causes secretion of the virus in the animal's saliva and promotes aggressive behavior ("mad dog"). This in turn promotes transmission of the virus. The virus can also be transmitted through the inhalation of aerosolized virus, in transplanted infected tissue (e.g., cornea), and by inoculation through intact mucosal membranes.

Virus may directly infect nerve endings by binding to **nicotinic acetylcholine receptors** or muscle at the site of inoculation. The virus remains at the site for days to months (Figure 58-2) before progressing to the central nervous system (CNS). Rabies virus travels by retrograde axoplasmic transport to the dorsal root ganglia and to the spinal cord. Once the virus gains access to the spinal cord, the brain becomes rapidly infected. The affected areas include the hippocampus, brainstem, ganglionic cells of the pontine nuclei, and Purkinje's cells of the cerebellum. The virus then disseminates from the CNS via afferent neurons to highly innervated sites, such as the skin of the head and neck, salivary glands, retina, cornea, nasal mucosa, adrenal medulla, renal parenchyma, and pancreatic acinar cells. After the virus invades the brain and spinal cord, an encephalitis develops, and neurons degenerate. Despite the extensive CNS involvement and impairment of CNS function, little histopathological change can be observed in the affected tissue.

With rare exception (three known cases), rabies is fatal once clinical disease is apparent. The length of the incubation period is determined by the concentration of the virus in the inoculum, the proximity of the wound to the brain, the severity of the wound, the host's age, and the host's immune status.

BOX 58-3   Epidemiology of Rabies Virus

DISEASE/VIRAL FACTORS

Virus-induced aggressive behavior in animals promotes spread.

Disease has long, asymptomatic incubation period.

TRANSMISSION

Zoonosis:

   Reservoir: wild animals.

   Vector: wild animals and unvaccinated dogs and cats.

Source of virus:

   Major: saliva in bite of rabid animal.

   Minor: aerosols in bat caves containing rabid bats.

WHO IS AT RISK?

Veterinarians and animal handlers.

Person bitten by a rabid animal.

Inhabitants of countries with no pet vaccination program.

GEOGRAPHY/SEASON

Virus is found worldwide, except in some island nations.

There is no seasonal incidence.

MODES OF CONTROL

Vaccination program is available for pets.

Vaccination is available for high-risk personnel.

Future vaccination program is needed for control of rabies in forest mammals.

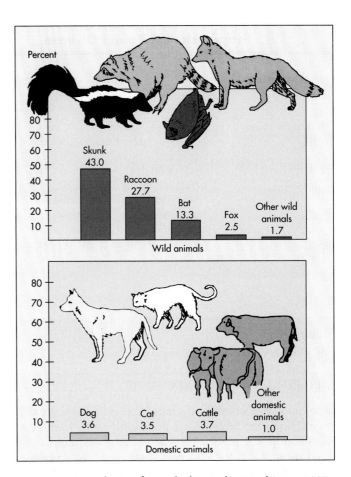

FIGURE 58-3 Distribution of animal rabies in the United States, 1987. The percentages relate to the total number of cases of animal rabies. (Redrawn from Centers for Disease Control: Rabies surveillance, United States, 1987 [CDC surveillance summaries], *MMWR* 37:SS-4, 1988.)

In contrast with other viral encephalitis syndromes, inflammatory lesions are rarely observed in patients with rabies. Neutralizing antibodies are not apparent until after the clinical disease is well established. Little antigen is released, and the infection probably remains hidden from the immune response. Cell-mediated immunity appears to play little or no role in protection against rabies virus infection.

Antibody can block the spread of virus to the CNS and to the brain if administered or generated during the incubation period. The incubation period is usually long enough to allow generation of a **therapeutic protective antibody** response after active immunization with the rabies vaccine.

EPIDEMIOLOGY

Rabies is the classic **zoonotic** infection, spread from animals to humans (Box 58-3). It is endemic worldwide in a variety of animals. Rabies is maintained and spread in two ways: In urban rabies, dogs are the primary transmitter, and in sylvatic (forest) rabies, many species of wildlife can serve as the transmitter. The principal **reservoir** for rabies in most of the world, however, is the **dog.** In Latin America this is a particular problem because of the existence of many stray, unvaccinated dogs and the

absence of rabies-control programs. These two factors are responsible for thousands of rabies cases in dogs each year in these countries. Because of the excellent vaccination program in the United States, sylvatic rabies accounts for most of the cases of animal rabies. Statistics for animal rabies are collected by the Centers for Disease Control and Prevention, which in 1992 recorded more than 8000 documented cases of rabies in skunks, raccoons, bats, and farm animals, in addition to dogs and cats (Figure 58-3). Badgers and foxes are also major carriers of rabies in Western Europe. In South America vampire bats transmit rabies to cattle, resulting in millions of dollars in losses each year.

The distribution of human rabies approximates the distribution of animal cases in each country. It is estimated that rabies accounts for at least 25,000 deaths annually in India, with the virus transmitted by dogs in 96% of the cases. In Latin America, cases of human rabies primarily results from contact with rabid dogs in urban areas. In the United States the incidence of human rabies is approximately 1 case per year because of effective dog

TABLE 58-1   Progression of Rabies Disease

DISEASE PHASE	SYMPTOMS	TIME	VIRAL STATUS	IMMUNOLOGICAL STATUS
Incubation phase	Asymptomatic	60-365 days after bite	Low titer, virus in muscle	—
Prodrome phase	Fever, nausea, vomiting, loss of appetite, headache, lethargy, pain at site of bite	2-10 days	Low titer, virus in CNS and brain	—
Neurological phase	Hydrophobia, pharyngeal spasms, hyperactivity, anxiety, depression; CNS symptoms: loss of coordination, paralysis, confusion, delirium	2-7 days	High titer, virus in brain and other sites	Detectable antibody in serum and CNS
Coma	Coma: cardiac arrest, hypotension, hypoventilation, secondary infections	0-14 days	High titer, virus in brain and other sites	—
Death	—	—	—	—

vaccination programs and limited contact with skunks, raccoons, and bats. Even so, annual costs for rabies prevention exceed $300 million.

CLINICAL SYNDROMES

Rabies is almost always a fatal disease unless treated by vaccination. After a long but highly variable incubation period, the prodrome phase of rabies ensues (Table 58-1) and includes symptoms such as fever, malaise, headache, pain or paresthesia (itching) at the site of the bite, gastrointestinal symptoms, fatigue, and anorexia. The prodrome usually lasts 2 to 10 days, after which the neurological symptoms specific to rabies appear. **Hydrophobia** (fear of water), the most characteristic symptom of rabies, occurs in 20% to 50% of patients. It is triggered by the pain associated with the patient's attempts to swallow water. Focal and generalized seizures, disorientation, and hallucinations are also common during the neurological phase. From 15% to 60% of patients exhibit paralysis as the only manifestation of rabies. The paralysis may lead to respiratory failure.

The patient becomes comatose after the neurological phase, which lasts from 2 to 10 days. This phase almost universally leads to death resulting from neurological and pulmonary complications.

LABORATORY DIAGNOSIS

The occurrence of neurological symptoms in a person who has been bitten by an animal generally establishes the diagnosis of rabies. Laboratory tests are usually performed to confirm the diagnosis and to determine whether a suspected animal is rabid (postmortem). Unfortunately, **evidence of infection, including symptoms and the detection of antibody, does not occur until it is too late for intervention.**

The diagnosis of rabies is made by detection of viral antigen in the CNS or skin, isolation of the virus, and

serological findings. The hallmark diagnostic finding has been the detection of intracytoplasmic inclusions consisting of aggregates of viral nucleocapsids (**Negri bodies**) in affected neurons (see Figure 48-3). Although a finding diagnostic of rabies, Negri bodies are seen in only 70% to 90% of brain tissue of infected humans.

Antigen detection using immunofluorescence has become the most widely used method for diagnosing rabies. Brain biopsy or autopsy material, impression smears of corneal epithelial cells, and skin biopsy material from the nape of the neck are the specimens most frequently used for this purpose. The test has a high degree of sensitivity and specificity in experienced hands.

Rabies can also be grown in cell culture or intracerebrally inoculated infant mice. Inoculated cell cultures or brain tissues are subsequently examined by direct immunofluorescence.

Rabies antibody titers in serum and cerebrospinal fluid is usually measured by a rapid fluorescent focus inhibition test. Antibody usually is not detectable until late in the disease, however.

TREATMENT AND PROPHYLAXIS

With the exception of three documented cases of humans who survived, clinical rabies is invariably fatal unless treated. Once the symptoms have appeared, little other than supportive care can be given.

Postexposure prophylaxis is the only hope for preventing overt clinical illness in the affected person. Although human cases of rabies are rare, approximately 20,000 people receive rabies prophylaxis each year in the United States alone. Prophylaxis should be initiated for anyone exposed by bite or by contamination of an open wound or mucous membrane to the saliva or brain tissue of an animal suspected to be infected with the virus, unless the animal is tested and shown not to be rabid.

The first protective measure is local treatment of the wound. The wound should be washed immediately with soap and water, detergent, or another substance that inactivates the virus. The World Health Organization Expert Committee on Rabies also recommends the instillation of antirabies serum around the wound.

Subsequently, immunization with vaccine in combination with administration of one dose of equine antirabies serum or human rabies immune globulin (HRIG) is recommended. Passive immunization with HRIG provides antibody until the patient produces antibody in response to the vaccine. A series of five immunizations is then administered over the course of a month. The slow course of rabies disease allows active immunity to be generated in time to afford protection.

The rabies vaccine is a killed-virus vaccine prepared by the chemical inactivation of rabies-infected tissue culture human diploid cells (HDCV) or fetal rhesus lung cells. These vaccines cause fewer negative reactions than older vaccines (Semple or Fermi), which were prepared in the brains of adult or suckling animals. The HDCV is administered intramuscularly on days 0, 3, 7, 14, and 28 after exposure.

Preexposure vaccination of animal workers, laboratory workers who handle potentially infected tissue, and people traveling to areas where rabies is endemic should be performed. HDCV administered intramuscularly or intradermally in three doses is recommended and provides 2 years of protection.

Ultimately the prevention of human rabies hinges on the effective control of rabies in domestic and wild animals. Its control in domestic animals depends on the removal of strays and unwanted animals and the vaccination of all dogs and cats. A variety of attenuated oral vaccines have also been used successfully to immunize foxes. A live recombinant vaccinia virus vaccine expressing the rabies virus G protein has been developed and is being tested for animal use.

CASE STUDY AND QUESTIONS

An 11-year-old boy was brought to a hospital in California after falling; the symptoms were treated, and he was released. The following day he refused to drink water with his medicine, and he became more anxious. That night he began to act up and hallucinate. He also was salivating and had difficulty breathing. Two days later, he had a fever of 40.8° C (105.4° F) and experienced two episodes of cardiac arrest. Although rabies was sus-

pected, no remarkable data were obtained from a computed tomographic image of the brain or cerebrospinal fluid analysis. A skin biopsy from the nape of the neck was negative for viral antigen on day 3 but was positive for rabies on day 7. His condition continued to deteriorate, and he died 11 days later. When the parents were questioned, it was learned that the child had been bitten on the finger by a dog 6 months earlier while on a trip to India.

1. What clinical features of this case suggested rabies?
2. Why does rabies have such a long incubation period?
3. What treatment should have been given immediately after the dog bite? As soon as the diagnosis was suspected?
4. How do the clinical aspects of rabies differ from those of other neurological viral diseases?

Bibliography

Anderson LJ et al: Human rabies in the United States, 1960-1979: epidemiology, diagnosis, and prevention, *Ann Intern Med* 100:728-735, 1984.

Baer GM, Bellini WJ, Fishbein DB: *Rhabdoviruses.* In Fields BN, Knipe DM, editors: *Virology,* New York, 1990, Raven.

Centers for Disease Control: Rabies surveillance, United States, 1987 (CDC surveillance summaries), *MMWR* 37:SS-4, 1988.

Centers for Disease Control: Rabies vaccine, adsorbed: a new rabies vaccine for use in humans, *MMWR* 37:217-218, 223, 1988.

Fields BN, Knipe DM, Howley PM, editors: *Virology,* ed 3, New York, 1996, Lippincott-Raven.

Fishbein DB: Rabies, *Infect Dis Clin North Am* 5:53-71, 1991.

Immunization Practices Advisory Committee: Rabies prevention: supplementary statement on the preexposure use of human diploid cell rabies vaccine by the intradermal route, *MMWR* 35:767-768, 1986.

Robinson PA: *Rabies virus.* In Belshe RB, editor: *Textbook of human virology,* ed 2, St Louis, 1991, Mosby.

Steele JH: Rabies in the Americas and remarks on the global aspects, *Rev Infect Dis* 10(suppl 4):S585-S597, 1988.

Warrell DA, Warrell MJ: Human rabies and its prevention: an overview, *Rev Infect Dis* 10(suppl 4):S726-S731, 1988.

Winkler WG, Badoel K: Control of rabies in wildlife, *Sci Am* June 1992.

Wunner WH et al: The molecular biology of rabies viruses, *Rev Infect Dis* 10(suppl 4):S771-S784, 1988.

Togaviruses and Flaviviruses

The members of the Togaviridae and Flaviviridae families are enveloped, positive, single-stranded RNA viruses (Box 59-1). Most are transmitted by arthropods and are therefore **arboviruses.** For this reason, the flaviviruses were included in the Togaviridae family. However, differences in their size, morphology, gene sequence, and replication strategy necessitated their being classified as an independent virus family.

The togaviruses can be classified into three major genera (Table 59-1): *Alphavirus, Rubivirus,* and *Arterivirus.* No known arteriviruses cause disease in humans, and these are therefore not discussed further here. **Rubella** virus is the only member of the *Rubivirus* group; it is discussed separately, however, because its disease presentation **(German measles)** and its means of spread differ from those of the alphaviruses. The Flaviviridae include the flaviviruses, *Pestivirus,* and hepatitis C and G virus. Hepatitis C and G are discussed in Chapter 62. *Alphavirus* and *Flavivirus* are discussed together because of similarities in the diseases that they cause and their epidemiology.

ALPHAVIRUSES AND FLAVIVIRUSES

The alphaviruses and flaviviruses were classified as arboviruses because they are usually spread by arthropod vectors. These viruses have a very **broad host range,** including vertebrates (e.g., mammals, birds, amphibians, reptiles) and invertebrates (e.g., mosquitoes, ticks).

Viruses spread by animals or with an animal reservoir are called **zoonoses.** Examples of pathogenic alphaviruses and flaviviruses are listed in Table 59-2. The hepatitis C and G viruses are classified as flaviviruses on the basis of their genomic structure. They are not likely to prove to be arboviruses.

Structure and Replication of Alphaviruses

The alphaviruses are similar to the picornaviruses in that they have an **icosahedral capsid** and a **positive-sense, single-strand RNA** genome that resembles messenger RNA (mRNA). They differ from picornaviruses by being slightly larger (45 to 75 nm in diameter) and are surrounded by an **envelope** (Latin *toga,* meaning "cloak"). In addition, the togavirus genome encodes **early and late proteins.** The envelope consists of lipids obtained from the host cell membranes and glycoprotein spikes that protrude from the surface of the virion. Alphaviruses have two or three glycoproteins that associate to form a single spike. The COOH-terminus of the glycoproteins is anchored in the capsid, forcing the envelope to wrap tightly ("shrink-wrap") and take on the shape of the capsid (Figure 59-1). The capsid proteins of all the alphaviruses are similar in structure and are antigenically cross-reactive as well. The envelope glycoproteins express unique antigenic determinants that distinguish the different viruses and also express antigenic determinants that are shared by a group, or "complex," of viruses.

BOX 59-1 Unique Features of Togaviruses and Flaviviruses

Viruses have enveloped single-stranded positive-sense RNA.

Togavirus replication includes early (nonstructural) and late (structural) protein synthesis.

Togaviruses replicate in the cytoplasm and bud at the plasma membrane.

Flaviviruses replicate in the cytoplasm and bud at the internal membranes.

TABLE 59-1 Togaviruses and Flaviviruses

VIRUS GROUP	HUMAN PATHOGENS
Togaviruses	
Alphavirus	Arboviruses
Rubivirus	Rubella virus
Pestivirus	None
Arterivirus	None
Flaviviruses	Arboviruses
	Hepatitis C virus

FIGURE 59-1 Alphavirus morphology. **A,** The outline of the envelope and the glycoprotein spikes of the Sindbis virus are visualized by negative staining. **B,** More detail on the morphology of the virion is obtained from electron microscopy. **C,** Surface representation of the Sindbis virus obtained by image processing of the cryoelectron micrographs indicates that the envelope is held tightly and conforms to the shape and symmetry of the capsid. (From Fuller SD: *Cell* 48:923-934, 1987.)

TABLE 59-2 Arboviruses

DISEASE	VECTOR	HOST	DISTRIBUTION	DISEASE
ALPHAVIRUSES				
Sindbis*	*Aedes* and other mosquitoes	Birds	Africa, Australia, India	Subclinical
Semliki Forest*	*Aedes* and other mosquitoes	Birds	East and West Africa	Subclinical
Venezuelan equine encephalitis	*Aedes, Culex*	Rodents, horses	North, South, and Central America	Mild systemic; severe encephalitis
Eastern equine encephalitis	*Aedes, Culiseta*	Birds	North and South America, Caribbean	Mild systemic; encephalitis
Western equine encephalitis	*Culex, Culiseta*	Birds	North and South America	Mild systemic; encephalitis
Chikungunya	*Aedes*	Humans, monkeys	Africa, Asia	Fever, arthralgia, arthritis
FLAVIVIRUSES				
Dengue*	*Aedes*	Humans, monkeys	Worldwide, especially tropics	Mild systemic; break-bone fever, dengue hemorrhagic fever, and shock syndrome
Yellow fever*	*Aedes*	Humans, monkeys	Africa, South America	Hepatitis, hemorrhagic fever
Japanese encephalitis	*Culex*	Pigs, birds	Asia	Encephalitis
West Nile encephalitis	*Culex*	Birds	Africa, Europe, Central Asia	Fever, encephalitis, hepatitis
St. Louis encephalitis	*Culex*	Birds	North America	Encephalitis
Russian spring-summer encephalitis	*Ixodes* and *Dermacentor* ticks	Birds	Russia	Encephalitis
Powassan encephalitis	*Ixodes* ticks	Small mammals	North America	Encephalitis

*Prototypical viruses.

FIGURE 59-2 Replication of a togavirus: Semliki Forest virus. *1,* Semliki Forest virus binds to cell receptors, is shuttled into a coated pit, and is internalized in a coated vesicle. *2,* The virus is transferred to an endosome, and the viral envelope fuses with the endosomal membrane on acidification to release the nucleocapsid into the cytoplasm. *3,* Ribosomes bind to the positive-sense RNA genome, and the p230 or p270 (full-length) early polyproteins are made. *4,* The polyproteins are cleaved to produce nonstructural proteins 1 to 4 (NSP$_1$ to NSP$_4$), which include a polymerase to transcribe the genome into a minus-sense RNA template. *5,* The template is used to produce a full-length 42S positive-sense mRNA genome and a late 26S mRNA for the structural proteins. *6,* The C (capsid) protein is translated first, exposing a protease cleavage site and then a signal peptide for association with the endoplasmic reticulum. *7,* The E glycoproteins are then synthesized, glycosylated, processed in the Golgi apparatus, and transferred to the plasma membrane. *8,* The capsid proteins assemble on the 42S genomic RNA and then associate with regions of cytoplasmic and plasma membranes containing the E$_1$ to E$_3$ spike proteins. *9,* Budding from the plasma membrane releases the virus.

The alphaviruses attach to specific receptors expressed on many different cell types from many different species (Figure 59-2). The host range for these viruses includes vertebrates such as humans, monkeys, horses, birds, reptiles, and amphibians and invertebrates such as mosquitoes and ticks. However, the individual viruses have different tissue tropisms, which can account somewhat for the different disease presentations.

The virus enters the cell by means of receptor-mediated endocytosis (Figure 59-2). The viral envelope then fuses with the membrane of the endosome on acidification of the vesicle to deliver the capsid and genome into the cytoplasm.

Once released into the cytoplasm, the alphavirus genomes bind to ribosomes as mRNA. The alphavirus genome is translated in early and late phases. The initial two thirds of the alphavirus RNA is translated into a polyprotein, which is subsequently cleaved by proteases into four nonstructural early proteins (NSP 1-4). These proteins include a protease activity and an RNA-dependent RNA polymerase. A full-length 42S negative-sense RNA is synthesized as a template for replication of the genome, and more 42S positive-sense mRNA is produced. In addition, a 26S mRNA, corresponding to one third of the genome, is transcribed from the template.

The 26S RNA encodes the capsid (C) and envelope (E$_{1-3}$) proteins. Late in the replication cycle, viral mRNA can account for as much as 90% of the mRNA in the infected cell. The abundance of late mRNAs allows the production of a large amount of structural proteins required for packaging the virus.

The structural proteins are produced by protease cleavage of the late polyprotein produced from the 26S mRNA. The C protein is translated first and cleaved from the polyprotein (Figure 59-2). A signal sequence is then made that associates the nascent polypeptide with the endoplasmic reticulum. The envelope glycoproteins are then translated, glycosylated, and cleaved from the remaining portion of the polyprotein to produce the E$_1$, E$_2$, and E$_3$ glycoprotein spikes. The E$_3$ is released from most alphavirus glycoprotein spikes. The glycoproteins are processed by the normal cellular machinery in the endoplasmic reticulum and Golgi apparatus and are also acetylated and acylated with long-chain fatty acids (Figure 59-2). Alphavirus glycoproteins are then transferred efficiently to the plasma membrane.

The C proteins associate with the genomic RNA soon after their synthesis and form an icosahedral capsid. Once this is completed, the capsid associates with portions of the membrane expressing the viral glycoproteins.

Togavirus genome (Sindbis virus)

Flavivirus genome (Yellow fever virus)

FIGURE 59-3 Comparison of the togavirus (alphavirus) and flavivirus genomes. Alphavirus: The enzymatic activities are translated from the 5' end of the input genome, promoting their early rapid translation. The structural proteins are translated later from a smaller mRNA transcribed from the genomic template. Flavivirus: The genes for the structural proteins of the flaviviruses are at the 5' end of the genome/mRNA, and only one species of polyprotein is made, which represents the entire genome. *Poly A,* Polyadenylate. (Redrawn from Hahn CS, Galler R, Rice CM: *Annu Rev Microbiol* 44:649-688, 1990.)

The alphavirus capsid has binding sites for the C-terminus of the glycoprotein spike, which pulls the envelope tightly around itself in a manner similar to a form-fitting wrapper (Figures 59-1 and 59-2). Alphaviruses are released on budding from the plasma membrane.

Structure and Replication of Flaviviruses

The flaviviruses also have positive-strand RNA and an envelope. However, the virions are slightly smaller than those of the alphaviruses (37 to 50 nm in diameter), the RNA does not have a polyadenylate sequence, and a capsid structure is not visible within the virion. All the flaviviruses are serologically related, and antibodies to one virus may neutralize another virus.

The attachment and penetration of the flaviviruses occur in the same way as described for the alphaviruses, but the flaviviruses can also attach to the Fc receptors on macrophages, monocytes, and other cells when they are coated with antibody. The antibody actually enhances the infectivity of these viruses by providing new receptors for the virus and by promoting viral uptake into these target cells.

The major differences between alphaviruses and flaviviruses are in the organization of their genomes and their mechanisms of protein synthesis. In contrast to the alphaviruses, the entire flavivirus genome is translated into a single polyprotein (Figure 59-3). As a result, there is no temporal distinction in the translation of the different viral proteins. The polyprotein produced from the

yellow fever genome contains four to eight nonstructural proteins, including a protease and an RNA-dependent RNA polymerase, plus the capsid and envelope structural proteins.

Unlike the alphaviruses, the structural genes are at the 5' end of the genome. As a result, the portions of the polyprotein containing the structural (not the catalytic) proteins are synthesized first and with the greatest efficiency. This may allow the production of more structural proteins, but it decreases the efficiency of nonstructural protein synthesis and the initiation of viral replication. This may contribute to the long latent period that precedes the detection of flavivirus replication.

Another distinction of the flaviviruses is that they acquire their envelope by budding into intracellular vesicles rather than at the cell surface. The virus is then released by exocytosis or cell lysis.

Pathogenesis and Immunity

Because the arboviruses are acquired from the bite of an arthropod such as a mosquito, a knowledge of the course of infection in both the vertebrate host and the invertebrate vector is important for an understanding of the diseases. These viruses can cause lytic or persistent infections of both vertebrate and invertebrate hosts (Box 59-2). Infections of invertebrates are usually persistent, with continued virus production.

The death of the cell results from a combination of virus-induced insults. The large amount of viral RNA produced on the replication and transcription of the genome blocks cellular mRNA from binding to ribosomes. Increased permeability of the target cell membrane and changes in ion concentrations can alter enzyme activities and favor the translation of viral mRNA over cellular mRNA. The displacement of cellular mRNA from the protein synthesis machinery prevents rebuilding and maintenance of the cell and is a major cause of the death of the virus-infected cell. Some alphaviruses, such as western equine encephalitis (WEE) virus, make a nucleotide triphosphatase that degrades deoxyribonucleotides, depleting even the substrate pool for DNA production.

Female mosquitoes acquire the alphaviruses and flaviviruses by taking a blood meal from a **viremic vertebrate host.** A sufficient viremia must be maintained in the vertebrate host to allow acquisition of the virus, however. The virus then infects the epithelial cells of the midgut of the mosquito, spreads through the basal lamina of the midgut to the circulation, and infects the salivary glands. The virus sets up a persistent infection and replicates to high titers in these cells. The salivary glands can then release virus into the saliva. Not all arthropod species support this type of infection, however. For example, the normal vector for the WEE virus is the *Culex tarsalis* mosquito, but certain strains of virus are limited to the midgut of the mosquito, cannot infect its salivary glands, and therefore cannot be transmitted to humans.

BOX 59-2   Disease Mechanisms of Togaviruses and Flaviviruses

Viruses are cytolytic, except for rubella.
Viruses establish systemic infection and viremia.
Viruses are good inducers of interferon, which can account for the influenza-like symptoms of infection.

Viruses, except rubella and hepatitis C, are arboviruses.
Flaviviruses infect cells of the monocyte-macrophage lineage.
Nonneutralizing antibody can enhance flavivirus infection via Fc receptors on the macrophage.

	INFLUENZA-LIKE SYNDROME	ENCEPHALITIS	HEPATITIS	HEMORRHAGE	SHOCK
Dengue	+		+	+	+
Yellow fever	+		+	+	+
St. Louis encephalitis	+	+			
Venezuelan encephalitis	+	+			
Western equine encephalitis	+	+			
Eastern equine encephalitis	+	+			
Japanese encephalitis	+	+			

On biting a host, the female mosquito regurgitates virus-containing saliva into the victim's bloodstream. The virus then circulates freely in the host's plasma and comes into contact with susceptible target cells such as the endothelial cells of the capillaries, macrophages, monocytes, and the reticuloendothelial system.

The nature of alphavirus and flavivirus disease is determined primarily by the specific tissue tropisms of the individual virus type, the concentration of infecting virus, and individual responses to the infection. These viruses are associated with **mild systemic disease, encephalitis, arthrogenic disease,** or **hemorrhagic disease.**

The initial viremia produces systemic symptoms such as fever, chills, headaches, backaches, and other influenza-like symptoms within 3 to 7 days of infection. Some of these symptoms can be attributed to the effects of the interferon produced after infection of the host cells. This is considered a mild systemic disease, and most viral infections do not progress beyond this point.

After replication in cells of the reticuloendothelial system, a secondary viremia may result. This viremia can produce sufficient virus to infect target organs such as the brain, liver, skin, and vasculature, depending on the tissue tropism of the virus (Figure 59-4). The virus gains access to the brain by infecting the endothelial cells lining the small vessels of the brain or the choroid plexus.

The primary target cells of the flaviviruses are of the monocyte-macrophage lineage. Although these cells are found throughout the body and may have different characteristics, they express Fc receptors for antibody and release lymphokines on challenge. Flavivirus infection is enhanced 200-fold to 1000-fold by nonneutralizing antiviral antibody that promotes binding of the virus to the Fc receptors and uptake into the cell.

Immune Response

Both humoral and cellular immunity are elicited and are important to the control of primary infection and the prevention of future infections with the alphaviruses and flaviviruses.

Replication of the alphaviruses and flaviviruses produces a double-stranded RNA replicative intermediate that is a good inducer of interferon-alpha and interferon-beta. The interferon is released into the bloodstream and limits replication of the virus; it also stimulates the immune response but in doing so causes the rapid onset of the influenza-like symptoms characteristic of mild systemic disease.

Circulating IgM is produced within 6 days of infection, followed by the production of IgG. The antibody blocks the viremic spread of the virus and the subsequent infection of other tissues. Immunity to one flavivirus can provide some protection against infection with other flaviviruses through recognition of the type-common antigens expressed on all viruses in the family. Cell-mediated immunity is also important in controlling the primary infection.

Immunity to these viruses is a double-edged sword in that the inflammation resulting from the cell-mediated immune response can destroy tissue and significantly contribute to the pathogenesis of encephalitis. Hypersensitivity reactions such as delayed-type hypersensitivity, the formation of immune complexes with virions and viral antigens, and the activation of complement can also occur. This can weaken the vasculature and cause it to rupture, leading to hemorrhagic symptoms.

A nonneutralizing antibody can enhance the uptake of flaviviruses into macrophages and other cells that express Fc receptors. Such an antibody can be generated to a related strain of virus in which the neutralizing epitope is not expressed or is different.

Epidemiology

Alphaviruses and flaviviruses are prototypical arboviruses (*ar*thropod-*bo*rne viruses) (Box 59-3). To be an arbovirus, the virus must be able to (1) infect both verte-

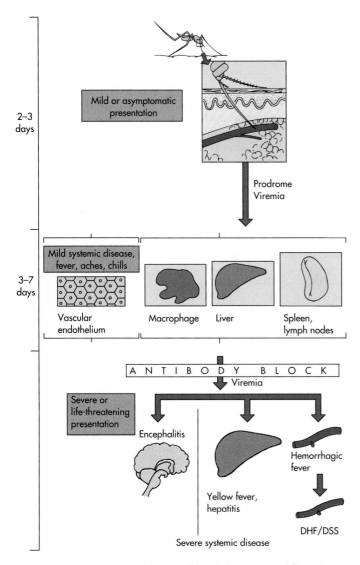

2–3 days

Mild or asymptomatic presentation

Prodrome Viremia

3–7 days

Mild systemic disease, fever, aches, chills

Vascular endothelium   Macrophage   Liver   Spleen, lymph nodes

A N T I B O D Y   B L O C K
Viremia

Severe or life-threatening presentation

Encephalitis

Yellow fever, hepatitis

Hemorrhagic fever

DHF/DSS

Severe systemic disease

FIGURE 59-4 Disease syndromes of the alphaviruses and flaviviruses. Primary viremia may be associated with mild systemic disease. Most infections are limited to this. If sufficient virus is produced during the secondary viremia to escape immune protection and to reach critical target tissue, severe systemic disease or encephalitis may result. For dengue virus, rechallenge with another strain can result in severe dengue hemorrhagic fever *(DHF)*, which can cause dengue shock syndrome *(DSS)* because of the loss of fluids from the vasculature.

BOX 59-3   **Epidemiology of Togavirus and Flavivirus Infection**

DISEASE/VIRAL FACTORS

Enveloped virus must stay wet and can be inactivated by drying, soap, and detergents.
Virus can infect mammals, birds, reptiles, and insects.
Asymptomatic or nonspecific (flulike fever or chills), encephalitis, hemorrhagic fever, or arthritis.

TRANSMISSION

Togaviruses and flaviviruses: specific arthropods characteristic of each virus (zoonosis: arbovirus).

WHO IS AT RISK?

People who enter ecological niche of arthropod: arboviruses.

GEOGRAPHY/SEASON

Endemic regions for each arbovirus are determined by habitat of mosquito or other vector.
Aedes mosquito, which causes dengue and yellow fever, is found in urban areas and in pools of water.
Culex mosquito, which causes St. Louis encephalitis, is found in forest and urban areas.
Disease is more common in summer.

MODES OF CONTROL

Mosquito breeding sites and mosquitoes should be eliminated.
Live attenuated vaccines are available for yellow fever virus and Japanese encephalitis virus.

The vectors, natural hosts, and geographical distribution of representative alphaviruses and flaviviruses are given in Table 59-2.

These viruses are usually restricted to a specific arthropod vector, its vertebrate host, and their ecological niche. The most common vector is the mosquito, but some arboviruses are also spread by ticks and sandflies. Even in a tropical region overrun with mosquitoes, the spread of these viruses is still restricted to a specific genus of mosquitoes. Not all arthropods can act as good vectors for each virus. For example, *Culex quinquefasciatus* is resistant to infection by the WEE virus (alphavirus) but is an excellent vector for St. Louis encephalitis virus (flavivirus).

Birds and small mammals are the usual **reservoir** hosts for the alphaviruses and flaviviruses, but reptiles and amphibians can also act as hosts. A large population of viremic animals can develop in these species to continue the infection cycle of the virus.

Arbovirus diseases occur during the **summer months** and rainy seasons when the arthropods breed and the arboviruses are cycled between a host/reservoir (bird), an arthropod (e.g., mosquito), and human hosts. This

brates and invertebrates, (2) initiate a sufficient viremia in a vertebrate host for a sufficient time to allow acquisition of the virus by the invertebrate vector, and (3) initiate a persistent productive infection of the salivary gland of the invertebrate to provide virus for the infection of other host animals. Humans are usually **"dead-end" hosts** in that they cannot spread the virus back to the vector because a persistent viremia is not maintained. If the virus is not in the blood, the mosquito cannot acquire it. A full cycle of infection occurs when the virus is transmitted by the arthropod vector and amplified in a susceptible, immunologically naive host **(reservoir)** that allows the reinfection of other arthropods (Figure 59-5).

maintains and increases the amount of virus in the environment. In the winter, neither the normal host nor the vector remain to maintain the virus. The virus may persist in arthropod larvae or eggs or in reptiles or amphibians that remain in the locale, or it may migrate with the birds and then return during the summer.

When humans travel into the ecological niche of the mosquito vector, they risk being infected by the virus. For example, as many as half the Indians living in the Everglades come into contact with *Culex* and *Aedes* mosquitoes carrying Venezuelan equine encephalitis (VEE) virus and are seropositive for the virus. Pools of standing water, drainage ditches, and dumps in cities can also provide breeding grounds for mosquitoes such as *Aedes aegypti*, the vector for yellow fever, dengue, and chikungunya. An increase in the population of these mosqui-

toes therefore puts the human population at risk for infection.

Humans can be reservoir hosts for yellow fever, dengue, and chikungunya viruses (Figure 59-5). These viruses are maintained by *Aedes* mosquitos in a **sylvatic or jungle cycle** in which monkeys are the natural host and also in an **urban cycle** in which humans are the host. *A. aegypti* is a vector for each of these viruses and is a household mosquito. It breeds in pools of water, open sewers, and other accumulations of water in cities. St. Louis encephalitis virus can also establish an urban cycle of spread using its vector, *Culex* mosquitoes, which prefer stagnant water such as sewage. The occurrence of numerous inapparent infections in high-density populations provides sufficient viremic human hosts for the continued spread of these viruses.

Clinical Syndromes

More humans are infected with alphaviruses and flaviviruses than show significant, characteristic symptoms. The incidence of arbovirus disease is sporadic. Alphavirus disease is usually characterized as low-grade disease, and influenza-like symptoms (chills, fever, rash, aches) correlate with systemic infection during the initial viremia. Eastern equine encephalitis (EEE), WEE, and VEE virus infections can progress to encephalitis (as the names imply) in humans and horses, with EEE causing the most severe disease. These viruses are usually more of a problem to livestock than to humans, however. The name *chikungunya* refers to the crippling arthritis associated with serious disease. Although predominant in South America and western Africa, this disease may spread to the United States because of the return of the *A. aegypti* mosquito, its vector.

Most infections with flaviviruses are relatively benign, but serious encephalitic or hemorrhagic disease can occur. The encephalitis viruses include St. Louis, Japanese, Murray Valley, and Russian spring-summer viruses. Hundreds to thousands of cases of St. Louis encephalitis virus disease are noted in the United States annually. The hemorrhagic viruses are dengue and yellow fever viruses.

Dengue virus is a major worldwide problem, with up to 100 million cases of dengue fever and 250,000 cases of dengue hemorrhagic fever (DHF) occurring per year. The incidence of the more serious DHF has quadrupled since 1985. Dengue fever is also known as *break-bone fever*, with the symptoms and signs consisting of high fever, headache, rash, and back and bone pain that last 6 to 7 days. On rechallenge with another of the four related strains, **dengue** can also cause DHF and dengue shock syndrome (**DSS**). Nonneutralizing antibody promotes uptake of the virus into macrophages, which causes memory T cells to become activated, release inflammatory lymphokines, and initiate hypersensitivity reactions. These result in weakening and rupture of the vasculature, internal bleeding, and loss of plasma, leading to shock symptoms and internal bleeding. In 1981 in Cuba, dengue-2 virus infected a population previously

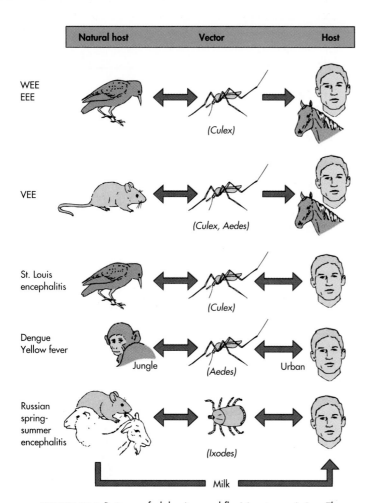

FIGURE 59-5 Patterns of alphavirus and flavivirus transmission. The cycle of arbovirus transmission maintains and amplifies the virus in the environment. Host-vector relationships that can provide this cycle are indicated by the double arrow. "Dead-end" infections with no transmission of the virus back to the vector are indicated by the single arrow. For St. Louis encephalitis, yellow fever, and dengue viruses, humans are not dead-end hosts and support an urban cycle. The Russian spring-summer encephalitis virus can be transmitted to humans by a tick bite and in milk form from infected goats. *EEE*, Eastern equine encephalitis; *VEE*, Venezuelan equine encephalitis.

exposed to dengue-1 virus between 1977 and 1980, leading to an epidemic in which there were more than 100,000 cases of DHF/DSS and 168 deaths.

Yellow fever infections are characterized by severe systemic disease, with degeneration of the liver, kidney, and heart and hemorrhage. Liver involvement causes the jaundice from which the disease gets its name, but massive gastrointestinal hemorrhages ("black vomit") may also occur. The mortality rate associated with yellow fever during epidemics is as high as 50%.

Laboratory Diagnosis

The alphaviruses and flaviviruses can be grown in both vertebrate and mosquito cell lines, but most are difficult to isolate. Infection can be detected by cytopathological studies, immunofluorescence, and the hemadsorption of avian erythrocytes. After isolation, the viruses can be distinguished by RNA "fingerprints" of the genomic RNA. Monoclonal antibodies to the individual viruses have become a useful tool for distinguishing the individual species and strains of viruses.

A variety of serological methods can be used to diagnose infections, including hemagglutination inhibition, enzyme-linked immunosorbent assays, and latex agglutination. The presence of specific IgM or a fourfold increase in titer between acute and convalescent sera is used to indicate a recent infection. The serological cross-reactivity between viruses in a group or complex limits identification of the actual viral species in many cases, however.

Treatment, Prevention, and Control

No treatments exist for arbovirus diseases other than supportive care.

The easiest means to prevent the spread of any arbovirus is elimination of its vector and breeding grounds. After 1900, when Walter Reed and his colleagues discovered that yellow fever was spread by *A. aegypti*, the number of cases was reduced from 1400 to none within 2 years purely by controlling the mosquito population. Avoidance of the breeding grounds of a mosquito vector is also a good preventive measure.

Vaccination is one of the best means of protection. A live vaccine against yellow fever virus and killed vaccines against EEE, WEE, Japanese, and Russian spring-summer encephalitis viruses are available. These vaccines are meant for people working with the virus or at risk for contact, however. A live vaccine against VEE virus is available but only for use in domestic animals. A vaccine against dengue virus has not been developed because of the potential risk for immune enhancement of the disease on subsequent challenge.

The yellow fever vaccine is prepared from the 17D strain isolated from a patient in 1927 and grown for long periods in monkeys, mosquitos, embryonic tissue culture, and embryonated eggs. The vaccine is administered intradermally and elicits lifelong immunity to yellow fever and possibly other cross-reacting flaviviruses.

RUBELLA VIRUS

Rubella virus shares the structural properties and mode of replication with the other togaviruses, as described earlier. Unlike the other togaviruses, however, rubella is a **respiratory virus** and **does not cause readily detectable cytopathology.**

Rubella is one of the five **classic childhood exanthems,** with measles, roseola, fifth disease, and chickenpox the other four. Rubella, meaning "little red" in Latin, was first distinguished from measles and other exanthems by German physicians, thus the common name for the disease, **German measles.** An astute Australian ophthalmologist, Norman McAlister Gregg, recognized in 1941 that maternal rubella infection was the cause of congenital cataracts. Maternal rubella infection has since been correlated with several other **severe congenital defects.** This prompted the development of a unique program to vaccinate children to prevent infection of pregnant women and neonates.

Pathogenesis and Immunity

Rubella virus is not cytolytic but does cause limited cytopathological effects in certain cell lines, such as Vero and RK13. The replication of rubella prevents (**heterologous interference**) the replication of superinfecting picornaviruses. This property allowed the first isolations of rubella virus in 1962.

Rubella infects the upper respiratory tract and then spreads to local lymph nodes, which coincides with a period of lymphadenopathy (Figure 59-6). This is followed by establishment of viremia, which spreads the virus throughout the body. Infection of other tissues and the characteristic mild rash result. The prodromal period lasts approximately 2 weeks (Figure 59-7). The person can shed virus in respiratory droplets during the prodromal period and for as long as 2 weeks after the onset of the rash.

Immune Response

Antibody is generated after the viremia, and its appearance correlates with the appearance of the rash. The antibody limits viremic spread, but cell-mediated immunity plays an important role in resolving the infection. Only one serotype of rubella exists, and natural infection produces lifelong protective immunity. Most important, serum antibody in a pregnant woman prevents spread of the virus to the fetus. Immune complexes most likely cause the rash and arthralgia associated with rubella infection.

Congenital Infection

Rubella infection in a pregnant woman can result in serious congenital abnormalities in the child. If the mother does not have antibody, the virus can replicate in the placenta and spread to the fetal blood supply and throughout the fetus. Rubella can replicate in most tissues of the fetus. The virus may not be cytolytic, but the normal

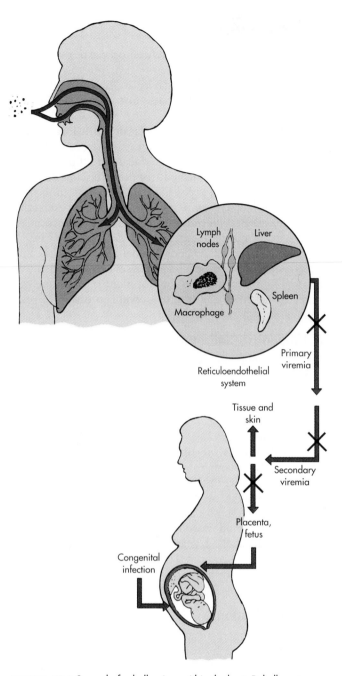

FIGURE 59-6 Spread of rubella virus within the host. Rubella enters and infects the nasopharynx and lung and then spreads to the lymph nodes and reticuloendothelial system. The resulting viremia spreads the virus to other tissues and the skin. Circulating antibody can block the transfer of virus at the indicated points *(X)*. In an immunologically deficient pregnant woman, the virus can infect the placenta and spread to the fetus.

growth, mitosis, and chromosomal structure of the fetus' cells can be altered by the infection. This can lead to improper development of the fetus, small size of the infected baby, and the **teratogenic** effects associated with congenital rubella infection. The nature of the disorder is determined by the affected tissue and the stage of development that is disrupted. The virus may persist in tis-

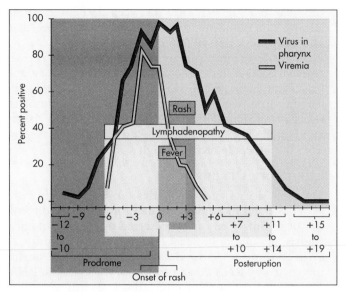

FIGURE 59-7 Time course of rubella disease. Rubella production in the pharynx precedes the appearance of symptoms and continues throughout the course of the disease. The onset of lymphadenopathy coincides with the viremia. Fever and rash occur later. The person is infectious as long as the virus is produced in the pharynx. (Redrawn from Plotkin SA: *Rubella vaccine.* In Plotkin SA, Mortimer EA, editors: *Vaccines,* Philadelphia, 1988, WB Saunders.)

sues, such as the lens of the eye, for 3 to 4 years and may be shed up to a year after birth. The presence of the virus during the development of the baby's immune response may even have a tolerative effect on the system, preventing effective clearance of the virus after birth. Immune complexes that produce further clinical abnormalities may also form in the neonate or infant.

Epidemiology

Humans are the only host for rubella (Box 59-4). The virus is spread in respiratory secretions and is generally acquired during childhood. The virus is less communicable than measles or varicella, but crowded conditions such as day-care centers promote contagion.

Approximately 20% of women of childbearing age escape infection during childhood and are susceptible to infection unless vaccinated. Programs in many U.S. states ensure that expectant mothers have antibodies to rubella.

Before the development and use of the rubella vaccine, cases of rubella in school children would be reported every spring, and major epidemics of rubella occurred at regular 6- to 9-year intervals. The severity of the 1964 to 1965 epidemic in the United States is indicated in Table 59-3. Congenital rubella occurred in as much as 1% of all the children born in cities such as Philadelphia during this epidemic. Since the development of the vaccine, however, the incidence of rubella and congenital rubella is now less than 1 and 0.1 per 100,000 pregnancies, respectively.

FIGURE 59-8 Close-up of the rubella rash. Small erythematous macules are visible. (From Hart CA, Broadwell RL: *A color atlas of pediatric infectious disease,* London, 1992, Wolfe.)

TABLE 59-3 Estimated Morbidity Associated with the 1964-1965 U.S. Rubella Epidemic

CLINICAL EVENTS	NUMBER AFFECTED
Rubella cases	12,500,000
Arthritis-arthralgia	159,375
Encephalitis	2,084
Deaths	
Excess neonatal deaths	2,100
Other deaths	60
TOTAL DEATHS	2,160
Excess fetal wastage	6,250
Congenital rubella syndrome	
Deaf children	8,055
Deaf-blind children	3,580
Mentally retarded children	1,790
Other congenital rubella syndrome symptoms	6,575
TOTAL CONGENITAL RUBELLA SYNDROME	20,000
Therapeutic abortions	5,000

From National Communicable Disease Center: *Rubella surveillance,* US Department of Health, Education and Welfare, no 1, June 1969.

Clinical Syndromes

Rubella disease is normally benign in children. The symptoms in children consist of a 3-day rash and swollen glands (Figures 59-8). Infection in adults, however, can be more severe and include problems such as bone and joint pain (arthralgia and arthritis) and (rarely) thrombocytopenia or postinfectious encephalopathy. Immunopathology resulting from cell-mediated immunity and hypersensitivity reactions is a major cause of the more severe forms of rubella in adults.

Congenital disease is the most serious outcome of rubella infection. The fetus is at major risk until the twentieth week of pregnancy. Maternal immunity to the virus resulting from prior exposure or vaccination prevents spread of the virus to the fetus. The most common manifestations of congenital rubella infection include cataracts, mental retardation, and deafness (Table 59-3 and Box 59-5). The mortality in utero and within the first year of birth is high for these babies.

Laboratory Diagnosis

It is difficult to isolate the rubella virus, and for this reason it is rarely attempted. The diagnosis is usually confirmed by the presence of anti-rubella-specific IgM. A fourfold increase in specific IgG antibody titer between acute and convalescent sera is also used to indicate a recent infection. Antibodies to rubella are assayed early in pregnancy to determine the immune status of the woman. This test is required in many states.

When isolation of the virus is necessary, the virus is usually obtained from urine and is detected by interference with ECHO 11 virus replication in primary African green monkey kidney cell cultures.

Treatment, Prevention, and Control

No treatment has been found for rubella. The best means of preventing rubella is vaccination with the

Rubella cases per 100,000 population | CRS cases per 100,000 live births

- Rubella, total
- Rubella, ≥15-year-old
- CRS

Vaccine licensed

Year

FIGURE 59-9 Effect of rubella virus vaccination on the incidence of rubella and congenital rubella syndrome *(CRS)*. (Redrawn from Williams MN, Preblud SR: *MMWR* 33:1SS, 1984.)

live cold-adapted RA27/3 vaccine strain of virus (Figure 59-9). The live rubella vaccine is usually administered with the measles and mumps vaccines (MMR vaccine). The triple vaccine is included routinely in well-baby care. Vaccination promotes both humoral and cellular immunity.

The primary reason for the rubella vaccination program is to prevent congenital infection by decreasing the number of susceptible people in the population, especially children. There are then fewer seronegative mothers and less chance of their exposure to the virus. Because **only one serotype** for rubella exists and **humans are the only reservoir,** vaccination of a large proportion of the population can significantly reduce the likelihood of exposure to the virus. Unlike smallpox, with rubella, vaccination programs will not eliminate the disease because the virus can be transmitted by people with asymptomatic infections.

CASE STUDIES AND QUESTIONS

A 27-year-old businessman experienced a high fever, serious retroorbital headache, and severe joint and back pain 5 days after he and his family returned from a trip to Malaysia. The symptoms lasted for 4 days, and then a rash appeared on his palms and soles and lasted for 2 days. His 5-year-old son experienced mild influenza-like symptoms and then collapsed after 2 to 5 days. His hands were cold and clammy, his face was flushed, and his body was warm. There were petechiae on his forehead and ecchymoses elsewhere. He bruised very easily. He was breathing rapidly and had a weak rapid pulse. He then rapidly recovered after 24 hours.

1. What features of these cases pointed to the diagnosis of dengue virus infection?
2. Of what significance was the trip to Malaysia?
3. What was the source of infection in the father and son?
4. What was the significance of and the pathogenic basis for the petechiae and ecchymoses in the child?

Two weeks after returning from a trip to Mexico, a 25-year-old man had arthralgia (joint aches) and a mild rash that started on his face and spread to his body. He recalled that he felt as though he had the "flu" a few days before the onset of the rash. The rash disappeared in 4 days.

1. What features of this case pointed to the diagnosis of rubella infection?
2. Why is it significant that the symptoms started after a trip outside the United States?
3. What precaution could he have taken to prevent this infection?
4. How was this infection transmitted?
5. Who was at risk for a serious outcome of this infection?
6. If this disease is normally mild in children, why is their immunization so important?

Bibliography

Belshe RB, editor: *Textbook of human virology,* ed 2, St Louis, 1991, Mosby.

Fields BN, Knipe DM, Howley PM, editors: *Virology,* ed 3, New York, 1996, Lippincott-Raven.

Freestone DS: *Yellow fever vaccine.* In Plotkin SA, Mortimer EA, editors: *Vaccines,* Philadelphia, 1988, WB Saunders.

Hahn CS, Galler R, Rice CM: Flavivirus genome organization, expression, and replication, *Annu Rev Microbiol* 44:649-688, 1990.

Johnson RT: *Viral infections of the nervous system,* New York, 1982, Raven.

Koblet H: The "merry-go-round": alphaviruses between vertebrate and invertebrate cells, *Adv Virus Res* 38:343-403, 1990.

Plotkin SA: *Rubella vaccine.* In Plotkin SA, Mortimer EA, editors: *Vaccines,* Philadelphia, 1988, WB Saunders.

Stollar V: *Approaches to the study of vector specificity for arboviruses: model systems using cultured mosquito cells.* In Maramorosch K, Murphy FA, Shatkin AJ, editors: *Advances in virus research,* vol 33, New York, 1987, Academic.

Tsai TF: *Arboviral infections in the United States, Infect Dis Clin North Am* 5:73-102, 1991.

60

Bunyaviridae

The Bunyaviridae constitute a "supergroup" of at least **200 enveloped, segmented, negative-strand RNA viruses.** The supergroup is further broken down into the following four genera on the basis of structural and biochemical features: *Bunyavirus, Phlebovirus, Nairovirus,* and *Hantavirus* (Table 60-1). Most of the Bunyaviridae are **arboviruses** (*ar*thropod *bo*rne) that are spread by mosquitoes, ticks, or flies and are endemic to the environment of the vector. The **hantaviruses** are the exception; they are carried by **rodents.**

STRUCTURE

The bunyaviruses are roughly spherical particles that are 90 to 120 nm in diameter (Box 60-1). The envelope of the virus contains two glycoproteins (G1 and G2) and encloses three unique negative-strand RNAs that are associated with the protein (nucleocapsids) (Table 60-2). The nucleocapsids include the large **(L),** medium **(M),** and small **(S)** RNA associated with the RNA-dependent RNA polymerase (L protein) and two nonstructural proteins (NS$_s$, NS$_m$) (Figure 60-1). Unlike other negative-strand RNA viruses, the Bunyaviridae **do not have a matrix protein.** Differences in the number and sizes of the virion proteins; the lengths of the L, M, and S strands of the genome; and their transcription distinguish the five genera of Bunyaviridae.

REPLICATION

The Bunyaviridae replicate in the same way as the enveloped, negative-strand viruses. Specifically, after interaction of the G1 glycoprotein with cell surface receptors, the virus is internalized by endocytosis and fuses with endosomal membranes on acidification of the vesicle. The release of the nucleocapsid into the cytoplasm allows mRNA and protein synthesis to begin.

The M strand encodes the NS$_m$ nonstructural protein and the G1 (viral attachment protein) and G2 proteins, and the L strand encodes the L protein (polymerase) (Table 60-2). The S strand of RNA encodes two nonstructural proteins, N and NS$_s$.

Replication of the genome by the L protein also provides new templates for transcription, thereby increasing the rate of mRNA synthesis. The glycoproteins are then synthesized and glycosylated in the endoplasmic reticulum, after which they are transferred to the Golgi apparatus and not translocated to the plasma membrane. Virions are assembled by **budding into the Golgi apparatus** and are released by cell lysis or exocytosis.

PATHOGENESIS

As **arboviruses,** Bunyaviridae possess many of the same pathogenic mechanisms as the togaviruses and flaviviruses (Box 60-2). For example, the virus is spread by an arthropod vector and is injected into the blood, which initiates a viremia. Progression past this stage to secondary viremia and further dissemination of the virus can deliver the virus to target sites typically involved in that particular viral disease, such as the central nervous system, liver, kidney, and vascular endothelium.

Bunyaviridae cause neuronal and glial damage and cerebral edema, leading to encephalitis. In certain viremic infections (e.g., Rift Valley fever), hepatic necrosis may occur. In others (e.g., Crimean hemorrhagic fever and Hantaan hemorrhagic disease), the primary lesion involves the leakage of plasma and erythrocytes through the vascular endothelium. In the latter infec-

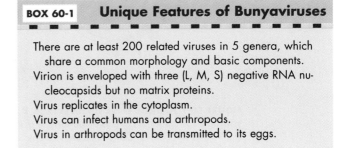

BOX 60-1   **Unique Features of Bunyaviruses**

There are at least 200 related viruses in 5 genera, which share a common morphology and basic components.

Virion is enveloped with three (L, M, S) negative RNA nucleocapsids but no matrix proteins.

Virus replicates in the cytoplasm.

Virus can infect humans and arthropods.

Virus in arthropods can be transmitted to its eggs.

TABLE 60-1   Notable Bunyaviridae Genera*

GENUS	MEMBERS	INSECT VECTOR	PATHOLOGICAL CONDITIONS	VERTEBRATE HOSTS
Bunyavirus	Bunyamwera virus, California encephalitis virus, LaCrosse virus, Oropouche virus; 150 members	Mosquito	Febrile illness, encephalitis, febrile rash	Rodents, small mammals, primates, marsupials, birds
Phlebovirus	Rift Valley fever virus, Sandfly fever virus; 36 members	Fly	Sandfly fever, hemorrhagic fever, encephalitis, conjunctivitis, myositis	Sheep, cattle, domestic animals
Nairovirus	Crimean-Congo hemorrhagic fever virus; 6 members	Tick	Hemorrhagic fever	Hares, cattle, goats, seabirds
Uukuvirus	Uukuniemi virus; 7 members	Tick	—	Birds
Hantavirus	Hantaan virus	None	Hemorrhagic fever with renal syndrome, adult respiratory distress syndrome	Rodents

*An additional 35 viruses possess several common properties with Bunyaviridae but are as yet unclassified.

TABLE 60-2   Genome and Proteins of California Encephalitis Virus

GENOME*	PROTEINS
L	RNA polymerase, 170 kD
M	Spike glycoprotein, 75 kD
	Spike glycoprotein, 65 kD
	Nonstructural protein, 15 to 17 kD
S	Nucleocapsid protein, 25 kD
	Nucleocapsid protein, 10 kD

*Negative-strand RNA.

BOX 60-2   Disease Mechanisms for Bunyaviruses

Virus is acquired from an arthropod bite (e.g., mosquito).

Initial viremia may cause influenza-like symptoms.

Establishment of secondary viremia may allow virus access to specific target tissues, including the central nervous system, organs, and vascular endothelium.

Antibody is important in controlling viremia; interferon and cell-mediated immunity may prevent the outgrowth of infection.

Glycoprotein (5-10 nm spikes)
Lipid envelope
Nucleocapsids

A

1. L RNA
2. M RNA
3. S RNA
Ⓛ polymerase

B

FIGURE 60-1 **A,** Model of bunyavirus particle. **B,** Electron micrograph of La Crosse variant of bunyavirus. Note the spike proteins at the surface of the virion envelope. (**A** redrawn from Fraenkel-Conrat H, Wagner RR, editors: *Comprehensive virology,* vol 14, New York, 1979, Plenum; **B** courtesy Centers for Disease Control and Prevention, Atlanta.)

tion, these changes are most prominent in the kidney and are accompanied by hemorrhagic necrosis of the kidney. Unlike most other bunyaviruses, the **hantavirus** initiates infection and remains in the lung, where it causes hemorrhagic tissue destruction and lethal pulmonary disease.

BOX 60-3   **Epidemiology of Bunyavirus Infections**

DISEASE/VIRAL FACTORS

Virus is able to replicate in mammalian and arthropod cells.
Virus is able to pass into ovary and infect arthropod eggs, allowing virus to survive during winter.

TRANSMISSION

Via arthropods through break in skin.
California encephalitis group: *Aedes* mosquito.
  Aedes mosquitoes are daytime feeders and live in forest.
  Aedes mosquitoes lay eggs in small pools of water trapped in places such as trees and tires.

WHO IS AT RISK?

People in habitat of arthropod vector.
California encephalitis group: campers, forest rangers, woodsmen.

GEOGRAPHY/SEASON

Disease incidence correlates with distribution of vector.
Disease is more common in summer.

MODES OF CONTROL

Elimination of vector or vector's habitat.
Avoidance of vector's habitat.

EPIDEMIOLOGY

Most bunyaviruses are transmitted by infected mosquitoes, ticks, or *Phlebotomus* flies to rodents, birds, and larger animals (Box 60-3). The animals then become the reservoir for the virus, thereby continuing the cycle of infection. Humans are infected when they enter the environment of the insect vector (Figure 60-2). Transmission occurs during the summer, but unlike many other arboviruses, many of the Bunyaviridae can survive a winter in the ova of the mosquito and stay in a locale.

Many of the members of this virus family are found in South America, southeastern Europe, Southeast Asia, and Africa and bear the exotic name of their ecological niche. Viruses of the **California encephalitis virus group (e.g., La Crosse virus)** are found in the **forests of North America** and cause human encephalitis in people dwelling in the United States (Figure 60-3). However, more people are infected than exhibit symptoms. These viruses are spread mainly by *Aedes triseriatus,* which breeds in the water in treeholes and discarded tires.

The hantaviruses do not have an arthropod vector but are maintained in a rodent species specific for each virus. Humans are infected by close contact with rodents or through the inhalation of aerosolized rodent urine. In May 1993, an outbreak of **hantavirus pulmonary syndrome** occurred in the Four Corners area of New Mexico. The outbreak is attributed to increased contact with the deer mouse vector during a season of unusually high rainfall, an increased availability of food, and an increase in the rodent population. The Sin Nombre and Convict Creek virus strains were isolated from the victims and rodents. Since this inci-

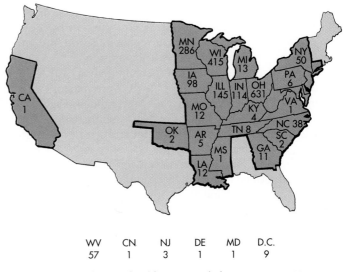

Squirrel (chipmunk) — *Aedes triseriatus* — Transovarial transmission — Human

FIGURE 60-2 Transmission of La Crosse (California) encephalitis virus.

FIGURE 60-3 Distribution of California encephalitis, 1964 to 1989. (Redrawn from Tsai TF: *Infect Dis Clin North Am* 5:73-102, 1991.)

dent, hantavirus has been associated with other outbreaks of respiratory tract disease.

CLINICAL SYNDROMES

Bunyaviridae, which are mosquito-borne viruses, usually cause a nonspecific febrile illness related to the viremia (Table 60-1) that is indistinguishable from illnesses caused by other viruses. The incubation period for these illnesses is approximately 48 hours, and the fevers last approximately 3 days. Most patients with infections, even those infected by agents known to cause severe illness (e.g., Rift Valley fever virus, La Crosse virus), have mild illness. **Encephalitis** illnesses (e.g., La Crosse virus) are sudden in onset after an incubation period of approximately 1 week, and symptoms at this time include fever, headache, lethargy, and vomiting. Seizures occur in 50% of patients with encephalitis, usually early in the illness. Signs of meningeal irritation are present in only one third of patients. The illness lasts an average of 7 days. Death occurs in less than 1% of patients, but seizure disorders may occur as sequelae in as much as 20%. **Hemorrhagic fevers** such as Rift Valley fever are characterized by petechial hemorrhages, ecchymosis, epistaxis, hematemesis, melena, and bleeding of the gums. Death occurs in as many as half of patients with hemorrhagic phenomena. The **hantavirus pulmonary syndrome** is a terrible disease that initiates with a prodrome of fever and muscle aches, which is followed rapidly by interstitial pulmonary edema, respiratory failure, and death within days.

LABORATORY DIAGNOSIS

Serological tests are generally performed to confirm a diagnosis of bunyavirus infection. Virus neutralization assays can be used to identify the virus. IgM-specific assays are useful in the documentation of acute infection. Seroconversion or a fourfold increase in the titer of the IgG antibody is used to document recent infection, but cross-reactions within viral genera are common.

Enzyme-linked immunosorbent assay (ELISA) may detect antigen in clinical specimens from patients with an intense viremia (e.g., Rift Valley fever, hemorrhagic fever with renal syndrome, Crimean hemorrhagic fever). ELISA tests that can detect viral antigen in mosquitoes have been developed.

The Sin Nombre and Convict Creek hantaviruses were identified using the reverse transcriptase polymerase chain reaction. Viral RNA from patient tissue was converted to complementary DNA using the reverse transcriptase of a retrovirus and then DNA primers representing conserved sequences of hantaviruses were used to promote synthesis of the characteristic hantavirus sequences.

TREATMENT, PREVENTION, AND CONTROL

No specific therapy for Bunyaviridae infections is available. Human disease is prevented by interrupting the contact between humans and the vector, whether arthropod or mammal. Arthropod vectors are controlled by eliminating the growth conditions for the vector and insecticide spraying and by netting or screening windows and doors, wearing protective clothing, and controlling the tick infestation of animals. Rodent control minimizes the transmission of many viruses, especially hantaviruses. Rift Valley fever vaccines have been developed for use in humans and animals (sheep and cattle).

CASE STUDY AND QUESTIONS

A 15-year-old summer camp counselor in Ohio suddenly complained of a headache, nausea, and vomiting; had a fever; and developed a stiff neck. She was admitted to the hospital, where a spinal tap revealed inflammatory cells. She became lethargic over the next day but became alert again after 4 to 5 days.

1. The physician suspected La Crosse encephalitis virus as the agent. What clues pointed to La Crosse virus?
2. What other agents would also be considered in the differential diagnosis?
3. How was the patient infected?
4. How would the transmission of this agent be prevented?
5. How could the local public health department determine the prevalence of La Crosse virus in the environment of the summer camp? What samples would they obtain and how would they test them?

Bibliography

Bishop DHL, Shope RE: *Bunyaviridae.* In Fraenkel-Conrat H, Wagner RR, editors: *Comprehensive virology,* vol 14, New York, 1979, Plenum.

Fields BN, Knipe DM, Howley PM, editors: *Virology,* ed 3, New York, 1996, Lippincott-Raven.

Kolakofsky D: Bunyaviridae, *Curr Top Microbiol Immunol* 169:1-256, 1991.

McKee KT, LeDuc JW, Peters CJ: *Hantaviruses.* In Belshe RB, editor: *Textbook of human virology,* ed 2, St Louis, 1991, Mosby.

Peters CJ, LeDuc JW: *Bunyaviruses, phleboviruses and related viruses.* In Belshe RB, editor: *Textbook of human virology,* ed 2, St Louis, 1991, Mosby.

Tsai TF: Arboviral infections in the United States, *Infect Dis Clin North Am* 5:73-102, 1991.

Wrobel S: Serendipity, science and a new hantavirus, *FASEB J* 9:1247-1254, 1995.

Retroviruses

The retroviruses are probably the most studied group of viruses in molecular biology. These viruses are **enveloped, positive-strand RNA** viruses with a unique morphology and means of replication. In 1970, Baltimore and Temin showed that the retroviruses encode an RNA-dependent DNA polymerase (**reverse transcriptase**) and replicate through a DNA intermediate. The DNA copy of the viral genome is then integrated into the host chromosome to become a cellular gene. This discovery, which earned the Nobel Prize, contradicted the central dogma of molecular biology—that genetic information passed from DNA to RNA and then to protein.

The first retrovirus to be isolated was the Rous sarcoma virus, shown by Peyton Rous to produce solid tumors (sarcomas) in chickens. Like most retroviruses, the Rous sarcoma virus proved to have a very limited host and species range. Cancer-causing retroviruses have since been isolated from other animal species and are classified as RNA tumor viruses or oncornaviruses. Many of these viruses alter cellular growth by expressing analogues of cellular growth–controlling genes (**oncogenes**). Not until 1981, however, when Robert Gallo and his associates isolated human T-lymphotropic virus (HTLV-1) from a person with adult human T-cell leukemia, was a human retrovirus isolated and associated with human disease.

In the late 1970s and early 1980s an unusual number of young homosexual men, Haitians, heroin addicts, and hemophiliacs (the initial "4H club" of risk groups) were noted to be dying of normally benign opportunistic infections. Their symptoms defined a new disease, acquired immunodeficiency syndrome (AIDS). However, as is now known, AIDS proved not to be limited to these groups but can occur in anyone exposed to the virus. Now approximately 8 million men, women, and children around the world have AIDS, and a further 22 million are infected with the virus that causes AIDS. Montagnier and associates in Paris and Gallo and co-workers in the United States reported the isolation of the **human immunodeficiency virus (HIV-1)** from patients with lymphadenopathy and AIDS. A variant of HIV-1, designated **HIV-2,** was isolated later and is prevalent in West

Africa. Understanding this disease and its agents has become the infectious disease challenge of the 1990s.

Our understanding of the retroviruses has paralleled progress in molecular biology. In turn, the retroviruses have provided a major tool for molecular biology, the reverse transcriptase enzyme, and through the study of viral oncogenes have also provided a means of advancing our understanding of cell growth, differentiation, and oncogenesis.

The three subfamilies of human retroviruses are the **Oncornavirinae,** or oncovirus (HTLV-1, HTLV-2, HTLV-5); the **Lentivirinae** (HIV-1, HIV-2); and the **Spumavirinae** (Table 61-1). Although spumavirus was the first human retrovirus to be isolated, no such virus has been associated with human disease. **Endogenous retroviruses,** the ultimate parasite, have integrated and are transmitted vertically as part of the host chromatin. Although they may not replicate, their gene sequences have been detected in many animal species and in humans.

The pathogenic human retroviruses include **HTLV-1** and **HTLV-2,** which as just noted are oncoviruses, and **HIV-1** and **HIV-2,** which are lentiviruses. HTLV-1 and HIV-1 infect CD4 T cells, are spread by similar means, and have long latency periods. Nonetheless they cause very different diseases because of the way in which they interact with the infected host cell.

CLASSIFICATION

The retroviruses are classified by the diseases they cause, tissue tropism and host range, virion morphology, and genetic complexity (Table 61-1). The oncoviruses include the only retroviruses that can immortalize or transform target cells. These viruses are also categorized by the morphology of their core and capsid as type A, B, C, or D, as seen in electron micrographs (Table 61-1 and Figure 61-1). The lentiviruses are slow viruses associated with neurological and immunosuppressive diseases. The spumaviruses, represented by a foamy virus, cause a distinct cytopathological effect but as already noted do not seem to cause clinical disease.

TABLE 61-1   Classification of Retroviruses

SUBFAMILY	CHARACTERISTICS	EXAMPLES
Oncovirinae	Are associated with cancer and neurological disorders	—
B	Have eccentric nucleocapsid core in mature virion	Mouse mammary tumor virus
C	Have centrally located nucleocapsid core in mature virion	Human T-lymphotropic virus* (HTLV-1, HTLV-2, HTLV-5), Rous sarcoma virus (chickens)
D	Have nucleocapsid core with cylindrical form	Mason-Pfizer monkey virus
Lentivirinae	Have slow onset of disease: cause neurological disorders and immunosuppression; are viruses with D-type, cylindrical nucleocapsid core	Human immunodeficiency virus* (HIV-1, HIV-2), visna virus (sheep), caprine arthritis/encephalitis virus (goats)
Spumavirinae	Cause no clinical disease but characteristic vacuolated "foamy" cytopathology	Human foamy virus*
Endogenous viruses	Have retrovirus sequences that are integrated into human genome	Human placental virus

*Also classified as complex retroviruses because of the requirement for accessory proteins for replication.

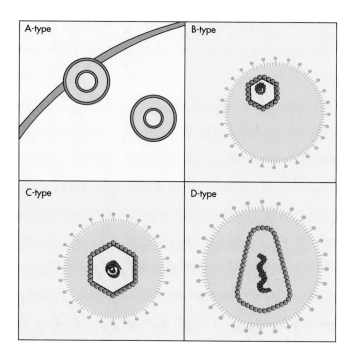

FIGURE 61-1 Morphological distinction of retrovirions. The morphology and position of the nucleocapsid core are used to classify the viruses. A-type particles are immature intracytoplasmic forms that bud through the plasma membrane into mature B-type, C-type, and D-type particles.

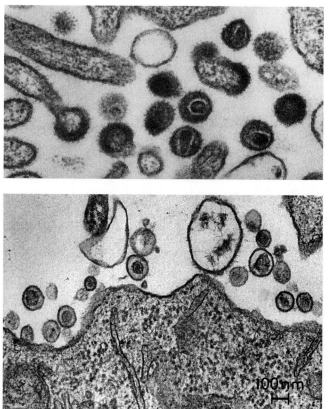

FIGURE 61-2 Electron micrographs of two retroviruses. **A,** HIV-1. Note the cone-shaped nucleocapsid in several of the virions. **B,** HTLV. Note the C-type morphology characterized by a central symmetrical nucleocapsid. (From Belshe RB, editor: *Textbook of human virology,* ed 2, St Louis, 1991, Mosby.)

STRUCTURE

The retroviruses are roughly spherical, enveloped RNA viruses with a diameter of 80 to 120 nm (Figure 61-2 and Box 61-1). The envelope contains viral glycoproteins and is acquired by budding from the plasma membrane. The envelope surrounds a capsid that contains **two identical copies of the positive-strand RNA genome** inside an electron-dense core. The virion also contains 10 to 50 copies of the **reverse transcriptase** and **integrase** enzymes and **two cellular transfer RNAs (tRNAs)**. These tRNAs are base-paired to each copy of the genome to be used as a primer for the reverse transcriptase. The morphology of the core differs for different viruses and is used as a means of classifying the retroviruses (Figure 61-1). The HIV virion core resembles a truncated cone (Figure 61-3).

The retrovirus genome has a 5′ cap and is polyadenylated at the 3′ end (Figure 61-4 and Table 61-2). Although the genome resembles a messenger RNA (mRNA), it is not infectious because it does not encode a polymerase that can directly generate more mRNA. The genome of the *simple retroviruses* consists of **three major genes** that encode polyproteins for the following enzymatic and structural proteins of the virus: **gag** (group-specific antigen, *capsid proteins*), **pol** (*polymerase, protease, and integrase*), and **env** (envelope, glycoproteins). At each end of the genome are **long-terminal repeat (LTR)** sequences. The LTR sequences contain promoters, enhancers, and other gene sequences used for binding different cellular transcription factors. Oncogenic

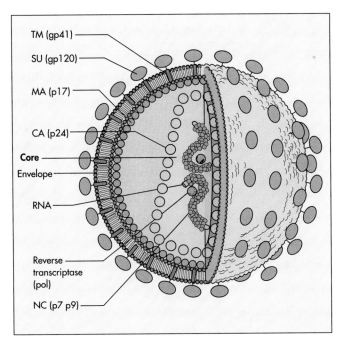

FIGURE 61-3 Cross section of HIV. The enveloped virion contains two identical RNA strands, RNA polymerase, integrase, and two tRNAs base-paired to the genome within the protein core. This is surrounded by proteins and a lipid bilayer. The envelope spikes are the glycoprotein (gp) 120 attachment protein and gp41 fusion protein. (Redrawn from Gallo RC, Montagnier L: *Sci Am* 259:41-51, 1988.)

FIGURE 61-4 Genomic structure of human retroviruses. **A,** HTLV-1. **B,** HIV-1. The genes are defined in Table 61-2 and Figure 61-7. Unlike the other genes of these viruses, production of the messenger RNA for tax and rex (HTLV-1) and tat and rev (HIV) requires the excision of two intron units. HIV-2 has a similar genome map. The vpu for HIV-2 is termed *vpx*. LTR, Long-terminal repeat. Protein nomenclature for HIV: *ma*, matrix protein; *ca*, capsid protein; *nc*, nucleocapsid protein; *pr*, protease; *rt*, reverse transcriptase; *in*, integrase; *su*, surface glycoprotein component; *tm*, transmembrane glycoprotein component. (Redrawn from Belshe RB, editor: *Textbook of human virology*, ed 2, St Louis, 1991, Mosby.)

TABLE 61-2 Retrovirus Genes and Their Function

GENE	VIRUS	FUNCTION
gag	All	Group-specific antigen: core and capsid proteins
pol	All	Polymerase: reverse transcriptase, protease, integrase
env	All	Envelope: glycoproteins
tax	HTLV	Transactivation of viral and cellular genes
tat	HIV-1	Transactivation of viral and cellular genes
rex	HTLV	Regulation of RNA splicing and promotion of export to cytoplasm
rev	HIV-1	Regulation of RNA splicing and promotion of export to cytoplasm
nef	HIV-1	Alteration of cell activation signals; progression to AIDS (essential)
vif	HIV-1	Virus infectivity, promotion of assembly
vpu	HIV-1	Facilitation of release of virus, decrease of cell surface CD4
vpr (vpx*)	HIV-1	Transport of complementary DNA to nucleus, arresting of cell growth
LTR	All	Promoter, enhancer elements

LTR, Long-terminal repeat (sequences).
*In HIV-2.

viruses may also contain a growth-regulating oncogene that operates at the expense of other sequences. The *complex retroviruses*, HTLV, and the lentiviruses (including HIV) also encode several regulatory proteins that require more complex transcriptional processing (splicing) than the simple retroviruses.

The viral glycoproteins are produced by proteolytic cleavage of the polyprotein encoded by the env gene. The size of the glycoproteins differs for each group of viruses. For example, the (glycoprotein) gp62 of HTLV1 is cleaved into a gp46 and p21, and the gp160 of HIV is cleaved into gp41 and gp120. These glycoproteins form lollipop-like trimer spikes that are visible on the surface of the virion. The larger of the glycoproteins is responsible for producing the tissue tropism of the virus and is recognized by neutralizing antibody. The smaller subunit (gp41 in HIV) forms the lollipop stick and promotes cell-cell fusion. The gp120 of HIV is extensively glycosylated, and its antigenicity can drift during the course of a chronic HIV infection. Both of these factors impede immune clearance of the virus. Detection of these glycoproteins is a useful marker of infection.

REPLICATION

Replication of the retroviruses is initiated by the binding of the viral glycoprotein spikes to specific cell surface receptor proteins (Figure 61-5). *The presence of virus receptors is the initial determinant of the tissue and host tropism of the virus.*

The gp120 of HIV binds with the CD4 surface molecule expressed on T-helper cells and cells of the macrophage lineage (e.g., macrophage, dendritic cells, microglial cells). A second receptor, a 7-transmembrane G-protein–coupled chemokine receptor (fusin [CXCR4] on T cells and CCR5 on macrophages), is also required and further defines the type of target cell (Figure 61-6). HIV enters the cell by fusion of the envelope with the cellular plasma membrane; other retroviruses may enter the cell by receptor-mediated endocytosis.

Once released into the cytoplasm, the reverse transcriptase uses the virion tRNA as a primer and synthesizes a complementary, negative-strand DNA. The reverse transcriptase also acts as a ribonuclease H, degrades the RNA genome, and then synthesizes the positive strand of DNA (**complementary DNA [cDNA]**) (Figure 61-7). During the synthesis of the virion DNA (**provirus**), sequences from each end of the genome (U3 and U5) are duplicated, which attaches the LTRs to both ends. This process creates sequences necessary for integration and also creates enhancer and promoter sequences for the regulation of transcription. The DNA copy of the genome is larger than the original RNA.

Reverse transcriptase is very error prone. For example, the error rate for the reverse transcriptase from HIV is 1 error per 2000 base pairs, or approximately 5 errors per genome (HIV, 9000 base pairs). This genetic instability of HIV is responsible for promoting the generation of new strains of virus during a person's disease, a property that may alter the pathogenicity of the virus and promote immune escape.

The double-stranded cDNA is then delivered to the nucleus and spliced into the host chromosome with the aid of a virus-encoded, virion-carried enzyme, **integrase.** HIV and other lentiviruses produce an abundance of nonintegrated circular DNA, which is not transcribed efficiently but may play a role in the cytopathogenesis of the virus.

Once integrated, the viral DNA is **transcribed as a cellular gene** by the host RNA polymerase II. Transcription of the genome produces a full-length RNA, which for simple retroviruses is processed to produce several mRNAs containing either the gag, gag-pol, or env gene sequences. The full-length transcripts of the genome can also be assembled into new virions.

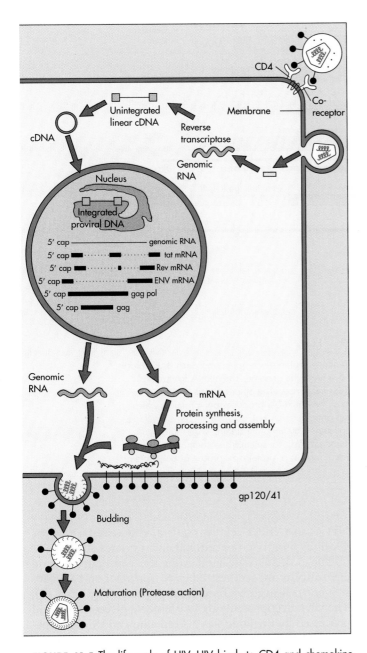

FIGURE 61-5 The life cycle of HIV. HIV binds to CD4 and chemokine co-receptors and enters by fusion. The genome is reverse transcribed into DNA in the cytoplasm and integrated into the nuclear DNA. Transcription and translation of the genome occurs in a fashion similar to that of HTLV-1 (see Figure 61-7). The virus assembles at the plasma membrane and matures after budding from the cell. *cDNA,* Complementary DNA. (Redrawn from Fauci AS: *Science* 239:617-622, 1988.)

FIGURE 61-6 Target cell binding of HIV. (Redrawn from *Science* 274:1988, 1996.)

Because the virus acts as a cellular gene, its replication depends on the ability of the cell to use the enhancers and promoter sequences encoded in the LTR region, the extent of methylation of the viral DNA, and the cell's growth rate. Stimulation of the cell by mitogens, certain lymphokines, or infection with exogenous viruses (e.g., herpesviruses) produces transcription factors that also bind to the LTR and can activate transcription of the

virus. Viral oncogenes (if present) promote cell growth and as a result stimulate transcription and viral replication. *The efficiency of viral transcription is the second major determinant of retroviral tissue tropism and the host range of the virus.*

HTLV and HIV are complex retroviruses. HTLV-1 encodes two proteins, **tax** and **rex,** that regulate viral replication. Unlike the other viral mRNAs, the mRNA for tax and rex requires more than one splicing step. The rex gene encodes two proteins that bind to a structure on the viral mRNA and thereby prevent further splicing and promote mRNA transport to the cytoplasm. The

FIGURE 61-7 Transcription and translation of HTLV-1. (A similar but more complex approach is used for HIV.) All HTLV-1 and HIV mRNA initiate and include the 5' end of the genome. The mRNA for tax and rex requires excision of two sequences, the gag-pol and env sequences. The other mRNAs, including the env mRNA, require excision of one sequence. Translation of these mRNAs produces polyproteins, which are subsequently cleaved. Gene nomenclature: *gag*, group antigen gene; *pol*, polymerase; *env*, envelope glycoprotein gene; *tax*, transactivator; *rex*, regulator of splicing. Protein nomenclature: *MA*, matrix; *CA*, capsid; *NC*, nucleocapsid; *PR*, protease; *SU*, surface component; *TM*, transmembrane component of envelope glycoprotein; *N*, N-terminus; *C*, C-terminus of peptide. Prefixes: *p*, protein; *Pr*, precursor polyprotein; *gp*, glycoprotein; *gPr*, glcosylated precursor polyprotein.

doubly spliced tax/rex mRNA is expressed early (low concentration of rex), and structural proteins are expressed late (high concentration of rex). Late in the infection, rex selectively enhances the expression of the singly spliced structural genes, which are required in abundance. The tax protein is a transcriptional activator *(in trans)*. Tax enhances transcription of the viral genome from the promoter gene sequence in the 5' LTR, as well as other genes, including the lymphokine genes for interleukin-2 (IL-2), IL-3, and granulocyte-macrophage colony-stimulating factor and the receptor for IL-2. Activation of these genes leads to activation and growth of the infected T cell.

HIV replication is regulated by as many as six "accessory" gene products (Table 61-2). The **tat,** like tax, is a transactivator of the transcription of viral and cellular genes. The **rev** acts like the rex protein. The **nef** protein reduces cell surface CD4 expression, alters T-cell signaling pathways, regulates the cytotoxicity of the virus, and is required to maintain high viral loads. The nef protein appears to be essential for causing the infection to progress to AIDS. The **vif** protein promotes assembly and maturation. The **vpu** reduces cell surface CD4 expression and enhances virion release. The **vpr** (vpx in HIV-2) is required to give the virus a growth advantage.

HIV is also under cellular control, and activation of the T cell by a mitogen or antigen also activates the virus.

The proteins translated from the gag, gag-pol, and env mRNAs are synthesized as polyproteins and are subsequently cleaved to functional proteins (Figure 61-7). The viral glycoproteins are synthesized, glycosylated, and processed by the endoplasmic reticulum and Golgi apparatus. These glycoproteins are then cleaved into a membrane spanning and an extracellular region and associate to form trimers that migrate to the plasma membrane.

The gag and the gag-pol polyproteins are acylated and then bind to the plasma membrane containing the envelope glycoprotein. The association of two copies of the genome and cellular tRNA molecules promotes budding of the virion. After its envelopment and release from the cell, the **viral protease** cleaves the gag and gag-pol polyproteins. This action releases the reverse transcriptase and forms the virion core and is *required* for the production of infectious virions. The protease is a target for antiviral drugs.

The envelopment and release of retroviruses occur at the cell surface. HIV can also spread from cell to cell through the production of multinucleated giant cells, or syncytia. Syncytia are fragile, and their formation enhances the cytolytic activity of the virus.

Disease Mechanisms of HIV

HIV primarily infects CD4 T cells and cells of the macrophage lineage (e.g., monocytes, macrophages, alveolar macrophages of the lung, dendritic cells of the skin, and microglial cells of the brain).

Virus causes lytic infection of CD4 T cells and persistent low-level productive infection of macrophage lineage cells.

Virus causes syncytia formation, with cells expressing large amounts of CD4 antigen (T cells) with subsequent lysis of the cells.

Virus alters T-cell and macrophage cell function.

TABLE 61-3	**Means of HIV Escape from the Immune System**

CHARACTERISTIC	FUNCTION
Infection of lymphocytes and macrophages	Inactivation of key element of immune defense
Inactivation of CD4 helper cells	Loss of activator of the immune system and DTH response
Antigenic drift of gp120	Evasion of antibody detection
Heavy glycosylation of gp120	Evasion of antibody detection

HUMAN IMMUNODEFICIENCY VIRUS
Pathogenesis and Immunity

The major determinant in the pathogenesis and disease caused by HIV is the virus tropism for **CD4-expressing T cells and macrophages** (Box 61-2 and Figure 61-8). HIV-induced immunosuppression (AIDS) results from a reduction in the number of CD4 T cells, which decimates the helper and delayed-type hypersensitivity (DTH) functions of the immune response.

Initially, infection occurs in macrophages with a macrophage tropic virus directed toward the CD4 molecule and the CC CKR5 chemokine receptor. T-cell tropic strains, which recognize CD4 and the fusin chemokine receptor, evolve later in the infection. Chemokines are small peptides involved in promoting inflammatory reactions, and their receptors are guanosine triphosphate–binding, protein-coupled receptors. A small percentage of people are resistant to infection because they are genetically deficient in these co-receptors.

The course of the disease parallels the CD4 T-cell numbers and the amount of virus in the blood (Figure 61-9). Initially, there is a large burst of virus production and viremia, which corresponds to the occurrence of a mononucleosis-like syndrome. Virus levels in the blood decrease during a clinically latent period, but viral replication continues in the lymph nodes. Late in the disease, CD4 levels are significantly decreased, the structure of the lymph nodes is destroyed, and the patient becomes immunosuppressed.

The initial challenge by HIV-1 occurs on filtration through the follicular-dendritic cell network of the germinal centers of the lymph nodes, where **macrophage-lineage cells** become infected. Macrophages are persistently infected with HIV. In fact, monocytes and macrophages are probably the major reservoirs and means of distribution of HIV. Circulating macrophages, microglial cells of the brain, pulmonary alveolar macrophages, dendritic cells, and other cells of the monocyte-macrophage lineage can spread the virus and

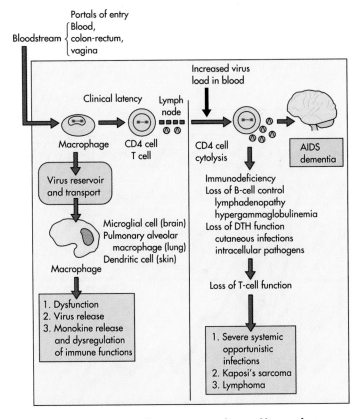

FIGURE 61-8 Pathogenesis of HIV. HIV causes lytic and latent infection of CD4 T cells and persistent infection of cells of the monocyte/macrophage family and disrupts neurons. The outcomes of these actions are immunodeficiency and AIDS dementia. *DTH,* Delayed type hypersensitivity. (Redrawn from Fauci AS: *Science* 239:617-622, 1988.)

potentially contribute to the clinical manifestation of HIV disease.

HIV induces several cytopathological effects that may kill the cell (Table 61-3). These include an accumulation of nonintegrated circular DNA copies of the genome, increased permeability of the plasma membrane, syncytial formation, and the induction of apoptosis (programmed cell death). The relative ability of HIV to kill the target cell correlates with the amount of CD4 expressed by the cell. Macrophages may be spared the cytolytic action of HIV because they express less CD4 than T cells. The accessory proteins of HIV are important for replication and virulence. As noted earlier, the **nef** protein appears to be essential for promoting the progression of HIV infection to AIDS. Individuals infected with natural mutants of nef and primates infected with the simian immunodeficiency virus (SIV), which lacks nef, have lived beyond their expected lifetimes.

Continual replication of the virus occurs in the lymph nodes, with subsequent release of the virus and infected T cells into the blood. **Reductions in the numbers of CD4 T cells may result from HIV-induced cytolysis, cytotoxic T-cell immune cytolysis, or the natural terminal differentiation of T cells, which would occur in response to the large HIV antigen challenge.** The increased release of virus into the blood as the numbers of CD4 cells decrease correlates directly with the development of the symptoms of AIDS (Figure 61-9).

The central role of the CD4 helper T cells in the initiation of an immune response and DTH is indicated by the extent of immunosuppression induced by HIV infection (Figure 61-10). Activation of the CD4 T cells is one of the first steps in the initiation of a normal immune response. Helper T cells then release lymphokines and the interferon-gamma required for the activation of macrophages, other T cells, B cells, and natural killer cells. When CD4 T cells are unavailable or not functional, antigen-specific immune responses (especially cellular immune responses) are incapacitated, and humoral responses are uncontrolled. The loss of the CD4 T cells responsible for producing DTH allows the outgrowth of many of the opportunistic intracellular infections characteristic of AIDS.

In addition to immunosuppressive disorders, HIV can also cause neurological abnormalities. The microglial cell and macrophage are the predominant cell type of the brain infected with HIV, but neurons and glial cells may also be infected. Infected monocytes and microglial cells may release neurotoxic substances or chemotactic factors that promote inflammatory responses in the brain. Direct cytopathological effects of the virus on neurons are also possible.

The immune response to HIV restricts viral infection but contributes to pathogenesis. For example, neutraliz-

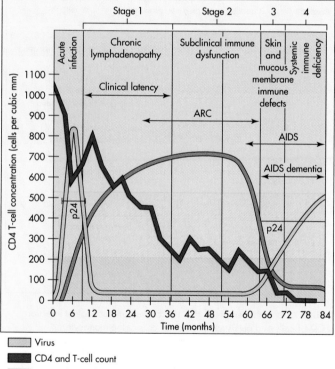

FIGURE 61-9 Time course and stages of HIV disease. A long clinical latency period follows the initial mononucleosis-like symptoms. The progressive decrease in the number of CD4 T cells, even during the latency period, allows opportunistic infections to occur. The stages (World Health Organization and Centers for Disease Control and Prevention) in HIV disease are defined by the CD4 T-cell levels and occurrence of opportunistic diseases. *ARC,* AIDS-related complex. (Redrawn from Redfield RR, Buske DS: *Sci Am* 259:90-98, 1988, updated 1996.)

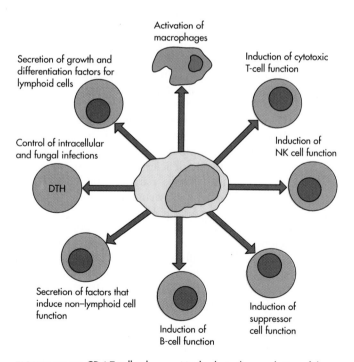

FIGURE 61-10 CD4 T cells play a critical role in the regulation of the human immune response by mediating the release of soluble factors and the DTH response toward intracellular pathogens. HIV-induced loss of the CD4 T cells results in loss of the functions shown, especially the DTH responses and the lymphokine control of immune responses. (Redrawn from Fauci AS: *Science* 239:617-622, 1988.)

ing antibodies are generated against gp120 and also participate in antibody-dependent cellular cytotoxicity responses. Antibody-coated virus is infectious, however, and is taken up by macrophages.

In addition, CD8 T cells generated in response to the HIV-infected CD4 T cells produce suppressive factors that restrict viral replication, including chemokines that also block the binding of virus to its co-receptor. CD8 T cells promote direct cytotoxic activity, which reduces the number of HIV-infected cells but also reduces the number of CD4 T cells. Other cell-mediated and cytokine responses may suppress the replication of HIV and limit the progression of disease after the initial acute phase of infection. However, the ability of HIV to incapacitate the immune system, persist in macrophages and lymphocytes, and alter its antigenicity allows the virus to escape immune clearance and prevents resolution of the disease (Table 61-3).

Epidemiology

AIDS was first noted in male homosexuals in the United States but has spread in epidemic proportions through-out the population (Box 61-3). As of mid-1996, an estimated 28 million people have been infected with HIV, with an estimated 7.7 million cases of AIDS since 1970 (according to UNAIDS-WHO data) (Figures 61-11 and 61-12). All HIV-infected people whose disease has progressed to AIDS are expected to die of the complications of the disease.

HIV is thought to be derived from an SIV, and in fact HIV-2 is similar to SIV. The initial human infection may have occurred in Africa relatively recently but went unnoticed in rural areas. The migration of infected people to the cities after the 1960s brought the virus into population centers; cultural acceptance of prostitution promoted its transmission throughout the population.

Transmission

The presence of HIV in the **blood, semen,** and **vaginal secretions** of infected people and the long incubation period are factors that have promoted the spread of the disease through sexual contact and exposure to contaminated blood and blood products (Table 61-4). The virus can also be transmitted perinatally to newborns. HIV is *not*, however, transmitted by casual contact, touching, hugging, kissing, coughing, sneezing, insect bites, water,

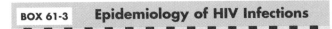

BOX 61-3 Epidemiology of HIV Infections

DISEASE/VIRAL FACTORS

Enveloped virus is easily inactivated and must be transmitted in body fluids.

Disease has long prodromal period.

Virus can be shed before development of identifiable symptoms.

TRANSMISSION

Virus is present in blood, semen, and vaginal secretions.

See Table 61-4 for modes of transmission.

WHO IS AT RISK?

Intravenous drug abusers; sexually active people with multiple partners (homosexual and heterosexual); prostitutes; newborns of HIV-positive mothers.

Blood and organ transplant recipients and hemophiliacs: before 1985.

GEOGRAPHY/SEASON

There is an expanding epidemic worldwide.

There is no seasonal incidence.

MODES OF CONTROL

Antiviral drugs limit progression of disease.

Vaccines for prevention and treatment are in trials.

Safe, monogamous sex helps limit spread.

Sterile injection needles should be used.

Large-scale screening programs have been developed for blood for transfusions, organs for transplants, and clotting factors used by hemophiliacs.

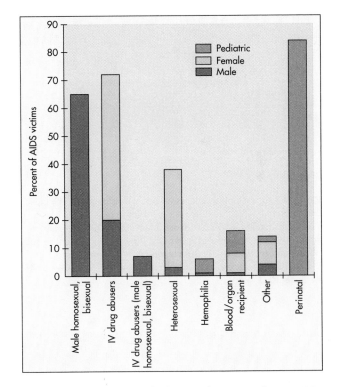

FIGURE 61-11 AIDS statistics for the United States as of June 1992. The percentages of AIDS cases are presented by exposure category for men, women, and children under 13. Unlike Africa and many other parts of the world, in the United States, male homosexuals are the largest exposure category. However, intravenous *(IV)* drug abusers and heterosexual partners are becoming more prevalent. (Data reported by the Centers for Disease Control and Prevention and published in *AIDS* 6:1229-1233, 1992.)

TABLE 61-4 Transmission of HIV Infection

ROUTES	SPECIFIC TRANSMISSION
KNOWN ROUTES OF TRANSMISSION	
Inoculation in blood	Transfusion of blood and blood products
	Needle sharing among intravenous drug abusers
	Needlestick, open wound, and mucous membrane exposure in health care workers
	Tattoo needles
Sexual transmission	Anal and vaginal intercourse
Perinatal transmission	Intrauterine transmission
	Peripartum transmission
	Breast milk
ROUTES NOT INVOLVED IN TRANSMISSION	
Close personal contact	Household members
	Health care workers not exposed to blood

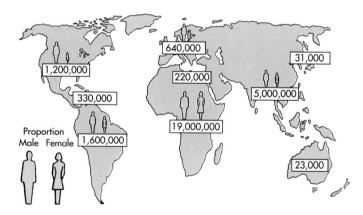

FIGURE 61-12 Estimated cumulative global distribution of HIV infections as of mid-1996. The estimated cumulative global total of HIV-infected adults in 1996 is about 27.9 million. Infection rates vary widely in different regions of the world. The highest rates are in sub-Saharan Africa, where 1 in 20 men and 1 in 20 women are estimated to be infected. (Modified from UNAIDS/COS/SG96017-fbw, June 30, 1996.)

food, or utensils or in toilets, swimming pools, or public baths.

Populations at Highest Risk

Sexually active people (homosexual *and* heterosexual), intravenous drug abusers and their sexual partners, and the newborns of HIV-positive mothers are at highest risk for HIV infections, with blacks and Hispanics disproportionally represented in the HIV-positive population.

As already noted, AIDS was initially observed in young, promiscuous male homosexuals and is still preva-

lent in the gay community. Anal intercourse is an efficient means of viral transmission. However, heterosexual transmission by vaginal intercourse and intravenous drug abuse have become the major routes by which HIV is being spread in the population. Its prevalence in drug abusers stems from the sharing of contaminated syringe needles, a common practice in "shooting galleries." In New York City alone more than 80% of intravenous drug abusers are positive for the HIV antibody, and these people are now the major source of heterosexual and congenital transmission of the virus.

Before 1985, people receiving blood transfusions or organ transplants and hemophiliacs receiving clotting factors from pooled blood were at high risk for HIV infection. Now, however, screening of the blood supply in the United States has practically eliminated the danger of HIV being transmitted in blood transfusions. Hemophiliacs who receive pooled clotting factors are protected further by the proper handling of the factor (prolonged heating) to kill the virus. However, as much as 60% of hemophiliacs may be positive for the HIV antibody as the result of prior exposure to HIV-contaminated factor VIII pooled from thousands of donors.

Relatively few health care workers have contracted HIV infection from accidental needlesticks or cuts or through the exposure of broken skin to contaminated blood. Prospective studies of needlestick victims have shown that seroconversion occurs in fewer than 1% of those exposed to HIV-positive blood. Tattoo needles and contaminated inks are other potential means by which HIV can be transmitted.

Geographical Distribution

HIV-1 infections are spreading worldwide, with the largest number of AIDS cases in sub-Saharan Africa, but with a growing number of cases in Asia, the United States, and the rest of the world (Figure 61-11). HIV-2 is more prevalent in Africa (especially West Africa) than in the United States. Heterosexual transmission is the major means of spread of HIV-1 and HIV-2 in Africa, and both men and women are equally affected by these viruses. HIV-2 produces a disease similar to but less severe than AIDS.

Clinical Syndromes

AIDS is one of the most devastating epidemics ever recorded. Most HIV-infected people will become symptomatic, and the overwhelming majority of these will ultimately succumb to the disease. HIV disease may be viewed as a continuum ranging from an asymptomatic infection to profound immunosuppression, sometimes referred to as *full-blown AIDS* (Figure 61-12). The diseases related to AIDS mainly consist of opportunistic infections, cancers, and the direct effects of HIV on the central nervous system (Table 61-5). Although rare, there are cases of long-term survivors, but these result from infection with HIV strains that lack a functional nef protein. Resistance to the virus correlates with a lack of

TABLE 61-5	Indicator Diseases of AIDS*
INFECTION	**DISEASE**
Opportunistic infections	
Protozoal	Toxoplasmosis of the brain
	Cryptosporidiosis with diarrhea
	Isosporiasis with diarrhea
Fungal	Candidiasis of the esophagus, trachea, and lungs
	Pneumocystis carinii pneumonia
	Cryptococcosis (extrapulmonary)
	Histoplasmosis (disseminated)
	Coccidioidomycosis (disseminated)
Viral	Cytomegalovirus disease
	Herpes simplex virus infection (persisting or disseminated)
	Progressive multifocal leukoencephalopathy
	Hairy leukoplakia caused by Epstein-Barr virus
Bacterial	*Mycobacterium avium-intracellulare* complex (disseminated)
	Any "atypical" mycobacterial disease
	Extrapulmonary tuberculosis
	Salmonella septicemia (recurrent)
	Pyogenic bacterial infections (multiple or recurrent)
Opportunistic neoplasias	Kaposi's sarcoma
	Primary lymphoma of the brain
	Other non-Hodgkin's lymphomas
Others	HIV wasting syndrome
	HIV encephalopathy
	Lymphoid interstitial pneumonia

Modified from Belshe RB: editor: *Textbook of human virology*, ed 2, St Louis, 1991, Mosby.

*Manifestations of HIV infection–defining AIDS according to criteria of Centers for Disease Control and Prevention.

expression of the chemokine co-receptor for the virus.

The symptoms of initial HIV infection may resemble those of influenza or infectious mononucleosis, with an "aseptic" meningitis or a rash occurring up to 3 months after infection. As in mononucleosis, the symptoms stem from immune responses triggered by a widespread infection of lymphoid cells. These symptoms subside spontaneously after 2 to 3 weeks and are followed by a period of asymptomatic infection or a persistent generalized lymphadenopathy that may last for years. During this period, the virus is replicating in the lymph nodes.

A deterioration of the immune response is indicated by an increased susceptibility to opportunistic pathogens, especially those controlled by CD4 T-cell DTH responses (e.g., yeasts, herpesviruses). The onset of symptoms correlates with a reduction in the number of CD4

T cells to less than 450/μl and increased levels of virus and protein p24 in the blood. Full-blown AIDS occurs when the CD4 T-cell counts are less than 200/μl and involves the onset of more significant diseases, including HIV wasting syndrome (weight loss and diarrhea for more than 1 month) and the occurrence of indicator diseases such as **Kaposi's sarcoma** or specific opportunistic diseases, especially *Pneumocystis carinii* **pneumonia,** *Mycobacterium avium-intracellulare* **complex infection,** and severe **cytomegalovirus** disease (Table 61-5).

AIDS may manifest in one of several different ways, including lymphadenopathy and fever, opportunistic infections, malignancies, and AIDS-related dementia.

Lymphadenopathy and Fever

Lymphadenopathy and fever can occur, and this combination of clinical findings has been called the *AIDS-related complex (ARC)*. It is a process that develops insidiously and may be accompanied by weight loss and malaise. These findings may persist indefinitely or may progress. Symptoms may also include opportunistic infections, diarrhea, night sweats, and fatigue. The wasting disease is termed *slim disease* in Africa.

Opportunistic Infections

Normally benign infections caused by agents such as yeast and other fungi, DNA viruses capable of recurrent disease, parasites, and intracellular-growing bacteria cause significant disease after the HIV depletion of CD4 T cells. *Pneumocystis carinii* pneumonia is a major sign of AIDS. Oral candidiasis (thrush), cerebral toxoplasmosis, and cryptococcal meningitis also often occur, as do prolonged and severe infections caused by the herpesviruses (e.g., herpes simplex virus; varicella-zoster virus; Epstein-Barr virus [induced hairy leukoplakia of the mouth]; cytomegalovirus [especially retinitis, pneumonia, and bowel disease]; papovaviruses [JC virus causing progressive multifocal leukoencephalopathy]). Tuberculosis and other mycobacterial diseases and diarrhea caused by common pathogens (*Salmonella, Shigella,* and *Campylobacter* species) and uncommon agents (cryptosporidia, mycobacteria, *Amoeba* species) are also frequent problems.

Malignancies

The most notable malignancy to develop in patients with AIDS is Kaposi's sarcoma, an otherwise benign skin cancer that disseminates to involve visceral organs in immunodeficient patients. Non-Hodgkin's lymphoma and Epstein-Barr virus–related lymphomas are also prevalent.

AIDS-Related Dementia

AIDS-related dementia may result from HIV infection of the microglial cells and neurons of the brain. Patients with this condition may undergo a slow deterioration of their intellectual abilities and other signs of a neurological disorder, similar to the signs of the early stages of Alzheimer's disease. Neurological deterioration could also result from infection with one of the many opportunistic infections.

Laboratory Diagnosis

Tests for HIV infection are performed for one of three reasons: to identify those with the infection so that antiviral drug therapy can be initiated, to identify carriers who may transmit infection to others (specifically blood or organ donors, pregnant women, and sex partners), and to confirm the diagnosis of AIDS (Table 61-6). The chronic nature of the disease allows the use of serological tests to document HIV infection. Unfortunately, serological tests cannot identify recently infected people. The finding of the p24 viral antigen, virus, reverse transcriptase, or viral RNA indicates the presence of recent infection or late-stage disease (Figure 61-12). The virus is not routinely isolated. Viral RNA in blood can be detected by the reverse transcriptase–polymerase chain reaction (RT-PCR) method.

Serology

Enzyme-linked immunosorbent assays (ELISAs) or agglutination procedures are used for routine screening. The ELISA test, however, can yield false-positive results. More specific procedures, such as the Western blot analysis, are subsequently used to confirm seropositive results. The Western blot assay (see Figure 53-13), on the other hand, determines the presence of antibody to the viral antigens (p24 or p31) and glycoproteins (gp41 and gp120/160). HIV antibody may develop slowly, taking 4 to 8 weeks in most patients; however, it may take 6 months or more in as much as 5% of those infected (Figure 61-12).

Culture

It is more difficult to culture HIV than many other viruses of human importance, so culture is not done routinely. The virus is cell associated, and for this reason co-culture of the patient's peripheral blood mononuclear cells with those from non–HIV-infected donors in the presence of IL-2 is necessary. Culture appears to detect even latent virus. Characteristic cytopathological effects include syncytia formation and cytolysis.

Immunological Studies

The status of an HIV infection can be determined from an analysis of the T-cell subsets. The absolute **number of CD4 lymphocytes** and the ratio of helper to inducer lymphocytes (**CD4:CD8 ratio**) are abnormally low in HIV-infected people. The particular concentration of CD4 lymphocytes identifies the stage of AIDS.

Treatment, Prevention, and Control

Treatment

An extensive effort to develop antiviral drugs and vaccines effective against HIV has been initiated worldwide. The principal (as of summer 1997) anti-HIV therapies are listed in Box 61-4. The anti-HIV drugs approved by the U.S. Food and Drug Administration can be classified as **nucleoside analogue reverse transcriptase inhibitors, nonnucleoside reverse transcriptase inhibitors,** or **protease inhibitors.** Azidothymidine (AZT), dideoxyinosine (ddI), and dideoxycytidine (ddC) and the other nucleotide analogues are phosphorylated by cellular enzymes, inhibit the reverse transcriptase, and after incorporation into DNA, cause chain termination. Nonnucleoside reverse transcriptase inhibitors (nevirapine) inhibit the enzyme by other mechanisms. Protease inhibitors block the morphogenesis of the

---

TABLE 61-6   Laboratory Analysis for HIV

TEST	PURPOSE
Serology	
ELISA	Initial screening
Latex agglutination	Initial screening
Western blot analysis	Confirmation test
Immunofluorescence	Confirmation test
Virion RNA RT-PCR	Detection of virus in blood
p24 antigen	Early marker of infection
Isolation of virus	Test not readily available
CD4:CD8 T-cell ratio	Correlate of HIV disease

RT-PCR, Reverse transcriptase–polymerase chain reaction.

BOX 61-4   Potential Antiviral Therapies for HIV Infection

NUCLEOSIDE ANALOGUE REVERSE TRANSCRIPTASE INHIBITORS
Azidothymidine (AZT) (Zidovudine)
Dideoxycytidine (ddC) (Zalcitabine)
Dideoxyinosine (ddI) (Didanosine)
d4T (Stavudine)
3TC (Lamivudine)

NONNUCLEOSIDE REVERSE TRANSCRIPTASE INHIBITORS
Nevirapine
Delavirdine

PROTEASE INHIBITORS
Saquinavir
Ritonavir
Indinavir
Nelfinavir

COMBINATION THERAPY
Indinavir/AZT/3TC
Ritonavir/AZT/3TC
Nelfinavir/AZT/3TC
Nevirapine/AZT/ddI
Nevirapine/indinavir/3TC

virion by inhibiting the cleavage of the gag and gag-pol polyproteins. This prevents activation of the virion.

Other anti-HIV drugs being developed include different nucleotide analogues and other inhibitors of reverse transcriptase, receptor antagonists (CD4 and gp120 analogues), inhibitors of tat function (Ro 24-7429), glycoprotein glycosylation inhibitors, interferon and interferon inducers, and antisense DNA to essential genome sequences (see Chapter 47).

In the current guidelines, AZT is recommended for the treatment of asymptomatic or mildly symptomatic people with CD4 counts of less than 500/μl and for the treatment of infected pregnant women to reduce the likelihood of transmission of the virus to the fetus. The significant toxic side effects associated with high-dose AZT therapy can be minimized by administering AZT early in the disease and in smaller, multiple doses. Unfortunately, the high mutation rate of HIV promotes the development of **resistance** to these drugs. **A cocktail of several antiviral drugs** (e.g., *AZT, 3TC, protease inhibitor*), each with different mechanisms of action, has less potential to breed resistance and has become a recommended therapy. Multidrug therapy can reduce blood levels of virus to nearly zero and reduce morbidity and mortality in many AIDS patients with advanced disease.

Education

The principal way in which HIV infection can be controlled is by educating the population regarding the methods of transmission and the measures that may curtail viral spread. For instance, monogamous relationships, the practice of safe sex, and the use of condoms reduce the possibility of exposure. Because contaminated needles are a major source of HIV in intravenous drug abusers, people must be taught that needles must not be shared. The reuse of contaminated needles in clinics was the source of outbreaks of AIDS in the former Soviet Bloc and other countries. In some places, efforts have been launched to provide sterile equipment to intravenous drug abusers.

Blood and Blood Product Screening

Potential blood donors are screened before they donate blood, and blood products are screened before use. People testing positive for HIV must not donate blood. People who anticipate a future need for blood, such as those awaiting elective surgery, should consider donating blood beforehand. To limit the worldwide epidemic, blood screening must be initiated in underdeveloped nations as well.

Infection Control

The infection-control procedures for HIV infection are the same as those for the hepatitis B virus. They include the use of universal blood and body fluid precautions, which were founded on the assumption that all patients are infectious for HIV and other blood-borne pathogens. The precautions include the wearing of protective clothing (e.g., gloves, mask, gown) and the use of other barriers to prevent exposure to blood products. Contaminated surfaces should be disinfected with 10% household bleach, 70% ethanol or isopropanol, 2% glutaraldehyde, 4% formaldehyde, or 6% hydrogen peroxide. The washing of laundry in hot water with detergent should be sufficient to inactivate HIV.

Vaccine Development

No vaccine against HIV is available. A successful vaccine would prevent acquisition of the virus by adults and transmission of the virus to infants of HIV-positive mothers and also block the progression of the disease.

Most HIV vaccines being investigated use gp120 or its precursor, gp160, as the immunogen. The gene for this protein has been cloned, expressed in different eukaryotic cell systems (e.g., yeast, baculovirus), and developed as a subunit vaccine. The env gene has also been incorporated into the vaccinia virus to create a hybrid vaccine. Specific epitopes and T-cell antigens are also being investigated as possible peptide vaccines. DNA vaccines consisting of eukaryotic expression vectors (plasmids) containing the gene for gp160 or other HIV genes is the newest approach to immunization.

The development of a vaccine against HIV is fraught, however, with several problems unique to the virus. For instance, initial protection would require the production of secretory antibody to prevent the sexual transmission and acquisition of the virus. Both antibody and cell-mediated immunity are necessary to protect against HIV infection. In addition, the antigenicity of the virus changes readily through mutation. A further problem is that the virus can be spread through syncytia and also remains latent, thereby hiding from antibody. HIV also infects and inactivates the cells required to initiate an immune response. Testing of the vaccine would be a problem because HIV is a human disease and long-term follow-up is required to monitor the efficacy of the vaccine.

HUMAN T-LYMPHOTROPIC VIRUS AND OTHER ONCOGENIC RETROVIRUSES

The Oncovirinae were originally called the *RNA tumor viruses* and have been associated with the development of leukemias, sarcomas, and lymphomas in many animals. These viruses are **not cytolytic**. The members of this family are distinguished by the mechanism of cell transformation and thus the length of the latency period between infection and the development of disease (Table 61-7).

The **sarcoma and acute leukemia viruses** have incorporated cellular genes (**protooncogenes**) encoding growth-controlling factors into their genome. These include genes that encode growth hormones, growth hormone receptors, protein kinases, guanosine triphosphate–binding proteins, and nuclear DNA-binding proteins. These viruses can cause transformation and are highly oncogenic. **No human virus** of this type has been identified.

At least 35 different viral oncogenes have been identified (Table 61-8). Transformation results from the overproduction or altered activity of the growth-stimulating oncogene product. Increased cell growth then promotes transcription, which also promotes viral replication. The incorporation of the oncogene into many of these viruses causes the coding sequences for the gag, pol, or env genes to be replaced, such that these viruses are defective and require helper viruses for replication. Many of these viruses remain endogenous and are transmitted vertically through the germ line of the animal.

The **leukemia viruses,** including **HTLV-1,** are competent in terms of replication but cannot transform cells in vitro. They cause cancer after a **long latency period** of at least 30 years. The leukemia viruses promote cell growth in more indirect ways than the oncogene-encoding viruses. Specifically, a transcriptional regulator, tax, is produced and is capable of activating promoters in the LTR region and specific cellular genes (including growth–controlling and lymphokine genes such as IL-2 and granulocyte-macrophage colony-stimulating factor) to promote the outgrowth of that cell. Alternatively, by integrating near cellular growth–controlling genes, the enhancer and promoter gene sequences encoded in the viral LTR region can promote the expression of growth-stimulating proteins. Uncontrolled cell growth may be sufficient to transform the cell neoplastically or may promote other genetic aberrations over a long period. These viruses are also associated with nonneoplastic neurological disorders and other diseases. For example, HTLV-1 causes **adult acute T-cell lymphocytic leukemia (ATLL)** and also **HTLV-1–associated myelopathy (tropical spastic paraparesis),** a nononcogenic neurological disease.

The human oncoviruses include HTLV-1, HTLV-2, and HTLV-5, but only HTLV-1 has been definitively associated with disease (i.e., ATLL). HTLV-2 was isolated from atypical forms of hairy cell leukemia, and HTLV-5 was isolated from a malignant cutaneous lymphoma. HTLV-1 and HTLV-2 share as much as 50% homology.

Pathogenesis and Immunity

HTLV-1 is cell associated and is spread in cells after **blood transfusion, sexual intercourse,** or breast-feeding. The virus enters the bloodstream and infects the CD4 helper and DTH T cells. These T cells have a tendency to reside in the skin, which contributes to the symptoms of ATLL. Neurons also express a receptor for HTLV-1.

HTLV is competent for replication, with the gag, pol, and env genes transcribed, translated, and processed as described earlier. In addition to its action on viral genes, the tax protein transactivates the cellular genes for the T-

| TABLE 61-7 | **Mechanims of Retrovirus Oncogenesis** |

DISEASE	SPEED	EFFECT
Acute leukemia or sarcoma	Fast: oncogene	Direct effect
		Provision of growth-enhancing proteins
Leukemia	Slow: transactivation	Indirect effect
		Transactivation protein (tax) or long-terminal repeat promoter sequences that enhance expression of cellular growth genes

| TABLE 61-8 | **Representative Examples of Oncogenes** |

FUNCTION	ONCOGENE	VIRUS
Tyrosine kinase	src	Rous sarcoma virus
	abl	Abelson murine leukemia virus
	fes	ST feline sarcoma virus
Growth factor receptors	erb-B (EGF receptor)	Avian erythroblastosis virus
	erb-A (thyroid hormone receptor)	Avian erythroblastosis virus
Guanosine triphosphate–binding proteins	Ha-ras	Harvey murine sarcoma virus
	Ki-ras	Kirsten murine sarcoma virus
Nuclear proteins	myc	Avian myelocytomatosis virus
	myb	Avian myeloblastosis virus
	fos	Murine osteosarcoma virus FBJ
	jun	Avian sarcoma virus 17

Based on data from Jawetz E et al: *Medical microbiology,* ed 18, Los Altos, Calif, 1989, Appleton & Lange.

cell growth factor, IL-2 and its receptor (IL-2R), which activates growth in the infected cell. The virus may remain latent or replicate slowly for many years but may also induce the clonal outgrowth of particular T-cell clones. There is a long latency period (approximately 30 years) before the onset of leukemia.

Although the virus can induce a polyclonal outgrowth of T cells, the HTLV-1–induced **adult T-cell leukemia** is usually monoclonal. Chromosomal aberrations and rearrangements in the T-cell antigen receptor beta gene may accumulate in the HTLV growth-stimulated cells, and it may be this that causes the leukemia.

Antibodies are elicited to the gp46 and other proteins of HTLV-1. The presence of these antibodies in infected people may down-regulate the expression of viral antigens. This would prevent the cell-mediated immune clearance of virally infected cells. HTLV-1 infection also causes immunosuppression.

Epidemiology

HTLV-1 is transmitted and acquired by the same routes as HIV. It is endemic in southern Japan and is also found in the inhabitants of the Caribbean and among blacks in the southeastern United States. In the endemic regions of Japan, the children acquire HTLV-1 in breast milk from their mothers, whereas the adults are infected sexually. The number of seropositive people in some regions of Japan may be as high as 35% (Okinawa), with the mortality resulting from leukemia double that seen in other regions. Intravenous drug abuse and blood transfusion are becoming the most prominent means of transmitting the virus in the United States. In the United States, the high-risk groups for HTLV-1 infection are the same as those for HIV infection, and the seroprevalence of HTLV-1 is approaching or is surpassing that of HIV.

Clinical Syndromes

HTLV infection is usually asymptomatic but can progress to ATLL in approximately 1 in 20 persons over a 30- to 50-year period. ATLL caused by HTLV-1 is a neoplasia of the CD4 helper T cells that can be acute or chronic. The malignant cells have been termed *flower cells* because they are pleomorphic and contain lobulated nuclei. In addition to an elevated white blood cell count, this form of ATLL is characterized by skin lesions similar to those seen in another leukemia, Sézary syndrome. Acute ATLL is usually fatal within a year of diagnosis, regardless of treatment.

Laboratory Diagnosis

HTLV-1 infection is detected immunologically (ELISA) by the finding of virus-specific antigens in blood, using RT-PCR for viral RNA or using ELISA serologically to detect specific antibodies.

Treatment, Prevention, and Control

A combination of AZT and interferon-alpha has been effective in some patients with ATLL. However, no particular treatment has been approved for the management of HTLV-1 infection.

The measures used to limit the spread of HTLV-1 are the same as those used to limit the transmission of HIV. Sexual precautions, screening of the blood supply, and increased awareness of the potential risks and diseases are all ways to prevent transmission of the virus. Maternal infection of children is very difficult to control, however. The use of routine screening procedures for HTLV would limit spread of the virus, but such measures have not been instituted.

ENDOGENOUS RETROVIRUSES

Different retroviruses have integrated into and become a part of the chromosomes of humans and animals. In fact, retrovirus sequences may make up as much as 0.1% of the human genome. Complete and partial provirus sequences with gene sequences similar to those of HTLV, mouse mammary tumor virus, and other retroviruses can be detected in humans. These endogenous viruses generally lack the ability to replicate because of deletions or the insertion of termination codons or because they are poorly transcribed. One such retrovirus can be detected in placental tissue and is activated by pregnancy. This virus may facilitate placental function.

CASE STUDY AND QUESTIONS

A 28-year-old man had several complaints. He had a bad case of thrush (oral candidiasis) and low-grade fever, had serious bouts of diarrhea, had lost 20 pounds in the past year without dieting, and, most seriously, complained of difficulty breathing. His lungs showed a bilateral infiltrate on x-ray examination, which is characteristic of *Pneumocystis carinii* pneumonia. A stool sample was positive for *Giardia* organisms. He was a heroin addict and admitted to sharing needles at a "shooting gallery."

1. What laboratory tests should have been done to support and confirm a diagnosis of HIV infection and AIDS?
2. How did this man acquire the HIV infection? What are other high-risk behaviors for HIV infection?
3. What was the immunological basis for the increased susceptibility of this patient to opportunistic infections?
4. What precautions should have been taken in handling samples from this patient?
5. Several forms of HIV vaccines are being developed. What are possible components of an HIV vaccine? Who would be appropriate recipients of an HIV vaccine?

Bibliography

AIDS: Ten years later, *FASEB J* 5:2338-2455, 1991.

Anderson RM: Understanding the AIDS pandemic, *Sci Am* May 1992, pp 58-66.

Antiretroviral therapy for HIV infection in 1996: consensus statement, *JAMA* 276:146-154, 1996.

Arts EJ, Wainberg MA: Human immunodeficiency virus type 1 reverse transcriptase and early events in reverse transcription, *Adv Virus Res* 46:99-166, 1996.

Caldwell JC, Caldwell P: The African AIDS epidemic, *Sci Am* March 1996.

Fauci AS: The human immunodeficiency virus: infectivity and mechanisms of pathogenesis, *Science* 239:617-622, 1988.

Fields BN, Knipe DM, Howley PM, editors: *Virology,* ed 3, New York, 1996, Lippincott-Raven.

Guidelines for prevention of transmission of human immunodeficiency virus and hepatitis B virus to health-care and public-safety workers, *MMWR* 38:S-6, 1989.

Hehlmann R: *Human retroviruses.* In Belshe RB, editor: *Textbook of human virology,* ed 2, St Louis, 1991, Mosby.

Hehlmann R, Erfle V: *Introduction to retroviruses: human retroviruses.* In Belshe RB, editor: *Textbook of human virology,* ed 2, St Louis, 1991, Mosby.

Kräusslich HG: Morphgenesis and maturation of retroviruses, *Curr Top Microbiol Immunol* 214:1-344, 1996.

The new face of AIDS, *Science* 272:1879-1890, 1996.

Ng VL, McGrath MS: Human T-cell leukemia virus involvement in adult T-cell leukemia, *Cancer Bull* 40:276-280, 1988.

Oldstone MBA, Vitkovic L: HIV and dementia, *Curr Top Microbiol Immunol* 202:1-279, 1995.

Pantaleo G, Fauci AS: Immunopathology of HIV infection, *Annu Rev Microbiol* 50:825-854, 1996.

The science of AIDS 1989: readings from Scientific American, New York, Scientific American Books.

Williams AO: *AIDS: an African perspective,* Boca Raton, Fla, 1992, CRC.

Hepatitis Viruses

There are at least six viruses, A through E and a newly discovered G, that are considered hepatitis viruses (Table 62-1). Although the target organ for each of these viruses is the liver, they differ greatly in their structure, mode of replication, and mode of transmission and in the course of the disease they cause. The hepatitis A (HAV) and B (HBV) viruses are the best known, but in recent years three non-A, non-B hepatitis (NANBH) viruses (C, G, and E) have been described, as has hepatitis D virus (HDV), the delta agent. Additional non-A, non-B agents also exist.

Each of the hepatitis viruses infects and damages the liver, causing the classic **icteric symptoms of jaundice** and **the release of liver enzymes.** The specific course, nature, and serology of the disease differ for each virus. These viruses are readily spread because infected people are contagious before, or even without, showing symptoms.

Hepatitis A, which is sometimes known as *infectious hepatitis,* (1) is caused by a picornavirus, an RNA virus; (2) is spread by the fecal-oral route; (3) has an incubation period of approximately 1 month, after which icteric symptoms start abruptly; (4) does not cause chronic liver disease; and (5) rarely causes fatal disease.

Hepatitis B, previously known as *serum hepatitis,* (1) is caused by a **hepadnavirus** with a DNA genome; (2) is spread parenterally by blood or needles, by sexual contact, and perinatally; (3) has a median incubation period of approximately 3 months, after which icteric symptoms start insidiously; (4) is followed by chronic hepatitis in 5% to 10% of patients; and (5) is causally associated with primary hepatocellular carcinoma. An estimated 300,000 cases of hepatitis B occur in the United States each year, with 4000 deaths caused by the agent. However, the incidence of HBV is decreasing, especially in infants, because of the development and use of the **HBV subunit vaccine.**

NANBH viruses include hepatitis C, G, E, and other undefined hepatitis viruses. **Hepatitis C** virus (HCV) is spread by the same routes as HBV and can also cause chronic disease, but it is a flavivirus with an RNA genome. HCV differs in the general course of the disease it causes. Hepatitis G virus is also a flavivirus; it can be

identified only by polymerase chain reaction (PCR) techniques. **Hepatitis E** virus (HEV) is an enteric virus.

Hepatitis D, or delta hepatitis, is unique in that it requires actively replicating HBV as a "helper virus" and occurs only in patients who have active HBV infection. HBV provides an envelope for HDV RNA and its antigen or antigens. Delta agent exacerbates the symptoms caused by hepatitis B virus.

HEPATITIS A VIRUS

As just noted, HAV causes infectious hepatitis and is spread by the fecal-oral route. HAV infections often result from the consumption of contaminated water, shellfish, or other food. HAV is a picornavirus and has been renamed **enterovirus 72.**

Structure

HAV has the structural characteristics of a **picornavirus** (Figure 62-1). It has a 27-nm, naked icosahedral capsid surrounding a positive-sense, single-stranded RNA genome consisting of approximately 7470 nucleotides. The HAV genome has a VPg protein attached to the 5′ end and polyadenosine attached to the 3′ end. The capsid is even more stable than other picornaviruses to acid and other treatments (Box 62-1). There is only **one serotype** of HAV.

Replication

HAV replicates like other picornaviruses (see Chapter 54). It interacts specifically with a receptor expressed on liver cells and a few other cell types. Unlike other picornaviruses, however, HAV is not cytolytic and is released by exocytosis. Laboratory isolates of HAV have been adapted to growth in primary and continuous monkey kidney cell lines, but clinical isolates are very difficult to grow in cell culture.

Pathogenesis

HAV is ingested and probably enters the bloodstream through the oropharynx or the epithelial lining of the intestines to reach its target, the parenchymal cells of the liver (Figure 62-2). The virus can be localized by im-

TABLE 62-1 Comparative Features of Hepatitis Viruses

FEATURE	HEPATITIS A	HEPATITIS B	HEPATITIS C	HEPATITIS D	HEPATITIS E
Common name	"Infectious"	"Serum"	"Non A, non B–posttransfusion"	"Delta agent"	"Enteric non A, non B"
Virus structure	Picornavirus; capsid, RNA	Hepadnavirus; envelope, DNA	Flavivirus; envelope, RNA	Viroidlike; envelope, circular RNA	Calicivirus-like; capsid, RNA
Transmission	Fecal-oral	Parenteral, sexual	Parenteral, sexual	Parenteral, sexual	Fecal-oral
Onset	Abrupt	Insidious	Insidious	Abrupt	Abrupt
Incubation period (days)	15-50	45-160	14-180	15-64	15-50
Severity	Mild	Occasionally severe	Usually subclinical	*Co-infection* with HBV occasionally severe; *superinfection* with HBV often severe	Normal patients, mild, pregnant women, severe
Mortality	<0.5%	1%-2%	0.5%-1%	High to very high	Normal patients, 1%-2%; pregnant women, 20%
Chronicity/carrier state	No	Yes	Yes	Yes	No
Other disease associations	None	Primary hepatocellular carcinoma, cirrhosis	Primary hepatocellular carcinoma, cirrhosis	Cirrhosis, fulminant hepatitis	None
Laboratory diagnosis	Symptoms and anti-HAV IgM	Symptoms and serum levels of HBsAg, HBeAg, and anti-HBc IgM	Symptoms and anti-HCV ELISA	Anti-HDV ELISA	—

IgM, Immunoglobulin M; *HAV,* hepatitis A virus; *HCV,* hepatitis C virus; *ELISA,* enzyme-linked immunosorbent assay; *HDV,* hepatitis D virus.

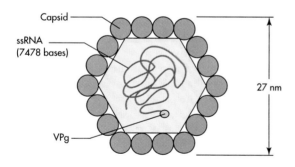

FIGURE 62-1 The picornavirus structure of the HAV. The icosahedral capsid is made up of four viral polypeptides (VP1 to VP4). Inside the capsid is a single-stranded, positive-sense RNA *(ssRNA)* that has a genomic viral protein (VPg) on the 5′ end.

BOX 62-1 Characteristics of HAV

Stable to:
    Acid at pH 1
    Solvents (ether, chloroform)
    Detergents
    Saltwater, groundwater (months)
    Drying (stable)
    Temperature
        4° C: weeks
        56° C for 30 minutes: stable
        61° C for 20 minutes: partial inactivation
Inactivated by:
    Chlorine treatment of drinking water
    Formalin (0.35%, 37° C, 72 hours)
    Peracetic acid (2%, 4 hours)
    B-propiolactone (0.25%, 1 hour)
    Ultraviolet radiation (2 μW/cm²/min)

munofluorescence in hepatocytes and Kupffer's cells. Virus is produced in these cells and is released into the bile and from there into the stool. Virus is shed into the stool approximately 10 days before symptoms appear or antibody can be detected.

HAV replicates slowly in the liver without producing apparent cytopathological effects (CPEs). In the absence of cytolysis, the virus readily establishes a persistent infection. Although interferon limits viral replication, natural killer cells and cytotoxic T cells are required to lyse

infected cells. Antibody, complement, and antibody-dependent cellular cytotoxicity also facilitate clearance of the virus and the induction of immunopathology. Icterus, resulting from damage to the liver, occurs when antibody is detected and cell-mediated immune re-

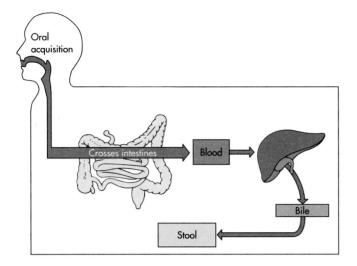

FIGURE 62-2 Spread of HAV within the body.

BOX 62-2 **Epidemiology of HAV and HEV Infections**

DISEASE/VIRAL FACTORS

Capsid viruses are very resistant to inactivation.
Contagious period extends from before to after symptoms.
Virus may cause asymptomatic shedding.

TRANSMISSION

Virus can be transmitted via fecal-oral route.
Ingestion of contaminated food and water can cause infection.
HAV in shellfish is from sewage-contaminated water.
Virus can be transmitted by food handlers, day-care workers, and children.

WHO IS AT RISK?

People in overcrowded, unsanitary areas.
Children: mild disease, possibly asymptomatic; day-care centers: major source of spread of HAV.
Adults: abrupt-onset hepatitis.
Pregnant women: high mortality associated with HEV.

GEOGRAPHY/SEASON

Virus is found worldwide.
There is no seasonal incidence.

MEANS OF CONTROL

Good hygiene.
HAV: passive antibody protection for contacts.
Killed vaccine.

sponses to the virus occur. Antibody protection against reinfection is lifelong.

The liver pathology caused by HAV infection is indistinguishable histologically from that caused by HBV. It is most likely caused by immunopathology and not virus-induced cytopathology. However, unlike HBV, HAV cannot initiate a chronic infection and is not associated with hepatic cancer.

Epidemiology

Approximately 40% of the acute cases of hepatitis are caused by HAV (Box 62-2). HAV is released into stool in high concentrations, especially during the 2 weeks before the onset of jaundice. The virus then spreads readily in a community because most infected people are contagious before symptoms occur and 90% of infected children and 25% to 50% of infected adults have inapparent but productive infections.

The virus is spread via the fecal-oral route: in contaminated water, in food, and by dirty hands. HAV is resistant to detergents, acid (pH of 1), and temperatures as high as 60° C, and it can survive for many months in freshwater and saltwater. Raw or improperly treated sewage can taint the water supply and contaminate shellfish. Shellfish, especially clams, oysters, and mussels, are important sources of the virus because they are very efficient filter feeders and can therefore concentrate the viral particles, even from dilute solutions. This is exemplified by an epidemic of HAV that occurred in Shanghai, China, in 1988 in which 300,000 people were infected with the virus as the result of eating clams obtained from a polluted river.

HAV outbreaks usually originate from a common source (e.g., water supply, restaurant, day-care center). Day-care settings are a major source of spread of the virus, with the virus spreading among classmates and to their parents. A further problem is posed by the fact that, because the children and personnel in day-care centers

may be transient, the number of contacts at risk for HAV infection from a single day-care center can be great.

A relatively high incidence of HAV infection is directly related to poor hygienic conditions and overcrowding. Most people infected with HAV in developing countries are children who have mild illness and then lifelong immune protection against reinfection. In the populations of more highly developed countries, infection occurs later in life. The seropositivity rate of adults ranges from a low of 13% of the adult population in Sweden to a high of 88% in Taiwan and 97% in Yugoslavia, with a 41% to 44% rate in the United States.

Clinical Syndromes

The symptoms caused by HAV are very similar to those caused by HBV and stem from immune-mediated damage to the liver. As already noted, disease in children is generally milder than that in adults and is usually asymptomatic. The symptoms occur **abruptly** 15 to 50 days after exposure and intensify for 4 to 6 days before the icteric (jaundice) phase (Figure 62-3). Initial symptoms include fever, fatigue, nausea, loss of appetite, and abdominal pain. Jaundice is observed in 2 of 3 adults but only 1 or 2 of 10 children. Symptoms generally wane

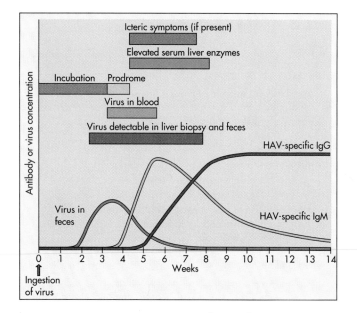

FIGURE 62-3 Time course of HAV infection.

during the jaundice period. Viral shedding in the stool precedes the onset of symptoms by approximately 14 days but stops before the cessation of symptoms. Complete recovery occurs 99% of the time.

Fulminant hepatitis in HAV infection occurs in 1 to 3 persons per 1000 and is associated with an 80% mortality rate. Unlike HBV, immune complex–related symptoms (e.g., arthritis, rash) rarely occur in people with HAV disease.

Laboratory Diagnosis

The diagnosis of HAV infection is generally made on the basis of the time course of the clinical symptoms, the identification of a known infected source, and, most reliably, the results yielded by specific serological tests. The best way to demonstrate an acute HAV infection is by the finding of anti-HAV immunoglobulin M (IgM), as measured by an enzyme-linked immunosorbent assay (ELISA) or radioimmunoassay (RIA). Virus isolation is not routinely performed because efficient tissue culture systems for growing the virus are not available.

Treatment, Prevention, and Control

The spread of HAV is reduced by interrupting the fecal-oral spread of the virus. This includes the avoidance of potentially contaminated water or food, especially uncooked shellfish. Proper handwashing, especially in daycare centers, mental hospitals, and other care facilities, is very important. Chlorine treatment of drinking water is generally sufficient to kill the virus.

Prophylaxis with immune serum globulin given before or early in the incubation period (i.e., less than 2 weeks after exposure) is 80% to 90% effective in preventing clinical illness.

A killed HAV vaccine has been approved by the U.S. Food and Drug Administration and is available for use in children and adults at high risk for infection, especially travelers to endemic regions. A live HAV vaccine has been developed in China. There is only one serotype of HAV, and HAV infects only humans, factors that help ensure the success of an immunization program.

HEPATITIS B VIRUS

HBV is the major member of the **hepadnaviruses.** Other members of this family (Box 62-3) include woodchuck, ground squirrel, and duck hepatitis viruses. These viruses have very limited tissue tropisms and host ranges. HBV infects the liver and, to a lesser extent, the kidney and pancreas of only humans and chimpanzees. Advances in molecular biology have made it possible to study HBV despite the limited host range of the virus and the lack of a cell culture system in which to grow it.

Structure

HBV is a **small, enveloped DNA** virus with several unusual properties (Figure 62-4). Specifically, the genome is a **small, circular, partly double-stranded DNA** of only 3200 bases. Although a DNA virus, it encodes a **reverse transcriptase** and replicates through an RNA intermediate.

The virion, also called the **Dane particle,** is 42 nm in diameter. The virions are unusually stable for an enveloped virus. They resist treatment with ether, a low pH, freezing, and moderate heating. This assists transmission from one person to another and hampers disinfection.

The HBV virion includes a polymerase with reverse transcriptase, ribonuclease H activity, and a P protein attached to the genome, which is surrounded by the hepatitis B core antigen (**HBcAg**) and an envelope containing the glycoprotein hepatitis B surface antigen (**HBsAg**). A hepatitis B e antigen (**HBeAg**) protein is a minor component of the virion. The HBeAg and HBcAg proteins share most of their protein sequence. However, the HBeAg is processed differently by the cell, is primarily secreted into serum, does not self-assemble like a capsid antigen, and expresses different antigenic determinants.

HbsAg-containing particles are released into the serum of infected people and outnumber the actual virions. These particles can be spherical (but smaller than the Dane particle) or filamentous (Figure 62-4). They are immunogenic and were processed into the first commercial vaccine against HBV.

The HBsAg, originally termed the **Australia antigen,** includes three glycoproteins (L, M, and S) encoded by the same gene and read in the same frame but translated into protein from different AUG start codons. The S (gp27; 24 to 27 kD) glycoprotein is completely contained in the **M** (gp36; 33 to 36 kD) glycoprotein, which is contained in the **L** (gp42; 39 to 42 kD) glycoprotein; all share the same C-terminal amino acid se-

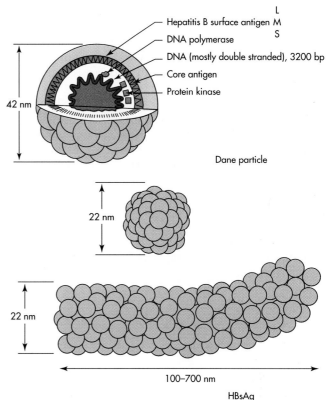

FIGURE 62-4 HBV (Dane particle) and HBsAg particles. The spherical HBsAg consists mainly of the S form of HBsAg with some M. The fiber HBsAg has S, M, and L forms. *bp*, Base pair; *L*, gp42; *M*, gp36; *S*, gp27.

BOX 62-3 Unique Features of Hepadnaviruses

Virus has **enveloped** virion containing **partially double-stranded, circular DNA** genome.

Replication is through a circular **RNA intermediate.**

Virus encodes and carries a **reverse transcriptase.**

Virus encodes several proteins (HBsAg [L, M, S], HBe/HBc) that share genetic sequences but with different in-frame start codons (AUG).

HBV has a strict tissue tropism to the liver.

HBV-infected cells produce and release large amounts of HBsAg particles lacking DNA.

The HBV genome can integrate into the host chromosome.

quences. All three forms of HBsAg are found in the virion. The **S** glycoprotein is the major component of HBsAg particles. It self-associates into **22-nm spherical particles** that are released from the cells. The **filamentous particles** of HBsAg found in serum contain mostly S but also small amounts of the M and L glycoproteins and other proteins and lipids. The L glycoprotein is an essential component for virion assembly and promotes filament formation and the retention of these structures in the cell. The glycoproteins of HBsAg contain the group-specific (termed *a*) and type-specific determinants of HBV (termed *d* or *y* and *w* or *r*). Combinations of these antigens (e.g., ady, adw) result in eight subtypes of HBV that are useful epidemiological markers.

Replication

The replication of HBV is unique for several reasons (Box 62-1). First, HBV has a very defined tropism for the liver. Its small genome also necessitates economy, as illustrated by the pattern of its transcription and translation. In addition, HBV replicates through an RNA intermediate and produces and releases antigenic decoy particles (HBsAg) (Figure 62-5).

The attachment of HBV to hepatocytes is mediated by the HBsAg glycoproteins. Although the actual receptor and mechanism of entry are not known, it is known that HBsAg binds to polymerized human serum albumin and other serum proteins, and this interaction may target the virus to the liver.

On penetration into the cell, the partial DNA strand of the genome is completed by being formed into a complete double-stranded DNA circle, and the genome is delivered to the nucleus. Transcription of the genome is controlled by cellular transcription elements found in hepatocytes. The DNA is transcribed into three major classes (2100, 2400, and 3500 bases) and two minor classes (900 bases) of overlapping messenger RNAs (mRNAs) (Figure 62-6). The 3500-base mRNA is larger than the genome. It encodes the HBc and HBe antigens, the polymerase, and a protein primer for DNA replica-

tion and also acts as the template for replication of the genome. The HBe and HBc are related proteins that are translated from different in-phase start codons of closely related mRNA. This causes differences in their processing, structure, and distribution in the cell and virion. Similarly, the 2100-base mRNA encodes the small and medium glycoproteins from different in-phase start codons. The 2400-base mRNA, which encodes the large glycoprotein, overlaps the 2100-base mRNA. The 900-base mRNA encodes the X protein, which promotes viral replication as a transactivator of transcription and as a protein kinase.

Replication of the genome occurs in the cytoplasm. To begin, the 3500-base mRNA is packaged into the core nucleocapsid that contains the RNA-dependent DNA polymerase. This polymerase has **reverse transcriptase** and ribonuclease H activity but lacks the integrase activity of the retrovirus enzyme. Negative-strand DNA is then synthesized on a protein primer, which remains covalently attached to the 5' end. After this, the RNA is degraded by the ribonuclease H activity as the positive-strand DNA is synthesized from the negative-sense DNA template. However, this process is interrupted by envelopment of the nucleocapsid at HBsAg-containing membranes of the endoplasmic reticulum or Golgi apparatus, thereby capturing genomes containing RNA-DNA circles with different lengths of RNA. Continued degradation of the remainder of the RNA in the virion yields a partly double-stranded DNA genome. The virion is then released from the hepatocyte by exocytosis and not by cell lysis.

The entire genome can also be integrated into the host cell chromatin. HBsAg, but not other proteins, can often be detected in the cytoplasm of cells containing integrated HBV DNA. The significance of the integrated DNA in the replication of the virus is not known, but integrated viral DNA has been found in hepatocellular carcinomas.

Pathogenesis and Immunity

HBV can cause acute or chronic, symptomatic or asymptomatic disease. Which of these occurs seems to be determined by the person's immune response to the infection. Detection of both the HBsAg and the HBeAg components of the virion in the blood indicates the existence of an ongoing active infection (Figure 62-7). HBsAg particles continue to be released into the blood even after virion release has ended and until the infection resolves.

The major source of infectious virus is blood, but HBV can be found in semen, saliva, milk, vaginal and menstrual secretions, and amniotic fluid. The most efficient way to acquire HBV is through injection of the virus into the bloodstream. Common but less efficient routes of infection are sexual contact and birth.

The virus starts to replicate within 3 days of its acquisition, but as already noted, symptoms may not be observed for 45 days or longer, depending on the infectious

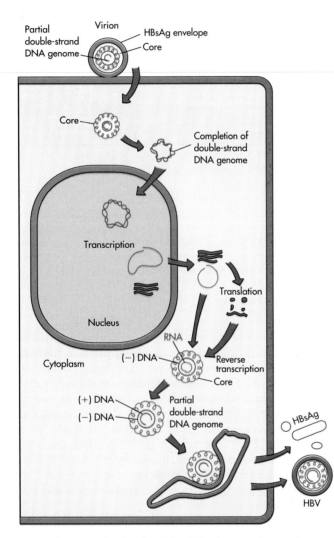

FIGURE 62-5 Proposed pathway for the replication of HBV. After entry into the hepatocyte and uncoating of the nucleocapsid core, the partially double-stranded DNA genome is completed by enzymes in the core and then delivered to the nucleus. Transcription of the genome produces four messenger RNAs, including an mRNA larger than the genome (3500 bases). The mRNA then moves to the cytoplasm and is translated into protein. Core proteins assemble around the 3500-base messenger RNA, and negative-sense DNA is synthesized by a reverse transcriptase activity in the core. The RNA is then degraded as a positive-sense (+) DNA is synthesized. The core is enveloped before completion of the positive-sense DNA and then released by exocytosis.

FIGURE 62-6 mRNA transcripts and proteins of HBV. Diagram depicts the mRNA and proteins encoded by the HBV genome. Note that several proteins share the same coding sequences but start at different AUG codons and that different mRNAs overlap. The 3500-base transcript is larger than the genome and is the template for replication of the genome. DR1 and DR2 are direct repeat sequences of DNA and are important for the replication and integration of the genome. The genome is black with the nucleotide number in the central circle. E, E protein (HBeAg); C, C protein (HBcAg); P, polymerase-protein primer for replication; S, S protein (HBsAg); l, large glycoprotein; m, medium glycoprotein; s, small glycoprotein; X, X protein; AAA, 3' polyA at end of mRNA. (Redrawn from Blum HE et al: *Trends Gen* 5:154-158, 1989.)

dose, the route of infection, and the person. The virus replicates in hepatocytes with minimal CPE, after which infection proceeds for a relatively long time without causing liver damage (i.e., elevation of liver enzyme levels) or symptoms. During this time, copies of the HBV genome integrate into the hepatocyte chromatin and remain latent. The intracellular buildup of filamentous forms of HBsAg can produce the ground-glass hepatocyte cytopathology characteristic of HBV infection.

Cell-mediated immunity and inflammation are responsible for causing the symptomatology and effecting resolution of the HBV infection. Interferon most likely initiates the response by enhancing major histocompatibility complex antigen expression and the display of peptides from the HBs, HBc, and HBe antigens to cytotoxic killer T cells. An insufficient T-cell response to the infection generally results in the occurrence of mild symptoms, an inability to resolve the infection, and the development of chronic hepatitis (Figure 62-8). Antibody (as generated by vaccination) can protect against infection. However, serum HBsAg binds to and blocks the action of neutralizing antibody, which limits the antibody's capacity to resolve an infection. Immune complexes formed between HBsAg and anti-HBs contribute to the development of hypersensitivity reactions, leading to problems such as vasculitis, arthralgia, rash, and renal damage.

Infants and young children have an immature cell-mediated immune response and exhibit less tissue damage and milder symptoms. As many as 90% of infants infected perinatally become chronic carriers. Viral replication persists in these people for long periods.

During the acute phase of infection, the liver parenchyma shows degenerative changes consisting of cellular swelling and necrosis, especially in hepatocytes surrounding the central vein of a hepatic lobule. The inflammatory cell infiltrate is mainly composed of lymphocytes. Resolution of the infection allows the parenchyma to regenerate. Fulminant infections, the activation of chronic infections, or co-infection with the delta agent can lead to permanent liver damage and cirrhosis.

Epidemiology

In the United States more than 300,000 persons are infected with HBV each year. However, even more people are infected in underdeveloped nations, with as much as 15% of the population infected during birth or childhood. High rates of seropositivity are observed in Italy, Greece, Africa, and Southeast Asia (Figure 62-9). In

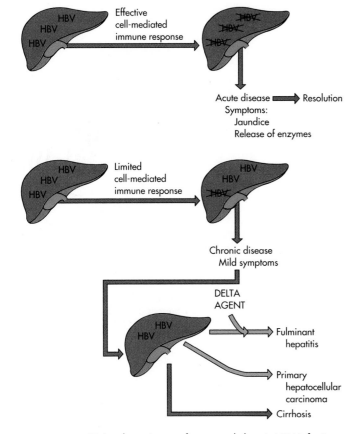

FIGURE 62-7 Major determinants of acute and chronic HBV infection. HBV infects the liver but does not cause direct cytopathology. Cell-mediated immune lysis of infected cells, potentially triggered by interferon action, produces the symptoms and resolves the infection. Insufficient immunity can lead to chronic disease. Chronic HBV disease predisposes a person to more serious outcomes. Purple arrows indicate symptoms; green arrows indicate a possible outcome.

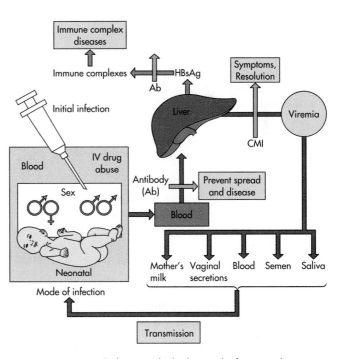

FIGURE 62-8 Spread of HBV in the body. Initial infection with HBV occurs through injection, heterosexual and homosexual sex, and birth. The virus then spreads to the liver, replicates, induces a viremia, and is transmitted in various body secretions in addition to blood to start the cycle again. Symptoms are caused by cell-mediated immunity (*CMI*) and immune complexes between antibody and HBsAg. *IV,* Intravenous.

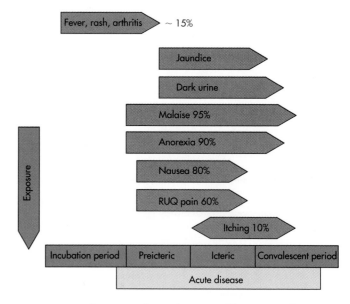

FIGURE 62-9 Worldwide prevalence of hepatitis B carriers and primary hepatocellular carcinoma. (Courtesy Centers for Disease Control and Prevention, Atlanta.)

BOX 62-4 **High-Risk Groups for HBV Infection**

People from endemic regions (i.e., China, parts of Africa, Alaska, Pacific islands)
Babies of mothers with chronic HBV
Intravenous drug abusers
People with multiple sex partners: homosexual and heterosexual
Hemophiliacs and other patients requiring blood and blood product treatments
Health care personnel who have contact with blood
Residents and staff members of institutions for the mentally retarded

FIGURE 62-10 Symptoms of typical acute viral hepatitis B infection are correlated with the four clinical periods of this disease. *RUQ*, Right upper quadrant. (Redrawn from Hoofnagle JH: *Lab Med* 14:705-716, 1983.)

some areas of the world (southern Africa and southeastern Asia), the seroconversion rate is as high as 50%. **Primary hepatocellular carcinoma (PHC),** a long-term sequela of the infection, is also endemic in these regions.

The many asymptomatic chronic carriers capable of secreting virus in blood and other body secretions foster the spread of the virus. In the United States, 0.1% to 0.5% of the general population are chronic carriers. Carrier status may be lifelong.

The virus is spread mainly by the percutaneous routes (e.g., needle sharing, acupuncture, ear piercing, tattooing) and through very close personal contact involving the exchange of blood or secretions (e.g., sex, childbirth). People at particular risk are listed in Box 62-4. Sexual promiscuity and drug abuse are major risk factors for HBV infection. HBV can be transmitted to babies

through contact with the mother's blood at birth and in mother's milk. Babies born to chronic HBV-positive mothers are at highest risk for infection. The serological screening of donor units in blood banks has greatly reduced the risk of acquisition of the virus from contaminated blood or blood products. Safer sex habits adopted to prevent HIV transmission and the administration of the HBV vaccine have also been responsible for decreasing the transmission of HBV.

One of the major concerns about HBV is its association with PHC. This type of carcinoma probably accounts for 250,000 to 1 million deaths per year worldwide; in the United States, approximately 5000 deaths per year are attributed to PHC.

Clinical Syndromes

Acute Infection

As already noted, the clinical presentation of HBV in children is less severe than that in adults, and infection may even be asymptomatic. Clinically apparent illness occurs in as many as 25% of those infected with HBV (Figures 62-10 to 62-12).

HBV infection is characterized by a long incubation period and an insidious onset. Symptoms during the prodromal period may include fever, malaise, and anorexia, followed by nausea, vomiting, abdominal discomfort, fever, and chills. The classic icteric symptoms of liver damage (e.g., jaundice, dark urine, pale stools) follow soon thereafter. Recovery is indicated by a decline in the fever and renewed appetite.

Fulminant hepatitis occurs in approximately 1% of icteric patients and may be fatal. It has more severe symptoms and indications of severe liver damage, such as ascites and bleeding.

HBV infection can promote hypersensitivity reactions that are due to immune complexes of HBsAg and antibody. These may produce rash, polyarthritis, fever, acute necrotizing vasculitis, and glomerulonephritis.

Chronic Infection

Chronic hepatitis occurs in 5% to 10% of people with HBV infections, usually after mild or inapparent initial disease. It may be detected only by the finding of elevated liver enzyme levels on a routine blood chemistry profile, but as many as 10% of patients with chronic hepatitis may develop cirrhosis and liver failure. Chronically infected people are the major source for spread of the virus and are at risk for fulminant disease if they become co-infected with the HDV.

Primary Hepatocellular Carcinoma

The World Health Organization estimates that 80% of all cases of PHC can be attributed to chronic HBV infections. The HBV genome is integrated into these PHC cells, and the cells express HBV antigens. PHC is usually fatal and is one of the three most common causes of cancer mortality in the world. In Taiwan, at least 15% of the population are HBV carriers, and nearly half die of PHC or cirrhosis. PHC may become the first vaccine-preventable human cancer.

HBV may induce PHC by promoting continued liver repair and cell growth in response to tissue damage or by integrating into the host chromosome and stimulating cell growth directly. Such integration could stimulate genetic rearrangements or juxtapose viral promoters next to cellular growth–controlling genes. Alternatively, a protein encoded by the HBV X gene may transactivate

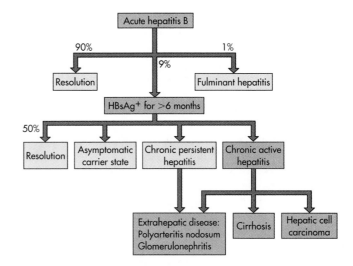

FIGURE 62-11 Clinical outcomes of acute hepatitis B infection. (Redrawn from White DO, Fenner F: *Medical virology*, ed 3, New York, 1986, Academic.)

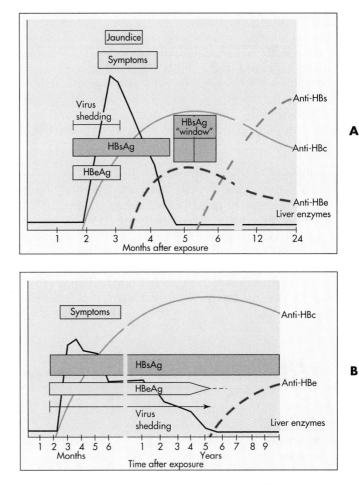

FIGURE 62-12 A, The serological events associated with the typical course of acute hepatitis B disease. **B,** Development of the chronic HBV carrier state. Routine serodiagnosis is difficult during the HBsAg window when HBs and anti-HBs are undetectable. *anti-HBs,* Antibody to HBsAg; *anti-HBc,* antibody to HBcAg; *anti-HBe,* antibody to HBeAg. (Redrawn from Hoofnagle JH: *Annu Rev Med* 32:1-11, 1981.)

(turn on) the transcription of cellular proteins and stimulate cell growth. The presence of the HBV genome may allow a subsequent mutation to promote carcinogenesis. The latency period between HBV infection and PHC may be as short as 9 years or as long as 35 years.

Laboratory Diagnosis

The initial diagnosis of hepatitis can be made on the basis of the clinical symptoms and the presence of liver enzymes in the blood (Figure 62-12). However, the serology of HBV infection describes the course and the nature of the disease (Table 62-2). Acute and chronic HBV infections can be distinguished by the presence of HBsAg and HBeAg in the serum and the pattern of antibodies to the individual HBV antigens. The serological pattern of HBV infection is better understood if one remembers that antibody bound into an antibody-antigen complex cannot be detected in routine laboratory tests.

HBsAg, HBcAg, and HBeAg are secreted into the blood during viral replication. The detection of HBeAg is the best correlate to the presence of infectious virus. A chronic infection can be distinguished by the continued finding of HBeAg, HBsAg, or both and a lack of detectable antibody to these antigens.

During the symptomatic phase of infection, detection of antibodies to HBeAg and HBsAg is obscured because the antibody is complexed with antigen in the serum. The best way to diagnose a recent acute infection, especially during the period when neither HBsAg nor anti-HBs can be detected (the window), is to measure IgM anti-HBc.

Treatment, Prevention, and Control

No specific treatment exists for HBV infection. Interferon-alpha may be effective for treating a chronic HBV infection. **Hepatitis B immune globulin** may be administered within a week of exposure and to newborn infants of HBsAg-positive mothers.

The transmission of HBV in blood or blood products has been greatly reduced through the screening of donated blood for the presence of HBsAg and anti-HBc.

Additional efforts to prevent the transmission of HBV consist of avoiding intimate personal contact with a carrier of HBV and avoiding the life-styles that facilitate spread of the virus. Household contacts and sexual partners of HBV carriers are at increased risk, as are hemodialysis patients, recipients of pooled plasma products, health care workers exposed to blood, and babies born of HBV-carrier mothers.

Vaccination is recommended for infants, children, and especially people in high-risk groups known to be anti-HBsAg negative (Box 62-4). Vaccination is useful even after exposure for newborns of HBsAg-positive mothers and people accidentally exposed either percutaneously or permucosally to blood or secretions from an HBsAg-positive person. Immunization of mothers should decrease the incidence of transmission to babies and older children, which will also reduce the number of chronic HBV carriers. Prevention of chronic HBV will most likely prevent PHC.

The HBV vaccines are **subunit vaccines.** The initial HBV vaccine was derived from the 22-nm HBsAg particles in human plasma obtained from chronically infected people. The current vaccine was genetically engineered and is produced by the insertion of a plasmid containing the **S** gene for HBsAg into a yeast, *Saccharomyces cerevisiae.*

The vaccine must be given in a series of three injections, with the second and third given 1 and 6 months after the first. More than 95% of individuals receiving the full 3-dose course will develop protective antibody. The single serotype and limited host range (humans) help ensure the success of an immunization program.

The objectives of **universal blood and body fluid precautions** are to limit exposure to and inactivate HBV. Gloves are required for handling blood and body fluids; wearing protective clothing and eyeglasses may also be necessary. Special care should be taken with needles and sharp instruments. HBV-contaminated materials can be disinfected with 10% bleach solutions, but unlike most enveloped viruses, detergents are not sufficient for the inactivation of HBV.

TABLE 62-2	**Interpretation of Serological Markers of HBV Infection**						
		DISEASE STATE				**HEALTHY STATE**	
SEROLOGICAL REACTIVITY	**EARLY (PRESYMPTOMATIC)**	**EARLY ACUTE**	**ACUTE**	**CHRONIC**	**LATE ACUTE**	**RESOLVED**	**VACCINATED**
Anti HBc	−	−	−*	+	+/−	+	−
Anti HBe	−	−	−	−	+/−	+/−†	−
Anti HBs	−	−	−	−	−	+	+
HBeAg	−	+	+	+	−	−	−
HBsAg	+	+	+	+	+	−	−
Infectious virus	+	+	+	+	+	−	−

*Anti-HBc IgM should be present.

†Anti-HBe may be negative after chronic disease.

HEPATITIS C VIRUS

HCV accounts for 90% of the cases of NANBH virus infection and is the major cause of posttransfusion hepatitis. HCV is a **flavivirus** with a positive-sense RNA genome and is enveloped. The genome of HCV (9100 nucleotides) has been cloned and sequenced. As a flavivirus, HCV has an inclination to establish noncytolytic, persistent infections and therefore **chronic disease.**

Epidemiology

The existence of NANBH viruses in serum was indicated by the incidence of HBV-negative, posttransfusion hepatitis (Box 62-5). HCV is spread parenterally and sexually. Intravenous drug abusers, transfusion and organ recipients, and hemophiliacs receiving factor VIII or IX are at highest risk for infection.

HCV infection once occurred in 5% to 10% of transfusion recipients (150,000 cases per year), causing chronic hepatitis in half and leading to cirrhosis in at least 20% of those with acute cases. The high incidence of chronic asymptomatic infections (1% of American blood donors) promotes the spread of the virus in the blood supply. However, new screening procedures for

---

BOX 62-5	**Epidemiology of HBV, HCV, and HDV**

DISEASE/VIRAL FACTORS

Enveloped virus is labile to drying. HBV is less sensitive to detergents than other enveloped viruses.
Virus is shed during asymptomatic periods.
Virus causes chronic disease with potential shedding.

TRANSMISSION

In blood, semen, and vaginal secretions (HBV: saliva and mother's milk).
Via transfusion, needlestick injury, shared drug paraphernalia, sex, and breast-feeding.

WHO IS AT RISK?

Children: mild asymptomatic disease with establishment of chronic infection.
Adults: insidious onset of hepatitis.
HBV-infected people co-infected or superinfected with HDV: abrupt, more severe symptoms with possible fulminant disease.
Adults with chronic HBV: at high risk for primary hepatocellular carcinoma.

GEOGRAPHY/SEASON

Viruses are found worldwide.
There is no seasonal incidence.

MODES OF CONTROL

Avoidance of high-risk behavior.
HBV: **vaccine** and screening of blood supply.

---

donors has led to a reduction in the levels of transmission. Non–transfusion-related sporadic cases also occur.

Clinical Syndromes

HCV can cause acute infections but is more likely to establish chronic infections. A viremia can be detected within 1 to 3 weeks of a transfusion of HCV-contaminated blood. The viremia lasts 4 to 6 months in people with an acute infection and longer than 10 years in those with a persistent infection. In its acute form, NANBH virus infection is similar to acute HAV and HBV infection, but the inflammatory response is less intense, and the symptoms are usually milder. **Chronic persistent hepatitis** caused by HCV is even more prevalent than that caused by HBV, often progressing to chronic active hepatitis, **cirrhosis** (20% of chronic cases), and finally **liver failure** (20% of cirrhotic cases). Cell-mediated immunopathology is responsible mainly for producing the tissue damage. It has been suggested that the continual liver repair and induction of cell growth occurring during chronic HCV infection are predisposing factors in the development of PHC. Antibody to HCV is not protective, and findings yielded by experimental infection of chimpanzees indicate that immunity to HCV may not be lifelong.

Laboratory Diagnosis

The diagnosis of HCV infection is based on the ELISA detection of antibody. Seroconversion occurs within 7 to 31 weeks of infection. However, antibody is not always present in viremic people. This suggests that serological assays may be useful for identifying only chronic and not acute HCV disease. The presence of the virion RNA in serum is a better indicator of disease. The reverse transcriptase–polymerase chain reaction technique, a variation of the PCR technique, can detect HCV RNA in seronegative people and may become a key tool in the diagnosis of HCV infection.

Treatment, Prevention, and Control

Recombinant interferon-alpha is the only known effective treatment for HCV. There are no other treatments for infection with HCV or the other NANBH viruses, except supportive therapy.

Illicit drug abuse and transfusion are the most identifiable sources of NANBH viruses. Unlike HBV, the tests available for detecting HCV cannot detect a current acute case of HCV, and tests for other NANBH viruses are not available. This limits the efficacy of screening procedures for the protection of the nation's blood supply.

HEPATITIS D VIRUS

Approximately 15 million people in the world are infected with HDV (delta agent), and the virus is responsible for causing 40% of the **fulminant hepatitis** infections. HDV is unique in that it uses HBV and target cell proteins to replicate and produce its one protein. It is a viral parasite, proving that "even fleas have fleas." The

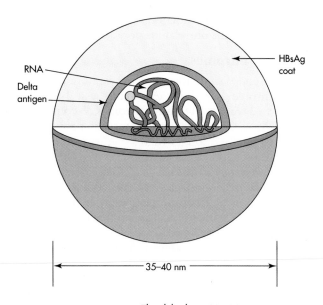

FIGURE 62-13 The delta hepatitis virion.

FIGURE 62-14 Consequences of delta virus infection. Delta virus (δ) requires the presence of HBV infection. Superinfection of a person already infected with HBV (carrier) causes a more rapid, severe progression than co-infection (*shorter arrow*).

HBsAg is essential for packaging the virus. The delta agent resembles plant virus satellite agents and viroids in its size, genomic structure, and requirement for a helper virus for replication (Figure 62-13).

Structure and Replication

The HDV RNA genome is very small (approximately 1700 nucleotides), and unlike other viruses, the **single-stranded RNA is circular** and forms a rod shape as a result of its extensive base pairing. The virion is approximately the same size as the HBV virion (35 to 37 nm in diameter). The genome is surrounded by the delta antigen core, which in turn is surrounded by an HBsAg-containing envelope. The **delta antigen** exists as a small (24 kD) or large (27 kD) form; the small form is predominant.

The delta agent binds to and is internalized by hepatocytes in the same manner as HBV because it has HBsAg in its envelope. Transcription and replication of the HDV genome are unusual. Specifically, the host cell's RNA polymerase II makes an RNA copy, replicates the genome, and makes mRNA. The genome then forms an RNA structure called a *ribozyme*, which cleaves the RNA circle to produce an mRNA. The gene for the delta antigen is mutated by a cellular enzyme (double-stranded RNA–activated adenosine deaminase) during infection, thereby allowing the production of the large delta antigen. The production of this antigen limits replication of the virus and cell destruction, which promotes persistent infection. The genome, delta antigen, and HBsAg associate and are then released from the cell.

Pathogenesis

Similar to HBV, the delta agent is spread in blood, semen, and vaginal secretions. However, it can replicate and cause disease only in people with active HBV infections. Because the two agents are transmitted by the same routes, a person can be **co-infected** with HBV and the delta agent. A person with chronic HBV can also be **superinfected** with the delta agent. A more rapid, severe progression occurs in HBV carriers superinfected with HDV than in people co-infected with HBV and the delta agent because during co-infection, the HBV must first establish its infection before HDV can replicate (Figure 62-14), whereas superinfection of an HBV-infected person allows the delta agent to replicate immediately.

Replication of the delta agent results in cytotoxicity and liver damage. A persistent delta agent infection is often established in HBV carriers even after symptoms have disappeared. Although antibodies are elicited against the delta agent, protection probably stems from the immune response to HBsAg because it is the external antigen and viral attachment protein for HDV. Unlike HBV disease, damage to the liver occurs as a result of the direct CPE of the delta agent combined with the underlying immunopathology of the HBV disease.

Epidemiology

The delta agent infects children and adults with underlying HBV infection (Box 62-5), and people who are persistently infected with both HBV and HDV are a source for the virus. The agent has a worldwide distribution and is endemic in southern Italy, the Amazon basin, parts of Africa, and the Middle East. Epidemics of HDV infection occur in North America and Western Europe, usually in illicit drug users.

HDV is spread by the same routes as HBV, and the same groups are at risk for infection, with parenteral drug abusers and hemophiliacs those at highest risk.

Clinical Syndromes

The delta agent increases the severity of HBV infections. **Fulminant hepatitis** is more likely to develop in people infected with the delta agent than in those infected with the other hepatitis viruses. This type of hepatitis can result in hepatic encephalopathy (with altered mental capacity) and massive hepatic necrosis, which is fatal in 80%

of cases. Chronic infection with the delta agent can occur in people with chronic HBV.

Laboratory Diagnosis

The only way to determine the presence of the agent is by detecting the delta antigen or antibodies. ELISA and RIA procedures are available for doing this. The delta antigen can be detected in the blood during the acute phase of disease in a detergent-treated serum sample.

Treatment, Prevention, and Control

There is no known specific treatment for HDV hepatitis. Because the delta agent depends on HBV for replication and is spread by the same routes, the prevention of infection with HBV will prevent HDV infection. Immunization with HBV vaccine protects against subsequent delta virus infection. If a person has already acquired HBV, delta agent infection may be prevented by reducing exposure to illicit intravenous drugs, carriers of the virus, or HDV-contaminated blood products.

HEPATITIS E VIRUS

HEV (E-NANBH) *(the E stands for "enteric" or "epidemic")* is predominantly spread by the fecal-oral route, especially in contaminated water (Box 62-2). It resembles calicivirus or the Norwalk agent in size (27 to 34 nm) and structure. Although HEV is found throughout the world, it is most problematic in developing countries. Epidemics have been reported in India, Pakistan, Nepal, Burma, North Africa, and Mexico.

The symptoms and course of HEV disease are very similar to those of HAV disease; it causes only acute disease. However, the symptoms for HEV may occur later than those of HAV disease, and there may be a poor serum immunoglobulin G response. The mortality rate associated with HEV disease is 1% to 2%, approximately 10 times that associated with HAV disease. HEV infection is especially serious in pregnant women (mortality rate of approximately 20%).

CASE STUDIES AND QUESTIONS

Patient A. A 55-year-old man was admitted to the hospital with fatigue, nausea, and abdominal discomfort. He had a slight fever, his urine was dark yellow, and his abdomen was distended and tender. He had returned from a trip to Thailand within the previous month.

Patient B. A 28-year-old woman was admitted to the hospital complaining of vomiting, abdominal discomfort, nausea, anorexia, dark urine, and jaundice. She admitted that she was a former heroin addict and that she had shared needles. She was also 3 months pregnant.

Patient C. A 65-year-old man was admitted with jaundice, nausea, and vomiting 6 months after undergoing coronary artery bypass grafting.

1. What clinical or epidemiological clues would have assisted in the diagnosis of hepatitis A, B, and C?
2. What laboratory tests would have been helpful in distinguishing the different hepatitis infections?
3. What was the most likely means of viral acquisition in each case?
4. What personal and public health precautions should have been taken to prevent the transmission of virus in each case?
5. Which of the patients was susceptible to chronic disease?
6. What laboratory tests distinguish acute from chronic HBV disease?
7. How can HBV disease be prevented? Treated?

Bibliography

Blum HE, Gerok W, Vyas GN: The molecular biology of hepatitis B virus, *Trends Genet* 5:154-158, 1989.

Bradley DW, Krawczynski K, Kane MA: *Hepatitis E.* In Belshe RB, editor: *Textbook of human virology,* ed 2, St Louis, 1991, Mosby.

Fallows DA, Goff AP: Hepadnaviruses: current models of RNA encapsidation and reverse transcription, *Adv Virus Res* 46:167-196, 1996.

Fields BN, Knipe DM, Howley PM, editors: *Virology,* ed 3, New York, 1996, Lippincott-Raven.

Frosner G: *Hepatitis A virus.* In Belshe RB, editor: *Textbook of human virology,* ed 2, St Louis, 1991, Mosby.

Hadler SC, Fields HA: *Hepatitis delta virus.* In Belshe RB, editor: *Textbook of human virology,* ed 2, St Louis, 1991, Mosby.

Hoofnagle JH: Type A and type B hepatitis, *Lab Med* 14:705-716, 1983.

Lennette EH, Halonen P, Murphy FA, editors: *Laboratory diagnosis of infectious diseases: principles and practice,* New York, 1988, Springer-Verlag.

Lutwick LI: *Hepatitis B virus.* In Belshe RB, editor: *Textbook of human virology,* ed 2, St Louis, 1991, Mosby.

Mason WS, Seeger C, editors: Hepadnaviruses: molecular biology and pathogenesis, *Curr Top Microbiol Immunol* 162:1-206, 1991.

Plageman PGW: Hepatitis C virus, *Arch Virol* 120:165-180, 1991.

Reyes GR, Baroudy BM: Molecular biology of NANBH agents: hepatitis C and hepatitis E viruses, *Adv Vir Res* 40:57-102, 1991.

Robinson W, Koike K, Will H, editors: *Hepadnavirus,* New York, 1987, Liss.

Tam AW et al: Hepatitis E virus: molecular cloning and sequencing of the full-length viral genome, *Virology* 185:120-131, 1991.

Unconventional Slow Viruses: Prions

The unconventional slow viruses cause spongiform encephalopathies, which are slow neurodegenerative diseases. These include the human diseases kuru, Creutzfeldt-Jakob disease (CJD), Gerstmann-Sträussler-Scheinker (GSS) disease, and fatal familial insomnia (FFI) and the animal diseases scrapie, bovine spongiform encephalopathy (mad cow disease), chronic wasting disease (in mule, deer, and elk), and transmissible mink encephalopathy (Box 63-1). **CJD, FFI, and GSS disease are also genetic human disorders.**

Slow virus agents are filterable and can transmit disease but otherwise do not conform to the standard definition of a virus (Table 63-1). Unlike conventional viruses, no virion structure or genome has been detected, no immune response is elicited, and the agents are extremely resistant to inactivation by heat, disinfectants, and radiation. The slow virus agent appears to be a modified host protein known as a **prion** (a small proteinaceous infectious particle), which can transmit the disease.

After long incubation periods, these agents cause damage to the central nervous system, which leads to a subacute spongiform encephalopathy. The long incubation period, which can last 30 years in humans, has made study of these agents difficult. Carlton Gajdusek won the Nobel Prize for showing that kuru has an infectious etiology and also for showing the means for initially analyzing the agent. The major breakthroughs came when the kuru agent was transmitted to monkeys and when it was recognized that the scrapie agent induced a characteristic cytopathology in hamsters long before the disease was evident. These studies provided a useful means for assaying this agent and identifying its biological properties.

STRUCTURE AND PHYSIOLOGY

The slow virus agents were suspected to be viruses because they can pass through filters that block the passage of particles greater than 100 nm in diameter and still transmit disease. The agents are resistant to a wide range of chemical and physical treatments, such as formaldehyde, ultraviolet radiation, and heat to 80° C.

BOX 63-1	Slow Virus Diseases

HUMAN

Kuru
Creutzfeldt-Jakob disease (CJD)
Gerstmann-Sträussler-Scheinker (GSS disease)
Fatal familial insomnia (FFI)

ANIMAL

Scrapie (sheep and goats)
Transmissible mink encephalopathy
Bovine spongiform encephalopathy (mad cow disease)
Chronic wasting disease (mule, deer, and elk)

TABLE 63-1	Comparision of Classic Viruses and Prions

	VIRUS	PRION
Filterable, infectious agents	Yes	Yes
Presence of nucleic acid	Yes	No?
Defined morphology (electron microscopy)	Yes	No
Presence of protein	Yes	Yes
Disinfection by:		
Formaldehyde	Yes	No
Proteases	Some	No
Heat (80° C)	Most	No
Ionizing and ultraviolet radiation	Yes	No
DISEASE		
Cytopathological effect	Yes	No
Incubation period	Depends on virus	Long
Immune response	Yes	No
Interferon production	Yes	No
Inflammatory response	Yes	No

The prototype of these agents is scrapie, which has been adapted so that it can infect hamsters. Scrapie-infected hamsters have scrapie-associated fibrils in their brain. These fibrils are infectious and contain the prion.

The prion lacks detectable nucleic acids and consists of aggregates of a protease-resistant, hydrophobic glycoprotein, which for scrapie is termed **PrP^Sc** (scrapie prion protein) (27,000 to 30,000 daltons). Humans and other animals encode a protein PrP^c (cellular prion protein) that is closely related to PrP^Sc in its protein sequence but differs in many of its other properties (Table 63-2). Differences in posttranslational modifications cause the two proteins to behave very differently. PrP^Sc is protease resistant, aggregates into amyloid rods (fibrils), is found in cytoplasmic vesicles in the cell, and is secreted. The normal PrP^c, on the other hand, is protease sensitive and appears on the cell surface.

Many theories have been proposed to explain how an aberrant protein could cause disease. Stanley Prusiner suggested one model in which he conjectures that the PrP^Sc binds to the normal PrP^c on the cell surface, then causes it to be processed into PrP^Sc, released from the cell, and aggregated as amyloid-like plaques in the brain. After this, the cell replenishes the PrP^c, and the cycle continues. The fact that these plaques consist of host protein may explain the lack of an immune response to these agents in patients with the spongiform encephalopathies.

Although there is strong evidence indicating that the prion is infectious and can cause scrapie and that similar proteins are responsible for causing CJD and kuru, other possibilities remain. For example, the protein may be a component of an undiscovered virus or may be induced by a viral infection.

PATHOGENESIS

The term **spongiform encephalopathy** is derived from the characteristic degeneration of neurons and axons of the gray matter that occurs in affected patients (Box 63-2). Vacuolation of the neurons, the formation of amyloid-containing plaques and fibrils, a proliferation and hypertrophy of astrocytes, and the fusion of neurons and adjacent glial cells are observed (Figure 63-1). In addition, prions reach high concentrations in the brain, further contributing to the tissue damage. Prions can also be isolated from tissue other than the brain, but only the brain shows any pathology. No inflammation or immune response to the agent is generated, which distinguishes this disease from a classic viral encephalitis.

The incubation period for CJD and kuru may be as long as 30 years, but once the symptoms become evident, the patient dies within a year.

EPIDEMIOLOGY

CJD is transmitted predominantly by injection, the transplantation of contaminated tissue (e.g., corneas), or contact with contaminated medical devices (e.g., brain electrodes) (Box 63-3). CJD, FFI, and GSS disease are also inheritable, and families with genetic histories of these diseases have been identified. These diseases are rare but occur worldwide.

Kuru, however, was limited to a very small area of the New Guinea highlands. The name of the disease means "shivering" or "trembling," and the disease was related to the cannibalistic practices of the Fore tribe of New Guinea. Before Gajdusek intervened, it was the custom of these people to eat the bodies of their deceased kinsmen. When Gajdusek began his study, he noted that women and children in particular were the most susceptible to the disease, and he deduced that this was because the women and children prepared the food and because they were given the less desirable viscera and brains to eat. That is, their risk for infection was increased because they handled the contaminated tissue, making it possible for the agent to be introduced through the conjunctiva or cuts in the skin, and they ingested the neural tissue, which contains the highest concentrations of the kuru agent. Cessation of this cannibalistic custom has stopped the spread of kuru.

An epidemic of mad cow disease and the unusual incidence of CJD in younger people (younger than 45

TABLE 63-2   Comparision of PrP^Sc and PrP^c*

	PRP^SC	PRP^C
Structure	Globular	Extended
Protease resistance	Yes	No
Presence in scrapie fibrils	Yes	No
Location in or on cells	Cytoplasmic vesicles	Plasma membrane
Turnover	Days	Hours

*PrP^Sc is the prion scrapie agent, and PrP^c is the natural cellular homologue.

BOX 63-2   Pathogenic Characteristics of Slow Viruses

No cytopathological effect in vitro
Long doubling time of at least 5.2 days
Long incubation period
Cause of vacuolation of neurons (spongiform), amyloid-like plaques, gliosis
Symptoms that include loss of muscle control, shivering, tremors, dementia
Lack of antigenicity
Lack of inflammation
Lack of immune response
Lack of interferon production

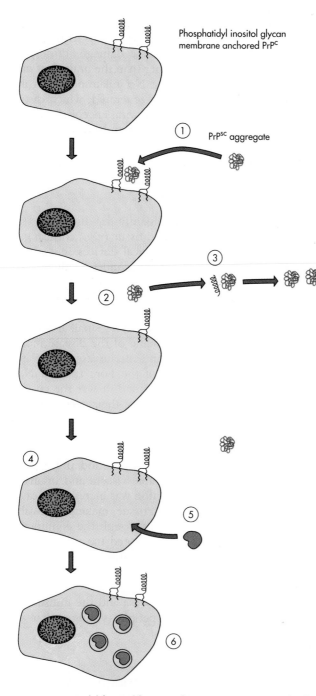

Phosphatidyl inositol glycan
membrane anchored PrP^c

① PrP^{sc} aggregate

②

③

④

⑤

⑥

FIGURE 63-1 Model for proliferation of prions. PrP^c is a normal cellular protein that is anchored in the cell membrane by phosphatidyl inositol glycan. PrP^{sc} is a hydrophobic globular protein that aggregates with itself and with PrP^c on the cell surface *(1)*. This causes the release of PrP^c *(2)* and its conversion to PrP^{sc} *(3)*. The cell synthesizes new PrP^c *(4)*, and the cycle is repeated. A form of PrP^{sc} is internalized by neurons *(5)* and accumulates *(6)*, giving the cell a spongiform appearance. Other models have been proposed.

Infection   Incubation period   Prodrome   Dementia/
                                              Myoclonic stage
                                                              → Death
              1–30 years   3.5 months   4 months

FIGURE 63-2 Progression of transmissible CJD.

years old) prompted concern that contaminated beef was the source of this new variant of CJD. The association between the bovine and human diseases has not been proved, however.

CLINICAL SYNDROMES

As already noted, the slow virus agents cause a progressive, degenerative neurological disease with a long incubation period but with rapid progression to death after the onset of symptoms (Figure 63-2). The spongiform encephalopathies are characterized by a loss of muscle control, leading to shivering, myoclonic jerks, tremors, loss of coordination, and rapidly progressive dementia.

LABORATORY DIAGNOSIS

There are no methods for directly detecting virus in tissue using electron microscopy, antigen detection, or nucleic acid probes. Also, no serological tests can detect viral antibody. The diagnosis must be made on clinical grounds, with confirmation by the characteristic histological changes in brain tissue described in the section on pathogenesis.

TREATMENT, PREVENTION, AND CONTROL

No treatment exists for kuru or CJD. The causative agents are also impervious to the disinfection procedures used for other viruses, including formaldehyde, detergents, and ionizing radiation. Autoclaving at 15 psi for 1 hour instead of 20 minutes or treatment with 5% hypochlorite solution or 1.0 M sodium hydroxide can be used for decontamination. Because these agents can be transmitted on instruments and brain electrodes, such items should be carefully disinfected before reuse.

CASE STUDY AND QUESTIONS

A 70-year-old woman complained of severe headaches and appeared dull and apathetic with a constant tremor in the right hand. One month later, she suffered memory loss and moments of confusion. The patient's condition continued to deteriorate, and an abnormal electroencephalograph tracing showing periodic biphasic and triphasic slow-wave complexes was obtained 2 months later. By 3 months, the patient was in a comalike state. She also had occasional spontaneous clonic twitching of the arms and legs and a startle myoclonic jerking response to a loud noise. The patient died of pneumonia 4 months after the onset of symptoms. No gross abnor-malities were noted at autopsy. Astrocytic gliosis of the cerebral cortex with fibrils and intracellular vacuolation throughout the cerebral cortex were seen microscopically. There was no swelling and no inflammation.

1. What viral neurological diseases would have been considered in the differential diagnosis formulated on the basis of the symptoms described? What other diseases?
2. What key features of the postmortem findings were characteristic of the diseases caused by unconventional slow virus agents (spongiform encephalopathies, prions)?
3. What key features distinguish the unconventional slow virus diseases from more conventional neurological viral diseases?
4. What precautions should the pathologist have taken for protection against infection during the postmortem examination?

Bibliography

Chesebro B: *Spongiform encephalopathies: the transmissible agents.* In Fields BN, Knipe DM, editors: *Virology,* ed 2, New York, 1990, Raven.

Fields BN, Knipe DM, Howley PM: editors: *Virology,* ed 3, New York, 1996, Lippincott-Raven.

Prusiner SB: Molecular biology and genetics of neurodegenerative diseases caused by prions, *Adv Virus Res* 41:241-280, 1992.

Prusiner SB: Prions, prions, prions, *Curr Top Microbiol Immunol* 207:1-162, 1996.

64

Miscellaneous Viruses

CORONAVIRUSES

Coronaviruses are named for the solar corona–like appearance (the surface projections) of their virion when viewed with an electron microscope (Figure 64-1). Coronaviruses are the second most prevalent cause of the **common cold** (rhinovirus is the first). Electron microscopy findings have also linked coronaviruses to gastroenteritis in children and adults. Only two strains of virus have been isolated from humans; however, other strains are believed to exist.

Structure and Replication

Coronaviruses are **enveloped** virions with long helical nucleocapsids that measure 80 to 160 nm (Box 64-1). The glycoproteins on the surface of the envelope appear as club-shaped projections that are 20 nm long and 5 to 11 nm wide. The virion is normally sensitive to acid, ether, and drying, but some strains are capable of traversing the gastrointestinal tract.

The genome is composed of a **plus-stranded RNA** (27,000 to 30,000 bases). On infection, the genome is translated to produce an RNA-dependent RNA polymerase (**L** [225,000 daltons]). The polymerase generates a negative-sense template RNA. The L protein then uses the template RNA to replicate new genomes and produce individual messenger RNAs (mRNAs) encoding the other viral proteins. This is similar to the mode of replication for togaviruses.

Virions contain the glycoproteins **E1** (20,000 to 30,000 daltons) and **E2** (160,000 to 200,000 daltons) and a core nucleoprotein (**N** [47,000 to 55,000 daltons]); some strains also contain a hemagglutinin-neuraminidase (**E3** [120,000 to 140,000 daltons]) (Table 64-1). The E2 glycoprotein is responsible for mediating viral attachment and membrane fusion and is the target of neutralizing antibodies. The E1 glycoprotein is a transmembrane matrix protein. The replication scheme for coronaviruses is shown in Figure 64-2.

Pathogenesis and Clinical Syndromes

Coronaviruses inoculated into the respiratory tracts of human volunteers have been found to infect epithelial cells. Infection remains localized to the upper respiratory tract because the *optimum temperature for viral growth is 33° to 35° C* (Box 64-2).

The virus is most likely spread by aerosols and in large droplets (e.g., sneezes). Coronaviruses cause an upper respiratory tract infection similar to the colds caused by rhinoviruses but with a longer incubation period (average, 3 days). The infection may exacerbate a preexisting chronic pulmonary disease such as asthma and bronchitis. Although the infection is usually mild, pneumonia may occur in children and adults.

BOX 64-1 **Unique Features of Coronaviruses**

Virus has medium-sized virions with a solar corona–like appearance.

Single-stranded, positive-sense RNA genome is enclosed in an envelope containing the E2 viral attachment protein, E1 matrix protein, and N nucleocapsid protein.

Translation of genome occurs in two phases: Early phase produces an RNA polymerase (L). Late phase, from a negative-sense RNA template, yields structural and nonstructural proteins.

Virus assembles at the rough endoplasmic reticulum.

Virus is difficult to isolate and grow in routine cell culture.

BOX 64-2 **Disease Mechanisms of Human Coronaviruses**

Virus infects epithelial cells of upper respiratory tract.

Virus replicates best at 33° to 35° C; therefore it is restricted to upper respiratory tract.

Reinfection occurs in presence of serum antibodies.

Enveloped virus may be able to survive the gastrointestinal tract.

FIGURE 64-1 A, Electron micrograph of the human respiratory coronavirus. (× 90,000.) **B,** Model of a coronavirus. The viral nucleocapsid is a long, flexible helix composed of the plus-strand genomic RNA and many molecules of the phosphorylated nucleocapsid protein N. The viral envelope includes a lipid bilayer derived from the intracellular membranes of the host cell and two viral glycoproteins (E1 and E2). (**A** Courtesy Centers for Disease Control and Prevention, Atlanta; **B** redrawn from Fields BF, Knipe DM, editors: *Virology,* New York, 1985, Raven.)

FIGURE 64-2 Replication of human coronaviruses. The E2 glycoprotein interacts with receptors on epithelial cells, the virus fuses or is endocytosed into the cell, and the genome is released into the cytoplasm. Protein synthesis is divided into early and late phases similar to that of the togaviruses. The genome binds to ribosomes, and an RNA-dependent RNA polymerase is translated. This enzyme generates a full-length, negative-sense RNA template for the production of new virion genomes and six individual mRNAs for the other coronavirus proteins. The genome associates with rough endoplasmic reticulum membranes modified by virion proteins and buds into the lumen of the rough endoplasmic reticulum. Vesicles that contain virus migrate to the cell membrane and are released by exocytosis. (Redrawn from Balows A et al, editors: *Laboratory diagnosis of infectious diseases: principles and practice,* New York, 1988, Springer-Verlag.)

TABLE 64-1	Major Human Coronavirus Proteins		
PROTEINS	**MOLECULAR WEIGHT (kD)**	**LOCATION**	**FUNCTIONS**
E2 (peplomeric glycoprotein)	160-200	Envelope spikes (peplomer)	Binding to host cells; fusion activity
H1 (hemagglutinin protein)	60-66	Peplomer	Hemagglutination
N (nucleoprotein)	47-55	Core	Ribonucleoprotein
E1 (matrix glycoprotein)	20-30	Envelope	Transmembrane proteins
L (polymerase)	225	Infected cell	Polymerase activity

Modified from Balows A et al, editors: *Laboratory diagnosis of infectious diseases: principles and practice,* New York, 1988, Springer-Verlag.

Infections, which occur mainly in infants and children, appear either sporadically or in outbreaks in the winter and spring. Usually, one strain predominates in an outbreak. On the basis of findings from serological studies, coronaviruses are known to cause approximately 10% to 15% of upper respiratory tract infections and pneumonias in humans. Antibodies to coronaviruses are uniformly present by adulthood, but reinfections are common despite the preexisting serum antibodies.

Coronavirus-like particles have also been seen in electron micrographs of stool specimens obtained from adults and children with diarrhea and gastroenteritis and infants with neonatal necrotizing enterocolitis.

Laboratory Diagnosis

Laboratory tests are not routinely done to diagnose coronavirus infections. However, enzyme-linked immunosorbent assay (ELISA) can be used to evaluate acute and convalescent serum. Electron microscopy has also been used to detect coronavirus-like particles in stool specimens.

Treatment, Prevention, and Control

Control of the respiratory transmission of coronaviruses would be difficult and is probably unnecessary because of the mildness of the infection. No vaccine or specific antiviral therapy is available.

CALICIVIRUS AND OTHER SMALL, ROUND GASTROENTERITIS VIRUSES

Norwalk agent was discovered by electron microscopy in stool from adults during an epidemic of an acute gastroenteritis in Norwalk, Ohio. Norwalk agent and other small, round gastroenteritis viruses include the caliciviruses, astroviruses, and unclassified viruses bearing the names of the geographical locations where they were identified (Box 64-3).

Structure and Replication

Caliciviruses, including Norwalk agent, are approximately the same size as picornaviruses. Their **positive-sense RNA genome** (approximately 7500 bases) is contained in a 27-nm **naked capsid** consisting of one 60,000-dalton capsid protein. Norwalk virions are round with a ragged outline, whereas other calicivirions have cup-shaped indentations and a six-pointed star shape. The virions of the astroviruses have a five- or six-pointed star shape on the surface but no indentations. Antibodies from seropositive people can also be used to distinguish these viruses.

Caliciviruses and astroviruses can be grown in cell culture, but the Norwalk viruses cannot. These viruses replicate in the cytoplasm, with release of viral particles on cell destruction.

Pathogenesis

The virus compromises the function of the intestinal brush border, which prevents proper absorption of water and nutrients. Although no histological changes occur in the gastric mucosa, gastric emptying may be delayed. Examination of jejunal biopsy specimens from human volunteers infected with caliciviruses has revealed the existence of blunted villi, cytoplasmic vacuolation, and infiltration with mononuclear cells, but viral particles are not detected on electron micrographs of epithelial cells.

Epidemiology

Norwalk and related viruses typically cause **outbreaks of gastroenteritis** as a result of a **common source of contamination** (e.g., water, shellfish, food service). These viruses are transmitted by the fecal-oral and possibly airborne routes. Outbreaks in developed countries may occur year-round and have been described in schools, resorts, hospitals, nursing homes, restaurants, and cruise ships. The importance of these agents is indicated by the fact that almost 10% of all outbreaks of gastroenteritis and almost 60% of those that are nonbacterial in origin are attributed to Norwalk viruses. Immunity is generally short lived at best and may not be protective.

Approximately 3% of the cases of gastroenteritis in children in **day-care centers** in the United States are at-

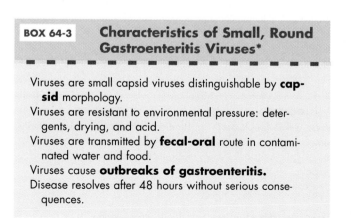

BOX 64-3   Characteristics of Small, Round Gastroenteritis Viruses*

Viruses are small capsid viruses distinguishable by **capsid** morphology.
Viruses are resistant to environmental pressure: detergents, drying, and acid.
Viruses are transmitted by **fecal-oral** route in contaminated water and food.
Viruses cause **outbreaks of gastroenteritis.**
Disease resolves after 48 hours without serious consequences.

*Includes Norwalk agent and calicivirus.

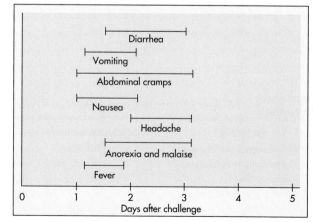

FIGURE 64-3 Response to ingestion of Norwalk virus. Symptoms may vary in severity.

tributed to caliciviruses. As many as 70% of children have antibodies to the astroviruses by the age of 7.

Clinical Syndromes

Norwalk and related viruses cause symptoms similar to those caused by the rotaviruses. Infection causes **diarrhea with nausea and vomiting,** especially in children (Figure 64-3). **Bloody stools do not occur.** Fever may occur in as many as one third of the patients. The incubation period is 24 to 48 hours, and the illness resolves within 12 to 60 hours without problems. Astroviruses cause diarrhea without vomiting and are less likely to cause disease in adults.

Laboratory Diagnosis

Immune electron microscopy can be used to concentrate and identify the virus from stool. The addition of an antibody directed against the suspected agent causes the virus to aggregate, thereby facilitating recognition. Radioimmunoassay (RIA) and ELISA have been developed to detect the virus and viral antigen.

Serology is the method used to identify most infections. Antibody to the Norwalk agent may be detected by RIA or ELISA. Antibodies to the other calicivirus-like agents are more difficult to detect.

Treatment, Prevention, and Control

No specific treatment for infection with the calicivirus or other small, round gastroenteritis viruses is available. Bismuth subsalicylate may reduce the severity of the gastrointestinal symptoms. Outbreaks may be minimized by handling food carefully and by maintaining the purity of the water supply.

FILOVIRUSES

The Marburg and Ebola viruses (Figure 64-4) were classified as members of the Rhabdoviridae but are now classified as filoviruses. They are **filamentous, enveloped, negative-strand RNA viruses.** These agents cause **severe or fatal hemorrhagic fevers** and are **endemic in**

FIGURE 64-4 Electron micrograph of the Ebola virus. (Courtesy Centers for Disease Control and Prevention, Atlanta.)

Africa. Increased awareness of Ebola occurred after an outbreak of the disease in Zaire in 1995 and in Gabon in 1996 and also after the release of the movie *Outbreak,* based on the book by Robin Cook, and the book *The Hot Zone* by Richard Preston.

Structure and Replication

Filoviruses have a **single-stranded RNA genome** (4.5×10^6 daltons), which encodes seven proteins. The virions form **enveloped filaments** with a diameter of 80 nm but may also assume other shapes. They vary in length from 800 nm to as long as 14,000 nm. The nucleocapsid is helical and enclosed in an envelope containing one glycoprotein. The virus replicates in the cytoplasm in a manner similar to that of the rhabdoviruses.

Pathogenesis

The filoviruses replicate efficiently, producing large amounts of virus and causing extensive tissue necrosis in parenchymal cells of the liver, spleen, lymph nodes, and lungs. The widespread hemorrhage that occurs in affected patients causes edema and hypovolemic shock.

Epidemiology

Marburg virus infection was first detected among laboratory workers in Marburg, Germany, who had been exposed to tissues from apparently healthy African green monkeys. Rare cases of Marburg virus infection have been seen in Zimbabwe and Kenya.

Outbreaks of Ebola virus disease have occurred in Zaire and the Sudan. During an outbreak, the Ebola virus is so lethal that it eliminates the susceptible population before it can be spread extensively. However, in rural areas of central Africa as much as 18% of the population have antibody to this virus, indicating that subclinical infections do occur.

The mechanisms of natural transmission are unknown. These viruses may be endemic in wild monkeys but can be spread from monkeys to humans and between humans. Laboratory contact with infected monkeys obtained from a questionable source was a source of human infection and death. These viruses have been transmitted by accidental injection and through the use of contaminated syringes. Virus may also be passed to a person who comes into close contact with body fluids.

Clinical Syndromes

Marburg and Ebola viruses are the most severe causes of viral hemorrhagic fevers. The illness usually begins with influenza-like symptoms such as headache and myalgia. Nausea, vomiting, and diarrhea occur within a few days; a rash also may develop. Subsequently, hemorrhage from multiple sites, especially the gastrointestinal tract, and death occur in as many as 90% of patients with clinically evident disease.

Laboratory Diagnosis

All specimens from patients with a suspected filovirus infection must be handled with extreme care to prevent accidental infection. Handling of these viruses requires level 4 isolation procedures that are not routinely available. Marburg virus may grow rapidly in tissue culture (Vero cells), but animal (e.g., guinea pig) inoculation may be necessary to recover Ebola virus.

Infected cells have large eosinophilic cytoplasmic inclusion bodies. Viral antigens in tissues can be detected by direct immunofluorescence analysis.

IgG and IgM antibody to filovirus antigens can be detected by immunofluorescence, ELISA, or RIA. Seroconversion or a fourfold increase in the IgG antibody levels may be diagnostic of active infection, as may the detection of specific IgM antibody.

Treatment, Prevention, and Control

Antibody-containing serum and interferon therapies have been tried in patients with these infections. Infected patients should be quarantined, and contaminated animals should be sacrificed. Handling of the viruses or contaminated materials requires very stringent isolation procedures (level 4).

ARENAVIRUSES

The arenaviruses include lymphocytic choriomeningitis (LCM) and hemorrhagic fever viruses such as the Lassa, Junin, and Machupo viruses. These viruses cause persistent infections in specific **rodents** and can be transmitted to humans as **zoonoses.**

Structure and Replication

Arenaviruses are seen in electron micrographs to be pleomorphic, **enveloped** viruses (diameter, 120 nm) that have a sandy appearance (the name comes from the Greek word *arenosa,* meaning "sandy") because of the **ribosomes in the virion** (Box 64-4). Although functional, the ribosomes do not seem to serve a purpose. Virions contain a beaded nucleocapsid with **two single-stranded RNA circles** (S, 3.2×10^6 daltons; L, 4.8×10^6 daltons) and a transcriptase. The L strand is a negative-sense RNA and encodes the polymerase. The S strand encodes the nucleoprotein (N protein) and the glycoproteins but is **ambisense.** Whereas the mRNA for

the N protein is transcribed directly from the ambisense S strand, the mRNA for the glycoprotein is transcribed from a full-length template of the genome. As a result, the glycoproteins are produced as late proteins after genome replication. Arenaviruses replicate in the cytoplasm and acquire their envelope by budding from the host cell plasma membrane.

Arenaviruses readily cause persistent infections. This may result from inefficient transcription of the glycoprotein genes.

Pathogenesis

Arenaviruses are able to infect macrophages and possibly cause the release of mediators of cell and vascular damage. Tissue destruction is significantly exacerbated by T-cell immunity. Persistent infection of rodents results from neonatal infection and the induction of immune tolerance. The incubation period for arenavirus infections averages 10 to 14 days.

Epidemiology

Most arenaviruses, except for the virus that causes LCM, are found in the tropics of Africa and South America. The arenaviruses infect specific rodents and are endemic to the rodents' habitats. Chronic asymptomatic infection is common in these animals and leads to a chronic viremia and long-term viral shedding in saliva, urine, and feces. Humans may become infected through the inhalation of aerosols, the consumption of contaminated food, or contact with fomites. Bites are not a usual mechanism of spread.

The virus that causes LCM infects hamsters and house mice *(Mus musculus).* In Washington, D.C., it was found in 20% of mice. LCM disease in the United States is associated with contact with pet hamsters and with the animals in rodent-breeding facilities. Lassa fever virus infects *Mastomys natalensis,* an African rodent. The Lassa fever virus is spread from human to human through contact with infected secretions or body fluids, but the viruses that cause LCM or other hemorrhagic fevers are rarely if ever spread in this way.

Clinical Syndromes

Lymphocytic Choriomeningitis

The name of the virus that causes LCM suggests that meningitis is a typical clinical event, but actually LCM causes a febrile illness with influenza-like myalgia more often than meningeal illness. It is estimated that approximately 25% of infected persons exhibit clinical evidence of a central nervous system infection. The meningeal illness, if it occurs, may be subacute and persist for several months. Perivascular mononuclear infiltrates may be seen in neurons of all sections of the brain and in the meninges.

Lassa and Other Hemorrhagic Fevers

Lassa fever, which is endemic to west Africa, is the best known of the hemorrhagic fevers caused by the are-

---

BOX 64-4 **Characteristics of Arenaviruses**

Virus has **enveloped** virion with two **circular, negative RNA** genome segments (L, S). Virion appears **sandy because of ribosomes.**
S genome segment is ambisense.
Arenavirus infections are zoonoses, establishing persistent infections in rodents.
Pathogenesis of arenavirus infections is largely attributed to T-cell immunopathogenesis.

navirus. Other agents, however, such as the Junin and Machupo viruses, cause similar syndromes in the inhabitants of different geographical areas (Argentina and Bolivia, respectively).

Clinical illness is characterized by fever, coagulopathy, petechiae, and occasional visceral hemorrhage, as well as liver and spleen necrosis, but not vasculitis. Hemorrhage and shock also occur, as does occasional cardiac and liver damage. In contrast to LCM, no lesions are present in the central nervous system of patients with hemorrhagic fevers. Pharyngitis, diarrhea, and vomiting may be prevalent, especially in patients with Lassa fever. Death occurs in as many as 50% of those with Lassa fever and in a smaller percentage of those infected with the other arenaviruses that cause hemorrhagic fevers. The diagnosis is suggested by recent travel to endemic areas.

Laboratory Diagnosis

An arenavirus infection is usually diagnosed on the basis of serological findings. These viruses are too dangerous for routine isolation. Throat specimens can yield arenaviruses; urine is often positive for the Lassa fever virus but negative for the LCM virus. Substantial risk for infection is present for laboratory workers handling body fluids. Therefore if the diagnosis is suspected, laboratory personnel should be so warned and specimens processed only in facilities that specialize in the isolation of contagious pathogens (level 3 for LCM and level 4 for Lassa fever and other arenaviruses).

Treatment, Prevention, and Control

The antiviral drug ribavirin has limited activity against arenaviruses and can be used to treat Lassa fever. However, supportive therapy is usually all that is available for patients with arenavirus infections.

These rodent-borne infections can be prevented by limiting contact with the vector. For example, improved hygiene to limit contact with mice reduced the incidence of LCM in Washington, D.C. In the geographical areas where hemorrhagic fever occurs, trapping rodents and carefully storing food may decrease exposure to the virus.

The incidence of laboratory-acquired cases can be reduced if samples submitted for arenavirus isolation are processed in at least type 3 or 4 biosafety facilities and not in the usual clinical virology laboratory.

CASE STUDIES AND QUESTIONS

A 58-year-old woman complained of influenza-like symptoms, severe headache, stiff neck, and photophobia. She was lethargic and had a mild fever. Her cerebrospinal fluid contained 900 white blood cells, mostly lymphocytes, and LCM virus. She recovered after a week. Her home was infested with gray mice *(Mus musculus)*.

1. What were the significant symptoms of this disease?
2. How was the virus transmitted?
3. What type of immune response is most important in controlling this infection?

Several adults complained of serious diarrhea, nausea, vomiting, and a mild fever 2 days after visiting Le Cafe Grease. The symptoms were too severe to result from food poisoning or a routine gastroenteritis but lasted only 24 hours.

1. What characteristics distinguished this disease from a rotavirus infection?
2. What was the most likely means of viral transmission?
3. What physical characteristics of the virus allowed it to be transmitted by these means?
4. What public health measures could be followed to prevent such outbreaks?

Bibliography

Balows A, Hausler WJ Jr, Lennette EH: *Laboratory diagnosis of infectious diseases: principles and practice,* New York, 1988, Springer-Verlag.

Belshe RB, editor: *Textbook of human virology,* ed 2, St Louis, 1991, Mosby.

Bishop RF: *Other small virus-like particles in humans.* In Tyrrell DAJ, Kapikian AZ, editors: *Virus infections of the gastrointestinal tract,* New York, 1982, Marcel Dekker.

Blacklow NR, Greenberg HB: Viral gastroenteritis, *N Engl J Med* 325:252-264, 1991.

Christensen ML: Human viral gastroenteritis, *Clin Microbiol Rev* 2:51-89, 1989.

Fields BN, Knipe DM, Howley PM: editors: *Virology,* ed 3, New York, 1996, Lippincott-Raven.

Oldstone MBA: Arenaviruses, *Curr Top Microbiol Immunol* 133:1-116, 134:1-242, 1987.

Preston R: *The hot zone,* New York, 1994, Random House.

Sodhi A: Ebola virus disease, *Postgrad Med* 99:75-76, 1996.

ter Meulen V, Siddell S, Wege H, editors: *Biochemistry and biology of coronaviruses,* New York, 1981, Plenum.

Xi JN et al: Norwalk virus genome cloning and characterization, *Science* 250:1580-1583, 1990.

Role of Viruses in Disease

Most viral infections cause mild or no symptoms and do not require extensive treatment. The common cold, influenza, influenza-like syndromes, and gastroenteritis are common viral diseases. Other viral infections, which cause significant tissue damage or target essential tissues and organs, can cause serious and even life-threatening disease. In general the symptoms and severity of a viral infection are determined by two things: (1) the victim's ability to prevent or rapidly resolve the infection before the virus can reach important organs or cause significant damage and (2) the ability of the body to repair the damage. Previous chapters stressed the viral characteristics that promote disease. In this chapter, viral diseases are discussed with respect to their symptoms, the organ system they target, and the host factors that influence their presentation.

VIRAL DISEASES

The major sites of viral disease are the respiratory tract; the gastrointestinal tract; the epithelial, mucosal, and endothelial linings of the skin, mouth, and genitalia; the lymphoid tissue; the liver and other organs; and the central nervous system (CNS) (Figure 65-1).

Oral and Respiratory Tract Infections

The oropharynx and respiratory tract are the **most common sites** of viral infection and disease (Table 65-1). The viruses are spread in respiratory droplets and aerosols, food and water, and saliva; by close contact; and on hands. Similar respiratory symptoms may be caused by several different viruses. For example, bronchiolitis may be caused by respiratory syncytial or parainfluenza virus. Alternatively, one virus may cause different symptoms in different people. For example, influenza virus may cause a mild upper respiratory tract infection in one person and life-threatening pneumonia in another.

The symptoms and severity of a respiratory viral disease depend on the nature of the virus, the site of infection (upper or lower respiratory tract), and the immune status and the age of the person. Conditions such as cystic fibrosis and smoking, which compromise the ciliated

and mucoepithelial barriers to infection, increase the risk of serious disease.

Pharyngitis and oral disease are common viral presentations. Most enteroviruses infect the oropharynx and then progress by way of a viremia to other target tissues. For example, symptoms such as acute-onset pharyngitis, fever, and oral **vesicular lesions** are characteristic of coxsackie A virus **(herpangina, hand-foot-and-mouth disease)** and some *coxsackie B virus* and *echovirus* infections. Herpesviruses cause local primary infections of the oral mucosa and face. A latent neuronal infection follows *gingivostomatitis* caused by herpes simplex virus (HSV) and recurs in the form of **herpes labialis** (cold sores, fever blisters). HSV is also a common cause of pharyngitis. *Epstein-Barr virus* (EBV) and *human herpesvirus 6* (HHV6) initiate and may cause symptoms in the oropharynx and then establish infection of the lymphocytes. Vesicular lesions on the buccal mucosa **(Koplik's spots)** are an early diagnostic feature of *measles* infection.

Although **upper respiratory tract viral infections,** including the **common cold** and pharyngitis, are generally benign, they still account for at least 50% of absenteeism from schools and the workplace. *Rhinoviruses* and *coronaviruses* are the predominant causes of upper respiratory tract infections. A runny nose (rhinitis) followed by congestion, cough, sneezing, conjunctivitis, headache, and sore throat are typical symptoms of the common cold. Other causes of the common cold and pharyngitis include specific serotypes of *echoviruses* and *coxsackieviruses, adenoviruses, influenza viruses, parainfluenza viruses,* and *respiratory syncytial virus.*

Tonsillitis, laryngitis, and **croup (laryngotracheobronchitis)** may accompany certain respiratory tract viral infections. *Adenovirus* and the early stages of *EBV* disease are characterized by sore throat and tonsillitis with an exudative membrane. *HSV* and *coxsackie A viruses* may also involve the tonsils but with vesicular lesions. Laryngitis (adults) and croup (children) are caused by inflammatory responses to the viral infection that cause the trachea to narrow below the vocal cords (subglottic area). This causes loss of voice; a hoarse, barking cough;

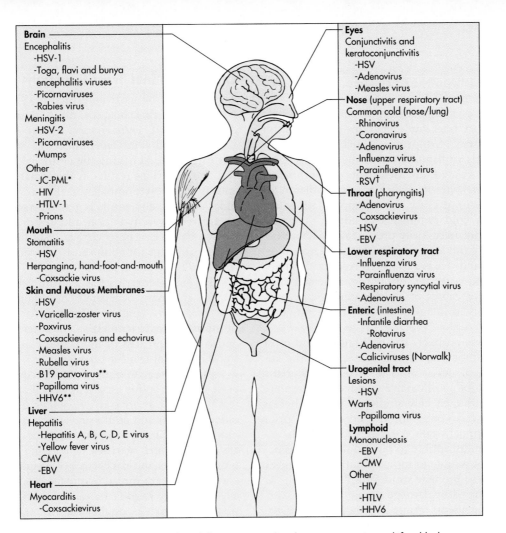

Brain
Encephalitis
-HSV-1
-Toga, flavi and bunya encephalitis viruses
-Picornaviruses
-Rabies virus
Meningitis
-HSV-2
-Picornaviruses
-Mumps
Other
-JC-PML*
-HIV
-HTLV-1
-Prions
Mouth
Stomatitis
-HSV
Herpangina, hand-foot-and-mouth
-Coxsackie virus
Skin and Mucous Membranes
-HSV
-Varicella-zoster virus
-Poxvirus
-Coxsackievirus and echovirus
-Measles virus
-Rubella virus
-B19 parvovirus**
-Papilloma virus
-HHV6**
Liver
Hepatitis
-Hepatitis A, B, C, D, E virus
-Yellow fever virus
-CMV
-EBV
Heart
Myocarditis
-Coxsackievirus

Eyes
Conjunctivitis and keratoconjunctivitis
-HSV
-Adenovirus
-Measles virus
Nose (upper respiratory tract)
Common cold (nose/lung)
-Rhinovirus
-Coronavirus
-Adenovirus
-Influenza virus
-Parainfluenza virus
-RSV†
Throat (pharyngitis)
-Adenovirus
-Coxsackievirus
-HSV
-EBV
Lower respiratory tract
-Influenza virus
-Parainfluenza virus
-Respiratory syncytial virus
-Adenovirus
Enteric (intestine)
-Infantile diarrhea
-Rotavirus
-Adenovirus
-Caliciviruses (Norwalk)
Urogenital tract
Lesions
-HSV
Warts
-Papilloma virus
Lymphoid
Mononucleosis
-EBV
-CMV
Other
-HIV
-HTLV
-HHV6

FIGURE 65-1 Major target tissues of viral disease. Asterisk indicates progressive multifocal leukoencephalopathy, and dagger indicates respiratory syncytial virus. Infection by viruses indicated by two asterisks results in an immune-mediated rash.

TABLE 65-1	**Oral and Respiratory Diseases**

DISEASE	ETIOLOGICAL AGENT	DISEASE	ETIOLOGICAL AGENT
Common cold (including pharyngitis)	Rhinovirus* Coronavirus* Influenza viruses Parainfluenza viruses Respiratory syncytial virus Adenovirus Enteroviruses	Bronchiolitis	Respiratory syncytial virus* (infants) Parainfluenza virus 3* (infants and children) Parainfluenza viruses 1 and 2
Pharyngitis	Herpes simplex virus Epstein-Barr virus Adenovirus* Coxsackie A virus* (herpangina, hand-foot-and-mouth disease) and other enteroviruses	Pneumonia	Respiratory syncytial virus* (infants) Parainfluenza virus* (infants) Influenza virus* Adenovirus Varicella-zoster virus (primary infection of adults or immunocompromised hosts) Cytomegalovirus (infection of immunocompromised host) Measles
Croup, tonsillitis, laryngitis, and bronchitis (children younger than 2 years)	Parainfluenza virus 1* Parainfluenza virus 2 Influenza virus Adenovirus Epstein-Barr virus		

*Most common causal agents.

and the risk, especially in young children, for a blocked airway and choking. Children infected with *parainfluenza viruses* are especially at risk for croup.

Lower respiratory tract viral infections can also result in more serious disease. Symptoms of such infections include **bronchiolitis** (inflammation of the bronchioles), **pneumonia,** and related diseases. The *parainfluenza* and *respiratory syncytial viruses* are major problems for infants and children but cause only asymptomatic infections or common cold symptoms in adults. Infection early in life does not necessarily prevent rechallenge because protection of the lung requires the presence of secretory antibody, and this is a transient response. Parainfluenza 3 virus and especially respiratory syncytial virus infections are major causes of life-threatening pneumonia or bronchiolitis in infants who are younger than 6 months old.

Influenza virus is probably the best known and most feared of the common respiratory viruses, with the annual introduction of new strains of virus ensuring the presence of immunologically naive victims. Children are universally susceptible to new strains of virus, whereas older people may have been immunized during a prior outbreak of the annual strain. Despite the latter, the elderly are especially susceptible to new strains of virus because they may not be able to mount a sufficient primary immune response to the new strain of influenza virus or be able to repair the tissue damage caused by the disease. Other possible viral agents of pneumonia include *adenovirus, paramyxoviruses, and primary varicella-zoster virus (VZV)* infections of adults.

Many viral infections start in the oropharynx or respiratory tract, infect the lung, and spread without causing significant symptoms. *VZV* and *the measles virus* initiate infection in the lung and can cause pneumonia but generally cause systemic infections resulting in an **exanthem (rash).** Other viruses that establish primary infection of the oropharynx or respiratory tract and then progress to other sites include *rubella, mumps, enteroviruses,* and several human herpesviruses (HSV, VZV, EBV, cytomegalovirus [CMV], and HHV6).

Influenza-Like and Systemic Symptoms

Many viral infections cause classic **influenza-like symptoms** (fever, malaise, anorexia, headache, and body aches) during a viremic phase of disease because of the release of interferon and lymphokines. In addition to the *respiratory viruses,* influenza-like symptoms may accompany infections by *arboencephalitis viruses, herpes simplex virus type 2 (HSV-2),* and other viruses.

Arthritis and other inflammatory diseases may result from immune hypersensitivity responses to the infection. For example, *B19* parvovirus infection of adults, *rubella,* and infection with several *other togaviruses* elicit arthritis. Immune-complex disease that is associated with chronic *hepatitis B virus (HBV)* can result in various presentations, including arthritis and nephritis.

Gastrointestinal Tract Infections

Infections of the gastrointestinal tract can result in **gastroenteritis, diarrhea,** or no symptoms (Box 65-1). *Norwalk virus, caliciviruses, astroviruses, adenoviruses, reoviruses,* and *rotaviruses* infect the small intestine but not the colon, damaging the epithelial lining and the absorptive villi. This results in the malabsorption of water and an electrolyte imbalance. The resultant diarrhea in older children and adults is generally self-limited and can be treated by rehydration and restoration of the electrolyte balance. These viruses, especially *rotavirus,* are major problems for adults and children in regions where there is drought and starvation.

Viral gastroenteritis has a more significant effect on infants and may necessitate hospitalization. *Rotavirus and adenovirus serotypes 40* and *41* are the major causes of **infantile gastroenteritis.** The extent of tissue damage and consequent loss of fluids and electrolytes is a more significant problem for infants.

Fecal-oral spread of the enteric viruses is promoted by poor hygiene and is especially prevalent in day-care centers. *Norwalk virus* and *calicivirus* outbreaks affecting older children and adults are generally linked to a common contaminated food or water source. Vomiting usually accompanies diarrhea in patients infected with the Norwalk virus and rotavirus. Although *enteroviruses* (picornaviruses) are spread by the fecal-oral route, they usually cause only *mild* or *no* gastrointestinal symptoms. Instead these viruses establish a viremia, spread to other target organs, and then cause clinical disease.

Exanthems and Hemorrhagic Fevers

Virus-induced skin disease (Table 65-2) can result from infection through the mucosa or small cuts or abrasions in the skin (HSV), as a secondary infection after establishment of a viremia (VZV and smallpox), or as a result of the inflammatory response mounted against viral antigens (measles rash). The major forms of rashes are classified as maculopapular, vesicular, nodular, and hemorrhagic. **Macules** are flat, colored spots. **Papules** are slightly raised areas of the skin and may result from immune or inflammatory responses rather than the direct effects of the virus. **Vesicular lesions** are blisters and are likely to contain virus. Papillomaviruses cause warts, and molluscum contagiosum causes wartlike growths by stimulating the growth of skin cells.

BOX 65-1	**Gastrointestinal Viruses**
INFANTS	**INFANTS, CHILDREN, AND ADULTS**
Rotavirus A*	Norwalk virus
Adenovirus 40, 41	Calicivirus
Coxsackie A24 virus	Astrovirus
	Rotavirus B (outbreaks in China)
	Reovirus

*Most common cause.

The classic **childhood exanthems** include *roseola infantum (exanthem subitum [HHV6]), fifth disease (erythema infectiosum [B19 parvovirus]),* and, in unvaccinated children, varicella, *measles and rubella.* The rash follows a viremia and is accompanied by fever. Except for measles, exanthems are not serious diseases. Rashes are also caused by enterovirus infections, dengue, and other infections caused by flaviviruses or alphaviruses and are occasionally seen in patients with infectious mononucleosis.

The *yellow fever virus, dengue virus,* and other *hemorrhagic fever* viruses establish a viremia and infect the endothelial cell lining of the vasculature, which may compromise the structure of the blood vessel. Viral or immune cytolysis may then lead to increased permeability or rupture of the vessel, producing a **hemorrhagic rash** with **petechiae** (pinpoint hemorrhages under the skin) and **ecchymoses** (massive bruises) and hence internal bleeding, the loss of electrolytes, and shock.

Infections of the Eye

Infections of the eye result from direct contact with a virus or from viremic spread (Box 65-2). **Conjunctivitis** (pinkeye) is a normal feature of many childhood infections and is a characteristic of infections caused by specific *adenovirus* serotypes (3, 4a, and 7), the *measles virus,* and the *rubella virus.* **Keratoconjunctivitis** caused by *adenovirus* (8, 19a, and 37), *HSV,* or *VZV* involves the cornea and can cause severe damage. *Enterovirus 70* and *coxsackie A24* viruses can cause an **acute hemorrhagic conjunctivitis.** **Cataracts** are classic features of babies born with *congenital rubella syndrome.* **Chorioretinitis** is associated with *congenital CMV* in-

fection and CMV infection in immunosuppressed people (e.g., those who have acquired immunodeficiency syndrome [AIDS]).

Infections of the Organs and Tissues

Infection of the major organs may cause significant disease or result in further spread or secretion of the virus (Box 65-2). The symptoms may result from tissue damage or inflammatory responses.

The **liver** is a prominent target for many viruses that reach the liver by means of a viremia or the mononuclear phagocyte (reticuloendothelial) system. The liver acts as a source for a secondary viremia but can also be damaged by the infection. The classic symptoms of **hepatitis** result from infections with *hepatitis A, B, C, D,* and *E viruses* and *yellow fever virus* and are often associated with EBV infectious mononucleosis and CMV infections. The liver is also a major target in disseminated HSV infection of neonates and infants.

The heart and other muscles are also susceptible to viral infection and damage. *Coxsackievirus* can cause **myocarditis** or pericarditis in newborns, children, and adults. *Coxsackie B virus* can infect muscle and cause **pleurodynia** (Bornholm disease). Other viruses (e.g., influenza virus, CMV) may also infect the heart.

Infection of the secretory glands, accessory sexual organs, and mammary glands results in contagious spread of the virus (CMV). An inflammatory response to the infection, as occurs in mumps **(parotitis, orchitis),** may be the cause of the symptoms. CMV infection of the kidney and reactivation are problems for immunosuppressed people and a predominant reason for kidney transplant failure.

TABLE 65-2	**Viral Exanthems**
CONDITION	**ETIOLOGICAL AGENT**
RASH	
Rubeola	Measles virus
German measles	Rubella virus
Roseola infantum	HHV6
Erythema infectiosum	Human parvovirus B19
Boston exanthem	Echovirus 16
Infectious mononucleosis	EBV, CMV
VESICLES	
Oral or genital herpes	HSV*
Chickenpox/shingles	VZV*
Hand-foot-and-mouth disease, herpangina	Coxsackie A virus*
PAPILLOMAS	
Warts	Papilloma virus*
Molluscum	Molluscum contagiosum

*Most common cause.

BOX 65-2	**Infections of the Organs and Tissues**
LIVER	**MUSCLE**
Hepatitis A,* B,* C, D, and E viruses	Coxsackie B virus (pleurodynia)
Yellow fever virus	
EBV	**GLANDS**
Hepatitis in the neonate or immunocompromised person:	CMV
CMV	Mumps virus
HSV	
VZV	**EYE**
Rubella virus (congenital rubella syndrome)	HSV
	Adenovirus*
HEART	Measles virus
Coxsackie B virus	Rubella virus
	Enterovirus 70
KIDNEY	Coxsackie A24 virus
CMV	

*Most common cause.

BOX 65-3   CNS Infections

MENINGITIS

Enteroviruses
   Echoviruses
   Coxsackievirus*
   Poliovirus
HSV-2
Adenovirus
Mumps virus
Lymphocytic choriomen-
   ingitis virus
EBV
Arboencephalitis viruses

PARALYSIS

Poliovirus
Enteroviruses 70 and 71
Coxsackie A7 virus

ENCEPHALITIS

HSV-1*
VZV
Arboencephalitis viruses*
Rabies virus
Coxsackie A and B
   viruses
Polioviruses

POSTINFECTIOUS ENCEPHALITIS (IMMUNE MEDIATED)

Measles virus   VZV
Mumps virus   Influenza viruses
Rubella virus

OTHER

JC virus (progressive multifocal leukoencephalopathy [in
   immunosuppressed people])
Measles variant (subacute sclerosing panencephalitis)
Prion (encephalopathy)
HIV (AIDS dementia)
HTLV-1 (tropical spastic paraparesis)

*Most common cause.

Infections of the Central Nervous System

Viral infections of the brain and CNS may cause the most serious viral diseases because of the importance of the CNS and its very limited capacity to repair damage (Box 65-3). Tissue damage is usually caused by a combination of viral pathogenesis and immunopathogenesis. However, most neurotropic viral infections do not result in disease because the virus does not reach the CNS or does not cause sufficient tissue damage to produce symptoms.

Virus may spread to the CNS in blood *(arboviruses)* or in macrophages *(human immunodeficiency virus [HIV]);* it may spread from a peripheral infection of the neurons (olfactory), or it may first infect skin *(HSV)* or muscle *(rabies)* and then progress to the innervating neurons. The virus then infects the neuronal cells that express a viral receptor. For example, the temporal lobe is targeted in *HSV* encephalitis, Ammon's horn in *rabies,* and the anterior horn of the spinal cord and motor neurons in paralytic *poliomyelitis.*

Viral infections of the CNS are usually distinguished from bacterial infections by the finding of mononuclear cells, low numbers of polymorphonuclear leukocytes, and normal or slightly reduced levels of glucose in the cerebrospinal fluid. Immunoassay detection of specific antigen or isolation of the virus from the cerebrospinal fluid or a biopsy specimen confirms the diagnosis and identifies the viral agent. The season of the year also facilitates the diagnosis in that enteroviral and arboviral diseases generally occur during the summer, whereas HSV encephalitis and other viral syndromes may be observed year-round.

Aseptic meningitis is caused by an inflammation and swelling of the meninges enveloping the brain and spinal cord in response to infection with *enteroviruses* (especially *echoviruses and coxsackieviruses*), *HSV-2,* the *mumps virus,* or the *lymphocytic choriomeningitis virus.* The disease is usually self-limited and, unlike bacterial meningitis, resolves without sequelae unless the virus gains access to and infects neurons or the brain (meningoencephalitis). The viruses gain access to the meninges by means of a viremia.

Encephalitis and **myelitis** result from a combination of viral pathogenesis and immunopathogenesis in brain tissue and neurons and either are fatal or cause significant damage and permanent neurological sequelae. *HSV, VZV, rabies virus, California encephalitis viruses, St. Louis encephalitis virus,* and *measles virus* are potential causes of encephalitis. *Poliovirus* and several other *enteroviruses* cause paralytic disease (myelitis).

HSV and *VZV* are ubiquitous and usually cause asymptomatic latent infections of the CNS but can also cause encephalitis. Most *arboencephalitis virus* infections result in influenza-like symptoms rather than encephalitis. *Postmeasles encephalitis* and subacute sclerosing panencephalitis were rare sequelae of measles in the prevaccine era.

Other virus-induced neurological syndromes include *HIV dementia, human T-lymphotropic virus type 1 (HTLV-1) tropical spastic paraparesis, JC papovavirus–induced, progressive multifocal leukoencephalopathy* in immunosuppressed people, and the *spongiform encephalopathies (kuru, Creutzfeldt-Jakob disease, Gerstmann-Sträussler-Scheinker disease),* which are postulated to be caused by prions.

Hematological Diseases

Lymphocytes and macrophages are not very permissive for viral replication but are targets for several viruses that establish persistent infections. Transient viral replication of *EBV, HIV,* or *CMV* elicits a large T-cell response, resulting in mononucleosis-like syndromes. In addition, *CMV, measles virus,* and *HIV infections* of T cells are immunosuppressive. HIV reduces the numbers of CD4 helper and delayed-type hypersensitivity T cells, which further compromises the immune system. HTLV-1 infection causes little disease on infection but may lead to adult T-cell leukemia or tropical spastic paraparesis much later in life.

Macrophages and cells of the macrophage lineage can be infected by many viruses. Macrophages act as vehicles for spreading the virus throughout the body because viruses replicate inefficiently in them and the cells are generally not lysed by the infection. This promotes per-

BOX 65-4   Sexually Transmitted Viruses

Human papillomavirus 6, 11, 42
Human papillomavirus 16 and 18 (associated with human cervical carcinoma)
HSV (predominantly HSV-2)
CMV
HBV, HCV, HDV
HIV
HTLV-1

sistent and chronic infections. The macrophage is the primary target cell for the dengue virus. Nonneutralizing antibody can promote *dengue* uptake into the cell through Fc receptors. Macrophages and cells of the macrophage lineage infected with *HIV* provide a reservoir for the virus and access to the brain. AIDS dementia is thought to result from the actions of HIV-infected microglial cells in the brain.

Sexually Transmitted Viral Diseases

Although **sexual transmission** is not a very efficient route of viral spread, it is a major route for the spread of *papillomavirus, HSV, CMV, HIV, HTLV-1, HBV, hepatitis C virus (HCV),* and *hepatitis D virus (HDV)* (Box 65-4). These viruses establish chronic and latent-recurrent infections, with asymptomatic shedding into the semen and vaginal secretions. These viral properties foster dissemination via a route of transmission that is used relatively infrequently and would be avoided during symptomatic disease. These viruses can also be transmitted neonatally or perinatally to infants. *Papillomaviruses* and *HSV-2* establish local primary infections with recurrent disease at the same site. Lesions and asymptomatic shedding are sources for sexual transmission and for perinatal transmission to the newborn. *CMV* and *HIV* enter the bloodstream and infect lymphoid cells, whereas *HBV* is delivered to the liver. These viruses are present in blood, semen, and vaginal secretions, in which the virus can be transmitted to sexual partners and neonates.

Viruses Spread by Transfusion and Transplantation

HBV, HCV, HDV, HIV, HTLV-1, and *CMV* are transmitted by blood and organ transplants. These viruses are also present in semen and therefore are sexually transmitted. The chronic nature of the infection, the persistent asymptomatic release of the virus, or the infection of macrophages and lymphocytes promotes transmission by these routes. Screening of the blood supply for HBV and HIV has controlled transmission of these viruses in blood transfusions. Large-scale procedures for screening the other viruses have not been developed, so the risk remains for the spread of HCV, HTLV, and CMV by these routes.

Syndromes of Possible Viral Etiology

Several diseases produce symptoms or have epidemiological or other characteristics that resemble those of viral infections, or they may be the sequelae of viral infections (e.g., inflammatory responses to a persistent viral infection). These include **multiple sclerosis, Kawasaki disease, arthritis, diabetes,** and **chronic fatigue syndrome.**

CHRONIC AND POTENTIALLY ONCOGENIC INFECTIONS

Chronic infections occur when the immune system has difficulty resolving the infection. The DNA viruses (except parvovirus and poxvirus) and the retroviruses cause latent infections with the potential for recurrence. *CMV and other herpesviruses; hepatitis B, C,* and *D viruses; and retroviruses* cause **chronic productive infections.**

HBV, EBV, papillomavirus, and HTLV-1 are associated with human cancers. Cofactors, chromosomal aberrations, or both enable a clone of virus-containing cells to grow out into a cancer. Immunosuppression in patients who have AIDS, patients undergoing cancer chemotherapy, or transplant recipients also promotes lymphomagenesis by EBV.

EBV normally causes **infectious mononucleosis** but is also associated with African Burkitt's lymphoma and nasopharyngeal carcinoma; *HTLV-1* is associated with human adult T-cell leukemia. Many *papillomaviruses* induce a simple hyperplasia characterized by the development of a wart; however, several other strains of papillomaviruses have been associated with human cancers (e.g., type 16 and 18 associated with cervical carcinoma). *Chronic HBV* infection has been associated with primary hepatocellular carcinoma. *HSV-2* has been associated with human cervical carcinoma, most likely as a cofactor.

Development of a worldwide vaccine program for HBV not only would reduce the spread of viral hepatitis but would also prevent the occurrence of primary hepatocellular carcinoma. Vaccination should also prevent the occurrence of EBV- and papillomavirus-associated cancers.

INFECTIONS IN IMMUNOCOMPROMISED PATIENTS

Patients with deficient cell-mediated immunity are generally more susceptible to infection with enveloped viruses (especially the *herpesviruses, measles virus,* and even the *vaccinia virus* used for smallpox vaccinations) and to recurrences of infections with latent viruses (herpesviruses and papovaviruses). Severe T-cell deficiencies also affect the antiviral antibody response. Cell-mediated immunodeficiencies can be congenital or acquired. They may result from genetic defects (e.g., Duncan's disease, DiGeorge syndrome, Wiskott-Aldrich syndrome), leukemia or lymphoma, infections (e.g., AIDS), or immunosuppressive therapy.

Viruses cause atypical and more severe presentations in immunosuppressed people. For example, herpesvirus *(HSV, CMV, VZV)* infections, which are normally benign and localized, can progress locally or disseminate and cause visceral and neurological infections that may be life threatening. A measles infection can cause a giant cell (syncytial) pneumonia rather than the characteristic rash.

Immunoglobulin A–deficient and hypogammaglobulinemic people (antibody deficient) have more problems with respiratory and gastrointestinal viruses. For instance, hypogammaglobulinemic people are more likely to suffer significant disease after infection by the live polio vaccine, echovirus, or VZV.

CONGENITAL, NEONATAL, AND PERINATAL INFECTIONS

The development and growth of the fetus are so ordered and rapid that a viral infection may damage or prevent the appropriate formation of important tissues, leading to miscarriage or congenital abnormalities. Infection may occur in utero **(prenatal)** (rubella, parvovirus B19, CMV, HIV), during transit through the birth canal **(neonatal)** *(HSV-2, HBV, CMV), or soon after birth (postnatal)* (HIV, CMV, HBV, HSV, coxsackie B virus, echovirus).

Neonates depend on the mother's immunity to protect them from viral infections. They receive maternal antibodies through the placenta and then in the mother's milk. This type of passive immunity can remain effective for 6 months to a year after birth. Maternal antibodies can protect against viral spread to the fetus during a viremia (e.g., *rubella, B19*), protect against many enteric and respiratory tract viral infections, and reduce the severity of other viral diseases after birth. However, despite this and because the cell-mediated immune system is not mature at birth, newborns are susceptible to syncytia-forming viruses such as *HSV* and to other viruses that spread by cell-to-cell contact (e.g., *VZV, CMV, HIV*).

Rubella virus and CMV are examples of teratogenic viruses that can cause congenital infection and severe congenital abnormalities. HIV infection that is acquired in utero or from mother's milk initiates a chronic infection leading to lymphadenopathy, failure to thrive, or encephalopathy within 2 years of birth. HSV can be acquired during passage through an infected birth canal and result in life-threatening disseminated disease. Nosocomial infection of newborns can result in a similar out-

come. The B19 virus is acquired in utero and can cause spontaneous abortion.

INFECTION CONTROL

Infection control is essential in hospital and health care settings, with the spread of respiratory viruses the most difficult to prevent. Viral spread can be controlled in the following ways:

1. By limiting contact with sources of infection (i.e., wearing gloves, mask, goggles; using quarantine)
2. By improving hygiene, sanitation, and disinfection
3. By ensuring that all personnel are immunized against common diseases
4. By educating all personnel regarding points 1, 2, and 3 and in the ways to decrease high-risk behaviors

Methods for disinfection differ for each virus and depend on the structure of the virus. Most viruses are inactivated by 70% ethanol, 10% chlorine bleach, 2% glutaraldehyde, 4% formaldehyde, or autoclaving (as per the Centers for Disease Control guidelines for HIV and HBV [*MMWR* 38:S-6, 1989]). Most enveloped viruses are deactivated by soap and detergents. Other means of disinfection are also available.

Special "universal" precautions are required for the handling of human blood. That is, all blood should be assumed to be contaminated with HIV or HBV and handled with caution. In addition to these procedures, special care must be taken with syringe needles and surgical tools contaminated with blood to prevent needlesticks or cuts. Specific guidelines are available from the Centers for Disease Control and Prevention.

Control of an outbreak usually requires identification of the source or reservoir of the virus, followed by clean-up, quarantine, immunization, or a combination of these measures. The first step in controlling an outbreak of gastroenteritis or hepatitis A is identification of the food, water, or possibly day-care center that may be the source of the outbreak.

Education programs can promote compliance with immunization programs and help people change life-styles associated with viral transmission. Such programs have had a significant impact in reducing the prevalence of vaccine-preventable diseases such as smallpox, polio, measles, mumps, and rubella. It is hoped that educational programs will also promote changes in life-styles and habits that will restrict the spread of the bloodborne and sexually transmitted HBV and HIV.

QUESTIONS

1. What disinfection procedures are sufficient for inactivating the following viruses: hepatitis A virus, HBV, HSV, and rhinovirus?

2. What precautions should health care workers take to protect themselves from infection with the following viruses: HBV, influenza A virus, HSV (whitlow), and HIV?

3. What predisposing conditions would exacerbate an infection with influenza A virus, VZV, or rotavirus?

4. Describe and compare the nature and mechanism of exanthem development for measles, VZV, HSV (primary and recurrence), and yellow fever.

5. A kidney transplant recipient undergoing immunosuppressive therapy has a lymphoma that regresses in response to a reduction in immunosuppressive therapy. The lymphoma cells are found to contain EBV. How might EBV be involved in this lymphoma? Why does the lymphoma regress in response to the reduction in the immunosuppressive therapy? For what other viral infections would this person be at increased risk during the immunosuppressive therapy?

Bibliography

Belshe RB, editor: *Textbook of human virology,* ed 2, St Louis, 1991, Mosby.

Ellner PD, Neu HC: *Understanding infectious disease,* St Louis, 1992, Mosby.

Emond RTD, Rowland HAK: *Color atlas of infectious diseases,* ed 2, St Louis, 1987, Mosby.

Gorbach SL, Bartlett, JG, Blacklow NR: *Infectious diseases,* Philadelphia, 1992, WB Saunders.

Hart CA, Broadhead RL: *Color atlas of pediatric infectious diseases,* St Louis, 1992, Mosby.

Haukenes G, Haaheim LR, Pattison JR: *A practical guide to clinical virology,* New York, 1989, John Wiley & Sons.

Krugman S et al: *Infectious diseases of children,* ed 9, St Louis, 1992, Mosby.

Mandell GL, Douglas RG Jr, Bennett JE: *Principles and practice of infectious disease,* ed 3, New York, 1990, Churchill Livingstone.

Mims CA, White DO: *Viral pathogenesis and immunology,* Cambridge, Mass, 1984, Blackwell.

Shulman ST, Phair JP, Sommers HM: *The biologic and clinical basis of infectious diseases,* ed 4, Philadelphia, 1992, WB Saunders.

White DO, Fenner FJ: *Medical virology,* ed 4, Orlando, Fla, 1994, Academic.

SECTION VI

Mycology

CHAPTER 66

Mechanisms of Fungal Pathogenesis

Fungi are extremely common in nature, where they exist as free-living saprobes. They are major pathogens of plants and frequently damage foods and other commodities. They often reside on body surfaces as transient environmental colonizers but obtain no obvious benefit from this relationship. Because they are so ubiquitous, they are occasionally cultured from clinical specimens. Determining their role in an infection, however, may be difficult. Their effects on humans are numerous. Three major categories are of medical importance (Box 66-1).

MYCOTOXICOSES

Fungi are metabolically versatile organisms and sources of innumerable secondary metabolites such as alkaloids and other toxic compounds. The mycotoxicoses are most often the result of the accidental or recreational ingestion of fungi that produce these compounds. The source of the toxin is determined by obtaining the patient's clinical history. Unfortunately, because the patient is often comatose or delirious, a history cannot be obtained. When the fungi are ingested, emesis (vomiting) should be induced, and supportive measures should be instituted consistent with the physiological signs exhibited by the patient. The clinical situation and laboratory diagnosis are complicated when fungal material has been injected intravenously.

Ergot Alkaloids

The pharmacological properties of ergot alkaloids, which are produced when grain is infected with *Claviceps purpurea,* have been known throughout history. During the Middle Ages, epidemics known as St. Anthony's fire were associated with the consumption of bread and other bakery products made with contaminated rye and other grains. Symptoms consisted of inflammation of the infected tissues (cellular response to injury), followed by necrosis (cell death), and gangrene (death of large masses of tissue). Pharmacologically, the ergot alkaloids produce an alpha-adrenergic blockade, which inhibits certain responses to epinephrine and 5-hydroxytryptamine. These inhibited responses create marked peripheral vasoconstriction, which, if not corrected, restricts the blood flow, resulting in necrosis and gangrene.

Another property of the ergot alkaloids is their ability to directly stimulate smooth muscle contraction. They have been used as oxytocic agents, promoting labor during childbirth by increasing the force and frequency of uterine contractions. The ergot alkaloids also affect the central nervous system by stimulating the hypothalamus and other sympathetic portions of the midbrain.

Psychotropic Agents

Toxic metabolites produced by fungi have been used by primitive tribes for religious, magical, and social purposes. In recent times, problems involving toxins of fungi have been seen with the recreational use of psychotropic agents such as psilocybin and psilocin, as well as the semisynthetic derivative, lysergic acid diethylamide (LSD).

Aflatoxins

Among the mycotoxicoses, contamination with *Aspergillus flavus* has had a profound economic impact on society. Toxic metabolites produced by these fungi resulted in the outbreak of Turkey X disease in the early 1960s in England, which nearly destroyed the turkey industry. Turkey poults consumed contaminated feed and developed lethargy, anorexia, and muscle weakness, followed by spasms and death. Postmortem studies of the animals revealed gross hemorrhage and necrosis of the liver. Further histopathological examination showed parenchymal cell degeneration and extensive proliferation of the bile duct epithelial cells. Biochemical and pharmacological studies showed that the etiological agents of the disease were *A. flavus* toxins that belonged to a group of compounds that are called the **bisfuranocoumarin metabolites.** These compounds, called *aflatoxins,* have become known as potent carcinogens, but they have not been shown to play a specific role in human carcinogenesis.

Other Mycotoxicoses

Several other mycotoxicoses that have caused human illness have also been described. Two of these are yellow rice toxicosis in Japan and alimentary toxic aleukia in the former Soviet Union.

HYPERSENSITIVITY DISEASES

One index used to measure the degree of air pollution is the fungal spore count because fungal spores are ubiquitous in nature, supply a good index of environmental contamination, and carry medical relevance. Airborne spores and other fungal elements constantly bombard people. They can be an antigenic stimulus and may induce, depending on an individual's immunological status, hypersensitivity from the production of immunoglobulins or sensitized lymphocytes. Clinical manifestations of **hypersensitivity pneumonitis** include rhinitis, bronchial asthma, alveolitis, and various forms of atopy. However, growth of the fungus in the tissues is not required for the development of hypersensitivity, and clinical manifestations of the disease are seen only in sensitized persons after subsequent exposure to the fungus, its metabolites, or other cross-reactive materials. Symptomatic patients can have their skin tested with various crude and purified fungal extracts (allergens) to identify the allergen or allergens responsible for inducing the hypersensitivity.

COLONIZATION AND DISEASES

Virtually all of the fungal organisms implicated in human disease processes are free living. In general, people have a high level of innate immunity to fungi. Most fungal infections are mild and self-limiting. Intact skin serves as a primary barrier to any infection caused by fungi that primarily colonize the superficial, cutaneous, and subcutaneous layers of skin. Mucosal surfaces discourage colonization by organisms that cause pulmonary infections. Fatty acid content, pH, epithelial turnover, and the normal bacterial flora of the skin appear to contribute to host resistance. Humoral factors such as transferrin restrict the growth of several fungi by limiting the amount of available iron, but the role they play in resistance has not been established.

A few fungi can cause disease in otherwise healthy people. Once established, the infection can be classified according to the tissue layers infected (Box 66-2).

Fungal diseases of another category have gained significance because of their association with acquired immunodeficiency syndrome and the increased use of immunosuppressive therapy. They can be the result of infection with low pathogenic potential and produce disease only under unusual circumstances, mostly involving host debilitation. Fungi once thought to be innocuous saprobes have gained prominence as etiological agents of disease because of many medical advances. Some circumstances that lead to infection by these fungi are changes in the normal intestinal flora by the use of broad-spectrum antibacterial drugs, debilitation of the host by the use of therapeutic measures (e.g., cytotoxins, x-ray irradiation, steroids, and other immunosuppressive drugs), and alteration of the host's immune system by underlying endocrine disorders (e.g., uncontrolled diabetes mellitus, suppression such as that caused by acquired immunodeficiency syndrome). Fungal infections caused by fungi that infect because of compromising situations are categorized as **opportunistic mycoses.** If they are not rapidly diagnosed and aggressively managed and if the underlying disorders are not controlled, the infections become life threatening. *Candida albicans,* a yeast that is part of the normal flora of the mouth, buccal mucosa, gastrointestinal tract, and vaginal vault; *Malassezia furfur,* a lipophilic yeast often isolated from areas rich in sebaceous glands; and other environmental fungi (e.g., *Aspergillus* species and *Mucor* species) can all be etiological agents of opportunistic mycoses.

CHARACTERISTICS OF FUNGAL PATHOGENESIS

A great deal is known concerning the molecular genetic basis of bacterial virulence and factors that contribute to plant pathogenesis. However, there is a paucity of information concerning the genes and the genetic factors that control and influence the virulence of human fungal pathogens. Generally, healthy, immunocompetent persons have a high innate resistance to fungi, even though they are constantly exposed to the infectious propagules produced by these organisms. Infection and disease occur when there are disruptions in the protective barriers of the skin and mucous membranes or when defects in the immune system allow fungi to penetrate, colonize,

---

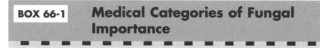

BOX 66-1   Medical Categories of Fungal Importance

Mycotoxicoses
Hypersensitivity diseases
Colonization of the host and resultant disease

BOX 66-2   Classification of Fungal Disease According to Primary Sites of Infections

Superficial mycoses—infections limited to the outermost layers of the skin and hair
Cutaneous mycoses—infections that extend deeper into the epidermis as well as invasive hair and nail diseases
Subcutaneous mycoses—infections involving the dermis, subcutaneous tissues, muscle, and fascia
Systemic mycoses—infections that originate primarily in the lung but that may spread to many organ systems

and reproduce in the host. Although most exposures are accidental, many fungi that cause disease have developed mechanisms that ease their survival and reproduction within this hostile environment. For example, dermatophytes (colonizers of the skin, hair, and nails) elaborate the enzyme keratinase, which hydrolyzes the structural protein keratin. Yeasts of the genus *Candida* become filamentous when they invade tissues, but the role of morphogenesis in virulence is unknown. Several agents that cause systemic mycoses are dimorphic; they are molds in nature but adapt to a unicellular morphology when they parasitize tissues. Those that cannot undergo the transition from mold to yeast, such as shown with *Histoplasma capsulatum,* are not virulent. *Cryptococcus neoformans* elaborates an acidic mucopolysaccharide capsule, a virulence factor.

The characteristics of human fungal pathogens allow them to be categorized into groups according to the primary tissues that they colonize. The agents causing superficial infections **(superficial mycoses),** for example, tend to grow only on the outermost layers of the skin or cuticle of the hair shaft, rarely inducing an immune reaction. The cutaneous mycoses (dermatophytes) are also limited to keratinized tissues of the epidermis, hair, and nails, but the fungi that cause cutaneous mycoses have greater invasive properties, and they may, depending on the species involved, evoke a highly inflammatory reaction from the host. The fungi that cause subcutaneous mycoses generally have a low degree of infectivity, and infections caused by these organisms are usually associated with some form of traumatic injury. All the systemic mycoses involve the respiratory tract, and the agents possess unique morphological features that contribute to their ability to survive within the host.

Bibliography

Cutler JE: Putative virulence factors of *Candida albicans, Ann Rev Microbiol* 454:187-218, 1991.

Lincoff G, Mitchel DH: *Toxic and hallucinogenic mushroom poisoning,* New York, 1977, Van Nostrand Reinhold.

Maresca B, Kobayashi GS: *HSPs in fungal infections.* In van Eden W, Young D, editors: *Stress proteins in medicine,* New York, 1996, Marcel Dekker.

Perfect, JR: Fungal virulence genes as target for antifungal chemotherapy, *Antimicrob Agents Chemother* 40:1577-1583, 1996.

Antifungal Agents

The etiological agent and the tissues involved in fungal disease as well as the immune status of the patient must be considered when deciding on a therapeutic strategy for infection management. The fungal pathogens that colonize humans and cause disease possess features that allow them to be categorized into groups according to the primary tissues that they colonize (see Box 66-2). These facts and the immunological status of the patient dictate the best clinical approach for disease management.

The agents causing **superficial infections** tend to grow only on the outermost layers of the skin or on the cuticles of the hair shafts, rarely inducing an immune reaction. These infections cause minimal destructive disease, are cosmetic in nature, and are readily diagnosed. In general, excellent clinical responses result from the use of topical antifungals combined with good personal hygiene.

The agents causing **cutaneous infections** (tineas or dermatophytes) are limited to keratinized tissues of the epidermis, hair, and nails. However, they have greater invasive properties than the agents that cause superficial infections, and they may, depending on the species involved, cause chronic disease or evoke a highly inflammatory reaction from the host. Although these infections respond well to topical agents, systemic therapy may occasionally be required, particularly with widespread involvement of the skin, scalp, or nails (see description of griseofulvin).

The agents that cause **subcutaneous** disease generally have a low degree of infectivity, and infections caused by these organisms are usually associated with some form of traumatic injury. The strategies used to treat the infection depend on the organism and the degree of tissue involvement. The drug of choice in treating lymphocutaneous sporotrichosis, for example, is a saturated solution of potassium iodide. Some forms of chromoblastomycosis, depending on the etiological agent, respond to high doses of orally administered 5-fluorocytosine (see the discussion of 5-fluorocytosine later in this chapter). Other infections in this group are refractory to antifungal therapy and may require amputation or surgical excision of the involved area.

All **systemic** agents of disease involve the respiratory tract, and they possess unique morphological features that appear to contribute to the organism's ability to survive within the host. Depending on the immune status of the patient and other underlying host factors, these diseases can be life threatening. They require rapid diagnosis and aggressive therapy with systemic antifungal compounds.

Whereas a large number of antibiotics are available to treat bacterial infections, only a few exist for therapy of systemic fungal infections. Several reasons can be given for this difference. There is not a great impetus for the development of antifungal agents because systemic fungal infections are less common than bacterial infections. Furthermore, fungal cells, like mammalian cells, are eukaryotic, and development of compounds that are highly specific for fungal cells but nontoxic to the parasitized host cells is difficult.

The antifungals presently used in treating systemic fungal infections fall into three major classes of compounds: polyenes, azoles, and nucleoside derivatives (Table 67-1). The polyenes affect cytosolic membranes, the azole derivatives inhibit ergosterol biosynthesis, and the fluorinated pyrimidine analogue 5-fluorocytosine interferes with DNA and RNA synthesis. The increasing incidence of life-threatening fungal infections has created a need to develop newer antifungals that are safer and more effective. This is particularly important in patients with acquired immunodeficiency syndrome (AIDS) or in other immunosuppressed patients who are receiving radiation or chemotherapy for various cancers or who are candidates for organ transplants. In most cases the patient's defective immunity must be corrected for successful antifungal treatment.

ANTIFUNGALS USED TO TREAT SYSTEMIC INFECTIONS
Polyenes

The polyenes are secondary metabolites produced by various species of *Streptomyces*. More than 150 have been isolated and chemically characterized. They are cyclic macrolide lactones containing a variable number of hy-

TABLE 67-1	Antifungal Agents and Primary Sites of Activity	

AGENT	TARGET
Polyenes (e.g., amphotericin B, nystatin)	Membrane sterols (bind to ergosterol)
Azole derivatives (e.g., miconazole, ketoconazole, fluconazole, itraconazole)	Ergosterol biosynthesis (inhibit cytochrome P450–dependent enzymes)
Nucleotide (e.g., 5-fluorocytosine)	DNA and RNA synthesis (inhibit synthesis)
Grisans (e.g., griseofulvin)	Microtubules (inhibits microtubular function)
Allylamines (e.g., naftifine, terbinafine)	Squalene epoxidase
Morpholines (e.g., amorolfine)	Ergosterol biosynthesis (inhibit delta$_{14}$-reductase and delta$_7$-delta$_8$-isomerase)
Potassium iodide (e.g., saturated solution)	Unknown (possibly activates lyosomal enzymes and breaks down granulomas)

A Amphotericin B (polyene)

B Ketoconazole (imidazole)

C Fluconazole (triazole)

D 5-Fluorocytosine (nucleotide)

FIGURE 67-1 Chemical structures of systemic antifungal agents.

droxyls and from two to seven conjugated double bonds (Figure 67-1). These compounds are classified by their amount of ring structure unsaturation (e.g., diene, triene, tetraene, pentaene, hexaene, heptaene). Although the mechanism of their action is complex, it is based primarily on the ability of these compounds to bind to sterols in the cytosolic membranes of susceptible cells. Because fungal membranes contain ergosterol, mammals contain cholesterol, plants contain sitosterol, and certain protozoa contain ergosterol, all are susceptible to the action of polyenes. This fact is the basis for the toxicity of these compounds when they are used to treat patients with systemic fungal infections.

Amphotericin B, a heptaene macrolide, is the only clinically useful polyene because its potency for damage is greater for fungal cells than for mammalian cells (Figure 67-1, *A*). It is selective because it preferentially binds to ergosterol-containing membranes rather than cholesterol-containing membranes. Although the structural aspects of the polyene-sterol binding are unclear, experimental evidence indicates that the amphotericin B molecule inserts into the cytoplasmic membrane of susceptible cells. Several molecules of the drug orient themselves parallel to the acyl side chains of the membrane phospholipids to form a cylindrical channel (Figure 67-2). The pores that are formed by amphotericin B increase the permeability of the membrane in a dose-dependent manner, leading to leakage of essential ions from the cytosol at low concentrations and destruction of the cell at high doses. Amphotericin B also has immunomodulatory properties that may play a role in its biological activity in vivo. Amphotericin B is insoluble in water at pH 6 to 7. A mixture of amphotericin B, deoxycholate, and phosphate buffer is used clinically. In aqueous solutions, amphotericin B dissociates from deoxycholate and forms, depending on its concentration, self-associated or monomeric species. When injected intravenously, it interacts with plasma proteins and binds

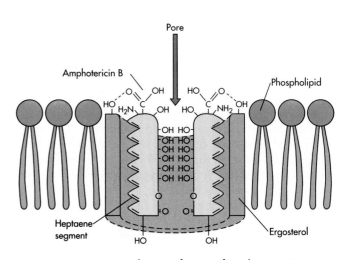

FIGURE 67-2 Mechanism of action of amphotericin B.

to cholesterol in lipoproteins, whereupon it is delivered mainly to tissues of the liver, spleen, lung, and kidney.

Nystatin (formerly called *fungicidin*) is a structural analogue of amphotericin B. The only difference between the two polyenes is the stretch of conjugated double bonds. The nystatin ring is interrupted to yield a diene-tetraene chromophore. Nystatin resembles amphotericin B in its permeabilizing and lethal effects on eukaryotic cells; however, little research has been done on its potential use as a systemic agent. At present, it is available only in topical, cream, suspension, or suppository form, primarily for the treatment of mucocutaneous, oropharyngeal, and vaginal candidiasis.

Azole Derivatives

The development of antifungal azole derivatives has rapidly progressed over the past 20 years with discoveries of benzimidazole and the antiparasitic compound thiabendazole. The azole derivatives constitute the largest group of antifungals that are commercially available. They have a broad spectrum of activity against fungi and, to some extent, gram-positive bacteria. These compounds are fungistatic and act by inhibiting the 14-alpha-demethylation of 24-methylenedihydrolanosterol, a precursor of ergosterol. The 14-alpha-demethylation step in ergosterol biosynthesis is a cytochrome P450-dependent process. The azoles are highly selective and act by binding to the heme moiety of cytochrome P450, thereby interfering with certain mixed oxidase reactions. As a result, synthesis of ergosterol is blocked and 14-alpha-methyl sterols accumulate.

These compounds are divided into two major groups characterized by five-membered azole rings with an *N*-linked methyl group derived by the addition of various halogenated phenyl or other complex chemical groups. The imidazoles (e.g., clotrimazole, miconazole, econazole, ketoconazole) (Figure 67-1, *B*) are derivatives that have two nitrogens in the ring, and the triazoles (e.g., fluconazole, itraconazole, terconazole) (Figure 67-1, *C*) are those with three nitrogens in the ring.

Nucleoside Analogues

5-Fluorocytosine (Figure 67-1, *D*) is a polar fluorinated pyrimidine that has a narrow spectrum of activity. It is used orally for the treatment of systemic infections caused by specific fungi mainly in the *Candida, Cryptococcus,* and *Aspergillus* genera and by certain fungi that cause chromoblastomycosis. It is well absorbed from the gastrointestinal tract, is low protein binding, is metabolically stable, and exhibits high bioavailability in humans. Unfortunately, it has a narrow spectrum of antifungal activity and rapidly induces resistance in susceptible organisms. In susceptible fungi, 5-fluorocytosine is taken up by a cytosine permease and is rapidly deaminated to 5-fluorouracil. This compound is then converted to either 5-fluorouridylic acid monophosphate, which inhibits RNA function, or 5-fluorodeoxyuridine monophosphate, a potent inhibitor of DNA synthesis.

ANTIFUNGALS USED TO TREAT DERMATOPHYTE INFECTIONS

Griseofulvin, an orally administered antifungal agent used to manage dermatophyte infections, is a grisan derivative produced by *Penicillium griseofulvum* (Figure 67-3, *A*). Griseofulvin interacts specifically with the tubulin of susceptible fungi, acting as a mitotic poison. The exact mechanism of action is unknown, but it appears to alter the function of tubulin rather than disaggregate or assemble tubulin subunits. Griseofulvin is active against dermatophytes but inactive against *Candida albicans* and the agents causing systemic mycoses. The mechanism of resistance appears to be lack of uptake, since griseofulvin reacts in vitro with tubulins isolated from a variety of sources (e.g., mammalian, dermatophyte, and amphibian cells).

The allylamines include the topical agent naftifine and the orally active antifungal agent terbinafine. The allylamines inhibit squalene epoxidase, a complex, membrane-bound system that requires phospholipids and oxygen as a source of reducing equivalents (Figure 67-3, *B*). These compounds are very active in vitro against dermatophytes and are effective against filamentous and dimorphic fungi but are ineffective against yeasts.

A Griseofulvin (grisan)

B Naftifine (allylamine)

C Tolnaftate (thiocarbamate)

D Amorolfine (morpholine)

FIGURE 67-3 Chemical structures of agents used primarily for dermatophyte infections.

Tolnaftate and tolciclate are thiocarbamates whose mechanisms of action are similar to those of the allylamines (Figure 67-3, C). They inhibit ergosterol biosynthesis in dermatophytes at the level of squalene epoxidase but are less active against yeasts. They are used topically in the management of dermatophyte infections.

Amorolfine, a morpholine derivative, is highly active against dermatophytes, and it exhibits moderate activity against yeasts, but its response in filamentous fungi is variable (Figure 67-3, D). Amorolfine has no effect on DNA, RNA, protein, or carbohydrate synthesis, but it appears to inhibit delta$_{14}$-reductase and delta$_7$-delta$_8$-isomerase in the pathway of ergosterol biosynthesis.

Other preparations, such as those containing 10-undecenoic (undecylenic acid), caprylic, or propionic acid as active ingredients, have also been used in the management of ringworm infections. These compounds do not possess fungicidal properties, and their role in eradicating fungi from the skin has not been established. Good hygienic practices in addition to the use of preparations containing these compounds are undoubtedly important to favorable clinical responses.

FUTURE CONSIDERATIONS
Identification of Novel Targets for the Development of Agents

The development of antifungals has primarily focused on the cytostolic membrane. Unfortunately the antifungals in use are toxic to host cells or are fungistatic and have a limited spectrum of activity. Clearly, there is a need to look for other targets. The cell wall is a major constituent of the fungal envelope. It determines the shape of the cell, serves as a protective permeability barrier to large molecules, and is essential for survival of the fungus. The fungal wall structure is multilayered and composed mainly of glucan, mannoproteins, and chitin. Chitin and beta-glucans are absent in host cells and unique to fungi. Thus the cell wall is an attractive target for antifungal drug development, and several efforts have been made to design compounds that interfere with its synthesis. Polyoxins are analogues of uridine diphosphate-N-acetylglucosamine, a class of compounds that are specific competitive inhibitors of chitin synthase. Antifungal activity has been demonstrated in vitro against *C. albicans*, but only a limited number of studies have been conducted in vivo. There is some question about uptake of these analogues by medically important fungi. As a result, development of the polyoxins has not progressed. The nikkomycins, a related group of compounds that are structurally similar to the polyoxins, are more promising. Like the polyoxins, nikkomycin Z is a competitive inhibitor of chitin

synthase. It is highly effective against murine coccidioidomycosis, blastomycosis, and histoplasmosis and prolongs the life of mice infected with *C. albicans*.

There have been efforts to find compounds that inhibit the synthesis of beta-glucan. Echinocandin B, a compound that was discovered about 20 years ago, is very effective against yeast. It is a cyclic lipopeptide metabolite produced by *Aspergillus nidulans*. Cilofungin (LY121019), a recently synthesized compound, is a derivative of echinocandin B that is produced by enzymatic deacylation using *Actinoplanes utahensis* with p-octyl-oxo-benzoic acid. It is less toxic and more potent than its parent compound. Promising results with cilofungin in vitro and in vivo have led to clinical trials for invasive candidiasis and esophageal disease. Unfortunately, its development has been abandoned because of toxicity from the vehicle used for its delivery.

In Vitro Susceptibility Testing

Paralleling the development and discovery of newer antifungal compounds has been the increasing use of these agents to treat the growing number of common and exotic fungal infections. This situation has brought about demands for in vitro antifungal testing methods that will accurately predict in vivo activity. Unfortunately, in vitro susceptibility testing with fungi has not been standardized yet, so the results of the current tests are not always predictive of clinical responses, particularly with the azole derivatives and, to some extent, 5-fluorocytosine. Efforts are being expended to develop standardized methods for in vitro susceptibility testing and to develop animal models of infection to evaluate these agents.

Complications of Therapy for Certain Populations

Although therapy for life-threatening fungal infections is far from ideal, progress has been made. Despite these advances, significant problems still exist in the treatment of fungal infections, particularly in patients who have AIDS or who are otherwise severely immunosuppressed. None of the agents in use appears to be curative in these patient populations. Lifelong suppressive therapy is often necessary to prevent recurrence of disease but poses a significant problem for these patients because they are taking a variety of medications to suppress the AIDS virus and other opportunistic organisms. Some of the available antifungals may interact with these drugs. In patients being treated with combinations of drugs, monitoring plasma levels and relevant pharmacological parameters may be necessary so that adverse drug effects can be minimized. Another complication of therapy is drug-resistant fungi, which may explain the emergence of recurrent disease.

QUESTIONS

1. What is the current thought on the mechanism of action of amphotericin B?
2. How do the azoles work?
3. How does 5-fluorocytosine work? What major problem is encountered with its use?
4. If you were to design an antifungal agent that specifically targeted fungi, what strategy would you use?

Bibliography

Anker van den JN, Popele van NML, Sauer PJJ: Antifungal agents in neonatal candidiasis, *Antimicrob Agents Chemother* 39:1391-1397, 1995.

Georgopapadakou NH, Walsh TJ: Antifungal agents: chemotherapeutic targets and immunological strategies, *Antimicrob Agents Chemother* 40:279-291, 1996.

Perfect, JR: Fungal virulence genes as targets for antifungal chemotherapy, *Antimicrob Agents Chemother* 40:1577-1583, 1996.

Yamaguchi H, Kobayashi GS, Takahashi H, editors: *Recent advances in antifungal chemotherapy*, New York, 1992, Marcel Dekker.

Laboratory Diagnosis of Fungal Diseases

DIAGNOSTIC PROCEDURES

The diagnosis of fungal infections caused by primary pathogens (e.g., *Histoplasma capsulatum, Blastomyces dermatitidis, Coccidioides immitis, Paracoccidioides brasiliensis, Cryptococcus neoformans*) can be made microscopically by visualizing the parasitic phase of the organism in clinical specimens or by growing the organism from tissues taken from the lesion. Diagnosis is more complicated when the fungal infections are caused by ubiquitous opportunistic agents (e.g., *Aspergillus, Candida,* and *Mucor* species) because these fungi, which are common in the environment, are frequently found as contaminants in the cultures. In this case, isolates of the same organism must be cultured repeatedly from lesion specimens that have been sampled at different time intervals. The validity of the isolates is further supported when fungal elements are seen in material taken from the site of infection.

The methods used in collecting and handling clinical specimens are of considerable importance in the isolation and identification of fungi. The sampling procedures vary according to the area and type of tissue involved. Although selective media are available for the isolation and culture of most pathogenic fungi, it is important to use sterile techniques whenever possible, especially with skin surfaces, nails, and hair that may be contaminated with saprobic fungi, bacteria, dirt, and epithelial debris. The skin surface should be swabbed with 70% ethanol and allowed to air-dry before sampling. The surface is scraped to remove skin scales or hair that contain the fungus. The specimen is treated with 10% potassium hydroxide to destroy tissue elements. A portion of the treated specimen should be examined microscopically to determine whether hyphal elements are present. Because fungi contain chitin and various complex polysaccharides in their cell wall, they are refractory to the alkali treatment, making it easy to visualize them by light microscopy (Figure 68-1). Several histological procedures that specifically stain fungi in tissue sections, such as Gomori's methenamine silver and periodic acid–Schiff stains, are based on the presence of chitin and polysaccharides in their cell wall.

When an infectious etiology is suspected, a portion of diseased tissue should be submitted to the pathologist for microscopic examination. Fungi can be stained preferentially because of the polysaccharide-rich properties of their cell walls. Preferential staining only tells the clinician whether fungi are present in the tissue. For definitive identification of the organism, the fungi must be cultured on suitable media and incubated at 25° to 30° C. Specimens taken from the blood, from the cerebrospinal fluid, and by surgical biopsy must be examined microscopically and cultured rapidly because dessication, autolytic processes, and bacterial contamination can make the specimen unsuitable for diagnostic procedures.

A variety of media support the growth of fungi. Sabouraud's dextrose agar, which is composed of 4% dextrose, 1% peptone, and 2% agar adjusted to a pH of 5.5, is the most conventional medium used in diagnostic laboratories for the growth of fungi. It is selective for the growth of fungi because of its acidic pH and high sugar concentration. Unfortunately, saprobic fungi grow rapidly on this medium and often overgrow the surface, obscuring any pathogens that might be present. Therefore a medium containing 2% glucose, 1% neopeptone, and 2% agar that is supplemented with cycloheximide and chloramphenicol and adjusted to a pH of 7.0 is often used for the primary isolation of dermatophytes and other pathogens. Chloramphenicol inhibits most bacteria, and cycloheximide inhibits the growth of most saprobic fungi. Some pathogens, such as *C. neoformans,* do not grow on this medium. Furthermore, the parasitic phase of some primary pathogens, such as *H. capsulatum,* do not grow on this medium at 37° C, so all cultures should be incubated at 25° to 30° C. Because the number of opportunistic fungal infections caused by saprobic fungi has increased tremendously, clinical specimens taken from deep tissues should be cultured on media with and without antibiotics.

In general, the techniques used for the laboratory identification of yeast are similar to those used to identify bacteria. These techniques are based on the biochemical and physiological properties of the organism. Gram stain, however, plays no role in identifying fungi because all fungi are gram positive. Yeasts are unicellular, grow rapidly, and can be uniformly suspended in broth. On the other hand, molds are filamentous, produce specialized conidia, and grow slowly. They are identified microscopically according to the size and shape of the conidia and the way they develop. The morphological features of specialized structures (e.g., chlamydospores, hyphae) also aid in the identification of molds. Identification of fungi requires a basic understanding and knowledge of different morphological features of fungi. (See Chapters 69 through 71 and the Bibliography for detailed descriptions of their identifying features.)

PROGRESSION OF MEDICAL MYCOLOGY

The study of fungi is in the process of transition, and advances in medicine have placed a great deal of importance on the organisms' role in human infections. Traditionally, medical mycology was almost entirely descriptive and taxonomically oriented, a result of its close and historical associations with botany and dermatology. At present, medical mycology is enjoying a period of rapid growth and interest. Fungi are being used as models for the elucidation of many molecular, genetic, and biological processes common to all living things. They are also being used as models to study cellular differentiation and adaptation, particularly host-parasite interactions. The need for rapid identification of fungi in clinical material has been partially met with the development of specific molecular probes, and there is now an emphasis on discovering newer antifungal agents and novel therapeutic strategies to treat the increasing number of fungal infections.

QUESTIONS

1. Fungi can be visualized in tissue sections by specific staining methods. What is the basis behind this technique?
2. Why are cultures for fungi held for at least 4 weeks before they are discarded as negative, whereas bacterial cultures are usually discarded after 2 to 5 days?
3. The laboratory procedure used to identify yeasts differs from that for molds. Why?
4. When clinical material is processed, why are media with and without antibiotics used?
5. In contrast to bacteria, why is it unnecessary to use ×1000 magnification to visualize fungi in clinical material?
6. Why is a strong alkaline solution used to treat tissue specimens when the presence of fungi is suspected?
7. In certain situations, fungal cultures are incubated at 25° and 37° C. Why?

FIGURE 68-1 Skin scraping treated with 10% potassium hydroxide. Fungi are refractory to alkali treatment and appear as septa that branch hyphal fragments.

Bibliography

Kreger-van Rij NJW, editor: *The yeasts: a taxonomic study*, ed 3, Amsterdam, 1984, Elsevier Science.

Kwon-Chung KJ, Bennett JE: *Medical mycology*, Philadelphia, 1992, Lea & Febiger.

Larone DH: *Medically important fungi: a guide to identification*, ed 3, Washington, DC, 1995, American Society for Microbiology.

Merz WG, Roberts GD: *Detection and recovery of fungi from clinical specimens*. In Murray PR et al, editors: *Manual of clinical microbiology*, ed 6, Washington, DC, 1995, American Society for Microbiology.

Wilson ML: General principles of specimen collection and transport, *Clin Infect Dis* 22:766-777, 1996.

CHAPTER 69

Superficial, Cutaneous, and Subcutaneous Mycoses

Fungal infections can be classified according to the tissues that are initially colonized (see Box 66-2). Infections classified as (1) the **superficial mycoses** are limited to the outermost layers of the skin and hair; (2) the **cutaneous mycoses** include infections that are deeper in the epidermis and its integuments, the hair and nails; and (3) the **subcutaneous mycoses** involve the dermis, subcutaneous tissues, muscle, and fascia.

In general, intact skin and mucosal surfaces serve as barriers to infection caused by superficial, cutaneous, and subcutaneous mycoses. Fatty acid content, pH, epithelial turnover of the skin, and normal bacterial flora contribute to host resistance. The mucosa and the ciliary action of cells lining the respiratory tract help eliminate organisms that are accidentally inhaled. Humoral factors such as transferrin restrict the growth of several fungi in vitro by limiting the amount of available iron. Such factors may restrict the growth of dermatophytes to the outer layers of skin.

SUPERFICIAL MYCOSES

Superficial fungal infections are usually cosmetic problems that are easily diagnosed and treated. Four infections fall into this classification: pityriasis versicolor and tinea nigra, both involving the skin, and black piedra and white piedra, both involving the hair (Figure 69-1). Skin infections are limited to the outermost layers of the stratum corneum. Hair infections involve only the cuticle. In general, these superficial fungal organisms do not elicit a cellular response from the host because they colonize tissues that are not living. Furthermore, these infections cause no physical discomfort to the patient. They are generally brought to the attention of the physician as an incidental finding or for cosmetic reasons. They are easy to diagnose, and specific therapeutic measures usually result in good clinical responses (Table 69-1).

Etiology, Clinical Syndromes, and Diagnosis

Pityriasis Versicolor

Pityriasis versicolor (Figure 69-1, *A*) is caused by *Malassezia furfur* (Pityrosporum orbiculare), a lipophilic, yeastlike organism. The organism is found in ar-

eas of the body that are rich in sebaceous glands, and it is part of the normal flora of the skin. The organism requires a medium supplemented with saturated or unsaturated fatty acids to support its growth. It grows as a budding yeast, although the hyphal form is occasionally seen.

The lesions of pityriasis versicolor occur most commonly on the upper torso, arms, and abdomen as discrete, hyperpigmented or hypopigmented macular lesions (Figure 69-2). They scale very easily, giving the affected area a dry, chalky appearance. On rare occasions the lesions take on a papular (elevated) appearance, and in some cases where the hair follicle is involved, the lesions can cause folliculitis.

Clinical diagnosis of pityriasis versicolor is made microscopically by visualizing the characteristic "spaghetti and meatballs" appearance of the organism in potassium hydroxide–treated specimens (Figure 69-3). Cultures are not routinely done to confirm the diagnosis, since the organism requires a special medium containing fatty acids.

FIGURE 69-1 Schematic illustration of superficial fungal infection and tissue involvement. **A,** Pityriasis versicolor. **B,** Tinea nigra. **C,** Black piedra. **D,** White piedra.

FIGURE 69-2 Clinical presentation of pityriasis versicolor.

FIGURE 69-3 Skin scrapings stained with periodic acid–Schiff stain showing typical yeastlike and hyphal fragments of *M. furfur,* the etiological agent of pityriasis versicolor.

TABLE 69-1	**Features of the Organisms Causing Superficial Mycoses**			
ORGANISM	**DISEASE**	**TISSUE**	**CLINICAL FEATURES**	**DIAGNOSTIC PROCEDURES**
Malassezia furfur	Pityriasis versicolor	Skin	Hyperpigmented or hypopigmented macular lesions that scale readily, giving it chalky-branny appearance, and that occur most frequently on the upper torso of the body	Direct microscopic examination of skin scrapings treated with alkali stain* reveals fungal elements having the classical "spaghetti and meatballs" appearance. Cultures are not routinely done to confirm the diagnosis. Organism requires fatty acid–supplemented medium for growth.
Exophiala werneckii	Tinea nigra	Skin	Gray to black, well-demarcated macular lesions most frequently occurring on the palms	Direct microscopic examination of skin scrapings treated with alkali-stain* is done. Culture on Sabouraud's dextrose agar yields pigmented (brown to black) yeasts and hyphae (dimorphic).
Piedraia hortae	Black piedra	Hair	Hard, gritty, brown to black concretions that develop along the hair shaft and that house the sexual phase (asci and ascospores) of the fungus	Direct microscopic examination of hairs is done. Culture yields asexual phase of the fungus.
Trichosporon beigelii	White piedra	Hair	Soft, white to creamy yellow granules that form a sleevelike collarette along the hair shaft	Direct microscopic examination of hairs is done. Culture on Sabouraud's dextrose agar is done. Growth is dimorphic: hyphae, arthroconidia, and blastoconidia.

From Swartz JH, Lamkin B: *Arch Dermatol* 80:89, 1964.

*A useful alkaline dye containing clearing agent can be made from Parker Super Quink permanent blue-black ink by adding 10 g of potassium hydroxide/100 ml of ink. The solution is centrifuged to sediment the amorphous precipitate that forms. The clear blue supernatant should be decanted and stored in a plastic container to prevent insoluble carbonate precipitates from forming.

Tinea Nigra

The etiological agent of tinea nigra (Figure 69-1, *B*), *Exophiala werneckii,* is a dimorphic fungus that produces melanin, imparting a brown to black color to the organism. On primary isolation from clinical material, it grows as a yeast with many cells in various stages of cell division, producing characteristic two-celled oval structures (Figure 69-4). As the colony ages, elongate hyphae develop, and in older cultures, mycelia and conidia predominate.

The clinical manifestations of tinea nigra are usually asymptomatic and consist of well-demarcated macular lesions (discolored spots on the skin that are not raised above the surface) that enlarge by peripheral extension (Figure 69-5). The brown to black lesions are most often seen on the palms and soles but may occur on other areas of the body.

The diagnosis is made by visualizing the characteristic darkly pigmented, yeastlike cells and hyphal fragments during microscopic examination of potassium hydroxide–treated scrapings taken from the affected areas; it is confirmed by culture of the organism.

Black Piedra

The cause of black piedra (Figure 69-1, *C*), a superficial hair infection, is *Piedraia hortae,* an organism that exists in the perfect (teleomorphic) state when it colonizes the hair shaft. Cultures from clinical material usually yield only the asexual (anamorphic) state of the fungus, which consists of slow-growing, brown to reddish-black mycelia. The teleomorphic state is a state in which asci, which contain spindle-shaped ascospores, develop within specialized structures. This state is occasionally found in older cultures.

The major clinical feature of black piedra is the presence of hard nodules, found along the infected hair shaft (Figure 69-6). The nodules have a hard, carbonaceous consistency and contain asci. The differential diagnosis includes ruling out nits of pediculosis and abnormal hair growth.

The infection is easily diagnosed by microscopic examination of affected hairs.

White Piedra

White piedra (Figure 69-1, *D*), an infection of the hair, is caused by the yeastlike organism *Trichosporon beigelii* (Figure 69-7). The organism grows well on all laboratory media except those containing cycloheximide, an antibiotic used in some media (e.g., Mycosel agar) for the selective isolation of most pathogenic fungi. Young cultures are white and have a pasty consistency. As the culture ages, colonies develop deep, radiating furrows and become yellow and creamy. Microscopic examination reveals septate hyphae that fragment rapidly to form arthroconidia (Figure 69-7). The arthroconidia rapidly become round, and many cells form blastoconidia.

White piedra affects the hair of the scalp, mustache, and beard. It is characterized by the development of a soft, pasty, cream-colored growth along infected hair shafts (Figure 69-8). The growth occurs as a sleeve or collarette around the hair shaft and consists of mycelia that rapidly fragment into arthroconidia.

The organism is identified by various biochemical tests and its ability to assimilate certain carbohydrates.

FIGURE 69-4 Yeastlike cells of *E. werneckii,* the causative agent of tinea nigra.

FIGURE 69-5 Clinical presentation of tinea nigra. Note the dark pigmentation in the center of the palm.

FIGURE 69-6 Hair infected with *Piedraia hortae.* The hard black nodule contains asci and ascospores, the sexual phase of the fungus.

The differential diagnosis includes trichomycosis axillaris (caused by *Corynebacterium tenuis*) and the nits of pediculosis. The infection is diagnosed by microscopic examination of infected hairs and confirmed by culture of the organism.

Treatment

These infections generally are cosmetic and easily diagnosed. When proper therapy is instituted, the infections respond well, with no consequences. The general approach to treating pityriasis versicolor and tinea nigra is removal of the organism from the skin. This is accomplished by the topical use of keratolytic agents (chemicals that lyse keratin). Preparations containing selenium disulfide, hyposulfite, thiosulfate, or salicylic acid remove the organism, but the disease may recur. Topical preparations containing miconazole nitrate, an antifungal agent that inhibits ergosterol synthesis (see Chapter 67), are used effectively in eradicating the disease.

Effective therapy of hair infections caused by *P. hortae* and *T. beigelii* is achieved by shaving or cropping the infected hairs close to the scalp surface. These infections will not recur if proper personal hygiene is practiced.

FIGURE 69-7 Hyphae, arthroconidia, and blastospores of *T. beigelii*. The dimorphic characteristics of the agent of white piedra are shown.

FIGURE 69-8 Clinical presentation of white piedra.

CUTANEOUS MYCOSES

The cutaneous mycoses are diseases of the skin, hair, and nails. They are generally restricted to the keratinized layers of the integument and its appendages (Figure 69-9). Unlike the superficial infections, in cutaneous infections, various cellular immune responses may be evoked, causing pathological changes in the host that may be expressed in the deeper tissues of the skin. The severity of the response appears to be directly related to the immune status of the host and the strain or species of fungus involved in the infection. The term *dermatophyte* has been used traditionally to describe these agents. However, the suffix *-phyte,* which implies that these organisms are plants, is misleading because fungi are not phylogenetically related to plants. However, for historical reasons the term *dermatophyte* is used in this section in reference to the organisms causing these diseases.

The clinical manifestations of these diseases are also referred to as *ringworm* or *tinea*. The term *tinea* comes from Latin and means "worm" or "moth." It describes the serpentine (snakelike) and annular (ringlike) lesions on the skin that resemble a worm burrowing at the margin (Figure 69-10). A modifying term indicates the anatomical site involved: tinea pedis, feet; tinea capitis, scalp; tinea manus, hands; tinea unguium, nails; and tinea corporis, body. In some cases, the cutaneous mycoses are given special names that indicate the clinical appearance of the infection or the origin of the organism causing the disease: Favus ("honeycomb"), which is caused by *Trichophyton schoenleinii*, has a honeycomb appearance, and tokelau (Tokelau, a South Pacific atoll) is caused by *T. concentricum*, which is geographically restricted to the Pacific islands of Oceania, Southeast Asia, and Central and South America.

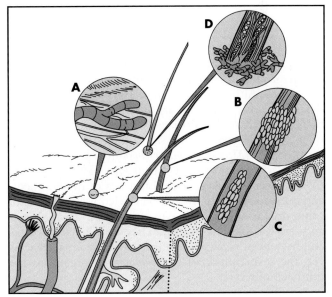

FIGURE 69-9 Schematic of tissues colonized by dermatophytes. **A,** Stratum corneum. **B,** Ectothrix hair infection. **C,** Endothrix hair infection. **D,** Favic hair infection.

FIGURE 69-10 Clinical presentation of tinea corporis.

Etiology

The cutaneous mycoses are caused by a homogeneous group of closely related organisms known as the *dermatophytes*. Although more than 100 species have been described, only about 40 are considered valid and less than half of these are associated with human disease (Box 69-1). In the anamorphic state, they are classified in three genera (*Microsporum, Trichophyton,* and *Epidermophyton*) according to their sporulation patterns (Figure 69-11), certain morphological features of development, and nutritional requirements. The teleomorphic state of some organisms belonging to the genera *Microsporum* and *Trichophyton* are known. They are all Ascomycetes and have been reclassified in the genus *Arthroderma*. As yet, the sexual phase of *Epidermophyton* organisms has not been observed.

Ecology and Epidemiology

The isolation of different species of dermatophytes varies markedly from one ecological niche to another. Some species are frequently isolated from the soil and have been grouped as geophilic dermatophytes. Other species have been found most often in association with domestic and wild animals and birds. These are referred to as *zoophilic dermatophytes*. A third group, the anthropophilic dermatophytes, has been found almost exclusively in association with humans and their habitats. Box 69-2 summarizes the groupings of the various species that are common throughout the world.

The clinical purpose of identifying species of dermatophytes is to determine the possible source of infection. There are also some considerations of prognostic value. The anthropophilic group tends to cause chronic infections and may be difficult to cure. The zoophilic and geophilic dermatophytes tend to cause inflammatory lesions, respond well to therapy, and may occasionally heal spontaneously.

Some species of dermatophytes are endemic in certain parts of the world and have a limited geographical distribution. *T. yaoundei, T. gourvilli,* and *T. soudenense* are geographically restricted to Central and West Africa; *M. ferrugineum* predominates in Japan and its surrounding areas; and *T. concentricum* is confined to islands in the South Pacific and a small area of Central and South America. However, the increasing mobility of the world's population is disrupting several of these patterns. In recent times, *T. tonsurans* has replaced *M. audouinii* as the principal agent of tinea capitis in the United States because of the mass migration of individuals from Mexico and other Latin American countries where *T. tonsurans* predominates. Less understood are the epidemics of ringworm that occasionally occur.

FIGURE 69-11 Sporulation pattern and identifying features of some dermatophytes. **A,** Macroconidia of *Microsporum canis.* **B,** Macroconidia of *M. gypseum.* **C,** Macroconidia of *Epidermophyton floccosum.* **D,** Microconidia and macroconidia of *Trichophyton mentagrophytes.* **E,** Favic chandelier of *Trichophyton schoenleinii.*

The prevalence of dermatophytes and the incidence of disease are difficult to determine because they are not reportable. Fragmentary surveys from epidemiological studies and case reports indicate that the cutaneous mycoses are the most common among human diseases. Reports estimate that they are the third most common skin disorder in children younger than 12 years of age and the second most common in older populations. The occurrence of these diseases varies with age, gender, ethnic group, and cultural and social habits of the population.

The incidence of the cutaneous mycoses and the clinical manifestations of the disease among various age groups depend on the anatomical site of involvement and the dermatophyte species involved in disease. Tinea capitis is a problem of the pediatric population until puberty, when it spontaneously ceases to be a major infectious disorder. On the other hand, tinea pedis, which is rarely a disease in childhood, gradually becomes the predominant infection with age and remains so into adulthood.

The incidence of tinea capitis in black children in the United States is disproportionately high. In India, tinea capitis occurs more often in the native children than in Europeans, whereas the Europeans have a higher incidence of tinea pedis. Clinical surveys conducted during the war in Southeast Asia revealed that people from the United States had a higher incidence of tinea pedis caused by *T. mentagrophytes* than the native population. The indigenous population appeared to be highly susceptible to a distinctive strain of *T. rubrum*. Tinea capitis, tinea pedis, and tinea cruris are more common in men than women, whereas tinea unguium (infections of the nail plate) of the hand is more common in women. For nails of the feet, tinea unguium is seen more often in men.

The reasons for these differences are poorly understood. The incidence of cutaneous mycoses is related to customs associated with the type of clothing and footwear worn. Studies on institutionalized populations and family outbreaks of dermatophyte infections indicate that close and crowded living conditions are a factor in the spread of infections. There is evidence that natural resistance to these infections exists in certain individuals. Certain humoral factors are fungistatic, and cell-mediated immunity appears to be important in resistance to dermatophyte infections.

Pathogenesis

A delicate balance appears to operate between the host and parasite in dermatophyte infections. Some fungi show an evolutionary development toward a parasitic existence. Those that have achieved a high level of coexistence with humans also exhibit a degree of specificity for the tissues that are colonized. These fungi are often referred to as **keratinophilic fungi** because they can use keratin as a substrate. Keratinases have been isolated from some of these fungi, but keratin is not an essential metabolite for them. The tissues containing this protein are highly selective for the growth of dermatophytes, but the reason is unknown. As versatile as these fungi may appear, they seem unable to invade organs other than the keratinized layers of skin, hair, and nails.

Laboratory Diagnosis

The diagnosis of disease requires that fungal elements be seen in clinical specimens of the lesion or that they be confirmed by culture of the organism. Skin and nail scrapings or hair taken from areas suspected to be infected are examined microscopically. The procedure for processing these specimens is similar to those described previously for examining clinical material from superficial fungal infections. The specimen is treated with an alkali solution to clear the epithelial cells and other debris. Dermatophytes resist the caustic solution and appear as branching, septate hyphal elements in specimens taken from cutaneous lesions or nails. Examination of fungal elements in infected hair reveals spores inside (endothrix infection) (Figure 69-12, *A*) or surrounding (ectothrix infection) (Figure 69-12, *B*) the hair shaft.

An exception to this type of sporulation is the hair infection caused by *T. schoenleinii.* Disease caused by this organism is called *favus,* and the infected hair has a waxy mass of hyphal elements (scutulum) surrounding the base of the hair follicle at the scalp line (Figure 69-9, *D*). Microscopic examination of the hair reveals degenerated hyphal elements coursing throughout the hair shaft (Figure 69-9, *D*). Such hairs are called *favic* and are diagnostic of the infection.

FIGURE 69-12 Fungal infections of the hair. **A,** Endothrix infection. **B,** Ectothrix infection.

Direct microscopic examination of clinical material confirms only the diagnosis of a fungal infection. Cultures must be taken to identify the specific etiological agent.

The skin surface harbors many bacterial species and saprobic fungi as part of the normal flora or transient colonizers. Thus media such as Sabouraud's dextrose agar are not routinely used for primary culture because these organisms overgrow the culture and inhibit the growth of the more slow-growing dermatophytes. For this reason, selective media containing antibiotics are recommended when culturing specimens from the skin. A medium commonly used for the isolation of dermatophytes from clinical material contains cycloheximide to suppress saprobic fungal growth and chloramphenicol to inhibit the growth of bacteria. Clinical material is seeded directly onto the medium and is incubated at 25° C. Dermatophytes and most pathogenic fungi grow well on this medium when incubated at 25° C, whereas saprobic fungi and bacteria are inhibited.

Cultures are examined periodically, and all fungi that grow are identified by microscopic examination and physiological tests. In general, the mycelia of these fungi are undifferentiated, and species identification is based primarily on the conidia produced (Table 69-2). The conidia may be large (5 to 100 × 6 to 8 mm) and mul-

TABLE 69-2	**General Characteristics of Macroconidia and Microconidia of Dermatophytes**	
GENUS	**MACROCONIDIA**	**MICROCONIDIA**
Microsporum	Numerous, thick-walled, rough*	Rare
Epidermophyton	Numerous, smooth-walled	Absent
Trichophyton	Rare, thin-walled, smooth	Abundant†

*M. audouinii is an exception.
†T. schoenleinii is an exception.

ticellular (macroconidia), or they may be small (3 × 10 mm) and unicellular (microconidia).

In addition to conidia, some dermatophytes produce spiral hyphae, chlamydospores, nodular bodies, racquet hyphae, and chandeliers. These structures are produced commonly by some species of dermatophytes and infrequently by others; however, they should not be considered distinguishing features of the species. Figure 69-11 illustrates the identifying features of some dermatophytes. All cultures are routinely held for 4 weeks before being discarded as negative.

Treatment

The clinical nature of the dermatophyte infections frequently poses a challenge to the clinician. Skin infections generally are approached conservatively with topical treatment. The discovery of azole derivatives as effective antifungal agents has provided several new drugs that can be used topically (e.g., miconazole, clotrimazole, econazole). All of the azole derivatives appear to work by interfering with the cytochrome P450–dependent enzyme systems at the demethylation step from lanosterol to ergosterol.

For hair infections, griseofulvin, a secondary metabolite of the fungus *Penicillium griseofulvum,* is a safe, effective drug prescribed orally for the management of tinea capitis. This compound is fungistatic and appears to work by affecting the microtubular system of fungi. It interferes with the mitotic spindle and cytoplasmic microtubules. The molecular action of griseofulvin is different from that of other inhibitors, such as colchicine and the vinca alkaloids, which bind to receptors on tubulin and inactivate the free subunits of microtubules.

SUBCUTANEOUS MYCOSES

The subcutaneous mycoses include a wide spectrum of fungal infections characterized by the development of lesions, usually at sites of trauma where the organism is implanted in the tissue (Figure 69-13). The infections initially involve the deeper layers of the dermis, subcuta-

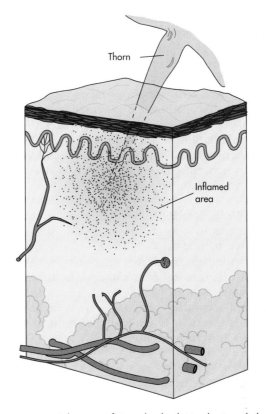

FIGURE 69-13 Schematic of tissue level colonized primarily by agents causing subcutaneous mycoses. The fungus gains access to the deeper layers of skin by traumatic implantation. The organisms implicated in these disease processes are usually common fungi found in the soil.

neous tissue, or bone. Most infections have a chronic and insidious growth pattern that eventually extends into the epidermis and are expressed clinically as lesions on the skin surface.

This group of infections has several features in common. The patient can usually remember trauma (e.g., a splinter, a thorn, a bite, the implantation of other foreign bodies) at the infection sites; then the lesions develop. The infections occur on parts of the body that are most prone to be traumatized (e.g., feet, legs, hands, arms, buttocks). The etiological agents are commonly found in the soil or on decaying vegetation.

Several bacterial infections (e.g., actinomycotic mycetoma, botryomycosis, atypical acid-fast disease) mimic the subcutaneous fungal infections. It is extremely important to establish the etiological agent because most of the bacterial infections can be managed with antibiotics. Finally, with one or two exceptions, the subcutaneous mycoses are difficult to treat, and surgical intervention (e.g., excision or amputation) may be indicated.

Etiology and Clinical Syndromes

Most subcutaneous fungal infections, with the exception of lymphocutaneous sporotrichosis, are rare and are considered exotic in the United States and other highly developed countries. The diseases less frequently or rarely seen are chromoblastomycosis, phaeohyphomycosis, chronic subcutaneous zygomycosis, and eumycotic mycetoma. Two diseases, lobomycosis and rhinosporidiosis, are considered to be caused by fungi, but culture fails to isolate the etiological agent.

The causative agents are a heterogeneous group of organisms with low pathogenic potential that are commonly isolated from soil or decaying vegetation. The clinical manifestations of these diseases appear to be an interplay between the etiological agent and host responses. In general, patients who develop disease have no underlying immunological defect.

Lymphocutaneous Sporotrichosis

Lymphocutaneous sporotrichosis, a chronic infection characterized by nodular and ulcerative lesions, develops along the lymphatic glands that drain the primary site of inoculation (Figure 69-14). Other infrequently seen forms of sporotrichosis include fixed cutaneous lesions, primary and secondary pulmonary sporotrichosis, and disseminated disease. The etiological agent is the dimorphic fungus *Sporothrix schenckii*.

Chromoblastomycosis

Chromoblastomycosis is characterized by the development of verrucous (warty) nodules that appear at sites of inoculation (Figure 69-15). As lesions progress, they appear to vegetate and take on a cauliflower-like appearance. The organisms responsible for chromoblastomycosis are common soil inhabitants collectively called the **dematiaceous fungi.** The term *dematiaceous* is used to describe fungi that have brown to black melanin pigments in their cell wall (see also the section on tinea nigra).

Phaeohyphomycosis

Another clinical disease caused by various dematiaceous fungi is phaeohyphomycosis, a heterogeneous group of cutaneous diseases caused by various dematiaceous fungi. The most common form described is phaeohyphomycotic cyst. The disease does not exhibit the intense hyperplasia seen in chromoblastomycosis, and when organisms are seen during histopathological examination of tissue, they usually appear as pigmented, septate hyphal fragments.

The taxonomy of the dematiaceous agents is undergoing careful scrutiny, and as yet complete agreement has not been reached. The dematiaceous fungi most often associated with chromoblastomycosis are *Fonsecaea pedrosoi, Fonsecaea compacta, Cladosporium carrionii,* and *Phialophora verrucosa.* These organisms are identified according to the pattern and type of sporulation exhibited by the isolate. In many cases the isolate may exhibit more than one pattern of sporulation, and for this reason, confusion and conflicts often arise concerning the correct taxonomic placement of the organism.

Similar taxonomic problems exist in the identification of agents implicated in phaeohyphomycosis, for which about 40 different organisms have been identified. Included in this large number of etiological agents are some rare fungi that undoubtedly reflect the exotic nature of some of these clinical entities.

Eumycotic Mycetoma

The term **mycetoma** is clinically descriptive and includes a wide spectrum of manifestations of the skin and deeper tissues of the dermis and subcutaneous tissues. The disease is characterized by indolent, deforming, swollen lesions that contain numerous draining sinus tracts.

Other Subcutaneous Mycoses

Zygomycosis, lobomycosis, and rhinosporidiosis are rare clinical entities. A detailed description of these diseases is contained in the references listed in the Bibliography at the end of this chapter.

Laboratory Diagnosis
Lymphocutaneous Sporotrichosis

In tissue and in cultures incubated at 37° C, *S. schenckii* is a budding yeast cell. Cultures at 25° C develop as delicate, radiating colonies that appear within 3 to 5 days on most media. The colonies are initially moist and white;

![FIGURE 69-14 and 69-15]

FIGURE 69-14 Clinical case of lymphocutaneous sporotrichosis. The characteristic pattern of lesions along the lymphatic system that drain the site of the original lesion is shown.

FIGURE 69-15 Clinical case of chromoblastomycosis. The characteristic verrucous vegetative lesions are illustrated.

they slowly develop a brown to black pigmentation with prolonged incubation. Microscopic examination reveals delicate branching hyphae about 2 μm in diameter, with numerous conidia developing in a rosette pattern at the ends of conidiophores (Figure 69-16). Laboratory confirmation is established by converting the mycelial growth to the yeast morphology by subculture at 37° C.

Chromoblastomycosis

The diagnosis of chromoblastomycosis is usually made by histopathological examination of clinical material taken from the lesions. A characteristic tissue response of the disease is pseudoepitheliomatous hyperplasia, an epithelial overgrowth caused by an abnormal multiplication in the number of normal cells in normal arrangement in the tissue. In addition to the histopathology, copper-colored, spherical cells in various stages of cell division are seen (Figure 69-17). These structures, called **sclerotic** or **Medlar bodies**, are the tissue forms of the fungus.

Eumycotic Mycetoma

Examination of the purulent fluid from the sinus tracts in eumycotic mycetoma often reveals small grains of fungal tissue. These elements may be white, brown, yellow, or black and can be well demonstrated on histopathological examination of lesion biopsies (Figure 69-18). The etiological agents causing these diseases consist of various actinomycetes belonging to the genera *Actinomyces*, *Nocardia*, *Streptomyces*, and *Actinomadura* as well as a whole host of fungi, including *Pseudallescheria boydii* and *Madurella grisea*. It is important to establish the cause of the disease by culturing specimens because the clinical management of the infection varies depending on the causative organism.

Treatment

Subcutaneous lymphangitic sporotrichosis responds dramatically to a saturated solution of potassium iodide given orally. Adverse side effects include gastrointestinal upset and dermatological problems that are rapidly reversed by discontinuing therapy. Extracutaneous sporotrichosis invariably requires systemic therapy with amphotericin B.

Cautery and surgical removal of early lesions are used in the treatment of chromoblastomycosis; however, most patients who seek help have advanced disease. The extensive tissue involvement is often not amenable to surgical intervention and requires chemotherapy. The drug of choice for treating chromoblastomycosis is 5-fluorocytosine. This drug is given orally and acts by inhibiting RNA and DNA synthesis.

As stated previously, the clinical treatment of eumycotic mycetoma varies with the causative agent. In the case of actinomycotic mycetomas, several antibacterial antibiotics can be used. For example, infections caused by *Actinomyces israelii* respond to high doses of penicillin, and those caused by *Nocardia asteroides* respond to sulfa drugs and streptomycin. However, if a fungal organism is the causative agent, the physician frequently resorts to total excision of the lesion or amputation of an affected limb when the disease is extensive, since antifungal therapy in general is unsuccessful.

FIGURE 69-17 Tissue section taken from a case of chromoblastomycosis. The characteristic "sclerotic" cells are shown.

FIGURE 69-16 Microscopic examination illustrating the rosette pattern of conidia in *S. schenckii*.

FIGURE 69-18 Histopathological section of tissue taken from mycetoma. A microcolony (often referred to as a *granule*) is illustrated.

CASE STUDY AND QUESTIONS

The school nurse was informed that three first-grade boys had scaly, patchy alopecia. She examined them for nits but found none, so she sent them home with instructions for them to be seen by their pediatrician. The pediatrician confirmed that nits were not the problem.

1. What should the pediatrician have done to confirm the diagnosis of tinea capitis?
2. Should their siblings and the rest of the classroom have been examined?
3. What are some interesting epidemiological and clinical features of the pathophysiology of tinea capitis, tinea pedis, and tineas caused by anthropophilic, zoophilic, and geophilic fungi?

Two healthy construction laborers were seen by a dermatologist after developing painless bilateral ulcerative lesions along the lymphatics of the forearms. On examination, they were afebrile. There was regional lymphadenopathy, and the lesions extended up the lymphatics as tender erythematous subcutaneous nodules, some of which were fluctuant. Histories taken from the patients revealed that these lesions began to appear 2 to 3 weeks after they had demolished an attic as part of an urban renewal project. Both stated that they got splinters from carrying salvaged wood from the rafters. They also commented that bats and pigeons had roosted in the attic and that a lot of dust was raised during the salvage.

1. What was the most likely diagnosis and how should the diagnosis have been confirmed?
2. What generalizations can you make about subcutaneous mycotic infections?
3. What are the therapeutic strategies used in the various subcutaneous mycoses?

Bibliography

Kwon-Chung KJ, Bennett JE: *Medical mycology,* Philadelphia, 1992, Lea & Febiger.

Larone DH: *Medically important fungi: a guide to identification,* ed 2, New York, 1987, Elsevier Science.

McGinnis MR: *Laboratory handbook of medical mycology,* New York, 1980, Academic.

Rebell G, Taplin D: *Dermatophytes: their recognition and identification,* Coral Gables, Fla, 1979, University of Miami.

Systemic Mycoses

The organisms classified as systemic mycotic agents are inherently virulent and cause disease in healthy humans. Five fungi are included in this group: *Histoplasma capsulatum, Blastomyces dermatitidis, Paracoccidioides brasiliensis, Coccidioides immitis,* and *Cryptococcus neoformans.* Each of these fungi exhibits biochemical and morphological features that enable it to evade host defenses.

Four of these pathogens *(H. capsulatum, B. dermatitidis, P. brasiliensis,* and *C. immitis)* are dimorphic. They grow as filamentous molds as saprobes and in culture at 25° C; however, when they infect humans or are cultured at 37° C, they transform to a unicellular morphology (Figure 70-1, *A* to *D*). Tissue infections caused by *H. capsulatum, B. dermatitidis,* and *P. brasiliensis* are characterized by the presence of budding yeast cells (Figure 70-1, *A* through *C*), whereas *C. immitis* infections are characterized by the presence of spherules (sporangium-like structures filled with endospores) (Figure 70-1, *D*).

Unlike the dimorphic pathogens, *C. neoformans* is monomorphic, growing as a yeast within infected tissue and culture at 25° or 37° C (Figure 70-1, *E*). A characteristic feature of *C. neoformans* is that it possesses an acidic mucopolysaccharide capsule.

The primary focus of infection for the systemic fungi is the lung. In most cases the respiratory infections are asymptomatic or of very short duration, resolve rapidly without therapy, and are accompanied by a high degree of specific resistance to reinfection in the host. In some cases the infection spreads to a secondary organ. Each organism exhibits its own characteristic pattern of secondary organ involvement. Frequently the secondary spread of systemic disease causes the patient to seek medical attention. The etiological agent and the host's immune status determine the severity of infection. The infection can be life threatening if therapy is not rapidly instituted and the underlying disorder not corrected for patients whose immune status is compromised because of underlying disease or immunosuppressive therapy. In addition, immunosuppression may cause reactivation of latent infection.

Four of the systemic mycoses (**histoplasmosis, blastomycosis, paracoccidioidomycosis,** and **coccidioidomycosis**) tend to be restricted to particular geographical regions. However, the ease of travel and increases in reactivation disease are starting to blur these distinctions.

HISTOPLASMOSIS

Histoplasmosis results from the inhalation of conidia or hyphal fragments of *H. capsulatum* (Figure 70-2). It occurs worldwide and is particularly common in the midwestern United States (Figure 70-3). In most cases, it is asymptomatic, but in about 5% of the cases, clinical symptoms of an acute pneumonia occur, followed less often by a progressive disseminated disease. Histoplasmosis also known as *Darling's disease, reticuloendothelial cytomycosis, cave disease,* and **spelunker's disease** (Box 70-1).

Morphology

The mold phase of *H. capsulatum* is characterized by thin, branching, septate hyphae that produce microconidia and tuberculate macroconidia (Figure 70-4). The parasitic or tissue phase of *H. capsulatum* is a small, budding yeast cell that is 2 to 5 µm in diameter and found almost exclusively within macrophages (Figure 70-5). The sexual state of *H. capsulatum* is designated *Ajellomyces capsulatus* and is classified as an ascomycete.

Epidemiology

The etiological agent of histoplasmosis, *H. capsulatum* var. *capsulatum,* grows in soil with a high nitrogen content, especially in areas contaminated with the excreta of bats and birds (starlings and chickens, in particular). Birds are not infected, whereas natural infection does occur in bats. The fungi are isolated from soil samples taken from various bird and bat habitats (e.g., chicken coops, attics, barns, wood piles, caves, roosting areas such as city parks and even school yards). Numerous well-documented epidemics of respiratory histoplasmosis have occurred when environments harboring the fungi have been disturbed by activities such as exploring

Saprobic phase
(25° C)

Parasitic phase
(37° C)

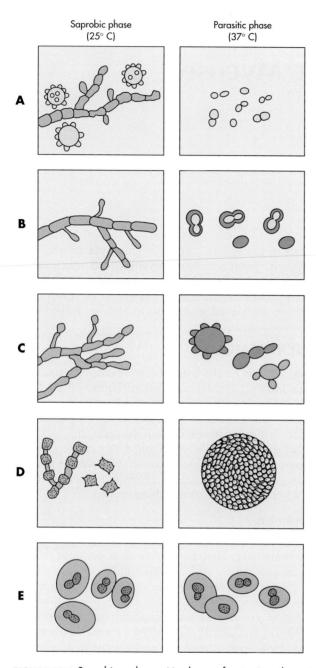

FIGURE 70-1 Saprobic and parasitic phases of systemic pathogenic fungi. **A,** *H. capsulatum.* **B,** *B. dermatitidis.* **C,** *P. brasiliensis* exhibits mold-to-yeast transition when infecting susceptible species. **D,** *C. immitis* exhibits mold-to-spherule transition when it infects susceptible species. **E,** *C. neoformans* is an encapsulated yeast at 25° or 37° C or in infected tissues.

FIGURE 70-2 Natural history of the saprobic and parasitic cycles of *H. capsulatum.*

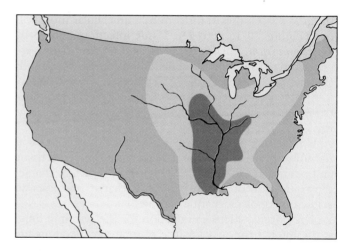

FIGURE 70-3 Endemic areas of histoplasmosis in North America. Dark purple shading indicates area of high endemicity. Light purple shading indicates area of moderate endemicity.

caves (spelunking), demolishing old buildings during urban renewal, cleaning chicken coops, and setting up campsites. Researchers and epidemiologists, from their efforts to document the outbreaks, have accidentally acquired the disease while exploring suspected sites for soil samples.

Histoplasmosis is widely distributed throughout the temperate, subtropical, and tropical zones of the world. Some areas within these zones are highly endemic, including the Ohio and Mississippi Valley regions of the United States, the southern fringes of the provinces of Ontario and Quebec in Canada, and scattered areas of Central and South America (Figure 70-3). Surveys of skin test reactivity to histoplasmin indicate that at least 80% of the long-term residents of the Ohio and Missis-

BOX 70-1 Summary of Histoplasmosis

ETIOLOGICAL AGENT

Asexual phase: *Histoplasma capsulatum.*
Sexual phase: *Ajellomyces capsulatus.*

MYCOLOGY

Dimorphic; mycelia at 25° C; typical tuberculate macro-
    conidia (8-14 μm in diameter); microconidia (2-4 μm
    in diameter).
At 37° C and in tissue, this organism is a budding yeast
    (2-3 × 3-4 μm in diameter).
Organism is found predominantly in histocytes.

EPIDEMIOLOGY AND ECOLOGY

Organism occurs throughout temperate, subtropical, and
    tropical areas of the world. Endemic areas include the
    Ohio and Mississippi River Valleys and parts of Central
    and South America.
The organism has been isolated from numerous soil sam-
    ples, particularly those contaminated by bat, chicken,
    and starling droppings. Bats are naturally infected, but
    birds are not.
A unique clinical form occurs in Africa; it is caused by
    H. capsulatum var. *duboisii.*

CLINICAL DISEASE

The clinical symptoms vary depending on the degree of
    individual exposure and immunological state of the pa-
    tient.
About 95% of all primary cases are not referable to spe-
    cific symptomology.
Less than 1% of infections become progressive and re-
    quire therapy. In this case, an underlying condition of
    debilitation or immunosuppression usually makes these
    people prone to life-threatening disease.

FIGURE 70-4 Tuberculate macroconidia and microconidia of *H. cap-sulatum.*

FIGURE 70-5 Yeast cells of *H. capsulatum* phagocytised by bone mar-row mononuclear cells (Giemsa-stained section).

sippi River Valleys have been infected with *H. capsula-tum.* Serial studies of individuals living in endemic areas show that skin test reactivity can be lost and reacquired, suggesting that the high incidence of reactivity in these areas results from reinfection.

Cases of histoplasmosis have also been reported in Europe and Asia. A variant form of histoplasmosis occurs in Africa; the etiological agent of this disease has been designated *H. capsulatum* var. *duboisii.*

Clinical Syndromes

The lung is the usual portal of entry for infection. Coni-dia or hyphal fragments of *H. capsulatum* are inhaled, are phagocytised by pulmonary macrophages, and then convert to yeasts, which are able to replicate in macrophages (Figure 70-5). In the immunocompetent host, macrophages acquire fungicidal activity, thereby containing the infection. Transient fungemia occurring

before the development of immunity accounts for the distribution of calcified granulomas in the liver and spleen that are frequently seen at autopsy of patients from endemic areas. Viable organisms may persist in the host after resolution of uncomplicated histoplasmosis; they are the presumed source of disseminated disease in immunocompromised patients who do not have a his-tory of recent exposure. The major clinical syndromes as-sociated with *H. capsulatum* infection are summarized in Table 70-1.

An estimated 500,000 people in the United States are exposed to *H. capsulatum* each year; however, most peo-ple infected with *H. capsulatum* have a high degree of natural resistance to the organism. Few, if any, overt symptoms appear, and the disease resolves rapidly. Ap-proximately 5% of infections result in symptomatic dis-ease, usually as an acute, self-limited, influenza-like ill-ness with varying degrees of pulmonary involvement.

TABLE 70-1	Classification of Histoplasmosis	
TYPE OF OF INFECTION	**SPECIFIC DISORDER**	**COMMENTS**
Histoplasmosis in normal hosts	Asymptomatic or mild influenza-like illness	Occurrence with normal exposure
	Acute pulmonary histoplasmosis	Occurrence with heavy exposure
	Rare complications	Pericarditis, mediastinal fibrosis
Opportunistic infection	Disseminated histoplasmosis	Occurrence in people with immune defects
	Chronic pulmonary histoplasmosis	Occurrence in people with structural defects

Symptoms usually resolve without specific antifungal therapy. Occasionally an overly vigorous host immune response can result in complications such as mediastinal fibrosis, which is the development of hard fibrous tissue in the upper mediastinum that causes compression, distortion, or obliteration of the superior vena cava and sometimes constriction of the bronchi and large pulmonary vessels.

H. capsulatum can also cause progressive and potentially fatal disease when host defenses are impaired. In a small number of cases the initial infection is not cleared, and the disease progresses to disseminated histoplasmosis. This condition is characterized by continued intracellular replication of *H. capsulatum* yeasts within macrophages, presumably caused by a defect in cell-mediated immunity. Clinically, infection ranges from acute, life-threatening, disseminated histoplasmosis to chronic, mild, disseminated histoplasmosis, depending on the extent of parasitization of the mononuclear phagocytic system. Patients frequently complain of fever, night sweats, and weight loss. Mucosal lesions are also common and may be the primary clinical finding in an otherwise healthy-appearing individual.

Severe, progressive, disseminated histoplasmosis is reported with increasing frequency in adults who have hematological malignancies and who are receiving immunosuppressive therapy (particularly chronic corticosteroid therapy) or who have acquired immunodeficiency syndrome (AIDS). In these settings, disseminated histoplasmosis is best described as an opportunistic infection. Infection with the human immunodeficiency virus (HIV-1) may trigger reactivation of dormant *H. capsulatum*. Central nervous system involvement, an unusual complication of disseminated histoplasmosis, has also been reported in association with HIV infection.

Chronic pulmonary histoplasmosis is most often seen in patients with underlying chronic obstructive pulmonary disease. Because of structural defects in the lung, *H. capsulatum* can escape normal defense mechanisms and cause progressive, destructive lesions similar to tuberculosis.

In Africa a distinct clinical form of histoplasmosis is seen. It involves primarily the bone and subcutaneous tissues.

Laboratory Diagnosis

The diagnosis of histoplasmosis is based on serological findings, direct histopathological examination of infected tissue, and culture of the etiological agent. Diagnosis of disseminated histoplasmosis requires demonstration of the organism in extrapulmonary sites. This is best accomplished by a combination of culture and histopathological examination of tissue.

The antigenic reagents used in the serological tests for histoplasmosis are derived from two sources: the cell-free culture filtrate from the mycelial phase of growth (histoplasmin) and inactivated, whole **yeast phase** cells. Both reagents are used because neither type of antigen detects antibodies in all cases.

In general, delayed skin test reactivity to histoplasmin develops within 2 weeks after exposure. This test is of little diagnostic or prognostic value and may be misleading because in a significant percentage of the hypersensitive patients, serological titers may become elevated as a result of skin testing with the reagent (anamnestic response). For this reason the skin test should not be used in the diagnostic workup of a patient.

Two serological tests are frequently used to diagnose histoplasmosis. The complement fixation test is the standard test, and the results are positive later in disease (6 weeks or longer after symptoms occur). Complement fixation tests, which measure antibodies directed against *H. capsulatum,* are performed using histoplasmin and intact formalin-treated yeast as the antigens. Serum complement fixation titers of at least 16 or a fourfold rise in titer suggest histoplasmosis; however, false-positive reactions can occur because of cross-reactive antibodies associated with other fungal infections and tuberculosis. Complement fixation titers decline after infection in normal hosts. Fewer than 5% of individuals have a positive complement fixation reaction in areas where the rate of positive skin tests is high. A single serological test does not allow a reliable diagnostic or prognostic interpretation and might cause a delay in instituting specific therapeutic measures. However, serological tests of two or more serum specimens taken at suitable intervals during the acute and convalescent phases of infection yield information of great diagnostic and prognostic value.

The immunodiffusion test detects antibodies to the H and M antigens of *H. capsulatum* (Figure 70-6) and is more specific but less sensitive than complement fixation. Serological tests can aid in the diagnosis of histoplasmosis but do not distinguish disseminated disease from other forms of histoplasmosis. Furthermore, the results of these tests can be negative in 25% or more of patients who have disseminated histoplasmosis.

In contrast to traditional serological tests, direct detection of *H. capsulatum* antigens in blood or urine may prove valuable for the rapid diagnosis of disseminated disease. Intracellular yeast can often be seen by histopathological examination of infected tissue, especially bone marrow, blood, and lung, using special stains, thus permitting rapid diagnosis. *H. capsulatum* can be cultured from bone marrow or blood in more than 75% of cases of disseminated histoplasmosis. Sputum cultures are useful in the diagnosis of chronic pulmonary histoplasmosis but are usually negative in cases of acute, self-limited disease. *H. capsulatum* usually takes 1 to 2 weeks to grow in culture. Preliminary identification of the isolate is based on morphological features, including delicate septate hyphae with tuberculate macroconidia (Figure 70-4).

In the past, confirmation was based on the ability to convert the culture morphology from the mycelial phase to the yeast phase, a process that can require weeks to months. Use of an **exoantigen test** now permits confirmation as soon as sufficient growth occurs. In the exoantigen test, antigens are extracted from the agar medium that supports fungal growth and are tested for their reaction against antihistoplasma antibody in an immunodiffusion test. A positive identification is made when precipitin lines of identity form with control histoplasmin antigens.

More recently a rapid DNA probe test has been developed; it uses nucleic acid hybridization for the rapid identification of *H. capsulatum* grown from clinical material. The test is based on the ability of complementary nucleic acid strands to specifically align and associate to form stable, double-stranded complexes. A commercially available test uses a chemiluminescent-labeled, single-stranded DNA probe that is complementary to the ribosomal RNA isolated from the unidentified culture. The test is read in a luminometer, which allows for the differentiation between hybridized and nonhybridized probes.

Treatment

Amphotericin B remains the mainstay of treatment for disseminated histoplasmosis and other severe forms of the disease. However, in AIDS patients, relapses after the completion of therapy are a significant problem, and lifelong suppressive therapy must be considered.

BLASTOMYCOSIS

Blastomycosis, also called **Chicago disease, Gilchrist's disease,** and **North American blastomycosis,** is caused by the inhalation of conidia of *B. dermatitidis* (Figure 70-7). Primary pulmonary infections are often inapparent and difficult to document, even radiologically. The forms of disease most often seen clinically are ulcerative lesions of the skin and lytic bone lesions, both of which represent systemic or disseminated disease (Box 70-2).

Morphology

B. dermatitidis is closely related biochemically and serologically to *H. capsulatum*. The sexual phase of *B. dermatitidis* has been discovered. It is classified as an ascomycete and designated *Ajellomyces dermatitidis*, the same genus as the sexual state of *H. capsulatum*.

Epidemiology

The geographical distribution of blastomycosis is limited to the North American continent and parts of Africa. Blastomycosis, like histoplasmosis, is endemic in the

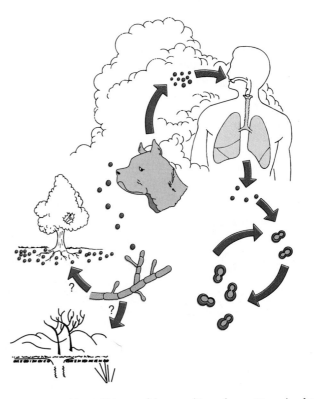

FIGURE 70-7 Natural history of the saprobic and parasitic cycle of *B. dermatitidis.*

FIGURE 70-6 Immunodiffusion illustrating H *(short arrow)* and M *(long arrow)* precipitin bands that form when histoplasmin is tested against sera containing reactive antibodies.

Ohio and Mississippi Valley regions and to a lesser extent the Missouri and Arkansas River basins. Additional endemic sites have been found in Minnesota, Southern Manitoba, and Southwest Ontario, including the St. Lawrence River basin. Epidemics have occurred in Wisconsin, Minnesota, Illinois, and in the eastern states of Virginia and North Carolina. It has also been reported in a wide geographical area of Africa. In endemic areas, natural disease exists among dogs and horses and is an important veterinary problem. The veterinary picture is similar to the clinical and pathological disease seen in human infections. Untreated, blastomycosis in animals may have a rapid and fatal course.

The natural reservoir for the agent of blastomycosis is unknown. Unlike *H. capsulatum*, *B. dermatitidis* is rarely cultured from soil in endemic areas. The organism is believed to be present in the soil but flourishes only in a narrow, as yet undefined, ecological niche.

Clinical Syndromes

The natural history of *B. dermatitidis* infections is not as well documented as that of *H. capsulatum* infections because of the lack of reliable serological tests and characteristic radiographic findings. Manifestations of symptomatic blastomycosis, an uncommon disease, often indicate systemic spread. Large numbers of asymptomatic infections presumably occur, analogous to histoplasmosis.

BOX 70-2   Summary of Blastomycosis

ETIOLOGICAL AGENT

Asexual phase: *Blastomyces dermatitidis.*
Sexual phase: *Ajellomyces dermatitidis.*

MYCOLOGY

Dimorphic; mycelia at 25° C; typical pyriform microconidia (2-4 μm in diameter).
At 37° C and in tissue, this organism is a yeast (8-15 μm in diameter).
Buds produced singly are attached to the parent cell by a broad base.

EPIDEMIOLOGY AND ECOLOGY

Geographically, the organism is limited to the North American continent and parts of Africa. The area of endemism in the United States overlaps that for histoplasmosis.
Blastomycosis is an important veterinary problem, and dogs develop a disease similar to that in humans.
There are few reports of successful isolation of this organism from soil.

CLINICAL DISEASE

Primary infection in the lung is often inapparent, although epidemics of respiratory blastomycosis have been documented.

Inhalation of *B. dermatitidis* conidia produces a primary pulmonary infection in the host. As with *H. capsulatum*, *B. dermatitidis* conidia convert to yeast and are phagocytised by macrophages, which may carry them to other organs. The initial infection can be symptomatic or asymptomatic. Chest x-ray films may show nonspecific pulmonary infiltrates; however, unlike histoplasmosis, resolution of these lesions is not accompanied by calcifications. Primary pulmonary disease can have three outcomes: resolution without involvement of other organs, progressive pulmonary disease, or resolution of the pulmonary infection followed by systemic disease.

Laboratory Diagnosis

Serological and immunological findings for blastomycosis are unclear. Two antigenic preparations are used in tests to detect the immune response to infection by *B. dermatitidis*: cell-free culture filtrate of the **mycelial phase (blastomycin)** and inactivated whole yeast phase cells. The data obtained from skin testing and serological studies are difficult to interpret because the antigenic preparations are poorly defined. The reagents tend be highly cross-reactive with etiological agents of other mycoses, particularly those of histoplasmosis and coccidioidomycosis.

An immunodiffusion test that appears to be specific for blastomycosis has been developed. It is based on a yeast phase culture filtrate, designated *A antigen*. Suitable control sera containing antibodies that react with A antigen must be included with patient sera in immunodiffusion studies.

The diagnosis of blastomycosis requires identification of the organism in infected tissue or isolation in culture. Microscopic examination reveals characteristic broad-based, budding yeast cells (Figure 70-8) in purulent abscess fluid that has been treated with potassium hydroxide or biopsies of stained skin lesions. The organism grows readily in culture. It is identified by its conversion from the mycelial phase to the yeast phase or by the exoantigen test.

FIGURE 70-8 Broad-based budding yeast cells of *B. dermatitidis* seen in purulent material expressed from a microabscess.

Treatment

Amphotericin B remains the mainstay of therapy for patients with systemic disease or serious pulmonary disease, particularly in immunocompromised patients. Uncomplicated pulmonary disease may respond to fluconazole.

PARACOCCIDIOIDOMYCOSIS

Paracoccidioidomycosis is a pulmonary disease resulting from the inhalation of infectious conidia of *P. brasiliensis* (Figure 70-9). Pulmonary infections are often asymptomatic. The most common form exhibits ulcerative lesions of the oral and nasal cavity. The disease is also called *South American blastomycosis* and *Lutz-Splendore-Almeida disease* (Box 70-3).

Morphology

P. brasiliensis is dimorphic, growing as a mold in the environment and as budding yeast in infected tissue. The yeast phase is characterized by multiple budding from a single cell (Figure 70-10). The transition from mold to yeast can be induced in vitro by raising the temperature from 25° to 37° C. Recent studies show that as little as 10^{-10} *M*-17-beta-estradiol significantly inhibits the transformation of mycelia to yeast at 37° C. Testosterone, corticosterone, and 17-alpha-estradiol have no inhibitory effect on the transition of the mycelia phase to the yeast phase at 37° C. The findings may have clinical significance (see the discussion on epidemiology). A sexual state for *P. brasiliensis* has not been described.

Epidemiology

Paracoccidioidomycosis is geographically restricted to Central and South America, having a high incidence in Brazil, Venezuela, and Colombia. The endemic areas have been delineated by data taken from extensive skin test surveys and case reports. Like *B. dermatitidis*, *P. brasiliensis* cannot routinely be cultured from soil in endemic areas. Careful, retrospective epidemiological studies and data from a report on the isolation of *P. brasilien-*

FIGURE 70-9 Natural history of the saprobic and parasitic cycle of *P. brasiliensis*.

FIGURE 70-10 Multipolar budding characteristic of the yeast phase of *P. brasiliensis*.

sis from soil samples suggest that the fungi reside in environments that have high humidity and average temperatures around 23° C.

Results of skin test surveys indicate an equal distribution of reactors between male and female patients. However, analysis of data from clinically significant disease indicates that the number of male patients affected is disproportionate to the number of female patients (9:1). This difference has been attributed to high risk factors, underlying disease, malnourishment, and hormonal differences. Inhibition of the mycelia to yeast transition by beta-estradiol may also account for the lower incidence of disseminated paracoccidioidomycosis in women.

Clinical Syndromes

The prominence of oral and nasal lesions led to the belief that infection resulted from local inoculation. However, primary infection of paracoccidioidomycosis, like the other systemic mycoses, is now known to occur in the lungs as a result of inhaling conidia. Primary pulmonary paracoccidioidomycosis is frequently asymptomatic but can develop into progressive pulmonary disease or disseminated disease.

Laboratory Diagnosis

Diagnosis of paracoccidioidomycosis, as with histoplasmosis and coccidioidomycosis, is based on detection of specific antibodies, visualization of the organism in histopathological material, and isolation of the organism in culture. Two antigenic preparations of *P. brasiliensis* are used for serological diagnosis: a cell-free culture filtrate of the mycelial phase (paracoccidioidin) and an inactivated whole yeast phase preparation. These serological reagents are not routinely available in the United States. Specific antibodies are measured by complement fixation and immunodiffusion.

The organism can be seen in potassium hydroxide preparations of infected material or in silver-stained histological sections. The presence of multiple small, budding cells arranged around a large, mature cell *(ship's wheel pattern)* is diagnostic of *P. brasiliensis* (Figure 70-10). However, in the absence of buds the yeast of *P. brasiliensis* may be confused with immature spherules of *C. immitis* or the nonbudding yeast of *B. dermatitidis* or *H. capsulatum.* Clinical material that is cultured on medium incubated at 25° C yields a slow-growing, white mold after 10 to 14 days of incubation. Microscopic examination of the growth is usually not diagnostic because *P. brasiliensis* does not sporulate readily. Transfer of the culture to incubation at 37° C yields a yeastlike growth with characteristic multipolar budding cells.

Treatment

Successful treatment of paracoccidioidomycosis generally requires long-term therapy. Amphotericin B is effective against all forms of paracoccidioidomycosis, but because of toxicity and difficulty of long-term administration, it is usually reserved for severe cases. Sulfa drugs have been used for decades to treat disease; however, treatment failures can occur despite therapy that lasts for years. Ketoconazole (and the newer azole agents) are very active in vitro against *P. brasiliensis* and appear to be clinically effective.

COCCIDIOIDOMYCOSIS

Inhalation of the arthroconidia of *C. immitis* causes an acute, self-limited, and usually benign respiratory infection. The condition may be asymptomatic, or it may vary in severity from the mildness of a common cold to the severity of a disseminated life-threatening disease (Figure 70-11). Coccidioidomycosis has also been called *Posadas-Wernicke disease, San Joaquin Valley fever,* and *desert rheumatism* (Box 70-4).

Morphology

C. immitis is a dimorphic fungus that grows as a filamentous mold in the environment. The mycelia fragment to produce cylindrical arthroconidia (Figure 70-12). The tissue phase of *C. immitis* is the spherule (Figure 70-13), a multinucleated structure that undergoes internal cleavage to produce uninucleate endospores that can then generate new spherules. A sexual state has not been observed for *C. immitis.*

Epidemiology

Coccidioidomycosis, which can be described as a disease of the "New World," is geographically limited to the North, Central, and South American continents (Figure 70-14). The areas of highest endemicity have a semiarid climate and include the central San Joaquin Valley in California, Maricopa and Pima Counties in Arizona, and several western and southwestern counties in Texas. The disease is also endemic in the northern states of Mexico and parts of Venezuela, Paraguay, and Argentina. Cases of coccidioidomycosis have also been reported in Central America. The organism can be routinely isolated from soil in areas of high endemicity. Although geographically restricted, the organism has on occasion spread extensively as a result of large dust storms.

Clinical Syndromes

The natural history of coccidioidomycosis has been well characterized because large groups of nonimmune individuals who have migrated to endemic areas could be studied (e.g., military personnel stationed in the San Joaquin Valley during World War II). Exposure to *C. immitis,* compared with *H. capsulatum,* causes a greater percentage of individuals to undergo a mild febrile to moderately severe respiratory disease. However, a high degree of innate immunity generally exists in the adult population. Approximately 40% of individuals develop a symptomatic pulmonary infection after exposure to the organism. These primary infections are usually self-limited, but in a small proportion of patients, *C. immitis* causes progressive pulmonary disease or disseminates to

Summary of Coccidioidomycosis

ETIOLOGICAL AGENT

Asexual phase: *Coccidioides immitis.*
Sexual phase: Not known.

MYCOLOGY

Dimorphic; mycelia at 25° C.

As the culture ages, the septate hyphae mature such that alternate cells develop into arthroconidia separated by vacuolized cells.

The arthroconidia separate readily and have a barrel-shaped appearance.

In tissue and at 37° C, the organism develops into large, spherical structures (10-60 μm in diameter) called *spherules* (sporangia) that are filled with endospores 2-5 μm in diameter.

EPIDEMIOLOGY AND ECOLOGY

This disease is geographically restricted to North, Central, and South America, where there are areas of high endemism. In North America, the disease is highly endemic in the San Joaquin Valley of California, the Southwestern part of the United States, and the northern states of Mexico.

Natural infection occurs in domestic and wild animals.

The organism has been repeatedly isolated form soil samples taken from an endemic area.

CLINICAL DISEASE

Approximately 60% of these infections are asymptomatic.

The most common symptoms of primary disease are cough, fever, and chest pain. Night sweats and joint pain are not unusual.

An epidemiological history should be taken to determine whether the patient has been in an endemic area.

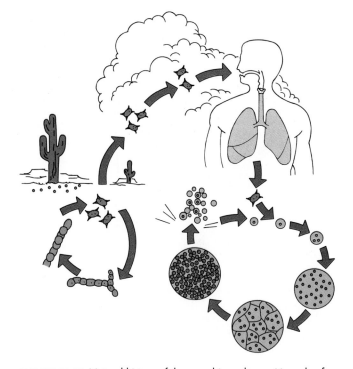

FIGURE 70-11 Natural history of the saprobic and parasitic cycle of *C. immitis.*

FIGURE 70-12 Hyphae and arthroconidia of *C. immitis.*

produce extrapulmonary disease that mainly involves the meninges, skin, or both.

Laboratory Diagnosis

Two sources of antigens, both of which are cell-free culture filtrates, are used in the preparation of serological reagents: the **mycelial phase** of growth (**coccidioidin**) and the **spherule phase (spherulin).** Skin test reactivity to coccidioidin develops 2 to 4 weeks after symptoms. The tube precipitin and the complement fixation tests are the time-honored serological procedures used to diagnose coccidioidomycosis. Precipitins appear early, between 2 and 4 weeks after symptoms, followed by the appearance of complement-fixing antibodies.

Other methods of detecting specific antibodies, such as latex particle agglutination and agar immunodiffusion, are now available. These tests largely replace the tube precipitin and complement fixation tests as routine screening methods because they are more sensitive in de-

FIGURE 70-13 Spherule phase of *C. immitis* as seen in stained tissue section.

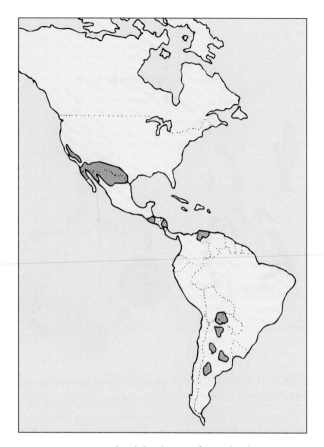

FIGURE 70-14 Geographical distribution of coccidioidomycosis in North, Central, and South America *(shaded)*.

> **BOX 70-5   Summary of Cryptococcosis**
>
> **ETIOLOGICAL AGENT**
>
> Asexual phase: *Cryptococcus neoformans.*
> Sexual phase: *Filobasidiella neoformans.*
>
> **MYCOLOGY**
>
> Monomorphic.
> This organism is a yeast at 25° and 37° C. The unique feature of the yeast is the acidic mucopolysaccharide capsule.
>
> **EPIDEMIOLOGY AND ECOLOGY**
>
> This disease is worldwide in distribution. This yeast has been repeatedly isolated from sites inhabited by pigeons, particularly their roosts and droppings. Pigeons are not naturally infected.
>
> **CLINICAL DISEASE**
>
> Primary pulmonary cryptococcosis is usually inapparent but may be chronic, subacute, or acute.
> The clinical entity most often seen is cryptococcal meningitis.
> Osseous and cutaneous disease can be present without apparent neurological involvement.

tecting specific antibodies of infected individuals, are commercially available, and are easily performed. In the immunodiffusion test, two lines of precipitation are significant: one line associated with the antigen that detects precipitin and agglutinating antibodies and another line associated with the complement-fixing antibodies. Once the presence of an infection has been established, complement fixation titers can yield important prognostic information. High, persistent, or rising titers indicate a high probability of disseminated disease. *C. immitis* spherules can be seen on infected tissue stained with hematoxylin and eosin. The organism can be cultured on conventional media; however, it must be handled with caution because *C. immitis* is a leading cause of laboratory-acquired infections. Although the mold phase of *C. immitis* is highly suggestive of the organism, arthroconidia are found in several saprobic fungi; therefore definitive identification is based on conversion to spherules or a specific exoantigen test.

Treatment

Amphotericin B is the drug of choice for the treatment of serious coccidioidal infections. Meningeal infections are particularly difficult to treat, partly because of the poor penetration of amphotericin B into cerebrospinal fluid. Fluconazole is effective in suppressing infections, but relapses occur after ceasing therapy.

CRYPTOCOCCOSIS

Cryptococcosis, also called **Busse-Buschke disease, torulosis,** or **European blastomycosis,** is a chronic to acute infection caused by *C. neoformans* (Box 70-5). There are two varieties of *C. neoformans*: *C. neoformans* var. *neoforman* (serotypes A and D) and *C. neoformans* var. *gatti* (serotypes B and C). In contrast to the other systemic mycotic agents, dimorphism does not play a role in the pathogenesis of *C. neoformans* because the organism is an encapsulated yeast in culture at 25° and 37° C and in tissues. Several putative virulence factors of *C. neoformans* have been identified. The capsular polysaccharide, for example, inhibits phagocytosis. Another virulence factor appears to be phenoloxidase, an enzyme that converts phenolic compounds to melanin. The lung is the primary site of infection; however, the organism has a high predilection for systemic spread to the brain and meninges (Figure 70-15). *C. neoformans* is the leading cause of fungal meningitis and is an important cause of morbidity and mortality in AIDS patients and transplant recipients. *C. neoformans* also produces systemic disease in patients who have no apparent underlying immunological disorder.

Morphology

Unlike the other systemic mycotic agents the asexual phase of *C. neoformans* is not dimorphic. The organism grows as a budding yeast in infected tissue and in culture at 25° C and 37° C. The most distinctive feature of

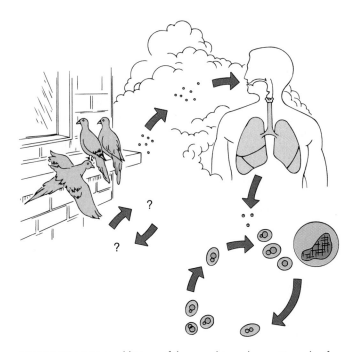

FIGURE 70-15 Natural history of the saprobic and parasitic cycle of *C. neoformans*.

C. neoformans is the presence of an acidic mucopolysaccharide capsule. This capsule is required for pathogenicity and is important diagnostically, both in terms of antigen detection and specific histological staining. The sexual phase of *C. neoformans* has been discovered; it is *Filobasidiella neoformans* and is classified as a basidiomycete (see Chapter 7). There is speculation that the basidiospore may be the infectious propagule, but it has not been identified.

Epidemiology

C. neoformans serotypes A and D are recovered in large numbers from the excreta and debris of pigeons. Thus the organism appears to survive well in a desiccated, alkaline, nitrogen-rich, and hypertonic environment. It has a close relationship with the habitats of pigeons, but the organism does not appear to naturally infect the bird. The natural reservoir of *C. neoformans* var. *gatti* (serotype B) was unknown until it was isolated recently from the tree sap of *Eucalyptus camaldulensis* (red gum). Cryptococcosis occurs throughout the world. The true prevalence of infection is unknown because of the lack of a reliable skin test or another serological screening test, but subclinical infections are believed to be common. Symptomatic cryptococcal disease, mainly meningitis, is frequently seen in individuals who are debilitated, immunosuppressed, or otherwise compromised. However, many patients who develop cryptococcal meningitis have no underlying immune or metabolic defects.

Clinical Syndromes

Primary pulmonary infections are frequently asymptomatic and may be detected as incidental findings on a routine chest x-ray examination A solitary pulmonary nodule that can mimic a carcinoma is most commonly observed; the correct diagnosis is usually made when the mass is resected. *C. neoformans* can also produce a symptomatic pneumonia characterized by diffuse pulmonary infiltrates.

Cryptococcal meningitis, which is caused by the hematogenous spread of yeast from the lungs to the meninges surrounding the brain, is the most frequently diagnosed form of cryptococcosis. Symptoms usually include the combinations of headache, mental status changes, and fever lasting several weeks. Occasionally, cryptococcal disease of the central nervous system may take the form of an expanding intracerebral mass that causes focal neurological deficits. Other common manifestations of disseminated cryptococcosis include skin lesions and osteolytic bone lesions.

Laboratory Diagnosis

Unlike the serological procedures used to diagnose the other systemic mycoses, the serologic procedures used in the diagnosis of cryptococcosis are based on the detection of antigens, not antibodies. The latex agglutination test for the detection of cryptococcal polysaccharide antigens in cerebrospinal fluid and serum is routinely used in clinical laboratories; it is sensitive, specific, and simple to perform. The test involves the use of latex particles coated with a rabbit anticryptococcal antibody. The capsular polysaccharide present in a clinical specimen binds to the antibodies, thereby agglutinating the latex particles. Because the latex particles are coated with antibodies, false-positive reactions can be caused by rheumatoid factor (immunoglobulin M antibodies that bind immunoglobulin G). Therefore an appropriate control test must be performed in which the clinical specimen is mixed with latex particles coated with nonimmune rabbit antibodies. In addition, the patient's serum can be treated with a protease to destroy any proteins that might cause nonspecific agglutination of the latex particles. Rare cross-reactions occur with sera from patients with disseminated infections caused by *Trichosporon beigelii*. To evaluate the clinical progress of a patient during therapy, serial samples of cerebrospinal fluid are examined for the presence of cryptococcal antigen. A favorable prognosis is indicated by a decrease in the titer of antigen.

A rapid diagnosis of cryptococcal meningitis can often be made by examination of an India ink preparation of cerebrospinal fluid. *C. neoformans* appears as a single cell or budding yeast surrounded by a clear halo because of the exclusion of the ink particles by the polysaccharide capsule (Figure 70-16).

Although diagnosis may be rapid with the India ink preparation, its results are positive in only half of cryptococcal meningitis cases. Culture remains the definitive method for documenting infection. The organism grows well on standard, nonselective mycological media but is inhibited by cycloheximide, an antibiotic used to suppress the growth of saprobes. The identification of

FIGURE 70-16 Encapsulated budding yeast cells of *C. neoformans* highlighted with India ink.

C. neoformans is based on the presence of a capsule, the production of the enzyme urease, the assimilation pattern of carbon substrates, and other specific biochemical reactions.

Treatment

Whereas pulmonary cryptococcosis is frequently a self-limited infection or can be cured by surgical excision of a solitary nodule, disseminated cryptococcosis is almost always fatal if untreated. Cryptococcal meningitis remains the model for combination therapy with antifungal agents. Amphotericin B is active against *C. neoformans* but exhibits relatively poor penetration into cerebrospinal fluid. Although 5-fluorocytosine has good cerebrospinal fluid penetration, the development of resistant cryptococci is a problem. Controlled clinical trials have shown that combination therapy with amphotericin B and 5-fluorocytosine for 6 weeks is as effective as amphotericin B alone for 10 weeks. Nonetheless, relapses after either treatment regimen remain a problem, particularly in AIDS patients.

CASE STUDY AND QUESTIONS

About 7 to 10 days after exploring a bat cave in Missouri, three of five members of a spelunkers' club who had gone on the expedition complained of influenza-like symptoms and made appointments to see their internist. Patient A was febrile and had a nonproductive cough but was otherwise fine. Patient B, who is HIV-positive, was febrile, had a very deep cough, and complained of night sweats, chest pains, and tender joints. Patient C could not see his internist immediately and waited a week for his appointment. When this patient was seen, he was asymptomatic and said that after taking a couple of aspirin with a lot of water and getting 3 days of rest, he felt "fit as a fiddle." The remaining two spelunkers said that they felt fine and did not experience any of the described symptoms. During the course of examination, all of the spelunkers remarked that bats had roosted in the cave and a great deal of dust was raised during their exploration.

1. What was the diagnosis, and what should have been done to confirm it?
2. What are the geographical distributions of and the endemic areas for (a) coccidioidomycosis, (b) histoplasmosis, (c) blastomycosis, (d) paracoccidioidomycosis, and (e) cryptococcosis?
3. What are the distinguishing morphological features of the etiological agents of the systemic mycoses (a) in nature and (b) in tissue?
4. What is interesting about the epidemiology of (a) paracoccidioidomycosis, (b) coccidioidomycosis, (c) histoplasmosis, (d) blastomycosis, and (e) cryptococcosis?
5. What concern should have been shown for the patient who was also HIV positive?

Bibliography

Drutz DJ, editor: Systemic fungal infections: diagnosis and treatment. I. *Med Clin North Am* vol 3, 1988 (entire issue).

Drutz DJ, editor: Systemic fungal infections: diagnosis and treatment. II. *Med Clin North Am* vol 4, 1989 (entire issue).

Kwon-Chung KJ, Bennett JE: *Medical mycology,* Philadelphia, 1992, Lea & Febiger.

Sarosi GA, Davies SF, editors: *Fungal diseases of the lung,* Orlando, Fla, 1986, Grune & Stratton.

Szaniszlo PJ, editor: *Fungal dimorphism: with emphasis on fungi pathogenic for humans,* New York, 1985, Plenum.

Opportunistic Mycoses

Humans are constantly exposed to viable fungal propagules. Most tolerate these exposures with no resulting sequelae, but some develop an allergic hypersensitivity (see Chapter 66). There are at least two reasons for this. First, healthy, immunologically competent people have a high degree of innate resistance to fungal colonization. Second, the majority of fungi have a low inherent virulence. However, under conditions that lead to host debilitation, many people become susceptible to fungi. If the infection is not diagnosed rapidly and treated aggressively and if the underlying conditions causing host debilitation are not brought under control, the fungal infection may become life threatening. These infections, once considered rare and exotic, have become more common and of great medical significance. This is because of acquired immunodeficiency syndrome (AIDS) and the increased use of radiation and cytotoxic drug therapy to treat patients who are recipients of organ transplants or who have malignancies. Because these fungi become pathogens by taking advantage of the host's debilitated condition, they are commonly called **opportunistic fungi.**

A growing list of exotic and rare fungi have been implicated in opportunistic infections, but the majority are caused by various species of *Candida* (e.g., *C. albicans*), *Aspergillus* (e.g., *A. fumigatus*), and various Zygomycetes (e.g., *R. arrhizus*). Although *opportunistic pathogens* is the term used to define these organisms, it is based on the clinical setting and has no taxonomic significance. Two of the most common ones, *C. albicans* and *A. fumigatus,* have very different biological properties and host interactions. In addition, pathogenicity is not an all-or-nothing phenomenon. Individual species within both *Candida* and *Aspergillus* genera exhibit a range of pathogenicity.

It is noteworthy to mention *Pneumocystis carinii* as an etiological agent of opportunistic infections. It is a unicellular eukaryotic organism that causes a severe interstitial plasma cell pneumonia. Until recently, this organism was classified as a protozoan; however, ultrastructural studies with immunological and molecular genetic evidence indicate that it is closely related phylogenetically to fungi. However, this parasitic organism is unique because it possesses features (in particular, its putative life cycle) that distinguish it from other fungi.

Numerous other fungi have been implicated as etiological agents of opportunistic infections of humans. A cursory examination of the literature supports the contention that the list of exotic and rare species of fungi causing infectious problems is large and continues to grow. For further details, see the Bibliography at the end of this chapter.

CANDIDIASIS

Several species of *Candida* are implicated in candidiasis (Box 71-1). Candidiasis is a major disease problem of immunocompromised hosts. The clinical spectrum of manifestations ranges from superficial infections of the skin to systemic life-threatening infections. Under various conditions, *C. albicans, C. tropicalis, C. kefyr* (formerly *C. pseudotropicalis*), *C. glabrata* (formerly *Torulopsis glabrata*), and *C. parapsilosis* are part of the normal flora of humans. They can be isolated from healthy mucosal surfaces of the oral cavity, vagina, gastrointestinal tract, and rectal area. As many as 80% of people may show colonization of these sites in the absence of disease.

In contrast the organism is rarely isolated from the surface of normal human skin except sporadically from certain intertriginous areas (i.e., skin surfaces that appose each other) such as the groin. Under certain circumstances, these organisms gain hematogenous access from the oropharynx or gastrointestinal tract when the mucosal barrier is breached (e.g., inflammation of mucous membranes secondary to chemotherapy) or when intravenous catheters and syringes are contaminated. The organs most often involved include the lungs, spleen, kidneys, liver, heart, and brain. *Candida* organisms may produce endophthalmitis (inflammation involving the eyes), indicating a hematogenous dissemination of *C. albicans* and the possibility of multiple organ involvement. Skin lesions may occur in 10% to 30% of patients who have disseminated infections. The early recognition of such lesions is important in diagnosis because antemortem blood cultures are negative in a high percentage of patients with autopsy-proven systemic candidiasis.

BOX 71-1   *Candida* Species

ETIOLOGICAL AGENTS

C. albicans
C. stellatoidea
C. tropicalis
C. parapsilosis
C. kefyr*

C. guilliermondi
C. krusei
C. glabrata†
C. viswanathii
C. lusitaniae

CLINICAL CATEGORIES

Cutaneous: intertrigo, paronychia, onychomycosis
Mucocutaneous: perlèche, thrush, perianal disease
Chronic: mucocutaneous candidiasis, granulomatous disease
Systemic: fungemia, endocarditis, pulmonary infection, urinary tract infection, meningitis, endophthalmitis

UNDERLYING CONDITIONS

Variable causes, mostly mechanical (e.g., trauma, occlusion); broad-spectrum antibacterial therapy; oral contraceptives
AIDS; avitaminosis; pregnancy
Defects in T-cell lymphocytes and macrophages
Various conditions leading to immunosuppression (e.g., endocrinopathies, diabetes mellitus, burns); intravascular catheters; intravenous drug abuse

*Formerly called *Candida pseudotropicalis*.
†Formerly called *Torulopsis glabrata*.

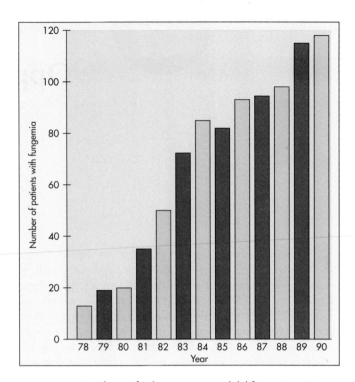

FIGURE 71-1 Incidence of culture-proven candidal fungemia at Barnes Hospital (St. Louis) from 1978 to 1990.

Morphology

With one exception a striking morphological feature of the yeasts in the genus *Candida* is that they multiply by forming blastospores, pseudohyphae, and septate hyphae (see Chapter 7). *Candida glabrata*, a yeast implicated in urinary tract infections and systemic disease in debilitated people, is the exception, producing only yeast cells.

Clinical Syndromes

The spectrum of infections caused by organisms in the genus *Candida* includes localized diseases of the skin and nails; diseases that affect the mucosal surfaces of the mouth, vagina, esophagus, and bronchial tree; and diseases that disseminate and involve multiple organ systems. The diseases involving the skin and nails frequently mimic those seen with the dermatophytes. In all cases the diagnosis must be supported by microscopically observing fungi in lesion specimens and must be confirmed by culture of the organism. Factors leading to a predisposition to the various candidal infections are summarized in Box 71-1.

Chronic mucocutaneous candidiasis (CMC) is a heterogeneous group of clinical syndromes characterized by chronic, treatment-resistant superficial *Candida* infections of the skin, nails, and oropharynx (see the discussion on immunity and host factors). Despite extensive cutaneous involvement, there is virtually no propensity for disseminated visceral candidiasis. In many cases, there are narrow but specific abnormalities in T-cell–mediated immunity. In others the defects are more general. Various underlying conditions, such as hypoparathyroidism, hypoadrenalism, hypothyroidism, and the presence of circulating autoimmune antibodies have been associated with CMC. In adults, CMC is frequently associated with thymoma. When cutaneous candidiasis indicates the possibility of an immunological or endocrine disorder, efforts must be made to uncover and to correct the underlying defect so that the fungal infection can be properly treated.

Disseminated candidiasis is usually spread through the bloodstream and therefore involves many organs. Severe neutropenia is considered to be the most significant predisposing factor for life-threatening infections. The incidence of this form of candidiasis is steadily rising as more patients with serious hematological malignancies are treated aggressively with potent immunosuppressive drugs and as more patients undergo bone marrow and organ transplants (Figure 71-1).

Whereas disseminated candidiasis continues to be a major problem in immunocompromised hosts, this is not the case in patients with AIDS, who develop serious infections of the oropharynx and upper gastrointestinal tract but rarely experience systemic disease. The development of oral candidiasis in previously healthy adults not receiving corticosteroid therapy or broad-spectrum antibiotic therapy should strongly alert the physician to consider infection with human immunodeficiency virus.

FIGURE 71-2 Sputum specimen illustrating budding yeast cells and pseudohyphae of *Candida* organisms.

FIGURE 71-3 Development of germ tubes by *C. albicans* yeast cells after incubation in serum for 2 hours at 37° C.

Immunity and Host Factors

Innate immunity to these organisms in the healthy adult human appears to be very good. The immune mechanisms responsible for protection against candidal infections include humoral and cell-mediated processes. Based on experiments with CMC indicating that a defect in cell-mediated immunity leads to extensive superficial candidiasis despite normal or exaggerated humoral defenses, cell-mediated processes are considered to be more important immune mechanisms.

Production of serum antibody to the principal wall glycoprotein antigens of the *Candida* species occurs in low titers in healthy people. The protective role of these antibodies, however, is controversial, and their presence may reflect only an immunological response to colonization of the gastrointestinal tract early in life. For this reason the serodiagnosis of candidiasis is not routinely performed. In certain experimental studies, such as the passive transfer of serum, a slight degree of protection may be provided. Yet in the clinical setting, it is clear that patients with primarily B-cell deficiency states are not at high risk for infection by *Candida* organisms. Evidence for the role of secretory immunoglobulin A in limiting mucosal infections is confusing. It is probable that various innate, nonimmune host factors in conjunction with cell-mediated immunity and complement activation contribute more to host defense against *Candida* organisms than humoral immunity.

Laboratory Diagnosis

The species most often responsible for these infections include *C. albicans, C. tropicalis, C. kefyr, C. glabrata, C. krusei,* and *C. parapsilosis.* In histopathological sections and sputum, they may produce budding yeast cells, pseudohyphae, and septate hyphae (Figure 71-2). On solid media the organisms produce yeast and pseudohyphal cells, and the gross appearance of the colony is opaque, cream colored, and pasty. The species of all yeasts cultured from blood, cerebrospinal fluid, and sur-

gical specimens should be identified. Laboratory standards should be set for identification of yeasts from sputum, urine, and other nonsterile sources, since yeasts may be part of the normal flora or transient colonizers. Several procedures are available for identification, most of which combine morphological, physiological, and biochemical tests. A rapid and reliable test to identify *C. albicans* is the germ tube test. Blastospores of *C. albicans* produce hyphal outgrowths (germ tubes) when they are suspended in serum and incubated at 37° C (Figure 71-3).

For the test to be valid the suspension must be examined within 2 to 3 hours after incubation because other species may form similar structures with longer incubation. A few isolates of *C. albicans* do not form germ tubes under these conditions. Therefore other tests are performed based on biochemical and physiological properties of the organisms, such as the ability to assimilate various sugars or produce morphological structures (e.g., chlamydospores) (Figure 71-4) under certain growth conditions.

Treatment, Prevention, and Control

In the immunologically competent patient, topical treatment is usually preferred for cutaneous and mucocutaneous disease, and except for disease of the nails, a good clinical response generally results when proper therapy is instituted. Therapy for systemic disease varies depending on the organ involvement and immune status of the patient. For systemic disease, amphotericin B alone or combined with 5-fluorocytosine may be indicated. Alternative therapy includes the use of the azole derivatives. Ketoconazole and fluconazole are preferred because they are active when given orally and less toxic than amphotericin B. However, the azole derivatives are fungistatic, and in many cases the disease recurs after therapy is discontinued. Fungal infections in immunosuppressed patients pose a problem because the underlying conditions leading to immunosuppression must be corrected to ob-

FIGURE 71-4 Formation of chlamydospores by *C. albicans* when cultured on cornmeal agar at 25° C.

tain maximal response from the antifungal treatment. Patients who are intubated or are connected to various support catheters must be monitored closely; lines must be changed frequently so that they do not become contaminated and serve as foci for fungal colonization. See Chapter 67 for further details regarding treatment, prevention, and control.

ASPERGILLOSIS

The spectrum of medical problems caused by various species of *Aspergillus* is broad (Table 71-1). Organisms belonging to this genus are extremely common in the environment. In contrast to most infections caused by *Candida* organisms, aspergillosis is acquired from exogenous sources. As a result, assessing the significance of culture reports may be difficult unless the organism is seen in histopathological specimens.

Morphology

These organisms are identified in culture by their morphological features, the pattern of conidiophore development, and the color of the formed conidia (Figure 71-5). Species of *Aspergillus* are extremely common in the environment, and several have been implicated as etiological agents. Of the approximately 900 described species, *A. fumigatus* and *A. flavus* have been most frequently associated with invasive disease.

Clinical Syndromes

The normal healthy individual is not susceptible to systemic aspergillosis. It is purely an opportunistic infection. As with candidiasis the type of disease evoked depends on the local or general physiological and immunological state of the host. Factors that lead to host

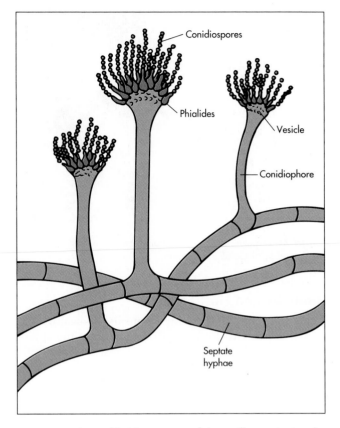

FIGURE 71-5 Asexual fruiting structure of *Aspergillus* species in culture. Septate hyphae, conidiophore, vesicle, phialides, and conidiospores are illustrated.

TABLE 71-1	Diseases Associated with *Aspergillus* Species
DISEASE	**ETIOLOGICAL AGENT**
Mycotoxicoses	Ingestion of contaminated food products
Hypersensitivity pneumonitis	Allergic bronchopulmonary disease
Secondary colonization	Fungal colonization of preexisting cavity (e.g., pulmonary abscess) without invasion into contiguous tissues
Systemic disease	Invasive disease involving multiple organs

debilitation are also important in aspergillosis. In contrast to candidiasis, the etiological agents implicated in aspergillosis are ubiquitous in the environment and are not part of the normal flora of humans, although transient colonization may occur. These agents are involved in many animal diseases, such as mycotic abortion of sheep and cattle and pulmonary infections of birds, and their metabolites serve as carcinogenic agents in animals that have ingested contaminated feed. Because of their

FIGURE 71-6 Chest film illustrating a cavity in the upper right lobe (arrow) with an organizing fungus ball.

FIGURE 71-7 Dichotomous branching septate hyphae of *A. fumigatus* in tissue specimen.

diverse involvement in both human and animal disease, these agents pose a great economic problem.

Allergic aspergillosis may initially occur as a benign process and then become severe as the patient grows older. Respiratory distress increases with age, leading to bronchiectasis (chronic dilatation of the air passages). Collapse of a segment of the lung eventually results in fibrosis (scarring).

In secondary colonization, a chronic clinical situation may exist with little distress, except occasional bouts of hemoptysis (coughing up of blood) and pathological changes in the lung that lead to the formation of a "fungus ball" (Figure 71-6). Histopathologically, the fungus ball is a spherical mass of intertwined, branching, septate hyphal elements. These structures can also be visualized radiologically as space-occupying spherical structures that move within the cavity as the patient's position is changed.

Systemic aspergillosis is an extremely serious disorder that is usually rapidly fatal unless diagnosed early and treated aggressively. In the immunosuppressed host the organism spreads from its primary site to contiguous tissues without regard to tissue planes, and lesions frequently contain hyphae within blood vessels, causing infarcts and hemorrhage. As in disseminated candidiasis

the physiological and immunological conditions that contribute to the host's increased susceptibility to the infection must be reversed for proper management.

Laboratory Diagnosis

The diagnosis of invasive aspergillosis is considered when septate hyphae that branch at regular intervals and that tend to be oriented in the same direction are seen in clinical specimens (Figure 71-7). Confirmation of invasive aspergillosis is sometimes difficult because cultures are not always performed or are often negative. Because these organisms exist everywhere in the environment, the clinical and histopathological diagnosis of invasive aspergillosis is strongly supported by repeated isolation of the organism in culture.

ZYGOMYCOSIS

Fungi belonging to the Zygomycetes are very common in the environment. The clinical entity zygomycosis, also termed *mucormycosis* or *phycomycosis,* encompasses a spectrum of infections similar to aspergillosis. As with candidiasis and aspergillosis, several underlying factors lead to the host's increased susceptibility to fungi belonging to the class Zygomycetes. Most notable are metabolic acidosis, diabetes mellitus, leukopenia, and hyperglycemia.

Morphology

Fungi causing the zygomycoses grow rapidly on all laboratory media not containing cycloheximide. *Rhizopus, Absidia,* and *Mucor* species have been implicated in zygomycosis. They form coenocytic hyphae (i.e., not separated by cross walls) and reproduce asexually by producing sporangia, within which develop sporangiospores (Figure 71-8). These organisms are ubiquitous in the environment and frequently are encountered as contaminants. The relevance of the isolate may be difficult to establish if coenocytic hyphal elements are not seen in the

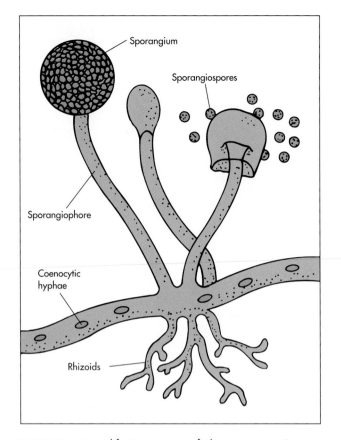

FIGURE 71-8 Asexual fruiting structure of *Rhizopus* species. Sporangium, sporangiophore, sporagiospores, coenocytic hyphae, and rhizoids are shown.

histopathological section. Repeated isolation of the organism from consecutive specimens provides strong evidence that the organism may be relevant, even though coenocytic hyphal elements are not seen in histopathological examination of tissue. A point to remember is that all fungi having coenocytic hyphae are classified as Zygomycetes, but not all Zygomycetes are coenocytic.

Clinical Syndromes

Various diseases are caused by organisms belonging to the class Zygomycetes order Mucorales. Rhinocerebral zygomycosis is the most common of the diseases. This infection originates in the paranasal sinuses and can involve the ocular orbit and palate with extension into the brain. It usually occurs as a terminal event in patients with acidosis who have metabolic disorders or uncontrolled diabetes mellitus. Other forms of zygomycosis seen in immunosuppressed or otherwise debilitated patients involve the lungs, gastrointestinal tract, and subcutaneous tissues. In severely burned patients, these organisms colonize the damaged tissues and tend to become invasive. In disseminated disease the organism shows a marked predilection for invading major blood vessels. The emboli (clots) that result cause ischemia (obstruction of blood vessels) and necrosis of adjacent tissues.

FIGURE 71-9 Histological section from a case of zygomycosis. Ribbonlike, broad, nonseptate (coenocytic) hyphae (stained with Gomori's methenamine silver) are illustrated.

Laboratory Diagnosis

These organisms are filamentous, and their distinct morphology helps identify them in microscopic examination of pathological material. The hyphal filaments are coenocytic and have a ribbonlike appearance in tissue specimens (Figure 71-9). Cultures grown on medium not containing antibiotics are dense and have a hairy appearance. Microscopic examination of this growth confirms the coenocytic nature of the hyphae, and sporulating species produce characteristic sporangia (asexual fruiting bodies) (Figure 71-8) that contain sporangiospores. The most frequently encountered agents of zygomycosis are *R. arrhizus* and *A. corymbifera*. Assessing reports on the number and variety of species that may cause disease is often difficult because culture frequently fails to isolate the organism. Therefore the diagnosis is often based on histopathological examination of tissue.

PNEUMOCYSTIS CARINII PNEUMONIA

Disease caused by *P. carinii* is associated with a variety of clinical conditions of debilitation, particularly those associated with age, congenital and iatrogenically induced immunosuppression, and AIDS. It is seen primarily in premature and malnourished children in crowded institutions such as orphanages and hospitals. It is also seen in adults in chronic disease wards and is the most common opportunistic infection in patients with AIDS and other immune deficiencies. As many as 85% of patients with AIDS develop pneumonia caused by *P. carinii*, which is a cosmopolitan organism in humans and other mammals. Although rodents are infected with this organism, they probably do not serve as a reservoir for its transmission to humans because comparison of surface antigens and nucleic acid sequences of various genes of rat and human isolates are distinct from each other. Transmission from host to host is apparently by droplet inhalation and close contact. This opportunistic organism is present in many persons whose disease is completely asymptomatic. Symptomatic disease develops when some imbalance or debilitating illness (e.g., AIDS) is present, suggesting reactivation of latent infection or a long-term carrier state.

Morphology and Taxonomic Status

Morphological and molecular genetic evidence indicate that phylogenetically *P. carinii* is closely related to fungi. The cyst wall closely resembles that of fungi; there is excellent homology of the conserved domains of the 16S rRNA subunit with that of ascomycetes, the 5S rRNA with that of primitive zygomycetous fungi, and the protein synthesis elongation factor (EF-3) with that of *Saccharomyces cerevisiae*. The respiratory tract appears to be the portal of entry, since primary infection is in the lung. Various stages of the organism's life cycle may be found in Giemsa- and methenamine-stained clinical specimens. The organism may appear in a trophic form (1.5 to 5.0 μm), as a uninucleated sporocyst (4.0 to 5.0 μm), or as a mature spore case (5.0 μm) containing eight spherical, oval to fusiform spores (1.0 to 3.0 μm). After the mature spore case ruptures to release the intracystic bodies, the cyst wall remains and may be seen as empty oval or as collapsed structures. *P. carinii* is atypical when it is compared with other fungi in terms of phenotypic features, the different morphological forms found in infected tissue, and the refractoriness toward most antifungal antibiotics.

Clinical Syndromes

Evidence from serological studies indicate that infection with *P. carinii* occurs at an early age and that it is very common in the environment. Subclinical infections in healthy people are probably frequent, and the organism may remain dormant for a long time. Alveolar macrophages and CD4+ T cells play an important role in host defense against *P. carinii*. Patients with AIDS are at high risk to develop disease when their CD4+ T cell count falls below 200 cells/ml³. The onset of disease is insidious, but it can be suspected in patients who are malnourished or immunocompromised and who develop fever and pneumonitis that are not otherwise explainable.

Interstitial pneumonitis with plasma cell infiltrates is a hallmark of *P. carinii* infections. As the disease progresses, the patient experiences weakness, dyspnea, and tachypnea, leading to cyanosis. Radiology of the lungs shows infiltrations spreading from hilar areas, giving the lungs a so-called ground-glass appearance. In these cases the arterial oxygen tension is low, and carbon dioxide tension is normal or low. Death results from asphyxiation.

In the past few years, extrapulmonary infections with *P. carinii* have been described in patients with AIDS. Multiple sites of involvement have been observed, including the ear, eye, liver, and bone marrow. Most patients have received aerosolized pentamidine as a prophylactic to prevent *P. carinii* pneumonia.

FIGURE 71-10 Gomori's methenamine silver–stained section of lung biopsy specimen demonstrates groups of rounded, cup-shaped organisms, 4-5 μm in diameter within the intraalveolar exudate. The staining of the cyst wall and intracystic bodies helps distinguish these organisms from yeast. The cuplike forms and indented shapes are characteristic of *P. carinii*.

Laboratory Diagnosis

The diagnosis of *P. carinii* pneumonia is done by morphological identification of the organism in clinical material. Typical *P. carinii* organisms are revealed by examination of stained slides of impression smears of lung tissue obtained by brush biopsy (Figure 71-10), material obtained by percutaneous transthoracic needle aspiration, aspirates of bronchial washings, and sputum. Bronchoalveolar lavage alone is adequate for demonstration of organisms in more than 90% of AIDS patients. Induced sputum specimens may also be useful for diagnosing *P. carinii* pneumonia in AIDS patients because of the tremendous number of organisms. The parasites can be stained by Gomori's methenamine silver or the Giemsa method or with calcofluor or specific fluorescein-labeled antibodies. Radiology is of value in establishing the typical appearance of lungs infected with *P. carinii*. Serological tests have been used for epidemiological surveys but are not useful as a diagnostic procedure.

Treatment, Prevention, and Control

The treatment of choice includes trimethoprim-sulfamethoxazole or pentamidine isethionate; both may have toxic side effects. Supportive measures such as oxygen and antibiotics may also be indicated. Treatment with amphotericin B or the azole derivatives are not clinically effective in patients with this infection.

Education regarding transmission of the organism, avoidance of close contact with infected patients, and elimination of possible contact with droplet transmission are all critical, as are prompt diagnosis and treatment. The organism and its transmission are difficult to control because of the extended carrier state and its presence as an opportunistic pathogen. Prophylaxis with trimethoprim-sulfamethoxazole or aerosolized pentamidine may be useful in people with AIDS.

CASE STUDY AND QUESTIONS

A 42-year-old man with end-stage liver disease secondary to hepatitis B underwent orthoptic liver transplantation. Immunosuppression was maintained with cyclosporine and prednisone therapy. Four months after the surgical procedure the patient was admitted to the hospital because of persistent fever and hypotension. Examination of the skin revealed ecchymotic lesions over the abdominal surface. Biopsies were taken for histological examination and culture. Microscopic examination revealed granulomatous inflammation of the deep dermis, and dichotomously branching septate hyphae were seen on special stains. Cultures grew *A. flavus*.

1. What are some of the predisposing factors of opportunistic fungal infections?
2. Why are epidemics of fungal infections rare?
3. Which is more important in opportunistic fungal infections: humoral-mediated or cell-mediated immunity? Why?
4. Is contagion a problem (i.e., should a patient be placed on isolation)?
5. What is the current taxonomic status of *P. carinii* and why is it classified as such?

Bibliography

Anker van den JN, Popele van NML, Sauer PJJ: Antifungal agents in neonatal candidiasis, *Antimicrob Agents Chemother* 39:1391-1397, 1995.

Dixon DM et al: Fungal infections: a growing threat, *Pub Health Reports* 111:226-235, 1996.

Gradon JD, Timpone JG, Schnittman SM: Emergence of unusual opportunistic pathogens in AIDS: a review, *Clin Infect Dis* 15:134-157, 1992.

Hadley KW, Ng VL: *Pneumocystis.* In Murray PR et al, editors: *Manual of clinical microbiology,* ed 6, Washington, DC, 1995, American Society for Microbiology.

Kwon-Chung KJ, Bennett JE: *Medical mycology*, Philadelphia, 1992, Lea & Febiger.

Perfect JR, Schell WA: The new fungal opportunists are coming, *Clin Infect Dis* 22:S112-S118, 1996.

SECTION VII

Parasitology

Pathogenesis of Parasitic Disease

Given the wide diversity that exists among human parasites, it is not surprising that the pathogenesis of protozoan and helminthic disease is highly variable. Although the various human parasites exhibit a wide range of **direct** pathogenic mechanisms, in most instances the organisms themselves are not highly virulent, are unable to replicate within the host, or have both reactions. Thus the severity of illness caused by many parasites is related to the infecting dose and the number of organisms acquired over time. Unlike many bacterial and viral infections, parasitic infections are often chronic, lasting months to years. Repeated exposures result in an ever-increasing parasite burden. When infection with a particular organism is associated with a strong immune response, there is undoubtedly a considerable immunopathological contribution to the disease manifestations attributed to the infection.

Important factors to consider when discussing parasite pathogenicity are listed in Box 72-1. Parasites are almost always exogenous to the human host and thus must enter the body through ingestion or direct penetration of anatomical barriers. Inoculum size and duration of exposure greatly influence the disease-causing potential of an organism. Likewise, the route of exposure is critical for most organisms. For example, pathogenic strains of *Entamoeba histolytica* are unlikely to cause disease on exposure to intact skin but may cause severe dysentery after oral ingestion. Many parasites have active, self-directed means of invading the human

host. Once they have invaded, parasites attach to specific host cells or organs, avoid immune detection, replicate (most protozoa and some helminths), produce toxic substances that destroy tissue, and cause disease secondary to the host's own immunologic response (Box 72-1). In addition, some parasites physically obstruct and damage organs and tissues because of their size alone. This chapter discusses factors that are important for parasite pathogenicity and provide examples of organisms and disease processes related to each factor.

EXPOSURE AND ENTRY

Although many infectious diseases are caused by **endogenous** organisms that are part of the normal flora of the human host, this is not the case with most diseases caused by protozoan and helminthic parasites. These organisms are virtually always acquired from an **exogenous** source and as such have evolved numerous ways to enter the body of the human host. The most common modes of entry are oral ingestion or direct penetration through the skin or other surfaces (Table 72-1). Transmission of parasitic diseases is frequently facilitated by environmental contamination with human and animal wastes. This is most applicable to diseases transmitted by the fecal-oral route but also applies to helminthic infections such as hookworm disease and strongyloidiasis, which rely on larval penetration of the skin.

Many parasitic diseases are acquired via the bites of arthropod vectors. Transmission of disease in this manner is extraordinarily effective, as evidenced by the widespread distribution of diseases such as malaria, trypanosomiasis, and filariasis. Examples of parasites and their ports of entry are listed in Table 72-1. This compilation should not be considered exhaustive; rather, the list provides examples of some of the more common parasites and the means by which they enter the human body.

Additional factors that determine the outcome of the interaction between parasite and host are **route of exposure** and **inoculum size.** Most human parasites have a limited range of organs or tissues in which they can

---

BOX 72-1 Factors Associated with Parasite Pathogenicity

Infective dose and exposure
Penetration of anatomical barriers
Attachment
Replication
Cell and tissue damage
Disruption, evasion, and inactivation of host defenses

replicate or survive. For example, simple skin contact with most intestinal protozoa does not result in disease; rather, the organisms must be ingested for the disease process to be initiated. Likewise, a minimum number of organisms is required to establish infection. Although some parasitic diseases may be acquired by the ingestion or inoculation of only a few organisms, a sizable inoculum is usually required. Whereas an individual may acquire malaria by a single bite of an infected female mosquito, large inocula are usually necessary to produce diseases such as amebiasis in humans.

ADHERENCE AND REPLICATION

Most infections are initiated by the attachment of the organism to host tissues, followed by replication to establish colonization. The life cycle of a parasite is based on species and tissue tropisms, which determine the organs or tissues of the host in which a parasite can survive. The attachment of the parasite to host cells or tissue can be relatively nonspecific, can be mediated by mechanical or biting mouthparts, or can result from the interaction between structures on the parasite surface known as **adhesins** and specific glycoprotein or glycolipid receptors found on some cell types but not on others. Specific surface structures that facilitate parasite adhesion include surface glycoproteins such as glycophorin A and B, complement receptors, adsorbed components of the complement cascade, fibronectin and *N*-acetylglucosamine conjugates. Examples of some of the adherence mechanisms identified in human parasites are listed in Table 72-2.

E. histolytica is a good model for the importance of adhesins in virulence. The pathogenesis of invasive amebiasis requires adherence of amoebae to the colonic mucous layer, parasite attachment to and lysis of colonic epithelium and acute inflammatory cells, and resistance of the amoebic trophozoites to host humoral and cell-mediated immune defense mechanisms. Amoebic adherence to colonic mucins, epithelial cells, and leukocytes is mediated by a surface lectin inhibitable by galactose (gal) or *N*-acetyl-D-galactosamine (GalNAc). Binding of the galactose-inhibitable adherence lectin to carbohydrates on the host cell surface is required for *E. histolytica* trophozoites to exert their cytolytic activity. The presence of the galactose-inhibitable adherence lectin is one feature that distinguishes pathogenic from nonpathogenic strains of *E. histolytica*.

Various attachment mechanisms have been associated with specific infections. For example, the Duffy blood group antigen acts as an attachment site for *Plasmodium vivax*. Red blood cells from most West Africans, in contrast to those from Europeans, lack the Duffy antigen. Accordingly, malaria resulting from *P. vivax* is almost unknown in West Africa. The physical structures of parasites may act with adhesion molecules to promote attachment to host cells. *Giardia lamblia* is a protozoan parasite that uses a ventral disk to attach to the intestinal epithelium by a clasping or suctionlike mechanism. Two recently identified adhesins, trypsin-activated *G. lamblia* lectin (taglin) and *G. lamblia* adherence molecule–1 (GLAM-1), may also be important in attachment to en-

TABLE 72-1	**Parasite Ports of Entry**
ROUTE	**EXAMPLES**
Ingestion	*Giardia* species, *E. histolytica*, *Cryptosporidium* species, cestodes, nematodes
Direct penetration	
Arthropod bite	Malaria, *Babesia* species, filaria, *Leishmania* species, trypanosomes
Transplacental penetration	*Toxoplasma gondii*
Organism-directed penetration	Hookworm, *Strongyloides* species, schistosomes

| TABLE 72-2 | **Examples of Parasitic Adherence Mechanisms** |

ORGANISM	DISEASE	TARGET	MECHANISM OF ATTACHMENT AND RECEPTOR
Plasmodium vivax	Malaria	Red blood cell	Merozoite (non–complement-mediated attachment), Duffy antigen
Plasmodium falciparum	Malaria	Red blood cell	Merozoite and glycophorin A and B
Babesia species	Babesiosis	Red blood cell	Complement-mediated C3b receptor
Giardia lamblia	Diarrhea	Duodenal and jejunal epithelium	Trypsin-activated *G. lamblia* lectin and mannose 6-phosphate *G. lamblia* adherence molecule–1 on disk
Entamoeba histolytica	Dysentery	Colonic epithelium	Lectin and *N*-acetylglucosamine conjugates
Trypanosoma cruzi	Chagas' disease	Fibroblast	Penetrin, fibronectin, and fibronectin receptor
Leishmania major	Leishmaniasis	Macrophage	Adsorbed C3bi and CR3
Leishmania mexicana	Leishmaniasis	Macrophage	Surface glycoprotein (gp63) and CR2
Necator americanus *Ancylostoma duodenale*	Hookworm	Intestinal epithelium	Mechanical and biting mouthparts

terocytes. It is believed that initial contact of the parasite with the intestinal surface is facilitated by taglin, which is distributed over the surface of the parasite, and that the disk-specific GLAM-1 is responsible for the avid attachment of the disk to the enterocyte surface.

After attachment to the specific cell or tissue type, the parasite may undergo replication as the next step in establishing infection. Most protozoan parasites replicate intracellularly or extracellularly in the human host, whereas replication is generally not observed with the helminths capable of establishing human infection.

Temperature may also play an important role in the ability of parasites to infect a host and cause disease. This is well illustrated by the *Leishmania* species. *Leishmania donovani* replicates well at 37° C and causes **visceral** leishmaniasis involving the bone marrow, liver, and spleen. In contrast, *L. tropica* grows well at 25° to 30° C but poorly at 37° C and causes an infection of the **skin** without involvement of deeper organs.

CELL AND TISSUE DAMAGE

Although some microorganisms may cause disease by localized multiplication and elaboration of potent microbial toxins, most organisms initiate the disease process by invading normally sterile tissue with subsequent replication and destruction. Parasitic protozoa and helminths are generally not known to produce toxins with potencies comparable to those of classic bacterial toxins such as anthrax toxin and botulinum toxin; however, parasitic disease can be established by the elaboration of toxic products, mechanical tissue damage, and immunopathologic reactions (Table 72-3).

Numerous authors have suggested that toxic products elaborated by parasitic protozoa are responsible for at least some aspects of pathology (Table 72-3). Proteases and phospholipases may be secreted and are released on the destruction of the parasites. These enzymes can cause host cell destruction, inflammatory responses, and gross tissue pathology. For example, the intestinal parasite *E. histolytica* produces proteinases that can degrade epithelial basement membrane and cell-anchoring proteins, disrupting epithelial cell layers. Furthermore, the amoebae produce phospholipases and an ionophore-like protein that lyse the responding host neutrophils, resulting in the release of neutrophil constituents that are toxic to host tissues. The expression of certain proteinases increases relative to the virulence of the strain of *E. histolytica*.

In contrast to the protozoan parasites, many of the pathogenic consequences of helminthic infections are related to the size, movement, and longevity of the parasites. The host is exposed to long-term damage and immune stimulation as well as the sheer physical consequences of being inhabited by large foreign bodies. The most obvious forms of **direct damage** from helminthic parasites are those resulting from **mechanical blockage**

TABLE 72-3	**Some Pathological Mechanisms in Parasitic Diseases**
MECHANISM	**EXAMPLES**
TOXIC PARASITE PRODUCTS	
Hydrolytic enzymes, proteinases, collagenase, elastase	Schistosomes (cercariae), *Strongyloides* species, hookworm, *E. histolytica*, African panosomes, *Plasmodium falciparum*
Amoebic ionophore	*E. histolytica*
Endotoxins	African trypanosomes, *Plasmodium falciparum*
Indole catabolites	Trypanosomes
MECHANICAL TISSUE DAMAGE	
Blockage of internal organs	*Ascaris* species, tapeworms, schistosomes, filaria
Pressure atrophy	*Echinococcus* species, *Cysticercus* species
Migration through tissue	Helminthic larvae
IMMUNOPATHOLOGY	
Hypersensitivity	See Table 72-4
Autoimmunity	See Table 72-4
Protein-losing enteropathies	Hookworm, tapeworm, *Giardia* species, *Strongyloides* species
Metaplastic changes	*Opisthorchis* species (liver flukes), schistosomes

of internal organs or from the effects of pressure exerted by growing parasites. Large adult *Ascaris* organisms can physically block the intestine and the bile ducts. Likewise, blockage of lymph flow, leading to elephantiasis, is associated with the presence of adult *Wuchereria* organisms in the lymphatic system. Some neurological manifestations of cysticercosis are due to the pressure exerted by the slowly expanding larval cysts of *Taenia solium* on the central nervous system (CNS) and eyes. Migration of helminths (usually larval forms) through body tissues such as the skin, lungs, liver, intestines, eyes, and CNS can damage the tissues directly and initiate hypersensitivity reactions.

As with many infectious agents, the manifestations of parasitic disease are due not only to the mechanical or chemical tissue damage produced by the parasite, but also to the host responses to the presence of the parasite. Cellular hypersensitivity is observed in protozoan and helminthic disease (Table 72-4). During a parasitic infection, host cell products such as cytokines and lymphokines are released from activated cells. These mediators influence the action of other cells and may contribute directly to the pathogenesis of parasite infections. Immunopathologic reactions range from acute anaphylactic reactions to cell-mediated delayed

TABLE 72-4   Immunopathological Reactions and Parasitic Diseases

REACTION	MECHANISM	RESULT	EXAMPLE
Type 1: anaphylactic	Antigen + IgE antibody attached to most cells: histamine release	Anaphylactic shock; bron–chospasm; local inflammation	Helminth infection, African trypanosomiasis
Type 2: cytotoxic	Antibody + antigen on cell surface: complement activation or antibody-dependent cellular cytotoxicity	Lysis of cell-bearing microbial antigens	*Trypanosoma cruzi* infection
Type 3: immune complex	Antibody + extracellular antigen complex	Inflammation and tissue damage; complex deposition in glomeruli, joints, skin vessels, brain; glomeru-lonephritis, and vasculitis	Malaria, schistosomiasis, trypanosomiasis
Type 4: cell-mediated (delayed)	Sensitized T cell reaction with antigen, liberation of lym-phokines, triggered cytotoxicity	Inflammation, mononuclear accumu-lation, macrophage activation; tissue damage	Leishmaniasis, schistoso-miasis, trypanosomiasis

Modified from Mims C et al: *Mims' pathogenesis of infectious disease,* ed 4, London, 1995, Academic.

TABLE 72-5   Microbial Interference with or Avoidance of Immune Defenses

TYPE OF INTERFERENCE OR AVOIDANCE	MECHANISM	EXAMPLE
Antigenic variation	Variation of surface antigens within the host	African trypanosomes, *Plasmodium* species, *Babesia* species, *Giardia* species
Molecular mimicry	Microbial antigens mimicking host antigens, leading to poor antibody response	*Plasmodium* species, trypanosomes, schistosomes
Concealment of anti-genic site (masking)	Acquisition of coating of host molecules	Hydatid cyst, filaria, schistosomes, trypanosomes
Intracellular location	Failure to display microbial antigen on host cell surface	*Plasmodium* species (RBC), trypanosomes, *Leishmania* species, *Toxoplasma* species
	Inhibition of phagolysosomal fusion	*Toxoplasma* species
	Escape from phagosome into cytoplasm with subsequent replication	*Leishmania* species, *Trypanosoma cruzi*
Immunosuppression	Suppression of parasite-specific B- and T-cell responses	Trypanosomes, *Plasmodium* species
	Degradation of immunoglobulins	Schistosomes

hypersensitivity reactions (Table 72-4). The fact that many parasites are long lived means that many inflammatory changes become irreversible, producing functional changes in tissues. Examples include hyperplasia of the bile ducts secondary to the presence of liver flukes and extensive fibrosis leading to genitourinary and hepatic dysfunction in chronic schistosomiasis. Migration of larval helminths through tissues such as the skin, lungs, liver, intestine, CNS, and eyes produces immune-mediated inflammatory changes in these structures. Finally, chronic inflammatory changes around parasites such as *Opisthorchis sinensis* and *Schistosoma haematobium* have been linked to the induction of carcinomatous changes in the bile ducts and the bladder, respectively.

DISRUPTION, EVASION, AND INACTIVATION OF HOST DEFENSES

Although the processes of cell and tissue destruction are often sufficient to **initiate** clinical disease, the parasite must be able to evade the host's immune defense system for the disease process to be maintained. Like other organisms, parasites elicit humoral and cell-mediated immune responses; however, parasites are particularly adept at interfering with or avoiding these defense mechanisms (Table 72-5).

Organisms can shift antigenic expression, such as that observed with the African trypanosomes. Rapid variation of expression of antigens in the glycocalyces of these organisms occurs each time that the host exhibits a new humoral response. Similar changes have been observed with *Plasmodium*, *Babesia*, and *Giardia* species. Some organisms may produce antigens that mimic host antigens (mimicry) or acquire host molecules that conceal the antigenic site (masking), thus preventing immune recognition by the host.

Many protozoan parasites evade the immune response by assuming an intracellular location in the host. The organisms that reside in macrophages have developed a variety of mechanisms to avoid intracellular killing. These include prevention of phagolysosome fusion, resistance to killing after exposure to lysosomal enzymes, and escape of phagocytosed cells from the phagosome into the cytoplasm with subsequent replication of the organism (Table 72-5).

Immunosuppression of the host is often observed during the course of parasitic infections. The immunosuppression may be parasite specific or generalized, involving a response to various nonparasite and parasite antigens. Proposed mechanisms include antigen overload, antigenic competition, induction of suppressor cells, and production of lymphocyte-specific suppressor factors. Certain helminths such as *Schistosoma mansoni* may also produce proteinases that can degrade immunoglobulins.

QUESTIONS

1. What are the most common modes of entry of parasites into the human host?
2. Name two factors that determine the outcome of the interaction between parasite and host.
3. Give an example of an adhesin that is directly related to the virulence of a parasite.
4. Name three pathological mechanisms thought to be important in parasitic diseases.
5. How can parasites resist immunological clearance? Give at least one example of each mechanism.
6. Name the four types of immunopathological reactions that occur in parasitic diseases and provide examples of each.

Bibliography

England PT, Sher A, editors: *The biology of parasitism: a molecular and immunological approach*, New York, 1988, Alan R Liss.

Mims C et al, editors: *Mims' pathogenesis of infectious disease*, ed 4, London, 1995, Academic.

Ravdin JL: Amebiasis, *Clin Infect Dis* 20:1453-1466, 1996.

Rose ME, McLaren JD, editors: *Pathophysiological responses to parasites*, London, 1986, British Society for Parasitology.

Turner M: *Antigenic variation in the parasitic protozoa*. In Birbeck TH, Penn CW, editors, *Antigenic variation in infectious diseases*, Oxford, 1986, IRL.

Antiparasitic Agents

The chemotherapeutic approach to the management of infectious diseases has clearly changed the face of medicine. Unfortunately, few of the antiinfective agents that have proved so successful against bacterial pathogens have been effective against parasites. In many instances, clinicians continue to rely on antiparasitic agents from the preantibiotic era. These and some newer agents remain limited in effectiveness and are relatively toxic. Many antiparasitic agents require prolonged or parenteral administration and may be effective only in certain disease states. Fortunately, in the last 5 to 10 years, several new agents have appeared that constitute significant advances in the treatment of parasitic diseases. In each case the previously available drugs were toxic and often ineffective.

In large part the difficulties in the treatment of parasitic diseases stem from the fact that parasites are eukaryotic organisms and thus are more similar to the human host than the more successfully treated prokaryotic bacterial pathogens. Furthermore, the chronic and prolonged course of infection and the complex life cycles and multiple developmental stages of many parasites add to the difficulties of effective chemotherapeutic intervention. Additional complicating factors in developing countries, where the majority of parasitic diseases occurs, include (1) the presence of multiple infections and the high probability of reinfection, (2) the large number of persons immunocompromised by malnutrition and human immunodeficiency virus infection, and (3) the overwhelming influence of poverty and poor sanitation, which facilitate the transmission of many parasitic infections. Although chemotherapeutic approaches may be used effectively to treat and prevent many parasitic infections, some agents have adverse effects or eventually meet with resistance (microbial and social). Most antiparasitic agents are too expensive for widespread use in developing countries. Thus the global approach to the prevention and treatment of parasitic diseases must involve several strategies, including improved hygiene and sanitation, control of the disease vector, use of vaccinations if available (largely unavailable for parasitic diseases), and prophylactic and therapeutic administration of safe and effective chemotherapy. These strategies now must also include efforts to decrease the transmission of infection by the human immunodeficiency virus.

TARGETS FOR ANTIPARASITE DRUG ACTION

As mentioned previously, parasites are eukaryotic organisms and thus have more similarities than differences with the human host. Consequently, many antiparasitic agents act on pathways (nucleic acid synthesis, carbohydrate metabolism) or targets (neuromuscular function) shared by both the parasite and the host. For this reason, developing safe and effective antiparasitic drugs based on biochemical differences between the parasite and host has been difficult. Differential toxicity is commonly achieved by preferential uptake, metabolic alteration of the drug by the parasite, or differences in the susceptibility of functionally equivalent sites in the parasite and host. Fortunately, as our understanding of the basic biology and biochemistry of parasites and the mechanism of action of antimicrobial agents has improved, so has our recognition of potential parasite-specific targets for chemotherapeutic attack. Examples of the chemotherapeutic strategies that exploit the differences between parasite and host are provided in Table 73-1. These are discussed in greater detail as we deal with the specific agents.

DRUG RESISTANCE

Resistance to antimicrobial agents is an important consideration in the treatment of infections resulting from bacteria and fungal pathogens and certainly plays a role in the chemotherapy of parasitic diseases. Unfortunately, our understanding of the molecular and genetic basis for resistance to most antiparasitic agents is quite limited. Most of the information regarding the molecular mechanisms of drug resistance in parasites has come from studies in plasmodia. Resistance to chloroquine, a major antimalarial agent, is most likely due to the presence of an active chloroquine efflux mechanism similar to that producing the rapid efflux of anticancer drugs observed in multidrug-resistant mammalian cancer cells. In addition, the development of plasmodial resistance to antifo-

TABLE 73-1 Chemotherapeutic Strategies That Exploit Differences Between Parasite and Host

UNIQUE SITE OF ATTACK	DRUG	ORGANISM
Drug-concentrating mechanism unique to parasite	Chloroquine	*Plasmodium* species
Folic acid pathway (parasite unable to use exogenous folate)	Pyrimethamine or trimethoprim sulfa	*Plasmodium* or *Toxoplasma* species
Inhibitor of trypanothion-dependent mechanism for reducing oxidized thiol groups	Arsenicals, difluoromethylornithine	Trypanosomes
Interference with neuro-mediators unique to parasites piperazine	Pyrantel pamoate,	*Ascaris* species
Inhibitors of GABA-mediated conduction in peripheral nervous system of parasites	Ivermectin	Filaria
Interaction with tubulin unique to parasites	Benzimidazoles	Many helminths
Inhibition of topoisomerase II fluoroquinolones	Pentamidine,	Trypanosomes

GABA, Gamma-aminobutyric acid.

late compounds such as pyrimethamine is due to a series of mutations in the parasite's combined dihydrofolate reductase–thymidylate synthetase enzyme. Further insights into the mechanisms of action and resistance to antiparasitic agents are necessary to optimize the effectiveness of antiparasite chemotherapy.

ANTIPARASITIC AGENTS

Although the number of effective antiparasitic agents is small relative to the vast array of antibacterial agents, the list is expanding (Table 73-2). Certainly in many cases the goal of antiparasitic therapy is similar to that of antibacterial therapy: to eradicate the organism rapidly and completely. In many cases, however, the agents and treatment regimens used for parasitic diseases are designed simply to decrease the parasite burden, to prevent the systemic complications of chronic infection, or both actions. Thus the goals of antiparasitic therapy, particularly as applied in endemic areas, may be quite different from those usually considered for therapy of microbial infection in the United States or other developed countries. Given the significant toxicity of many of these agents, in every case the need for treatment must be weighed against the toxicity of the drug. A decision to withhold therapy may often be correct, particularly when the drug can cause severe adverse effects.

Immunocompromised individuals pose a particular problem with respect to antiparasitic chemotherapy. On the one hand, prophylaxis, such as that administered for toxoplasmosis, may be effective in preventing infection. However, once infection is established, radical cure may not be possible, and long-term suppressive therapy may be indicated. In some diseases, such as cryptosporidiosis and microsporidiosis, effective (curative) therapy is not available, and care must be taken to avoid unnecessary toxicity while providing supportive care for the patient.

The remainder of this chapter provides an overview of the major classes of antiprotozoal and antihelminthic agents. These and additional antiparasitic agents, their mechanisms of action, and their clinical indications are listed in Table 73-2. Treatment of specific infections is discussed in the chapters that deal with the parasites. The Bibliography lists several excellent reviews for more complete information and for discussions of the antiparasitic agents that are available.

Antiprotozoal Agents

Similar to antibacterial and antifungal agents, the antiprotozoal agents are generally targeted at relatively rapidly proliferating, young, growing cells. Most commonly these agents target nucleic acid synthesis, protein synthesis, or specific metabolic pathways (e.g., folate metabolism) unique to the protozoan parasites.

Heavy Metals

The heavy metals used for the treatment of parasitic infections include arsenical (melarsoprol) and antimonial compounds (sodium stibogluconate, meglumine antimonate). These agents are thought to oxidize sulfhydryl groups of enzymes, which are essential catalysts in carbohydrate metabolism. Melarsoprol inhibits parasite pyruvate kinase, causing decreased concentrations of adenosine triphosphate (ATP), pyruvate, and phosphoenolpyruvate. Arsenicals also inhibit *sn*-glycerol 3-phosphate oxidase, which is needed for the regeneration of nicotinamide adenine dinucleotide in trypanosomes but is not found in mammalian cells. The antimonials, sodium stibogluconate and meglumine antimonate, inhibit the glycolytic enzyme phosphofructokinase and certain Krebs cycle enzymes in *Leishmania* organisms. In each instance the inhibition of parasite metabolism is parasiticidal. Unfortunately, the heavy metal compounds are toxic to the host, as well as the parasite. The toxicity is greatest on cells that are most metabolically active, such as neuronal, renal tubular, intestinal, and bone marrow stem cells. Their differential toxicity and therapeutic value are largely related to enhanced uptake by the parasite and its intense metabolic activity.

Melarsoprol is the drug of choice for trypanosomiasis involving the central nervous system. It can penetrate the blood-brain barrier and is effective in all stages of trypanosomiasis. The antimonial compounds are restricted to the management of leishmaniasis. Meglumine antimonate and sodium stibogluconate are the drugs of

TABLE 73-2   Mechanisms of Action and Clinical Indications for the Major Antiparasitic Agents

DRUG CLASS	MECHANISM OF ACTION	EXAMPLES	CLINICAL INDICATION
ANTIPROTOZOAL AGENTS			
Heavy metals: arsenicals and antimonials	Inactivate sulfhydril groups	Melarsoprol Sodium stibogluconate Meglumine antimonate	Trypanosomiasis Leishmaniasis
Aminoquinoline analogues	Accumulate in parasitized cells; interfere with DNA replication; bind to ferriprotoporphyrin IX; raise intravesicular pH; interfere with hemoglobin digestion	Chloroquine Mefloquine Quinine Primaquine	Malaria prophylaxis and therapy Radical cure (exoerythrocytic-primaquine only)
Folic acid antagonists	Inhibit dihydropteroate synthetase and dihydrofolate reductase	Sulfonamides Pyrimethamine Trimethoprim	Toxoplasmosis Malaria Cyclosporiasis
Inhibitors of protein synthesis	Block peptide synthesis at level of ribosome	Clindamycin Spiramycin Paromomycin Tetracycline Doxycycline	Malaria Babesiosis Amebiasis Cryptosporidiosis
Diamidines	Bind DNA Interfere with uptake and function of polyamines	Pentamidine	Pneumocystosis Leishmaniasis Trypanosomiasis
Nitroimidazoles	Unclear; interact with DNA Inhibit metabolism of glucose and interfere with mitochondrial function	Metronidazole Benzimidazole Tinidazole	Amebiasis Giardiasis Trichomoniasis
Quinolones	Inhibit DNA gyrase	Ciprofloxacin	Malaria
Sesquiterpenes	React with heme, causing free-radical damage to parasite membranes	Artemisinin	Malaria
Ornithine analogue	Inhibits ornithine decarboxylase Interferes with polyamine metabolism	Difluoromethylornithine	African trypanosomiasis
Inhibitors of nucleic acid synthesis	Inhibit enzymes in purine salvage pathway	Allopurinol	Leishmaniasis
Acetanilide	Unknown	Diloxanide furoate	Intestinal amebiasis
Sulfated naphthylamine	Inhibits sn-glycerol phosphate oxidase and glycerol 3-phosphate dehydrogenase, causing decreased ATP synthesis	Suramin	African trypanosomiasis
Phenanthrenemethanols	Bind to ferriprotoporphyrin IX; affect mitochondria	Halofantrine	Malaria
ANTIHELMINTHIC AGENTS			
Benzimidazoles	Inhibit fumarate reductase Inhibit glucose transport Disrupt microtubular function	Mebendazole Thiabendazole Albendazole	Broad-spectrum antihelminthics Nematodes Cestodes
Tetrahydropyrimidine	Blocks neuromuscular action Inhibits fumarate reductase	Pyrantel pamoate	Ascariasis Pinworm Hookworm
Piperazines	Are GABA agonists Cause neuromuscular paralysis Stimulate phagocytic cells	Piperazine Diethylcarbamazine	Ascaris and pinworm infections Filarial infections
Avermectins	Block neuromuscular action Are GABA antagonists Inhibit filarial reproduction	Ivermectin	Filarial infections
Pyrazinoisoquinoline	Is calcium agonist; causes tetanic muscular contractions; cause tegumental disruption; provides synergy with host defenses	Praziquantel	Broad-spectrum antihelminthics Cestodes Trematodes
Phenol	Uncouples oxidative phosphorylation	Niclosamide	Intestinal tapeworm

ATP, Adenosine triphosphate; *GABA,* gamma-aminobutyric acid.

Continued

TABLE 73-2	Mechanisms of Action and Clinical Indications for the Major Antiparasitic Agents—cont'd		
DRUG CLASS	**MECHANISM OF ACTION**	**EXAMPLES**	**CLINICAL INDICATION**
ANTIHELMINTHIC AGENTS—cont'd			
Quinolone	Alkylates DNA; inhibits DNA, RNA, and protein synthesis	Bithionol	Paragonimiasis
Organophosphate	Is anticholinesterase; blocks neuromuscular action	Oxamniquine	Schistosomiasis
		Metrifonate	Schistosomiasis
Sulfated naphthylamidine	Inhibits glycerophosphate oxidase and dehydrogenase	Suramin	Onchocerciasis

choice for leishmaniasis and are active against all forms of the disease. Prolonged therapy is usually required for disseminated leishmaniasis, and relapses are common.

Aminoquinoline Analogues

The aminoquinoline analogues include the 4-aminoquinolines (chloroquine), the 8-aminoquinolines (primaquine), and the 4-quinolinemethanols (mefloquine). Additional quinoline analogues include quinine, quinidine, quinacrine, and amodiaquine. These compounds all have antimalarial activity and accumulate preferentially in parasitized red blood cells. Several potential mechanisms of action have been proposed, including (1) binding to DNA and interfering with DNA replication; (2) binding to ferriprotoporphyrin IX released from hemoglobin in infected erythrocytes, producing a toxic complex; and (3) raising the pH of the parasite's intracellular acid vesicles, thus interfering with its ability to degrade hemoglobin. Quinine, the 4-aminoquinolines, and 4-quinolinemethanols rapidly destroy the erythrocytic stage of malaria and thus may be used prophylactically to suppress clinical illness or therapeutically to terminate an acute attack. The 8-aminoquinolines (e.g., primaquine) accumulate in tissue cells and destroy the extraerythrocytic (hepatic) stages of malaria, resulting in a radical cure of the infection.

Chloroquine remains the drug of choice for the prophylaxis and treatment of susceptible malaria strains. Chloroquine is active against all four *Plasmodium* species (*P. falciparum, P. vivax, P. ovale, P. malariae*) and is well tolerated, inexpensive, and effective orally. Unfortunately, resistance of *P. falciparum* to chloroquine is widespread in Asia, Africa, and South America, greatly limiting the use of this agent. Recently, resistance of *P. vivax* to chloroquine has been reported from Papua New Guinea, the Solomon Islands, Indonesia, and Brazil.

Quinine is used primarily to treat chloroquine-resistant *P. falciparum* infection. Presumably, it is active against the rare chloroquine-resistant strains of *P. vivax* as well. Quinine is used orally only to treat mild attacks and by the intravenous route to treat acute attacks of multidrug-resistant *P. falciparum*. Quinine is quite toxic and not rapidly parasiticidal; thus it is never used alone

but is often used with a sulfonamide or tetracycline antibiotic with antimalarial activity.

Mefloquine is a new 4-quinolinemethanol antimalarial agent used for the prophylaxis and treatment of falciparum malaria. It displays a high level of activity against most chloroquine-resistant parasites. Unfortunately, mefloquine-resistant strains of falciparum malaria have already been reported from Southeast Asia.

Folic Acid Antagonists

Similar to other organisms, protozoan parasites require folic acid for the synthesis of nucleic acids and ultimately DNA. Protozoa are unable to absorb exogenous folate and thus are susceptible to drugs that inhibit folate synthesis. The folic acid antagonists that are useful in treating protozoan infections include the diaminopyrimidines (pyrimethamine and trimethoprim) and the sulfonamides. These compounds block separate steps in the folic acid pathway. The sulfonamides inhibit the conversion of aminobenzoic acid to dihydropteroic acid. The diaminopyrimidines inhibit dihydrofolate reductase, which effectively blocks the synthesis of tetrahydrofolate, a precursor necessary for the formation of purines, pyrimidines, and certain amino acids. These agents are effective at concentrations far below those needed to inhibit the mammalian enzyme, so selectivity can be attained. When a diaminopyrimidine is used with a sulfonamide, a synergistic effect is achieved via the blockade of two steps in the same metabolic pathway, resulting in very effective inhibition of protozoan growth.

The diaminopyrimidine trimethoprim is used with sulfamethoxazole to treat toxoplasmosis. Another diaminopyrimidine, pyrimethamine, has a high affinity for sporozoan dihydrofolate reductase and has been very effective when combined with a sulfonamide in the treatment of malaria and toxoplasmosis. Resistance to antifolates is due to specific point mutations at the active site of the parasite's dihydrofolate reductase and has been largely confined to species of plasmodia.

Inhibitors of Protein Synthesis

Several antibiotics that inhibit protein synthesis in bacteria also exhibit antiparasitic activity in vitro and in vivo.

These agents include clindamycin, spiramycin, tetracycline, and doxycycline.

Clindamycin and the tetracyclines are active against *Plasmodia* species, *Babesia* species, and amoebae. Doxycycline is used for the chemoprophylaxis of chloroquine-resistant *P. falciparum* malaria, and tetracycline may be used with quinine for the treatment of chloroquine-resistant *P. falciparum* infection. Clindamycin may be useful in the treatment of central nervous system toxoplasmosis. Spiramycin is recommended as an alternative to the antifolates in the treatment of toxoplasmosis. Although spiramycin appears active against *Cryptosporidium* species in vitro, it has not been shown to be effective clinically for human cryptosporidiosis. Recent studies suggest that paromomycin, an older aminoglycoside, may be at least partially effective in treating cryptosporidiosis. Paromomycin, which is not systemically absorbed, is also used as a secondary drug in amebiasis and in giardiasis.

Diamidines

Pentamidine, a diamidine, is a relatively toxic agent. Pentamidine is a polycation and may interact with DNA, or it may interfere with the uptake and function of polyamines.

Pentamidine is effective in treating the tissue forms of leishmania and the early (pre–central nervous system) forms of African trypanosomiasis. Pentamidine does not penetrate the central nervous system and therefore is not useful in the late stages of infection with *Trypanosoma brucei gambiense*. Recent information suggests that pentamidine may inhibit kinetoplast topoisomerase II activity and may act against trypanosomes in part by this mechanism.

Nitroimidazoles

The nitroimidazoles include the well-known antibacterial agent metronidazole as well as benzimidazole and tinidazole. The mechanism of action of these compounds is unclear. It has been suggested that they inhibit DNA and RNA synthesis and also inhibit the metabolism of glucose and interfere with mitochondrial function. Metronidazole binds to parasite guanine and cytosine residues, causing the loss of helical structure and breakage of DNA strands.

The nitroimidazoles have excellent penetration into body tissues and therefore are particularly effective for the treatment of disseminated amebiasis. Metronidazole is the drug of choice for trichomoniasis and is effective in the treatment of giardiasis. Tinidazole appears to be more effective and less mutagenic than metronidazole; however, it is not yet available for use in the United States.

Other Antiprotozoal Agents

A number of additional agents used in therapy, their mechanism of action (if known), and clinical use are listed in Table 73-2.

Antihelminthic Agents

The strategy for the use of antihelminthic drugs is quite different from that for the use of drugs for treating most protozoal infections. Most antihelminthic drugs are targeted at nonproliferating adult organisms, whereas with protozoa the targets are generally younger, more rapidly proliferating cells. The helminthic life cycle is frequently quite complex, and the adaptation to survival in the human host depends strongly on (1) neuromuscular coordination for feeding movements and for maintenance of a favorable location of the worm within the host; (2) carbohydrate metabolism as the major source of energy, with glucose the primary substrate; and (3) microtubular integrity, since egg laying and hatching, larval development, glucose transport, and enzyme activity and secretion are impaired when microtubules are modified. Most antihelminthic agents are targeted at one of these biochemical functions in the adult organism.

The mechanisms of action and clinical indications for common antihelminthic agents are listed in Table 73-2.

Benzimidazoles

The benzimidazoles are broad-spectrum antihelminthic agents and include mebendazole, thiabendazole, and albendazole (not available in the United States). The basic structure of these agents consists of linked imidazole and benzene rings. Three mechanisms of action have been proposed for the benzimidazoles: (1) inhibition of fumarate reductase; (2) inhibition of glucose transport, resulting in glycogen depletion, cessation of ATP formation, and paralysis or death; and (3) disruption of microtubular function. Benzimidazoles block the assembly of tubulin dimers into tubulin polymers in a process mimicked by colchicine, a powerful antimitotic and embryotoxic drug. Because tubulin is important for parasite motility, drugs such as the benzimidazoles, which bind to parasite tubulin, are thought to act against nematode parasites by reducing or eliminating their motility.

The benzimidazoles have a wide spectrum of activity, including intestinal nematodes (*Ascaris, Trichuris, Necator,* and *Ancylostoma* species; *Enterobius vermicularis*), as well as a number of cestodes (*Taenia, Hymenolepis,* and *Echinococcus* species). Thiabendazole acts against larval and adult nematodes and is useful in the management of cutaneous larval migrans, trichinosis, and most intestinal nematode infections. Mebendazole is active against the intestinal nematodes and the cestodes previously listed. Albendazole has a spectrum similar to that of mebendazole and may have greater activity against *Echinococcus* species. In addition to its broad-spectrum antihelminthic activity, albendazole also has activity against *Giardia* species and appears promising in the treatment of intestinal microsporidiosis in patients with acquired immunodeficiency syndrome.

Tetrahydropyrimidines

Pyrantel pamoate, a tetrahydropyrimidine, is a cholinergic agonist that has a powerful effect on nematode muscle cells by binding to cholinergic receptors, which results in cell depolarization and muscle contraction. This paralytic action on intestinal nematodes leads to expulsion of the worm from the host intestinal tract.

Pyrantel pamoate is not readily absorbed from the intestine and is active against *Ascaris* species, pinworm, and hookworm. An analogue of pyrantel, oxantel, may be used with pyrantel to provide effective therapy for the three major soil-transmitted nematodes: *Ascaris* species, hookworm, and *Trichuris* species.

Piperazines

The piperazine antihelmintics include piperazine and diethylcarbamazine. Piperazine is thought to act by hyperpolarization of the muscle membrane, producing a flaccid paralysis. The current hypothesis is that piperazine acts against nematodes as a low-potency gamma-aminobutyric acid (GABA) agonist. Diethylcarbamazine may act by stimulating cholinergic receptors and depolarizing muscle cells, with subsequent paralysis of the worms. However, additional evidence suggests that it enhances the adherence of leukocytes to microfilariae and thus may act by altering the parasite surface membrane or by directly stimulating phagocytic cells.

The piperazines are active against *Ascaris* species and pinworm (*E. vermicularis*). In addition, diethylcarbamazine is active against the filariae that produce river blindness (*Onchocerca volvulus*) and lymphatic filariasis (*Wuchereria bancrofti* and *Brugia malayi*). Unfortunately, destruction of the microfilariae in the tissues may increase the pathology because of the host inflammatory response to the parasite antigens released on exposure to diethylcarbamazine. Recent information suggests that single-dose treatment with diethylcarbamazine may produce antiparasitic effects similar to those obtained with 14- to 21-day courses without the severe side effects observed with the multidose regimens.

Avermectins

Ivermectin, an avermectin, acts by interacting with the chloride channel on the helminth GABA receptor complex, thus inhibiting GABA-ergic synapses in the peripheral nervous system of nematode parasites. As a result, the parasites become paralyzed and may be eliminated by the host. The drug also inhibits the reproductive function of the adult female *O. volvulus* and alters the ability of the *O. volvulus* microfilariae to evade the host immune system.

Although ivermectin is used extensively to control gut-dwelling nematode infections in domestic and farm animals, its use in humans is limited primarily to treating ocular and lymphatic filariasis. Ivermectin is effective in the treatment of strongyloidiasis as well as several common intestinal parasitic nematodes including *Ascaris*, *Trichuris*, and *Enterobius* species. When used to treat filariasis, ivermectin has fewer side effects than diethylcarbamazine, and a single dose can eliminate microfilariae

for up to 6 months. Ivermectin has a dramatic effect on the tissue-dwelling microfilariae of *O. volvulus* and reduces the severity of the ocular pathology seen in onchocerciasis. Because of its ability to markedly reduce the number of microfilariae in the skin of people with onchocerciasis, ivermectin has been effective in reducing the transmission of onchocerciasis in endemic areas.

Pyrazinoisoquinolines

Praziquantel, a pyrazinoisoquinoline, is an antihelminthic active used against a broad spectrum of trematodes and cestodes. The drug is rapidly taken up by susceptible helminths in which it acts as a calcium agonist. The entry of calcium into various cells results in elevated intracellular calcium levels, tetanic muscular contraction, and destruction of the tegument. Praziquantel appears to act with the host immune system to produce a synergistic antihelminthic effect. The drug causes disruption of the parasite surface and tegument, allowing antibodies to attack parasite antigens not normally exposed on the surface (Figure 73-1). Irreversible damage to the parasite

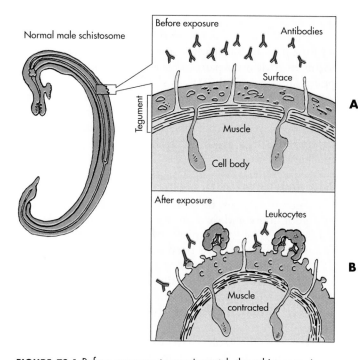

FIGURE 73-1 Before exposure to praziquantel, the schistosome is capable of avoiding the numerous antibodies directed toward surface and internally located antigens. **A,** Cross section of the dorsal surface of a normal male schistosome. Within 1 to 2 seconds after exposure to praziquantel, the muscles of the schistosome contract because of a drug-induced influx of calcium ions into the schistosome tegument. **B,** The change in permeability of the schistosome surface toward external ions initiates the appearance of small holes and balloonlike structures, making the parasite vulnerable to antibody-mediated adherence of host leukocytes that kill the helminth. (From Wingard LB Jr et al: *Human pharmacology: molecular to clinical*, St Louis, 1991, Mosby.)

probably occurs when complement or host leukocytes are recruited to the sites where antibody is bound.

Praziquantel has extremely broad-spectrum activity against trematodes including *Fasciolopsis, Fasciola, Clonorchis, Opisthorchis, Paragonimus,* and *Schistosoma* species. It is also active against cestodes including *Echinococcus, Taenia,* and *Dipylidium* species. Praziquantel is the drug of choice for the treatment of schistosomiasis, clonorchiasis, opisthorchiasis, and neurocysticercosis. There is now reliable evidence that praziquantel reduces hepatosplenomegaly and portal hypertension in schistosomiasis. Effective activity has also been demonstrated against other common trematode and cestode infections.

Phenols

Niclosamide, a phenol, is a nonabsorbable antihelminthic with selective activity against intestinal tapeworms. The drug is absorbed by gut-dwelling cestodes but not by nematodes. It acts by uncoupling oxidative phosphorylation in mitochondria, resulting in a loss of helminth ATP that ultimately immobilizes the parasite so that it is expelled with the feces. Niclosamide is effective in the treatment of intestinal tapeworms in humans and animals.

Other Antihelminthic Agents

Additional antihelminthic agents, including oxamniquine, metrifonate, and suramin, are described in Table 73-2. These agents are generally considered secondary agents for the treatment of trematode (oxamniquine and metrifonate) and filarial (suramin) infections.

QUESTIONS

1. What are the obstacles to effective treatment and prophylaxis of parasitic diseases in developing countries?
2. What are the goals of antiparasitic therapy and how are they different from antibacterial therapy?
3. What is the importance of aminoquinoline analogues?
4. How does the strategy for the use of antihelminthic agents differ from that for the use of drugs for protozoal infections?

Bibliography

Cook GC: Antihelminthic agents: some recent developments and their clinical application, *Postgrad Med J* 67:16-22, 1991.

Drugs for parasitic infections, *Med Lett Drugs Ther* 32:23-32, 1990.

Khaw M, Panosian CB: Human antiprotozoal therapy: past, present, and future, *Clin Microbiol Rev* 8:427-439, 1995.

Krogstad DJ: *Antiparasitic drugs: mechanisms of action and resistance, pharmacokinetics, pharmacodynamics, and in vitro and in vivo assays of drug activity.* In Lorian V, editor: *Antibiotics in laboratory medicine,* ed 3, Baltimore, 1991, Williams & Wilkins.

Liu LX, Weller PF: Antiparasitic drugs, *New Engl J Med* 334:1178-1184, 1996.

Rosenblatt JE: Antiparasitic agents, *Mayo Clin Proc* 67:276-287, 1992.

Schwartz IK: Prevention of malaria, *Infect Dis Clin North Am* 6:313-331, 1992.

Wingard LB Jr et al, editors: *Human pharmacology: molecular to clinical,* St Louis, 1991, Mosby.

CHAPTER 74

Laboratory Diagnosis of Parasitic Diseases

The diagnosis of parasitic infections may be very difficult, particularly in the nonendemic setting. The clinical manifestations of parasitic diseases are seldom specific enough to raise the possibility of these processes in the mind of the clinician, and routine laboratory tests are seldom helpful. Although peripheral eosinophilia is widely recognized as a useful indicator of parasitic disease, this phenomenon is characteristic only of helminthic infection and even in these cases is frequently absent. Thus the physician must maintain a heightened index of suspicion and must rely on detailed travel, food intake, transfusion, and socioeconomic history to raise the possibility of parasitic disease. Proper diagnosis requires that (1) the physician consider the possibility of parasitic infection, (2) appropriate specimens be obtained and transported to the laboratory in a timely fashion, (3) the laboratory competently perform the appropriate procedures for the recovery and identification of the etiological agent, (4) the laboratory results be effectively communicated to the physician, and (5) the results be correctly interpreted by the physician and applied to the care of the patient. In addition, for most parasitic diseases, appropriate test selection and interpretation is based on an understanding of the life cycle of the parasite as well as the pathogenesis of the disease process in humans.

Numerous methods for diagnosing parasitic diseases have been described (Box 74-1). Some are useful in detecting a wide variety of parasites, and others are particularly useful for one or a few parasites. Although the mainstay of diagnostic clinical microbiology is the isolation of the causative pathogen in culture, the diagnosis of parasitic diseases is accomplished almost entirely by morphological (usually microscopic) demonstration of parasites in clinical material. Occasionally, demonstration of a specific antibody response (serodiagnosis) helps in establishing the diagnosis. The detection of parasite antigens in serum, urine, or stool may provide a rapid and sensitive means of diagnosing infection with certain organisms. Likewise, the recent development of nucleic acid probe–based assays may prove to be an excellent means of detecting and identifying a number of parasites in biological samples such as blood, stool, urine, sputum,

and tissue biopsies obtained from infected patients. In general, it is better for the laboratory to offer a limited number of competently performed procedures than to offer a wide variety of infrequently and poorly performed tests.

This chapter provides a general description of the principles of specimen collection and processing necessary to diagnose most parasitic infections. Specific details of these and other procedures of general and limited usefulness may be found in several reference texts listed in the Bibliography.

PARASITE LIFE CYCLE AS AN AID IN DIAGNOSIS

Parasites may have complex life cycles involving single or multiple hosts. Understanding the life cycle of parasitic organisms is a key to understanding important features of geographical distribution, transmission, and pathogenesis of many parasitic diseases. The life cycles of parasites often suggest useful clues for diagnosis as well. For example, in the life cycle of filariae that infect humans, certain species such as *Wuchereria bancrofti* have a "nocturnal periodicity" in which greater numbers of microfilariae are found in the peripheral blood at night. Sampling the blood of such patients during daytime hours may fail to detect the microfilariae, whereas blood specimens collected between 10 PM and 4 AM may demonstrate many microfilariae. Likewise, intestinal nematodes such as *Ascaris lumbricoides* and hookworm, which reside in the lumen of the intestine, produce large numbers of eggs that can be detected easily in the stool of an infected patient. In contrast, another intestinal nematode, *Strongyloides stercoralis,* lays its eggs in the bowel wall rather than in the intestinal lumen. As a result, the eggs are rarely seen on stool examination; to make the diagnosis, the parasitologist must be alert for the presence of larvae. Finally, parasites may cause clinical symptoms at a time when diagnostic forms are not yet present in the usual site. For example, in certain intestinal nematode infections the migration of larvae through the tissues may cause intense symptomatology weeks before the characteristic eggs are present in the feces.

GENERAL DIAGNOSTIC CONSIDERATIONS

The importance of appropriate specimen collection, the number and timing of specimens, timely transport to the laboratory, and prompt examination by an experienced microscopist cannot be overemphasized. Because the majority of parasitological examinations and identifications are based entirely on recognizing the characteristic morphology of the organisms, any condition that may obscure or distort the morphological appearance of the parasite may result in an erroneous identification or missed diagnosis. As noted previously and in Box 74-1, there may be alternatives to microscopy for the detection and identification of certain parasites. These tests (e.g., antigen detection, nucleic acid probes), although presently uncommon, may become more widely applied in the future. They offer the promise of more rapid, sensitive, and specific diagnostic testing for parasitic diseases. These diagnostic test options may expand the testing capabilities of many laboratories, allowing laboratories with limited proficiency in parasitology to offer diagnostic testing for certain parasitic diseases. A list of common and uncommon diagnostic procedures and specimens to be collected for selected parasitic infections is provided in Table 74-1.

Intestinal and Urogenital Parasitic Infections

Protozoa and helminths may colonize or infect the intestinal and urogenital tract of humans. Most commonly these parasites are amoebae, flagellates, or nematodes (Table 74-2). However, infection with trematodes, cestodes, ciliate, coccidian, or microsporidian parasites may also be encountered.

In intestinal and urogenital infections, a simple wet mount or stained smear is often inadequate. Repeated specimen collection and testing are often necessary to optimize the detection of organisms that are shed inter-

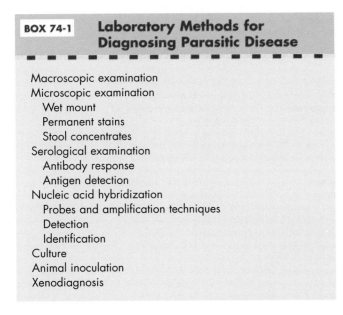

BOX 74-1   Laboratory Methods for Diagnosing Parasitic Disease

Macroscopic examination
Microscopic examination
   Wet mount
   Permanent stains
   Stool concentrates
Serological examination
   Antibody response
   Antigen detection
Nucleic acid hybridization
   Probes and amplification techniques
   Detection
   Identification
Culture
Animal inoculation
Xenodiagnosis

mittently or in fluctuating numbers. Concentration of specimens by sedimentation or flotation techniques may be required to detect low numbers of ova (worms) or cysts (protozoa) in fecal specimens.

Occasionally, specimens other than stool or urine must be examined (Table 74-1). Optimal detection of small bowel pathogens such as *Giardia lamblia* and *S. stercoralis* may require the aspiration of duodenal contents or even small bowel biopsy. Likewise, the detection of colonic parasites such as *Entamoeba histolytica* and *Schistosoma mansoni* may necessitate proctoscopic or sigmoidoscopic examination with aspiration or biopsy of mucosal lesions. Sampling of the perianal skin is a useful means of recovering the eggs of *Enterobius vermicularis* (pinworm) or *Taenia* species (tapeworm).

Fecal Specimen Collection

Patients, clinicians, and laboratory personnel must be properly instructed on collection and handling of specimens. Fecal specimens should be collected in clean, wide-mouthed, waterproof containers with a tight-fitting lid to ensure and maintain adequate moisture. Specimens must not be contaminated with water, soil, or urine because water and soil may contain free-living organisms that can be mistaken for human parasites and urine can destroy motile trophozoites and may cause helminth eggs to hatch. Stool specimens should not contain barium, bismuth, or medications containing mineral oil, antibiotics, antimalarials, or other chemical substances because such specimens compromise the detection of intestinal parasites. Specimen collection should be delayed for 5 to 10 days to allow barium to clear and for at least 2 weeks to allow intestinal parasites to recover from the toxic (but not curative) effects of antibiotics such as tetracycline.

Purged specimens may be collected when organisms are not detected in normally passed fecal specimens; however, only certain purgatives (sodium sulfate and buffered sodium biphosphate [Phospho-Soda]) are satisfactory. One series of purged specimens may be examined in place of, or in addition to, a series of normally passed specimens.

Unpreserved formed fecal specimens should arrive in the laboratory within 2 hours after passage. If the stool is liquid and thus more likely to contain trophozoites, it should reach the laboratory for examination within 30 minutes. Soft or loose stools should be examined within 1 hour of passage. All fresh fecal samples should be placed into preservatives such as 10% formalin, polyvinyl alcohol (PVA), merthiolate-iodine-formalin (MIF), or sodium acetate–formalin (SAF) if examination is not possible within the recommended time limits. Fecal specimens may be stored at 4° C but should not be incubated or frozen.

The number of specimens required to demonstrate intestinal parasites varies depending on the quality of the specimen submitted, the accuracy of the examination performed, the severity of the infection, and the purpose

| TABLE 74-1 | **Body Sites, Specimen Collection, and Diagnostic Procedures for Selected Parasitic Infections** |

INFECTING ORGANISM	SPECIMEN OPTIONS	COLLECTION METHODS	DIAGNOSTIC PROCEDURE
BLOOD			

Plasmodium species, *Babesia* species, filiaria	Whole blood, anticoagulated	Venipuncture	Microscopic examination (Giemsa stain)
			  Thin film
			  Thick film
			Blood concentration (filaria)
			Serology
			  Antibody
			  Antigen

BONE MARROW			
Leishmania species	Aspirate Serum	Sterile Venipuncture	Microscopic examination (Giemsa stain) Culture Serology (antibody)
CENTRAL NERVOUS SYSTEM			

Acanthamoeba species, *Naegleria* species, trypanosomes
Angiostrongylus cantonensis
	Spinal fluid
	Serum
		Sterile
		Venipuncture
			Microscopic examination
			  Wet mount
			  Permanent stain
			Culture
			Serology (antibody)

CUTANEOUS ULCERS			
Leishmania species	Aspirate Biopsy Serum	Sterile plus smears Sterile, nonsterile to histology Venipuncture	Microscopic examination (Giemsa stain) Culture Serology (antibody)
EYE			

Acanthamoeba species	Corneal scrapings	Sterile saline, air-dried smear	Microscopic examination
			  Wet mount
			  Permanent stain

INTESTINAL TRACT			

Entamoeba histolytica	Corneal biopsy
	Fresh stool
	Preserved stool
	Sigmoidoscopy material
	Serum
		Sterile saline
		Waxed container
		Formalin, PVA
		Fresh PVA
		Schaudinn's smears
		Venipuncture
			Culture
			Microscopic examination
			  Wet mount
			  Permanent stains
			Serology
			  Antigen (stool)
			  Antibody (serum)
			Culture

Giardia species	Fresh stool
	Preserved stool
	Duodenal contents
		Waxed container
		Formalin, PVA
		Entero-Test or aspirate
			Microscopic examination
			  Wet mount
			  Permanent stains
			Antigen
			  IFA
			  EIA
			Culture

Cryptosporidium species	Fresh stool
	Preserved stool
	Biopsy
		Waxed container
		Formalin, PVA
		Saline
			Microscopic examination (acid-fast)
			Antigen
			  IFA
			  EIA

PVA, Polyvinyl alcohol; *IFA,* immunofluorescent assays; *EIA,* enzyme immunoassay.

TABLE 74-1   **Body Sites, Specimen Collection, and Diagnostic Procedures for Selected Parasitic Infections—cont'd**

INFECTING ORGANISM	SPECIMEN OPTIONS	COLLECTION METHODS	DIAGNOSTIC PROCEDURE
INTESTINAL TRACT—cont'd			
Microsporidia	Fresh stool	Waxed container	Microscopic examination
	Preserved stool	Formalin, PVA	Giemsa stain
	Duodenal contents	Aspirate	Gram stain
	Biopsy	Saline	Chromotrope stain
Pinworm	Anal impression smear	Cellophane tape	Macroscopic examination
			Microscopic examination (eggs)
Helminths	Fresh stool	Waxed container	Macroscopic examination (adults)
	Preserved stool	Formalin, PVA	Microscopic examination (larvae and eggs)
	Serum	Venipuncture	Serology (antibody)
			Culture (*Strongyloides* species)
LIVER, SPLEEN			
E. histolytica, Leishmania species	Aspirates	Sterile, collected in four separate aliquots (liver)	Microscopic examination
			Wet mount
	Biopsy	Sterile; nonsterile to histology	Permanent stains
	Serum	Venipuncture	Serology
			Antigen
			Antibody
			Culture
LUNG			
Rarely: amoebae	Sputum	Induced, no preservative	Microscopic examination
(*E. histolytica*), trematodes	Lavage	No preservative	Giemsa stain
(*P. westermani*),	Transbronchial aspirate	Air-dried smears	Gram stain
larvae (*S. stercoralis*), or		Same as above	Hematoylin and eosin
cestode hooklets	Brush biopsy	Fresh squash preparation, non-sterile to histology	Antigen
	Open lung biopsy		IFA
			EIA
			Serum (antibody)
MUSCLE			
Trichinella spiralis	Biopsy	Nonsterile to histology	Microscopic examination
Trypanosoma cruzi	Serum	Venipuncture	Permanent stains
			Serology
			Antibody
			Antigen
SKIN			
Onchocerca volvulus, Leishmania species	Scrapings	Aseptic, smear, or vial	Microscopic examination
	Skin snip	No preservative	Wet mount
Cutaneous larval migrans	Biopsy	Nonsterile to histology	Permanent stains
	Serum	Venipuncture	Serology (antibody)
			Culture (*Leishmania* species)
UROGENITAL SYSTEM			
Trichomonas vaginalis	Vaginal discharge	Saline swab, culture medium	Microscopic examination
	Urethral discharge		Wet mount
	Prostatic secretions	Same as above	Permanent stains
			Antigen
			IFA
			Culture (*T. vaginalis*)
			Serology (antibody)
			Nucleic acid probes (*T. vaginalis*)
Schistosoma haematobium	Urine	Single, unpreserved specimen	Microscopic examination
	Biopsy	Nonsterile to histology	

TABLE 74-2	**Most Commonly Identified Intestinal Parasites in U.S. Laboratories (1995)**

ORGANISM	POSITIVE SPECIMENS	PATIENTS
Giardia lamblia	896	723
Cryptosporidium species	114	81
Dientamoeba fragilis	102	77
Ascaris lumbricoides	73	59
Entamoeba histolytica	66	52
Trichuris trichiura	58	44
Hookworm	53	45
Enterobius vermicularis	52	49
Strongyloides stercoralis	51	36
Hymenolepis nana	23	17
Isospora species	12	7
Microsporidia	8	6
Clonorchis or *Opisthorchis* species	5	4
Other helminths	24	22

Modified from Valenstein P, Pfaller M, Yungbluth M: *Arch Pathol Lab Med* 120:206-211, 1996.

TABLE 74-3	**Number of Specimens Required to Detect Intestinal Parasites**

SPECIMENS PER PATIENT	PERCENT OF INFECTED PATIENTS DETECTED*
1	91.9
2	97.6
3	99.8
4	99.9

Modified from Valenstein P, Pfaller M, Yungbluth M: *Arch Pathol Lab Med* 120:206-211, 1996.
*n = 1159.

for which the examination is made. If the physician is interested only in determining the presence or absence of helminths, one or two examinations may suffice, provided that concentration methods are used. For a routine parasitic examination, a total of three fecal specimens is recommended. The examination of three specimens using a combination of techniques ensures detection of more than 99% of infections. In a recent survey, examination of three specimens detected 99.8% of infected patients, and examination of four specimens detected an additional 0.1% (Table 74-3).

It is inappropriate for multiple specimens to be collected on the same patient on the same day. It is also not recommended for the three specimens to be submitted, one each day for 3 consecutive days. The series of three specimens should be collected within no more than 10 days. Many parasites do not appear in fecal specimens in consistent numbers on a daily basis; therefore collection of specimens on alternate days tends to yield a higher percentage of positive findings.

In recent years, it has become apparent that in the United States submission of stool for parasitological examination from patients with hospital-acquired diarrhea (onset more than 3 days after admission) is usually inappropriate. This is because the frequency of acquisition of protozoan or helminthic parasites in a hospital is vanishingly rare. A request for stool examination for ova and parasites in a hospitalized patient should be accompanied by a clear statement of clinical indications and only after the more common causes of hospital-acquired diarrhea (e.g., antibiotic induced) have been ruled out.

Techniques of Stool Examination

Specimens should be examined systematically by a competent microscopist for helminth eggs and larvae as well as intestinal protozoa. For optimal detection of these various infectious agents a combination of several techniques of examination is required.

Macroscopic examination. The fecal specimen should be examined for consistency and for the presence of blood, mucus, worms, and proglottids.

Direct wet mount. Fresh stools should be examined under the microscope using the saline and iodine wet-mount technique to detect motile trophozoites or larvae (*Strongyloides* species). The saline and iodine wet mounts are also used to detect helminth eggs, protozoan cysts, and host cells such as leukocytes and red blood cells. This approach is also useful in examining material from sputum, urine, vaginal swabs, duodenal aspirates, sigmoidoscopy, abscesses, and tissue biopsies.

Concentration. All fecal specimens should be placed in 10% formalin to preserve parasite morphology and should be concentrated using a procedure such as formalin–ethyl acetate (or formalin-ether) sedimentation or zinc sulfate flotation. These methods separate protozoan cysts and helminth eggs from the bulk of fecal material and thus enhance their ability to detect small numbers of organisms usually missed by the use of only a direct smear. After concentration, the material is stained with iodine and examined microscopically.

Permanently stained slides. The detection and correct identification of intestinal protozoa often depend on the examination of the permanently stained smear. These slides provide a permanent record of the protozoan organisms that are identified. The cytological detail revealed by one of the permanent staining methods is essential for accurate identification, and most identification should be considered tentative until confirmed by the permanently stained slide. The common permanent stains used are trichrome, iron hematoxylin, and phosphotungstic acid–hematoxylin. Slides are made either by preparing smears of fresh fecal material and placing them in Schaudinn's fixative solution or by fixing a small amount of fecal material in PVA fixative.

Collection and Examination of Specimens Other Than Stool

Frequently, specimens other than fecal material must be collected and examined to diagnose infections caused by intestinal pathogens. These specimens include perianal samples, sigmoidoscopic material, aspirates of duodenal contents and liver abscesses, sputum, urine, and urogenital specimens.

Perianal specimens. The collection of perianal specimens is frequently necessary to diagnose pinworm (*E. vermicularis)* and occasionally *Taenia* (tapeworm) infections. The methods include the preparation of a clear cellulose tape slide or an anal swab. The cellulose tape slide preparation is the method of choice for the detection of pinworm eggs. Specimens collected by either method should be obtained in the morning before the patient bathes or goes to the bathroom. The tape method requires that the adhesive surface of the tape be pressed firmly against the right and left perianal folds and then spread onto the surface of a microscope slide. Likewise, the anal swab should be rubbed gently over the perianal area and transported to the laboratory for microscopic examination. With either collection method the slides or swabs should be kept at 4° C if transport to the laboratory is to be delayed.

Sigmoidoscopic material. Material from sigmoidoscopy can be helpful in the diagnosis of *E. histolytica* infection that has not been detected by routine fecal examinations. The specimens consist of scraped or aspirated material from the mucosal surface. At least six areas should be sampled. After collection, the material should be placed in a tube containing 0.85% saline and should be kept warm during transport to the laboratory. The specimens should be examined immediately for motile trophozoites.

Duodenal aspirates. Sampling and examination of duodenal contents is a means of recovering *Strongyloides* larvae; the eggs of *Clonorchis, Opisthorchis,* and *Fasciola* species; and other small bowel parasites such as *Giardia, Isospora,* and *Cryptosporidium* organisms. Specimens may be obtained by endoscopic intubation or by the use of the enteric capsule or string test (Entero-Test). Endoscopic biopsy of the small intestinal mucosa may reveal *Giardia* organisms, *Cryptosporidium* organisms, and microsporidia as well as *Strongyloides* larvae. Specimens should be collected in saline and transported directly to the laboratory for microscopic examination.

Liver abscess aspirate. Suppurative lesions of the liver and subphrenic spaces may be caused by *E. histolytica* (extraintestinal amebiasis). Extraintestinal amebiasis may occur in the absence of any history of symptomatic intestinal infection. The specimen should be collected from the liver abscess margin instead of the necrotic center. The first portion removed is usually yellowish white in appearance and seldom contains amoebae. Later portions, which are reddish, are more likely to contain organisms. A minimum of two separate portions of exudative material should be removed. After aspiration, the collapse of the abscess and the subsequent inflowing of blood often release amoebae from the tissue. Subsequent aspirations may have a greater chance of revealing organisms. The aspirated material should be transported immediately to the laboratory.

Sputum. Occasionally, intestinal parasites may be detected in sputum. These organisms include the larvae of *Ascaris* species, *Strongyloides* species, and hookworm; cestode hooklets; and intestinal protozoa such as *E. histolytica* and *Cryptosporidium* species. The specimen should be a deep sputum rather than primarily saliva, and it should be delivered immediately to the laboratory. Microscopic examination should include saline wet-mount and permanent stain preparations.

Urine. Examination of urine specimens may be useful in diagnosing infections caused by *Schistosoma haematobium* (occasionally other species as well) and *Trichomonas vaginalis.* Detection of eggs in urine can be accomplished using direct detection or concentration using the sedimentation centrifugation technique. Eggs may be trapped in mucus or pus and are more frequently present in the last few drops of the specimen rather than the first portion. The production of *Schistosoma* eggs fluctuates; therefore examinations should be performed over several days. *T. vaginalis* may be found in the urinary sediment of male and female patients.

Urogenital specimens. Urogenital specimens are collected if infection with *T. vaginalis* is suspected. Identification is based on wet-mount preparation examinations of vaginal and urethral discharges, prostatic secretions, or urine sediment. Specimens should be placed in a container with a small amount of 0.85% saline and sent immediately to the laboratory for examination. If no organisms are detected by direct wet mounts, culture may be used.

Blood and Tissue Parasitic Infections

Parasites localized within the blood or tissues of the host are more difficult to detect than intestinal and urogenital parasites. Microscopic examination of blood films is a direct and useful means of detecting malarial parasites, trypanosomes, and microfilariae. Unfortunately, the concentration of organisms often fluctuates; thus the collection of multiple specimens over several days is required. The preparation of both wet mounts (microfilariae and trypanosomes) and permanently stained thick and thin blood films is the mainstay of diagnosis. Examination of sputum may reveal helminth ova (lung flukes) or larvae (*Ascaris Strongyloides* species) after appropriate concentration techniques. Biopsy of skin (onchocerciasis) or muscle (trichinosis) may be required for the diagnosis of certain nematode infections (Table 74-1).

Blood Films

The clinical diagnosis of parasitic diseases such as malaria, leishmaniasis, trypanosomiasis, and filariasis largely rests on the collection of appropriately timed blood samples and the expert microscopic examination of properly prepared and stained thick and thin blood films. The optimal time for obtaining blood for parasitological examination varies with the particular parasite expected.

Because malaria is one of the few parasitic infections that can be life threatening, blood collection and examination of blood films should be performed immediately as soon as the diagnosis is suspected. Laboratories offering this service should be prepared to do so on a 24-hour basis, 7 days a week. Because the levels of parasitemia may be low or fluctuating, it is recommended that repeat blood films be obtained and examined at 6, 12, and 24 hours after the initial sample. Detection of trypanosomes in blood is occasionally possible during the early acute phase of the disease. *Trypanosoma cruzi* (Chagas' disease) may also be detected during subsequent febrile periods. After several months to a year, the trypomastigotes of African trypanosomiasis (*Trypanosoma brucei rhodesiense* and *T. b. gambiense*) are better demonstrated in spinal fluid than blood. Blood films for the detection of nocturnal microfilariae (*W. bancrofti* and *Brugia malayi*) should be prepared between 10 PM and 4 AM, whereas for the diurnal *Loa loa*, films are prepared around noon.

Two types of blood films are prepared for the diagnosis of blood parasite infections: thin films and thick films. Although wet-mount preparations of blood films can be examined for motile parasites (microfilariae and trypanosomes), most laboratories proceed directly to the preparation of thick and thin films for staining. In the **thin film** the blood is spread over the slide in a thin (single cell) layer, and the red blood cells remain intact after staining. In the **thick film** the red cells are lysed before staining, and only the white blood cells, platelets, and parasites (if present) are visible. Thick films allow a larger amount of blood to be examined, which increases the possibility of detecting light infections. Unfortunately, increased distortion of the parasites makes species identification using the thick film particularly difficult. Proper use of this technique usually requires a great deal of expertise and experience.

Occasionally, other blood-concentration procedures may be used to detect light infections. Alternative concentration methods for detecting blood parasites include the use of microhematocrit centrifugation, the examination of buffy coat preparations, a triple centrifugation technique for the detection of low numbers of trypanosomes, and a membrane filtration technique for the detection of microfilariae.

Once prepared, blood films must be stained. The most dependable staining of blood parasites is obtained with Giemsa stain buffered to pH 7.0 to 7.2, although special stains may be occasionally used to identify species of microfilariae. Giemsa stain is particularly useful for the staining of protozoa (malaria and trypanosomes); however, the sheath of microfilariae may not always stain with Giemsa. In this case, hematoxylin-based stains may be used.

Specimens Other Than Blood

Examination of tissue and body fluids other than blood may be necessary based on clinical presentation and epidemiological considerations. Smears and concentrates of cerebrospinal fluid are necessary to detect trophozoites of *Naegleria* species, trypanosomes, and larvae of *Angiostrongylus cantonensis* within the central nervous system. Cerebrospinal fluid must be promptly examined because the trophozoite forms of these parasites are very labile (trypanosomes) or tend to round up and become nonmotile (*Naegleria* species). Examination of tissue impression smears of lymph nodes, liver biopsy material, spleen, or bone marrow stained with Giemsa stain is very useful in detecting intracellular parasites such as *Leishmania* and *Toxoplasma* species. Likewise, biopsies of various tissues are an excellent means of detecting localized or disseminated infections caused by protozoan and helminthic parasites. Saline mounts of superficial skin snips are very useful in detecting the microfilariae of *Onchocerca volvulus*. Examination of sputum (induced) is indicated when there is a question of pulmonary paragonimiasis (lung fluke) or abscess formation with *E. histolytica*. *Strongyloides* larvae may be detected in sputum in hyperinfection syndrome.

Alternatives to Microscopy

In the majority of cases the diagnosis of parasitic disease is made in the laboratory by microscopic detection and morphological identification of the parasite in clinical specimens. In some cases the parasite cannot be detected despite a careful search because of low or absent levels of organisms in readily available clinical material. In such cases the clinician may need to rely on alternative methods based on the detection of parasite-derived material (antigens or nucleic acids) or by the host response to parasitic invasion (antibodies). Additional approaches used in selected infections include culture, animal inoculation, and xenodiagnosis.

Immunodiagnostics

Immunodiagnostic methods have long been used as aids in the diagnosis of parasitic diseases. The majority of these serological tests are based on the detection of specific antibody responses to the presence of the parasite. The analytical approaches include the use of classical agglutination, complement fixation, and gel diffusion methods and more recently include immunofluorescence, enzyme immunoassay (EIA), and Western blot assays. Antibody detection is useful and indicated in the diagnosis of many protozoan diseases (e.g., extraintestinal amebiasis, South American trypanosomiasis, leishmaniasis, transfusion-acquired malaria, toxoplasmosis) and helminthic diseases (e.g., clonorchiasis, cysticercosis, hydatidosis, lymphatic filariasis, schistosomiasis, trichinellosis, toxocariasis). There is a problem with the detection of antibody as a means of diagnosis: Because of the persistence of antibody for months to years after the acute infection, demonstration of antibody can rarely differentiate between acute and chronic infection.

In contrast to antibody detection, the measurement of circulating parasite antigen in serum, urine, or feces may provide a more appropriate marker for the presence of active infection and may also indicate parasite load. Likewise, demonstrations of specific parasite antigen in lesion fluid, such as material from an amoebic abscess or fluid from a hydatid cyst, may provide a definitive diagnosis of the infecting organism. Most common antigen-detection assays use an EIA format; however, immunofluorescence, radioimmunoassay, and immunoblot methods have also proved useful. Several commercial assays for the detection of parasite antigens are now available in kits. These include EIA for the detection of *Giardia* and *Cryptosporidium* species in stool, EIA for the detection of *T. vaginalis* in urogenital specimens, and immunofluorescent assays (IFA) for the detection of *Giardia*, *Cryptosporidium*, and *Trichomonas* species. The reported sensitivity and specificity for most of these kits are quite good. The advantages to these approaches are labor savings and a potential increase in sensitivity. The disadvantages are the loss of parasitological expertise and the fact that in each case the available assay tests for only a single organism, whereas conventional microscopic examination provides the opportunity to recognize many different parasites. Although antigen-detection assays have been described for many other parasites, they are not widely available. The availability of a broader panel of antigen-detection assays would make the use of an antigen screen a viable alternative to tedious microscopic examination.

Molecular Diagnostic Approaches

In addition to immunodiagnostic methods, the diagnosis of parasitic diseases has been enhanced considerably by the application of molecular diagnostic methods based on nucleic acid hybridization. This approach takes advantage of the fact that all organisms contain nucleic acid sequences that may be used in a hybridization assay to distinguish among strains, species, and genera. Thus parasites may be simultaneously detected and identified in clinical material depending on the specificity of the nucleic acid probe used. Another advantage of nucleic acid–based detection systems is that they are independent of the patients' immunological status or previous infection history, thereby identifying active infection. Finally, the development of target amplification techniques such as the polymerase chain reaction provides exquisite sensitivity, allowing the detection of as little as one organism in a biological sample (Table 74-4).

Nucleic acid probes can be used to detect parasites not only in clinical samples of blood, stool, or tissue from infected patients but also in their natural vector. The application of DNA "fingerprinting" allows precise identification of the parasite or vector to the subspecies or strain level and has considerable value in epidemiological studies. Assay formats using nucleic acid probes range from dot blot and Southern hybridization methods to in situ hybridization in tissue to PCR amplification coupled with solid or solution phase hybridization. The use of nonisotopic DNA labeling techniques greatly expands the potential applicability of these assays worldwide. Diagnostic kits based on these methods are not widely available; however, several are under development and may be available for clinical use in the near future. A simple nucleic acid probe assay for *T. vaginalis* in urogenital specimens is now available commercially in kit form for use in clinics and physicians' offices.

Irrespective of the assay format, nucleic acid probes and amplification techniques are now being used on a research basis for the detection and identification of numerous species and strains, including *Plasmodium* species, *Leishmania* species, *T. cruzi*, *E. histolytica*, and *Toxoplasma gondii* (Table 74-4). It must be understood that the application of nucleic acid hybridization methods to the diagnosis of parasitic diseases is still in its infancy. The widespread use of these techniques requires further development of simple procedures for sample handling and preparation and will require extensive clinical and field testing before they can be applied broadly to aid in clinical diagnosis.

TABLE 74-4	**Examples of PCR-Based Detection of Parasitic Infections**		
ORGANISM	**GENE TARGET**	**SENSITIVITY**	**COMMENT**
Plasmodium vivax	Circumsporozoite gene	91%-96%	Dried blood–spotted filter paper samples are used.
Leishmania species	kDNA minicircle sequence	87%-100%	Results are compared to culture and microscopy of biopsy specimens.
Trypanosoma cruzi	kDNA minicircle sequence	100%	Results are compared to serology and xenodiagnosis of blood samples.
Toxoplasma gondii	B1 repetitive gene P30 major surface antigen Recombinant DNA sequences	46%-99%	PCR of BAL, blood, cerebrospinal fluid, and amniotic fluid show great potential for diagnosis of toxoplasmosis.
Entamoeba histolytica	P145 tandem repeat sequence	96%	Results are compared to microscopic diagnosis of stool samples. Test may distinguish pathogenic from nonpathogenic strains.

PCR, Polymerase chain reaction; *BAL,* bronchoalveolar lavage.

Culture

Although culture is the standard for the diagnosis of most infectious diseases, it is not commonly used in the parasitology laboratory. Certain protozoan parasites such as *T. vaginalis,* *E. histolytica,* *Acanthamoeba* species, *Naegleria* species, *Leishmania* species, *T. cruzi,* and *Toxoplasma* species can be cultured with relative ease. However, culture of other parasites has not been successful or is too difficult or cumbersome to be of practical value in routine diagnostic efforts.

Animal Inoculation

Animal inoculation is a sensitive means of detecting infection caused by blood and tissue parasites such as *T. b. gambiense,* *T. b. rhodesiense,* *T. cruzi,* *Leishmania* species, and *T. gondii.* Although useful, this approach is not practical for most diagnostic laboratories and is largely confined to research settings.

Xenodiagnosis

The technique of xenodiagnosis employs the use of laboratory-raised arthropod vectors to detect low levels of parasites in infected individuals. Classically, this approach was used to diagnose Chagas' disease by allowing an uninfected reduviid bug to feed on an individual suspected of having the disease. Subsequently, the bug was dissected and examined microscopically for evidence of developmental stages of *T. cruzi.* Although this technique may be used in endemic areas, it is obviously not practical for most diagnostic laboratories.

QUESTIONS

1. Why is it important to understand the life cycle of parasites when diagnosing parasitic diseases?
2. What factors may confound the use of microscopy in the diagnosis of parasitic disease?
3. Describe the important considerations in collecting and submitting a fecal specimen for parasitological examination.
4. Which parasites can be detected in blood?
5. What are the alternatives to microscopy for the diagnosis of parasitic infections?

Bibliography

Barker RH: DNA probe diagnosis of parasitic infections, *Exp Parasitol* 70:494-499, 1990.

Baron EJ, Peterson LR, Finegold SM: *Bailey & Scott's diagnostic microbiology,* ed 9, St Louis, 1994, Mosby.

Garcia LS et al: *Slide preparation and staining of blood films for the laboratory diagnosis of parasitic diseases,* National Committee for Clinical Laboratory Standards document M15-T, Villanova, Penn, 1992.

Hommel M: Impact of modern technologies on tropical medicine, *Trans Royal Soc Trop Med Hyg* 85:151-155, 1991.

Maddison SE: Serodiagnosis of parasitic diseases, *Clin Microbiol Rev* 4:457-469, 1991.

Markell EK, Voge M, John DT: *Medical parasitology,* ed 7, Philadelphia, 1992, WB Saunders.

Valenstein P, Pfaller M, Yungbluth M: The use and abuse of routine stool microbiology: a College of American Pathologists Q-Probes study of 601 institutions, *Arch Pathol Lab Med* 120:206-211, 1996.

Weiss JB: DNA probes and PCR for diagnosis of parasitic infections, *Clin Microbiol Rev* 8:113-130, 1995.

Intestinal and Urogenital Protozoa

Protozoa may colonize and infect the oropharynx, duodenum and small bowel, colon, and urogenital tract of humans. The majority of these parasites belong to the amoebae and flagellates; however, infection with ciliate, coccidian, or microsporidian parasites may also be encountered (see Table 74-2). These organisms are transmitted by the fecal-oral route. In the United States, transmission of intestinal protozoa is particularly problematic in day-care centers, where several outbreaks of diarrhea caused by *Giardia* or *Cryptosporidium* species have been documented. In other parts of the world the spread of enteric protozoal infections may be controlled in part by improved sanitation and by chlorination and filtration of water supplies; however, this may be difficult or impossible in many developing countries.

AMOEBAE

The amoebae are primitive unicellular microorganisms. Their life cycle is relatively simple and divided into two stages: the actively motile feeding stage **(trophozoite)** and the quiescent, resistant, infective stage **(cyst).** Replication is accomplished by binary fission (splitting the trophozoite) or by the development of numerous trophozoites within the mature multinucleated cyst. Motility is accomplished by extension of a pseudopod ("false foot") with extrusion of the cellular ectoplasm and then drawing up of the rest of the cell in a snail-like movement to meet this pseudopod. The amoebic trophozoites remain actively motile as long as the environment is favorable. The cyst form develops when the environmental temperature or moisture level drops.

Most amoebae found in humans are commensal organisms (*Entamoeba coli, Entamoeba hartmanni, Entamoeba gingivalis, Endolimax nana, Iodamoeba bütschlii*). However, *Entamoeba histolytica* is an important human pathogen. Other amoebae, particularly *Entamoeba polecki*, can cause human disease but are rarely isolated. Some free-living amoebae (*Naegleria fowleri, Acanthamoeba* species) are present in soil and in warm freshwater ponds or swimming pools and can be opportunistic human pathogens, causing meningoencephalitis or keratitis.

Entamoeba histolytica

Physiology and Structure

Cyst and trophozoite forms of *E. histolytica* are detected in fecal specimens from infected patients (Figure 75-1). Trophozoites can also be found in the crypts of the large intestine. In freshly passed stools, actively motile trophozoites can be seen, whereas in formed stools the cysts are usually the only form recognized. For the diagnosis of amebiasis, distinguishing between the *E. histolytica* trophozoites and cysts and those of commensal amoebae is important.

Pathogenesis

After ingestion, the cysts pass through the stomach, where exposure to gastric acid stimulates the release of the pathogenic trophozoite in the duodenum. The trophozoites divide and produce extensive local necrosis in the large intestine. The basis for this tissue destruction is incompletely understood, although it is attributed to production of a cytotoxin. Attachment of *E. histolytica* trophozoites to host cells via a galactose-inhibitable adherence protein is required for cytolysis and tissue necrosis to occur. The lysis of colonic epithelial cells, human neutrophils, lymphocytes, and monocytes by trophozoites is associated with a lethal alteration of host cell membrane permeability, resulting in an irreversible increase in intracellular calcium levels. The release of toxic neutrophil constituents after the lysis of neutrophils may contribute to the tissue destruction.

Recently, lectin binding, zymodeme analysis, genome DNA analysis, and staining with specific monoclonal antibodies have been used as markers to identify invasive strains of *E. histolytica*. Flask-shaped ulcerations of the intestinal mucosa are present with inflammation, hemorrhage, and secondary bacterial infection. Invasion into the deeper mucosa with extension into the peritoneal cavity may occur. This can lead to secondary involvement of other organs, primarily the liver but also the lungs, brain, and heart. Extraintestinal amebiasis is associated with trophozoites. Amoebae are found only in environments that have a low oxygen pressure because the protozoa are killed by ambient oxygen concentrations.

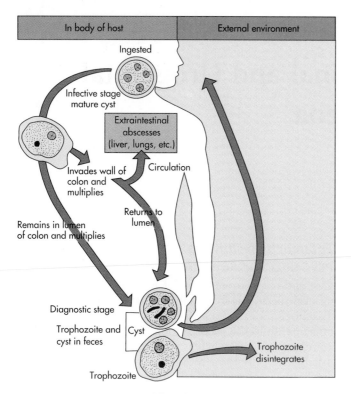

FIGURE 75-1 Life cycle of *E. histolytica.*

Epidemiology

E. histolytica has a worldwide distribution. Although it is found in cold areas such as Alaska, Canada, and Eastern Europe, its incidence is highest in tropical and subtropical regions that have poor sanitation and contaminated water. The average prevalence of infection in these areas is 10% to 15%, with as many as 50% of the population infected in some areas. Many of the infected individuals are asymptomatic carriers, who represent a reservoir for the spread of *E. histolytica* to others. The prevalence of infection in the United States is 1% to 2%.

Patients infected with *E. histolytica* pass noninfectious trophozoites and the infectious cysts in their stools. The trophozoites cannot survive in the external environment or in transport through the stomach if ingested. Therefore the main source of water and food contamination is the asymptomatic carrier who passes cysts. This is a particular problem in hospitals for the mentally ill, military and refugee camps, prisons, and crowded day-care centers. Flies and cockroaches can also serve as vectors for the transmission of *E. histolytica* cysts. Sewage containing cysts can contaminate water systems, wells, springs, and agricultural areas where human waste is used as fertilizer. Finally, cysts can be transmitted by oral-anal sexual practices, with amebiasis prevalent in homosexual populations. Direct trophozoite transmission in sexual encounters can produce cutaneous amebiasis.

Clinical Syndromes

The outcome of infection may result in a carrier state, intestinal amebiasis, or extraintestinal amebiasis. If the strain of *E. histolytica* has a low virulence, if the inoculum is low, or if the patient's immune system is intact, the organisms may reproduce, and cysts may be passed in stool specimens with no clinical symptoms. Noninvasive strains of *E. histolytica* have been characterized by specific isoenzyme profiles (zymodemes), their susceptibility to complement-mediated lysis, and their failure to agglutinate in the presence of the lectin concanavalin A. Detection of carriers in areas with a low endemicity is important for epidemiological purposes.

Patients with intestinal amebiasis develop clinical symptoms related to the localized tissue destruction in the large intestine. These include abdominal pain, cramping, and colitis with diarrhea. More severe disease is characterized by numerous bloody stools per day. Systemic signs of infection (fever, leukocytosis, rigors) are present in patients with extraintestinal amebiasis. The liver is primarily involved because trophozoites in the blood are removed as they pass through this organ. Abscess formation is common. The right lobe is most commonly involved. Pain over the liver with hepatomegaly and elevation of the diaphragm is observed.

Laboratory Diagnosis

The identification of *E. histolytica* trophozoites (Figure 75-2) and cysts in stools and trophozoites in tissue is diagnostic of amoebic infection. Care must be taken to distinguish between these amoebae and commensal amoebae as well as between these amoebae and polymorphonuclear leukocytes. Microscopic examination of stool specimens is inherently insensitive because the protozoa are not usually distributed homogeneously in the specimen and the parasites are concentrated in the intestinal ulcers and at the margins of the abscess, not in the stool or the necrotic center of the abscess. For this reason, multiple stool specimens should be collected. Extraintestinal amebiasis is sometimes diagnosed using scanning procedures for the liver and other organs. Specific serological tests, together with microscopic examination of the abscess material, can confirm the diagnosis. Virtually all patients with hepatic amebiasis and most patients (more than 80%) with intestinal disease have positive serological findings at the time of clinical presentation. This may be less useful in endemic areas where the prevalence of positive serological results is higher. Examinations of stool specimens are frequently negative in extraintestinal disease. In addition to conventional microscopic and serological tests, researchers have developed several immunological tests for the detection of fecal antigen as well as polymerase chain reaction and DNA-probe assays for the detection of pathogenic strains of *E. histolytica.* These newer diagnostic approaches are promising but as yet are not widely available.

Treatment, Prevention, and Control

Acute, fulminating amebiasis is treated with metronidazole followed by iodoquinol. Asymptomatic carriage can be eradicated with iodoquinol, diloxanide furoate, or paromomycin. As already noted, human infection results

A

B

FIGURE 75-2 *E. histolytica* trophozoite **(A)** and cyst **(B)**. Trophozoites are motile and vary in size from 12 to 60 μm (average, 15 to 30 μm). The single nucleus in the cell is round with a central dot (karyosome) and an even distribution of chromatin granules around the nuclear membrane. Ingested erythrocytes may be in the cytoplasm. The cysts are smaller (10 to 20 μm with an average size of 15 to 20 μm) and contain one to four nuclei (usually four). Round chromatoidal bars may be in the cytoplasm. (**A** from Lennette EH et al: *Manual of clinical microbiology,* ed 5, Washington, DC, 1991, American Society for Microbiology; **B** from Markell EK, Voge M, John DT: *Medical parasitology,* ed 7, Philadelphia, 1992, WB Saunders.)

from the ingestion of food or water contaminated with human feces or as a result of specific sexual practices. The elimination of the cycle of infection requires the introduction of adequate sanitation measures and education about the routes of transmission. The chlorination and filtration of water supplies may limit the spread of these and other enteric protozoal infections but are not possible in many developing countries. Physicians should alert travelers to developing countries of the risks associated with the consumption of water (including ice cubes), unpeeled fruits, and raw vegetables. Water should be boiled and fruits and vegetables thoroughly cleaned before consumption.

TABLE 75-1	**Morphological Identification of *E. histolytica* and *E. coli***	
	E. HISTOLYTICA	**E. COLI**
Size (diameter)		
Trophozoite	12-50 μm	20-30 μm
Cyst	10-20 μm	10-30 μm
Pattern of peripheral nuclear chromatin	Fine, dispersed ring	Coarse, clumped
Karyosome	Central, sharp	Eccentric, coarse
Ingested erythrocytes	+	0
Cyst structure		
Nuclei	1-4	1-8
Chromatoidal bars	Rounded ends	Splintered, frayed ends

Other Intestinal Amoebae

Other amoebae that can parasitize the human gastrointestinal tract include *E. coli, E. hartmanni, E. polecki, E. nana,* and *I. bütschlii.* Only *E. polecki,* which is primarily a parasite of pigs and monkeys, can cause human disease, a mild, transient diarrhea. The diagnosis of *E. polecki* infection is confirmed by the microscopic detection of cysts in stool specimens. Treatment is the same as for *E. histolytica* infections.

The nonpathogenic intestinal amoebae are important because they must be differentiated from *E. histolytica* and *E. polecki.* This is particularly true for *E. coli,* which is frequently detected in stool specimens collected from patients exposed to contaminated food or water. Accurate identification of intestinal amoebae requires careful microscopic examination of the cyst and trophozoite forms present in stained and unstained stool specimens (Table 75-1).

Free-Living Amoebae

Naegleria species, *Acanthamoeba* species, and other free-living amoebae are found in soil and in contaminated lakes, streams, and other water environments. Most human infections with these amoebae are acquired during the warm summer months by people exposed to the amoebae while swimming in contaminated water. Inhalation of cysts present in dust may account for some infections, whereas ocular infections with *Acanthamoeba* species are associated with the contamination of contact lenses with nonsterile cleaning solutions.

Clinical Syndromes

Naegleria are opportunistic pathogens. Although colonization of the nasal passages is usually asymptomatic, these amoebae can invade the nasal mucosa and extend into the brain. Destruction of brain tissue is characterized by a fulminant, rapidly fatal **meningoencephalitis.** Symptoms include intense frontal headache, sore throat, fever, blocked nose with altered senses of taste and smell, stiff neck, and Kernig's sign. The cerebrospinal fluid is purulent and may contain many erythrocytes and motile amoebae. Clinically, the course of the disease is rapid, with death usually occurring within 4 or 5 days. Post-mortem findings show *Naegleria* trophozoites present in the brain but no evidence of cysts. Although all cases were fatal before 1970, survival has now been reported in a few cases in which the disease was rapidly diagnosed and treated.

In contrast to *Naegleria*, *Acanthamoeba* organisms produce granulomatous amoebic encephalitis primarily in immunocompromised individuals. The course of the disease is slower, with an incubation period of at least 10 days. The resulting disease is a chronic granulomatous encephalitis with edema of the brain tissue.

Eye and skin infection caused by *Acanthamoeba* organisms may also occur. **Keratitis** is usually associated with eye trauma that occurred before contact with con-taminated soil, dust, or water. The use of improperly cleaned contact lenses is also associated with this disease. Invasion by *Acanthamoeba* species produces corneal ul-ceration and severe ocular pain. Cases of apparent dis-seminated cutaneous and subcutaneous infection with *Acanthamoeba* organisms recently have been described in patients with acquired immunodeficiency syndrome (AIDS). These infections include multiple soft tissue nodules, which on biopsy contain *Acanthamoeba* organ-isms. Central nervous system or deep tissue involvement may also be present with this form of infection.

Laboratory Diagnosis

For the diagnosis of *Naegleria* and *Acanthamoeba* infec-tions, nasal discharge, cerebrospinal fluid, and in the case of eye infections, corneal scrapings should be collected. The specimens should be examined using a saline wet preparation and iodine-stained smears. *Naegleria* and *Acanthamoeba* species are difficult to differentiate except by experienced microscopists. However, the observation of an amoeba in a normally sterile tissue is diagnostic (Figure 75-3). The clinical specimens can be cultured on agar plates seeded with live gram-negative enteric bacilli. Amoebae present in the specimens use the bacteria as a nutritional source and can be detected within 1 or 2 days by the presence of the trails that form on the agar surface as the amoebae move.

Treatment, Prevention, and Control

The treatment of choice for *Naegleria* infections is am-photericin B combined with miconazole and rifampin. Experimental infections with *Acanthamoeba* species ap-pear to respond to sulfadiazine. Amoebic keratitis and cutaneous infections may respond to topical miconazole, chlorhexidine gluconate, or propamidine isethionate. Treatment of amoebic keratitis may require repeated corneal transplantation or, rarely, enucleation of the eye. The wide distribution of these organisms in fresh and brackish waters makes the prevention and control of in-fection difficult. It has been suggested that known sources of infection be off-limits to bathing, diving, and

FIGURE 75-3 Numerous *Naegleria* trophozoites *(arrows)* in a section of spinal cord from a patient with amoebic meningoencephalitis. (From Rothrock JF, Buchsbaum HW: *JAMA* 243:2329-2330, 1980.)

water sports, although this is generally difficult to en-force. Swimming pools with cracks in the walls, allowing soil seepage, should be repaired to avoid creation of a source of infection.

FLAGELLATES

The flagellates of clinical significance include *Giardia lamblia, Dientamoeba fragilis,* and *Trichomonas vagi-nalis.* Nonpathogenic commensal flagellates such as *Chilomastix mesnili* (enteric) and *Trichomonas tenax* (oral) may also be observed. *Giardia* organisms, like *E. histolytica,* have cyst and trophozoite stages in their life cycles. In contrast, no cyst stage has been observed for *Trichomonas* or *Dientamoeba* species. Unlike the amoe-bae, most flagellates move by the lashing of flagella that pull the organisms through fluid environments. Diseases produced by flagellates are primarily the result of me-chanical irritation and inflammation. For example, *G. lamblia* attaches to the intestinal villi with an adhesive disk, resulting in localized tissue damage. The tissue in-vasion with extensive tissue destruction, as seen with *E. histolytica,* is rare with flagellates.

Giardia lamblia
Physiology and Structure

Both cyst and trophozoite forms of *G. lamblia* are de-tected in fecal specimens from infected patients (Figure 75-4).

Pathogenesis

Infection with *G. lamblia* is initiated by ingestion of cysts (Figure 75-5). The minimum infective dose for humans is estimated to be 10 to 25 cysts. Gastric acid stimulates excystation with the release of trophozoites in the duo-denum and jejunum, where the organisms multiply by binary fission. The trophozoites can attach to the intesti-nal villi by a prominent ventral sucking disk. Although

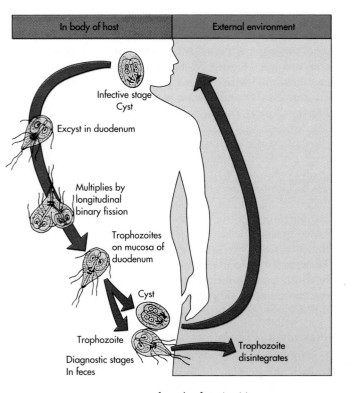

FIGURE 75-5 Life cycle of *G. lamblia.*

FIGURE 75-4 *G. lamblia* trophozoite **(A)** and cyst **(B).** Trophozoites are 9 to 12 μm long and 5 to 15 μm wide. Flagella are present, as are two nuclei with large central karyosomes, a large ventral sucking disk for attachment of the flagellate to the intestinal villi, and two ob-long parabasal bodies below the nuclei. The morphology gives the appearance that the trophozoites are looking back at the viewer. Cysts are smaller—8 to 12 μm long and 7 to 10 μm wide. Four nuclei and four parabasal bodies are present. (From Finegold SM, Baron EJ: *Bailey and Scott's diagnostic microbiology,* ed 7, St Louis, 1986, Mosby.)

the tips of the villi may appear flattened and inflammation of the mucosa with hyperplasia of lymphoid follicles may be observed, frank tissue necrosis does not occur. In addition, metastatic spread of disease beyond the gastrointestinal tract is very rare.

Epidemiology

Giardia species has a worldwide distribution, and this flagellate has a sylvatic or "wilderness" distribution in many streams, lakes, and mountain resorts. This sylvatic distribution is maintained in reservoir animals such as beavers and muskrats. Giardiasis is acquired by the consumption of inadequately treated contaminated water, ingestion of contaminated uncooked vegetables or fruits, or person-to-person spread by the fecal-oral or oral-anal route. The cyst stage is resistant to chlorine concentrations (1 to 2 parts per million) used in most

water-treatment facilities. Thus adequate water treatment should include chemicals with filtration.

Risk factors associated with *Giardia* infections include poor sanitary conditions, travel to known endemic areas, consumption of inadequately treated water (e.g., from contaminated mountain streams), day-care centers, and oral-anal sexual practices. Infections may occur in outbreak and endemic forms within day-care centers and other institutional settings and among family members of infected children. Scrupulous attention to handwashing and treatment of all infected individuals are important in controlling the spread of infection in these settings.

Clinical Syndromes

Giardia infection can result in either asymptomatic carriage (observed in approximately 50% of infected individuals) or symptomatic disease ranging from mild diarrhea to a severe malabsorption syndrome. The incubation period before symptomatic disease develops ranges from 1 to 4 weeks (average, 10 days). The onset of disease is sudden, with foul-smelling, watery diarrhea; abdominal cramps; flatulence; and steatorrhea. Blood and pus are rarely present in stool specimens, which is consistent with the absence of tissue destruction. Spontaneous recovery generally occurs after 10 to 14 days, although a more chronic disease with multiple relapses may develop. This is particularly a problem for patients with immunoglobulin A deficiency or intestinal diverticula.

Laboratory Diagnosis

With the onset of diarrhea and abdominal discomfort, stool specimens should be examined for cysts and trophozoites (Figure 75-4). *Giardia* species may occur in "showers," with many organisms present in the stool on a given day and few or none detected the next day. For this reason, the physician should never accept the results of a single negative stool specimen as evidence that the patient is free of intestinal parasites. One stool specimen per day for 3 days should be examined. If stools remain persistently negative in a patient in whom giardiasis is highly suspected, additional specimens can be collected by duodenal aspiration, Entero-Test or string test, or biopsy of the upper small intestine. In addition to conventional microscopy, several immunological tests for the detection of fecal antigen are available commercially. These tests include countercurrent immunoelectrophoresis, enzyme immunoassay, and indirect immunofluorescent staining. Reported sensitivities range from 88% to 98% and specificities from 87% to 100%.

Treatment, Prevention, and Control

It is important to eradicate *Giardia* species from asymptomatic carriers and diseased patients. The drug of choice is quinacrine, with metronidazole an acceptable alternative. The prevention and control of giardiasis involves the avoidance of contaminated water and food, especially by the traveler and outdoorsman. Protection is afforded by boiling drinking water from streams and lakes or in countries with a high incidence of endemic disease. Maintenance of properly functioning filtration systems in municipal water supplies is also required because cysts are resistant to standard chlorination procedures. Public health efforts should be made to identify the reservoir of infection to prevent spread of disease. In addition, high-risk sexual behavior should be avoided.

Dientamoeba fragilis

Physiology and Structure

Dientamoeba fragilis was initially classified as an amoeba; however, the internal structures of the trophozoite are typical of a flagellate. No cyst stage has been described.

Epidemiology

D. fragilis has a worldwide distribution. The transmission of the delicate trophozoite is not completely understood. Some observers believe the organism can be transported from person to person inside the protective shell of worm eggs such as *E. vermicularis*, the pinworm. Transmission by the fecal-oral and oral-anal routes does occur.

Clinical Syndromes

Most infections with *D. fragilis* are asymptomatic, with colonization of the cecum and upper colon. However, some patients may develop symptomatic disease with abdominal discomfort, flatulence, intermittent diarrhea, anorexia, and weight loss. There is no evidence of tissue invasion with this flagellate, although irritation of the intestinal mucosa occurs.

Laboratory Diagnosis

Infection is confirmed by the microscopic examination of stool specimens in which typical trophozoites can be seen. The trophozoite is small (5 to 12 μm), with one or two nuclei. The central karyosome consists of four to six discrete granules. The excretion of the parasite may fluctuate markedly from day to day, and thus collection of several stool samples may be necessary. Examination of a purged stool sample may also be useful.

Treatment, Prevention, and Control

The therapy of choice for *D. fragilis* infection is iodoquinol, with tetracycline and paromomycin acceptable alternatives. The reservoir for this flagellate and the organism's life cycle are unknown. Thus specific recommendations for prevention and control are difficult. However, infections can be avoided by maintaining adequate sanitary conditions. The eradication of infections with *Enterobius* organisms may also reduce the transmission of *Dientamoeba* infection.

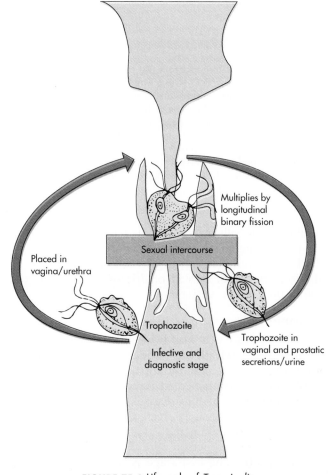

FIGURE 75-6 Life cycle of *T. vaginalis*.

Trichomonas vaginalis

Physiology and Structure

T. vaginalis is not an intestinal protozoan but rather the cause of urogenital infections. The flagellate's four flagella and short, undulating membrane are responsible for motility. *T. vaginalis* exists only as a trophozoite and is found in the urethras and vaginas of women and the urethras and prostate glands of men.

Epidemiology

This parasite has worldwide distribution, with sexual intercourse as the primary mode of transmission (Figure 75-6). Occasionally, infections have been transmitted by fomites (toilet articles, clothing), although this transmission is limited by the lability of the trophozoite form. Infants may be infected by passage through the mother's infected birth canal. The prevalence of this flagellate in developed countries is reported to be 5% to 20% in women and 2% to 10% in men.

Clinical Syndromes

Most infected women are asymptomatic or have a scant, watery vaginal discharge. Vaginitis may occur with more extensive inflammation and erosion of the epithelial lining that is associated with itching, burning, and painful urination. Men are primarily asymptomatic carriers who serve as a reservoir for infections in women. However, men occasionally experience urethritis, prostatitis, and other urinary tract problems.

Laboratory Diagnosis

The microscopic examination of vaginal or urethral discharge for characteristic trophozoites is the diagnostic method of choice (Figure 75-7). Stained (Giemsa, Papanicolaou) or unstained smears can be examined. The diagnostic yield may be improved by culturing the organism (93% sensitivity) or using monoclonal fluorescent antibody staining (86% sensitivity). A nucleic acid probe assay is also available commercially. Serological tests may be useful in epidemiological surveillance.

Treatment, Prevention, and Control

The drug of choice is metronidazole. Both male and female sex partners must be treated to avoid reinfection. Resistance to metronidazole has been reported and may require retreatment with higher doses. Personal hygiene, avoidance of shared toilet articles and clothing, and safe sexual practices are important preventive actions. Elimination of carriage in men is critical for the eradication of disease.

CILIATES

The intestinal protozoan *Balantidium coli* is the only member of the ciliate group that is pathogenic for humans. Disease produced by *B. coli* is similar to amebiasis because the organisms elaborate proteolytic and cytotoxic substances that mediate tissue invasion and intestinal ulceration.

Balantidium coli

Physiology and Structure

The life cycle of *B. coli* is simple, involving ingestion of infectious cysts, excystation, and invasion of trophozoites into the mucosal lining of the large intestine, cecum, and terminal ileum (Figure 75-8). The trophozoite is covered with rows of hairlike cilia that aid in motility. Morphologically more complex than amoebae, *B. coli* has a funnel-like primitive mouth called a *cytostome*, a large and small nucleus involved in reproduction, food vacuoles, and two contractile vacuoles.

Epidemiology

B. coli is distributed worldwide. Swine and (less commonly) monkeys are the most important reservoirs. Infections are transmitted by the fecal-oral route; outbreaks are associated with contamination of water supplies with pig feces. Person-to-person spread, including through food handlers, has been implicated in outbreaks. Risk factors associated with human disease include contact with swine and substandard hygienic conditions.

Clinical Syndromes

As with other protozoan parasites, asymptomatic carriage of *B. coli* can exist. Symptomatic disease is characterized by abdominal pain and tenderness, tenesmus, nausea, anorexia, and watery stools with blood and pus. Ulceration of the intestinal mucosa, as with amebiasis, can be seen; a secondary complication caused by bacterial invasion into the eroded intestinal mucosa can occur. Extraintestinal invasion of other organs is extremely rare in balantidiasis.

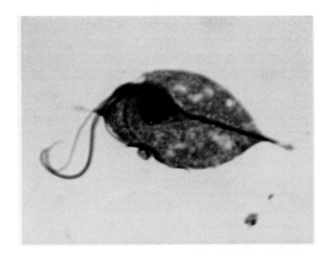

FIGURE 75-7 *T. vaginalis* trophozoite. The trophozoite is 7 to 23 μm long and 6 to 8 μm wide (average, 13 × 7 μm). The flagella and a short undulating membrane are present at one side, and an axostyle extends through the center of the parasite. (From Ash LR, Orihel TC: *Atlas of human parasitology*, ed 2, Chicago, 1984, American Society of Clinical Pathologists.)

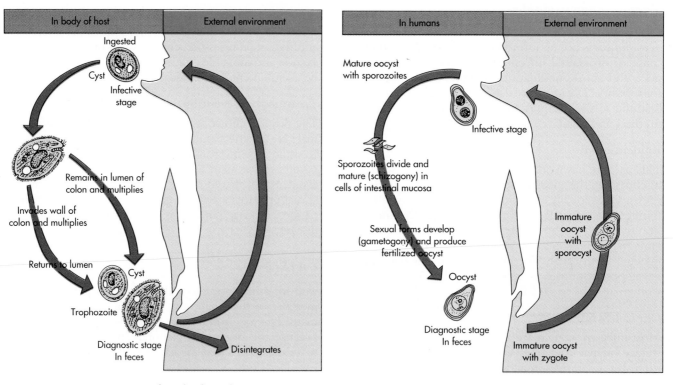

FIGURE 75-8 Life cycle of *B. coli*.

FIGURE 75-9 Life cycle of *Isospora* species.

Laboratory Diagnosis

Microscopic examination of feces for trophozoites and cysts is performed. The trophozoite is very large, varying in length from 50 to 200 μm and in width from 40 to 70 μm. The surface is covered with cilia, and the prominent internal structure is a macronucleus. A micronucleus is also present. Two pulsating, contractile vacuoles are also seen in fresh preparations of the trophozoites. The cyst is smaller (40 to 60 μm in diameter), is surrounded by a clear refractile wall, and has a single nucleus in the cytoplasm. *B. coli* is a large organism compared with other intestinal protozoa and is readily detected in fresh, wet microscopic preparations.

Treatment, Prevention, and Control

The drug of choice is tetracycline; iodoquinol and metronidazole are alternative antimicrobials. Actions for prevention and control are similar to those for amebiasis. Appropriate personal hygiene, maintenance of sanitary conditions, and the careful monitoring of pig feces are all important preventive measures.

COCCIDIA

Coccidia constitute a very large group called *Apicomplexa*, some members of which are discussed in this section with the intestinal parasites and others with the blood and tissue parasites. All coccidia demonstrate typical characteristics, especially the existence of asexual (schizogony) and sexual (gametogony) reproduction.

Most members of the group also share alternative hosts; for example, in malaria, mosquitoes harbor the sexual cycle and humans the asexual cycle. Coccidia discussed in this chapter are *Isospora, Sarcocystis, Cryptosporidium, Cyclospora,* and *Blastocystis* species.

Isospora belli

Physiology and Structure

I. belli is a coccidian parasite of the intestinal epithelium. Both sexual and asexual reproduction in the intestinal epithelium can occur, resulting in tissue damage (Figure 75-9). The end product of gametogenesis is the oocyst, which is the diagnostic stage present in fecal specimens.

Epidemiology

Isospora organisms are distributed worldwide but are infrequently detected in stool specimens. Recently, however, this parasite has been reported with increasing frequency in healthy and immunocompromised patients. This is probably due to the increased awareness of disease caused by *Isospora* species in patients with AIDS. Infection with this organism follows ingestion of contaminated food or water or oral-anal sexual contact.

Clinical Syndromes

Infected individuals may be asymptomatic carriers or suffer mild to severe gastrointestinal disease. Disease most commonly mimics giardiasis, with a malabsorption syndrome characterized by loose, foul-smelling stools. Chronic diarrhea with weight loss, anorexia, malaise, and

FIGURE 75-10 Immature oocyst of *Isospora* species. Oocysts are ovoid (approximately 25 μm long and 15 μm wide) with tapering ends. A developing sporocyst is seen within the cytoplasm. (From Lennette EH et al: *Manual of clinical microbiology,* ed 4, Washington, DC, 1985, American Society for Microbiology.)

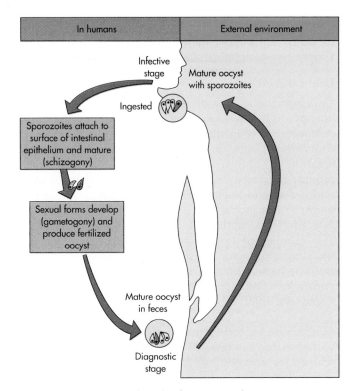

FIGURE 75-11 Life cycle of *Cryptosporidium* species.

fatigue can be seen, although it is difficult to separate this presentation from the patient's underlying disease.

Laboratory Diagnosis

Careful examination of concentrated stool sediment and special staining with iodine or a modified acid-fast procedure reveal the parasite (Figure 75-10). Small bowel biopsy has been used to establish the diagnosis when the results of tests on stool specimens are negative.

Treatment, Prevention, and Control

The drug of choice is trimethoprim-sulfamethoxazole, with the combination of pyrimethamine and sulfadiazine an acceptable alternative. Prevention and control are effected by maintaining personal hygiene and highly sanitary conditions and by avoiding oral-anal sexual contact.

Sarcocystis Species

Physician awareness of the genus *Sarcocystis* is important only in recognizing that it can be detected in stool specimens. *Sarcocystis* species can be isolated from pigs and cattle and are identical in all aspects to *Isospora* species with one exception: *Sarcocystis* oocysts rupture before passage in stool specimens, and only sporocysts are present.

Cryptosporidium Species
Physiology and Structure

The life cycle of *Cryptosporidium* species is typical of coccidians, as is the intestinal disease, but this species differs in the intracellular location in the epithelial cells. In contrast to the deep intracellular invasion observed with *Isospora* species, *Cryptosporidium* organisms are found just within the brush border of the intestinal epithelium. The coccidia attach to the surface of the cells and replicate by a process that involves schizogony (Figure 75-11).

Epidemiology

Cryptosporidium species are distributed worldwide. Infection is reported in a wide variety of animals, including mammals, reptiles, and fish. Waterborne transmission of cryptosporidiosis is now well documented as an important route of infection. The recent massive outbreak of cryptosporidiosis in Milwaukee (approximately 300,000 individuals infected) was linked to contamination of the municipal water supply. Cryptosporidia are resistant to the usual water-purification procedures (chlorination and ozone), and it is believed that runoff of local waste and surface water into municipal water supplies is an important source of contamination. Zoonotic spread from animal reservoirs to humans, as well as person-to-person spread by fecal-oral and oral-anal routes, is also common means of infection. Veterinary personnel, animal handlers, and homosexuals are at particularly high risk for infection. Many outbreaks have now been described in day-care centers where fecal-oral transmission is common.

Clinical Syndromes

As with other protozoan infections, exposure to *Cryptosporidium* organisms may result in asymptomatic carriage. Disease in previously healthy individuals is usually a mild, self-limiting enterocolitis characterized by watery diarrhea without blood. Spontaneous remission after an average of 10 days is characteristic. In contrast, disease in immunocompromised patients (e.g., patients with AIDS), characterized by 50 or more stools per day and tremendous fluid loss, can be severe and last for months to years. In some patients with AIDS, disseminated *Cryptosporidium* infections have been reported.

Laboratory Diagnosis

Cryptosporidium may be detected in large numbers in unconcentrated stool specimens obtained from immunocompromised individuals with diarrhea. Oocysts may be concentrated with the modified zinc sulfate centrifugal flotation technique or by Sheather's sugar flotation procedure. Specimens may be stained using the modified acid-fast method (Figure 75-12) or by an indirect immunofluorescence assay. An enzyme immunoassay for detecting fecal antigen is also commercially available. The number of oocysts shed in stool may fluctuate; therefore a minimum of three specimens should be examined. Serological procedures for diagnosing and monitoring infections are under investigation but are not yet widely available.

Treatment, Prevention, and Control

Unfortunately, no broadly effective therapy has been developed for managing *Cryptosporidium* infections in immunocompromised patients. No controlled studies have been published, and all therapeutic information is based on isolated reports and anecdotal information. Spiramycin may help control the diarrhea in some patients in the early stages of AIDS who have cryptosporidiosis but is ineffective in patients who have progressed to the later stages of AIDS. Spiramycin was no more effective than placebo in treating cryptosporidial diarrhea in infants. Reports concerning efficacy of oral paromomycin are promising, but these need confirmation. Therapy consists primarily of supportive measures to restore the tremendous fluid loss from the watery diarrhea.

Because of the widespread distribution of this organism in humans and other animals, preventing infection is difficult. The same methods of improved personal hygiene and sanitation used for other intestinal protozoa should be maintained for this disease. Contaminated water supplies should be treated with chlorination and filtration. In addition, avoidance of high-risk sexual activities is critical.

Cyclospora Species
Physiology and Structure

Cyclospora is a coccidian parasite that is taxonomically related to *Isospora* species and *Cryptosporidium parvum*. A single species infecting humans, *C. cayetanensis*, has been identified thus far.

Although the details of its life cycle have yet to be determined, *Cyclospora* organisms are similar to *Isospora* in that oocysts are excreted unsporulated and require a period of time outside the host for maturation to occur. The pathogenic mechanisms by which *Cyclospora* species causes clinical illness are unknown; however, the organism usually infects the upper small bowel and causes pronounced histopathological changes. The organism is found within vacuoles in the cytoplasm of jejunal epithelial cells, and its presence is associated with inflammatory changes, villous atrophy, and crypt hyperplasia.

The morphological characteristics of *Cyclospora* species are similar to those of *Isopora* species and *C. parvum* with a few exceptions. The oocysts of *Cyclospora* species are spherical and are 8 to 10 μm in diameter as opposed to the smaller oocysts of *C. parvum* (4 to 6 μm) and the much larger elliptical oocysts of *Isospora* species (20 to 30 × 10 to 19 μm). The oocysts of *Cyclospora* species contain two sporocysts, each of which contain two sporozoites, which in turn contain a membrane-bound nucleus and micronemes characteristic of the apicomplexans. In contrast, the *Cryptosporidium* oocyst contains four naked, or nonencysted, sporozoites, whereas the *Isospora* oocyst contains two sporocysts, each containing four sporozoites.

Epidemiology

As with *Cryptosporidium*, *Cyclospora* species is widely distributed throughout the world and infects a variety of reptiles, birds, and mammals. Although direct animal-to-human or person-to-person transmission has not been documented, there is now compelling evidence that *Cyclospora* infection is acquired through contaminated water. In areas of endemicity, such as Nepal, studies have documented an annual surge of cyclosporiasis that coincides with the rainy season. The prevalence of infection (symptomatic and asymptomatic) ranges from 2% to 18% in endemic areas and is estimated at 0.1% to 0.5% in developed countries. Recent outbreaks in the United States have occurred during the summer months, and although no source has been identified, transmission via contaminated water has been suggested. Like *Cryptosporidium*, *Cyclospora* species is resistant to chlorination and is not readily detected by methods used currently to ensure the safety of supplies of drinking water.

Clinical Syndromes

The clinical manifestations of cyclosporiasis resemble those of cryptosporidiosis and include mild nausea,

FIGURE 75-12 Acid-fast stained *Cryptosporidium* oocysts (approximately 5 to 7 μm in diameter).

anorexia, abdominal cramping, and watery diarrhea. Fatigue, malaise, flatulence, and bloating have also been reported. In immunocompetent hosts, diarrhea is self-limited but may be prolonged and last for weeks. Among immunocompromised people, specifically patients infected with the human immunodeficiency virus (HIV), clinical illness is typically prolonged and severe and is associated with a high rate of recurrence. Biliary tract infection with *Cyclospora* infection has been reported in two patients with AIDS.

Laboratory Diagnosis

The diagnosis of cyclosporiasis is based on the microscopic detection of oocysts in stool. Oocysts may be detected by light microscopic examination of unstained fecal material (wet mount), where they appear as nonrefractile, spherical to oval, slightly wrinkled bodies measuring 8 to 10 μm in diameter; they have an internal cluster of membrane-bound globules (Figure 75-13). In fresh specimens, *Cyclospora* organisms fluoresce when examined with an ultraviolet fluorescence microscope fitted with a 365-nm excitation filter.

Cyclospora oocysts may be concentrated with the modified zinc sulfate centrifugal flotation technique or by Sheather's sugar flotation procedure. Organisms are acid-fast and thus can be detected using one of the many acid-fast staining techniques, including the modified Ziehl-Neelsen stain or the Kinyoun acid-fast stain (Figure 75-14). A distinguishing feature of *Cyclospora* species is its variable appearance on acid-fast staining, which ranges from unstained to mottled pink to deep red.

The relative sensitivity, specificity, and predictive value of the various methods for diagnosing *Cyclospora* infection are not known. Currently, there are no immunodiagnostic techniques to aid in the diagnosis and monitoring of these infections. The rudimentary nature of the available diagnostic techniques and the incomplete understanding of the disease process may contribute to underrecognition of *Cyclospora* infection.

Treatment, Prevention, and Control

The effectiveness of trimethoprim-sulfamethoxazole has been demonstrated in anecdotal reports; in a large, open-label study of patients infected with HIV; and in a placebo-controlled trial. In HIV-infected patients, it appears that the high rate of recurrence can be attenuated with long-term suppressive therapy with trimethoprim-sulfamethoxazole. Although numerous additional agents, including metronidazole, norfloxacin, quinacrine, nalidixic acid, tinidazole, and diloxanide furoate, have been used in various trials, the effectiveness of any one of these agents has not been proved.

As with *Cryptosporidium* species, prevention of *Cyclospora* infection is difficult. Although *Cyclospora* organisms appear resistant to chlorination, the treatment of water supplies with chlorination and filtration remains a reasonable practice. In addition, the same methods of improved personal hygiene and sanitation used for other intestinal protozoa should be used as preventive measures for this disease.

Blastocystis hominis

Blastocystis hominis, previously regarded as a nonpathogenic yeast, is now the center of considerable controversy concerning its taxonomic position and its pathogenicity. The organism is found in stool specimens from asymptomatic individuals, as well as from persons with persistent diarrhea. It has been suggested that the presence of large numbers of these parasites (five or more per oil-immersion microscopic field) in the absence of other

FIGURE 75-13 Sporulated oocyst of *C. cayetanensis*. The oocysts measure 8 to 10 μm in diameter and contain two sporocysts with two sporozoites. (Saline wet mount; ×900.) (Courtesy Mr J Williams; from Peters W, Giles HM: *Color atlas of tropical medicine and parasitology,* ed 4, London, 1995, Mosby-Wolfe.)

FIGURE 75-14 Oocysts of *C. parvum (lower left)* and *Cyclospora cayetanensis (upper right)*. Both parasites stain red with Ziehl-Neelsen stain; however, *Cyclospora* organisms typically take up variable amounts of the stain, and the oocysts are larger (8 to 10 μm compared with 4 to 6 μm). (Courtesy Mr J Williams; from Peters W, Giles HM: *Color atlas of tropical medicine and parasitology,* ed 4, London, 1995, Mosby-Wolfe.)

intestinal pathogens indicates disease. Other investigators have concluded that "symptomatic blastocystosis" is attributable to an undetected pathogen or functional bowel problems. The organism may be detected in wet mounts or trichrome-stained smears of fecal specimens. Treatment with iodoquinol or metronidazole has been successful in eradicating the organisms from the intestine and alleviating symptoms. However, the definitive role of this organism in disease remains to be demonstrated.

MICROSPORIDIA

Physiology and Structure

Microsporidia are obligate intracellular pathogens belonging to the phylum Microspora. They are considered to be primitive eukaryotic organisms because they lack mitochondria, peroxisomes, Golgi membranes, and other typically eukaryotic organelles. The parasites are characterized by the structure of their spores, which have a complex tubular extrusion mechanism used for injecting the infective material (sporoplasma) into cells. Microsporidia have been detected in human tissues and implicated as participants in human disease. To date, five genera of microsporidia have been reported in humans: *Encephalitozoon, Pleistophora, Nosema, Septata,* and *Enterocytozoon.*

Pathogenesis

Infection with microsporidia is initiated by the ingestion of spores. After ingestion, the spores pass into the duodenum, where the sporoplasm with its nuclear material is injected into an adjacent cell in the small intestine. Once inside a suitable host cell, the microsporidia multiply extensively either within a parasitophorous vacuole or free within the cytoplasm. The intracellular multiplication includes a phase of repeated divisions by binary fission (merogony) and a phase culminating in spore formation (sporogony). The parasites spread from cell to cell, causing cell death and local inflammation. Although some species are highly selective in the cell type that they invade, collectively the Microspora are capable of infecting every organ of the body, and disseminated infections have been described in severely immunocompromised individuals. After sporogony the mature spores containing the infective sporoplasm may be excreted into the environment, thus continuing the cycle.

Epidemiology

Microsporidia are distributed worldwide and have a wide host range among invertebrate and vertebrate animals. Of the five genera, only *Enterocytozoon* and *Septata* are unique to humans. *Enterocytozoon bieneusi* and *Septata intestinalis* have gained increasing attention as causes of chronic diarrhea in patients with AIDS. Both *Encephalitozoon*-like and *Septata*-like organisms have been reported in the tissues of AIDS patients with hepatitis and peritonitis. *Pleistophora* organisms were the cause of myositis in an individual with AIDS. *Nosema* species has caused localized keratitis as well as dissemi-

FIGURE 75-15 Gram-positive spores of microsporidia *(arrow)* in jejunal biopsy. (Brown-Brenn stain; ×1750.) (From Weber R et al: *New Engl J Med* 326:161-166, 1992.)

nated infection in a child with severe combined immunodeficiency. *Microsporidium* species and *Encephalitozoon hellem* have caused infection of the human cornea.

Although the reservoir for human infection is unknown, transmission is likely accomplished by ingestion of spores that have been shed in the urine and feces of infected animals or individuals. As with cryptosporidial infection, individuals with AIDS and other cellular immune defects appear to be at increased risk for infection with microsporidia.

Clinical Syndromes

Clinical signs and symptoms of microsporidiosis are quite variable in the few human cases reported. Intestinal infection caused by *E. bieneusi* and *S. intestinalis* in patients with AIDS is marked by persistent and debilitating diarrhea similar to that seen in patients with cryptosporidiosis and isosporiasis. The clinical presentation of infection with other species of Microspora depends on the organ system involved and ranges from localized ocular pain and loss of vision (*Microsporidium* and *Nosema* species) to neurological disturbances and hepatitis *(Encephalitozoon cuniculi)* to a more generalized picture of dissemination with fever, vomiting, diarrhea, and malabsorption (*Nosema* species). In a report of disseminated infection with *Nosema connori*, the organism was observed involving the muscles of the stomach, bowel, arteries, diaphragm, and heart and the parenchymal cells of the liver, lungs, and adrenal glands.

Laboratory Diagnosis

Diagnosis of microsporidia infection may be made by detection of the organisms in biopsy material and by light microscopic examination of cerebrospinal fluid and urine. Spores measuring between 1.0 and 2.0 μm may be visualized by Gram (gram-positive), acid fast, periodic

FIGURE 75-16 Smear of formalin-fixed stool specimen showing pinkish-red–stained microsporidia spores, some with a distinct pinkish, beltlike stripe *(arrow)*. Bacteria are stained a faint green. (Chromotrope-based stain; ×1800.) (From Weber R et al: *New Engl J Med* 326:161-166, 1992.)

acid–Schiff, immunochemical, and Giemsa staining techniques (Figure 75-15). Recently a new chromotrope-based staining technique for light-microscopic detection of *E. bieneusi* and *S. intestinalis* spores in stool and duodenal aspirates was described (Figure 75-16). Electron microscopy is considered the gold standard for diagnostic confirmation of microsporidiosis; however, its sensitivity is unknown. Additional diagnostic techniques, including polymerase chain reaction, culture, and serological testing, are under investigation. These techniques are not yet considered reliable enough for routine diagnosis.

Treatment, Prevention, and Control

There is no known effective treatment for microsporidian infections. Treatment with metronidazole has resulted in temporary improvement in patients with intestinal microsporidiosis. Likewise, some patients treated with sulfa drugs have survived. Preliminary reports with albendazole also appear promising. In vitro studies have demonstrated activity of trimethoprim-sulfisoxazole and the antibiotic fumagillin against *E. cuniculi,* but these results have not been confirmed in vivo.

As with *Cryptosporidium,* preventing microsporidian infection is difficult. The same methods of improved personal hygiene and sanitation used for other intestinal protozoa should be maintained with this disease.

CASE STUDY AND QUESTIONS

A 31-year-old female veterinarian complained of diarrhea that she had experienced for 2 weeks. The diarrhea was described as thin, watery, and nonbloody. The patient described 10 to 14 diarrheal stools per day, the frequency of which was not influenced by a variety of over-the-counter antidiarrheal medications.

Physical examination revealed a well-developed, well-nourished woman who appeared somewhat fatigued and mildly dehydrated. The workup included a negative HIV serological test, a normal flexible sigmoidoscope examination, and a negative stool culture for bacterial pathogens. A microscopic examination of the stool for white blood cells was negative, as was a test for *Clostridium difficile* toxin. A stool specimen was sent for ova and parasite examination and, after appropriate concentration measures, demonstrated acid-fast oocysts.

1. Which parasite was found in the patient's stool?
2. What was the likely source of this individual's infection?
3. If this individual were HIV positive, what other intestinal pathogens would have been considered?
4. Other than conventional microscopy, what other methods could have been used to diagnose this infection?
5. Should this patient have received specific antimicrobial therapy? If so, what would have been prescribed? If not, why not?

Bibliography

Bruckner DA: Amebiasis, *Clin Microbiol Rev* 5:356-369, 1992.

Current WL, Garcia LS: Cryptosporidiosis, *Clin Microbiol Rev* 4:325-358, 1991.

Gay JD et al: *Entamoeba polecki* infections in Southeast Asian refugees: multiple cases of a rarely reported parasite, *Mayo Clin Proc* 60:523-530, 1985.

Hayes EB et al: Large community outbreak of cryptosporidiosis due to contamination of a filtered public water supply, *N Engl J Med* 320:1372-1376, 1989.

John DT, De Jonckheere JF: Isolation of *Naegleria australiensis* from an Oklahoma lake, *J Protozool* 32:571-575, 1985.

Markell EK, Voge M, John DT: *Medical parasitology,* ed 7, Philadelphia, 1992, WB Saunders.

May LP, Sidhu GS, Buchness MR: Diagnosis of *Acanthamoeba* infection by cutaneous manifestations in a man seropositive to HIV, *J Am Acad Dermatol* 26:352-355, 1992.

McLaren LC: Isolation of *Trichomonas vaginalis* from the respiratory tract of infants with respiratory disease, *Pediatrics* 71:888-890, 1983.

Ortega YR et al: *Cyclospora* spp.: a new protozoan pathogen of humans, *N Engl J Med* 328:1308-1312, 1993.

Osterholm MT et al: An outbreak of food-borne giardiasis, *N Engl J Med* 304:24-28, 1981.

Peters W, Giles HM: *Color atlas of tropical medicine and parasitology,* ed 4, London, 1995, Mosby-Wolfe.

Schwartz DA et al: Pathology of microsporidiosis: emerging parasitic infections in patients with acquired immunodeficiency syndrome, *Arch Pathol Lab Med* 120:173-188, 1996.

Soave R: Cyclospora: an overview, *Clin Infect Dis* 23:429-437, 1996.

Weber R et al: Improved light-microscopical detection of microsporidia spores in stool and duodenal aspirate, *N Engl J Med* 326:161-166, 1992.

Weber R et al: Human microsporidial infections, *Clin Microbiol Rev* 7:426-461, 1994.

Wolfe MS: Giardiasis, *Clin Microbiol Rev* 5:93-100, 1992.

Yang J, Scholten T: *Dientamoeba fragilis:* a review with notes on its epidemiology, pathogenicity, mode of transmission, and diagnosis, *Am J Trop Med Hyg* 26:16-22, 1977.

Blood and Tissue Protozoa

The protozoa of blood and tissues are closely related to the intestinal protozoan parasites in practically all aspects except for their sites of infection (Box 76-1). The malaria parasites (*Plasmodium* species) infect both blood and tissues.

PLASMODIUM SPECIES

Plasmodia are coccidian or sporozoan parasites of blood cells, and as seen with other coccidia, they require two hosts: the mosquito for the sexual reproductive stages and humans and other animals for the asexual reproductive stages.

The four species of plasmodia that infect humans are *P. vivax, P. ovale, P. malariae,* and *P. falciparum* (Table 76-1). These species share a common life cycle, as illustrated in Figure 76-1. Human infection is initiated by the bite of an *Anopheles* mosquito, which introduces infectious plasmodia sporozoites via its saliva into the circulatory system. The sporozoites are carried to the parenchymal cells of the liver, where asexual reproduction (schizogony) occurs. This phase of growth is termed the *exoerythrocytic cycle* and lasts 8 to 25 days, depending on the plasmodial species. Some species (e.g., *P. vivax, P. ovale*) can establish a dormant hepatic phase in which the sporozoites (called **hypnozoites** or *sleeping forms*) do not divide. The presence of these viable plasmodia can lead to the relapse of infections months to years after the initial clinical disease (**relapsing malaria**). The hepatocytes eventually rupture, liberating the plasmodia (termed **merozoites** at this stage), which in turn attach to specific receptors on the surface of erythrocytes and enter the cells, thus initiating the erythrocytic cycle.

Asexual replication progresses through a series of stages (ring, trophozoite, schizont) that culminates in the rupture of the erythrocyte, releasing up to 24 merozoites, which initiates another cycle of replication by infecting other erythrocytes. Some merozoites also develop within erythrocytes into male and female gametocytes. If a mosquito ingests mature male and female gametocytes during a blood meal, the sexual reproductive cycle of malaria can be initiated, with the eventual production of sporozoites infectious for humans. This sexual reproductive stage within the mosquito is necessary for the maintenance of malaria within a population.

Most malaria seen in the United States is acquired by visitors or residents of countries with endemic disease (**imported malaria**). However, the appropriate vector *Anopheles* mosquito is found in several sections of the United States, and domestic transmission of disease has been observed (**introduced malaria**). In addition to transmission by mosquitos, malaria can also be acquired by blood transfusions from an infected donor (**transfusion malaria**). This type of transmission can also occur among narcotic addicts who share needles and syringes (**"mainline" malaria**). Congenital acquisition, although rare, is also a possible mode of transmission (**congenital malaria**).

Plasmodium vivax

Physiology and Structure

P. vivax (Figure 76-2) is selective in that it invades only young, immature erythrocytes. In infections caused by *P. vivax,* infected red blood cells are usually enlarged and contain numerous pink granules or Schüffner's dots, the trophozoite is ring shaped but amoeboid in appearance, more mature trophozoites and erythrocytic schizonts containing up to 24 merozoites are present, and the gametocytes are round. These characteristics are helpful in identifying the specific plasmodial species, which is important for the treatment of malaria.

Epidemiology

P. vivax is the most prevalent of the human plasmodia with the widest geographical distribution, including the tropics, subtropics, and temperate regions.

Clinical Syndromes

After an incubation period (usually 10 to 17 days) the patient experiences vague influenza-like symptoms with headache, muscle pains, photophobia, anorexia, nausea, and vomiting.

As the infection progresses, increased numbers of rupturing erythrocytes liberate merozoites as well as toxic cellular debris and hemoglobin into the circulation. Together, these produce the typical pattern of chills, fever, and malarial rigors. These paroxysms usually reappear periodically (generally every 48 hours) as the cycle of infection, replication, and cell lysis progresses. The paroxysms may remain relatively mild or progress to severe attacks, with hours of sweating, chills, shaking, persistently high temperatures (103° to 106° F), and exhaustion.

P. vivax causes **"benign tertian malaria,"** which refers to the cycle of paroxysms every 48 hours (in untreated patients) and the fact that most patients tolerate the attacks and can survive for years without treatment. If left untreated, however, chronic *P. vivax* infections can lead to brain, kidney, and liver damage as a result of the malarial pigment, cellular debris, and capillary plugging of these organs by masses of adherent erythrocytes.

Laboratory Diagnosis

Microscopic examination of thick and thin films of blood is the method of choice for confirming the clinical diagnosis of malaria and identifying the specific species responsible for disease. The thick film is a concentration method and may be used to detect the presence of organisms. With training, thick films may be used to diagnose the species as well. The thin film is most useful for establishing species identification. Blood films can be taken at any time over the course of the infection, but the best time is midway between paroxysms of chills and fever, when the greatest number of intracellular organisms are present. It may be necessary to take repeated films at intervals of 4 to 6 hours.

Serological procedures are available, but they are used primarily for epidemiological surveys or for screening blood donors. Serological findings usually remain positive for approximately a year, even after complete treatment of the infection.

Treatment, Prevention, and Control

The treatment of *P. vivax* infection involves a combination of supportive measures and chemotherapy. Bed rest, relief of fever and headache, regulation of fluid balance, and in some cases, blood transfusion are supportive therapies.

The chemotherapeutic regimens are as follows:
1. Suppressive—aimed at avoiding infection and clinical symptoms (i.e., a form of prophylaxis)

BOX 76-1   Medically Important Blood and Tissue Protozoa

Plasmodium species	*Sarcocystis* species
Babesia species	*Leishmania* species
Toxoplasma species	*Trypanosoma* species

TABLE 76-1   Human Malarial Parasites

PARASITE	DISEASE
P. vivax	Benign tertian malaria
P. ovale	Benign tertian or ovale malaria
P. malariae	Quartan or malarial malaria
P. falciparum	Malignant tertian malaria

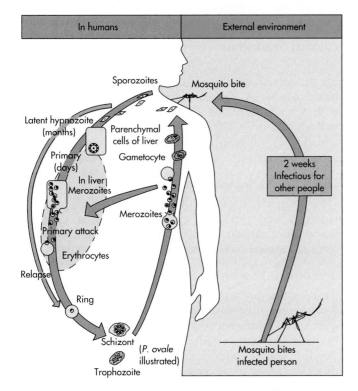

FIGURE 76-1 Life cycle of *Plasmodium* species.

FIGURE 76-2 *P. vivax* ring forms and young trophozoites. Note the multiple stages of the parasite seen in the peripheral blood smear, the enlarged parasitized erythrocytes, and the presence of Schüffner's dots with the trophozoite form. These are characteristic of *P. vivax* infections.

2. Therapeutic—aimed at eradicating the erythrocytic cycle
3. Radical cure—aimed at eradicating the exoerythrocytic cycle in the liver
4. Gametocidal—aimed at destroying erythrocytic gametocytes to prevent mosquito transmission

Chloroquine is the drug of choice for the suppression and therapeutic treatment of *P. vivax,* followed by primaquine for radical cure and elimination of gametocytes. Recent reports suggest the emergence of chloroquine-resistant forms of *P.* vivax in Indonesia, the Solomon islands, New Guinea, and Brazil. Patients infected with chloroquine-resistant *P. vivax* may be treated with other agents, including mefloquine, quinine, pyrimethamine-sulfadoxine (Fansidar), and doxycycline. Primaquine is especially effective in preventing a relapse from the latent forms of *P. vivax* in the liver. Because antimalarial drugs are potentially toxic, it is imperative that physicians carefully review the recommended therapeutic regimens.

Chemoprophylaxis and prompt eradication of infections are critical in breaking the mosquito-human transmission cycle. Control of mosquito breeding and protection of individuals by screening, netting, protective clothing, and insect repellents are also essential. Immigrants from and travelers to endemic areas must be carefully screened, using blood films or serological tests to detect possible infection. The development of vaccines to protect persons living in or traveling to endemic areas is under investigation.

Plasmodium ovale
Physiology and Structure

P. ovale is similar to *P. vivax* in many respects, including its selectivity for young, pliable erythrocytes. As a consequence, the host cell becomes enlarged and distorted, usually in an oval form. Schüffner's dots appear as pale pink granules, and the cell border is frequently fimbriated or ragged. The schizont of *P. ovale,* when mature, contains about half the number of merozoites seen in *P. vivax.*

Epidemiology

P. ovale is distributed primarily in tropical Africa, where it is often more prevalent than *P. vivax.* It is also found in Asia and South America.

Clinical Syndromes

The clinical picture of tertian attacks for *P.* ovale (**benign tertian or ovale malaria**) infection is similar to that for *P. vivax.* Untreated infections last only about a year instead of the several years for *P. vivax.* Both relapse and recrudescence phases are similar to *P. vivax.*

Laboratory Diagnosis

As with *P. vivax,* thick and thin blood films are examined for the typical oval host cell with Schüffner's dots and a ragged cell wall. Serological tests reveal cross-reaction with *P. vivax* and other plasmodia.

Treatment, Prevention, and Control

The treatment regimen, including the use of primaquine to prevent relapse from latent liver forms, is similar to that used for *P. vivax* infections. Preventing *P. ovale* infection involves the same measures as for *P. vivax* and other plasmodia.

Plasmodium malariae
Physiology and Structure

In contrast with *P. vivax* and *P. ovale, P. malariae* can infect only mature erythrocytes with relatively rigid cell membranes. As a result, the parasite's growth must conform to the size and shape of the red blood cell. This produces no red cell enlargement or distortion, as seen in *P. vivax* and *P. ovale,* but it does result in distinctive shapes of the parasite seen in the host cell: "band and bar forms" as well as very compact, dark-staining forms. The schizont of *P. malariae* shows no red cell enlargement or distortion and is usually composed of eight merozoites appearing in a rosette. Occasionally, reddish granules called *Ziemann's dots* appear in the host cell.

Unlike for *P. vivax* and *P. ovale,* hypnozoites for *P. malariae* are not found in the liver, and relapse does not occur. Recrudescence does occur, and attacks may develop after apparent abatement of symptoms.

Epidemiology

P. malariae infection occurs primarily in the same subtropical and temperate regions as the other plasmodia but is less prevalent.

Clinical Syndromes

The incubation period for *P. malariae* is the longest of the plasmodia, usually 18 to 40 days but possibly several months to years. The early symptoms are influenza-like, with fever patterns of 72 hours (**quartan** or **malarial malaria**) in periodicity. Attacks are moderate to severe and last several hours. Untreated infections may last as long as 20 years.

Laboratory Diagnosis

Observing the characteristic bar and band forms and the rosette schizont in thick and thin films of blood establishes the diagnosis of *P. malariae* infection. As noted serological tests cross-react with other plasmodia.

Treatment, Prevention, and Control

Treatment is similar to that for *P. vivax* and *P. ovale* infections and must be undertaken to prevent recrudescent infections. Treatment to prevent relapse caused by latent liver forms is not required because these forms do not develop with *P. malariae.* Preventive and controlling mechanisms are as discussed for *P. vivax* and *P. ovale.*

Plasmodium falciparum
Physiology and Structure

P. falciparum demonstrates no selectivity in host erythrocytes and invades any red blood cell at any stage in its existence. Also, multiple sporozoites can infect a single erythrocyte. Thus three or even four small rings may be seen in an infected cell. *P. falciparum* is often seen in the host cell at the very edge or periphery of the cell membrane, appearing almost as if it were "stuck" on the outside of the cell. This is called the *appliqué* or *accolé position* and is distinctive for this species.

Growing trophozoite stages and schizonts of *P. falciparum* are rarely seen in blood films because their forms are sequestered in the liver and spleen. Only in very heavy infections are they found in the peripheral circulation. Thus peripheral blood smears from patients with *P. falciparum* malaria characteristically contain only young ring forms and occasionally gametocytes. The typical crescentic gametocytes are diagnostic for the species. Infected red blood cells do not enlarge and become distorted like they do with *P. vivax* and *P. ovale.* Occasionally, reddish granules known as *Maurer's dots* are observed in *P. falciparum.*

P. falciparum, like *P. malariae*, does not produce hypnozoites in the liver. Relapses from the liver are not known to occur.

Epidemiology

P. falciparum occurs almost exclusively in tropical and subtropical regions.

Clinical Syndromes

The incubation period of *P. falciparum* is the shortest of all the plasmodia, ranging from 7 to 10 days, and does not extend for months to years. After the early influenza-like symptoms, *P. falciparum* rapidly produces daily (quotidian) chills and fever as well as severe nausea, vomiting, and diarrhea. The periodicity of the attacks then becomes tertian (36 to 48 hours), and fulminating disease develops. The term *malignant tertian malaria* is appropriate for this infection. Because the symptoms of this type of malaria are similar to those of intestinal infections, the nausea, vomiting, and diarrhea have led to the observation that malaria is "the malignant mimic."

Although any malaria infection may be fatal, *P. falciparum* is the most likely to result in death if left untreated. The increased numbers of erythrocytes infected and destroyed result in toxic cellular debris, adherence of red blood cells to vascular endothelium and to adjacent red blood cells, and formation of capillary plugging by masses of red blood cells, platelets, leukocytes, and malarial pigment.

Involvement of the brain (**cerebral malaria**) is most often seen in *P. falciparum* infection. Capillary plugging from an accumulation of malarial pigment and masses of cells can result in coma and death.

Kidney damage is also associated with *P. falciparum* malaria, resulting in an illness called **blackwater fever.** Intravascular hemolysis with rapid destruction of red blood cells produces a marked hemoglobinuria and can result in acute renal failure, tubular necrosis, nephrotic syndrome, and death. Liver involvement is characterized by abdominal pain, vomiting of bile, severe diarrhea, and rapid dehydration.

Laboratory Diagnosis

Thick and thin blood films are searched for the characteristic rings of *P. falciparum,* which frequently occur in multiples within a single cell, as well as in the accolé position (Figure 76-3). Also diagnostic are the distinctive crescentic gametocytes (Figure 76-4).

Laboratory personnel must perform a thorough search of the blood films because mixed infections can occur with any combination of the four species, but most often the combination is *P. falciparum* and *P. vivax.* The detection and proper reporting of a mixed infection directly affects the treatment chosen.

Treatment, Prevention, and Control

The treatment of malaria is based on the history regarding travel to endemic areas, prompt clinical review and differential diagnosis, accurate and rapid laboratory work, and correct use of antimalarial drugs.

Because chloroquine-resistant strains of *P. falciparum* are present in many parts of the world, physicians must review all current protocols for the proper treat-

FIGURE 76-3 Ring forms of *P. falciparum.* Note the multiple ring forms within the individual erythrocytes, which is characteristic this of organism.

FIGURE 76-4 Mature gametocyte of *P. falciparum.* The presence of this sausage-shaped form is diagnostic of *P. falciparum* malaria.

ment of *P. falciparum* infections, noting particularly where chloroquine resistance is known to occur. If the patient's history indicates that the origin is *not* from a chloroquine-resistant area, the drug of choice is either chloroquine or parenteral quinine. Patients infected with chloroquine-resistant *P. falciparum* (or *P. vivax*) may be treated with other agents, including mefloquine, quinine, quinidine, pyrimethamine-sulfadoxine (Fansidar), and doxycycline. Because quinine and pyrimethamine-sulfadoxine are potentially toxic, they are used more often for treatment than prophylaxis. Amodiaquine, an analogue of chloroquine, is effective against chloroquine-resistant *P. falciparum;* however, toxicity limits its use. Newer agents with promising activity against multidrug-resistant strains of *P. falciparum* include halofantrine, a phenanthrenemethanol, and artemisinin, a sesquiterpene derivative of qinghaosu. They are not yet available in the United States.

When there is uncertainty whether the *P. falciparum* is chloroquine resistant, it is advisable to assume that the strain is resistant and treat the patient accordingly. If the laboratory reports a mixed infection involving *P. falciparum* and *P. vivax,* the treatment must eradicate not only *P. falciparum* from the erythrocytes but also the liver stages of *P. vivax* to avoid relapses. Failure on the part of the laboratory to detect and report such a mixed infection can result in inappropriate treatment and unnecessary delay in accomplishing a complete cure.

P. falciparum infection can be prevented and controlled exactly as for *P. vivax* and the other human malarias. Chloroquine resistance complicates the management of these patients but can be overcome by the physician's awareness of appropriate regimens.

BABESIA SPECIES

Babesia are intracellular sporozoan parasites that morphologically resemble plasmodia. Babesiosis is a zoonosis infecting a variety of animals such as deer, cattle, and rodents; humans are accidental hosts. Infection is transmitted by *Ixodid* ticks. *Babesia microti* is the usual cause of babesiosis in the United States.

Physiology and Structure

Human infection follows contact with an infected tick (Figure 76-5). The infectious pyriform bodies are introduced into the bloodstream and infect erythrocytes. The intraerythrocytic trophozoites multiply by binary fission, forming tetrads, and then lyse the erythrocyte, releasing the merozoites. These can reinfect other cells to maintain the infection. Infected cells can also be ingested by feeding ticks, in which additional replication can take place. Infection in the tick population can also be maintained by transovarian transmission. The infected cells in humans resemble the ring forms of *P. falciparum,* but malarial pigment or other stages of growth characteristically seen with plasmodial infections are not seen with careful examination of blood smears.

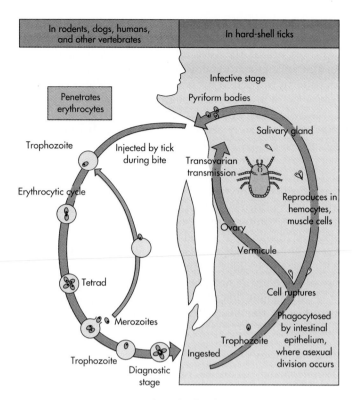

FIGURE 76-5 Life cycle of *Babesia* species.

Epidemiology

More than 70 different species of *Babesia* are found in Africa, Asia, Europe, and North America, with *B. microti* responsible for disease along the northeastern seaboard of the United States (e.g., Nantucket Island, Martha's Vineyard, Shelter Island). *Ixodes dammini* is the tick vector responsible for transmitting babesiosis in this area, and the natural reservoir hosts are field mice, voles, and other small rodents. Serological studies in endemic areas have demonstrated a high incidence of past exposure to *Babesia.* Presumably, most infections are asymptomatic or mild. *B. divergens,* which has been reported more frequently from Europe, causes severe, often fatal infections in people who have undergone splenectomies. Although most infections follow tick bites, transfusion-related infections have been demonstrated.

Clinical Syndromes

After an incubation period of 1 to 4 weeks, symptomatic patients experience general malaise, fever without periodicity, headache, chills, sweating, fatigue, and weakness. As the infection progresses with increased destruction of erythrocytes, hemolytic anemia develops, and the patient may experience renal failure. Hepatomegaly and splenomegaly can develop in advanced disease. Low-grade parasitemia may persist for weeks. Splenectomy or functional asplenia, immunosuppression, and advanced age increase a person's susceptibility to infections as well as to more severe disease.

Laboratory Diagnosis

Examination of blood smears is the diagnostic method of choice. Laboratory personnel must be experienced in differentiating *Babesia* and *Plasmodium* species. Infected patients may have negative smears because of the low-grade parasitemia. These infections can be diagnosed by inoculating samples of blood into hamsters, which are highly susceptible to infection. Serological tests are also available for diagnostic use.

Treatment, Prevention, and Control

The drugs of choice are clindamycin combined with quinine. Other antiprotozoal regimens, including chloroquine and pentamidine, have been used with variable results. However, most patients with mild disease recover without specific therapy. Exchange blood transfusion has also been successful in patients who have had splenectomies and who have severe infections caused by *B. microti* or *B. divergens*. The use of protective clothing and insect repellents can minimize tick exposure in endemic areas, which is critical for the prevention of disease. Ticks must feed on humans for several hours before the organisms are transmitted, so prompt removal of ticks can be protective.

TOXOPLASMA GONDII

T. gondii is a typical coccidian parasite related to *Plasmodium, Isospora,* and other members of the phylum Apicomplexa. *T. gondii* is an intracellular parasite, and it is found in a wide variety of animals, including birds and humans. Only one species exists, and there appears to be little strain-to-strain variation. The essential reservoir host of *T. gondii* is the common house cat and other felines.

Physiology and Structure

Organisms develop in the intestinal cells of the cat, as well as during an extraintestinal cycle with passage to the tissues via the bloodstream (Figure 76-6). The organisms from the intestinal cycle are passed in cat feces and mature into infective cysts within 3 to 4 days in the external environment. These oocysts are similar to those of *Isospora belli,* the human intestinal protozoan parasite, and can be ingested by mice and other animals (including humans) and produce acute and chronic infection of various tissues, including brain. Infection in cats is established when the tissues of infected rodents are eaten.

Some infective forms, or **trophozoites,** from the oocyst develop as slender, crescentic types called **tachyzoites.** These rapidly multiplying forms are responsible for the initial infection and the tissue damage. Slow-growing, shorter forms called **bradyzoites** also develop and form cysts in chronic infections.

Epidemiology

Human infection with *T. gondii* is ubiquitous; however, it is increasingly apparent that certain immunocompro-

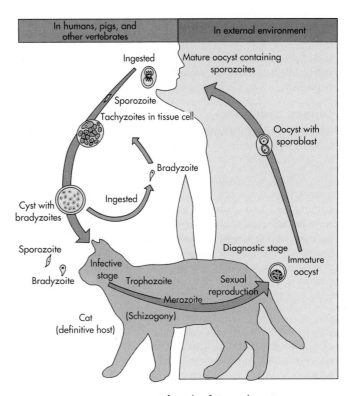

FIGURE 76-6 Life cycle of *T. gondii.*

mised individuals (patients with acquired immunodeficiency syndrome [AIDS]) are more likely to have severe manifestations. The wide variety of animals that harbor the organism—carnivores and herbivores as well as birds—accounts for the widespread transmission.

Humans become infected from two sources: (1) ingestion of improperly cooked meat from animals that serve as intermediate hosts and (2) the ingestion of infective oocysts from contaminated cat feces. Serological studies show an increased prevalence in human populations where the consumption of uncooked meat or meat juices is popular. It is noteworthy that serological tests of human and rodent populations are negative in the few geographical areas where cats have not existed. Outbreaks of toxoplasmosis in the United States are usually traced to poorly cooked meat (e.g., hamburgers) as well as contact with cat feces.

Transplacental infection can occur in pregnancy either from infection acquired from meat and meat juices or from contact with cat feces. Transfusion infection via contaminated blood can occur but is not common. Transplacental infection from an infected mother has a devastating effect on the fetus.

Although the rate of seroconversion is similar for individuals within a geographical location, the rate of severe infection is dramatically affected by the immune status of the individual. Patients with defects in cell-mediated immunity, especially those who are infected with the human immunodeficiency virus (HIV) or who have had an organ transplant or immunosuppressive therapy, are most likely to have disseminated or central nervous system (CNS) disease. Illness in this setting is generally believed to be caused by reactivation of previously latent infection rather than new exposure to the organism.

Clinical Syndromes

Most *T. gondii* infections are benign and asymptomatic, with symptoms occurring as the parasite moves in the blood to tissues, where it becomes an intracellular parasite. When symptomatic disease occurs, the infection is characterized by cell destruction, reproduction of more organisms, and eventual cyst formation. Many tissues may be affected; however, the organism has a particular predilection for cells of the lung, heart, lymphoid organs, and CNS, including the eye.

Symptoms of acute disease include chills, fever, headaches, myalgia, lymphadenitis, and fatigue; the symptoms occasionally resemble those of infectious mononucleosis. In chronic disease the signs and symptoms include lymphadenitis, occasionally a rash, evidence of hepatitis, encephalomyelitis, and myocarditis. In some of the cases, chorioretinitis appears and may lead to blindness.

Congenital infection with *T. gondii* also occurs in infants born to mothers infected during pregnancy. If infection occurs in the first trimester, the result is spontaneous abortion, stillbirth, or severe disease. Manifestations in the infant infected after the first trimester include epilepsy, encephalitis, microcephaly, intracranial calcifications, hydrocephalus, psychomotor or mental retardation, chorioretinitis, blindness, anemia, jaundice, rash, pneumonia, diarrhea, and hypothermia. Infants may be asymptomatic at birth only to develop disease months to years later. Most often these children develop chorioretinitis with or without blindness or other neurological problems, including retardation, seizures, microcephaly, and hearing loss.

In immunocompromised older patients a different spectrum of disease is seen. Reactivation of latent toxoplasmosis is a special problem for these people. The presenting symptoms of *Toxoplasma* infection in immunocompromised patients are usually neurological, most frequently consistent with diffuse encephalopathy, meningoencephalitis, or cerebral mass lesions. Reactivation of cerebral toxoplasmosis has emerged as a major cause of encephalitis in patients with AIDS. The disease is usually multifocal, with more than one mass lesion appearing in the brain at the same time. Symptoms are related to the location of the lesions and may include hemiparesis, seizures, visual impairment, confusion, and lethargy. Other sites of infection that have been reported include the eye, lung, and testes. Although disease is seen predominantly in patients with AIDS, it may also occur with similar manifestations in other immunocompromised patients, in particular those undergoing solid organ transplantation.

Laboratory Diagnosis

Serological testing is required for the diagnosis of acute active infection; the diagnosis is established by the finding of increasing antibody titers documented in serially collected blood specimens. Because contact with the organism is common, attention to increasing titers is essential to differentiate acute, active infection from previous asymptomatic or chronic infection. Currently the enzyme-linked immunoadsorbent assay (ELISA) for detecting immunoglobulin M antibodies appears to be the most reliable procedure because of its simplicity and rapidity in documenting acute infections. The test is not generally satisfactory in AIDS patients with latent or reactivated infections because they fail to produce an immunoglobulin M response or increasing immunoglobulin G titer.

Demonstration of these organisms as trophozoites and cysts in tissue and body fluids is the definitive method of diagnosis (Figure 76-7). Biopsy specimens from lymph nodes, brain, myocardium, or other suspected tissue as well as body fluids, including cerebrospinal fluid, amniotic fluid, or bronchoalveolar lavage fluid, can be directly examined for the organisms. Newer monoclonal antibody–based fluorescent stains may facilitate direct detection of *T. gondii* in tissue. Culture methods for *T. gondii* are largely experimental and not usually available in clinical laboratories. The two methods available are to inoculate potentially infected material into either mouse peritoneum or tissue culture. Advances in developing polymerase chain reaction–based detection methods are promising and may provide rapid and sensitive approaches for detecting the organism in blood, cerebrospinal fluid, amniotic fluid, and other clinical specimens.

Treatment, Prevention, and Control

The therapy for toxoplasmosis depends on the nature of the infectious process and the immunocompetence

FIGURE 76-7 Cyst of *T. gondii* in mouse brain. Hundreds of organisms may be present in the cyst, which may become active and initiate disease with decreased host immunity (e.g., immunosuppression in transplant patients and in diseases such as AIDS).

of the host. Most mononucleosis-like infections in normal hosts resolve spontaneously and do not require specific therapy. In contrast, disseminated or CNS infection in immunocompromised people must be treated. Before the association of *T. gondii* with HIV infection, immunocompromised patients with toxoplasmosis were treated for 4 to 6 weeks. In the setting of HIV infection, discontinuing therapy after 4 to 6 weeks is associated with a relapse rate of 25%. Such patients are currently treated with an initial high-dose regimen of pyrimethamine plus sulfadiazine and then continued on lower doses of both drugs indefinitely. Although this drug combination is the regimen of choice, toxicity (rash and bone marrow suppression) may necessitate changes to alternative agents. Clindamycin plus pyrimethamine is the best-studied alternative. Atovaquone and azithromycin (each alone or with pyrimethamine) also have some activity, although their efficacy and safety compared with those of clindamycin-pyrimethamine need to be assessed. Trimethoprim-sulfamethoxazole is not an acceptable alternative to pyrimethamine-sulfadiazine for treatment of disseminated or CNS toxoplasmosis. The use of corticosteroids is indicated as part of therapy of cerebral edema and ocular infections that involve or threaten the macula.

Infections in the first trimester of pregnancy are difficult to manage because of the teratogenicity of pyrimethamine in laboratory animals. Both clindamycin and spiramycin have been substituted with apparent success. Spiramycin does not appear to be effective for the treatment of toxoplasmosis in immunocompromised patients.

As more immunocompromised patients at risk for disseminated infection are identified, greater emphasis is placed on preventive measures and specific prophylaxis. Routine serological screening of patients before organ transplantation and early in the course of HIV infection is now being performed. Individuals with positive serological tests are at much higher risk for the development of disease and are now being considered for prophylaxis. Trimethoprim-sulfamethoxazole, which is also used as prophylaxis to prevent *Pneumocystis carinii* infections, also appears to be effective at preventing infections with *T. gondii*. Additional preventive measures for pregnant women and immunocompromised hosts should include avoiding the consumption and handling of raw or undercooked meat and avoiding exposure to cat feces.

SARCOCYSTIS LINDEMANNI

S. lindemanni is a typical coccidian closely related to the intestinal forms *S. suihominis*, *S. bovihominis*, and *Isospora belli* and the blood and tissue parasite *T. gondii*. *S. lindemanni* occurs worldwide in various animals, especially sheep, cattle, and pigs. Humans are accidentally infected only as the result of eating meat from these animals. Most infections are asymptomatic, but occasionally an infection may cause myositis, swelling of muscle, dyspnea, and eosinophilia. Infection of the myocardium has been observed but is extremely rare. There is no specific treatment for the muscle infection.

LEISHMANIA

The hemoflagellates are flagellated, insect-transmitted protozoa that infect blood and tissues. Three species of *Leishmania*, a protozoan hemoflagellate, produce human disease: *L. donovani*, *L. tropica*, and *L. braziliensis* (Table 76-2). The diseases are distinguished by the ability of the organism to infect deep tissues (**visceral leishmaniasis**) or replicate only in cooler superficial tissues (**cutaneous** or mucocutaneous leishmaniasis). The reservoir hosts and geographical distribution differ for the three species, but transmission by sandflies (belonging to the genera *Phlebotomus* or *Lutzomyia*) is common to all leishmanial species.

Leishmania donovani

Physiology and Structure

The life cycles of all leishmanial parasites differ in epidemiology, tissues affected, and clinical manifestations (Figure 76-8). The **promastigote** stage (long, slender form with a free flagellum) is present in the saliva of infected sandflies. Human infection is initiated by the bite of an infected sandfly, which injects the promastigotes into the skin, where they lose their flagella, enter the amastigote stage, and invade reticuloendothelial cells. Reproduction occurs in the amastigote stage, and as cells rupture, destruction of specific tissues (e.g., cutaneous tissues, visceral organs such as the liver and spleen) develops. The amastigote stage (Figure 76-9) is diagnostic for leishmaniasis, as well as the infectious stage for sandflies. Ingested amastigotes transform in the sandfly into the promastigote stage, which multiplies by binary fission in the fly midgut. After development, this stage migrates to the fly proboscis, where new human infection can be introduced during feeding.

Epidemiology

L. donovani infection of the classic kala-azar or **dumdum fever** type occurs in many parts of Asia, Africa, and Southeast Asia. Except for some rodents in Africa, there

TABLE 76-2	Leishmaniasis in Humans
PARASITE	**DISEASE**
L. donovani	Visceral leishmaniasis (kala-azar, dumdum fever)
L. tropica	Cutaneous leishmaniasis (Oriental sore, Delhi boil)
L. braziliensis	Mucocutaneous leishmaniasis (American leishmaniasis, espundia, chiclero ulcer)

are few reservoir hosts. The vector is the *Phlebotomus* sandfly. Variants of *L. donovani* are also recognized. *L. donovani infantum* is present in countries along the Mediterranean basin (European, Near Eastern, and African) and is found in parts of China and the former Soviet Union. Reservoir hosts of this organism include dogs, foxes, jackals, and porcupines. The vector is also

the *Phlebotomus* sandfly. *L. donovani chagasi* is found in South and Central America, especially Mexico and the West Indies. Reservoir hosts are dogs, foxes, and cats, and the vector is the *Lutzomyia* sandfly.

Clinical Syndromes

The incubation period for **visceral leishmaniasis** may be from several weeks to a year, with a gradual onset of fever, diarrhea, and anemia. Chills and sweating that may resemble malaria symptoms are common early in the infection. As organisms proliferate and invade cells of the liver and spleen, marked enlargement of these organs, weight loss, and emaciation occur. Kidney damage may also occur as cells of the glomeruli are invaded. With persistence of the disease, deeply pigmented, granulomatous areas of skin, referred to as *post–kala-azar dermal leishmaniasis,* occur. If untreated, visceral leishmaniasis develops into a fulminating, debilitating, and lethal disease in a few weeks or may persist as a chronic debilitating disease, leading to death in 1 or 2 years.

Laboratory Diagnosis

The amastigote stage can be demonstrated in tissue biopsy, bone marrow examination, lymph node aspiration, and thorough examination of properly stained smears. Culture of blood, bone marrow, and other tissues often demonstrates the promastigote stage of the organisms. Serological testing is also available.

Treatment, Prevention, and Control

Visceral leishmaniasis is treated with pentavalent antimonial compounds. The drug of choice is stibogluconate. Therapy is not uniformly successful, and relapse rates of 2% to 8% are seen. Alternative approaches include the addition of allopurinol or treatment with pentamidine or amphotericin B. Prompt treatment of human infections and control of reservoir hosts, along with insect control, help eliminate transmission of disease. Protection from sandflies by screening and insect repellents is also essential.

Leishmania tropica

Physiology and Structure

The life cycle of *L. tropica* is illustrated in Figure 76-8.

Epidemiology

Cutaneous leishmaniasis produced by *L. tropica* is present in many parts of Asia, Africa, Mediterranean Europe, and the southern region of the former Soviet Union. In these regions the reservoir hosts are dogs, foxes, and rodents, and the vector is the sandfly *Phlebotomus*. Two related species are also recognized. *L. aethiopica* is endemic in Ethiopia, Kenya, and Yemen, with dogs and rodents as reservoir hosts and the vector the *Phlebotomus* sandfly. *L. mexicana* occurs in South and Central America, especially in the Amazon basin, with sloths, rodents, monkeys, and raccoons as reservoir hosts. The vector is the *Lutzomyia* sandfly.

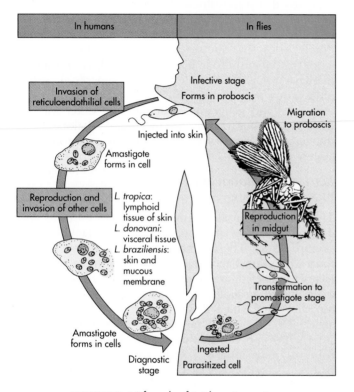

FIGURE 76-8 Life cycle of *Leishmania* species.

FIGURE 76-9 Giemsa-stained amastigotes (Leishman-Donovan bodies) of *L. donovani* present in bone marrow. A small, dark-staining kinetoplast can be seen next to the spherical nucleus in some parasites. (From Ash LR, Orihel TC: *Atlas of human parasitology,* ed 2, Chicago, 1984, American Society of Clinical Pathologists.)

Clinical Syndromes

The incubation period after a sandfly bite may be as short as 2 weeks or as long as 2 months. The first sign, a red papule, appears at the site of the fly's bite. This lesion becomes irritated, with intense itching, and begins to enlarge and ulcerate. Gradually, the ulcer becomes hard and crusted and exudes a thin, serous material. At this stage, secondary bacterial infection may complicate the disease. The lesion may heal without treatment in a matter of months but usually leaves a disfiguring scar. A disseminated nodular type of cutaneous leishmaniasis has been reported from Ethiopia, probably caused by an allergy to *L. aethiopica* antigens. A viscerotropic form of *L. tropica* has been described in people returning from the Persian Gulf.

Laboratory Diagnosis

Demonstration of the amastigotes in properly stained smears from touch preparations or ulcer biopsy specimens and cultures of ulcer tissue determines the diagnosis. Serological tests are also available. Recently, DNA probes have been developed for the direct examination of cutaneous lesions. There are no commercially available products for these tests, and careful studies to determine the accuracy of testing procedures have not yet been performed.

Treatment, Prevention, and Control

The drug of choice is stibogluconate, with an alternative treatment of applying heat directly to the lesion. Protection from sandfly bites using screening, protective clothing, and repellents is essential. Prompt treatment and eradication of the ulcers to prevent transmission, along with control of sandflies and reservoir hosts, reduce the incidence of human infection.

Leishmania braziliensis

Physiology and Structure

The life cycle of *L. braziliensis* is illustrated in Figure 76-8.

Epidemiology

Mucocutaneous leishmaniasis produced by *L. braziliensis* is seen from the Yucatan peninsula into Central and South America, especially in rain forests where workers are exposed to sandfly bites while harvesting the chicle sap for chewing gum (thus the name **chiclero ulcer**). There are many jungle reservoir hosts, and domesticated dogs serve as reservoirs as well. The vector is the *Lutzomyia* sandfly. The variant *L. braziliensis panamensis* is similar in all respects to *L. braziliensis* except for its more frequent occurrence in Panama and slight difference in growth in cultures. Reservoir hosts and the vector are similar to *L. braziliensis*.

Clinical Syndromes

The incubation period and appearance of ulcers for *L. braziliensis* are similar to those of *L. tropica*, requiring a few weeks to months for the papule to appear. The essential difference in clinical disease is the involvement and destruction of mucous membranes and related tissue structures. This is often combined with edema and secondary bacterial infection to produce severe and disfiguring facial mutilation.

Laboratory Diagnosis

The diagnostic tests are similar for all *Leishmania* infections. Organisms are demonstrated in ulcers or cultured tissue. Serological testing is also performed.

Treatment, Prevention, and Control

The drug of choice is stibogluconate; an alternative is amphotericin B. As with all the other *Leishmania* complexes, screening, protective clothing, insect repellents, and prompt treatment are needed to prevent transmission and control disease. The protection of forest and construction workers in endemic areas is most difficult, and disease in those places may be effectively controlled only by vaccination. Work to develop a vaccine is under way.

TRYPANOSOMES

Trypanosoma, another hemoflagellate, causes two distinctly different forms of disease (Table 76-3). One is called *African trypanosomiasis*, or **sleeping sickness,** and is produced by *Trypanosoma brucei gambiense* and *T. b. rhodesiense*. It is transmitted by tsetse flies. The second infection is called **American trypanosomiasis,** or Chagas' disease, produced by *T. cruzi*. It is transmitted by true bugs (triatomids, reduviids, also called *kissing bugs*).

Trypanosoma brucei gambiense

Physiology and Structure

The life cycle of the African forms of trypanosomiasis is illustrated in Figure 76-10. The infective stage of the organism is the **trypomastigote,** which is present in the salivary glands of transmitting tsetse flies. The organism in this stage has a free flagellum and an undulating membrane running the full length of the body. The trypomastigotes enter the wound created by the fly bite and find their way into blood and lymph, eventually invading the CNS. Reproduction of the trypomastigotes in blood,

TABLE 76-3	*Trypanosoma* Species Responsible for Human Diseases		
PARASITE		**VECTOR**	**DISEASE**
T. brucei subspecies *gambiense* and *rhodesiense*		Tsetse fly	African trypanosomiasis (sleeping sickness)
T. cruzi		Reduviids	American trypanosomiasis (Chagas' disease)

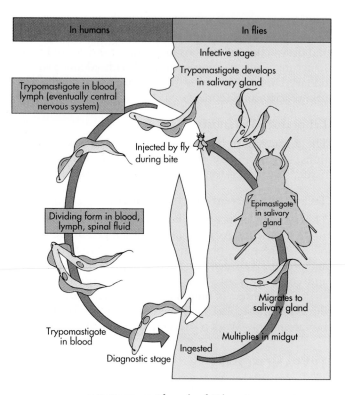

FIGURE 76-10 Life cycle of *T. brucei*.

FIGURE 76-11 Trypomastigote stage of *T. b. gambiense* in a blood smear. (From Ash LR, Orihel TC: *Atlas of human parasitology*, ed 2, Chicago, 1984, American Society of Clinical Pathologists.)

lymph, and spinal fluid is by binary or longitudinal fission. These trypomastigotes in blood are then infective for biting tsetse flies, where further reproduction occurs in the midgut. The organisms then migrate to the salivary glands where an **epimastigote** form (with a free flagellum but only a partial undulating membrane) continues reproduction to the infective trypomastigote stage. Tsetse flies become infective 4 to 6 weeks after feeding on blood from a diseased patient.

Epidemiology

T. b. gambiense is limited to tropical West and Central Africa, correlating to the range of the tsetse fly vector. The tsetse flies transmitting *T. b. gambiense* prefer shaded stream banks for reproduction and proximity to human dwellings. Persons who work in such areas are at greatest risk of infection. An animal reservoir has not been proved, although several species of animals have been infected experimentally.

Clinical Syndromes

The incubation period of Gambian sleeping sickness varies from a few days to weeks. *T. b. gambiense* produces chronic disease, often ending fatally, with CNS involvement after several years' duration. One of the earliest signs of disease is an occasional ulcer at the site of the fly bite. As reproduction of organisms continues, the lymph nodes are invaded, and fever, myalgia, arthralgia, and

lymph node enlargement result. Swelling of the posterior cervical lymph nodes is characteristic of Gambian disease and is called *Winterbottom's sign*. Patients in this acute phase often exhibit hyperactivity.

Chronic disease progresses to CNS involvement with lethargy, tremors, meningoencephalitis, mental retardation, and general deterioration. In the final stages of chronic disease, convulsions, hemiplegia, and incontinence occur, and the patient becomes difficult to arouse or respond, eventually progressing to a comatose state. Death is the result of CNS damage and other infections such as malaria or pneumonia.

Laboratory Diagnosis

Organisms can be demonstrated in thick and thin blood films, in concentrated anticoagulated blood preparations, and in aspirations from lymph nodes and concentrated spinal fluid (Figure 76-11). Methods for concentrating parasites in blood may be helpful. Approaches include centrifugation of heparinized samples and anion-exchange chromatography. Levels of parasitemia vary widely, and several attempts to visualize the organism over a number of days may be necessary. Preparations should be fixed and stained immediately to avoid disintegration of the trypomastigotes. Serological tests are also useful diagnostic techniques. Immunofluorescence, ELISA, precipitin, and agglutination methods have been used. Most reagents are not available commercially.

Treatment, Prevention, and Control

In the acute stages of the disease the drug of choice is suramin, with pentamidine as an alternative. In chronic disease with CNS involvement, the drug of choice is melarsoprol; alternatives are tryparsamide combined with suramin. Difluoromethylornithine has also been introduced and holds promise for the treatment of all stages of disease.

The most essential elements are control of breeding sites of the tsetse flies by clearing brush, using insecticides, and treating human cases to reduce transmission to flies. People going into known endemic areas should wear protective clothing and use screening, bed netting, and insect repellents.

Trypanosoma brucei rhodesiense

Physiology and Structure

The life cycle of *T. b. rhodesiense* is similar to that of *T. b. gambiense* (Figure 76-10), with both trypomastigote and epimastigote stages and transmission by tsetse flies.

Epidemiology

The organism is found primarily in East Africa, especially the cattle-raising countries where tsetse flies breed in the brush rather than along stream banks. *T. b. rhodesiense* also differs from *T. b. gambiense* in that domestic animal hosts (cattle and sheep) and wild game animals act as reservoir hosts. This transmission and vector cycle makes the organism more difficult to control than *T. b. gambiense*.

Clinical Syndromes

The incubation period for *T. b. rhodesiense* is shorter than that for *T. b. gambiense*. Acute disease (fever, rigors, and myalgia) occurs more rapidly and progresses to a fulminating, rapidly fatal illness. Infected persons are usually dead within 9 to 12 months if untreated.

This more virulent organism also develops in greater numbers in the blood. Lymphadenopathy is uncommon, and early in the infection, CNS invasion occurs with lethargy, anorexia, and mental disturbance. The chronic stages described for *T. b. gambiense* are not often seen because in addition to rapid CNS disease, the organism produces kidney damage and myocarditis, leading to death.

Laboratory Diagnosis

Examination of blood and spinal fluid is carried out as for *T. b. gambiense*. Serological tests are available; however, the marked variability of the surface antigens of trypanosomes limits the diagnostic usefulness of this approach.

Treatment, Prevention, and Control

The same treatment protocol applies as for *T. b. gambiense*, with early treatment for the more rapid neurological manifestations. Similar prevention and control measures are needed: tsetse fly control and use of protective

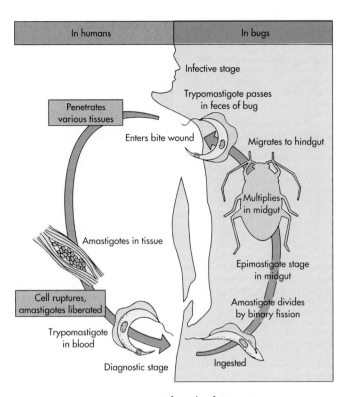

FIGURE 76-12 Life cycle of *T. cruzi.*

clothing, screens, netting, and insect repellent. In addition, early treatment is essential to control transmission, detect infection, and determine treatment in domestic animals. Control of infection in game animals is difficult, but infection can be reduced if measures to control the tsetse fly population, specifically eradication of brush and grassland breeding sites, are applied.

Trypanosoma cruzi

Physiology and Structure

The life cycle of *T. cruzi* (Figure 76-12) differs from *T. brucei* with the development of an additional form called an *amastigote* (Figure 76-13). The amastigote is an intracellular form with no flagellum and no undulating membrane. It is smaller than the trypomastigote, is oval, and is found in tissues. The infective trypomastigote, which is present in the feces of a reduviid bug ("kissing bug"), enters the wound created by the biting, feeding bug. The bugs have been called *kissing bugs* because they frequently bite people around the mouth and in other facial sites. They are notorious for biting, feeding on blood and tissue juices, and then defecating into the wound. The organisms in the feces of the bug enter the wound; penetration is usually aided when the patient rubs or scratches the irritated site.

The trypomastigotes then migrate to other tissues (e.g., cardiac muscle, liver, brain), lose the flagellum and undulating membrane, and become the smaller, oval, intracellular amastigote form. These intracellular amastigotes multiply by binary fission and eventually destroy the

FIGURE 76-13 Amastigote stage of *T. cruzi* in skeletal muscle. (From Ash LR, Orihel TC: *Atlas of human parasitology*, ed 2, Chicago, 1984, American Society of Clinical Pathologists.)

host cells. Then they are liberated to enter new host tissue as intracellular amastigotes or to become trypomastigotes infective for feeding reduviid bugs. Ingested trypomastigotes develop into epimastigotes in the midgut of the insect and reproduce by longitudinal binary fission. The organisms migrate to the hindgut of the bug, develop into metacyclic trypomastigotes, and then leave the bug in the feces after biting, feeding, and defecating, initiating a new human infection.

Epidemiology

T. cruzi occurs widely in both reduviid bugs and a broad spectrum of reservoir animals in North, Central, and South America. Human disease is found most often among children in South and Central America, where there is a direct correlation between infected wild animal reservoir hosts and the presence of infected bugs whose nests are found in human homes. Cases are rare in the United States because the bugs prefer nesting in animal burrows and because homes are not as open to nesting as those in South and Central America.

Clinical Syndromes

Chagas' disease may be asymptomatic, acute, or chronic. One of the earliest signs is development at the site of the bug bite of an erythematous and indurated area called a **chagoma.** This is often followed by a rash and edema around the eyes and face. The disease is most severe in children younger than 5 years of age and frequently is seen as an acute process with CNS involvement. Acute infection is also characterized by fever, chills, malaise, myalgia, and fatigue. Parasites may be present in the blood during the acute phase; however, they are sparse

in patients older than 1 year of age. Death may ensue a few weeks after an acute attack, the patient may recover, or the patient may enter the chronic phase as organisms proliferate and enter the heart, liver, spleen, brain, and lymph nodes.

Chronic Chagas' disease is characterized by hepatosplenomegaly, myocarditis, and enlargement of the esophagus and colon as a result of the destruction of nerve cells (e.g., Auerbach's plexus) and other tissues that control the growth of these organs.

Megacardia and electrocardiographic changes are commonly seen in chronic disease. Involvement of the CNS may produce granulomas in the brain with cyst formation and a meningoencephalitis. Death from chronic Chagas' disease results from tissue destruction in the many areas invaded by the organisms, and sudden death results from complete heart block and brain damage.

Laboratory Diagnosis

T. cruzi can be demonstrated in thick and thin blood films or concentrated anticoagulated blood early in the acute stage. As the infection progresses, the organisms leave the bloodstream and become difficult to find. Biopsy of lymph nodes, liver, spleen, or bone marrow may demonstrate the organisms in the amastigote stage. Culture of blood or inoculation into laboratory animals may be useful when the parasitemia is low. Serological tests are also available. In endemic areas, xenodiagnosis is widely used. Gene amplification techniques, such as polymerase chain reaction, have been used to detect the organism in the bloodstream. These approaches are not widely available and have not been adapted for use in the field.

Treatment, Prevention, and Control

Treatment of Chagas' disease is limited by the lack of reliable agents. The drug of choice is nifurtimox. Although it has some activity against the acute phase of disease, it has little activity against tissue amastigotes and has a number of side effects. Alternative agents include allopurinol and benzimidazole. Education regarding the disease, its insect transmission, and the wild animal reservoirs is critical. Bug control, eradication of nests, and construction of homes to prevent nesting of bugs are also essential. The use of dichlorodiphenyltrichloroethane (DDT) in bug-infested homes has demonstrated a drop in the transmission of malaria and Chagas' disease. Screening of blood by serological means or excluding blood donors from endemic areas prevents some infections that would otherwise be associated with transfusion therapy.

Development of a vaccine is possible because *T. cruzi* does not have the wide antigenic variation observed with the African trypanosomes.

CASE STUDY AND QUESTIONS

The patient, a 44-year-old heart transplant patient, complained to her primary physician about headache, nausea, and vomiting approximately 1 year after transplant. She had no skin lesions. A computed tomographic scan of the head demonstrated ring-enhancing lesions. A biopsy of the lesions was performed. All cultures (bacterial, fungal, viral) were negative. Special stains of the tissue revealed multiple cystlike structures of varying size.

1. What was the differential diagnosis of infectious agents in this patient? What was the most likely etiological agent?
2. What other tests would have been done to confirm the diagnosis?
3. What aspects of the medical history might suggest a risk for infection with this agent?
4. What were the therapeutic options and the likelihood that therapy would be successful?

Bibliography

Evans TG: Leishmaniasis, *Infect Dis Clin North Am* 7:527-546, 1993.

Garavelli PL, Corti E: Chloroquine resistance in *Plasmodium vivax:* the first case in Brazil, *Trans Roy Soc Trop Med Hyg* 86:128, 1992.

Gombert ME et al: Human babesiosis: clinical and therapeutic considerations, *JAMA* 248:3005-3007, 1982.

Kirchoff LV: Chagas' disease: American trypanosomiasis, *Infect Dis Clin North Am* 7:487-502, 1993.

Luft BJ Remington JS: Toxoplasmic encephalitis, *J Infect Dis* 157:1-6, 1988.

Markell EK, Voge M, John DT: *Medical parasitology,* ed 7, Philadelphia, 1992, WB Saunders.

McCabe R, Chirurgi V: Issues in toxoplasmosis, *Infect Dis Clin North Am* 7:587-604, 1993.

Murray PR et al: *Manual of clinical microbiology,* ed 6, Washington DC, 1995, American Society for Microbiology.

Rieckmann KH et al: *Plasmodium vivax* resistance to chloroquine? *Lancet* 2:1183-1184, 1989.

Zucker JR, Campbell CC: Malaria: principles of prevention and treatment, *Infect Dis Clin North Am* 7:547-567, 1993.

The most common helminths recognized in the United States are primarily intestinal nematodes, although in other countries nematode infections of blood and tissues can cause devastating disease. The nematodes are the most easily recognized form of intestinal parasite because of their large size and cylindrical, unsegmented bodies; hence the common name *roundworms*. These parasites live primarily as adult worms in the intestinal tract, and nematode infections are most commonly confirmed by detecting the characteristic eggs in feces. The identification of eggs should be approached in a systematic manner, taking into account the size and shape of the egg, the thickness of the shell, and the presence or absence of specialized structures such as polar plugs, knobs, spines, and opercula. The presence and characteristics of larvae within the eggs may also be useful. The most common nematodes of medical importance are listed in Table 77-1.

The filariae are long, slender roundworms that are parasites of blood, lymph, subcutaneous, and connective tissues. All of these nematodes are transmitted by mosquitoes or biting flies. Most produce larval worms called *microfilariae* that are demonstrated in blood specimens or in subcutaneous tissues and skin snips.

ENTEROBIUS VERMICULARIS

Physiology and Structure

E. vermicularis, the pinworm, is a small, white worm that is familiar to parents who find them in the perianal folds or vagina of an infected child. Infection is initiated by ingestion of embryonated eggs (Figure 77-1). Larvae hatch in the small intestine and migrate to the large intestine, where they mature into adults in 2 to 6 weeks. Fertilization of the female by the male produces the characteristic asymmetrical eggs. These eggs are laid in the perianal folds by the migrating female. As many as 20,000 eggs are deposited on the perianal skin. The eggs rapidly mature and are infectious within hours.

Epidemiology

E. vermicularis occurs worldwide but is most common in the temperate regions, where person-to-person spread is greatest in crowded conditions such as in day-care centers, schools, and mental institutions. An estimated 500 million cases of pinworm infection are reported worldwide, and this is the most common helminthic infection in North America.

Infection occurs when the eggs are ingested and the larval worm is free to develop in the intestinal mucosa.

TABLE 77-1	Nematodes of Medical Importance		
PARASITE	**COMMON NAME**	**DISEASE**
Enterobius vermicularis	Pinworm	Enterobiasis
Ascaris lumbricoides	Roundworm	Ascariasis
Toxocara canis	Dog ascaris	Visceral larva migrans
Toxocara cati	Cat ascaris	Visceral larva migrans
Trichuris trichiura	Whipworm	Trichuriasis
Ancylostoma duodenale	Old World hookworm	Hookworm infection
Necator americanus	New World hookworm	Hookworm infection
Ancylostoma braziliense	Dog or cat hookworm	Cutaneous larva migrans
Strongyloides stercoralis	Threadworm	Strongyloidiasis
Trichinella spiralis	—	Trichinosis
Wuchereria bancrofti	Bancroft's filariasis	Filariasis
Brugia malayi	Malayan filariasis	Filariasis
Loa loa	African eye worm	Loiasis
Mansonella species	Mansonelliasis	Filariasis
Onchocerca volvulus	River blindness	Onchocerciasis
Dirofilaria immitis	Dog heartworm	Filariasis
Dracunculus medinensis	Guinea worm	Dracunculosis

These eggs may be transmitted from hand to mouth by children scratching the perianal folds in response to the irritation caused by the migrating, egg-laying female worms, or the eggs may find their way to clothing and play objects in day-care centers. They can also survive long periods in the dust that accumulates over doors, on windowsills, and under beds in the rooms of infected people. Egg-laden dust can be inhaled and swallowed to produce infestation. In addition, **autoinfection** ("retrofection") can occur wherein eggs hatch in the perianal folds and the larval worms migrate into the rectum and large intestine. Infected individuals who handle food can also be a source of infection. No animal reservoir for *Enterobius* is known. Physicians should be aware of the related epidemiology of *Dientamoeba fragilis*; this organism correlates well with the presence of *E. vermicularis*, with *D. fragilis* transported in the pinworm eggshell.

Clinical Syndromes

Many children and adults show no symptoms and serve only as carriers. Patients who are allergic to the secretions of the migrating worms experience severe pruritus, loss of sleep, and fatigue. The pruritus may cause repeated scratching of the irritated area and lead to secondary bacterial infection. Worms that migrate into the vagina may produce genitourinary problems and granulomas.

Worms attached to the bowel wall may produce inflammation and granuloma formation around the eggs. Although the adult worms may occasionally invade the appendix, there remains no proven relationship between pinworm invasion and appendicitis. Penetration through the bowel wall into the peritoneal cavity, liver, and lungs has been infrequently recorded.

Laboratory Diagnosis

The diagnosis of enterobiasis is usually suggested by the clinical manifestations and confirmed by detection of the characteristic eggs on the anal mucosa. Occasionally, the adult worms are seen by laboratory personnel in stool specimens, but the method of choice for diagnosis involves use of an anal swab with a sticky surface that picks up the eggs (Figure 77-2) for microscopic examination. Sampling can be done with clear tape or commercially available swabs. The sample should be collected when the child arises and before bathing or defecation to pick up eggs laid by migrating worms during the night. Parents can collect the specimen and deliver it to the physician for immediate microscopic examination. Three swabbings, one per day for 3 consecutive days, may be required to detect the diagnostic eggs. The eggs are rarely seen in fecal specimens. Systemic signs of infection such as eosinophilia are rare.

Treatment, Prevention, and Control

The drug of choice is pyrantel pamoate; as an alternative drug, mebendazole is used. To avoid reintroduction of the organism and reinfection in the family environment, it is customary to treat the entire family simultaneously. Although cure rates are high, reinfection is common. Repeat treatment after 2 weeks may be useful in preventing reinfection.

Personal hygiene, clipping of fingernails, thorough washing of bed clothes, and prompt treatment of infected individuals all contribute to control. When housecleaning is done in the home of an infected family, dusting under beds, on window sills, and over doors should be done with a damp mop to avoid inhalation of infectious eggs.

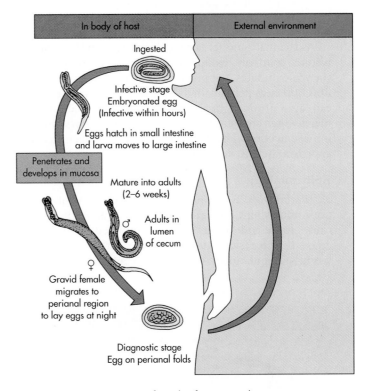

FIGURE 77-1 Life cycle of *E. vermicularis*.

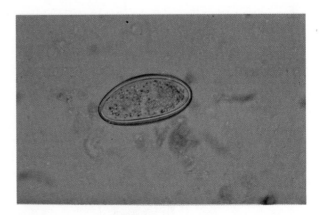

FIGURE 77-2 *E. vermicularis* egg. The thin-walled eggs are 50 to 60 × 20 to 30 μm, ovoid, and flattened on one side (not because children sit on them, but this is an easy way to correlate the egg morphology with the epidemiology of the disease).

ASCARIS LUMBRICOIDES

Physiology and Structure

A. lumbricoides are large (20 to 35 cm in length), pink worms that have a more complex life cycle than *E. vermicularis* (Figure 77-3) but are otherwise typical of an intestinal roundworm.

The ingested infective egg releases a larval worm that penetrates the duodenal wall, enters the bloodstream, is carried to the liver and heart, and then enters the pulmonary circulation. The larvae break free in the alveoli of the lungs, where they grow and molt. In about 3 weeks the larvae pass from the respiratory system to be coughed up, swallowed, and returned to the small intestine.

As the male and female worms mature in the small intestine (primarily jejunum), fertilization of the female by the male initiates egg production, which may amount to 200,000 eggs per day for as long as a year. Female worms can also produce unfertilized eggs in the absence of males. Eggs are found in the feces 60 to 75 days after the initial infection. Fertilized eggs become infectious after approximately 2 weeks in the soil.

Epidemiology

A. lumbricoides is prevalent in areas where sanitation is poor and where human feces are used as fertilizer. Because food and water are contaminated with *Ascaris* eggs, this parasite, more than any other, affects the world's population. Although no animal reservoir is known for *A. lumbricoides,* an almost identical species from pigs, *A. suum,* can infect humans. This species is seen in swine growers and is associated with the use of pig manure for gardening. *Ascaris* eggs are quite hardy and can survive extreme temperatures and persist for several months in feces and sewage. Ascariasis is the most common helminth worldwide, with an estimated 1 billion people infected.

Clinical Syndromes

Infections caused by the ingestion of only a few eggs may produce no symptoms; however, even a single adult *Ascaris* worm may be dangerous because it can migrate into the bile duct and liver and damage tissue. Furthermore, because the worm has a tough, flexible body, it can occasionally perforate the intestine, creating peritonitis with secondary bacterial infection. The adult worms do not attach to the intestinal mucosa but depend on constant motion to maintain their position within the bowel lumen.

After infection with many larvae, migration of worms to the lungs can produce pneumonitis resembling an asthmatic attack. Pulmonary involvement is related to the degree of hypersensitivity induced by previous infections and the intensity of the current exposure and may be accompanied by eosinophilia and oxygen desaturation. Also, a tangled bolus of mature worms in the intestine can result in obstruction, perforation, and occlusion of the appendix. As mentioned previously, migration into the bile duct, gallbladder, and liver can produce severe tissue damage. This migration can occur in response to fever, drugs other than those used to treat ascariasis, and some anesthetics. Patients with many larvae may also experience abdominal tenderness, fever, distention, and vomiting.

Laboratory Diagnosis

Examination of the sediment of concentrated stool reveals the knobby-coated, bile-stained, fertilized and unfertilized eggs. Eggs are oval, 55 to 75 μm long, and 50 μm wide. The thick-walled outer shell can be partially removed (decorticated egg). Occasionally, adult worms pass with the feces, which can be quite dramatic because of their large size (20 to 35 cm long). Roentgenologists may also visualize the worms in the intestine, and cholangiograms often disclose their presence in the biliary tract of the liver. The pulmonary phase of the disease may be diagnosed by the finding of larvae and eosinophils in sputum.

Treatment, Prevention, and Control

Treatment of symptomatic infection is highly effective. The drug of choice is mebendazole; pyrantel pamoate and piperazine are alternatives. Patients with mixed parasitic infections (*A. lumbricoides* and other helminths, *Giardia lamblia,* and *Entamoeba histolytica*) in the stool should be treated for ascariasis first to avoid provoking worm migration and possible intestinal perforation. Ed-

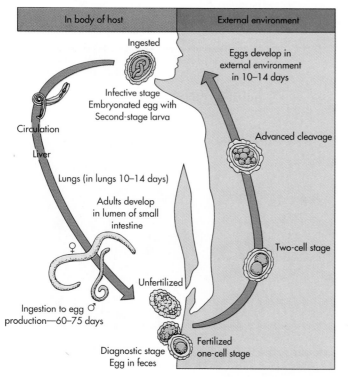

FIGURE 77-3 Life cycle of A. lumbricoides.

ucation, improved sanitation, and avoidance of human feces as fertilizer are critical. A program of mass treatment in highly endemic areas has been suggested, but this may not be economically feasible. Furthermore, eggs can persist in contaminated soil for 3 years or more. Certainly, improved personal hygiene among people who handle food is an important aspect of control.

TOXOCARA CANIS AND *TOXOCARA CATI*
Physiology and Structure

T. canis and *T. cati* are ascarid worms, naturally parasitic in the intestines of dogs and cats, that accidentally infect humans, producing a disease called **visceral larval migrans** or *toxocariasis*. When ingested by humans, the eggs of these worms can hatch into larval forms that cannot follow the normal developmental cycle as in the natural dog or cat host. They can penetrate the human gut and reach the bloodstream and then migrate as larvae to various human tissues. They do not develop beyond the migrating larval form.

Epidemiology

Wherever infected dogs and cats are present, the eggs are a threat to humans. This is especially true for children who are exposed more readily to contaminated soil and who tend to put objects in their mouths.

Clinical Syndromes

The clinical manifestations of toxocariasis in humans are related to the migration of the larvae through tissues. The larvae may invade any tissue of the body, where they can induce bleeding, the formation of eosinophilic granulomas, and necrosis. Patients may be asymptomatic and have only eosinophilia, but they can also have serious disease directly related to the number and location of the lesions caused by the migrating larvae as well as the degree to which the host is sensitized to the larval antigens. The organs most frequently involved are the lungs, heart, kidneys, liver, skeletal muscles, eyes, and central nervous system. Signs and symptoms include cough, wheezing, fever, rash, anorexia, seizures, fatigue, and abdominal discomfort. On examination, patients may have hepatosplenomegaly and nodular pruritic skin lesions. Death may result from respiratory failure, cardiac arrhythmia, or brain damage. Ocular disease can also occur with the movement of larvae through the eye and may be mistaken for malignant retinoblastoma. Prompt diagnosis is required to avoid unnecessary enucleation.

Laboratory Diagnosis

The diagnosis of visceral larval migrans is based on clinical findings, the presence of eosinophilia, known exposure to dogs or cats, and serological confirmation. Enzyme-linked immunosorbent assays are readily available and appear to offer the best serological marker for disease. The examination of feces from infected patients is not useful because egg-laying adults are not present.

However, examination of fecal material from infected pets often supports the diagnosis. Tissue examination for larvae may provide a definitive diagnosis but may be negative because of sampling error.

Treatment, Prevention, and Control

Treatment is primarily symptomatic, since antiparasitic agents are not of proven benefit. The drug of choice is diethylcarbamazine or thiabendazole. Mebendazole is an acceptable alternative. Corticosteroid therapy may be life saving if the patient has serious pulmonary, myocardial, or central nervous system involvement, since a major component of the infection is an inflammatory response to the organism. This zoonosis can be greatly reduced if pet owners conscientiously eradicate worms from their animals and clean up pet fecal material from yards and school playgrounds. Children's play areas and sandboxes should be carefully monitored.

TRICHURIS TRICHIURA
Physiology and Structure

Commonly called **whipworm** because it resembles the handle and lash of a whip, *T. trichiura* has a simple life cycle (Figure 77-4). Ingested eggs hatch into a larval worm in the small intestine and then migrate to the cecum, where they penetrate the mucosa and mature to adults. Some 3 months after the initial infection, the fertilized female worm starts laying eggs and may produce 3000 to 10,000 eggs per day. Female worms can live for

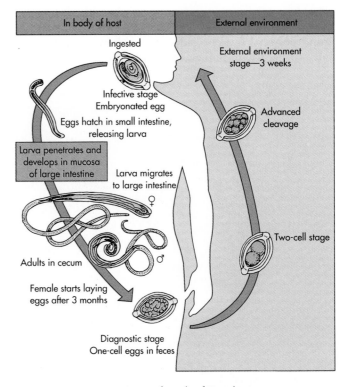

FIGURE 77-4 Life cycle of *T. trichiura*.

as long as 8 years. Eggs passed into the soil mature and become infectious in 3 weeks. *T. trichiura* eggs are distinctive, with dark bile staining, a barrel shape, and the presence of polar plugs in the egg shell (Figure 77-5).

Epidemiology

Similar to *A. lumbricoides,* with *T. trichiura,* distribution is worldwide and prevalence is directly correlated with poor sanitation and the use of human feces as fertilizer. No animal reservoir is recognized.

Clinical Syndromes

The clinical manifestations of trichuriasis are generally related to the intensity of the worm burden. Most infections are with small numbers of *Trichuris* organisms and are usually asymptomatic, although secondary bacterial infection may occur because the heads of the worms penetrate deep into the intestinal mucosa. Infections with many larvae may produce abdominal pain and distention, bloody diarrhea, weakness, and weight loss. Appendicitis may occur as worms fill the lumen, and prolapse of the rectum is seen in children because of the irritation and straining during defecation. Anemia and eosinophilia are also seen in severe infections.

Laboratory Diagnosis

Stool examination reveals the characteristic bile-stained eggs with polar plugs. Light infestations may be difficult to detect because of the paucity of eggs in the stool specimens.

Treatment, Prevention, and Control

The drug of choice is mebendazole. As with *A. lumbricoides,* prevention of *T. trichiura* depends on education, good personal hygiene, adequate sanitation, and avoidance of the use of human feces as fertilizer.

HOOKWORMS
Ancylostoma duodenale and *Necator americanus*
Physiology and Structure

The two human hookworms are *A. duodenale* (Old World hookworm) and *N. americanus* (New World hookworm). Differing only in geographical distribution, structure of mouthparts, and relative size, these two species are discussed together as agents of hookworm infection. The human phase of the hookworm life cycle is initiated when a **filariform** (infective form) larva penetrates intact skin (Figure 77-6). The larva then enters the circulation; is carried to the lungs; and like *A. lumbricoides,* is coughed up, swallowed, and develops to adulthood in the small intestine. The adult *N. americanus* has a hooklike head, which accounts for the name commonly used. Adult worms lay as many as 10,000 to 20,000 eggs per day, which are released into feces. Egg laying is initiated 4 to 8 weeks after the initial exposure and can persist for as long as 5 years. On contact with soil, the **rhabditiform** (noninfective) larvae are released from the eggs and within 2 weeks develop into filariform larvae. The filariform larvae can then penetrate exposed skin (e.g., bare feet) and initiate a new cycle of human infection.

Both species have mouthparts designed for sucking blood from injured intestinal tissue. *A. duodenale* has chitinous teeth, and *N. americanus* has shearing chitinous plates.

Epidemiology

Transmission of hookworm infection requires the deposition of egg-containing feces on shady, well-drained soil

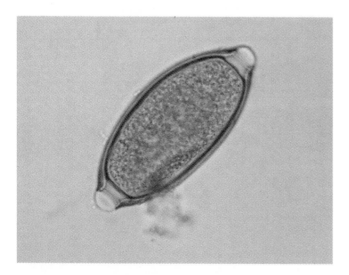

FIGURE 77-5 *T. trichiura* egg. The eggs are barrel shaped, measuring 50 × 24 μm, with a thick wall and two prominent plugs at the ends. Internally, an unsegmented ovum is present.

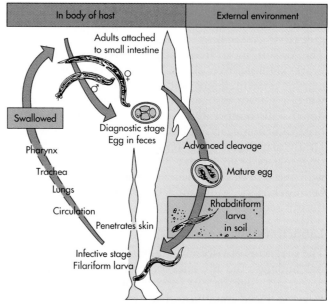

FIGURE 77-6 Life cycle of human hookworms.

and is favored by warm, humid (tropical) conditions. Hookworm infections are reported worldwide in places where direct contact with contaminated soil can lead to human disease, but they occur primarily in warm subtropical and tropical regions and in southern parts of the United States. It is estimated that more than 900 million individuals worldwide are infected with hookworms, including 700,000 in the United States.

Clinical Syndromes

Skin-penetrating larvae may produce an allergic reaction and rash at sites of entry, and larvae migrating in the lungs can cause pneumonitis. Adult worms produce the gastrointestinal symptoms of nausea, vomiting, and diarrhea. As blood is lost from feeding worms, a microcytic hypochromic anemia develops. Daily blood loss is estimated at 0.15 to 0.25 ml for each adult *A. duodenale* and 0.03 ml for each adult *N. americanus.* In severe chronic infections, emaciation and mental and physical retardation may occur related to anemia from blood loss and nutritional deficiencies. Also, intestinal sites may be secondarily infected by bacteria when the worms migrate along the intestinal mucosa.

Laboratory Diagnosis

Stool examination reveals the characteristic non–bile-stained segmented eggs shown in Figure 77-7. Larvae are not found in stool specimens unless the specimen was left at ambient temperature for a day or more. The eggs of *A. duodenale* and *N. americanus* cannot be distinguished. The larvae must be examined to identify these hookworms specifically, although this is clinically unnecessary.

Treatment, Prevention, and Control

The drug of choice is mebendazole; pyrantel pamoate is an alternative. In addition to eradication of the worms to stop blood loss, iron therapy is indicated to raise hemoglobin levels to normal. Blood transfusion may be necessary in severe cases of anemia. Education, improved sanitation, and controlled disposal of human feces are critical preventive measures. Wearing shoes in endemic areas helps reduce the prevalence of infection.

Ancylostoma braziliense
Physiology and Structure

A. braziliense, a species of hookworm, is naturally parasitic in the intestines of dogs and cats and accidentally infects humans. It produces a disease properly called **cutaneous larva migrans** but also called *ground itch* and *creeping eruption.* The filariform larvae of this hookworm penetrate intact skin but can develop no further in humans. The larvae remain trapped in the skin of the wrong host for weeks or months, wandering through subcutaneous tissue and creating serpentine tunnels.

Epidemiology

Similar to the situation with *Ascaris* worms, the threat of infection with *A. braziliense* is greatest among children coming into contact with soil or sandboxes contaminated with animal feces containing hookworm eggs. Infections are prevalent throughout the year on beaches in subtropical and tropical regions; in the summer, infection is reported as far north as the Canadian–U.S. border.

Clinical Syndromes

The migrating larvae may provoke a severe erythematous and vesicular reaction. Pruritus and scratching of the irritated skin may lead to secondary bacterial infection. About half of patients develop transient pulmonary infiltrates with peripheral eosinophilia (Löffler's syndrome), presumably resulting from pulmonary migration of the larvae.

Laboratory Diagnosis

Occasionally, larvae are recovered in skin biopsy or after freezing of the skin, but most diagnoses are based on the clinical appearance of the tunnels and a history of contact with dog and cat feces. The larvae are rarely found in sputum.

Treatment, Prevention, and Control

The drug of choice is thiabendazole. Antihistamines may be helpful in controlling pruritus. This zoonosis, as with animal *Ascaris* infection, can be reduced by educating pet owners to treat their animals for worm infections and to pick up pet feces from yards, beaches, and sandboxes. In endemic areas, shoes or sandals should be worn to prevent infection.

STRONGYLOIDES STERCORALIS
Physiology and Structure

Although the morphology of these worms and epidemiology of their infections are similar to the hookworm, the life cycle of *S. stercoralis* (Figure 77-8) differs in three aspects: (1) Eggs hatch into larvae in the intestine and before they are passed in feces, (2) larvae can mature into

FIGURE 77-7 Human hookworm egg. The eggs are 60 to 75 μm long and 35 to 40 μm wide, are thin shelled, and enclose a developing larva.

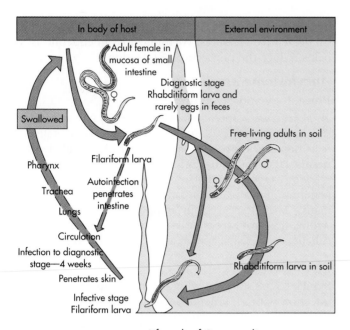

FIGURE 77-8 Life cycle of *S. stercoralis*.

filariforms in the intestine and cause autoinfection, and (3) a free-living, nonparasitic cycle can be established outside the human host.

In direct development, like the hookworm, a skin-penetrating *S. stercoralis* larva enters the circulation and follows the pulmonary course. It is coughed up and swallowed, and adults develop in the small intestine. Adult females burrow into the mucosa of the duodenum and reproduce parthenogenetically. Each female produces about a dozen eggs each day, which hatch within the mucosa and release rhabditiform larvae into the lumen of the bowel. The rhabditiform larvae are distinguished from the larvae of hookworms by their short buccal capsule and large genital primordium. The rhabditiform larvae are passed in the stool and may either continue the direct cycle by developing into infective filariform larvae or develop into free-living adult worms and initiate the indirect cycle.

In indirect development the larvae in soil develop into free-living adults that produce eggs and larvae. Several generations of this nonparasitic existence may occur before new larvae become skin-penetrating parasites.

Finally, in **autoinfection**, rhabditiform larvae in the intestine do not pass with feces but become filariform larvae. These penetrate the intestinal or perianal skin and follow the course through the circulation and pulmonary structures, are coughed up, and then are swallowed; at this point, they become adults, producing more larvae in the intestine. This cycle can persist for years and can lead to hyperinfection and massive or disseminated, often fatal infection.

Epidemiology

Similar to hookworms in its requirements for warm temperatures and moisture, *S. stercoralis* demonstrates low

prevalence but a somewhat broader geographical distribution, including parts of the northern United States and Canada. Sexual transmission also occurs. Animal reservoirs, such as domestic pets, are recognized.

Clinical Syndromes

Individuals with strongyloidiasis frequently are afflicted with pneumonitis from migrating larvae similar to that seen in ascariasis and hookworm infection. The intestinal infection is usually asymptomatic. However, heavy worm loads may involve the biliary and pancreatic ducts, the entire small bowel, and the colon, causing inflammation and ulceration leading to epigastric pain and tenderness, vomiting, diarrhea (occasionally bloody), and malabsorption. Symptoms mimicking peptic ulcer disease coupled with peripheral eosinophilia should strongly suggest the diagnosis of strongyloidiasis.

Autoinfection may lead to chronic strongyloidiasis that can last for years even in nonendemic areas. Although many of these chronic infections may be asymptomatic, as many as two thirds of patients have recurring episodic symptoms referable to the involved skin, lungs, and intestinal tract. Individuals with chronic strongyloidiasis are at risk of developing severe, life-threatening **hyperinfection** syndrome if the host-parasite balance is disturbed by any drug or illness that compromises the host's immune status. Hyperinfection syndrome is seen most commonly in individuals immunocompromised by malignancies (especially hematological malignancies), corticosteroid therapy, or both. Hyperinfection syndrome has also been observed in patients who have undergone solid organ transplantation and in malnourished people. Loss of cellular immune function may be associated with the conversion of rhabditiform larvae to filariform larvae, followed by dissemination of the larvae via the circulation to virtually any organ. Most commonly, extraintestinal infection involves the lung and includes bronchospasm, diffuse infiltrates, and occasionally cavitation. Widespread dissemination that involves the abdominal lymph nodes, liver, spleen, kidneys, pancreas, thyroid, heart, brain, and meninges is common. Intestinal symptoms of hyperinfection syndrome include profound diarrhea, malabsorption, and electrolyte abnormalities. Notably, hyperinfection syndrome is associated with a mortality rate of approximately 86%. Bacterial sepsis, meningitis, peritonitis, and endocarditis secondary to larval spread from the intestine are frequent and often fatal complications of hyperinfection syndrome.

Laboratory Diagnosis

The diagnosis of strongyloidiasis may be difficult because of the intermittent passage of low numbers of first-stage larvae in stool. Examination of concentrated stool sediment reveals the larval worms (Figure 77-9), but in contrast with hookworm infections, in *S. stercoralis* infections, eggs are generally not seen. Collecting samples from three stools, one per day for 3 days, as for *G. lamblia*, is recommended because *S. stercoralis* larvae may occur in "showers," with many present one day and few

FIGURE 77-9 *S. stercoralis* larvae. The larvae are 180 to 380 μm long and 14 to 24 μm wide. They are differentiated from hookworm larvae by the length of the buccal cavity and esophagus and by the structure of the genital primordium.

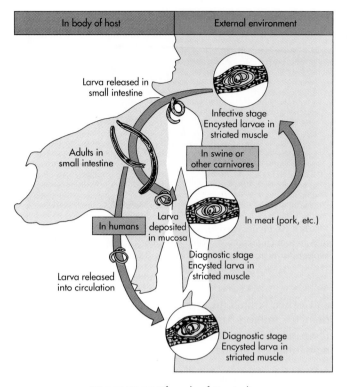

FIGURE 77-10 Life cycle of *T. spiralis*.

or none the next. Several authors favor the Baermann funnel gauze method of concentrating living *S. stercoralis* larvae from fecal specimens. This method uses a funnel with a stopcock and a gauze insert. The funnel is filled with lukewarm water to a level just covering the gauze, and a specimen of stool is placed on the gauze, partially in contact with the water. The larvae in the stool migrate through the gauze into the water and then sediment into the neck of the funnel where they may be detected by low-power microscopy. When absent from stool, larvae may be detected in duodenal aspirates or in sputum in the case of massive infection. Finally, culture of the larvae from stool using charcoal cultures or an agar plate method may be used, although these are not routine in most laboratories. Serological tests are generally not available.

Treatment, Prevention, and Control

All infected patients should be treated to prevent autoinfection and potential dissemination (hyperinfection) of the parasite. The drug of choice is thiabendazole, with mebendazole as an alternative. Patients in endemic areas who are preparing to undergo immunosuppressive therapy should have at least three stool examinations to rule out *S. stercoralis* infection and thus avoid the risks of autoinfection. Strict infection-control measures should be enforced when clinicians care for patients with hyperinfection syndrome because stool, saliva, vomitus, and body fluids may contain infectious filariform larvae. As with hookworm, control of *Strongyloides* species requires education, proper sanitation, and prompt treatment of existing infections.

TRICHINELLA SPIRALIS
Physiology and Structure

T. spiralis is the etiological agent of trichinosis. The adult form of this organism lives in the duodenal and jejunal mucosa of flesh-eating mammals worldwide. The infec-

tious larval form is present in the striated muscles of carnivorous and omnivorous mammals. Among domestic animals, swine are most frequently involved. Figure 77-10 illustrates the simple, direct life cycle, which terminates in the musculature of humans, where the larvae eventually die and calcify.

The infection begins when meat that contains encysted larvae is digested. The larvae leave the meat in the small intestine and within 2 days develop into adult worms. A single fertilized female produces more than 1500 larvae in 1 to 3 months. These larvae move from the intestinal mucosa into the bloodstream and are carried in the circulation to various muscle sites throughout the body, where they coil in striated muscle fibers and become encysted (Figure 77-11). The muscles invaded most frequently include the extraocular muscles of the eye; the tongue; the deltoid, pectoral, and intercostal muscles; the diaphragm; and the gastrocnemius muscle. The encysted larvae remain viable for many years and are infectious if ingested by a new animal host.

Epidemiology

Trichinosis occurs worldwide in humans, and its greatest prevalence is associated with the consumption of pork products. In addition to its transmission from pigs, many carnivorous and omnivorous animals harbor the organism and are potential sources of human infection. Notably, polar bears and walruses in the Arctic account for outbreaks in human populations, especially with a strain of *T. spiralis* that is more resistant to freezing than the *T. spiralis* strains found in the continental United States

FIGURE 77-11 Encysted larva of *T. spiralis* in a muscle biopsy specimen. (From Finegold SM, Baron EJ, editors: *Bailey and Scott's diagnostic microbiology,* ed 7, St Louis, 1986, Mosby.)

and other temperate regions. It is estimated that more than 1.5 million Americans carry live *Trichinella* cysts in their musculature and that 150,000 to 300,000 acquire new infection annually.

Clinical Syndromes

Trichinosis is one of the few tissue parasitic diseases still seen in the United States. As with other parasitic infections, most patients have minimal or no symptoms. The clinical presentation depends largely on the tissue burden of organisms and the location of the migrating larvae. Patients in whom no more than 10 larvae are deposited per gram of tissue are usually asymptomatic; those with at least 100 generally have significant disease; and those with 1000 to 5000 have a very serious course that occasionally ends in death. In mild infections with few migrating larvae, patients may experience only an influenza-like syndrome with slight fever and mild diarrhea. With more extensive larval migration, persistent fever, gastrointestinal distress, marked eosinophilia, muscle pain, and periorbital edema occur. "Splinter" hemorrhages beneath the nails, a common finding, are probably caused by vasculitis resulting from toxic secretions of the migrating larvae. In heavy infections, severe neurological symptoms, including psychosis, meningoencephalitis, and cerebrovascular accident, may occur.

Patients who survive the migration, muscle destruction, and encystment of larvae in moderate infections experience a decline in clinical symptoms in 5 or 6 weeks. Lethal trichinosis results when myocarditis, encephalitis, and pneumonitis combine; the patient dies 4 to 6 weeks after infection. Respiratory arrest often follows heavy invasion and muscle destruction in the diaphragm.

Laboratory Diagnosis

The diagnosis is usually established with clinical observations, especially when an outbreak can be traced to consumption of improperly cooked pork or bear meat. The laboratory may confirm the diagnosis if the encysted larvae are detected in the implicated meat or in a muscle biopsy specimen from the patient. Marked eosinophilia is characteristically presents in patients with trichinosis. Serological procedures are also available for confirmation of the diagnosis. Significant antibody titers are usually absent before the third week of illness but then may persist for years.

Treatment, Prevention, and Control

Treatment of trichinosis is primarily symptomatic, since there are no good antiparasitic agents for tissue larvae. Treatment of the adult worms in the intestine with mebendazole may halt the production of new larvae. Steroids, along with thiabendazole or mebendazole, are recommended for severe symptoms. Education regarding disease transmission from pork and bear meat is essential, especially the recommendation that pork and bear meat be cooked until the interior is gray. Microwave cooking and smoking or drying meat do not kill all larvae.

Laws regulating the feeding of garbage to pigs help control transmission, as may regulations controlling the foraging of bears in garbage pits and public parks. Freezing pork, as conducted in federally inspected meat packing plants, has reduced transmission. Quick freezing of pork at $-40°$ C effectively destroys the organisms, as does low-temperature storage at $-15°$ C for 20 days or more.

WUCHERERIA BANCROFTI AND *BRUGIA MALAYI*
Physiology and Structure

Because of their many similarities, *W. bancrofti* and *B. malayi* are discussed together. Human infection is initiated by the introduction of infective larvae, which is present in the saliva of a biting mosquito, into a bite wound (Figure 77-12). Various species of *Anopheles, Aedes,* and *Culex* mosquitoes are vectors of Bancroft's and Malayan filariasis. The larvae migrate from the location of the bite to the lymphatic system, primarily in the arms, legs, or groin, where larval growth to adulthood occurs. From 3 to 12 months after the initial infection, the adult male worm fertilizes the female, which in turn produces the sheathed larval microfilariae that find their way into the circulation. The presence of microfilariae in blood is diagnostic for human disease and is infective for feeding mosquitoes. In the mosquito the larvae move through the stomach and thoracic muscles in developmental stages and finally migrate to the proboscis. There, they become infective third-stage larvae and are transmitted by the feeding mosquito. The adult form in humans can persist for as long as 10 years.

Epidemiology

W. bancrofti occurs in tropical and subtropical areas and is endemic in central Africa, along the Mediterranean coast, and in many parts of Asia, including China,

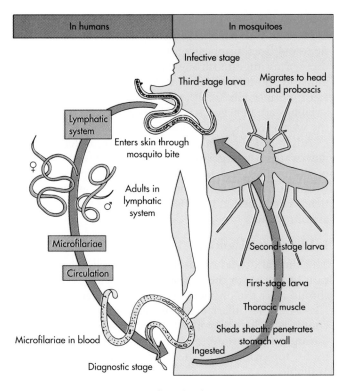

In humans	In mosquitoes

FIGURE 77-12 Life cycle of *W. bancrofti*.

FIGURE 77-13 *W. bancrofti* microfilaria in blood smear.

Korea, Japan, and the Philippines. It is also present in Haiti, Trinidad, Surinam, Panama, Costa Rica, and Brazil. No animal reservoir has been identified. *B. malayi* is found primarily in Malaysia, India, Thailand, Vietnam, and parts of China, Korea, Japan, and many Pacific islands. Animal reservoirs such as cats and monkeys are recognized.

Clinical Syndromes

In some patients, there is no sign of disease, even though blood specimens may show the presence of many microfilariae. In other patients, early acute symptoms are fever, lymphangitis and lymphadenitis with chills, and recurrent febrile attacks. The acute presentation is thought to result from the inflammatory response to the presence of molting adolescent worms and dead or dying adults within the lymphatic vessels. As the infection progresses, the lymph nodes enlarge, possibly involving many parts of the body, including the extremities, the scrotum, and the testes, with occasional abscess formation. This results from the physical obstruction of lymph in the vessels caused by the presence of adult worms and host reactivity in the lymphatic system. This process may be complicated by recurrent bacterial infections, which contribute to the tissue damage. The thickening and hypertrophy of tissues infected with the worms may lead to the enlargement of tissues, especially the extremities, progressing to **filarial elephantiasis.** Filariasis of this type is thus a chronic, debilitating, and disfiguring disease requiring prompt diagnosis and treatment. Occasionally, ascites

and pleural effusions secondary to rupture of the enlarged lymphatic vessels into the peritoneal or pleural cavity may be observed.

Laboratory Diagnosis

Eosinophilia is usually present during acute inflammatory episodes; however, demonstration of microfilariae in the blood is required for definitive diagnosis. As with malaria, microfilariae can be demonstrated in Giemsa-stained blood films in infections with *W. bancrofti* and *B. malayi* (Figure 77-13). Concentrations of anticoagulated blood specimens and urine specimens are also valuable procedures. Buffy coat films concentrate the white blood cells and are useful for the detection of microfilariae. The presence of small numbers of microfilariae in blood can be detected by a membrane-filtration technique in which anticoagulated blood is mixed with saline and forced through a 5-μm membrane filter. After several washes with saline or distilled water, the filter is examined microscopically for living microfilariae, or it is dried, fixed, and stained as for a thin blood film.

W. bancrofti and *B. malayi* have a periodicity in the production of microfilariae; it is called **nocturnal periodicity.** This results in greater numbers of microfilariae in blood at night. It is recommended that blood specimens be taken between 10 PM and 4 AM to detect infection.

W. bancrofti, as well as *B. malayi* and *Loa loa,* demonstrate a sheath on their microfilariae. This can be the first step in identifying the specific types of filariasis. Further identification is based on study of head and tail structures (Figure 77-14). Clinically, an exact species identification is not critical because treatment for all the filarial infections, except *Onchocerca volvulus,* is identical.

Serological testing is also available through reference laboratories so that a diagnosis can be reached. Detection of circulating filarial antigens is promising but is not widely available as a diagnostic test.

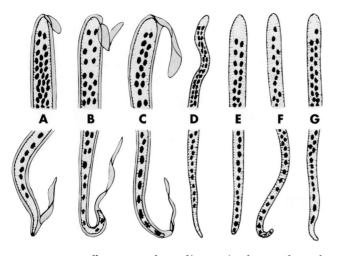

FIGURE 77-14 Differentiation of microfilariae. Identification of microfilariae is based on the presence of a sheath covering the larvae as well as the distribution of nuclei in the tail region. **A,** *W. bancrofti.* **B,** *B. malayi.* **C,** *L. loa.* **D,** *O. volvulus.* **E,** *Mansonella perstans.* **F,** *Mansonella streptocerca.* **G,** *Mansonella ozzardi.*

Treatment, Prevention, and Control

Treatment is of little benefit in most cases of chronic lymphatic filariasis. The drug of choice for treatment of *W. bancrofti* and *B. malayi* infections is diethylcarbamazine. Ivermectin appears promising, although controlled studies have not yet been performed. Supportive and surgical therapy for lymphatic obstruction may be of some cosmetic help. Education regarding filarial infections, mosquito control, use of protective clothing and insect repellents, and treatment of infections to prevent further transmission is essential. Control of *B. malayi* infections is more difficult because of the presence of disease in animal reservoirs.

LOA LOA

Physiology and Structure

The life cycle of *L. loa* is similar to that illustrated in Figure 77-12, except the vector is a biting fly called *Chrysops,* the mango fly. Approximately 6 months after infection, the production of microfilariae starts and can persist for 17 years or more. Adult worms can migrate through subcutaneous tissues, through muscle, and in front of the eyeball.

Epidemiology

L. loa is confined to the equatorial rain forests of Africa and is endemic in tropical West Africa, the Congo basin, and parts of Nigeria. Monkeys in these areas serve as reservoir hosts in the life cycle, with mango flies as vectors.

Clinical Syndromes

Symptoms usually do not appear until a year or so after the fly bite because the worms are slow in reaching adult-hood. One of the first signs of infection is the so-called fugitive or **Calabar swellings.** These swellings are transient and usually appear on the extremities, produced as the worms migrate through subcutaneous tissues, creating large, nodular areas that are painful and pruritic. Because eosinophilia (50% to 70%) is observed, Calabar swellings are believed to result from allergic reactions to the worms or their metabolic products.

Adult *L. loa* worms can also migrate under the conjunctiva, producing irritation, painful congestion, edema of the eyelids, and impaired vision. The presence of a worm in the eye can obviously cause anxiety in the patient. The infection may be long lived and in some cases asymptomatic.

Laboratory Diagnosis

The clinical observation of Calabar swellings or migration of worms in the eye, combined with eosinophilia, should alert the physician to consider infection with *L. loa.* The microfilariae can be found in the blood. In contrast to the other filariae, *L. loa* is primarily present during the daytime. Serological testing can also be useful for confirming the diagnosis but is not readily available.

Treatment, Prevention, and Control

Diethylcarbamazine is effective against adults and microfilariae; however, destruction of the parasites may induce severe allergic reactions that require treatment with corticosteroids. The role of ivermectin remains undefined for this infection. Surgical removal of worms migrating across the eye or bridge of the nose can be accomplished by immobilizing the worm with instillation of a few drops of 10% cocaine. Education regarding the infection and its vector, especially for people entering the known endemic areas, is essential. Protection from fly bites by using screening, appropriate clothing, and insect repellents, along with treatment of cases, is also critical in reducing the incidence of infection. However, the presence of disease in animal reservoirs (e.g., monkeys) limits the feasibility of controlling this disease.

MANSONELLA SPECIES

Filarial infections caused by *Mansonella* species are less important than those previously discussed, but physicians should be aware of the names because they may encounter patients with these infections. Infections caused by these organisms are generally asymptomatic but may cause dermatitis, lymphadenitis, hydrocele, and rarely, lymphatic obstruction resulting in elephantiasis.

All of the *Mansonella* species produce nonsheathed microfilariae in blood and subcutaneous tissues, and all are transmitted by biting midges (*Culicoides* species) or blackflies (*Simulium* species). As with previous filarial infections, infections from all of these species are treatable with diethylcarbamazine. Species identification, if desired, can be accomplished with blood smears, noting the structure of the microfilariae. Serological tests are also available.

Prevention and control require measures involving insect repellents, screening, and other precautions as for all insect-transmitted diseases.

Mansonella perstans

M. perstans occurs primarily in parts of tropical Africa and Central and South America. It may produce allergic skin reactions, edema, and Calabar swellings like those of *L. loa* infection. Reservoir hosts are chimpanzees and gorillas.

Mansonella ozzardi

M. ozzardi is found primarily in Central and South America and the West Indies. It may produce swelling of the lymph nodes and occasional hydrocele. There are no known reservoir hosts.

Mansonella streptocerca

M. streptocerca occurs primarily in Africa, especially in the Congo basin. It may produce edema in the skin and rarely, a form of elephantiasis. Monkeys serve as reservoir hosts.

ONCHOCERCA VOLVULUS

Physiology and Structure

Infection occurs after the introduction of *O. volvulus* larvae through the skin during the biting and feeding of the *Simulium* or blackfly vector (Figure 77-15). The larval worms migrate from the skin to subcutaneous tissue and develop into adult male and female worms. The adults become encased in fibrous subcutaneous nodules within which they may remain viable for as long as 15 years. The female worm, after fertilization by the male, begins producing as many as 2000 nonsheathed microfilariae each day. The microfilariae exit the capsule and migrate to the skin, the eyes, and other body tissues. These nonsheathed microfilariae appearing in skin tissue are infective for feeding blackflies.

Epidemiology

O. volvulus is endemic in many parts of Africa, especially in the Congo basin and the Volta River basin. In the western hemisphere, it occurs in many Central and South American countries. Onchocerciasis affects more than 50 million people worldwide and causes blindness in approximately 5% of infected people.

Several species of the blackfly genus *Simulium* serve as vectors but none so appropriately named as the principal vector, *Simulium damnosum* ("the damned blackfly"). These blackflies, or buffalo gnats, breed in fast-flowing streams, which makes control or eradication by insecticides almost impossible because the chemicals are rapidly washed away from the eggs and larvae.

There is a greater prevalence of infection in men than women in endemic areas because of their work in or near

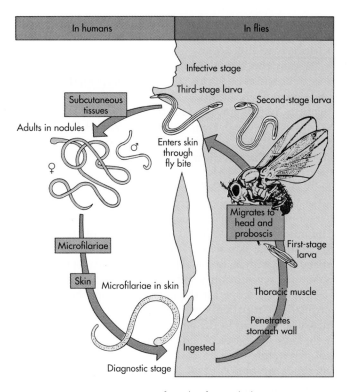

FIGURE 77-15 Life cycle of *O. volvulus*.

the streams where the blackflies breed. Studies in endemic areas in Africa have shown that 50% of men are totally blind before they reach 50 years of age. This accounts for the common term **river blindness,** which is applied to the disease onchocerciasis. This fear of blindness has created an additional problem in many parts of Africa because whole villages leave the area near streams and farmland that could produce food. The migrating populations then find themselves in areas where they face starvation.

Clinical Syndromes

Clinical onchocerciasis is characterized by infection involving the skin, subcutaneous tissue, lymph nodes, and eyes. The clinical manifestations of the infection are due to the acute and chronic inflammatory reaction to antigens released by the microfilariae as they migrate through the tissues. The incubation period from infectious larvae to adult worms is several months to a year. The initial signs of disease are fever, eosinophilia, and urticaria. As the worms mature, copulate, and produce microfilariae, subcutaneous nodules begin to appear on any part of the body. These nodules are most dangerous when they are present on the head and neck because the microfilariae may migrate to the eyes and cause serious tissue damage, leading to blindness. The mechanisms for development of eye disease are thought to be a combination of both direct invasion by the microfilaria and antigen-antibody complex deposition within the ocular tissues. Patients progress from conjunctivitis with photophobia to punctate and sclerosing keratitis. Internal eye disease with anterior uveitis, chorioretinitis, and optic neuritis may also occur.

Within the skin the inflammatory process results in loss of elasticity and areas of depigmentation, thickening, and atrophy. A number of skin conditions, including pruritus, hyperkeratosis, and myxedematous thickening, are related to the presence of this parasite. A form of elephantiasis called *hanging groin* also occurs when the nodules are located near the genitalia.

Laboratory Diagnosis

The diagnosis of onchocerciasis is made by the demonstration of microfilariae in skin snip preparations from the infrascapular or gluteal region. A sample is obtained by raising the skin with a needle and shaving the epidermal layer with a razor. The specimen is incubated in saline for several hours and is then inspected with a dissecting microscope for the presence of nonsheathed microfilariae. In patients with ocular disease, the organism may also be seen in the anterior chamber with the aid of a slit lamp. Serological and culture methods are not helpful, although efforts to develop serological detection methods are ongoing.

Treatment, Prevention, and Control

Surgical removal of the encapsulated nodule is often performed to eliminate the adult worms and stop production of microfilariae. In addition, treatment with ivermectin is recommended. A single oral dose of ivermectin (150 μg/kg) greatly reduces the number of microfilariae in the skin and eyes, thus diminishing the likelihood of developing a disabling onchocerciasis. In endemic areas, the dose of ivermectin can be repeated every 6 to 12 months to maintain suppression of dermal and ocular microfilariae. Suppression of dermal microfilariae reduces the transmission of this vector-borne disease, and thus mass chemotherapy may prove to be a successful strategy for the prevention of onchocerciasis.

Education regarding the disease and its transmission is essential. Protection from blackfly bites through the use of protective clothing, screening, and insect repellents, as well as prompt diagnosis and treatment of infections to prevent further transmission, are critical.

Although control of blackfly breeding is difficult because insecticides wash away in the streams, some form of biological control of this vector may reduce fly reproduction and disease transmission.

DIROFILARIA IMMITIS

Several mosquito-transmitted filariae infect dogs, cats, raccoons, and bobcats in nature and occasionally are found in humans. *D. immitis,* the dog heartworm, is notorious for forming a lethal worm bolus in the dog's heart. This nematode may also infect humans, producing a subcutaneous nodule called a *coin lesion* in the lung. Only very rarely have these worms been found in human hearts.

The coin lesion in the lung presents a problem for the radiologist and the surgeon because it resembles a malignancy requiring surgical removal. Unfortunately, no laboratory test can provide an accurate diagnosis of dirofilariasis. Peripheral eosinophilia is rare, and the radiographic features are insufficient to allow the clinician to distinguish pulmonary dirofilariasis from bronchogenic carcinoma. Serological tests are not sufficiently sensitive or specific to preclude the surgical intervention. A definitive diagnosis is made when a thoracotomy specimen is examined microscopically, revealing the typical cross sections of the parasite.

Transmission of the filarial infections can be controlled by mosquito control and the prophylactic use of the drug ivermectin in dogs.

DRACUNCULUS MEDINENSIS

The name *D. medinensis* means "little dragon of Medina." This is a very ancient worm infection thought by some scholars to be the "fiery serpent" noted by Moses with the Israelites at the Red Sea.

Physiology and Structure

D. medinensis is not a filarial worm but is a tissue-invading nematode of medical importance in many parts of the world. The worms have a very simple life cycle, depending on freshwater and a microcrustacean (copepod) of the genus *Cyclops* (Figure 77-16). When *Cyclops* species harboring larval *D. medinensis* are ingested in drinking water, the infection is initiated with

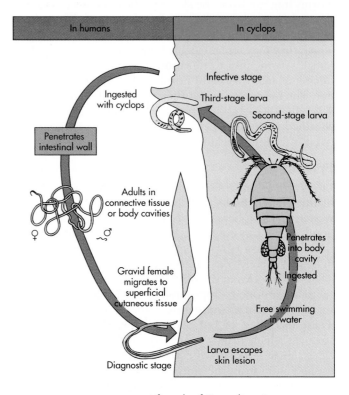

FIGURE 77-16 Life cycle of *D. medinensis.*

liberation of the larvae in the stomach. These larvae penetrate the wall of the digestive tract and migrate to the retroperitoneal space, where they mature. These larvae are not microfilariae and do not appear in the blood or other tissues. Male and female worms mate in the retroperitoneum, and the fertilized female then migrates to the subcutaneous tissues, usually in the extremities. When the fertilized female worm becomes gravid, a vesicle is formed in the host tissue, which will ulcerate. When the ulcer is completely formed, the worm protrudes a loop of uterus through the ulcer. On contact with water, the larval worms are released. The larvae are then ingested by the *Cyclops* species in freshwater, where they are then infective for humans or animals drinking the water containing the *Cyclops* species.

Epidemiology

D. medinensis occurs in many parts of Asia and equatorial Africa, infecting an estimated 10 million people. Reservoir hosts include dogs and many fur-bearing animals that come into contact with drinking water containing infective *Cyclops* species.

Human infections usually result from ingestion of water from so-called step wells where people stand or bathe in the water, at which time the gravid female worm discharges larvae from lesions on the arms, legs, feet, and ankles to infect *Cyclops* species in the water. Ponds and standing water are occasionally the source of infection when humans use them for drinking water.

Clinical Syndromes

Symptoms of infection usually do not appear until the gravid female creates the vesicle and the ulcer in the skin for the liberation of larval worms. This occurs usually 1 year after initial exposure. At the site of the ulcer, there are erythema and pain, as well as an allergic reaction to the worm. There is also the possibility of abscess formation and secondary bacterial infection, leading to further tissue destruction and inflammatory reaction with intense pain and sloughing of skin.

If the worm is broken in attempts to remove it, there may be toxic reactions, and if the worm dies and calcifies, there may be nodule formation and some allergic reaction. Once the gravid female worm has discharged all the larvae, it may retreat into deeper tissue, where it is gradually absorbed, or it may simply be expelled from the site.

Laboratory Diagnosis

Diagnosis is established by observing the typical ulcer and by flooding the ulcer with water to recover the larval worms when they are discharged. Occasionally, x-ray examination reveals worms in various parts of the body.

Treatment, Prevention, and Control

The ancient method of slowly wrapping the worm on a twig is still used in many endemic areas (Figure 77-17). Surgical removal is also a practical and reliable procedure

FIGURE 77-17 Removal of a *D. medinensis* adult from an exposed ulcer by winding the worm slowly around a stick. (From Binford CH, Conner DH: *Pathology of tropical and extraordinary diseases*, Washington DC, 1976, Armed Forces Institute of Pathology.)

for the patient. The drug of choice for treatment is niridazole; alternative drugs are metronidazole and thiabendazole. These drugs have an antiinflammatory effect and either eliminate the worm or make surgical removal easier.

Education regarding the life cycle of the worm and avoidance of water contaminated with *Cyclops* species are critical. Protection of drinking water by prohibiting bathing and washing of clothing in wells is essential. Persons who live in or travel to endemic areas should boil water before drinking it. The treatment of water with chemicals and the use of fish that consume *Cyclops* species as food also help control transmission. Prompt diagnosis and treatment of cases also limit further transmission. These preventive measures have been incorporated into an ongoing global effort to eliminate dracunculiasis.

CASE STUDY AND QUESTIONS

A 10-year-old boy was brought in by his father for evaluation of crampy abdominal pain, nausea, and mild diarrhea that had persisted for approximately 2 weeks. On the day before evaluation the boy reported to his parents that he passed a large worm into the toilet during a bowel movement. He flushed the worm before the parents could see it. Physical examination was completely unremarkable. The boy had no fever, cough, or rash and did not complain of anal pruritus. His travel history was unremarkable. Examination of a stool specimen revealed the diagnosis.

1. Which intestinal parasites of humans are nematodes?
2. Which nematode was likely in this case? What organisms may be found in stool?
3. What was the most likely means of acquisition of this parasite?
4. Was this patient at risk of autoinfection?
5. Describe the life cycle of this parasite.
6. Can this parasite cause extraintestinal symptoms? What other organs may be invaded and what might stimulate extraintestinal invasion?

Bibliography

Glickman LT, Magnaval JF: Zoonotic roundworm infections, *Infect Dis Clin North Am* 7:717-732, 1993.

Greene BM: Modern medicine versus an ancient scourge: progress toward control of onchocerciasis, *J Infect Dis* 199:15, 1992.

Liu LX, Weller PF: Strongyloidiasis and other intestinal nematode infections, *Infect Dis Clin North Am* 7:655-682, 1993.

Liu LX, Weller PF: Antiparasitic drugs, *New Engl J Med* 334:1178-1184, 1996.

Markell EK, Voge M, John DT: *Medical parasitology*, ed 7, Philadelphia, 1992, WB Saunders.

Ottesen EA: Filarial infections, *Infect Dis Clin North Am* 7:619-633, 1993.

Trematodes

The trematodes (**flukes**) are members of the Platy-helminthes and are generally flat, fleshy, leaf-shaped worms. In general, they are equipped with two muscular suckers: an oral type, which is the beginning of an incomplete digestive system, and a ventral sucker, which is simply an organ of attachment. The digestive system consists of lateral tubes that do not join to form an excretory opening. Most flukes are hermaphroditic, with both male and female reproductive organs in a single body. Schistosomes are the only exception; they have cylindrical bodies (like the nematodes), and separate male and female worms exist.

All flukes require intermediate hosts for the completion of their life cycles, and without exception the first intermediate hosts are mollusks (snails and clams). In these hosts an asexual reproductive cycle is a type of germ cell propagation. occurs Some flukes require various second intermediate hosts before reaching the final host and developing into adult worms. This variation is discussed in the sections on the individual species.

Fluke eggs are equipped with a "lid" at the top of the shell. Called an *operculum,* the lid opens to allow the larval worm to find its appropriate snail host. The schistosomes do not have an operculum; rather, the egg shell splits to liberate the larva. The medically significant trematodes are summarized in Table 78-1.

FASCIOLOPSIS BUSKI

A number of intestinal flukes are recognized, including *F. buski, Heterophyes heterophyes, Metagonimus yokogawai, Echinostoma ilocanum,* and *Gastrodiscoides hominis. F. buski* is the largest, most prevalent, and most important intestinal fluke. The other flukes are similar to *F. buski* in many respects (epidemiology, clinical syndromes, treatment) and are not discussed further. It is important only that physicians recognize the relationship among these different flukes.

Physiology and Structure

This large intestinal fluke has a typical life cycle (Figure 78-1). Humans ingest the encysted larval stage (metacercaria) when they peel the husks from aquatic vegeta-tion (e.g., water chestnuts) with the teeth. The metacercariae are scraped from the husk, swallowed, and develop into immature flukes in the duodenum. The fluke attaches to the mucosa of the small intestine with two muscular suckers, develops into an adult form, and undergoes self-fertilization. Egg production is initiated 3 months after the initial infection with the metacercariae. The operculated eggs pass in feces to water, where the operculum at the top of the egg shell pops open, liberating a free-swimming larval stage (miracidium). Glands at the pointed anterior end of the miracidium produce lytic substances that allow the penetration of the soft tissues of snails. In the snail tissue the miracidium develops through a series of stages by asexual germ cell propagation. The final stage (**cercaria**) in the snail is a free-swimming form that, after release from the snail, encysts on the aquatic vegetation, becoming the metacercariae, or infective stage.

Epidemiology

Because it depends on the distribution of its appropriate snail host, *F. buski* is found only in China, Vietnam, Thailand, parts of Indonesia, Malaysia, and India. Pigs, dogs, and rabbits serve as reservoir hosts in these endemic areas.

Clinical Syndromes

The symptomatology of *F. buski* infection relates directly to the worm burden in the small intestine. Attachment of the flukes in the small intestine can produce inflammation, ulceration, and hemorrhage. Severe infections produce abdominal discomfort similar to that of a duodenal ulcer, as well as diarrhea. Stools may be profuse, a malabsorption syndrome similar to giardiasis is common, and intestinal obstruction can occur. Marked eosinophilia is also present. Although death can occur, it is rare.

Laboratory Diagnosis

Stool examination reveals the large, golden, bile-stained eggs with an operculum on the top (Figure 78-2). The measurements and appearance of *F. buski* eggs are similar to that of the liver fluke *F. hepatica,* and differentia-

TABLE 78-1	Medically Significant Trematodes			
TREMATODE	**COMMON NAME**	**INTERMEDIATE HOST**	**BIOLOGICAL VECTOR**	**RESERVOIR HOST**
Fasciolopsis buski	Giant intestinal fluke	Snail	Water plants (e.g., water chestnuts)	Pigs, dogs, rabbits, humans
Fasciola hepatica	Sheep liver fluke	Snail	Water plants (e.g., watercress)	Sheep, cattle, humans
Opisthorchis (Clonorchis) sinensis	Chinese liver fluke	Snail, freshwater fish	Uncooked fish	Dogs, cats, humans
Paragonimus westermani	Lung fluke	Snail, freshwater crabs, crayfish	Uncooked crabs, crayfish	Pigs, monkeys, humans
Schistosome species	Blood fluke	Snail	None	Primates, rodents, domestic pets, livestock, humans

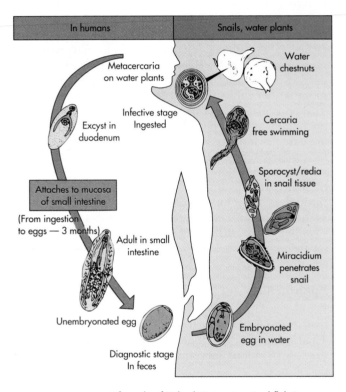

FIGURE 78-1 Life cycle of *F. buski* (giant intestinal fluke).

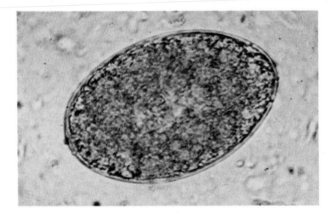

FIGURE 78-2 *F. buski* egg. The eggs are oval, large (75 to 100 × 130 to 150 μm), and surrounded by a thin shell. Although an operculum is present, it is rarely seen. (From Koneman EW et al: *Color atlas and textbook of diagnostic microbiology*, ed 2, Philadelphia, 1979, JB Lippincott.)

tion of the eggs of these species usually is not possible. Large (approximately 1.5 × 3.0 cm) adult flukes can rarely be found in feces or specimens collected at surgery.

Treatment, Prevention, and Control

The drug of choice is praziquantel, and the alternative is niclosamide. Education regarding the safe consumption of infective aquatic vegetation (particularly water chestnuts), proper sanitation, and control of human feces reduces the incidence of disease. In addition, the snail population may be eliminated with molluscacides. When infection occurs, treatment should be initiated promptly to minimize its spread. Control of the reservoir hosts also reduces transmission of the worm.

FASCIOLA HEPATICA

A number of liver flukes are recognized, including *F. hepatica*, *Opisthorchis sinensis*, *O. felineus*, and *Dicrocoelium dendriticum*. Only *F. hepatica* and *O. sinensis* are discussed in this chapter, although the eggs of other flukes are occasionally detected in the feces of patients in other geographical areas.

Physiology and Structure

Commonly called the **sheep liver fluke**, *F. hepatica* is a parasite of herbivores (particularly sheep and cattle) and humans. Its life cycle (Figure 78-3) is similar to that of *F. buski*, with human infection resulting from the ingestion of watercress that harbors the encysted metacercariae. The larval flukes then migrate through the duodenal wall and across the peritoneal cavity, penetrate the liver capsule, pass through the liver parenchyma, and enter the bile ducts to become adult worms. Approximately 3 to 4 months after the initial infection the adult flukes start producing operculated eggs that are identical to those of *F. buski*, as seen in stool examination.

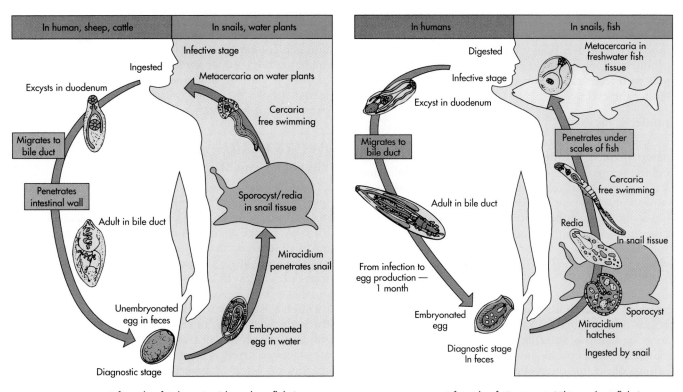

FIGURE 78-3 Life cycle of *F. hepatica* (sheep liver fluke).

FIGURE 78-4 Life cycle of *O. sinensis* (Chinese liver fluke).

Epidemiology

Infections have been reported worldwide in sheep-raising areas, with the appropriate snail as an intermediate host. These areas include the former Soviet Union, Japan, Egypt, and many Latin American countries. Outbreaks are directly related to human consumption of contaminated watercress in areas where infected herbivores are present. Human infection is rare in the United States, but several well-documented cases have been reported in travelers from endemic areas.

Clinical Syndromes

Migration of the larval worm through the liver produces irritation of this tissue, tenderness, and hepatomegaly. Pain in the right upper quadrant, chills, and fever with marked eosinophilia are commonly observed. As the worms take up residence in the bile ducts, their mechanical irritation and toxic secretions produce hepatitis, hyperplasia of the epithelium, and biliary obstruction. Some worms penetrate eroded areas in the ducts and invade the liver to produce necrotic foci referred to as *liver rot*. In severe infections, secondary bacterial infection can occur, and portal cirrhosis is common.

Laboratory Diagnosis

Stool examination reveals operculated eggs indistinguishable from the eggs of *F. buski*. Exact identification is a therapeutic problem because treatment is not the same for both infections. Whereas *F. buski* responds favorably to praziquantel, *F. hepatica* does not. When exact identification is desired, examination of a sample of the patient's bile differentiates the species; if the eggs are present in bile, they are *F. hepatica*, not *F. buski*, which is limited to the small intestine. Eggs may appear in stool samples from people who have eaten infected sheep or cattle liver. The spurious nature of this finding can be confirmed by having the patient refrain from eating liver and then rechecking the stool.

Treatment, Prevention, and Control

In contrast to *F. buski*, *F. hepatica* responds poorly to praziquantel. Treatment with bithionol or the benzimidazole compound triclabendazole has been effective. Preventive measures are similar to those for *F. buski* control; people who live in areas frequented by sheep and cattle should especially avoid ingestion of watercress and other uncooked aquatic vegetation.

OPISTHORCHIS SINENSIS
Physiology and Structure

O. sinensis, also referred to as *Clonorchis sinensis* in the older literature, is commonly called the *Chinese liver fluke*. Figure 78-4 illustrates its life cycle, which involves two intermediate hosts. This trematode differs from other fluke cycles because the eggs are eaten by the snail and then reproduction begins in the soft tissues of the snail. *O. sinensis* also requires a second intermediate host, freshwater fish, where the cercariae encyst and develop into infective metacercariae. When uncooked freshwater fish harboring metacercariae are eaten, flukes develop first in the duodenum and then migrate to the bile ducts where they become adults. The adult fluke undergoes self-fertilization and begins producing eggs. *O. sinensis* may survive in the biliary tract for as long as 50 years, producing approximately 2000 eggs per day. These eggs pass with feces and are once again eaten by snails, reinitiating the cycle.

Epidemiology

O. sinensis is found in China, Japan, Korea, and Vietnam, where it is estimated to infect approximately 19 million people. It is one of the most frequent infections seen among Asian refugees, and it can be traced to the consumption of raw, pickled, smoked, or dried freshwater fish that harbor the viable metacercariae. Dogs, cats, and fish-eating mammals can also serve as reservoir hosts.

Clinical Syndromes

Infection in humans is usually mild and asymptomatic. Severe infections with many flukes in the bile ducts produces fever, diarrhea, epigastric pain, hepatomegaly, anorexia, and occasionally jaundice. Biliary obstruction may occur, and chronic infection can result in adenocarcinoma of the bile ducts. Invasion of the gallbladder may produce cholecystitis, cholelithiasis, and impaired liver function, as well as liver abscesses.

Laboratory Diagnosis

The diagnosis is made by recovering the distinctive eggs from stool. The eggs measure 27 to 35 × 12 to 19 μm and are characterized by a distinct operculum with prominent shoulders and a tiny knob at the posterior (abopercular) pole (Figure 78-5). In mild infections, repeated examinations of stool or duodenal aspirates may be necessary. In acute symptomatic infection, there are usually eosinophilia and an elevation of serum alkaline phosphatase levels. Radiographic imaging procedures may detect abnormalities of the biliary tract.

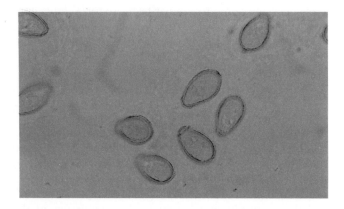

FIGURE 78-5 *O. sinensis* egg. These ovoid eggs are small (22 to 30 μm long and 12 to 19 μm wide) and have a yellowish brown, thick shell with a prominent operculum at one end and a small knob at the other.

Treatment, Prevention, and Control

The drug of choice is praziquantel. Prevention of infection is accomplished by not eating uncooked fish and by implementing proper sanitation policies, including the disposal of human, dog, and cat feces in adequately protected sites so that they cannot contaminate water supplies with the intermediate snail and fish hosts.

PARAGONIMUS WESTERMANI

Physiology and Structure

P. westermani, commonly called the *lung fluke*, is one of several species of *Paragonimus* that infect humans and many other animals. Figure 78-6 shows a familiar fluke life cycle from egg to snail to infective metacercaria. The infective stage occurs in a second intermediate host: the muscles and gills of freshwater crabs and crayfish. In humans who ingest infected meat, the larval worm hatches in the stomach and follows an extensive migration through the intestinal wall to the abdominal cavity, then through the diaphragm, and finally to the pleural cavity. Adult worms reside in the lungs and produce eggs that are liberated from ruptured bronchioles and appear in sputum or, when swallowed, in feces.

Epidemiology

Paragonimiasis occurs in many countries in Asia, Africa, India, and Latin America. It can be seen in refugees from

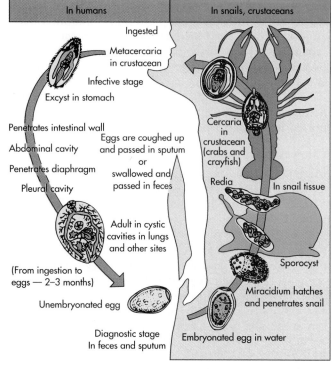

FIGURE 78-6 Life cycle of *P. westermani* (Oriental lung fluke).

Southeast Asia. Its prevalence is directly related to the consumption of uncooked freshwater crabs and crayfish. It is estimated that approximately 3 million people are infected with this lung fluke. As many as 1% of all Indochinese immigrants to the United States are infected with *P. westermani*. A wide variety of shore-feeding animals (e.g., wild boars, pigs, and monkeys) serve as reservoir hosts, and some human infections result from ingestion of meat containing migrating larval worms from these reservoir hosts. Human infections endemic to the United States are usually caused by a related species, *P. kellicotti*, which is found in crabs and crayfish in eastern and Midwestern waters.

Clinical Syndromes

The clinical manifestations of paragonimiasis may result from larvae migrating through tissues or from adults established in the lungs or other ectopic sites. The onset of disease coincides with larval migration and is associated with fever, chills, and high eosinophilia. The adult flukes in the lungs first produce an inflammatory reaction that results in fever, cough, and increased sputum. As the destruction of lung tissue progresses, cavitation occurs around the worms, sputum becomes blood tinged and dark with eggs (so-called rusty sputum), and patients experience severe chest pain. The resulting cavity may become secondarily infected with bacteria. Dyspnea, chronic bronchitis, bronchiectasis, and pleural effusion may be seen. Chronic infections lead to fibrosis in the lung tissue. The location of larvae, adults, and eggs in ectopic sites may produce severe clinical symptoms depending on the site involved. The migration of larval worms may result in invasion of the spinal cord and brain, producing severe neurological disease (visual problems, motor weakness, and convulsive seizures) referred to as **cerebral paragonimiasis**. Migration and infection may also occur in subcutaneous sites, the abdominal cavity, and the liver.

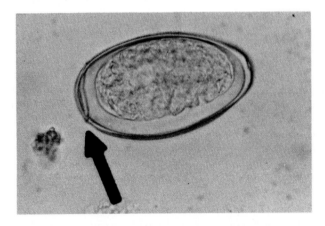

FIGURE 78-7 *P. westermani* egg. These large, ovoid eggs (80 to 120 μm long and 45 to 70 μm wide) have a thick, yellowish brown shell and a distinct operculum *(arrow)*. (From Koneman EW et al: *Color atlas and textbook of diagnostic microbiology,* ed 2, Philadelphia, 1979, JB Lippincott.)

Laboratory Diagnosis

Examination of sputum and feces reveals golden brown, operculated eggs (Figure 78-7). Pleural effusions, when present, should be examined for eggs. Chest x-ray films often show infiltrates, nodular cysts, and pleural effusion. Marked eosinophilia is common. Serological procedures are available through reference laboratories and can be helpful, particularly in cases with extrapulmonary (e.g., central nervous system) involvement.

Treatment, Prevention, and Control

The drug of choice is praziquantel; bithionol is an alternative. Education regarding the consumption of uncooked freshwater crabs and crayfish, as well as the flesh of animals found in endemic areas, is critical. Pickling and wine-soaking of crabs and crayfish do not kill the infective metacercarial stage. Proper sanitation and control of the disposal of human feces are essential.

SCHISTOSOMES

Schistosomiasis is a major parasitic infection of tropical areas, with some 200 million infections worldwide. The three schistosomes most frequently associated with human disease are *Schistosoma mansoni, S. japonicum,* and *S. haematobium.* They collectively produce the disease called **schistosomiasis,** also known as *bilharziasis* or **snail fever.** As discussed earlier, the schistosomes differ from other flukes: They are male and female rather than hermaphroditic, and their eggs do not have an operculum. They also are obligate intravascular parasites and are not found in cavities, ducts, and other tissues. The infective forms are skin-penetrating cercariae liberated from snails, and these differ from other flukes in that they are not eaten on vegetation, in fish, or in crustaceans.

Figure 78-8 illustrates the life cycle of the different schistosomes. Infection is initiated by ciliated, free-swimming cercaria in fresh water that penetrate intact skin, enter the circulation, and develop in the intrahepatic portal circulation (*S. mansoni* and *S. japonicum*) or in the vesical, prostatic, rectal, and uterine plexuses and veins *(S. haematobium)*. The female has a long, slender, cylindrical body, whereas the shorter male, which appears cylindrical, is actually flat. The cylindrical appearance derives from folding the sides of the body to produce a groove, the gynecophoral canal, in which the female resides for fertilization. Both sexes have oral and ventral suckers and an incomplete digestive system, which is typical of a fluke.

As the worms develop in the portal circulation, they elaborate a remarkable defense against host resistance. They coat themselves with substances that the host recognizes as itself; consequently, there is little host response directed against their presence in blood vessels. This protective mechanism accounts for chronic infections that may last 20 to 30 years or longer.

After developing in the portal vein, the male and female adult worms pair up and migrate to their final

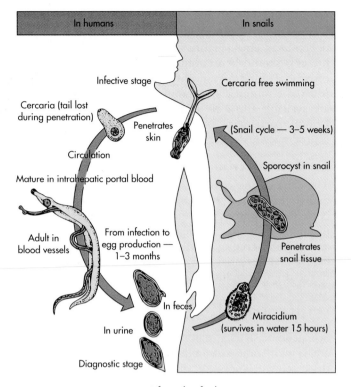

In humans	In snails

Infective stage

Cercaria free swimming

Cercaria (tail lost during penetration)

Penetrates skin

(Snail cycle — 3–5 weeks)

Circulation

Mature in intrahepatic portal blood

Sporocyst in snail

Adult in blood vessels

From infection to egg production — 1–3 months

Penetrates snail tissue

In feces

In urine

Miracidium (survives in water 15 hours)

Diagnostic stage

FIGURE 78-8 Life cycle of schistosomes.

FIGURE 78-9 *S. mansoni* egg. These eggs are 115 to 175 μm long and 45 to 70 μm wide, contain a miracidium, and are enclosed in a thin shell with a prominent lateral spine.

locations, where fertilization and egg production begin. *S. mansoni* and *S. japonicum* are found in mesenteric veins and produce **intestinal schistosomiasis;** *S. haematobium* occurs in veins around the urinary bladder and causes **vesicular schistosomiasis.** On reaching the submucosal venules of their respective locations, the worms initiate oviposition, which may continue at the rate of 300 to 3000 eggs daily for 4 to 35 years. Although the host inflammatory response to the adult worms is minimal, the eggs elicit an intense inflammatory reaction with mononuclear and polymorphonuclear cellular infiltrates and the formation of microabscesses. In addition, the larvae inside the eggs produce enzymes that aid in tissue destruction and allow the eggs to pass through the mucosa and into the lumen of the bowel and bladder, where they are passed to the external environment in the feces and urine, respectively.

The eggs hatch quickly on reaching fresh water to release motile miracidia. The miracidia then invade the appropriate snail host, where they develop into thousands of infectious cercariae. The free-swimming cercariae are released into the water, where they are immediately infectious for humans and other mammals.

The infection is similar in all three species of human schistosomes in that disease results primarily from the host's immune response to the eggs. The very earliest signs and symptoms are due to the penetration of the cercariae through the skin. Immediate and delayed hypersensitivity to parasite antigens result in an intensely pruritic papular skin rash.

The onset of oviposition results in a symptom complex known as *Katayama syndrome,* which is marked by fever, chills, cough, urticaria, arthralgias, lymphadenopathy, splenomegaly, and abdominal pain. This syndrome is typically seen 1 to 2 months after primary exposure and may persist for 3 months or more. It is thought to result from the massive release of parasite antigens with subsequent immune complex formation. Associated laboratory abnormalities include leukocytosis, eosinophilia, and polyclonal gammopathy.

The more chronic and significant phase of schistosomiasis is due to the presence of eggs in various tissues and the resulting formation of granulomas and fibrosis. The retained eggs induce extensive inflammation and scarring, the clinical significance of which is directly related to the location and number of eggs.

Because of differences in some aspects of disease and epidemiology, these worms are discussed as separate species.

Schistosoma mansoni
Physiology and Structure

S. mansoni usually resides in the small branches of the inferior mesenteric vein near the lower colon. The species of *Schistosoma* can be differentiated by their characteristic egg morphology (Figures 78-9 to 78-11). The eggs of *S. mansoni* are oval, possess a sharp lateral spine, and measure 115 to 175 × 45 to 70 μm (Figure 78-9).

Epidemiology

The geographical distribution of the various species of *Schistosoma* depends on the availability of a suitable snail host. *S. mansoni* is the most widespread of the schistosomes and is endemic in Africa, Saudi Arabia, and Madagascar. It has also become well established in the western hemisphere, particularly in Brazil, Surinam, Venezuela, parts of the West Indies, and Puerto Rico. Cases origi-

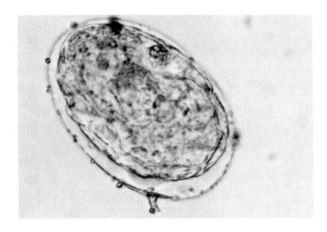

FIGURE 78-10 *S. japonicum* egg. These eggs are smaller than those of *S. mansoni* (70 to 100 μm long and 55 to 65 μm wide) and have a spine that is inconspicuous. (From Ash LR, Orihel TC: *Atlas of human parasitology,* ed 2, Chicago, 1984, American Society of Clinical Pathologists.)

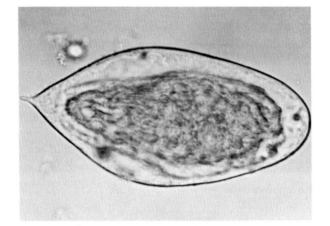

FIGURE 78-11 *S. haematobium* egg. These eggs are similar in size to those of *S. mansoni* but can be differentiated by the presence of a terminal spine. (From Ash LR, Orihel TC: *Atlas of human parasitology,* ed 2, Chicago, 1984, American Society of Clinical Pathologists.)

nating in these areas occur in the United States. In all of these areas, there are also reservoir hosts, specifically primates, marsupials, and rodents. Schistosomiasis may be considered a disease of economic progress; the development of massive land irrigation projects in desert and tropical areas has resulted in the dispersion of infected humans and snails to previously uninvolved areas.

Clinical Syndromes

As noted before, cercarial penetration of the intact skin may be seen as dermatitis with allergic reactions, pruritus, and edema. Migrating worms in the lungs may produce cough; as they reach the liver, hepatitis may appear.

Infections with *S. mansoni* may produce hepatic and intestinal abnormalities. As the flukes take up residence in the mesenteric vessels and egg laying begins, fever, malaise, abdominal pain, and tenderness of the liver may be observed. Deposition of eggs in the bowel mucosa results in inflammation and thickening of the bowel wall with associated abdominal pain, diarrhea, and blood in the stool. Eggs may be carried by the portal vein to the liver, where inflammation can lead to periportal fibrosis and eventually to portal hypertension and its associated manifestations.

Chronic infection with *S. mansoni* produces a dramatic hepatosplenomegaly with large accumulations of ascitic fluid in the peritoneal cavity. On gross examination, the liver is studded with white granulomas (**pseudotubercles**). Although *S. mansoni* eggs are primarily deposited in the intestine, eggs may appear in the spinal cord, lungs, and other sites. A similar fibrotic process occurs at each site. Severe neurological problems may follow when eggs are deposited in the spinal cord and brain. In fatal schistosomiasis caused by *S. mansoni,* fibrous tissue, reacting to the eggs in the liver, surrounds the portal vein in a thick, grossly visible layer ("clay pipestem fibrosis").

Laboratory Diagnosis

The diagnosis of schistosomiasis is usually established by the demonstration of characteristic eggs in feces. Stool examination reveals the large golden eggs with a sharp lateral spine (Figure 78-9). Concentration techniques may be necessary in light infections. Using rectal biopsy, the clinician can see the egg tracks laid by the worms in rectal vessels. Quantitation of egg output in stool is useful in estimating the severity of infection and in following the response to therapy. Serological tests are also available but are largely of epidemiological interest only. The development of newer tests using stage-specific antigens may allow the distinction of active from inactive disease and thus have greater clinical application.

Treatment, Prevention, and Control

The drug of choice is praziquantel, and the alternative is oxamniquine. Antihelminthic therapy may terminate oviposition but does not affect lesions caused by eggs already deposited in tissues. Schistosomal dermatitis and Katayama syndrome may be treated with the administration of antihistamines and corticosteroids. Education regarding the life cycles of these worms and control of snails using molluscacides are essential. Improved sanitation and control of human fecal deposits are critical. Mass treatment may one day be practical, and the development of a vaccine may be forthcoming.

Schistosoma japonicum

Physiology and Structure

S. japonicum resides in branches of the superior mesenteric vein around the small intestine and in the inferior mesenteric vessels. *S. japonicum* eggs (Figure 78-10) are smaller, are almost spherical, and possess a tiny spine. These eggs are produced in greater numbers than those of *S. mansoni* and *S. haematobium*. Because of the size, shape, and numbers of these eggs, they are carried to more sites in the body (liver, lungs, brain), and infection with a few *S. japonicum* adults can be more severe than infections involving similar numbers of *S. mansoni* or *S. haematobium.*

Epidemiology

This **Oriental blood fluke** is found only in China, Japan, the Philippines, and on the island of Sulawesi, Indonesia. Epidemiological problems correlate directly with a broad range of reservoir hosts, many of which are domestic (cats, dogs, cattle, horses, and pigs).

Clinical Syndromes

The initial stages of infection with *S. japonicum* are similar to those of *S. mansoni,* with dermatitis, allergic reactions, fever, and malaise, followed by abdominal discomfort and diarrhea. Katayama syndrome associated with the onset of oviposition is observed more commonly with *S. japonicum* than with *S. mansoni.* In chronic *S. japonicum* infection, hepatosplenic disease, portal hypertension, bleeding esophageal varices, and accumulation of ascitic fluid are commonly seen. Granulomas that appear as pseudotubercles in and on the liver are common, along with the clay pipestem fibrosis as described for *S. mansoni.*

S. japonicum frequently involves cerebral structures when eggs reach the brain and granulomas develop around them. The neurological manifestations include lethargy, speech impairment, visual defects, and seizures.

Laboratory Diagnosis

Stool examination demonstrates the small, golden eggs with tiny spines; usually, rectal biopsy is similarly revealing. Serological tests are available.

Treatment, Prevention, and Control

The drug of choice is praziquantel. Prevention and control may be achieved by measures similar to those for *S. mansoni,* especially education of populations in endemic areas regarding proper water purification, sanitation, and control of human fecal deposits. Control of *S. japonicum* must also involve the broad range of reservoir hosts and consider the fact that people work in rice paddies and on irrigation projects where infected snails are present. Mass treatment may offer help, and a vaccine may be developed someday.

Schistosoma haematobium
Physiology and Structure

After development in the liver, these blood flukes migrate to the vesical, prostatic, and uterine plexuses of the venous circulation; occasionally the portal bloodstream; and only rarely other venules.

Large eggs with a sharp terminal spine (Figure 78-11) are deposited in the wall of the bladder and occasionally in the uterine and prostatic tissues. Those deposited in the bladder wall can break free and are found in urine.

Epidemiology

S. haematobium occurs throughout the Nile Valley and in many other parts of Africa, including islands off the eastern coast. It also appears in Asia Minor, Cyprus, southern Portugal, and India. Reservoir hosts include monkeys, baboons, and chimpanzees.

Clinical Syndromes

Early stages of infection with *S. haematobium* are similar to those of infections involving *S. mansoni* and *S. japonicum,* with dermatitis, allergic reactions, fever, and malaise. Unlike the other two schistosomes, *S. haematobium* produces hematuria, dysuria, and urinary frequency as early symptoms. Associated with hematuria, bacteriuria is frequently a chronic condition. Egg deposition in the walls of the bladder may eventually result in scarring with loss of bladder capacity and the development of obstructive uropathy.

Patients with *S. haematobium* infections involving many flukes frequently demonstrate squamous cell carcinoma of the bladder. It is commonly stated that the leading cause of cancer of the bladder in Egypt and other parts of Africa is *S. haematobium.* The granulomas and pseudotubercles seen in the bladder may also be present in the lungs. Fibrosis of the pulmonary bed caused by egg deposition leads to dyspnea, cough, and hemoptysis.

Laboratory Diagnosis

Examination of urine specimens reveals the large, terminally spined eggs. Occasionally, bladder biopsy is helpful in establishing the diagnosis. *S. haematobium* eggs may appear in stool if worms have migrated to mesenteric vessels. Serological tests are also available.

Treatment, Prevention, and Control

The drug of choice is praziquantel. At present, education, possible mass treatment, and development of a vaccine are the best approaches to the control of *S. haematobium* disease. The basic problems of irrigation projects (e.g., dam building), migratory human populations, and multiple reservoir hosts make prevention and control extremely difficult.

CERCARIAL DERMATITIS

Several nonhuman schistosomes have cercariae that penetrate human skin, producing a severe dermatitis ("swimmer's itch"), but these schistosomes cannot develop into adult worms. The natural hosts are birds and other shore-feeding animals from freshwater lakes throughout the world and a few marine beaches. The intense pruritus and urticaria from this skin penetration may lead to secondary bacterial infection from scratching the sites of infection.

Treatment consists of oral trimeprazine and topical applications of palliative agents. When indicated, sedatives may be given. Control is difficult because of bird migration and the transfer of live snails from lake to lake. Molluscicides such as copper sulfate have produced some reduction in the snail populations. Immediate drying of the skin when people leave such waters offers some protection.

CASE STUDY AND QUESTIONS

A 45-year-old Egyptian man was referred for evaluation of hematuria and urinary frequency of 2 months' duration. This individual had lived in the Middle East for most of his life but for the past year lived in the United States. He denied previous renal or urological problems. His physical examination was unremarkable. A midstream urine specimen was grossly bloody.

1. What was the differential diagnosis of hematuria in this patient?
2. What was the etiological agent of this patient's urological process?
3. What exposures might put an individual at risk for this infection?
4. What are the major complications of this infection?
5. How is this disease treated?

Bibliography

Beaver PC, Jung RC, Cupp EW: *Clinical parasitology,* ed 9, Philadelphia, 1984, Lea & Febiger.

Burton K et al: Pulmonary paragonimiasis in Laotian refugee children, *Pediatrics* 70:246-248, 1982.

Harinasuta T, Pungpak S, Keystone JS: Trematode infections: opisthorchiasis, clonorchiasis, fascioliasis, and paragonimiasis, *Infect Dis Clin North Am* 7:699-716, 1993.

James SL: *Schistosoma* spp: progress toward a defined vaccine, *Exp Parasitol* 63:247-252, 1987.

Johnson RJ et al: Paragonimiasis: diagnosis and use of praziquantel in treatment, *Rev Infect Dis* 7:200-206, 1985.

Lucey DR, Maguire JH: Schistosomiasis, *Infect Dis Clin North Am* 7:635-653, 1993.

Markell EK, Voge M, John DT: *Medical parasitology,* ed 7, Philadelphia, 1992, WB Saunders.

Wongratanacheewin S et al: Characterization of humoral immune response in the serum and bile of patients with opisthorchiasis and its application in immunodiagnosis, *Am J Trop Med Hyg* 38:356-362, 1988.

Cestodes

The bodies of cestodes, **tapeworms,** are flat and ribbonlike, and the heads are equipped with organs of attachment. The head, or scolex, of the worm usually has four muscular, cup-shaped suckers and a crown of hooklets. An exception is *Diphyllobothrium latum,* the fish tapeworm, whose scolex is equipped with a pair of long, lateral muscular grooves and lacks hooklets.

The individual segments of tapeworms are called *proglottids,* and the chain of proglottids is called a *strobila.*

All tapeworms are hermaphroditic, with male and female reproductive organs present in each mature proglottid. The eggs of most tapeworms are nonoperculated and contain a six-hooked hexacanth embryo; the one exception, *D. latum,* has an unembryonated, operculated egg similar to fluke eggs. Tapeworms have no digestive system, and food is absorbed from the host intestine through the soft body wall of the worm. Most tapeworms found in the human intestine have complex life cycles involving intermediate hosts, and in some instances (cysticercosis, echinococcosis, sparganosis) humans serve as a form of intermediate host that harbors larval stages. The presence of extraintestinal larvae are at times more serious than that of adult worms in the intestine. The most common cestodes of medical importance are listed in Table 79-1.

TAENIA SOLIUM

Physiology and Structure

After a person ingests pork muscle containing a larval worm called a *cysticercus* ("bladder worm"), attachment of the scolex with its four muscular suckers and crown of hooklets initiates infection in the small intestine (Figure 79-1). The worm then produces proglottids until a strobila of proglottids is developed, which may be several meters in length. The sexually mature proglottids contain eggs, and as these proglottids leave the host in feces, they can contaminate water and vegetation ingested by swine. The eggs in swine become a six-hooked larval form called an **oncosphere** that penetrates the pig's intestinal wall, migrates in the circulation to the tissues, and becomes a cysticercus to complete the cycle.

Epidemiology

T. solium infection is directly correlated with eating insufficiently cooked pork and is prevalent in Africa, India, Southeast Asia, China, Mexico, Latin American countries, and Slavic countries. It is seen infrequently in the United States.

Clinical Syndromes

Adult *T. solium* in the intestine seldom causes appreciable symptoms. The intestine may be irritated at sites of attachment, and abdominal discomfort, chronic indigestion, and diarrhea may occur. Most patients become aware of the infection only when they see proglottids or a strobila of proglottids in their feces.

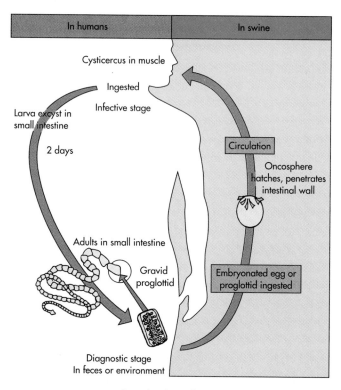

FIGURE 79-1 Life cycle of *T. solium* (pork tapeworm).

Laboratory Diagnosis

Stool examination may reveal proglottids and eggs, and treatment may produce the entire worm for identification. The eggs are spherical, are 30 to 40 μm in diameter, and possess a thick, radially striated shell containing a six-hooked hexacanth embryo (Figure 79-2). The eggs are identical to those of *T. saginata* (beef tapeworm), so eggs alone are not sufficient for species identification. Critical examination of the proglottids reveals their internal structure, which is important for the differentiation of *T. solium* and *T. saginata*. Gravid proglottids of *T. solium* are smaller than those of *T. saginata* and contain only 7 to 13 lateral uterine branches vs. 15 to 30 for the beef tapeworm.

Treatment, Prevention, and Control

The drug of choice is niclosamide; praziquantel, paromomycin, or quinacrine is an effective alternative. Prevention of pork tapeworm infections requires that pork be either cooked until the interior of the meat is gray or frozen at −20° C for at least 12 hours. Sanitation is critical; every effort must be made to keep human feces containing *T. solium* eggs out of water and vegetation ingested by pigs.

FIGURE 79-2 *Taenia* egg. The eggs are spherical, are 30 to 40 μm in diameter, and contain three pairs of hooklets internally. The eggs of the different *Taenia* species cannot be differentiated.

CYSTICERCOSIS

Physiology and Structure

Cysticercosis involves infection of people with the larval stage of *T. solium*, the cysticerci, which normally infect pigs (Figure 79-3). Human ingestion of water or vegetation contaminated with *T. solium* eggs from human feces initiates the infection. Autoinfection may occur when eggs from a person infected with the adult worm are transferred from the perianal area to the mouth on contaminated fingers. Once ingested, the eggs hatch in the stomach of the intermediate host, releasing the hexacanth embryo or oncosphere. The oncosphere penetrates the intestinal wall and migrates in the circulation to the tissues, where it develops into a cysticercus over 3

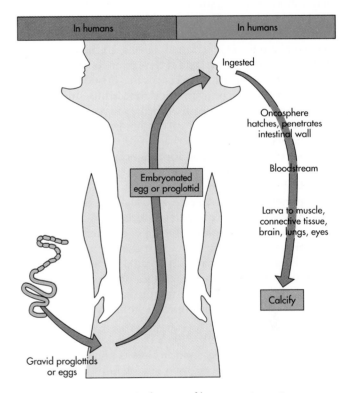

FIGURE 79-3 Development of human cysticercosis.

TABLE 79-1	Medically Important Cestodes		
CESTODE	**COMMON NAME**	**RESERVOIR FOR LARVAE**	**RESERVOIR FOR ADULTS**
Taenia solium	Pork tapeworm	Hogs	Humans
	Cysticercosis	Humans	—
Taenia saginata	Beef tapeworm	Cattle	Humans
Diphyllobothrium latum	Fish tapeworm	Freshwater crustaceans and fish	Humans, dogs, cats, bears
Echinococcus granulosus	Unilocular hydatid cyst	Herbivores, humans	Canines
Echinococcus multilocularis	Alveolar hydatid cyst	Herbivores, humans	Foxes, wolves, dogs, cats
Hymenolepis nana	Dwarf tapeworm	Rodents, humans	Rodents, humans
Hymenolepis diminuta	Dwarf tapeworm	Insects	Rodents, humans
Dipylidium caninum	Pumpkin seed tapeworm	Fleas	Dogs, cats

to 4 months. The cysticerci may develop in muscle, connective tissue, brain, lungs, and eyes and remain viable for as long as 5 years.

Epidemiology

Cysticercosis is found in the areas where *T. solium* is prevalent and is directly correlated with human fecal contamination. In addition to fecal-oral transmission, autoinfection may occur when a proglottid containing eggs is regurgitated from the small intestine into the stomach, allowing the eggs to hatch and release the infectious oncosphere.

Clinical Syndromes

A few cysticerci in nonvital areas (e.g., subcutaneous tissues) may not provoke symptoms, but serious disease may follow as the cysticerci lodge in vital areas such as the brain and eyes. In the brain, they may produce hydrocephalus, meningitis, cranial nerve damage, seizures, hyperactive reflexes, and visual defects. In the eye, loss of visual acuity may occur, and if the larvae lodge along the optic tract, visual field defects result. Tissue reaction to viable larvae may be only moderate, thus minimizing symptoms. However, death of the larvae results in the release of antigenic material that stimulates a marked inflammatory reaction; exacerbation of symptoms can result in fever, muscle pains, and eosinophilia.

Laboratory Diagnosis

The presence of cysticerci is usually established by the appearance of calcified cysticerci in soft tissue roentgenograms, surgical removal of subcutaneous nodules, and visualization of cysts in the eye. Central nervous system lesions may be detected by computed tomography, radioisotope scanning, or ultrasonography. Serological studies may be useful; false-positive results may occur in people with other helminthic infections.

Treatment, Prevention, and Control

The drug of choice for cysticercosis is praziquantel. Albendazole has also been used successfully in the treatment of parenchymal neurocysticercosis. Concomitant steroid administration may be necessary to minimize the inflammatory response to dying larvae. Surgical removal of cerebral and ocular cysts may be necessary. Critical to the prevention and control of human infection are the treatment of human cases harboring adult *T. solium* (to reduce egg transmission) and the controlled disposal of human feces. These measures also reduce the likelihood of infection in pigs.

TAENIA SAGINATA

Physiology and Structure

The life cycle of *T. saginata*, the **beef tapeworm**, is similar to that of *T. solium* (Figure 79-4), with infection resulting after cysticerci are ingested in insufficiently cooked beef. After excystment, the larvae develop into adults in the small intestine and initiate egg production in maturing proglottids. The adult worm may parasitize the jejunum and small intestine of humans for as long as 25 years, attaining a length of 10 m. In contrast with *T. solium* infections, cysticercosis produced by *T. saginata* does not occur in humans. The adult *T. saginata* worm also differs from *T. solium* because it lacks a crown of hooklets on the scolex and has a different proglottid uterine branch structure. These facts are important in differentiating between the two tapeworms but do not affect therapy.

Epidemiology

T. saginata occurs worldwide and is one of the most frequent causes of cestode infections in the United States. Humans and cattle perpetuate the life cycle: Human feces contaminate water and vegetation with eggs, which are then ingested by cattle. The cysticerci in cattle produce adult tapeworms in humans when rare or insufficiently cooked beef is eaten.

Clinical Syndromes

The syndrome that results from *T. saginata* infection is similar to the intestinal infection with *T. solium*. Patients are generally asymptomatic or may complain of vague abdominal pains, chronic indigestion, and hunger pains. Proglottids may pass out of the anus directly.

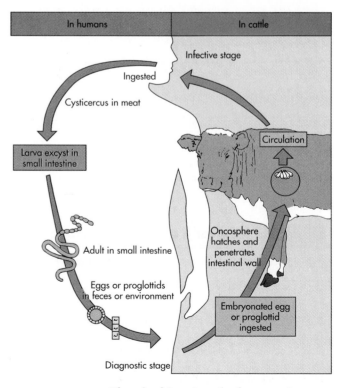

FIGURE 79-4 Life cycle of *T. saginata* (beef tapeworm).

Laboratory Diagnosis

The diagnosis of *T. saginata* infection is similar to that of *T. solium*, with recovery of proglottids and eggs or recovery of an entire worm whose scolex lacks hooklets. Study of the uterine branches in the proglottids differentiates *T. saginata* from *T. solium*.

Treatment, Prevention, and Control

Treatment is identical to that for the intestinal phase of *T. solium*. A single dose of niclosamide is highly effective in eliminating the adult worm. Education regarding cooking beef and controlling of the disposal of human feces is a critical measure.

DIPHYLLOBOTHRIUM LATUM

Physiology and Structure

One of the largest tapeworms (20 to 30 feet long), *D. latum* (**fish tapeworm**) has a complex life cycle involving two intermediate hosts: freshwater crustaceans and freshwater fish (Figure 79-5). The ribbonlike larval worm in the flesh of freshwater fish is called a **sparganum.** Ingestion of this sparganum in raw or insufficiently cooked fish initiates infection. The scolex of *D. latum* is shaped like a lance and has long, lateral grooves (bothria), which serve as organs of attachment. The proglottids of *D. latum* are broad, have a central uterine structure resembling a rosette, and produce eggs with an operculum, like fluke eggs, and a knob on the shell at the bottom of the egg. The adult worms may produce eggs for months or years. More than 1 million eggs per day are released into the fecal stream. On reaching fresh water, the unembryonated, operculate eggs require a period of 2 to 4 weeks to develop a ciliated, free-swimming larval form called a *coracidium*. The fully developed coracidium leaves the egg via the operculum and is ingested by tiny crustaceans that are called *copepods* (e.g., *Cyclops* and *Diaptomus* species); then the coracidium develops into a procercoid larval form. The crustacean harboring the larval stage is then eaten by a fish, and the infectious plerocercoid or sparganum larvae develop in the musculature of the fish. If the fish is in turn eaten by another fish, the sparganum simply migrates into the muscles of the second fish. Humans are infected when they eat raw or undercooked fish containing the larval forms.

Epidemiology

D. latum infection occurs worldwide, most prevalently in cool lake regions where raw or pickled fish is popular. Insufficient cooking over campfires and tasting and seasoning "gefilte fish" account for many infections. A reservoir of infected wild animals, such as bears, minks, walruses, and members of the canine and feline families that eat fish, are also sources for human infections. The practice of dumping raw sewage into freshwater lakes contributes to the propagation of this tapeworm.

Clinical Syndromes

Clinically, as is the case with most adult tapeworm infections, most *D. latum* infections are asymptomatic. Occasionally, people complain of epigastric pain, abdominal cramping, nausea, vomiting, and weight loss. As many as 40% of *D. latum* carriers may have low serum levels of vitamin B_{12}, presumably because of the competition between the host and the worm for dietary vitamin B_{12}. A small percentage (0.1% to 2%) of people infected with *D. latum* develop clinical signs of vitamin B_{12} deficiency, including megaloblastic anemia and neurological manifestations such as numbness, paresthesia, and loss of vibration sense.

Laboratory Diagnosis

Stool examination reveals the bile-stained, operculated egg with its knob at the bottom of the shell (Figure 79-6). Typical proglottids with the rosette uterine structure may also be found in stool specimens. Concentration techniques are usually not necessary because the worms produce large numbers of ova.

Treatment, Prevention, and Control

The drug of choice is niclosamide; praziquantel and paromomycin are acceptable alternatives. Vitamin B_{12} supplementation may be necessary in people with evidence of clinical vitamin B_{12} deficiency. The prevalence of this infection is reduced by avoiding the ingestion of insufficiently cooked fish; controlling the disposal of hu-

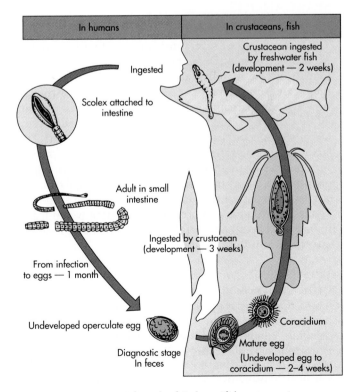

FIGURE 79-5 Life cycle of *D. latum* (fish tapeworm).

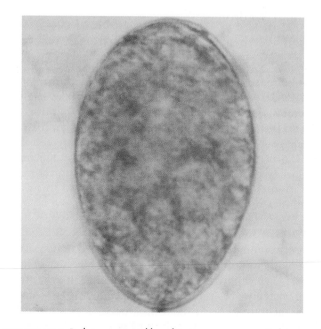

FIGURE 79-6 *D. latum* egg. Unlike other tapeworm eggs, *D. latum* eggs are operculated. They are 45 × 70 μm in size. (From Lennette EH et al: *Manual of clinical microbiology,* ed 4, Washington, DC, 1985, American Society for Microbiology.)

man feces, especially the proper treatment of sewage before disposal in lakes; and promptly treating infections.

SPARGANOSIS

Physiology and Structure

The larval forms of several tapeworms closely related to *D. latum* (most often *Spirometra* species) can produce human disease in subcutaneous sites and in the eye. In these cases, humans act as the end-stage host for the larval stage, or sparganum. Infections are acquired primarily by drinking pond or ditch water that contains crustaceans (copepods) that carry a larval tapeworm. This larval form penetrates the intestinal wall and migrates to various sites in the body, where it develops into a sparganum. Infections may also occur if tadpoles, frogs, and snakes are ingested raw or if the flesh of these animals is applied to wounds as a poultice. The larval worm leaves the relatively cold flesh of the dead animal and migrates into the warm human flesh.

Epidemiology

Cases have been reported from various parts of the world, including the United States, but the infection is most prevalent in the Orient. Regardless of location, drinking contaminated water and eating raw tadpole, frog, and snake flesh lead to infection.

Clinical Syndromes

In subcutaneous sites, sparganosis can produce painful inflammatory tissue reactions and nodules. In the eye the tissue reaction is intensely painful, and periorbital edema is common. Corneal ulcers may develop with ocular involvement. Ocular disease is frequently associated with the use of frog or snake flesh as a poultice over a wound near the eye.

Laboratory Diagnosis

Sections of tissue removed surgically show characteristic tapeworm features, including highly convoluted parenchyma and dark-staining calcareous corpuscles.

Treatment, Prevention, and Control

Surgical removal is the customary approach. The drug praziquantel may be used; however, no clinical data support its efficacy. Education regarding possible contamination of drinking water with crustaceans that harbor larval worms is essential, and contamination most likely occurs in pond and ditch water. Ingestion of raw frog and snake flesh or their use as poultices over wounds also should be avoided.

ECHINOCOCCUS GRANULOSUS

Physiology and Structure

Infection with *E. granulosus* is another example of accidental human infection, with humans serving as dead-end intermediate hosts in a life cycle that occurs naturally in other animals. *E. granulosus* adult tapeworms are found in nature in the intestines of canines (dog, fox, wolf, coyote, jackal, dingo); the larval cyst stage is present in the viscera of herbivores (sheep, cattle, swine, deer, moose, elk) (Figure 79-7). The worm consists of a *Taenia*-like scolex with four sucking disks and a double row of hooklets as well as a strobila containing three proglottids: one immature, one mature, and one gravid. Adult tapeworms in the canine intestine produce infective eggs that pass in feces. The eggs are identical in appearance to those of the *Taenia* species. When these eggs are ingested by humans, a six-hooked larval stage called an *oncosphere* hatches. The oncosphere penetrates the human intestinal wall and enters the circulation to be carried to various tissue sites, primarily the liver and lungs but also the central nervous system and bone. This same cycle occurs in the viscera of herbivores. When the herbivore is killed by a canine predator or viscera is fed to canines, the ingestion of cysts produces adult tapeworms in the canine intestine to complete the cycle and initiate new egg production. Adult tapeworms do not develop in the intestines of herbivores or humans.

In humans the larvae form a **unilocular hydatid cyst,** which is a slow-growing, tumorlike, and space-occupying structure enclosed by a laminated germinative membrane. This membrane produces structures on its wall called **brood capsules,** where tapeworm heads **(protoscolices)** develop. **Daughter cysts** may develop in the original mother cyst and also produce brood capsules and protoscolices. The cysts and daughter cysts accumulate fluid as they grow. This fluid is potentially toxic; if

FIGURE 79-7 Life cycle of *E. granulosus*.

spilled into body cavities, anaphylactic shock and death can result. Spillage and the escape of protoscolices can lead to the development of cysts in other sites because the protoscolices have the germinative potential to form new cysts. Eventually, the brood capsules and daughter cysts disintegrate within the mother cyst, liberating the accumulated protoscolices. These become known as **hydatid sand.** This type of echinococcus cyst is called a *unilocular cyst* to differentiate it from related cysts that grow differently. The unilocular cyst is generally about 5 cm in diameter, but some as large as 20 cm, containing almost 2 L of cyst fluid, have been reported. The cyst may die and become calcified over long periods.

Epidemiology

Human infection with *E. granulosus* unilocular cyst is directly correlated with raising sheep in many countries in Europe, South America, Africa, Asia, Australia, and New Zealand. It occurs in Canada and in the United States, with cases reported from Alaska, Utah, New Mexico, Arizona, California, and the lower Mississippi valley. Human infection follows ingestion of contaminated water or vegetation as well as hand-to-mouth transmission of canine feces carrying the infective eggs.

Clinical Syndromes

Because the unilocular cyst grows slowly, 5 to 20 years may pass before any symptoms appear. In many instances, it appears that the cyst is as old as its host. The

pressure of the expanding cyst in an organ is usually the first sign of infection. In the majority of cases the cysts are located in the liver or lung. In the liver the cyst may exert pressure on both bile ducts and blood vessels and create pain and biliary rupture. In the lungs cysts may produce cough, dyspnea, and chest pains. Rupture of the cysts may occur in 20% of cases, producing fever, urticaria, and occasionally anaphylactic shock and death, which are caused by the release of antigenic cyst contents. Cyst rupture may also lead to dissemination of infection resulting from the release of thousands of protoscolices. In bone the cyst is responsible for erosion of the marrow cavity and the bone itself. In the brain, severe damage may occur as a result of the cyst's tumorlike growth into brain tissue.

Laboratory Diagnosis

The diagnosis of hydatid disease is difficult and depends primarily on clinical, radiographic, and serological findings. Radiologic examination, scanning procedures, tomography, and ultrasound techniques are all valuable and may provide the first evidence of the cyst's presence. Aspiration of cyst contents may demonstrate the presence of the protoscolices (hydatid sand); however, it is contraindicated because of the risk of anaphylaxis and dissemination of the infection. Serological testing may be useful, but results are negative in 10% to 40% of infections.

Treatment, Prevention, and Control

Surgical resection of the cyst is the treatment of choice. In some instances the cyst is first aspirated to remove the fluid and hydatid sand, and then it is instilled with formalin to kill and detoxify remaining fluid; finally, it is rolled into a marsupial pouch and sewn shut. If the condition is inoperable because of the cyst's location, medical therapy with high-dose albendazole, mebendazole, or praziquantel may be considered. The most important factor in preventing and controlling echinococcosis is education regarding the transmission of infection and the role of canines in the life cycle. Proper personal hygiene and the washing of hands and cooking utensils in environments inhabited by dogs are critical. Dogs should not be allowed in the vicinity of animal slaughter and should never be fed the viscera of slain animals. In some areas the killing of stray dogs has reduced the incidence of infection.

ECHINOCOCCUS MULTILOCULARIS
Physiology and Structure

Like infection with *E. granulosus*, human infection with *E. multilocularis* is accidental (Figure 79-8). Adult *E. multilocularis* tapeworms are primarily found in foxes and wolves, although farm dogs and cats harbor them in some rural environments. The intermediate hosts that harbor the cyst stage are rodents (mice, voles, shrews, and lemmings). Humans become infected with the cyst

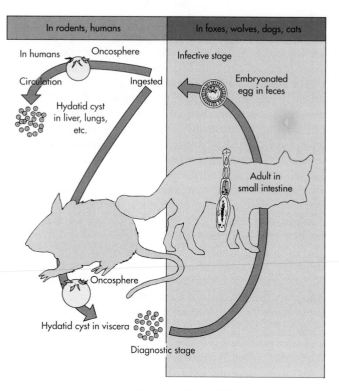

FIGURE 79-8 Life cycle of *E. multilocularis.*

and portal pathways. Often the growth metastasizes to the lungs and brain. Malnutrition, ascites, and portal hypertension produced by *E. multilocularis* create the appearance of hepatic cirrhosis. Among all of the worm infections of humans, *E. multilocularis* is one of the most lethal. If left untreated, the mortality rate is approximately 70% of infected people.

Laboratory Diagnosis

Unlike *E. granulosus,* the tissue form of *E. multilocularis* presents no protoscolices, and the material so resembles a neoplasm that even pathologists mistake it for carcinoma. Radiologic procedures and scanning techniques are helpful, and serological methods are available.

Treatment, Prevention, and Control

Surgical removal of the cyst is indicated, especially if an entire hepatic area can be resected. The same surgical approach applies to lesions in the lung wherein a lobe can be resected. Mebendazole and albendazole, as used for the treatment of *E. granulosus,* have produced clinical cures. As with *E. granulosus,* education, proper personal hygiene, and deworming of farm dogs and cats are critical. It is extremely important to treat animals that have contact with children.

HYMENOLEPIS NANA
Physiology and Structure

H. nana, the **dwarf tapeworm,** is only 2 to 4 cm in length, unlike *Taenia* organisms, which measure several meters. The life cycle is also simple and does not require an intermediate host (Figure 79-9), although mice and beetles may be infected and enter the cycle.

Infection begins when the embryonated eggs are ingested and develop in the intestinal villi into a larval cysticercoid stage. This cysticercoid larva attaches its four muscular suckers and crown of hooklets to the small intestine, and the adult worm produces a strobila of egg-laden proglottids. Eggs passing in the feces are then immediately and directly infective, initiating another cycle. Infection may also be acquired by ingesting infected insect intermediate hosts.

H. nana also can cause autoinfection, with a subsequent increased worm burden. Eggs are able to hatch in the intestine, develop into a cysticercoid larva, and then grow into adult worms without leaving the host. This can lead to hyperinfection with very heavy worm burdens and severe clinical symptoms.

Epidemiology

H. nana occurs worldwide in humans and is also a common parasite of mice. The most common tapeworm infection in North America, it occasionally develops its cysticercoid stage in beetles; humans and mice may ingest these beetles in contaminated grain and flour. Children are especially at risk of infection, and because of the simple life cycle of the parasite, families with children in day-

stage as a result of contact with fox, dog, or cat feces contaminated with eggs. Trappers and workers who handle fur pelts may become infected by inhaling fecal dust that carries eggs.

Infective eggs hatch in and penetrate the intestinal tract to become oncospheres. These forms enter the circulation and take up residence primarily in the liver and lungs but also possibly in the brain.

The **alveolar hydatid cyst** develops as an alveolar or honeycombed structure that is *not* covered by a unilocular-limiting mother cyst–laminated membrane. The cyst grows via exogenous budding, eventually resembling a carcinoma. In humans, individual cysts are said to be sterile and rarely produce protoscolices (hydatid sand).

Epidemiology

E. multilocularis is found primarily in northern areas such as Canada, the former Soviet Union, northern Japan, Central Europe, and Alaska, Montana, North and South Dakota, Minnesota, and Iowa in the United States. There is evidence that the life cycle may be extending to other Midwestern states, where foxes and mice transmit the organism to dogs and cats and eventually to humans.

Clinical Syndromes

E. multilocularis, because of its slow growth, may be present in human tissues for many years before symptoms appear. In the liver, cysts eventually mimic a carcinoma, with liver enlargement and obstruction of biliary

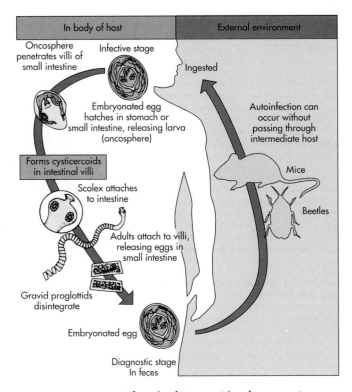

FIGURE 79-9 Life cycle of *H. nana* (dwarf tapeworm).

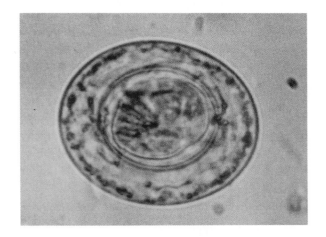

FIGURE 79-10 *H. nana* egg. The eggs are 30 to 45 μm in diameter and have a thin shell containing a six-hooked embryo. (From Lennette EH et al: *Manual of clinical microbiology,* ed 4, Washington, DC, 1985, American Society for Microbiology.)

care centers experience problems in controlling the transmission of this organism.

Clinical Syndromes

With only a few worms in the intestine, there are no symptoms. In heavy infections, especially if autoinfection and hyperinfection occur, patients experience diarrhea, abdominal pain, headache, anorexia, and other vague complaints.

Laboratory Diagnosis

Stool examination reveals the characteristic *H. nana* egg with its six-hooked embryo and polar filaments (Figure 79-10).

Treatment, Prevention, and Control

The drug of choice is praziquantel; an alternative is niclosamide. Treatment of cases, improved sanitation, and proper personal hygiene, especially in the family and institutional environments, are essential for controlling the transmission of *H. nana*.

HYMENOLEPIS DIMINUTA

Physiology and Structure

H. diminuta, closely related to *H. nana,* is primarily a tapeworm of rats and mice, but it is also found in humans. It differs from *H. nana* in length, measuring 20 to 60 cm. The scolex lacks hooklets, and the egg is larger, is bile-stained, and has no polar filaments. The life cycle of *H. diminuta* is more complex than that of *H. nana,* and it requires larval insects ("mealworms") to reach the infective cysticercoid stage.

Epidemiology

Infections have been found all over the world, including in the United States. Larval beetles and other larval insects become infected when they feed on rat feces that carry *H. diminuta* eggs. Humans are infected by ingesting the larval insects (mealworms) in contaminated grain products (e.g., flour, cereals).

Clinical Syndromes

Mild infections produce no symptoms, but heavier worm burdens produce nausea, abdominal discomfort, anorexia, and diarrhea.

Laboratory Diagnosis

Stool examination demonstrates the characteristic bile-stained egg that lacks polar filaments.

Treatment, Prevention, and Control

The drug of choice is niclosamide, with praziquantel an alternative. Rodent control in areas where grain products are produced or stored is essential. Thorough inspection of uncooked grain products to detect mealworms is also important.

DIPYLIDIUM CANINUM

Physiology and Structure

D. caninum, a small tapeworm averaging about 15 cm in length, is primarily a parasite of dogs and cats, but it can infect humans, especially children whose mouths are licked by infected pets. The life cycle involves the development of larval worms in dog and cat fleas. These fleas, when crushed by the teeth of the infected pet, are carried on the tongue to the child's mouth when the child kisses

FIGURE 79-11 *D. caninum* eggs. Free eggs are rarely seen. Instead, egg packets that contain 8 to 15 six-hooked oncospheres enclosed in a thin membrane are most commonly found in fecal specimens. (From Lennette EH et al: *Manual of clinical microbiology,* ed 4, Washington, DC, 1985, American Society for Microbiology.)

the pet or the pet licks the child. Swallowing the infected flea leads to intestinal infection.

Because of the size and shape of the mature and terminal proglottids, *D. caninum* is often called the *pumpkin seed tapeworm.* The eggs are distinctive because they occur in packets covered with a tough, clear membrane. There may be as many as 25 eggs in a packet, and a single egg free of the packet is seldom seen.

Epidemiology

D. caninum occurs worldwide, especially in children. Its distribution and transmission are directly correlated with dogs and cats infected with fleas.

Clinical Syndromes

Light infections are asymptomatic; heavier worm burdens produce abdominal discomfort, anal pruritus, and diarrhea. Anal pruritus results from the active migration of the motile proglottid.

Laboratory Diagnosis

Stool examination reveals the colorless egg packets (Figure 79-11), and proglottids may be in feces brought to physicians by patients.

Treatment, Prevention, and Control

The drug of choice is niclosamide; praziquantel and paromomycin are alternatives. Dogs and cats should be dewormed and not be allowed to lick the mouths of children. Pets should be treated to eradicate the fleas.

CASE STUDY AND QUESTIONS

A 30-year-old Hispanic man entered the emergency department after a focal neurological seizure. The patient had recently emigrated from Mexico and was in his usual state of good health before the seizure. Neurological examination revealed no focal findings. A computed tomographic scan of the head revealed multiple small cystic lesions in both cerebral hemispheres. Punctate calcification was noted in several of the lesions. A lumbar puncture revealed a glucose level of 65 mg/dl (normal) and a protein level of 38 mg/dl (normal) in cerebrospinal fluid. The white blood cell count was 20/mm³ (abnormal) with a differential of 5% neutrophils, 90% lymphocytes, and 5% monocytes. A purified protein derivative skin test was negative with positive controls. Serological test for human immunodeficiency virus was negative.

1. What was the differential diagnosis of this patient's neurological process?
2. Which parasite or parasites may have caused this condition?
3. What diagnostic tests were available for this infection?
4. What were the therapeutic options for this patient?
5. How do people become infected with this parasite?
6. What tissue sites (besides the central nervous system) may be involved? How would these additional foci of infection be documented.

Bibliography

Beaver PC, Jung RC, Cupp EW: *Clinical parasitology,* ed 9, Philadelphia, 1984, Lea & Febiger.

Botero D et al: Taeniasis and cysticercosis, *Infect Dis Clin North Am* 7:683-697, 1993.

Cook GC: Neurocysticercosis: parasitology, clinical presentation, diagnosis, and recent advances in management, *Q J Med* 68:575-583, 1988.

Desowitz RS: *New Guinea tapeworms and Jewish grandmothers,* New York, 1983, Avon/Discus.

Gottstein B: Molecular and immunologic diagnosis of echinococcosis, *Clin Microbiol Rev* 5:248-261, 1992.

Kammerer WS, Schantz PM: Echinococcal disease, *Infect Dis Clin North Am* 7:605-618, 1993.

Liu LX, Weller PF: Drug therapy: antiparasitic drugs, *New Engl J Med* 334:1178-1184, 1996.

Markell EK, Voge M, John DT: *Medical parasitology,* ed 7, Philadelphia, 1992, WB Saunders.

Schmidt GD Roberts LS: *Foundations of parasitology,* ed 4, St Louis, 1989, Mosby.

Arthropods

The arthropods are the largest of the animal phyla, with over 1 million species. The phylum Arthropoda comprises invertebrate animals with a segmented body, several pairs of jointed appendages, bilateral symmetry, and a rigid, chitinous exoskeleton that is molted periodically as the animal grows. Characteristically, arthropods develop from egg to adult by a process known as *metamorphosis*. As they mature, the organisms pass through several distinct morphological stages including egg, larvae or nymph, pupa (certain insects), and adult. Five classes of arthropods are of medical importance on the basis of the number or the severity of the illnesses they cause: the Chilopoda, Pentastomida, Crustacea, Arachnida, and Insecta (Table 80-1).

The arthropods or their larvae may affect human health in many ways. Most arthropods function indirectly in human disease; they transmit but do not produce disease. Arthropods may transmit disease mechanically, as when flies carry enteric bacterial pathogens from feces to human food. Of outstanding importance is the ability of many arthropods to act as biological vectors and intermediate hosts in the transmission and developmental cycle of viruses, bacteria, protozoa, and metazoa (Table 80-2). Certain arthropods may inflict direct injury by their bites or stings. Other species, such as lice, scabies mites, and tissue-invading maggots, may act as true parasites. Still other species may function as both parasites and vectors of disease.

It is not the purpose of this chapter to consider medical entomology in detail. Rather, our purpose is to provide a brief overview of several of the more important aspects of arthropods and their relationship to human disease. More detailed information on arthropods of medical importance and the therapy and control of arthropod infestations may be found in the references listed in the Bibliography.

CHILOPODA
Centipedes

Physiology and structure. The centipedes are elongated, multisegmented (15 to more than 181 segments), many-legged, tracheate arthropods. They possess a distinct head and trunk. The body is dorsoventrally flattened, and each trunk segment bears a single pair of legs. Maxillipeds or poison claws are situated on the first segment and are used for capturing prey. The centipedes are sometimes classified with the millipedes; however, millipedes lack the poison claws of centipedes and have two pairs of legs per segment.

Epidemiology. Most centipedes are predaceous insectivores and are commonly found in dark, damp environments such as the areas beneath logs, among rubbish, and inside old buildings. Human bites are almost invariably the result of accidental exposure to the organism during outdoor activities.

Clinical syndromes. Centipede bites may be extremely painful and cause swelling at the site of the bite. Reports of the effects of centipede bites on humans are conflicting. One species, *Scolopendra gigantea*, which is found in Central and South America and the Galapagos Islands, reportedly has caused several deaths. With the exception of *Scolopendra* and related tropical genera, the bite of most centipedes is harmless to humans.

Treatment, prevention, and control. Treatment of a centipede bite includes local measures such as the application of compresses of sodium bicarbonate or solutions of Epsom salts. Control consists of removing rubbish near dwellings.

| TABLE 80-1 | **Medically Important Classes of Arthropods** |

PHYLUM	CLASS	ORGANISMS
Arthrodpoda	Chilopoda	Centipedes
	Pentastomida	Tongue worms
	Crustacea	Copepods
		Decapods (crabs, crayfish)
	Arachnida	Spiders, scorpions, mites, ticks
	Insecta	Flies, mosquitoes, lice, fleas, bugs, stinging insects

TABLE 80-2	**Select Human Illnesses Transmitted by Arthropods**

PRIMARY VECTOR OR INTERMEDIATE HOST	DISEASE	ETIOLOGICAL AGENT
ARACHNIDA		
Mite: *Leptotrombidium* species	Scrub typhus (tsutsugamushi disease)	*Rickettsia tsutsugamushi*
Mite: *Liponyssoides sanguineus*	Rickettsial pox	*Rickettsia akari*
Tick: *Dermacentor* species	Tularemia	*Francisella tularensis*
Tick: *Dermacentor species* and other ixodid ticks	Rocky Mountain spotted fever	*Rickettsia rickettsii*
Tick: *Dermacentor* species, *Boophilus* species	Q fever	*Coxiella burnetii*
Tick: *Dermacentor* species	Colorado tick fever	Orbivirus
Tick: *Ornithodoros* species	Relapsing fever	*Borrelia* species
Tick: *Ixodes* species	Babesiosis	*Babesia microti*
Tick: *Ixodes* species	Lyme disease	*Borrelia burgdorferi*
Tick: *Dermacentor variabilis, Amblyomma americanum*	Ehrlichiosis	*Ehrlichia risticii*
CRUSTACEA		
Copepod: *Cyclops* species	Diphyllobothriasis	*Diphyllobothrium latum*
Copepod: *Cyclops* species	Dracunculiasis	*Dracunculus medinensis*
Crabs, crayfish: various freshwater species	Paragonimiasis	*Paragonimus westermani*
INSECTA		
Lice: *Pediculus humanus*	Epidemic typhus	*Rickettsia prowazekii*
Lice: *Pediculus humanus*	Trench fever	*Rickettsia quintana*
Lice: *Pediculus humanus*	Louse-borne relapsing fever	*Borrelia recurrentis*
Flea: *Xenopsylla cheopis*, various other rodent fleas	Plague	*Yersinia pestis*
Flea: *Xenopsylla cheopis*	Murine typhus	*Rickettsia typhi*
Flea: various species	Dipylidiasis	*Dipylidium caninum*
Bug: *Triatoma* species, *Panstrongylus* species	Chagas' disease	*Trypanosoma cruzi*
Beetles: flour beetle	Hymenolepiasis	*Hymenolepis nana*
Fly, gnat: *Glossina* species (tsetse flies)	African trypanosomiasis	*Trypanosoma brucei rhodesiense* and *T. b. gambiense*
Fly, gnat: *Simulium* species	Onchocerciasis	*Onchocerca volvulus*
Fly, gnat: *Chrysops* species	Tularemia	*Francisella tularensis*
Fly, gnat: *Phlebotomus* species, *Lutzomyia* species (sandflies)	Leishmaniasis	*Leishmania* species
Fly, gnat: *Phlebotomus* species	Bartonellosis	*Bartonella bacilliformis*
Mosquito: *Anopheles* species	Malaria	*Plasmodium* species
Mosquito: *Aedes aegypti*	Yellow fever	Flavivirus
Mosquito: *Aedes* species	Dengue fever	Flavivirus
Mosquito: *Culiseta melanura, Coquillettidia perturbans, Aedes vexans*	Eastern equine encephalitis	Alphavirus
Mosquito: *Aedes triseriatus*	La Crosse encephalitis	Bunyavirus
Mosquito: *Culex* species	St. Louis encephalitis	Flavivirus
Mosquito: *Culex* species	Venezuelan equine encephalitis	Alphavirus
Mosquito: *Culex tarsalis*	Western equine encephalitis	Alphavirus
Mosquito: various species	Bancroftian filariasis	*Wuchereria bancrofti*
Mosquito: various species	Malayan filariasis	*Brugia* species
Mosquito: various species	Dirofilariasis	*Dirofilaria immitis*

PENTASTOMIDA
Tongue Worms

The pentastomids, or tongue worms, are bloodsucking endoparasites of reptiles, birds, and mammals. Their taxonomic status is uncertain. Some scientists include pentastomids among the arthropods because their larvae superficially resemble those of mites. Others consider them annelids, and still others place them in an entirely separate phylum. For purposes of this discussion, they are considered with the arthropods.

Physiology and structure. Tongue worms are degenerate, wormlike arthropods that live primarily in the nasal and respiratory passages of reptiles, birds, and mammals. Adult pentastomids are white, cylindrical or flattened parasites that possess two distinct body regions: an anterior head, or cephalothorax, and an abdomen. The adults are elongated and may attain a length of 1 to 10 cm. The head has a mouth and two pairs of hooks. Although the abdomen may appear annulated, it is not segmented (Figure 80-1). The pentastomids possess digestive and reproductive organs; however, they lack circulatory and respiratory systems.

The adult pentastomids are found in the lungs of reptiles and the nasal passages of mammals. Many vertebrates, including humans, may serve as intermediate hosts. The embryonated eggs are discharged in the feces or respiratory secretions of the infected definitive host and contaminate vegetation or water, which is in turn ingested by one of several possible intermediate hosts (fish, rodents, goats, sheep, or humans). The eggs hatch in the intestine, and the primary larvae penetrate the intestinal wall and attach to the peritoneum. The larvae mature in the peritoneum and develop into infective larvae, encyst in viscera, or die and become calcified. In tissue sections, encysted larvae can be identified by acidophilic glands, a chitinous cuticle, and prominent hooks, which are present in the anterior end of the organism. Subcuticular glands and striated muscle fibers may also be observed beneath the cuticle.

Humans may also become infected by ingesting the inadequately cooked flesh of infected reptiles or other definitive hosts or by eating the infected flesh of intermediate hosts (e.g., goats, sheep) containing infective larvae. In the latter instance, the infective larvae migrate from the stomach to the nasopharyngeal tissues, where they develop into adult pentastomids and produce the symptoms of the *halzoun syndrome* (see section on clinical syndromes). In this case, the human host is considered a temporary definitive host.

Epidemiology. Most tongue worm infections are reported in Europe, Africa, and South and Central America. The infection is common in Malaysia, where autopsy studies reveal pentastomiasis in up to 45% of people. As previously described, the infection is acquired by ingesting raw vegetables or water contaminated with pentastome eggs or by consuming raw or undercooked flesh of infected animals.

Clinical syndromes. In most cases, infection is asymptomatic and is discovered accidentally during roentgenographic examination (calcified larvae), at surgery, or at autopsy. Pneumonitis, pneumothorax, peritonitis, meningitis, nephritis, and obstructive jaundice have all been ascribed to pentastomid infections; however, definitive proof of a causal relationship between disease and the presence of the parasite is frequently lacking. Localized infection of the eye has been reported, presumably secondary to direct inoculation.

Halzoun syndrome, caused by the attachment of adult pentastomes to the nasopharyngeal tissues, is characterized by pharyngeal discomfort, paroxysmal coughing, sneezing, dysphagia, and vomiting. Asphyxiation has been rarely reported.

Laboratory Diagnosis. The diagnosis is made by identifying a pentastomid in a biopsy specimen obtained at surgery or at autopsy. Occasionally, calcified larvae may be observed on x-ray films of the abdomen or chest, providing a presumptive diagnosis. There are no useful serological tests.

Treatment, prevention, and control. Treatment is not usually warranted. In symptomatic patients, surgical removal of free or encysted parasites should be attempted. Preventive measures include thorough cooking of meat and vegetables and avoidance of contaminated water.

FIGURE 80-1 Adult female pentastome *(Armillifer armillatus)* attached to the respiratory surface of the lung *(short arrow)* of a rock python. Note the short cephalothorax *(long arrow)* and a long, annulated abdomen. (From Binford CH, Connor DH: *Pathology of tropical and extraordinary diseases,* vol 2, Washington, DC, 1976, Armed Forces Institute of Pathology.)

CRUSTACEA

The crustaceans are primarily gill-breathing arthropods of fresh and salt water. Those of medical importance are found in fresh water and serve as intermediate hosts of various worms (Table 80-2).

The copepods, or water fleas, are represented by the genera *Cyclops* and *Diaptomus*. The larger crustaceans, called *decapods*, include crabs and crayfish. These crustaceans also serve as the second intermediate hosts of the lung fluke *Paragonimus westermani* (Table 80-2).

Copepods

Physiology and structure. Copepods are small, simple aquatic organisms. They lack a carapace, have one pair of maxillae, and have five pairs of biramous swimming legs. Free and parasitic forms exist. The genera *Diaptomus* and *Cyclops* are medically important.

Copepods are an intermediate host in the life cycle of several human parasites, including *Dracunculus medinensis* (dracunculiasis), *Diphyllobothrium latum* (diphyllobothriasis), *Gnathostoma spinigerum* (gnathostomiasis), and *Spirometra* species (sparganosis). Copepods have been associated with a single case of a perirectal abscess but generally are not considered a primary cause of human infection.

Epidemiology. Copepods have a worldwide distribution and serve as intermediate hosts for helminthic diseases in the United States and Canada as well as in Europe and the tropics. Human infection with these helminthic parasites results from ingesting water contaminated with copepods or from eating the raw or insufficiently cooked flesh of infected fish. Pseudooutbreaks of copepods present in human stool specimens submitted for ova and parasite examination have been reported from New York. As many as 40% of concentrated stools submitted for ova and parasite examination were found to contain copepods, presumably as a result of contamination of a hospital water supply. The single reported case of apparent human infection with copepods occurred in this hospital.

Clinical syndromes. The clinical signs and symptoms associated with helminthic infections in which copepods serve as intermediate hosts are described in Chapters 77 and 79. The single case of apparent human infection with copepods occurred in a 22-year-old man with Crohn's disease who had a perirectal abscess. Drainage of the abscess revealed purulent material that on microscopic examination contained numerous copepods surrounded by leukocytes. It was hypothesized that the copepods were introduced into preexisting perirectal lesions during sitz baths, which were prepared with unfiltered tap water and may have contained copepods. Although the copepods contained within the abscess material were viable and may have been successfully feeding on body tissue, it was felt that the copepods were unlikely to have been the primary cause of the abscess.

Laboratory diagnosis. The laboratory diagnosis of helminthic infections in which copepods serve as intermediate hosts are described in Chapters 77 and 79. In general, infection is demonstrated by detection of the infecting organism by microscopic examination of clinical material.

Treatment, prevention, and control. Specific treatment of copepod-associated helminthic infection is covered in Chapters 77 and 79. Prevention of these infections requires attention to standard public health measures such as the chlorination and filtration of water and thorough cooking of all fish. Infected people must not be allowed to bathe in water used for drinking, and suspected water should be avoided.

Decapods

The decapods include the prawns, shrimps, lobsters, crayfish, and crabs. The cephalothorax of these animals is always covered by a carapace. They have three anterior pairs of thoracic appendages that are modified into biramous maxillipeds and five posterior pairs that are developed into uniramous legs. Crabs and crayfish are medically important as the second intermediate hosts of the lung fluke *P. westermani*. The parasitic, epidemiological, and clinical aspects of infection with *P. westermani* are described in Chapters 77 and 79. Thorough cooking of crabs and crayfish is the most effective means of preventing infection with *P. westermani*.

ARACHNIDA
Spiders

Spiders have a number of characteristic features that permit easy identification. Specifically, they possess eight legs, no antennae, a body divided into two regions (cephalothorax and abdomen), and an unsegmented abdomen with spinnerets posteriorly. All true spiders produce venom and kill their prey by biting; however, few have fangs (chelicerae) powerful enough to pierce human skin or venom potent enough to produce more than a transitory local skin irritation. Venomous spiders may be classified as those that cause *systemic arachnidism* and those that cause *necrotic arachnidism*. This classification is based on the type of tissue damage produced.

Systemic arachnidism is primarily caused by tarantulas and black widow spiders. Tarantulas (family Theraphosidae) are large, hairy spiders of the tropics and subtropics. The tarantulas are of little importance because they are not very aggressive and avoid human habitations. Their bite causes intense pain and a phase of agitation, followed by stupor and somnolence. The black widow spider, *Latrodectus mactans*, is widespread through the southern and western United States. Related species of *Latrodectus* are found throughout temperate and tropical regions of all continents, but none is primarily domestic; thus their contact with humans is limited.

Necrotic arachnidism is produced by spiders that belong to the genus *Loxosceles*. The bites of these spiders may produce severe tissue reaction. *Loxosceles reclusa*, the brown recluse spider, is a medically important spider of this genus.

Black Widow Spiders

Physiology and structure. The female black widow spider (*L. mactans*) is easily recognized by the presence

FIGURE 80-2 Female black widow spider *(L. mactans).* (From Peters W: *A colour atlas of arthropods in clinical medicine,* London, 1992, Wolfe.)

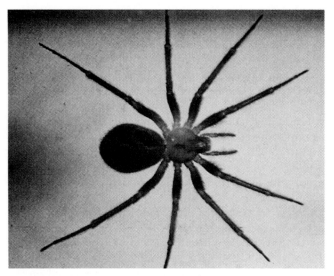

FIGURE 80-3 Female brown recluse spider *(L. laeta).* (Courtesy Professor H Schenone; from Peters W: *A colour atlas of arthropods in clinical medicine,* London, 1992, Wolfe.)

of a globose, shiny, black abdomen bearing the characteristic orange or reddish hourglass marking on the ventral surface (Figure 80-2). Females vary from 5 to 13.5 mm in body length, but the males are much smaller.

The venom of the black widow spider is a potent peripheral neurotoxin, which is delivered by a pair of jaw-like structures, or chelicerae. Only the female *Latrodectus* spider is dangerous to humans; the small, feeble male delivers an ineffective bite.

Epidemiology. These spiders frequent wood and brush piles, old wooden buildings, cellars, hollow logs, and privies. Given these locations, the bite is often located on the genitalia, buttocks, or extremities. Black widow spiders are common to the southern United States but are found throughout the temperate and tropical regions of both the New and Old World.

Clinical syndromes. As is true with most cases of envenomation, the clinical picture depends on factors such as the amount of the venom injected, the location of the bite, and the age, weight, and sensitivity of the patient. Shortly after the bite, there is a sharp pain but little or no immediate swelling. This is followed by local redness, swelling, and burning. Systemic signs and symptoms generally occur within an hour of the bite and include muscular cramps, chest pains, nausea, vomiting, diaphoresis, intestinal spasms, and visual difficulties. Abdominal tetanic cramps producing a "boardlike" abdomen are highly characteristic and may mimic an acute surgical abdomen. The acute symptoms usually subside within 48 hours; however, in severe cases, paralysis and coma may precede cardiac or respiratory failure. Mortality from the bite of the black widow spider is estimated at 4% to 5%.

Treatment, prevention, and control. Healthy adults usually recover, but small children or weakened people suffer considerably from these bites and may die

without treatment. Muscle spasms may be severe and may require the intravenous administration of calcium gluconate or other muscle relaxant agents. A specific antivenin is available and remains the treatment of choice. It is valuable if given shortly after the bite. Because it is prepared from the serum of hyperimmunized horses, patients must be tested for sensitivity to horse serum before administration. Hospitalization is advisable for the care of people with known or suspected bites.

Good housekeeping can be the simplest and most effective control for spiders in homes. This includes dusting webs and carefully removing debris from around homes and adjacent sheds. Children should be discouraged from playing on wood piles and in wood sheds.

Brown Recluse Spiders

Physiology and structure. Spiders producing necrotic arachnidism belong to the genus *Loxosceles*. These spiders are yellow to brown and are of medium size (5 to 10 mm long) with relatively long legs (Figure 80-3). They commonly display two distinguishing characteristics: a dark fiddle- or violin-shaped marking on the dorsal side of the cephalothorax, and six eyes arranged in three pairs forming a semicircle. The venom injected by the female or male spider is a necrotoxin that may also have hemolytic properties and that causes necrotic lesions with deep tissue damage.

Epidemiology. Four species of the genus *Loxosceles* are found in the Americas. *L. reclusa* is found in the south and central United States, *L. arizonica* is in the western states, and *L. laeta* is in South America. *L. reclusa* is found outdoors in wood piles and debris in warmer climates and in basements or storage areas in cooler regions. *L. laeta* is found in closets and corners of rooms. Humans are bitten only when the spider is threatened or disturbed.

Clinical syndromes. Initially the bite of *Loxosceles* species tends to be painless; however, several hours later, itching, swelling, and soreness may develop in the area of the bite. Frequently a vesicle or bleb may form at the site. General systemic symptoms are unusual but when present may include chills, headache, and nausea. Within 3 to 4 days the bleb sloughs and may be followed by ulceration and radiating necrosis, which does not heal but continues to spread for weeks or months.

Intravascular coagulation and hemolysis may occur and be accompanied by hemoglobinuria and cardiac and renal failure. This hemolytic syndrome may be life threatening and occurs more commonly after the bite of *L. laeta*. In South America, this syndrome is known as *visceral loxoscelism*.

Diagnosis. The discrimination of a species of spider is not possible from the appearance of the lesion alone; however, a working diagnosis is commonly based on the appearance of bleb formation around puncture marks and the nature of the developing lesion. The spider may be identified easily by the characteristic features previously described. An enzyme-linked immunosorbent assay has been developed to confirm the diagnosis of brown recluse spider bite but is not widely available.

Treatment, prevention, and control. The treatment of brown recluse spider bites is variable and based on the severity of the necrotic reaction. Most bites in the United States are inconsequential and require no specific therapy. Cleansing the bite wound and providing tetanus prophylaxis and antibiotics to prevent secondary infection may all be indicated. Healing is generally uncomplicated, and debridement or excision should not be performed for 3 to 6 weeks to allow natural healing to commence. Excision and skin grafting may be necessary for bites that have not healed in 6 to 8 weeks. Systemic therapy with corticosteroids may be useful in treating the hemolytic syndrome but are of little proven value in preventing or treating cutaneous necrosis. Although not available in the United States, an antivenin is used in South America for the treatment of visceral loxoscelism.

Preventive measures are similar to those recommended for black widow spiders. *Loxosceles* (and other) spiders may be controlled in dwellings with insecticide compounds.

Scorpions

Physiology and structure. The typical scorpion is elongated with conspicuous, pincherlike claws, or pedipalps, at the anterior end of the body; four pairs of walking legs; and a distinctly regimented abdomen that tapers to a curved, hollow, needlelike stinger (Figure 80-4). When the scorpion is disturbed, it uses the stinger for defense. Both male and female scorpions can sting. Venom is injected through the stinger from two venom glands in the abdomen. Most scorpions are unable to penetrate human skin or inject enough venom to cause real damage; however, a few species are capable of inflicting painful wounds that may cause death.

FIGURE 80-4 Scorpion (*Centruroides* species). (Courtesy Dr JC Cokendolpher; from Peters W: *A colour atlas of arthropods in clinical medicine,* London, 1992, Wolfe.)

Epidemiology. Scorpions considered dangerous may be found in the southwestern United States, Mexico, and Venezuela. This includes several species of the genus *Centruroides*, which accounts for as many as 1000 deaths annually. Also important are several species of *Tityus*, found in Trinidad, Argentina, Brazil, Guyana, and Venezuela. Children under the age of 5 years are most likely to be fatally stung by scorpions.

Scorpions are nocturnal, and during the day, they remain concealed under logs, rocks, and other dark, moist places. They invade human habitations at night, where they may hide in shoes, towels, clothing, and closets.

Clinical syndromes. The effect of a scorpion sting in a patient is highly variable and depends on factors such as the species and age of the scorpion, the kind and amount of venom injected, and the age, size, and sensitivity of the person who was stung. Although the sting of many scorpions is relatively nontoxic and produces only local symptoms, other stings may be quite serious. Scorpions produce two types of venom: a neurotoxin and hemorrhagic or hemolytic toxin. The hemolytic toxin is responsible for local reactions at the site of the sting, including radiating, burning pain; swelling; discoloration; and necrosis. The neurotoxin produces minimal local reaction but rather severe systemic effects, including chills, diaphoresis, excessive salivation, difficulty speaking and swallowing, muscle spasm, tachycardia, and generalized seizures. In severe cases, death may result from pulmonary edema and respiratory paralysis.

Diagnosis. Local or systemic signs and symptoms coupled with physical evidence of a single point of skin penetration are usually sufficient to establish the diagnosis. The patient may have observed the scorpion or brought it in for identification. Although scorpions are relatively easy to identify, it is important to realize that other nonpoisonous arachnids strongly resemble scorpions. An entomologist or parasitologist should be consulted if there is a taxonomic question.

Treatment, prevention, and control. The management of scorpion stings varies. In the absence of systemic symptoms, palliative treatment may be all that is necessary. Pain may be relieved by analgesics or local injection of xylocaine; however, opiates appear to increase toxicity. Local cryotherapy may reduce swelling and retard the systemic absorption of the toxin. Hot packs produce vasodilatation and may accelerate toxin distribution systemically and are therefore contraindicated. Antivenin is available and is effective if administered soon after the sting. Very young children with systemic symptoms should be treated as medical emergencies. Systemic symptoms and shock should be treated supportively.

Preventive measures include the use of chemical pesticides to reduce scorpion populations. Removal of debris around dwellings can reduce hiding and breeding places.

Mites

Mites are small, eight-legged arthropods characterized by a saclike body and no antennae. A large number of mite species are free-living or are normally associated with other vertebrates (e.g., birds, rodents) and may cause dermatitis in humans on rare occasions. The number of mites that are considered true human parasites or present real medical problems is quite small and include the human itch mite *(Sarcoptes scabiei)*, the human follicle mite *(Demodex folliculorum)*, and the chigger mite. Mites affect humans in three ways: by causing dermatitis, by serving as vectors of infectious diseases, and by acting as a source of allergens.

Itch Mites

Physiology and structure. The itch mite *(S. scabiei)* causes an infectious skin disease variably known as *scabies, mange,* or *the itch.* The adult mites average 300 to 400 μm in length with an oval, saclike body in which the first and second pairs of legs are widely separated from the third and fourth pairs (Figure 80-5). The body has dorsal transverse parallel ridges, spines, and hairs. The ova measure 100 to 150 μm.

Adult mites enter the skin, creating serpiginous burrows in the upper layers of the epidermis. The female mite lays her eggs in the skin burrows, and the larval and nymph stages that develop also burrow in the skin. The female mites live and deposit eggs and feces in epidermal burrows for up to 2 months. Characteristically, the preferred sites of infestation are the interdigital and popliteal folds, the wrist and inguinal regions, and the inframammary folds. The presence of the mites and their secretions cause intense itching of the involved areas. The mite is an obligate parasite and can perpetuate itself in a single host indefinitely.

Epidemiology. Scabies is cosmopolitan in distribution, with an estimated global prevalence of about 300 million cases. The mite is an obligate parasite of domestic animals and humans; however, it may survive for hours to days away from the host, thus facilitating its spread. Transmission is accomplished by direct contact or by contact with contaminated objects such as cloth-

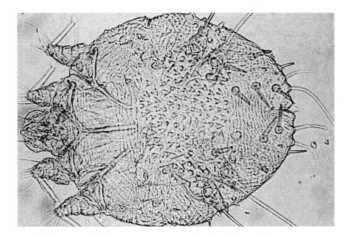

FIGURE 80-5 Scabies mite *(Sarcoptes* species). (From Peters W: *A colour atlas of arthropods in clinical medicine,* London, 1992, Wolfe.)

ing. Sexual transmission has been well documented. Spread of the infection to other areas of the body is accomplished by scratching and manual transfer of the mite by the affected person. Scabies may occur in epidemic fashion among people in crowded conditions such as day-care centers, nursing homes, military camps, and prisons.

Clinical syndromes. The outstanding clinical diagnostic symptom is intense itching, usually in the interdigital folds and sides of the fingers, buttocks, external genitalia, wrists, and elbows. The uncomplicated lesions appear as short, slightly raised cutaneous burrows. At the end of the burrow, there is frequently a vesicle containing the female mite. The intense pruritus usually leads to excoriation of the skin secondary to scratching, which in turn produces crusts and secondary bacterial infection. Patients experience their first symptoms within weeks to months after exposure; however, the incubation period may be as little as 1 to 4 days in persons sensitized by prior exposure. Host hypersensitivity (delayed or type IV) probably plays an important role in determining the variable clinical manifestations of scabies.

Some immunodeficient people may develop a variant of scabies, so-called Norwegian scabies, characterized by generalized dermatitis with extensive scaling and crusting and the presence of thousands of mites in the epidermis. This disease is highly contagious and suggests that host immunity also plays a role in suppressing *S. scabiei.*

Diagnosis. The clinical diagnosis of scabies is based on the characteristic lesions and their distribution. The definitive diagnosis of scabies depends on the demonstration of the mite in skin scrapings. Because the adult mite is most frequently found in the terminal portions of a fresh burrow, it is best to make scrapings in these areas. The scrapings are placed on a clean microscopic slide, cleared by the addition of 1 or 2 drops of a 20% solution of potassium hydroxide, covered with a coverslip, and examined under a low-power microscope. With experience, the mite and ova may be recognized. Skin biopsy may also reveal the mites and ova in tissue sections.

Treatment, prevention, and control. The standard, and very effective, treatment for scabies is 1% gamma benzene hexachloride (lindane) in a lotion base. One or two applications (head to toe) at weekly intervals is effective against scabies. Lindane is absorbed through the skin, and repeated applications may be toxic. For this reason, it is not advisable to use it in treating infants, small children, or pregnant or lactating women.

Recently, a 5% permethrin cream (Elimite) has replaced lindane lotions as the treatment of choice for scabies. Clinical trials have shown permethrin to be more effective and less toxic than lindane. Other precautions used to treat scabies include crotamiton, sulfur (6%) preparations, benzyl benzoate, and tetraethylthiuram monosulfide. The last two preparations are not available in the United States.

Primary prevention of scabies is best achieved with good hygiene habits, personal cleanliness, and routine washing of clothing and bed linens. Secondary prevention includes the identification and treatment of infected people and possibly their household and sexual contacts. In an epidemic situation, simultaneous treatment of all affected people and their contacts may be necessary. This is followed by thorough cleansing of the environment (e.g., boiling clothing and linens) and ongoing surveillance to prevent reoccurrence.

Human Follicle Mites

Physiology and structure. The human follicle mites include two species of the genus *Demodex, D. folliculorum* and *D. brevis*. These mites are minute (0.1 to 0.4 mm) organisms with a wormlike body, four pairs of stubby legs, and an annulate abdomen. *D. folliculorum* parasitizes the hair follicles of the face of most adult humans, whereas *D. brevis* is found in the sebaceous glands of the head and trunk.

Epidemiology. Organisms of the *Demodex* genus are obligate parasites of the human integument and are cosmopolitan in their distribution. Infestations are uncommon in young children and increase at the time of puberty. It is estimated that 50% to 100% of adults are infested with these mites.

Clinical syndromes. The role of *Demodex* species in human disease is uncertain. They have been associated with acne, blackheads, blepharitis, abnormalities of the scalp, and truncal rashes. More recently, extensive papular folliculitis resulting from *Demodex* infestation has been described in people with acquired immunodeficiency. Factors such as poor personal hygiene, increased sebum production, mite hypersensitivity, and immunosuppression may increase host susceptibility and enhance the clinical presentation of *Demodex* infestation. Most people infested with these mites remain asymptomatic.

Diagnosis. Mites may be demonstrated microscopically in material expressed from an infested follicle. They may be seen as incidental findings in histological sections of facial skin.

Treatment. Effective treatment consists of a single application of 1% gamma benzene hexachloride.

Chigger Mites

Physiology and structure. Chiggers are the larvae of mites of the family Trombiculidae. The adult trombiculid mites infest grass and bushes, and their larvae (i.e., chiggers) attack humans and other vertebrates, producing severe dermatitis. The larvae have three pairs of legs and are covered with characteristic branched, featherlike hairs.

The larvae appear as minute, barely visible, reddish dots attached to the skin where they use their hooked mouth parts to ingest tissue fluids. Chiggers typically attach to the skin areas where clothing is tight or restricted such as the wrists, ankles, armpits, groin, and waistline. After feeding, the engorged larvae fall to the ground where they molt and undergo development into nymphs and adults.

Epidemiology. Chiggers that are important in North America include the larvae of *Eutrombicula alfreddugesi* and *E. splendens*. In Europe the important species is the harvest mite, *Trombicula autumnalis*. Chiggers are a particular problem for outdoor enthusiasts such as campers and picnickers. In Europe and the Americas, they are associated with intensely pruritic lesions; however, in Asia, Australia, and the western Pacific rim, they serve as vectors of the rickettsial disease scrub typhus or tsutsugamushi fever *(Rickettsia tsutsugamushi)* (Table 80-2).

Clinical syndromes. Saliva injected into the skin at the time of mite attachment produces an intense pruritus and dermatitis. The skin lesions appear as small erythematous marks that progress to papules and may persist for weeks. Mite larvae may be visible in the center of the reddened swollen area. The irritation may be so severe that it causes fever and sleep disruption. Secondary bacterial infection of the excoriated lesions may occur.

Treatment, prevention, and control. Treatment for dermatitis caused by chiggers is largely symptomatic and consists of antipruritics, antihistamines, and steroids. The use of insect repellents such as *N,N'*-diethyl-m-toluamide (DEET) may be of some help in prevention for persons going into chigger-infested areas.

Ticks

Physiology and structure. Ticks are bloodsucking ectoparasites of a number of vertebrates, including humans. Ticks are opportunistic rather than host specific and tend to suck blood from a number of large and small animals. Ticks have a four-stage life cycle that includes the egg, larva, nymph, and adult. Although the larva, nymph, and adults are all bloodsuckers, it is the adult tick that usually bites humans.

Ticks comprise two large families, the Ixodidae, or hard ticks, and the Argasidae, or soft ticks. Soft ticks have a leathery body that lacks a hard dorsal scutum, and the mouthparts are located ventrally and are not visible from above (Figure 80-6). Hard ticks have a hard dorsal plate or scutum, and the mouthparts are clearly visible from above (Figure 80-7). Both hard and soft ticks serve as ectoparasites of humans. Soft ticks differ from hard ticks primarily in their feeding behavior. Soft ticks complete engorgement in a matter of minutes or at most a few hours; hard ticks feed slowly, taking 7 to 9 days to become engorged.

Epidemiology. Ticks are found in wooded and rural areas worldwide. In North America, the important species of hard ticks include *Dermacentor variabilis* (the American dog tick), *D. andersoni* (the Rocky Mountain wood tick), *Amblyomma americanum* (the lone star tick), *Rhipicephalus sanguineus* (the brown dog tick), and *Ixodes dammini* (the deer tick). These ticks are found variably throughout the United States and are important vectors of several infectious diseases, including Rocky Mountain spotted fever (*Dermacentor* species), tularemia (*Dermacentor* species), Q fever (*Dermacentor* species), Lyme disease (*Ixodes* species), babesiosis (*Ixodes* species), and ehrlichiosis *(D. variabilis* and *A. americanum)* (Table 80-2). Soft ticks of the genus *Ornithodoros* transmit relapsing fever spirochetes (*Borrelia* species) in limited areas in the West (Table 80-2). In general, people at risk for tick exposure are involved in outdoor activities in wooded areas. Tick exposure may also occur during stays in rural cabins inhabited by small rodents, which commonly serve as hosts for ticks and other ectoparasites.

Clinical syndromes. Tick bites are generally of minor consequence and are limited to small erythematous papules. More serious consequences of tick bite include the development of a type of paralysis resulting from substances released by ticks during feeding, and trans-

mission of a number of rickettsial, bacterial, viral, spirochetal, and protozoan diseases of humans and other animals.

Ticks may attach at any point on the body but typically favor the scalp hairline, ears, axillae, and groin. The initial bite is usually painless, and the presence of the tick may not be detected for several hours after contact. After the tick has dropped off or has been removed manually, the area may become reddened, painful, and pruritic. The wound may become secondarily infected and necrotic, particularly if the mouthparts remain attached after manual removal.

Three species of tick, *D. andersoni, D. variabilis,* and *A. americanum,* have all been reported to cause tick paralysis. This is characterized by an ascending flaccid paralysis, fever, and general intoxication, which may lead to respiratory compromise and death. The paralysis is due to toxic substances released in the saliva of the tick and may be reversed by tick removal. Tick paralysis is observed more commonly in young children and when tick attachment is in opposition to the central nervous system (e.g., scalp, head, neck).

Ticks are also involved in the transmission of infections such as Lyme disease, Rocky Mountain spotted fever, ehrlichiosis, Colorado tick fever, relapsing fever, tularemia, Q fever, and babesiosis (Table 80-2). The reader is referred to the appropriate sections of this book for discussion of the clinical and microbiological aspects of these infections.

Diagnosis. The diagnosis of tick bites and tick-borne diseases usually rests on the finding of a tick or a history of exposure to tick-infested areas. The identification of an organism as an adult tick is usually straightforward and based on the observations of an organism that is

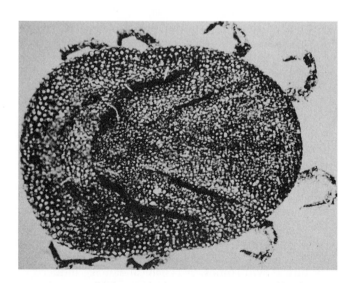

FIGURE 80-6 Soft tick (*Ornithodoros* species). (From Strickland GT: *Hunter's tropical medicine,* ed 7, Philadelphia, 1991, WB Saunders.)

FIGURE 80-7 Hard tick *(I. dammini).* (Courtesy Professor A Spielman; from Peters W: *A colour atlas of arthropods in clinical medicine,* London, 1992, Wolfe.)

dorsoventrally flattened and possesses four pairs of legs and no visible segmentation (Figures 80-6 and 80-7). An entomologist or parasitologist should be consulted if further identification is desired. The diagnosis of specific tick-borne infectious diseases is covered in the respective sections of this book.

Treatment, prevention, and control. Early removal of attached ticks is of primary importance and may be accomplished by steady traction on the tick body, grasped with forceps as close to the skin as possible. Care should be taken to avoid twisting or crushing the tick, which may leave the mouthparts attached to the skin or inject potentially infectious material into the wound. Steady traction is superior to noxious stimuli or occlusive techniques for the removal of ticks. After removal, the wound should be cleansed and observed for secondary infection. Because ticks may harbor highly infectious agents, the clinician should use appropriate infection-control precautions (e.g., use of gloves, handwashing, proper disposal of ticks and contaminated material) during tick removal.

Preventive measures used in tick-infested areas include the wearing of protective clothing that fits snugly about the ankles, wrists, waist, and neck so that ticks cannot gain access to the skin. Insect repellents such as N,N'-diethyl-m-toluamide (DEET) are generally effective. People and pets should be inspected for ticks after visits to tick-infested areas.

INSECTA

The insects, or hexapods, constitute the largest and most important of all the classes of arthropods, accounting for approximately 70% of all known species of animals. Insects include animals such as mosquitoes, flies, fleas, lice, roaches, bees, wasps, beetles, and moths to name just a few. The insect body is divided into three parts—head, thorax, and abdomen—and is equipped with one pair of antennae, three pairs of appendages, and one or two pairs of wings or no wings at all. The medical significance of any insect is related to its way of life, particularly its mouthparts and feeding habits. Insects may serve as vectors for a number of bacterial, viral, protozoan, and metazoan pathogens. Certain insects may serve merely as mechanical vectors for the transmission of pathogens, whereas in other insects the pathogens undergo multiplication or cyclic development within the insect host. The methods by which the insects transmit pathogens vary and are discussed here. Insects can also be pathogens themselves by causing mechanical injury through bites, chemical injury through the injection of toxins, and allergic reactions to materials transmitted by bites or stings. There are more than 30 orders of insects, but only those of major medical importance are discussed in this section.

Bloodsucking Diptera

Diptera is the large order of flying insects. All dipterans have a single pair of functional membranous wings and various modifications of the mouthparts, which have been adapted for piercing the skin and sucking blood or tissue juices. Their most important feature is their role as mechanical or biological vectors of a number of infectious diseases, including leishmaniasis, trypanosomiasis, malaria, filariasis, onchocerciasis, tularemia, bartonellosis, and the viral encephalitides (Table 80-2). The bloodsucking flies include mosquitoes, sandflies, and blackflies, all of which are capable of transmitting diseases to humans. Other dipterans such as horse flies and stable flies are capable of inflicting painful bites but are not known to transmit human pathogens. Although the common housefly does not bite, it certainly is capable of mechanical transmission of a number of viral, bacterial, and protozoan infections to human hosts. The infectious diseases transmitted by bloodsucking flies are well covered in other chapters of this book. The following section deals only with injury resulting from the bite of these insects and the effects of salivary substances introduced into the human skin and tissues.

Mosquitoes

Physiology and structure. Adult mosquitoes are small and have delicate legs, one pair of wings, long antennae, and greatly elongated mouthparts adapted for piercing and sucking. The two major families of mosquitoes (Culicidae), the Anophelinae and the Culicinae, share a number of similarities in their life cycles and development. They lay eggs on or near water, are good fliers, and feed on nectar and sugars. The females of most species also feed on blood, which they require for each clutch of 100 to 200 eggs. Females may take a blood meal every 2 to 4 days. In the act of feeding, the female mosquito injects saliva, which produces mechanical damage to the host but also may transmit disease and produce immediate and delayed immune reactions.

Epidemiology. Within the family Anophelinae, the genus *Anopheles* contains the species responsible for the transmission of human malaria. In the tropics, these mosquitoes breed continually in relation to rainfall. These species vary in their capacity for the transmission of malaria, and within each geographical area the number of species that serves as malaria vectors is small. *A. gambiae* is an important vector of malaria in sub-Saharan Africa.

Mosquitoes from *Aedes,* the largest genus of the subfamily Culicinae, are found in all habitats ranging from the tropics to the Arctic. This species may develop overwhelming populations in marsh or tundra and pasture or floodwater and have a severe impact on wildlife, livestock, and humans. *A. aegypti,* the yellow fever mosquito, usually breeds in man-made containers (flower pots, gutters, cans) and is the primary vector of yellow fever and dengue in urban environments throughout the world.

Clinical syndromes. Mechanical damage induced by the feeding mosquito is usually minor but may be accompanied by mild pain and irritation. The bite is usually followed within a few minutes by a small, flat weal surrounded by a red flare. The delayed reaction consists of itching, swelling, and reddening of the wound region. Secondary infection may follow as a result of scratching.

Treatment, prevention, and control. Medical attention is usually not sought for a bite unless secondary infection occurs. Local anesthetics or antihistamines may be useful in treating reactions to mosquito bites.

Preventive measures in mosquito-infested areas include the use of window screens, netting, and protective clothing. Insect repellents such as DEET are generally effective. Mosquito-control measures that involve the use of insecticides have been effective in some areas.

Gnats and Biting Midges

Physiology and structure. *Ceratopogonids* represent an assortment of tiny flies with names such as *gnats, midges,* and *punkies.* The majority of the flies that attack humans belong to the genus *Culicoides;* they are minute (0.5 to 4 mm long) and slender enough to pass through the fine mesh of ordinary window screens. The females suck blood and typically feed at dusk, when they may attack in large numbers.

Epidemiology. Biting midges may be important pests in beach and resort areas near salt marshes. Those of the genus *Culicoides* are the main vectors of filariasis in Africa and the New World tropics.

Clinical syndromes. The mouthparts of biting midges are lancetlike and produce a painful bite. Bites may produce local lesions lasting hours or days.

Treatment, prevention, and control. Local treatment is palliative with lotions, anesthetics, and antiseptic measures. The treatment of breeding sites with pesticides and repellents may be useful against some of the common species of these pests.

Sandflies

Physiology and structure. Sandflies, or moth flies, belong to a single subfamily of the Psychodidae, the Phlebotominae. They are small (1 to 3 mm), delicate, hairy, weak-flying insects that suck the blood of humans, dogs, and rodents. They transmit a number of infections, including leishmaniasis (Table 80-2). Female flies become infected when they feed on infected people.

Epidemiology. Phlebotomine larvae develop in nonaquatic habitats such as moist soil, stone walls, and rubbish heaps. In many areas, sandflies cause problems as pests. They also serve as vectors of infectious diseases such as leishmaniasis in the Mediterranean, the Middle East, Asia, India, and Latin America.

Clinical syndromes. The bite may be painful and pruritic around the local lesion. Sensitized people may have allergic reactions. Sandfly fever is characterized by severe frontal headaches, malaise, retroorbital pain, anorexia, and nausea.

Treatment, prevention, and control. Sandflies are very sensitive to insecticides, which should be applied to breeding sites and window screens. Various insect repellents may also be useful.

Blackflies

Physiology and structure. Members of the family Simuliidae are commonly called *blackflies* or *buffalo gnats.* They are 1 to 5 mm long, are hump-backed, and have mouthparts consisting of six "blades" that are capable of tearing skin (Figure 80-8). Blackflies are bloodsucking insects and breed in fast-flowing streams and rivers. They are of major importance as vectors of onchocerciasis (Table 80-2).

Epidemiology. Blackflies are common in Africa and South America, where they serve as vectors of onchocerciasis. In North America they are common around the lake regions of Canada and the northern United States. They are pests to hunters and fisherman in these areas. In large numbers they may cause significant blood loss and pose a major threat to wild and domestic animals.

Clinical syndromes. A variety of responses have been observed in humans after the bite of blackflies. The bite of the female can tear the skin surface and induce bleeding that continues for some time after the fly has departed. There is usually a distinct hemorrhagic spot at the site of the bite. Multiple bites may result in considerable blood loss. The bite is painful and is accompanied by local inflammation, itching, and swelling.

The local reaction may also be accompanied by a systemic response that varies according to the number of bites and the sensitivity of the person. This syndrome is known as *blackfly fever* and is marked by headache, fever, and adenitis. It usually subsides within 48 hours and is considered a hypersensitivity reaction to the salivary secretions of the fly.

In addition to local and systemic responses to blackfly bites, a hemorrhagic syndrome has been described after bites of blackflies in certain areas of Brazil. This syndrome resembles thrombocytopenic purpura and is characterized by local and disseminated cutaneous hemor-

FIGURE 80-8 Blackfly (*Simulium* species), the vector of onchocerciasis. (Courtesy Dr S Meredith; from Peters W: *A colour atlas of arthropods in clinical medicine,* London, 1992, Wolfe.)

rhages associated with mucosal bleeding. It is thought that this hemorrhagic syndrome may be produced by a hypersensitivity phenomenon or response to a toxin caused by multiple blackfly bites.

Diagnosis. The blackfly bite is marked characteristically by a point of dried blood and subcutaneous hemorrhage at the wound site. In people with the hemorrhagic syndrome, platelet counts are reduced; there is a prolonged bleeding time and poor clot retraction in about half of patients.

Treatment, prevention, and control. Treatment includes the usual palliative measures (e.g., anesthetics, antihistamines, lotions) to relieve local pruritus and swelling. Patients with the hemorrhagic syndrome have shown marked improvement with corticosteroid therapy.

Preventive measures include protective clothing. In general, insect repellents are ineffective against blackflies. Some control is achieved by pouring insecticides into rivers and streams.

Horse and Deer Flies

The family Tabanidae consists of species that attack mainly animals, including horse flies, deer flies, gadflies, and mango flies. They are large, ranging in length from 7 to 30 mm. The males feed on plant juices, the females on blood. In the act of biting, the female fly leaves a deep wound, causing blood to flow, which the fly laps up. The fly may serve as a mechanical vector of infectious diseases when the fly's mouthparts become contaminated on one host and transfer organisms to the next. These flies are not considered important vectors of infectious disease in humans.

Muscoid Flies

Physiology and structure. The muscoid flies include the important insects, the housefly, *Musca domestica;* the stable fly, *Stomoxys calcitrans;* and the tsetse flies of the genus *Glossina.* The stable fly, often mistaken for the housefly, is a true bloodsucker capable of serving as a short-term mechanical vector of a number of bacterial, viral, and protozoal infections. The tsetse fly (Figure 80-9) is also a biting fly and serves as the biological vector and intermediate host for the agents of African trypanosomiasis, *Trypanosoma brucei rhodesiense* and *T. b. gambiense.* The common housefly represents a host of genera that are nonpiercing or contaminating flies. Because of their living and feeding habits, they mechanically transmit diverse agents to humans.

Epidemiology. The tsetse fly is found in the eastern and central regions of Africa, where it is of major medical and veterinary importance as the intermediate host and biological vector of a number of trypanosomes that infect humans and animals. The housefly and stable fly are cosmopolitan in distribution and serve as indicators of poor sanitation. The housefly, *M. domestica,* lays eggs on any matter that will serve as food for developing fly larvae, or maggots (feces, garbage, decaying plant matter). Stable flies commonly lay eggs in moist, decaying

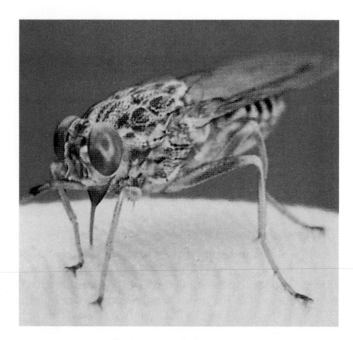

FIGURE 80-9 Tsetse fly, the vector of African trypanosomiasis. (Courtesy Wellcome Foundation, Ltd, Berkhamsted; from Peters W: *A colour atlas of arthropods in clinical medicine,* London, 1992, Wolfe.)

vegetable matter such as grass clippings or compost heaps found in suburban communities.

Prevention and control. Control of tsetse fly populations has been problematic because of their widespread distribution in primarily rural and undeveloped areas. Insect repellents and insecticides may be effective against adult flies. Improved sanitation is important in controlling houseflies. Plant refuse should be protected from rain or destroyed.

Myiasis-Causing Flies

Myiasis is the term applied to the disease produced by maggots that live parasitically in human tissues. Clinically, myiasis may be classified according to the body part involved (e.g., nasal, intestinal, or urinary myiasis). The number of myiasis-producing flies and the diversity in life-style requirements are enormous. Only the host-relations and sites of predilection of some of the more important species are covered in this section.

Specific myiasis refers to myiasis caused by flies that require a host for larval development. One important example is the human botfly, *Dermatobia hominis,* which is found in the humid regions of Mexico and Central and South America. The adult botfly attaches her eggs to the abdomen of bloodsucking flies or mosquitoes, which in turn distribute the eggs while obtaining a blood meal from an animal or human. The larvae enter the skin through the wound created by the biting insect. The larvae develop over 40 to 50 days, during which time a painful lesion known as a warble appears. When the larvae reach maturity, they leave the host to pupate. The resulting lesion may take weeks to months to heal and may become secondarily infected. If the larva dies before leaving the skin, an abscess forms.

Semispecific myiasis is caused by flies that normally lay their eggs on decaying animal or plant matter but develops in a host if entry is facilitated by the presence of wounds or sores. Representatives of this group include the green-bottle fly, *Phaenicia*; blue-bottle flies, *Cochliomyia;* and black-bottle flies, *Phormia*. These flies are worldwide in distribution, and their presence is encouraged by poor sanitation. They occasionally lay their eggs on the open sores or wounds of animal and humans. Another group that causes myiasis in humans is the flesh flies, or sarcophagids. These flies have a worldwide distribution and normally breed in decomposing matter. They may deposit their larvae on foods that, if ingested, may serve as a source of infection.

Flies that produce accidental myiasis have no requirement for development in a host. Accidental infection may occur when eggs are deposited on oral or genitourinary openings and the resulting larvae gain entry into the intestinal or genitourinary tract. Flies that may produce accidental myiasis include *M. domestica,* the common housefly.

Sucking Lice

Physiology and structure. Although several species of lice (Anoplura) infest humans as blood-feeding parasites, only the body louse is important in medicine as the vector of the rickettsia of typhus and trench fevers and the vector of the spirochetes of relapsing fever (Table 80-2). The body louse, *Pediculus humanus,* and the head louse, *P. humanus capitis,* are elongated, wingless, flattened insects with three pairs of legs and mouthpieces adapted for piercing flesh and sucking blood (Figure 80-10). The pubic or crab louse, *Phthirus pubis,* has a short, crablike abdomen with clawed second and third legs (Figure 80-11).

Epidemiology. Epidemics of head lice are reported frequently in the United States, particularly among school children. The head lice inhabit the hairs of the head and are transmitted by physical contact or sharing of hair brushes or hats. Crab lice survive on blood meals around the hairs of the pubic and perianal areas of the body. They are transmitted frequently from one person to another by sexual contact and contaminated toilet seats or clothing. Body lice are usually found on clothing. Unlike head or crab lice, they move to the body for feeding and return to the clothing after obtaining a blood meal. All of the lice inject salivary fluids into the body during the ingestion of blood, which causes varying degrees of sensitization in the human host.

Clinical syndromes. Intense itching is the usual characteristic of infestation by lice (pediculosis). The patient may have pruritic, red papules around the ears, face, neck, or shoulders. Secondary infection and regional adenopathy may be present.

Diagnosis. The diagnosis is made by demonstration of the lice or eggs from a patient complaining of pruri-

FIGURE 80-10 Body louse *(P. humanus).* (Courtesy Oxford Scientific Films, Ltd [Dr RJ Warren]; from Peters W: *A colour atlas of arthropods in clinical medicine,* London, 1992, Wolfe.)

FIGURE 80-11 Crab louse *(P. pubis).* (Courtesy Dr RV Southcott; from Peters W: *A colour atlas of arthropods in clinical medicine,* London, 1992, Wolfe.)

tus. Frequently the patient has noticed the insects, and the diagnosis may be made over the telephone. The eggs, or nits, are white, round objects that may be found attached to the hair shafts (head and crab lice) or on clothing (body lice).

Treatment, prevention, and control. Gamma benzene hexachloride (lindane) lotion applied to the entire body and left on for 24 hours is an effective treatment for lice. Shaving the hair of affected areas is a desirable

FIGURE 80-12 Flea. (From Peters W: *A colour atlas of arthropods in clinical medicine,* London, 1992, Wolfe.)

adjunct. Adult lice in clothing must be destroyed by the application of lindane or DDT powder or by boiling. Lice may survive in the environment for up to 2 weeks; thus items such as brushes, combs, and bedding must be treated with a pediculicide or by boiling.

The best strategy for primary prevention is education and practice of good hygiene habits. Secondary prevention may be practiced by a policy of routine surveillance (e.g., scalp inspections) in schools, day-care centers, military camps, and other institutions. Repellents may be necessary for people who run a high risk of exposure in crowded conditions.

Fleas

Physiology and structure. Fleas (Siphonaptera) are small, wingless insects with laterally compressed bodies and long legs adapted for jumping (Figure 80-12). Their mouthparts are adapted for sucking or "siphoning" blood from the host.

Epidemiology. Fleas are cosmopolitan in distribution. Most species are adapted to a particular host; however, they can readily feed on humans, particularly when deprived of their preferred host. Fleas are important as vectors of plague and murine typhus and as intermediate hosts for dog (*Dipylidium caninum*) and rodent (*Hymenolepis* species) tapeworms that occasionally infect humans.

In contrast to the majority of fleas that do not invade the human integument, the chigoe flea, *Tunga penetrans,* may cause considerable damage by actively invading the skin. The female chigoe flea burrows into the skin, often under the toenails or between the toes, where she sucks blood and lays her eggs. The chigoe flea is found in tropical and subtropical regions of America as well as in Africa and the Far East. It is not known to transmit human pathogens.

Clinical syndromes. As with the bites of other bloodsucking arthropods, flea bites result in pruritic, erythematous lesions of varying severity, which depends on the intensity of the infestation and the sensitivity of the bitten person. The irritation caused by the flea's saliva may produce physical findings that vary from small, red welts to a diffuse, red rash. Secondary infection may be a complication.

Cutaneous invasion by the chigoe flea produces an erythematous papule that is painful and pruritic. Infested tissue can become severely inflamed and ulcerated. Secondary infection is common. In severe cases the infestation may be complicated by tetanus or by gas gangrene, resulting in amputation.

Diagnosis. The diagnosis of flea infestation is inferred in a patient with annoying bites who is also a pet (dog or cat) owner. Examination of the patient and pet usually reveals the characteristic insect. Diagnosis of tungiasis is made by detecting the dark portion of the chigoe flea's abdomen as it protrudes from the skin surface in the center of an inflamed lesion.

Treatment, prevention, and control. Palliative treatment with antipruritics and antihistamines is indicated for most flea bites. Surgical removal of the chigoe flea is indicated.

Commercially available insecticides may control fleas at the source. Topically applied repellents can protect people against flea bites. Flea collars or powders on pets are also effective preventive measures.

Bugs

Physiology and structure. *Bugs* refer specifically to two bloodsucking insects: the bedbug and the triatomid bug (Figures 80-13 and 80-14). Both bugs are characterized by a long proboscis that is folded ventrally under the body when not in use. The bedbug (*Cimex lectularius*) is a reddish brown insect approximately 4 to 5 mm long. It has short wing pads but cannot fly. The triatomid, or "kissing" bug, has yellow or orange markings on the body and an elongated head. Triatomid bugs have wings and are aerial.

Epidemiology. Both bedbugs and triatomid bugs are nocturnal and feed indiscriminately on most mammals. Bedbugs are cosmopolitan in distribution, whereas triatomid bugs are limited to the Americas. Bedbugs hide during the day in cracks and crevices of wooden furniture, under loose wallpaper, in the tufts of mattresses, and in box springs. Triatomid bugs live in the cracks and crevices of walls and in thatched roofs. Bedbugs do not play a role in the transmission of human disease; how-

FIGURE 80-13 Bedbug *(C. lectularius).* (From Peters W: *A colour atlas of arthropods in clinical medicine,* London, 1992, Wolfe.)

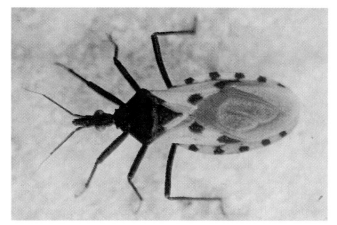

FIGURE 80-14 Triatomid bug. (Courtesy Dr D Minter; from Peters W: *A colour atlas of arthropods in clinical medicine,* London, 1992, Wolfe.)

ever, triatomid bugs are important vectors of Chagas' disease (Table 80-2 and Chapter 76).

Clinical syndromes. The bites of bedbugs and triatomid bugs produce lesions that range from small, red marks to hemorrhagic bullae. Bedbugs tend to bite in linear fashion on the trunk and arms, whereas triatomid bugs bite with higher frequency on the face. The classic periorbital edema secondary to a triatomid bite is known as *Romaña's sign.* The intensity of reaction to a bite depends on the degree of sensitization of the patient. In addition to causing local lesions, bedbugs may be associated with nervous disorders and sleeplessness in children and adults.

Diagnosis. The pattern and location of bites suggests bedbugs or triatomid bugs. The detection of tiny spots of blood on bedding or the dead insects themselves is frequently the first sign of bedbug infestation.

Treatment, prevention, and control. Topical palliatives are appropriate for the relief of pruritus. Antihistamines may be indicated if dermatitis is severe. Control consists of proper hygiene and the environmental applications of insecticides.

Stinging Insects

Physiology and structure. The order Hymenoptera comprises the bees, wasps, hornets, and ants. The modified ovipositor of the female, the apparatus for egg laying, serves as a stinging organ and is used for defense or to capture prey for food. Members of Hymenoptera are known for their complex social systems, castes, and elaborate hive or nest structures.

Epidemiology. Of the hymenopterans, the bees, or Apidae, live in complex social organizations such as hives or in less structured underground nests. Only honeybees

and bumblebees are of concern to humans because of their ability to sting. The Vespidae include wasps, hornets, and yellow jackets; all are aggressive insects and a major cause of stings in humans. In the act of stinging, the aroused insect inserts the sheath to open the wound. The thrust of the stylets and injection of venom immediately follow.

One group of ants of concern in the United States is the fire ant, *Solenopsis invicta.* Fire ants are particularly common in the southeastern states. They are well camouflaged in large, hard-crusted mounds and attack when disturbed. They bite their victim with strong mandibles and then sting repeatedly.

Clinical syndromes. An estimated 50 to 100 people die each year in the United States from reactions to stings of the hymenopterans. Severe toxic reactions such as fever and muscle cramps can be caused by as few as 10 stings. Allergic reactions are the most serious consequence, but others include pain, edema, pruritus, and a heat sensation at the site of the sting. Anaphylactic shock from bee stings has resulted in death in some instances.

Treatment, prevention, and control. No satisfactory treatment has been discovered for stings. If left in the wound, the sting apparatus should be removed immediately. The injection of epinephrine is sometimes necessary to counteract anaphylaxis. (Emergency kits are available by prescription for sensitive people.) For the relief of local discomfort, calamine lotion or a topical corticosteroid cream for more severe local lesions is helpful.

Although there are no effective repellents against these insects, their nests can be destroyed with any of several commercially available insecticidal compounds. General avoidance of areas inhabited by hymenopterans is advised for sensitive people.

CASE STUDY AND QUESTIONS

A 4-year-old child was brought in by her mother with a complaint of itchy hands. The child stayed at a day-care center during the day while her mother worked. The girl had intense itching and a rash on her hands and arms for about 2 weeks. The itching became more severe and interfered with the child's sleep. On physical examination, the child appeared well nourished and cared for. The skin on her hands, wrists, and forearms appeared red and excoriated. Raised, serpiginous "tracks" were noted on the sides of her fingers, on the ventral aspects of her wrists, and in the popliteal folds. Several of the tracks were inflamed and were beginning to form pustules. The mother stated that several other children at the day-care center were experiencing a similar problem.

1. What was the likely diagnosis?
2. How would this diagnosis have been confirmed?
3. How would this child have been treated and what advice would have been given to the mother regarding prevention?
4. Did this child require antibiotic therapy? If so, why?
5. What should have been done regarding the other children at the day-care center?

Bibliography

Binford CH, Connor DH: *Pathology of tropical and extraordinary diseases,* vol 3, Washington, DC, 1976, Armed Forces Institute of Pathology.

Blondell RD: Parasites of the skin and hair, *Primary Care* 8:167-183, 1991.

Markell EK, Voge M, John DT: *Medical parasitology,* ed 7, Philadelphia, 1992, WB Saunders.

Najarian HH: *Textbook of medical parasitology,* Baltimore, 1967, Williams & Wilkins.

Peters W: *A colour atlas of arthropods in clinical medicine,* London, 1992, Wolfe.

Pratt HD et al: *Arthropods of medical importance.* In Murray PR et al, editors: *Manual of clinical microbiology,* ed 6, Washington DC, 1995, American Society for Microbiology.

Strickland GT: *Hunter's tropical medicine,* ed 7, Philadelphia, 1991, WB Saunders.

Van Horn KG et al: Copepods associated with a perirectal abscess and copepod pseudo-outbreaks in stools for ova and parasite examinations, *Diagn Microbiol Infect Dis* 15:561-565, 1992.

Index

We Want To Hear From You!

To help us publish the most useful materials for students, we would appreciate your comments on this book. Please take a few moments to answer the questions below, and E-mail us your comments. Thank you for your input.

Murray: MEDICAL MICROBIOLOGY 3e
microbiology.medtext@mosby.com

1. How are you using this book? Please be specific: for a first-year medical school course, as part of a clerkship rotation, to refresh the material before a Board exam, etc.

2. Was this book useful to you? Why or why not?

3. What features of books are important to you?
   -color figures
   -summary tables and boxes
   -summaries
   -self-assessment questions
   -price
   -what else?

4. What influenced your decision to buy this book?
   -required/recommended by instructor
   -recommended by student
   -bookstore display
   -what else?

5. What other instructional materials did/would you find useful in this course?
   -computer-assisted instruction
   -slides
   -what else?

Are you interested in doing in-depth reviews of our textbooks?
If so, please send us your name, address and telephone number.

THANK YOU!